Ensure success in the classr[oom] the OR with these essential [resources!]

Surgical Instrumentation:
An Interactive Approach
Renee Nemitz, CST, RN, AAS
2010 • 320 pp., 530 illus.
ISBN: 978-1-4160-3702-6

Learn surgical instruments with an interactive combination of detailed text and video!

• **More than 500 full-color, high quality photographs** help you learn the most common surgical instruments for all surgical procedures.
• **Companion CD** provides an expansive image library with zooming and rotating capabilities, a glossary with sound pronunciations, and fun learning exercises.

Mosby's PDQ for Surgical Technology:
Necessary Facts at Hand
Robin Hueske, CST
2008 • 176 pp., 80 illus.
ISBN: 978-0-323-05261-0

Quickly reference essential information in the operating room!

• **Pocket size, spiral binding, and waterproof pages** enable instant access to pharmacology, supplies, sutures, etc. in the field.
• **80 full-color illustrations** demonstrate positioning, preparations, and important anatomy.

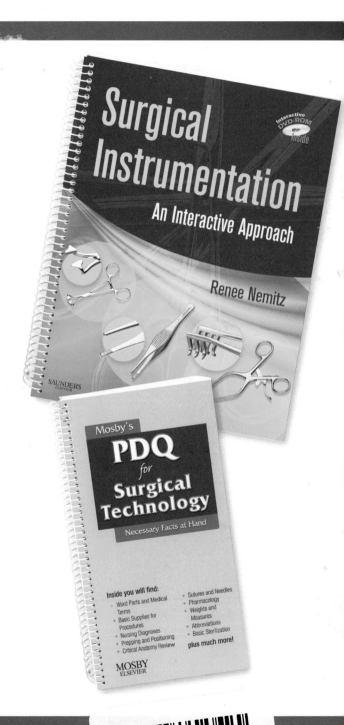

Get your copies today!

• Order securely [at] [.com]
• Call toll-free 1-800-545-2522
• Visit your local bookstore

FIFTH
EDITION

SURGICAL
TECHNOLOGY
PRINCIPLES AND PRACTICE

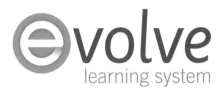

learning system

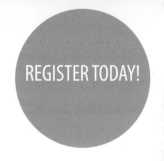

To access your Student Resources, visit:

http://evolve.elsevier.com/Fuller/surgical/

Register today and gain access to:

- ## *Review Questions for each Chapter*
  Review Questions presented in engaging activites will help students review key concepts quickly.

- ## Flashcards
  Quickly review important terminology from the textbook.

- ## Surgical Millionaire Game
  A comprehensive game that allows students to test their knowledge in a game show format.

- ## Mosby's Essential Drug List
  Detailed drug monographs, including full-color pill photos, for the top 200 dispensed drugs in the United States.

- ## Weblinks
  Links to places of interest on the web specifically for surgcial technologists.

- ## Content Updates
  Find out the latest information on relevant issues in the field of surgical technology.

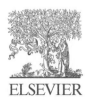

ELSEVIER

FIFTH EDITION

SURGICAL TECHNOLOGY

PRINCIPLES AND PRACTICE

Joanna Kotcher Fuller, BA, BSN, RN, RGN, MPH

Emergency Medical Coordinator
Medical Emergency Relief International, UK—Global

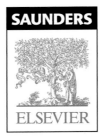

SAUNDERS

ELSEVIER

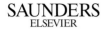

3251 Riverport Lane
St. Louis, Missouri 63043

SURGICAL TECHNOLOGY: PRINCIPLES AND PRACTICE ISBN: 978-1-4160-6035-2

Copyright © 2010 by Saunders, an imprint of Elsevier Inc.

Notice

Previous editions copyrighted 2005, 1994, 1986, 1981

ISBN: 978-1-4160-6035-2

Publishing Director: Andrew Allen
Acquisitions Editor: Jennifer Janson
Associate Developmental Editor: Kelly Brinkman
Publishing Services Manager: Julie Eddy
Project Manager: Rich Barber
Design Direction: Paula Catalano

Printed in China

Last digit is the print number: 9 8 7 6 5 4 3 2 1

Contributors

Rebecca Ferguson, RN, BSN, CNOR, ARNP
The FACE Clinic
Dothan Alabama
Chapter 27: Surgery of the Ear, Nose, Pharynx, and Larynx
Chapter 28: Oral and Maxillofacial Surgery
Chapter 29: Plastic and Reconstructive Surgery

Mary Grace Hensell, RN, BSN, CNOR
Allegheny General Hospital
Pittsburgh, Pennsylvania
Chapter 25: Genitourinary Surgery
Chapter 26: Ophthalmic Surgery

Donna R. McEwen, RN, BSN, CNOR
Sr. Instructional Designer, Care Solutions Training
OptumHealth Care/United Health Group
San Antonio, Texas
Chapter 35: Neurosurgery

Debra Penney CNM, MS, MPH
Associate Clinical Professor
University of Utah, College of Nursing
Salt Lake City, Utah
Chapter 24: Gynecological and Obstetrical Surgery

Patricia Seifert, RN, MSN, CRNFA, CNOR, FAAN
Inova Fairfax Hospital
Falls Church, Virginia
Chapter 32: Thoracic and Pulmonary Surgery
Chapter 33: Cardiac Surgery

Reviewers

Jeffrey Lee Bidwell CST, CFA, CSA, KCSA, MA
Surgical Assisting and Surgical Technology Program Director
Madisonville Community College
Madisonville, Kentucky

Becky Brodin RN, MA, CNOR
Program Director, Surgical Technology; Assistant Professor
Saint Mary's University of Minnesota
Minneapolis, Minnesota

Susan L Bugajsky BS, PA, RN
Coordinator of Surgical Technology
Prairie State College
Chicago Heights, Illinois

G. A. Candie Gagne, CST, MS
Surgical Technology Instructor
Sanford-Brown Institute—Monroeville
Pittsburgh, Pennsylvania

Tarek W. Halim, MD
Director of Education
Medical Career Institute
Ocean Township, New Jersey

Stacey May
Program Director and Instructor of Surgical Technology and Surgical Assisting
South Plains College
Levelland, Texas

Janet Anne Milligan, RN, CNOR, BS ed
Program Manager/Associate Professor Surgical Technology program
College of Southern Idaho
Twin Falls, Idaho

Dorothy L. Nichols, BBA, RN, CNOR
Surgical Technology Program Director
Southern Union State Community College
Opelika, Alabama

Elizabeth Slagle, MS, RN, CST
Associate Professor and Chair
Department of Surgical Technology
University of Saint Francis
Fort Wayne, Indiana

Al Smith, RN, BSN, M.Ed
Assistant Professor, Program Director
Surgical Technology
Bossier Parish Community College
Bossier City, Louisiana

Christallia I. Starks, RN, MSN, MA, CRCST
Director, Department of Surgical Technology
Baptist Health System School of Health Professions
San Antonio, Texas

Jeffrey B. Ware CST, CFA
Education/Accreditation Consultant
JBW Enterprise
Hagerstown, Maryland

Preface

Surgical Technology now represents one of the fastest growing health professions in the United States. Opportunities for surgical technologists are varied and challenging. Current trends include specialization in a particular focal area such as orthopedics, pediatrics, cardiology, maxillofacial and otolaryngological surgery, and many others. Professional development as a certified first assistant (CFA) is a common career goal for these specialists. The training and skills of the surgical technologist provide the basis for advancement in diverse careers such as health administration and management and biomedical technology. Nursing and medicine are logical career goals for many surgical technologists, and those individuals who have an interest in international humanitarian aid may pursue a career with an international non-governmental organization.

THE EVOLUTION OF SURGICAL TECHNOLOGY PRINCIPLES AND PRACTICE

Shortly after the historical entry of *operating room technician* as a civilian allied health profession, *Surgical Technology: Principles and Practice* was introduced as the first and only textbook written by a certified surgical technologist and intended solely for the study of surgical technology. Since that time this textbook has been in continuous publication, with succeeding editions that paralleled the growth of the profession.

This fifth edition of *Surgical Technology: Principles and Practice* represents a long-term partnership between educators and students that spans more than 20 years. Throughout this period there have been striking advances in biotechnology and associated demands for professional development of the surgical technologist. The Association of Surgical Technologists was instrumental in creating structures for course accreditation through a number of collaborating agencies. *Surgical Technology: Principles and Practice* has been there to support students throughout the growth and development of the profession. It has kept pace with technological advances in the profession but also with a wider role in patient care. These changes require students and practitioners to understand the ethical and legal implications of the professional role in surgery. The surgical technologist today is not only a team player but also a *decision* maker, a role that requires greater demands on personal as well as technical skills. *Surgical Tech-*

nology continues to provide authoritative information in a manner that encourages students to think strategically and creatively as they face new challenges as they provide patient care.

Who will benefit from this book?

This textbook has been written primarily for surgical technology students. The book's comprehensive approach covers all core content required for instruction in surgical technology programs that are accredited by both the Commission on Accreditation of Allied Health Education Programs (CAAHEP) and the American Board of Health Education Schools (ABHES). Although primarily a student textbook, the progressive technical discussions and comprehensive approach make it a standard reference book for central processing staff, surgical nurses, medical students, and interns working or rotating through surgery.

Why is this book important to the profession?

Surgical Technology: Principles and Practice is an important work, not only because it was the first textbook written for and by a surgical technologist, but because it is based in sound evidence-based practice and a high level of ethical scholarship. The principles of ethical textbook writing are based on the need for a text that is original and creative. Its standards must be soundly based in responsible scholarship. For students and instructors, this means that information—no matter what the form—must be thoroughly researched with appropriate recognition of sources. Standards of practice are established by the coordinated efforts of the many peer-reviewed professional and governmental organizations involved in medicine, nursing, environment safety, infectious disease, and patient protection. These practices are evidence-based. *Surgical Technology: Principles and Practice* presents these standards as the basis of practice using language and terms widely recognized by the medical and nursing community. One of the important goals of *Surgical Technology: Principles and Practice* has been to present facts and material without pretention or jargon—to make it accessible so that students can realize their personal career goals.

The fifth edition continues in these traditions.

Organization

Surgical Technology: Principles and Practice is organized to support teaching of 11- to 24-month surgical technology programs. Unit 1, Theory Techniques in Surgery, contains the foundational material. Unit 2, Surgery and Surgical Procedures, contains the surgical procedures organized by specialty. This format prepares the student to learn the core surgical procedures only after garnering a solid core knowledge. Each chapter includes a chapter outline, learning objectives, terminology, introduction, bulleted chapter summary, a review summary, and references and bibliography.

Distinctive Features

Surgical Technology Principles and Practice simplifies difficult concepts and mentors students through complex procedures. A dynamic, full-color design and layout are very student-friendly and accessible. Bullets, numbering, technique boxes, and the extensive use of tables and figures all draw attention to important facts and enhance learning. The NEW clinical skills DVD enables independent, interactive review of concepts best conceptualized through visual example.

New to this Edition

The fifth edition of *Surgical Technology Principles and Practice* presents important new chapters and information required for an expanded and more advanced role for the surgical technologist.

- Chapter 3: *Death and Dying* discusses the clinical, social, and interpersonal events following the death of a patient in surgery.

- Chapter 13: *Postoperative Recovery and Patient Discharge* introduces the student to the Postoperative Recovery Unit (PACU), the events during recovery, emergency situations, and discharge from the health facility.
- Chapter 18: *Biomechanics and Computer Technology* presents a new dimension of learning to the surgical technologist. The basis of biotechnology is explained through fundamental (qualitative) physics in simple terms and discussions. A section on elementary computer technology is also included in this chapter.
- Chapter 19: *Energy Sources in Surgery* provides a more complex discussion on the types and hazards of energy sources used in modern surgery. These include all forms of electrosurgery, ultrasound, radiofrequency ablation, laser, and cryosurgery. The chapter is authoritatively documented and includes extensive hazard and safety standards.
- Chapter 21: *Minimally Invasive, Endoscopic, and Robotic Assisted Surgery* introduces the student to the science, instruments, and principles of these advanced surgical techniques. Concise illustrations and explanations accompany each section.

In addition to these new chapters, additional student aids have been included. Each chapter is preceded by a chapter outline, learning objectives, and terminology relevant to the chapter. Terms essential to understanding the material have been reproduced in bold type in the body of the text. References, chapter questions, and a chapter review appear at the end of each chapter.

Learning Aids

A variety of pedagogical features are included in the book to aid learning:

- Chapter Outlines, Learning Objectives and Terminology with glossary-style definitions are the beginning of each chapter, set the stage for student learning

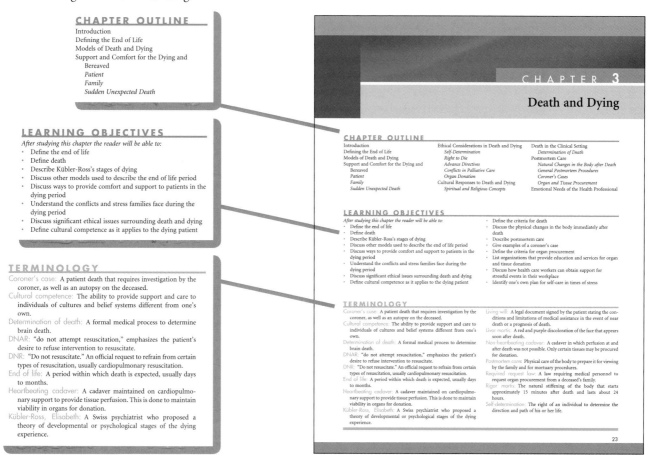

- Technique Boxes are included insight into the profession and practical information to apply to the concepts presented

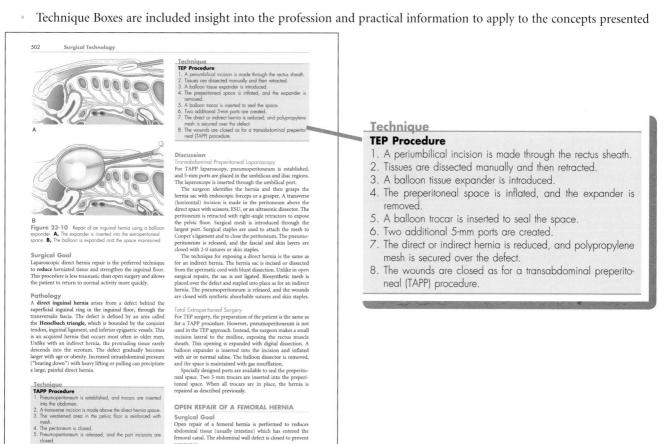

Technique
TEP Procedure
1. A periumbilical incision is made through the rectus sheath.
2. Tissues are dissected manually and then retracted.
3. A balloon tissue expander is introduced.
4. The preperitoneal space is inflated, and the expander is removed.
5. A balloon trocar is inserted to seal the space.
6. Two additional 5-mm ports are created.
7. The direct or indirect hernia is reduced, and polypropylene mesh is secured over the defect.
8. The wounds are closed as for a transabdominal preperitoneal (TAPP) procedure.

- Dynamic, full-color photos provide visual connection and promote student involvement with the material

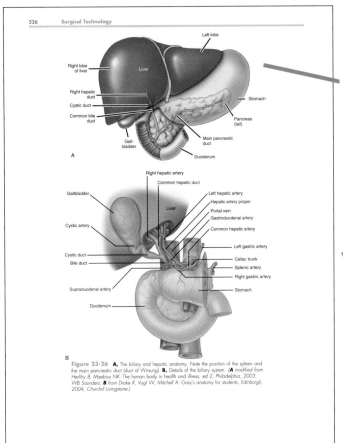

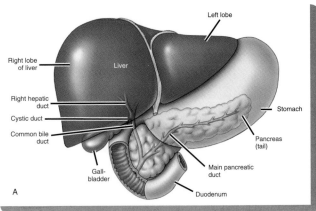

- Information is presented in an at-a-glance format through the use of lists, illustrations, and tables.

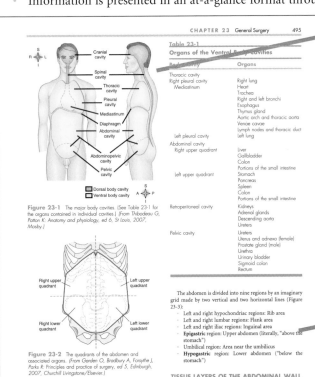

The abdomen is divided into nine regions by an imaginary grid made by two vertical and two horizontal lines (Figure 23-3):

- Left and right hypochondriac regions: Rib area
- Left and right lumbar regions: Flank area
- Left and right iliac regions: Inguinal area
- **Epigastric** region: Upper abdomen (literally, "above the stomach")
- Umbilical region: Area near the umbilicus
- **Hypogastric** region: Lower abdomen ("below the stomach")

- Step-by-step instructions with full color illustrations make it easy to learn skills and procedures.

214   Surgical Technology

Face
Apply only nonalcohol solutions to the face. Triclosan is a mild antiseptic commonly used in this area. The hair contains a high concentration of bacteria and is still considered a contaminated area.

Special Supplies
- Nonalcohol prep solution (e.g., triclosan)
- Warm normal saline
- Cotton swabs
- Cotton-tipped applicators
- Towels
- Comb and water-soluble hair gel (nonsterile supplies)

Procedure
1. Apply gel to the hair if necessary before combing it back away from the face. Use clips if necessary to hold the hair away from the face and ears.
2. Place a towel on each side of the neck to prevent the bed linen from becoming soaked.
3. Prep the face from the neck or chin upward to the hairline. The ears may be included in the face prep.
4. Use cotton-tipped applicators to cleanse the folds of the pinna. Do not allow prep solution to drain into the ear canal.
5. Prep the face from the incision area outward. Prep the incision site again with fresh sponges. No prep sponge that touches the hairline should be brought back over the skin. Rinse the skin with cotton swabs dipped in warm normal saline solution.

Neck
The neck and throat area is prepared for thyroid surgery, tracheotomy, carotid artery surgery, lymph node biopsy, or radical dissection of the mandible, shoulder plexus, and mediastinum. If radical dissection is anticipated or scheduled, the prep area extends from the chin to the nipple line or waist and around the side of the body to the operating table on each side (Figure 11-4).

Procedure
1. Turn the patient's gown down to several inches below the prep area.
2. Place sterile towels at the periphery of the prep site.
3. Begin the prep at the incision site, applying prep solution in a circular motion to the periphery of the site.

Breast and Thorax
The boundaries of the prep area for breast and thoracic procedures depend on the extent of the surgery and the patient's position. The prep area for radical breast or thoracic surgery extends from the chin to the umbilicus and includes the lateral thorax on each side.

When the surgery involves removal of a mass without the possibility of more extensive surgery, the breast is prepped from the clavicle to the midthorax and from the midline, including the sides of the thorax to the operating table on the affected side. The prep area is extended into

the axilla for lesions in the upper lateral quadrant of the breast.

Surgery that includes both biopsy of a mass and the possibility of mastectomy requires a much wider prep area. A radical mastectomy requires a prep boundary that encompasses the neck, shoulder of the affected side, thorax to the operating table surface, and midpelvic region (Figure 11-5).

Tissue that is suspected of being cancerous must be prepared gently. The area should be painted with as little friction and pressure as possible to prevent tumor cells from migrating into surrounding tissue. Skin prep for surgery of the thoracic cavity uses a bilateral extension of the boundaries for radical breast surgery.

Procedure
1. Square the prep boundary with sterile towels.
2. If the umbilicus is included in the prep, clean it with cotton-tipped applicators.
3. Prep the operative area, starting at the incision site.
4. If the shoulder is included in the prep, an assistant should abduct the arm so that solution can be applied circumferentially.

Shoulder
The shoulder prep includes the neck, shoulder, upper arm, and scapula on the affected side (Figure 11-6). One assistant is required to elevate the patient's arm. The subscapular and midback area also may be elevated on a pad.

Procedure
1. Remove the patient's gown to the umbilicus.
2. Place sterile prep towels at the periphery of the prep area.

Figure 11-4 Skin prep for neck and throat procedures. (Modified from Phillips N: Berry and Kohn's operating room technique, ed 10, St Louis, 2004, Mosby.)

Procedure
1. Turn the patient's gown down to several inches below the prep area.
2. Place sterile towels at the periphery of the prep site.
3. Begin the prep at the incision site, applying prep solution in a circular motion to the periphery of the site.

- More than 600 illustrations and photos have been revised to provide true-to-life full-color images that reflect the most current techniques and equipment.

FOR THE INSTRUCTOR

Evolve

Surgical Technology: Principles and Practice offers several assets on Evolve to aid instructors:
- Test bank: An Exam-View test bank of more than 1400 multiple choice questions that feature rationales, cognitive levels, and page number references to the text. This can be used as review in class or for test development.
- PowerPoint Presentations: One PowerPoint presentation has been developed for each chapter. These can be used "as is" or as a template to prepare chapter lectures.
- Image Collection: All of the images from the book are available as JPGs and can be downloaded into PowerPoint Presentations. These can be used during lecture to illustrate important concepts.
- Text Answer Key: All of the answers to the Review Questions from the text.

- Workbook Answer Key: All of the answers to the Workbook exercises.
- TEACH Instructors Resource: Including lesson plans, lecture outlines, and PowerPoint slides, all available via Evolve. The TEACH Instructors Resource provides instructors with customizable lesson plans and lecture outlines based on learning objectives. With these valuable resources, instructors will save valuable preparation time and create a learning environment that fully engages students in classroom participation. The lesson plans are keyed chapter-by-chapter and are divided into 50-minute units in a three-column format. In addition to the lesson plans, instructors will have unique lecture outlines in PowerPoint with talking points, thought-provoking questions, and unique ideas for lectures.

FOR THE STUDENT

Skills DVD

The student skills DVD includes:
- Provides students with a 70-minute visual interactive review of more than 40 key skills that they learn in the classroom.
- Broken down into three units including: The Role of the Surgical Technologist, Preparation for Surgery, and Preparing the Patient.

Student Workbook

The student workbook includes:

- Comprehensive review of terminology, anatomy, and chapter content that are reinforced by a variety of recall exercises.
- Application exercises that encourage students to put concepts into practice.
- Critical thinking exercises that take information to the next level and prepare students for the real world through patient case scenarios.

Evolve

The student resources on Evolve:

- Surgical Millionaire game to enhance review of key concepts
- Chapter activities that provide review of content covered in text for additional practice.
- Mosby's Essential Drugs for Surgical Technologists, which includes 200 detailed drug monographs for drugs commonly used in surgery.
- WebLinks for all Internet research activities, organized by chapter.
- Archie Animations that show various anatomy and procedure demonstrations discussed in the text.
- Flash cards to provide a quick review of terms found throughout the textbook.
- Content updates to keep the text current.

NOTE TO THE STUDENT

This fifth edition of *Surgical Technology: Principles and Practice* probably represents the greatest upward trend in technological expertise and patient care skills since the first edition was created in the 1980s. As a group, health care workers have tremendous power to change the public's health-seeking behaviors and contribute to an equitable quality of life for all people. In this edition you will see a holistic approach to health, which is turned outward to the patient. Surgical Technology should not focus on itself or its profession but on *people*—patients, families, and the community. You have the power to speak out about the goals of equality in patient care and improvements in public health in our own country and even abroad. *Surgical Technology: Principles and Practice* provides the academic and scientific tools to speak with authority and knowledge. Use the book as you would any text, but keep it as a reference to back up your own technical discussions and health advocacy for patients. Use the many clear illustrations and references to make your point. Continue with the difficult ethical and legal discussions, which affect a patient's well-being even after you have graduated. Use the book as a guide to your future aspirations. You have an exciting start in a profession that can lead to a multitude of goals. You can trust that *Surgical Technology Principle and Practice* gives you a sound foundation for achieving these goals. Enjoy the book and above all—enjoy your studies.

Acknowledgments

The fifth edition of *Surgical Technology: Principles and Practice* was created through the dedicated efforts of many people. I am most grateful to Jennifer Janson, Acquisitions Editor, for her continual support, sharp decision making, and positive approach to the many challenges that accompany a textbook of this dimension. I especially appreciate her respectful and professional attitude, which was evident in the team collaboration. Kelly Brinkman, Associate Developmental Editor, has been exceptional in formatting; tracking; and managing the manuscript, documents, art, and deadlines. I thank her for her efficiency and hard work that was often performed behind the scenes but was essential to a successful project. The layout for this edition stands out above all other editions in its organization, visual appeal, and quality of reproduction. I would like to thank everyone at Elsevier who contributed to this process.

A number of surgical equipment manufacturers provided technical illustrations and photographs, which are vital to any textbook. Many individuals devoted time and effort to provide high-quality reproductions. These companies deserve recognition for the value they place on education and for their continuing cooperation through many editions of *Surgical Technology: Principles and Practice*. I would specifically like to thank those who provided artwork from Zimmer Corporation, STERIS Corporation, Karl Storz USA, Olympus America, and Kimberly Clark. Sklar Instruments, ConMed Corporation, Covidien, Gyrus ACMI, and Katena Instruments contributed many high-quality images of surgical instruments and suture materials. Finally, Intuitive Corporation provided images of the da Vinci robotic system and was very cooperative and helpful during the development of this section of the book.

With slight modifications, Sandra McMahon's original illustrations, depicting surgical positions and aseptic technique, continue to demonstrate these topics with fluidity and precision. These illustrations have shown marked longevity and deserve high praise for her talent as a medical illustrator.

Contents

The Surgical Technologist

CHAPTER OUTLINE

LEARNING OBJECTIVES

After studying this chapter the reader will be able to:

- Understand the development of the role of the surgical technologist after World War II
- Describe the process of certification for the surgical technologist
- Discuss career opportunities available to the surgical technologist

- List the personal attributes needed for success as a surgical technologist
- Describe the process of certification
- Identify the duties of the surgical technologist

TERMINOLOGY

ACS: American College of Surgeons. A professional organization that establishes educational standards for surgeons and surgical residency programs.

Allied health profession: A profession that follows the principles of medicine and nursing but that focuses on an expertise set apart from those practices.

AORN: Association of periOperative Registered Nurses. The professional organization for surgical nurses; originally known as the Association of Operating Room Nurses.

ARC/STSA: Accreditation Review Council on Education in Surgical Technology and Surgical Assisting. The ARC/STSA establishes, maintains, and promotes quality standards for education programs in surgical technology and surgical first assisting.

AST: Association of Surgical Technologists. The professional association for surgical technologists (Web site: http://www.ast.org).

CAAHEP: Commission on Accreditation of Allied Health Education Programs. The CAAHEP is an organization that accredits health science programs, including those for surgical technology.

Certification: Acknowledgment by a private agency that a person has achieved a minimum level of knowledge and skill. Certification usually is established by graduation from an accredited institution and passing a written examination. Certification does not confer legal status.

Circulator: The nonsterile team member who assists in gathering additional supplies and equipment needed during the surgical procedure and advocates for the patient.

Continuing education: More formally called professional development. It demonstrates an ongoing learning process in an individual's profession. Continuing education credits are provided by a professional organization. Credits are earned by attending lectures and in-service presentations or by study and examination. Usually only peer-reviewed professional literature qualifies for CE credits.

CST: Certified surgical technologist. A surgical technologist who has successfully passed the National Board of Surgical Technology and Surgical Assisting certification examination.

CST-CFA: Certified surgical technologist–certified first assistant. A surgical technologist with advanced training who has successfully passed the certification examination for surgical first assistants and is credentialed by the National Board of Surgical Technology and Surgical Assisting.

Delegation: The transfer of responsibility for an activity from one person to another.

Dependent tasks: In medicine, nursing, and allied health, those tasks that are performed with the collaborative oversight of another professional. For example, the surgeon provides oversight to the surgical assistant during surgery.

Independent tasks: In medicine, nursing, and allied health, tasks for which a professional has full responsibility and accountability without the oversight of another professional.

Licensure: Professional status, granted by state government, that defines the limits (scope) of practice and regulates those who hold a license. Licensure is provided to protect the public and to ensure a legal minimum standard of professional and ethical conduct.

National Certifying Examination for Surgical Technologists: A comprehensive written examination required for official certification by the Association of Surgical Technologists.

NBSTSA: National Board of Surgical Technology and Surgical Assisting. The NBSTA (formerly the Liaison Council on Certification for the Surgical Technologist) is responsible for all decisions related to certification such as eligibility, renewal, and revocation.

NCCT: National Center for Competency Testing. A nonprofit organization that provides a certification examination for military and other trained surgical technologists whose programs are not recognized by the Association of Surgical Technologists.

Nonsterile team members: Surgical team members who handle only nonsterile equipment, supplies, and instruments. The circulator is the primary nonsterile team member.

ORTs: Operating room technicians. Former title of the surgical technologist (the title was changed in the early 1970s).

Proprietary school: Private, for-profit school.

Scrub: Role and name commonly applied to the surgical technologist or perioperative nurse who is part of the sterile team. The scrub participates in surgery and handles only sterile supplies, instruments, and equipment.

Sterile personnel: Members of the surgical team who have performed a surgical scrub or hand and arm antisepsis procedure. They don sterile gown and gloves and either perform the surgery or assist directly. Sterile personnel include the surgeon, assistant(s), and scrub. Other sterile personnel such as students and preceptors may also be part of the sterile team.

Surgical conscience: In surgery, professional and personal honesty about one's actions, mistakes, and abilities.

TS-C (NCCT): Tech in surgery–certified. A qualification awarded by the National Center for Competency Testing that is achieved by examination and specific entry requirements.

INTRODUCTION

Surgical technology is an **allied health profession.** Professionals in allied health follow the principles of medicine and nursing in that they participate in the health and well-being of people through specific tasks and expertise. However, allied health professionals have distinct expertise that is both humanistic and technical. Allied health professionals are highly trained and must have a global view of health, as well as the education and capability to focus on highly technical aspects of health care delivery. Other allied health professions include emergency medical technologists, nuclear medicine technicians, and specialists in the fields of medical physics, hemodialysis, bioengineering, dentistry, and respiratory therapy. In the past 2 decades, the number of allied health professionals has increased enormously, as have their educational requirements. Advances in technology and the need for specialist training has resulted in the development of new allied health professions and expanded the roles of those already in existence. Surgical technology has also followed this trend.

Whether the surgical technologist is trained in an intensive military program or through rigorous study and practice in a civilian health facility, the profession offers a variety of challenges and opportunities.

HISTORY OF SURGICAL TECHNOLOGY

Beginning with the development of effective anesthesia and antisepsis in the late nineteenth century, the role of the *nurse* in surgery has been easily defined and tracked. In the late 1800s, she prepared instruments for surgery, and in the early 1900s, she assisted in surgical procedures and in the administration of ether, called "etherizing." Her duties from about the 1920s to the 1940s were those of today's circulator. She also instructed student nurses in their surgical education. Often the operating room supervisor was the only graduate nurse in surgery, and it was her duty to oversee the student nurses as they completed their rotation in surgery.

The need for assistive personnel in surgery did not arise until World War II. During World War I, Army corpsmen worked on the battlefield to offer aid and comfort to the wounded, but they had no role in surgery. World War II dramatically changed that. With the development of antibiotics, such as penicillin and sulfa, war surgeons could operate on and save the lives of many more patients than previously was possible. Technological advances also created a need for trained personnel who could assist the surgeon.

The increase in battlefield survivors created a drastic shortage of nurses. In addition to the nurses needed to staff the field hospitals, many more were needed at base hospitals. At home, extra nurses were trained to attend the wounded who returned from battle. To supply the field hospitals in the Pacific and European theaters, the Army began training corpsmen to assist in surgery, a role that previously had been filled only by nurses. By this time, however, corpsmen were expected to administer anesthesia and also assistant the surgeon.

When nurses were not available, such as on combat ships, corpsmen worked under the direct supervision of the surgeon. In this way, a new profession was born, and the Army called these corpsmen *operating room technicians* (**ORTs**). From this time on, the military played a significant role in refining the position of the ORT. Each branch of the military provided specific training and job descriptions for the ORT, who received secondary training after becoming a medic.

After World War II, the Korean War resulted in a continued shortage of operating room nurses, and the need for fully trained nurses in the operating room was questioned. At this time, the operating room supervisors began to recruit former corpsmen to work in civilian surgery. Their primary function was that of a circulator. Registered nurses continued to fill the role of the scrub, or instrument, nurse until about 1965, when the roles were reversed. At this point, hospitals began training civilian ORTs.

In 1967, prompted by the need for guidelines and standards in the training of paramedical surgical personnel, the Association of Operating Room Nurses (**AORN**) published a book, *Teaching the Operating Room Technician.* In 1968 the AORN board of directors created the Association of Operating Room Technicians (AORT). Formal training for the civilian ORT began in proprietary schools across the United States.

Along with organizational independence came steps toward formalizing the technologist's education. The AORT created two new committees, the Liaison Council on Certification for the Surgical Technologist (LCC-ST) and the Joint Review Committee on Education. In 1970, the first certifying examination for operating room technicians was administered, and those who passed were given the title certified operating room technician (CORT). In 1973, the AORT became independent from the AORN, and the profession changed its title to Association of Surgical Technologists (**AST**). The certified technician became known as a certified surgical technologist (**CST**).

ASSOCIATION OF SURGICAL TECHNOLOGISTS

The AST is the surgical technologists' professional organization. The association promotes professional standards by providing services to its members, as well as legislative support to promote and formalize the status of surgical technologists. These services include the following:

- Establishing a code of ethics
- Regular conferences for surgical technologists and educators
- Continuing education credits
- Educational and training materials for professional development
- Career planning and job posting
- Scholarships for students
- Participation in legislative activities
- Participation in state assemblies
- Information on education for the surgical technologist and surgical first assistant
- An official Web site
- Community promotion of the professional

For the student or practicing surgical technologist, it is important to become an active member of the AST and to promote the standards of the profession. Participation in conferences and educational seminars ensures that the high standards set by the organization are maintained through a process of continuing education and public awareness.

The AST is an important link between surgical technologists and the public. The future direction of the profession is maintained through active participation by its members. The student forms commitment by keeping current with news and events, educational opportunities, and public campaigns to enhance public awareness of the profession. This develops into professionalism that maintains high standards of practice after graduation and long into a career.

❖ *The Web site of the Association of Surgical Technologists can be accessed at http://www.ast.org.*

AFFILIATE ORGANIZATIONS

As a body of professionals, surgical technologists are supported by a number of key organizations. Each has a designated role in promotion, certification, accreditation, and continuing education.

Accreditation Review Council on Education in Surgical Technology and Surgical Assisting

The Accreditation Review Committee on Education in Surgical Technology and Surgical Assisting (**ARC/STSA**) provides educational standards and recommendations required for accreditation of programs in surgical technology and surgical first assisting. The Commission on Accreditation of Allied Health Education Programs (**CAAHEP**) accredits programs upon recommendation of the ARC/STSA. Accreditation is granted only after a stringent on-site evaluation of compliance with ARC/STSA standards, including adherence to an approved curriculum. To date there are 449 accredited programs in the United States.

❖ *The ARC/STSA Web site can be accessed at http://www.arcst.org.*

National Board of Surgical Technology and Surgical Assisting

The National Board of Surgical Technology and Surgical Assisting (**NBSTSA**) (formerly the LCC-ST) oversees certification and credentialing of surgical technologists and surgical technologist–first assistants. The organization is responsible for the eligibility, granting, revoking, and denial of certification. The organization's policies, procedures, and certification test information can be found at the NBSTSA Web site.

❖ *The NBSTSA Web site can be accessed at http://www.lcc-st.org.*

ACCOUNTABILITY

Public and governmental (state) accountability of surgical technologists is currently in transition. It is important that surgical technologists, nurses, and even physicians understand the various levels of accountability and regulation.

Public safety is the primary goal of laws and regulations governing any profession. In medicine, nursing, and allied health, professionals perform their work in the interest of the patients they serve. Laws regulating practice are implemented to assure the public that the individuals caring for them are qualified to carry out their responsibilities. Surgical technologists are voluntarily regulated through their professional association and officially regulated in *selected states*. The Association of Surgical Technologists actively supports the profession and its members. Through its legislative mission, the AST advocates for graduation from an accredited program in surgical technology and credentialing as a Certified Surgical Technologist by the National Board of Surgical Technology and Surgical Assisting are a condition of employment. Surgical technologists must determine the level of regulation necessary in their states by contacting the AST or the Board of Health in their state. Not all health professionals are regulated through the Board of Health, but information about registration, certification, and licensure usually can be obtained through the board.

REGISTRATION

State registration means that the professional's name, address, and qualifications are recorded by a designated state authority (e.g., the Board of Health). Registration does not confer a legal status or imply competence in the profession. It is a method of tracking that person for accountability.

CERTIFICATION

Certification is a demonstration of competency to a particular standard, usually set by the professional organization. It is voluntary and is not required for practice in a profession. Only individuals who have achieved certification may use the title "certified."

LICENSURE

Licensure is a process in which the state government issues registration *and the right to practice*. This is accompanied by enforcement of specific state rules and laws pertaining to that particular profession, including its scope of practice. Licensure is usually not the same as registration in which professionals are only required to provide demographic information. Licensure is a protected status which is earned by demonstration of competetence, usually through proof of approved education and examination.

PROFESSIONAL STANDARDS OF PRACTICE

The surgical technologist is a member of the perioperative team which performs tasks within well-defined practice standards. Professional standards are evidence-based and informed by research. Many organizations such as the Centers for Disease Control (CDC), the Association for the Advancement of Medical Instrumentation (AAMI) conduct the research necessary to establish evidence-based standards. Two important professional organizations—the **Association of periOperative Registered Nurses** (**AORN**), and the **American College of Surgeons** (**ACS**) have historically provided extensive documentation of these standards and guidelines which are widely accepted by perioperative and other medical and nursing organizations.

TRAINING AND CERTIFICATION FOR SURGICAL TECHNOLOGISTS

PROGRAM ACCREDITATION

Surgical technologists are trained in, 2-year colleges, military facilities, and vocational and **proprietary** (for-profit) programs. The curriculum for surgical technologists is varied and intense. The educational requirements have expanded in recent years, and the 2-year program (associate degree) is now preferred. Students who want to become a Certified Surgical Technologist must graduate from a school approved by the ARC/STSA. NCCT certification is available for professional military staff and for those who fit the NCCT criteria (see the section on certification by the NCCT).

Surgical technology programs accredited by the ARC-STSA achieve this status through a formal process. The curricula for surgical technology programs are written in accordance with the educational guidelines developed by the AST. Programs are required to submit written documentation demonstrating that the guidelines have been met. On-site visits are required for initial and continuing accreditation.

CERTIFICATION

Certification demonstrates a standard of knowledge and understanding of the principles of surgical technology. It is an important commitment to establishing and maintaining quality assurance in patient care throughout the surgical technologist's career. Not all hospitals and health care facilities require certification for employment. However, most hospitals prefer to hire certified surgical technologists.

Graduates from the military or accredited surgical technology programs and previously certified surgical technologists are eligible to sit for a certification examination. A passing grade on the examination demonstrates entry level competency in the profession, and the surgical technologist earns the title of certified surgical technologist (CST).

Eligibility for Certification

To be eligible to take the certification examination, the applicant must meet one of the following criteria:

1. The individual must be a graduate of a surgical technology program accredited by CAAHEP (see earlier discussion) or by the Accrediting Bureau of Health Education Schools (ABHES).
2. The individual must currently be or previously have been a CST.

Students may apply to take the examination before graduation; however, the results of the examination are not released until proof of graduation is presented.

CERTIFICATION BY THE NATIONAL CENTER FOR COMPETENCY TESTING

The National Center for Competency Testing (**NCCT**) has developed certification examinations for surgical technologists; these examinations are separate from the AST certification process. The NCCT certification process is essential for highly trained medical military staff, whose educational programs are not recognized by the AST. For certification as a surgical technologist, the NCCT requires scrub experience from all applicants, with a minimum of 150 validated, documented surgical cases. The NCCT also requires applicants to have a high school diploma or equivalent, and they must meet any of the following eligibility requirements:

- Be a graduate of an operating room technician, surgical technician, or surgical technologist program offered by a school or college recognized by the U.S. Department of Education (DOE).
- Be a graduate of a formal operating room technician or surgical technology training program, with 1 year of validated work experience in the past 2 years or 2 years of work experience in the past 4 years.
- Have 7 years of validated scrub experience within the past 10 years.
- Be a medical doctor (MD), registered nurse (RN), licensed practical nurse (LPN), or licensed vocational nurse (LVN) with extensive, documented scrub experience.

Applicants must pass the certification examination to receive the credential tech in surgery–certified, or **TS-C (NCCT)**. The NCCT also requires individuals to maintain continuing education (CE) credits for certification. Those who pass the surgical assistant certification examination earn the credential assistant in surgery–certified, or AS-C (NCCT).

❖ *The NCCT Web site can be accessed at http://www.ncctinc. com.*

NATIONAL CERTIFYING EXAMINATION FOR SURGICAL TECHNOLOGISTS

The national certifying examination for surgical technologists is offered through the National Board of Surgical Technology and Surgical Assisting. This is a comprehensive examination covering the principles and basic practices of surgical technology, including basic sciences and patient care in the operating room. Students have the opportunity to take the examination before graduation. A passing grade on the examination confers the right to certification and the title Certified Surgical Technologist upon graduation from an accredited school.

CONTINUING EDUCATION

As mentioned earlier, **continuing education** provides an opportunity for professionals to improve their knowledge and competency throughout their career. Changes in practice, research, and the application of skills require ongoing study and demonstration of continuing competency. The AST provides resources for CE credits through its CE Resources. These are available directly from the AST, through on-line courses, or through *The Surgical Technologist*, the professional journal published by the AST. Credits are registered with the NBSTSA to maintain certification.

CLINICAL LADDER PROGRAM

The Clinical Ladder program was established by the Association of Surgical Technologists to provide incentives for surgical technologists to advance their clinical skills and competency in key areas. According to the AST, the program provides a "tool for measuring the ongoing progress of the surgical technologist from one level to another." (AST Recommended Clinical Ladder for the Surgical Technologist, http://www.ast. org/pdf/RecClinLad_ST.pdf) The stated goals of the Clinical Ladder are primarily to:

- Improve patient care
- Encourage employer recognition of the surgical technologist
- Promote accountability
- Increase the visibility of the surgical technologist's role in the health facility
- Encourage experienced surgical technologists to contribute to the professional growth of others

The Clinical Ladder program defines specific levels of practice (I through III) and provides clinical and learning objectives for each level. The levels are characterized by increasing technical ability and responsibilities for tasks involving patient care and management.

CAREERS FOR CERTIFIED SURGICAL TECHNOLOGISTS

HOSPITAL-BASED TECHNOLOGIST

The unique combination of health care and technological expertise opens the door to a wide range of roles and responsibilities. Most surgical technologists work in hospitals as members of the surgical team; this is the role that entry level CSTs are trained to fulfill. It is a complex job involving many disciplines, including:

- Basic patient care
- Organization, use, and care of surgical instruments and devices
- Team building skills
- Principles and practice of sterile technique
- Surgical procedures

Surgical technologists may also work as *agency* personnel. In this position, they are not permanent employees of a particular hospital, but rather work under short-term contracts in different hospitals. This provides a variety of experiences in different locations.

MILITARY PRACTICE

The military offers a surgical technology program for a specialized setting; this is referred to as the operating room specialist course. The educational program parallels civilian requirements, with additional training in combat and war surgery and in *golden hour* treatment (the golden hour is the first hour of treatment close to the front lines). The military program was the prototype for surgical technologists and remains dedicated to high standards, offering care to the war wounded and to other military personnel and civilians in combat areas where the armed forces are deployed. Opportunities in military surgery extend to more complex tasks associated with emergency settings and to licensure for operating room nursing.

SPECIALTY PRACTICE

The hospital-based surgical technologist may specialize in one or more surgical specialties, such as orthopedics, neurosurgery, cardiac surgery, obstetrics, or plastic surgery. CSTs at the midlevel and advanced stages of their career have the experience and knowledge to provide expert assistance in these specialties, and their work is in high demand.

Many surgical technologists work as private scrub assistants in the specialties in which they trained as hospital employees. These positions require middle and advanced level experience, as well as management and leadership skills. Surgical specialists may be required to provide preoperative education to patients in the office practice, and they may also fulfill that role in the hospital or health care facility.

Educational requirements for the role of specialist begin with certification in basic surgical technology. More advanced education in patient care and management may be required to provide care in the medical office.

SURGICAL FIRST ASSISTANT

The **Certified Surgical Technologist—Certified First Assistant (CST-CFA)** functions in an expanded role, which has been defined by the AST to include:

- Positioning the surgical patient
- Providing visualization of the operative site (retraction)
- Assisting in hemostasis
- Applying sutures or other techniques to close tissue layers

Surgical first assistants often are privately employed specialist assistants who are supervised by the surgeon who employs them, although the trend is moving to hospitals employing first assistants for specialty positions.

Preparation for this role includes certification in entry level surgical technology, additional training through an educational program, and demonstrated experience, which lead to certification of the surgical first assistant.

EDUCATOR AND CLINICAL INSTRUCTOR

The preferred educational pathway for the surgical technologist is a 2-year college degree. In the future, a 4-year bachelor of science (BS) degree may become the norm. In the field of education, certified surgical technologists currently work as formal instructors and as clinical department heads. They also design and develop the curriculum for their institutions and manage departments. These roles are becoming increasingly widespread, because the profession now is firmly established, and the need for quality instructors has greatly increased.

Entry level certification plus at least 2 years of experience in surgery are required for an educator position. A bachelor's degree in education is not required, although it may be in the future. Specific requirements depend on the type of institution (e.g., proprietary and state or community level).

MEDICAL INDUSTRY REPRESENTATIVE

An increasing number of CSTs with advanced training and experience work as representatives in the medical services and equipment industry. Service representatives are responsible for advising and training hospital and private clinical staff in their company's products. They often travel to clinical sites in their designated area and are available on call to answer questions and provide on-site assistance during surgery that involves the equipment. In this role, they promote their company's equipment, but they also have the technical expertise to troubleshoot problems.

The educational requirements for the role of medical services representative include entry level certification plus experience and additional training in management and service provision, which is provided by the company. More advanced positions in medical industry management might require a degree in business.

MATERIALS MANAGEMENT AND PROCESSING

Materials management is the processing of equipment and instruments in preparation for surgery. This field is growing in complexity and scope, requiring the expertise of instrument technology and a thorough knowledge about safety and health standards. The scope of duties and responsibilities includes disinfection and sterilization processes, assembly of surgical instrument sets, and management of complex instrument systems. It also may include managing and ordering other supplies used in surgery and maintaining accurate records of processing, use, and distribution. The surgical technologist may manage a materials processing department or function under the supervision of others.

The educational requirements for the role of materials management and processing are basic entry level certification plus at least 1 year of experience in operating room technology. Some hospitals may require certification as a Central Processing Technician. Management positions may also require supervisory experience or an advanced degree.

RESEARCH PRODUCT AND DEVELOPMENT

The surgical technologist is well prepared to work in research product and development in the area of surgical instruments, supplies, and devices. In this role, the technologist documents the results for new products and provides essential information for their further development and production. Basic entry level certification and additional education in research methodology are required.

ROLE OF THE SURGICAL TECHNOLOGIST

INTEGRATION OF ROLES

An important goal for surgical technology students and experienced professionals alike is role integration. Because the job is complex, it is easy to lose sight of the importance of connecting or integrating tasks and responsibilities. The work of the surgical technologist is never performed in a vacuum or in isolation. Every task and responsibility is an integral part of a larger domain of medicine.

> ❖ *The specific domain of surgical technology is patient care in the perioperative setting, focusing on the safe use of technology and the art of surgery to promote the patient's well-being.*

This larger picture casts the surgical technologist's role as a combination of four main areas of health care and technology:
- Assistant in surgical procedures as part of the surgical team
- Specialist in the preparation, handling, and use of surgical devices, equipment, and instruments
- Patient care provider in the perioperative setting
- Participant in leadership and management
- Educator and preceptor

Clearly, the surgical technologist has many roles and performs many tasks, ranging from the basic to the complex (see Chapter 16). In the perioperative setting, these usually are divided into time-oriented organization.

Assistant in Surgical Procedures

The surgical technologist is part of the surgical team, and most of the technologist's tasks and responsibilities culminate in this role. Before surgery, the surgical technologist helps position the patient and obtains appropriate equipment and supplies. During surgery, the surgical technologist is responsible for maintaining an orderly sterile field and is vigilant for any changes that require emergency action. Surgical technologists assist the surgeons in their work by pre-paring equipment and instruments and passing them in an approved, safe manner. At the close of surgery, the technologist assists in the application of dressings and removes sterile drapes. The technologist remains sterile and on standby until the patient is ready for transportation to the postanesthesia recovery unit.

Specialist in the Preparation, Handling, and Use of Instruments

In the role of specialist in the preparation, handling, and use of instruments, surgical technologists put into practice their specific knowledge about how instruments are used in surgery. This is one of the most important roles of the surgical technologist (ST), because the ST facilitates the surgical procedure by handing the right instrument at the right time. The ST knows how to clean and sterilize instruments and can troubleshoot problems with all types of equipment, from simple to complex. The ST maintains and protects instruments at all times so that they are safe to use.

Patient Care Provider in the Perioperative Setting

The surgical technologist is more than a technical adviser and manager of equipment. The technologist's role as a care provider has increased in scope and practice in the past 10 years. This domain of the integrated role demands the skills and duty of care similar to a nursing or medical assistant but includes specific considerations unique to the perioperative environment.

A surgical patient is exposed to numerous risks, and many of these are directly related to the technology used to accomplish the surgical goals. The direct care that the surgical technologist, nursing, and medical team provide helps mitigate or eliminate these risks. Psychosocial support is equally important to the patient's recovery and well-being. More advanced roles in direct patient care are included in surgical assisting in surgical specialties.

Leadership and Management

Unique opportunities in leadership and management are available to experienced surgical technologists. Specialty services such as orthopedics; ophthalmology; ear, nose, and throat (ENT); and plastic surgery need team leaders to facilitate and direct personnel and to manage equipment in specialty departments. Other leadership opportunities are available in facilitating safety and emergency protocols.

Surgical technologists may choose to pursue an advanced degree in hospital administration and management. At advanced levels, the integrated experience of both technology and patient care is an excellent springboard for a broader managerial career.

Educator

Surgical technologists are needed to provide mentoring and training at all levels of the profession. The ST educator is an instructor or department head of a surgical technology program. The demand for CST educators is increasing yearly, because more surgical technologists are being trained than ever before.

Preceptor

Surgical technologists often are asked to act as preceptors (personal tutors) while scrubbed. Some people enjoy this role and are natural teachers. Others are uncomfortable with the responsibility or are disappointed that they can no longer handle cases alone. Serving as preceptor requires patience and a willingness to share knowledge and experience.

TASKS AND RESPONSIBILITIES OF THE SURGICAL TECHNOLOGIST

The tasks of the surgical technologist are described as *sterile* or *nonsterile*. **Sterile personnel** are scrubbed and have donned a surgical gown and gloves. In this role, the surgical technologist assists in the surgery, handling only sterile instruments, equipment, and supplies. The scrubbed surgical technologist or registered nurse is commonly referred to as a **scrub**. This familiar term differentiates the sterile and non-sterile (circulator) roles. **Nonsterile personnel** do not wear sterile attire. The **circulator** is a nonsterile team member. Surgical technologists circulate under the direct supervision of a registered nurse. In this role, the technologist handles nonsterile equipment and supplies used in surgery. The circulating technologist also assists in patient care duties as defined by their state's practice laws. The specific tasks of the scrubbed and circulating surgical technologist are explained in Chapter 16 and also emphasized throughout the text.

DESIRABLE ATTRIBUTES OF THE SURGICAL TECHNOLOGIST

A successful surgical technologist has certain personal characteristics and aptitudes that contribute to good patient care and job satisfaction. Although most skills can be learned, certain characteristics, such as honesty, empathy, and caring, cannot be taught. Novices to the profession likely have many valuable untapped skills and attributes that develop with time and experience.

Success in the profession is defined by positive patient outcomes and a sense that one has contributed to successful care. The surgical technologist can achieve this goal in any setting, whether it is a high-profile institution, military post in a war zone, or a small, community-based setting. Everyone has unique talents to bring to the workplace. Some surgical technologists prefer a quiet workplace in which highly co-operative interpersonal relations are emphasized. Others prefer a highly technical, high-pressure environment in which many overtime hours are required and a wide variety of procedures are performed.

Perhaps the greatest skill surgical technologists acquire is an appreciation for their own professional niche, in which they can deliver the best possible patient care, feel challenged but not overwhelmed, achieve a high degree of satisfaction, and attain professional growth.

CARE AND EMPATHY

A person who chooses to enter a health care profession usually has the qualities of care and empathy. However, once the professional begins working, these qualities can be enhanced through personal growth, or they can be lost through job stress. Providing care in the health domain requires a devotion to human beings, in all their states and predicaments. It is nonjudgmental and requires the caregiver to look beyond the patient's external circumstances and take part in a privileged dialogue between health and illness.

Empathy is a response to the emotional or physical experience of another human being. It is the dual ability to comprehend another's feelings—grief, joy, sorrow, pain—and to convey that comprehension through words, actions, or body language. Trust is an essential component of care and empathy. Without trust, the patient cannot allow the caregiver to participate fully in the healing process.

Having the desire to contribute to the patient's well-being is the most important attribute of any health care worker. However, it is important to separate empathy from pity. Pity is a singular emotional reaction to another person's condition. Pity evokes strong feelings that may prevent therapeutic communication with the patient. Empathy involves communication between the caregiver and the patient that results in a healing response, whereas pity centers on the emotions of the caregiver only.

RESPECT FOR OTHERS

Respect for others is a quality that is universally recognized and admired in all environments. When people are respected, they feel accepted as they are. Lack of respect implies that a person has little worth as a human being. Simple expressions of thanks, acknowledging everyone's contribution to the work environment, and avoiding gossip are just a few ways that health care workers can demonstrate respect for each other. Respect for the patient is required of all health care workers. When coworkers do not show respect for each other in front of the patient, the patient may question or mistrust care received from those people.

EMOTIONAL MATURITY

The operating room environment can be stressful at times. The emotional maturity and self-control of operating room personnel contribute greatly to a professional and safe work environment. Emotional maturity is the ability to control strong feelings and to vent them appropriately in a constructive manner.

HONESTY AND ETHICAL BEHAVIOR

In surgery, professional and personal honesty about one's actions, mistakes, and abilities is called a **surgical conscience.** When any professional makes an error, the individual must admit the error at the time it is made. It is difficult to expose an error, particularly in front of others, but doing so and accepting responsibility are signs of professional and emotional maturity. It is a requirement for work in any health care profession.

MANUAL DEXTERITY

The surgical technologist must work quickly and deftly, sometimes with complex or very small instruments. Equipment must be assembled and handled efficiently and without confusion. This requires manual skills and keen observation. Excellent hand-eye coordination is required to master the skills needed to prepare for and assist during surgery. Speed is not always the most important skill; in fact, if the surgical technologist tries to work too fast, organization can break down, instruments can be dropped, and injuries can occur.

ORGANIZATIONAL SKILLS

Good organizational skills in surgery are expressed as the ability to prioritize tasks and equipment in a logical and efficient manner. For example, the surgical technologist is required to prepare, assemble, and physically arrange instruments and equipment in order of need. This requires overall knowledge of the surgical process and all the steps needed to complete the task. Any one procedure may require the organization of hundreds of items. Instruments, sutures, sponges, needles, electrosurgical devices, solutions, and medications all must be immediately available. Materials must be organized in a logical and methodical way so that they are readily at hand when needed. This skill is developed with practice and time.

ABILITY TO CONCENTRATE

Surgery requires constant, focused attention on both the operative site and the equipment. Although lulls in activity may occur, the surgical technologist is in motion during most of the procedure, preparing equipment or passing instruments in the correct spatial position. At the same time, the ST must anticipate the next step of the procedure. This requires moderate to intense levels of concentration. Lapses in focus can increase the risk to the patient and other team members. Many operative accidents, such as needle sticks, accidental cutting or burning, and loss of items in the surgical wound, are not the result of a lack of knowledge or skill but of a lack of attention. The short- and long-term problems that are the most common causes of lost concentration include:

* Stress
* Hunger (hypoglycemia)
* Lack of sleep
* Illness
* Substance abuse
* Exhaustion
* Lack of interest or burnout

PROBLEM-SOLVING SKILLS

The work of the surgical technologist is complex. Problems arise in every workday. Some problems require technical expertise, whereas others need a combination of "people skills" or environmental adjustments. A person with good problem-solving skills is able to:

* Prioritize activities when many must be accomplished
* Demonstrate genuine willingness to seek solutions to problems
* Use time wisely and anticipate problems
* Assess his or her own abilities (e.g., asking oneself, "Do I have what I need to solve this problem myself? If not, who can best assist?")
* Demonstrate flexibility (e.g., asking oneself, "If the problem cannot be solved with the time and resources available, what alternatives do I have?")
* Select the best alternative to achieve positive results
* Analyze the result and accept feedback from others as part of the learning experience

SENSE OF HUMOR

The ability to put events in perspective and enjoy the lighter side of work and life is a great asset. Humor, when expressed appropriately, can ease tension and promote good practice. Not all humor is appropriate. Humor that is sarcastic, mean spirited, prejudicial, or crude creates tension, disdain, and contempt among team members. A sense of humor can always be developed in a supportive environment.

SURGICAL TECHNOLOGIST'S SCOPE OF PRACTICE

In all work settings, the surgical technologist performs duties within task boundaries known as the *scope of practice*. The scope of practice is determined by several regulating agencies to protect the public and ensure high-quality medical care. Regulating bodies specify the type of activities that the surgical technologist can legally perform. Regulatory documents that may define the scope of practice include:

* State nursing practice acts
* State medical boards
* State business and professional codes
* Regulations of the Department of Health and Human Services
* Guidelines established by The Joint Commission

Surgical technologists often are confronted with situations in which they are asked to perform an activity they are prohibited from performing by state regulations. All members of the surgical team are responsible for knowing their state's practice acts. Many states specify certain tasks that the surgical technologist cannot perform even if a surgeon, a licensed nurse, or another licensed professional delegates the task. For example, the surgical technologist can never administer medications of any kind. Delegation does not imply permission. Because few states explicitly define the role of the surgical technologist, the ST's scope of practice is defined by professional organizations and, by default, by the part of state codes that applies to assistive personnel. Because cost cutting and efficiency are major concerns in hospitals, the role of the surgical technologist is constantly changing. Responsibility and accountability are increasing.

In most states the surgical technologist may not engage in the practice of medicine. The state of Washington, for example, defines the practice of medicine as follows:

A person is practicing medicine if he does one or more of the following:
1. *Offers or undertakes to diagnose, cure, advise, or prescribe for any human disease, ailment, injury, infirmity, deformity, pain or other condition, physical or mental, real or imaginary, by any means or instrumentality;*
2. *Administers or prescribes drugs or medicinal preparations to be used by any other person;*
3. *Severs or penetrates the tissue of human beings.*

As with the prohibition against the practice of medicine, in most states the surgical technologist may not practice nursing. Prohibited activities include but are not restricted to the following:

- Activities that require nursing assessment and judgment during their implementation
- Physical, psychological, and social assessments that require nursing judgment, referral, or intervention
- Design of a plan of nursing care and evaluation of that plan
- Administration of medications by any route
- As a general rule, patient or family health teaching is also a nursing duty that cannot be delegated. This includes giving advice about postoperative care.

TASKS AND DELEGATION

DEPENDENT AND INDEPENDENT TASKS

Surgery is a collaborative effort. Each member of the team has specific duties and tasks that all have a common goal. **Independent tasks** are tasks the surgical technologist performs without supervision. Activities such as preparing surgical equipment and maintaining the sterile field are independent tasks. Some tasks, however, may require supervision. **Dependent tasks** are tasks that require direct supervision by a surgeon, a licensed nurse, a dentist, a podiatrist, an anesthesiologist or, in some states, a physician assistant.

DELEGATION

Delegation is the transfer of responsibility for an activity from one person to another. In the health care setting, *delegation* refers to the assignment of tasks that normally are the responsibility of a licensed nurse or physician. An individual may delegate specific tasks to another person provided the delegee has the necessary training and knowledge and is legally permitted to carry out the delegated task.

❖ *Legal accountability for the outcome of a delegated task lies with the person who delegated it.*

For example, if the surgeon delegates the task of retraction to the surgical technologist during surgery, the surgeon is accountable for any tissue damage that may occur as a result of that retraction. A licensed health care professional can delegate a task to another individual only if that person:

- Can legally perform the task
- Has received the proper training
- Is competent to perform the task

Surgical technologists should be knowledgeable about what tasks can be delegated in their institution and state. This knowledge can protect them from situations that may result in conflict or injury.

CHAPTER SUMMARY

- The profession of surgical technologist developed out of a need for qualified personnel who were familiar with the technical aspects of surgery and could assist in intraoperative patient care.
- The U. S. military has trained surgical technologists since World War II and continues to do so today.
- The Association of Surgical Technologists is the professional organization for surgical technologists. It provides its members with opportunities for career planning, training materials, national conferences, and professional and legislative support.
- The NCCT provides certification by examination for surgical technologists with documented surgical experience and academic qualifications. This includes individuals trained in the armed forces.
- Surgical technology is one of the fastest growing professions in the United States. Many opportunities are available for career placement and advancement.
- Surgical technologists may be employed in a health care facility, hospital, or private clinic. Many develop expertise in specialty areas such as orthopedics, cardiac surgery, trauma, ophthalmic surgery, and plastic surgery.
- Other opportunities exist in education and marketing for surgical manufacturers and as central service managers (materials management).
- The surgical technologist assists in surgery as a sterile member of the team. In nonsterile roles, the surgical technologist assists in preparing the patient, supplies, and equipment needed for a surgical procedure.
- Surgical technologists are required to have the same professional attributes as any other health professional. Honesty, professionalism, respect for others, empathy for patients and other staff members, and the ability to work on a team are necessary.

REVIEW QUESTIONS

1. How can a surgical technologist become certified?
2. Why should a graduate technologist become certified?

3. How is certification maintained?
4. Why do you think the role and duties of the surgical technologist have expanded in recent years?
5. What kinds of job opportunities are available for the surgical technologist?
6. In your opinion, what skills and attributes of a good surgical technologist can be learned or acquired?
7. What does it mean to *delegate* a task? What are the requirements for delegation of a task?
8. What is surgical conscience?
9. What is the difference between *empathy* and *pity*?
10. What is meant by the phrase *scope of practice*?

BIBLIOGRAPHY

Accreditation Review Council on Education in Surgical Technology and Surgical Assisting (ARC/STSA): http://www.arcst.org.

Accreditation Review Council on Education in Surgical Technology and Surgical Assisting: ARC/STSA communiqué. Accessed October 17, 2007, at http://arcst.org/core_curriculum.htm.

Association of periOperative Registered Nurses (AORN): *Standards, recommended practices and guidelines, 2007 edition,* Denver, 2007, AORN.

Association of Surgical Technologists (AST): Standards of practice. Accessed October 22, 2007, at www.ast.org.

Association of Surgical Technologists: Surgical technology: a growing career. Accessed October 5, 2007, at http://www.ast.org.

National Board of Surgical Technology and Surgical Assisting (NBSTSA): http://www.lcc-st.org.

Peck M: "Golden hour" surgical units prove worth, *Military Medical Technology* 11:7, 2007. Accessed November 1, 2007, at www.military-medical-technology.com/article.cfm?DocID=176.

US Army Medical Department Center and School Portal: Operating room branch. Accessed November 1, 2007, at http://www.cs.armedd.army.mil/details.aspx?dt=165.

US Department of Labor: Occupational outlook: surgical technologists. Accessed October 22, 2007, at http://www.bls.gov/oco/ocos106.htm.

CHAPTER 2

The Patient in Surgery

CHAPTER OUTLINE

LEARNING OBJECTIVES

After studying this chapter the reader will be able to:

- Define patient-centered and outcome-oriented care
- List the domains of Maslow's hierarchy of human needs
- Describe the role of the technologist in each of the domains of Maslow's hierarchy of needs
- Discuss concepts of patient care that apply to the surgical technologist
- Describe some common patient fears and their origins
- Discuss why patients feel a loss of security as a result of illness and surgery
- Understand and apply the concept of body image to disfigurement
- Discuss and practice therapeutic communication

- Describe therapeutic touch in health care
- Define cultural competence and discuss its importance in ethics and health care
- Define spirituality as it applies to patient care
- Provide spiritual support to the patient
- List the developmental stages of the pediatric patient and describe pediatric patients' beliefs about surgery according to their developmental stage
- Discuss the physiological risks of the elderly patient
- Describe how to communicate with an elderly patient
- Discuss the impaired patient and how to provide support for this patient group
- List patient groups at high risk for surgery

TERMINOLOGY

Body image: The way individuals perceive themselves physically in the eyes of others.

Critical thinking: The process of analyzing information about the patient, comparing it with similar previous experience, and responding to the unique needs of that patient.

Cultural competence: The ability to communicate with people of other cultures and belief systems. Institutions are required to provide access to resources for achieving and promoting cultural competence.

Elimination: The physiological process of removing cellular and chemical waste products from the body.

Maslow's hierarchy of human needs: A model of human achievement and self-actualization developed by psychologist Abraham Maslow.

Mobility: The ability of an organism to move. As a protective mechanism, mobility allows an organism to move away from harmful stimuli.

Nutrition: Usually refers to the intake of food. On a cellular and tissue level, it may include the availability of nutrients, fluid, and electrolytes.

Outcome-oriented care: Care based on the predicted result of particular tasks and duties.

Patient-centered care: Therapeutic care, communication, and intervention provided according to the unique needs of the patient.

Physiological: A term that refers to the biochemical, mechanical, and physical processes of life.

Reflection: Communication with the patient that helps the individual connect current emotions with events in the environment.

Regression: An abnormal return to a former or earlier state, particularly infantile patterns of thought or behavior. In patients, this can result from feelings of helplessness and dependency.

Relational: A term that refers to a person's interactions with other individuals.

Respiration: Oxygen exchange at the cellular and molecular levels and the process of ventilation.

Self-actualization: An individual's ability to express and achieve personal goals.

Therapeutic communication: A purposeful method of communication in which the caregiver responds to explicit or implicit needs of the patient.

Thermoregulation: The body's ability to regulate the core (inner) temperature.

Ventilation: The physical mechanisms of lung expansion, accessory muscle action, and air intake during the process of respiration.

INTRODUCTION

This chapter presents an overview of the patient's needs and experiences in the perioperative environment. The discussion focuses on the basic physiological, social, and psychological needs of patients and the role of the surgical technologist (ST) in meeting those needs. The technologist's role is focused on safety, advocacy, and psychosocial support. This holistic approach to patient care requires a *patient-centered* and *outcome-oriented* way of thinking and acting.

In **patient-centered care,** the surgical team bases its assessments, planning, and interventions on the unique needs of the individual patient. These unique needs are revealed through information from others, astute observation, and good communication. **Outcome-oriented care** involves predicting the results of particular tasks and duties and choosing the correct course of action.

MASLOW'S HIERARCHY OF NEEDS

In the 1970s, psychologist Abraham Maslow developed a theory about human needs. His model, known as **Maslow's hierarchy of human needs,** is depicted as a triangular hierarchy in which the most important needs are at the base levels (Figure 2-1). The most basic of human needs are **physiological;** that is, they involve the biochemical, mechanical, and physical processes of life (Table 2-1). According to Maslow's model, if the most basic requirements for life are not met, the needs at the higher levels cannot be fulfilled. Maslow's model provides a guide for patient care and a method of prioritizing the patient's needs.

PHYSIOLOGICAL DOMAINS

Respiration

Respiration is not just breathing, which involves the mechanical functions of the lungs, diaphragm, and accessory muscles. It also is the process of oxygen exchange at the cellular and molecular level and many other complex physiological processes.

The surgical technologist is concerned with respiration in many ways. For example, in positioning the surgical patient, full **ventilation,** which is the physical expansion of the lungs and thoracic cavity, is a major goal. Without adequate ventilation, air exchange cannot occur. The surgical technologist helps protect the patient's airway when safety measures are

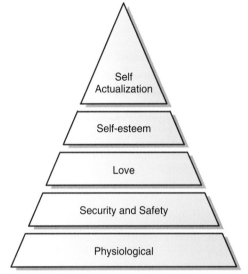

Figure 2-1 Maslow's hierarchy of human needs.

Table 2-1

Basic Physiological Needs of the Patient

Type of Need	How Needs Are Met in the Perioperative Environment
Nutrition, water	Administration of intravenous replacement fluids and nutritive or electrolyte fluids
Shelter	Control of temperature through cloth blankets, air heating, or cooling blankets
Air and oxygen	Maintenance of an open airway
	Provision of the proper mix of oxygen with anesthetic or room air
	Attention to signs of oxygen deficit
Rest and sleep	Protection from environmental stress such as noise, light, or cold
Elimination	Catheterization or opportunity to void as needed
	Medical attention to conditions that prevent elimination
Movement	Freedom from restraint and assistance with movement when patient is unable to move on his or her own
	Protecting the patient from harm
Freedom from pain	Observation of the patient for signs of pain
	Administration of pain medication
	Exercise of care when moving the patient

enforced during laser surgery of the upper respiratory tract. The surgical technologist has suction available at all times during airway surgery to prevent aspiration (inhalation) of blood or solutions into the bronchi and lungs.

Nutrition

At the physiological level, **nutrition** means supplying fluid, electrolytes, and organic substances to cells to maintain electrical activity and transport of materials into and out of the cells. It also refers to the breakdown of food into molecular components for tissue repair and growth. Fluid in the cells and vascular system is also maintained in equilibrium, and this is balanced with output, or excretion.

The surgical technologist contributes to information about fluid balance by tracking and reporting the amounts used for fluid irrigation during a procedure.

Temperature Control (Thermoregulation)

The body functions at an optimal level when the core temperature is maintained within a narrow range. Complex biological functions maintain the body within this range as long as the **thermoregulation** mechanisms are intact. As the core temperature drifts to the limits of this range, physiological function is greatly impaired. When the limits are exceeded, death occurs.

The surgical technologist contributes to temperature regulation in many ways. The surgical technologist maintains irrigation fluids at the correct temperature. Thermal (body warming) devices used during surgery are the responsibility of the registered nurse (RN) circulator and the surgical technologist who assists. The surgical technologist ensures that patients are covered with warm blankets while awaiting surgery or during transportation. This is not just a comfort measure; it also is important for maintaining the core temperature.

Mobility

Mobility is the body's way of avoiding painful or dangerous environments and stimuli. In surgery, *the anesthetized patient looses this ability.* The caregivers must be constantly alert for environmental dangers from which the patient normally would move away. This is a great responsibility, one that requires knowledge, vigilance, and care. In many circumstances, caregivers know instinctively that the patient is in danger. For example many obvious precautions are taken to prevent patient burns caused by fire or electrical malfunction.

However, many hundreds of dangers require **critical thinking** and knowledge. These are subtle dangers. Examples include nerve damage from a table accessory hidden by drapes or an unseen electrical burn caused by damaged insulation on a surgical instrument. The patient cannot move away from the pain and injury caused by these accidents. The surgical technologist is responsible for knowing the dangers and preventing them. For example, the surgical technologist maintains instruments to prevent patient injury. Surgical technologists are knowledgeable about electrosurgery and its many hazards. They help position the patient in such a way that no pressure points are created that can cause irreparable nerve and vascular damage.

Rest

In physiological terms, rest is the slowing down of metabolic functions. This is necessary for repair and growth and for maintaining alert mental functions that signal a person to respond when the body is in danger. Sleep is the body's natural response to fatigue. However, functions also slow down in illness and pain. If the body cannot slow down naturally, we experience physiological, emotional, or metabolic stress, which can lead to a cycle of illness and more stress on the body.

Major surgery can cause extreme physiological and psychological stress. Not only are patients deprived of normal activities, but they also experience pain, fatigue, and sometimes life-threatening metabolic changes. Hospital-acquired infection (HAI) increases these stressors to an even greater level. Death from HAI often is a result of the combination of the stress of surgery or the preexisting illness and the destructive effects of the infection itself.

The ST has a role in preventing metabolic stress. By following strict aseptic technique and sound surgical conscience, surgical technologists prevent postoperative infection. They provide comfort and reassurance to the patient, whose fear and anxiety about the process of surgery adds to the physical stress of the procedure.

Elimination

Elimination is the physiological process of removing cellular and chemical waste products from the body. During the processes of metabolism, both toxic and nontoxic by-products are produced, such as urea, carbon dioxide, and dead cells. The elimination process takes place at the cellular and tissue level. Waste products are finally shunted from the body in feces and urine. Without these systems, metabolic waste would soon create systemic toxicity and death, as is seen in kidney failure.

During surgery, the body continues to produce normal metabolites (the by-products of metabolism). The physiological process is maintained by adequate fluid balance and gentle handling of tissues. Kidney function is an important indicator of metabolism. Urinary catheterization and urine collection provide a method of monitoring kidney function during surgery.

PROTECTION

Safety and Security

Safety and security are both physical and psychological concepts. In the physical realm, people need to be safe from any threat to physical well-being. Threatening psychological events can contribute to physical stress and the ability to make decisions, have relationships with others, and care for one's self. In surgery, safety and security precautions for the patient are well defined. Although many patients are confident about the outcome of surgery and even feel relieved to be resolving a medical problem, most feel fear about their safety and security.

The surgical technologist contributes to the patient's physical safety and security by being knowledgeable about and observing for environmental dangers. These dangers are related to devices and equipment, procedures (e.g., positioning and transporting the patient), infection control, and many other activities. The surgical technologist responds to the patient's need to *feel* safe and secure through verbal and nonverbal communication.

RELATIONAL AND PERSONAL DOMAINS

Love and Belonging

Love and belonging are powerful needs. They determine our sense of well-being through others' acceptance and nurturing. Love and belonging affirm our humanity and provide emotional fulfillment.

Self-Actualization

Self-actualization is the individual's ability to express and achieve personal goals. Personal goals are whatever that person defines as a goal or an achievement. Personal goals are unique and valued by each individual. The frustration and grief many patients feel is related to their inability to achieve goals because of their illness. Surgical patients are vulnerable to this risk because of the added psychological burden of altered body image or loss of function. This can be related to the surgery itself or to the illness that requires the surgery. Perioperative caregivers can help their patients through this difficult situation by understanding the meaning of individual loss.

PSYCHOLOGICAL NEEDS OF THE PATIENT

Surgical technologists in different health care settings have varying levels of social and professional contact with patients. In some settings the surgical technologist may have only brief encounters with patients, whereas in others, contact is extensive. Regardless of how brief or extended the professional relationship is, the surgical technologist can understand and support a patient's psychological needs.

Patients may have many concerns and fears about surgery but may never have discussed them with perioperative personnel. If asked, they may admit that they are afraid, but they do not volunteer this information. The surgical technologist can support the patient by showing care and by acknowledging the patient's feelings rather than trying to minimize them.

An early treatise on patient care, written by Paul E. Johnson, describes the state of the seriously ill hospital patient with clarity and compassion:

> The hospital patient suffers from mental anguish more acute than his physical pain. His emotional condition is one of anxiety and insecurity as he dangles in a chasm of distress between a past he would gladly return to and a future he is reluctant to face. He has lost the values he once had of health, freedom, and power to do and be sufficient to the strenuous joys of active achievement. He can look back but with vain regret. Looking ahead he sees only poignant uncertainty. Am I to live or die? If I live, will I be disabled and have to live in restricted patterns of uncertain health, with faltering steps and hesitant, watchful caution? Can I ever be free again? . . . Am I on borrowed time from now on, costing more than I can earn, depriving my family of their necessities, turning over my work to stronger men, trying to look more cheerful than I feel, with a brave pose of gaiety that covers a hollow gulf of threatening insecurity?

As caregivers, we cannot presume to meet all the psychosocial needs of the patient, especially in the brief time that we interact with them. Human needs, both inner and demonstrated, are complex. However, we can be aware of those needs and be aware of our own feelings and attitudes about the complex psychosocial aspects of care. Knowledge of our own attitudes helps clarify and prepare our response to the patient. As professionals, we must never allow our own beliefs to interfere with care or cause judgment of another. The role of the caregiver is to support and heal.

FEAR

Many patients approach their surgery with anxiety and fear. Even though a patient may understand the process of the surgery and the goals, the emotional reactions to surgery can overwhelm this understanding.

Reassurance and open acknowledgement of the patient's fears are good methods of communicating empathy. Patients develop trust in caregivers who *demonstrate* their care through their actions. The patient feels greater security when team members explain, honestly and professionally, what is occurring and why. For example, the patient safety strap is secured as soon as the patient is transferred to the operating table. Rather than saying jokingly, "I'm putting this strap on so you don't get away" or "This strap is to keep you from falling off the table" (the latter introduces a new source of anxiety, because that event may never have occurred to the patient), the surgical technologist can use a more reassuring statement, such as, "The operating bed is very narrow. I'm putting this strap over your legs to remind you to stay centered on the bed." This statement explains that a safety issue exists and is being addressed.

Patients share many of the same fears:

- **Anesthesia.** Many patients fear that they will not awaken from the anesthetic or that they will be able to feel all the sensations of the procedure but will be unable to move or respond (called *anesthesia awareness*).
- **Death.** Fear of death during or after surgery is common among patients. This fear often is greater in a patient who is about to receive a general anesthetic. The concept of being held unconscious and in another's control increases feelings of impending death.
- **Pain.** Fear of pain is a normal protective mechanism. However, surgical patients sometimes have *extreme* fear of postoperative pain. They might not have sufficient information about their postoperative care, or they may have experienced severe pain in the past.
- **Disfigurement.** Patients undergoing radical or reconstructive surgery have realistic fears about disfigurement. Body image is a very important psychological consideration for patients. People identify themselves with their body image,

Box 2-1

Guidelines for Maintaining the Security of Electronic-Based Patient Records

The protection of sensitive information is of utmost importance in the health care setting. Safeguards have been created to prevent unauthorized access to patient-specific information. Violation of a patient's confidentiality can result in serious sanctions, including the termination of employment. Security measures include the use of passwords or terminal access keys.

Computer passwords and access keys must never be shared. When a computer password is selected, the individual should not use personal numbers, such as the user's birth date or telephone number, or names, such as the user's name or that of family members.

Computer users must log off any computer before leaving the terminal to prevent another person from viewing information by using another's password. Information that has been accessed is linked to the password of the person who was logged onto the computer at the time the information was accessed. Regardless of who actually accessed the information, the person who was logged on will be held responsible for any breach of patient confidentiality.

If a user forgets a password or if a computer access key has been lost or stolen, the authorized user must contact the system administrator or administrative supervisor as soon as possible.

which often influences their ability to relate to others. Disfigurement is attached to social stigma and rejection, which are powerful triggers for fear and anxiety.

- **Helplessness.** When patients enter the health care system, they often feel a loss of personal rights and control. For the surgical patient, these feelings are intensified. The anticipation of general anesthesia often triggers feelings of helplessness. The patient may also anticipate immobilization as a result of pain or loss of function.
- Fear that private information will be shared with others. Many patients are afraid that information about their health may not be held in confidence. They fear that the information may result in loss of employment or that it will injure their relationships with others. The ethical responsibility to hold all patient information in strict confidence cannot be overemphasized. The use of computer-based communication and patient charting presents particular risks. A review of computer security guidelines is provided in Box 2-1.

LOSS OF SECURITY

Many patients are very anxious about how their surgery will affect their self-reliance. This fear often is focused on employment and financial security. Patients undergoing surgery that limits their mobility, whether temporarily or permanently, may have profound concerns about their livelihood and ability to support their families. The cost of surgery may require substantial sacrifice in lifestyle or savings intended for future income, or both. This may cause fears of becoming dependent on family members for survival and accompanying anxiety over the need to be self-reliant and independent.

ROLE AND SELF-IMAGE

Illness and surgery can affect an individual's role in the family and the community. Loss of function and mobility as a result of surgery can alter the patient's roles or the person's perception of them. Patients may view their roles of responsibility as severely threatened or changed by their inability to carry out certain physical or mental functions as a result of surgery. Sexual and **relational** roles are often altered by surgery, and this can feel threatening or debilitating to the patient.

Self-image is closely associated with body image. **Body image** is the way we perceive ourselves physically in the eyes of others. When we are comfortable with our body image, we feel good about ourselves. When a person's body image is altered suddenly or is perceived to be altered, feelings of embarrassment, rejection, and isolation can arise. Many societies discriminate against those whose appearance is different from the "norm." Acceptance in society is a basic need of all people. Fear of losing acceptance can be overwhelming. Patients who need counseling to adjust to sudden changes in their appearance can be guided to support groups or trained specialists.

THERAPEUTIC COMMUNICATION

Today's health care system often requires that as many surgeries as possible be completed in each 24-hour period. The surgical patient lives in the center of a storm of activity, in a very busy environment that is frightening and authoritative. The patient has no control over what is happening and is handed from one person to the next, often with no knowledge about the roles of the people involved in the medical environment.

The types of communication in which surgical technologists are likely to engage focus on the surgical environment, the patient's physical (comfort) needs, and perhaps the way the patient is feeling. The surgical technologist can greatly affect the patient's well-being by showing focused, purposeful, and caring communication. Appropriate **therapeutic communication** requires a nonjudgmental and supportive attitude. Box 2-2 presents important guidelines for therapeutic communication.

CHARACTERISTICS OF THERAPEUTIC COMMUNICATION

Therapeutic communication has four primary characteristics:
- **It is goal directed.** It has a specific purpose. The purpose is to comfort the patient, gain information about the patient's needs, and respond in a way that meets or acknowledges those needs.
- **It is unique to each patient.** Every patient is a unique individual with particular hopes, fears, and concerns. Therapeutic relationships honor this uniqueness with spe-

Box 2-2
Guidelines for Therapeutic Communication

- Listen to the patient attentively. Show your interest by making eye contact (unless this is culturally inappropriate; for example, in traditional Islamic cultures, women do not make direct eye contact with men).
- Do not allow yourself to be distracted while communicating with the patient. If your attention is split, you will convey a lack of concern. Remember that your thoughts are revealed by your body language, actions, and expressions.
- Explain what you are doing in plain, simple language. Look for cues that the patient understands. Do not assume that because the message was given, it was also received and comprehended.
- Continual questioning can make a person feel uncomfortable. Therapeutic communication allows the patient to express needs and concerns. For example, "How are you feeling?" and "Do you have any concerns about your procedure?"
- Do not talk about yourself. It is inappropriate for team members to share personal information with the patient or with coworkers in the presence of the patient.
- Joking and offensive language can have serious effects on the patient's sense of security. Although it is not meant to offend the patient, it is not only disconcerting but also unprofessional. Would you want to hear the details of someone's date while waiting to have abdominal surgery for cancer?
- Refer questions when you do not know the answers. Be honest about what you do not know. Patients often are unaware of the professional roles of their caretakers. If you are asked a medical question or one that requires assessment or other nursing skills, refer the question to licensed personnel. Ask the patient if he or she has discussed the issue with the physician. It is better to delay an answer than to mislead or give information that is outside the scope of one's practice.

cific verbal and physical responses are more therapeutic than stock answers. Therapeutic communication is learned behavior.

- **It requires active engagement.** It is not accidental or haphazard.
- **It requires excellent observation and listening skills.** These are reinforced through experience and guidance. Listening is both an art and a skill. It requires patience, focus, and presence. One can learn important information by observing the patient. One can meet needs by recognizing the signs of discomfort, fear, anxiety, or other intense emotions.

THERAPEUTIC RESPONSES

Therapeutic responses include cue giving, clarification, restatement, paraphrasing, reflection, and touch. When these responses are used, communication becomes centered on the patient's needs.

Leads and cues are actions and words that encourage the patient to communicate. The goal is to prevent the patient from becoming self-conscious or afraid to express feelings and sensations. Leads and cues include nodding in affirmation and making comments such as "Really?" and "I see."

Example—Restatement
PATIENT: *"I should have had this surgery a long time ago, but I just couldn't face it."*
RESPONSE: *"Really?"* (A short verbal cue indicates that the listener cares and invites the patient to continue to share her feelings.)
PATIENT: *"I was so afraid."*
RESPONSE: *"It must have been very difficult for you."* (Acknowledges the patient's fear.)

Restatement is not simply parroting the patient, but rather restating the patient's comment in a way that takes in the underlying meaning.

Example—Paraphrasing
PATIENT: *"This is the fifth back surgery in 8 years for me. I just hope this surgeon knows what he is doing."*
RESPONSE: *"You've been through a lot of surgery; you're hopeful that this surgeon has the knowledge to help you?"*

In this case, the patient expresses doubts about the expertise of the surgeon. The caregiver acknowledges the patient's anxiety.

Paraphrasing is different from restatement in that the caregiver looks past the patient's stated words and addresses the underlying message. In paraphrasing, the caregiver demonstrates empathy about the unstated need for comfort and security.

Example—Reflection
PATIENT (nervously): *"Everyone here is so busy."*
RESPONSE: *"I know there is a lot of activity. It must seem really fast, but everyone is taking care of their patients. Is there anything I can do to help you feel more comfortable while we're waiting for the anesthesiologist?"* (Appropriately addresses the unstated meaning, which is, "I wonder if they will take good care of me; there is so much going on.")

Reflection allows the patient to connect his or her emotions with information provided in the immediate environment or from a different event or situation.

Example–Therapeutic Response
PATIENT: *"It's always so cold in these places. With all the money these hospitals make, the least they could do is turn up the heat."*
RESPONSE: *"It sounds as if you feel frustrated about being here. It's a difficult time. The temperature is low for safety reasons. I'll get you a warm blanket."*

A skilled caregiver understands that the patient is not only cold but also angry about being helpless in this situation and unable to meet his or her own environmental needs. The caregiver acknowledges the patient's frustration and responds appropriately.

Nontherapeutic responses are casual and do not help the patient cope with anxiety or conflict.

Example—Nontherapeutic Response

PATIENT: *"Are all those instruments for my surgery?"*

NONTHERAPEUTIC RESPONSE: *"Yeah, we have to have everything ready in case we need it. You never know what the doctor might want."*

PATIENT: *"Oh"* (unstated and unresolved fear). *"It must mean they think there will be complications. Maybe the surgery will be much more extensive than I thought. What if I have cancer and they didn't tell me?"*

CORRECT RESPONSE: *"Our instruments come in preassembled sets. We use only what we need from each set."* (This response conveys order, knowledge, and professionalism. It answers the question directly and addresses underlying fears.)

PATIENT: *"I'm relieved to hear that!"*

THERAPEUTIC TOUCH

Touch is an important part of therapeutic communication, but it must be used with caution and respect. Some patients do not want to be touched. There are many reasons a patient may not want to be touched, including cultural beliefs and previous experience. The caregiver may ask permission to touch a neutral area of the body, such as the hand, and watch for cues from the patient. If the patient is comforted by touch, the person's body language and facial expression will show relaxation and relief. If touch is rejected, the patient may pull back or show signs of distrust or fear. Every patient has the right to reject or refuse touch. In this case, the caregiver must seek other methods of offering reassurance and comfort. When touch is acceptable, it can convey deep empathy and caring.

CULTURAL COMPETENCE

Cultural competence is the ability to communicate and interact with people of different cultures and beliefs. Health care providers were among the first professionals to recognize the need for cultural competence. Meeting a patient's needs depends on good communication, trust, and respect for the other's values.

Cultural competence adheres to guiding values and principles. These apply to the individual, family, community, and organizations. The most effective way to approach a patient whose cultural beliefs are different from one's own is with knowledge of that culture. What may seem strange or "wrong" to one person often is cherished by a person of a different culture. Health care professionals have an ethical responsibility to honor and respect those beliefs, just as they would want their own beliefs to be honored in a different culture.

Language barriers often make health care more difficult and frustrating for both the patient and the caregiver. However, translators are available. When the patient cannot understand verbal or written communication, the results can be extremely frustrating or even harmful. Resources available

at the institutional level may fall short at the bedside because of understaffing.

Acquiring the skills to communicate effectively among different cultures takes time. It is a process grounded in the rights of all people to receive equal care. Classes and conferences in culturally appropriate health care are available from health care educational institutions.

SPIRITUAL NEEDS OF THE PATIENT

Spirituality is not necessarily the same as religion, although they often are expressed as one entity. Spirituality is a sense or understanding of something more profound than humanity that is not perceived by the physical senses. It is an awareness or belief in an energy or power greater than humankind. This power may be referred to as *creator, spirit,* or *God,* or the patient may have no name for it. In the religious setting, spiritual life is integrated into rituals (practices that have special meaning) and ceremonies common to those who practice a particular faith. Patients have the right to express their religious faith in the health care setting. Ritual defines life-changing events and is important to physical and mental healing. For many it *is* the healing force.

Examining one's own beliefs and broadening the definition of *spirituality* is the first step toward the development of spiritual care. These are challenging but rewarding goals that the surgical technologist must develop to be a holistic and patient-centered caregiver.

SPECIAL PATIENT POPULATIONS

PEDIATRIC PATIENTS

The pediatric patient presents particular challenges in both communication and the physiological response to surgery. Pediatric patient groups are defined according to approximate chronological age ranges. The age group reflects the developmental stage:

Infant	Birth to 18 months
Toddler	19 months to 3 years
Preschool	4 to 6 years
School age	7 to 12 years
Adolescent	13 to 16 years

Physiological Considerations

In pediatric patients, the size of anatomical structures, the relative fragility of the body, and the ratio of surface area to volume presents particular risks for surgery. Loss of even a small amount of blood or fluid is severe in the pediatric patient. The large surface area compared to mass predisposes the patient to chilling or overheating during surgery. This can result in excess fluid loss or hypoglycemia, especially in infants.

Developmental Stages and Surgery

Children of different developmental stages have predictable fears, responses, and reactions to hospitalization and the process of surgery. Knowledge of these stages can help the surgical technologist understand the behaviors exhibited by children in the operating room.

Infants need to be physically close to their caretakers. They should be held as much as possible until the procedure begins. Stress is high in infant patients. They have been separated from the familiar feel, smell, and sight of their primary caregiver, and feedings have been stopped before surgery. For these reasons, they are difficult to comfort and may cry continually.

Toddlers suffer frustration and loss of autonomy, as well as extreme anxiety, when separated from their primary caretaker. The operating room environment can be terrifying to a toddler, who expresses this by crying and screaming or through aggression and **regression.** Toddlers are especially difficult to restrain. They require patience and understanding from their caregivers. Stronger restraint (or more restrainers) usually causes more terror and increased resistance. Taking the time to instill calm is the humane way to provide medical intervention. When this is unsuccessful, rapid sedation may be required.

Preschoolers also suffer extreme fear in the operating room environment. These patients commonly view the hospital and surgical experience as a type of punishment or as deliberate abandonment. Prone to fantasy, they may imagine extreme mutilation as a result of surgery. Because they are unable to understand what the inside of the body actually looks like, they interpret descriptions of surgery literally. They are concrete thinkers and understand words such as *cut, bleed,* and *stick* in extreme, literal, and often exaggerated forms.

School-age children are more compliant and cooperative with health care personnel, but many tend to withdraw from their caregivers. They are curious about their bodies and often insist on "helping" with their own care. They are very sensitive about body exposure, which can be extremely stressful. For school-age children, receiving information is a way of coping with their fears. They welcome explanations and descriptions of how things work and how devices and equipment in the environment relate to their own bodies.

Adolescents are very sensitive about body image and changes in the body. They resent any intrusion on their privacy and bodily exposure. They also fear loss of control. At times stoic and curious, they are grateful for concrete information about the surgical environment and the procedure itself. Among their many concerns, potential loss of presence with their peers and fear of being "left out" because of illness or deformity are very important.

ELDERLY PATIENTS

The elderly patient faces significant risks in surgery. These are related to coexisting disease, emergency surgery, and risks associated with certain types of surgery (e.g., procedures involving major blood vessels and abdominal and thoracic conditions). Surgery that involves significant blood loss (e.g., hip replacement or repair) can also be high risk for the elderly patient.

The normal physiological alterations of aging (Table 2-2) often affect the decision on whether surgery should be performed, as well as the outcome. The cardiovascular system looses elasticity, and circulation is often decreased, particularly to vital organs such as the kidneys and heart. The lungs lose their ability to expand because of resistance. This can lead to infectious postoperative pneumonia, which is among the most common hospital-acquired infections. Decreased functioning of the digestive system can lead to poor nutritional status both before and after surgery.

Table 2-2
Physical Changes that Occur with Age

Body System	Changes
Respiratory	• Chest diameter decreases from front to back (anterior to posterior). • Blood oxygen level decreases. • Lungs become more rigid and less elastic. • Recoil of alveoli diminishes.
Gastrointestinal	• Peristalsis diminishes. • Liver loses storage capacity. • Motility of stomach muscles decreases. • Gag reflex diminishes.
Cardiovascular	• Capillary walls thicken. • Systolic blood pressure increases. • Cardiac output decreases.
Musculoskeletal	• Muscle strength decreases. • Range of motion decreases. • Cartilage decreases. • Bone mass decreases.
Sensory perception	• Progressive hearing loss occurs. • Sense of smell diminishes. • Pain threshold increases. • Night vision decreases. • Sensitivity to glare increases. • Sense of body position in space (proprioception) can decrease.

Genitourinary	• Bladder capacity diminishes.
	 • Stress incontinence in women occurs.
	 • Kidney filtration rate decreases.
	 • Reproductive changes occur in women:
	   • Vaginal secretions decrease.
	   • Estrogen levels decrease.
	   • Reproductive organs atrophy.
	   • Breast tissue decreases.
	 • Reproductive changes occur in men:
	   • Testosterone production decreases.
	   • Testicular size decreases.
	   • Sperm count decreases.

Skin	• Skin loses turgor (elasticity). • Sebaceous glands become less active. • Skin becomes thin and delicate. • Pigment changes occur.
Endocrine	• Cortisol production decreases. • Blood glucose level increases. • Pancreas releases insulin at a slower rate.

Kidney function may be significantly decreased in elderly patients. This can lead to electrolyte and fluid imbalance.

Elderly patients are at risk for skin, joint, muscle, and bone injury, especially during transfer and positioning. During the aging process, soft connective tissue loses tone, mass, and elasticity. This increases the risk of skeletal injury. The elderly patient's skin often is dry and extremely fragile. Decreased body fat increases the patient's risk for hypothermia.

These fragile conditions require increased vigilance and care in the perioperative environment. The surgical technologist must make sure that transportation, transferal, and positioning are performed slowly and deliberately. The patient's core temperature must be maintained before, during, and after surgery, and blood loss and urinary output must be monitored accurately. Box 2-3 lists the risk factors for elderly patients.

Box 2-3
Risk Factors in Elderly Patients

Surgical Risks
Emergency surgery
Surgical site
Duration of the procedure

Anesthetic Risks
Age older than 75
Preexisting conditions (e.g., hypertension; diabetes; kidney, liver, cardiac, or respiratory disease)

Disease Risks
Respiratory Disease
Bronchitis
Pneumonia

Cardiovascular Disease
Angina
Previous myocardial infarction
Congestive heart failure

Digestive Disease
Poor nutritional status
Protein deficiency
Cirrhosis
Peptic ulcer

Endocrine Disease
Adrenal insufficiency
Hypothyroidism

Other Factors
Dehydration
Anemia
Malignancy
Impaired mobility
Lack of social support
Emotional distress
Poverty

Modified from Rothrock J: *Care of the patient in surgery*, St Louis, 2007, Mosby.

Communicating with Elderly Patients

The following tips can be helpful when communicating with an elderly patient.

- **Do not use clichés.** Do not reach for the first available, easiest response. For example, if the patient says that she is a burden to others in her illness, do not respond with, "Oh, I'm sure you're no bother." Instead, support the patient in her feelings. For example, "It must be very difficult for you to have surgery right now."
- **Do not refer to the patient by diminutives such as "sweetie," or "honey."** These names are offensive to many patients. They convey a lack of respect for the patient as an adult with a lifetime of accomplishments and knowledge. Always address the patient by his or her proper name and demonstrate to others in your environment that you acknowledge the fullness of the patient's life.
- **Do not assume that the elderly patient is mentally impaired.** The normal aging process does not include dementia. Senile dementia is a disease state. Some elderly patients are slightly confused or disoriented in the hospital. Perioperative caregivers can help orient the patient by explaining procedures and identifying personnel in the environment. If there is evidence or knowledge of organic brain disease, it may be necessary to repeat questions and responses.

PATIENTS WITH SENSORY IMPAIRMENTS

Patients with sensory impairments have an altered sense of their environment or cannot interpret the environment. They may have difficulty understanding directions that aid their care. For example, they may not understand simple directions such as moving onto the operating bed or keeping their hands down. When communicating with a patient who is impaired, the surgical technologist should follow these guidelines:

- Speak clearly and slowly
- Face the patient while speaking
- Speak in a normal voice
- Provide additional communication cues, such as gestures

Surgical technologists must remember that the patient probably is extremely anxious, and they should provide emotional support through touch or body language.

MALNOURISHED PATIENTS

A malnourished patient lacks the necessary nutritional reserves to support the process of healing. Trauma to the body, whether intentional (e.g., surgery) or unintentional, requires high metabolic activity during the healing process. Protein and carbohydrates are in particularly high demand by the body to rebuild tissue and meet the physiological demands of organ systems. The patient who enters surgery *undernourished* (without enough food intake to support health) or *malnourished* (lacking the right kinds of food to support body functions) is at high risk. Cancer, alcoholism, metabolic disease, and advanced age are a few conditions that often result in malnutrition or undernutrition.

PATIENTS WITH DIABETES

Diabetes mellitus is an endocrine disease that disrupts the metabolism of carbohydrates, fats, and proteins. When diabetes is not controlled, severe damage to vascular and neurological tissues results. The risks associated with surgery in diabetic patients are complex. They arise from impairments in the healing properties of the vascular system and in the efficient use of glucose for tissue metabolism. Because many diabetic patients have a compromised vascular system, their risk of infection at the surgical site is higher than for other groups. They also are subject to prolonged wound healing, hypertension, and peripheral edema.

IMMUNOSUPPRESSED PATIENTS

The patient whose immune system is compromised or suppressed faces the threats of postoperative infection and delayed healing. The body requires a healthy immune system to respond to the trauma of surgery and to defend against pathogens that may have invaded during surgery. Patients being treated with immunosuppressants or antineoplastic agents for cancer are immunosuppressed. Patients undergoing organ transplantation receive immunosuppressants to depress the body's immune reaction to the new organ. Patients infected with the human immunodeficiency virus (HIV) and those who have developed acquired immunodeficiency syndrome (AIDS) or other conditions that affect the immune response are also at increased risk for nosocomial (hospital-acquired) infections.

Trauma Patients

The patient who is rushed into surgery because of physical trauma is at high risk for many reasons. With severe trauma, there may be no time to obtain a previous medical history or the patient may be physically unable to provide it. Pre-existing conditions may not be known, especially if the patient is unconscious. The patient may have eaten recently, which increases the risk of vomiting, aspiration, and subsequent pneumonia. There may be no witnesses to the trauma. Witnesses can supply important information about the nature of the trauma, which aids diagnosis. Injuries may be undetected, especially if the patient cannot answer questions. The trauma patient may arrive in surgery in a precarious physiological state, with extensive blood loss, severe shock, and fluid-electrolyte imbalance. Intoxication from alcohol or drugs can alter the physiological response to surgery and complicate the process and method of anesthesia.

Patients with HIV or AIDS

The patient with HIV or AIDS faces multiple barriers to a safe postoperative recovery. Because the patient does not have a healthy immune system, the potential for postoperative infection is high. The patient with AIDS has multiple co-morbid diseases, which deplete the body's reserves for healing. Skin integrity often is compromised by open sores and lesions. Bacterial or viral infection may already be present. During surgery, infectious microorganisms can gain access to the sterile surfaces of the body and create serious systemic disease. One of the most common disorders associated with AIDS is infection with *Pneumocystis carinii*, a pathogenic microorganism that causes lung disease. Drug-resistant tuberculosis is also common in these patients.

With the advent of highly active antiretroviral therapy (HAART), HIV is becoming recognized as a manageable illness. However, many of the medications currently used to treat HIV may have detrimental effects on a person's metabolism that may impair wound healing. Certain anti-HIV medications also may affect lipid levels in the blood, leading to an increased risk of heart disease and peripheral vascular disease.

CHAPTER SUMMARY

- The needs of human beings have been summarized in a theory known as Maslow's hierarchy of human needs. This theory, which is commonly used to identify areas of focus for patient care, includes physiological needs, protection, and relational and personal needs.
- Direct patient care prioritizes the physiological and emotional needs of the patient.
- Communication with the patient establishes the basis of all care.
- Therapeutic communication is a learned skill that all health care professionals must develop.
- Cultural competence is the ability to interact with all people regardless of their culture or belief.
- Cultural competence cannot be learned by reading or studying cultures. It is developed through training and experience with people.
- Health care workers must examine their own beliefs and prejudices to become truly culturally competent.
- Cultural competence includes respect and acknowledgement of another's faith or spiritual beliefs.
- Special patient populations have particular physiological and psychological needs.
- Special populations include pediatric patients, the elderly, patients with sensory deficits, and those who are immunosuppressed. Trauma patients and those with chronic diseases also have special needs that must be considered in their care.

REVIEW QUESTIONS

1. Define patient-centered care.
2. List the domains of Maslow's hierarchy.
3. What are the roles (not tasks) of the surgical technologist in the domain of professionalism?
4. What is body image? In what ways does body image influence a patient's anxieties about surgery?
5. What methods would you use in therapeutic communication?

6. Define cultural competence. Why is cultural competence important in health care?
7. What are the results of inadequate cultural competence?
8. What would you do to communicate with a patient who does not speak English? What if no interpreter is available?
9. Why is the patient with impairments particularly anxious in surgery?
10. What do you think are the postoperative risks for an impoverished patient? What needs does this patient have that might not be met?

CASE STUDIES

Case 1

You are transporting a patient with AIDS to the operating room on a stretcher. The patient is silent. She is cooperative, but her facial expression shows anxiety. What will you say to this patient while transporting her to the operating room? What psychosocial needs do you think this patient has? How can you meet these needs?

Case 2

You are preparing equipment for a cardiac procedure. The patient has been brought into surgery and is lying on the operating table. He says to you, "How long do you think this will take?" How will you respond? What possible concerns does this patient have? Is he expressing these concerns to you through his question?

Case 3

You are assisting the circulator with a 3-year-old patient about to have a tonsillectomy. The patient is screaming and kicking.

He is crying and saying he wants his mommy. The circulator calls for more help to restrain the child. When you attempt to soothe him, he kicks you. What will you do? What is this patient experiencing? What can you provide for this patient?

Case 4

The patient is a 20-year-old brought to the operating room for an emergency cesarean section. She is crying. She says to you, "I hope I don't lose the baby. When will my doctor be here?" What is your response?

Case 5

The patient is a 40-year-old woman from Southeast Asia. She does not speak English. You overhear a coworker mimicking her attempts to speak to staff members. The patient overhears this, too, and begins to cry silently. How will you respond to her? Will you respond to your coworker?

BIBLIOGRAPHY

Dreger V, Tremback T: Management of preoperative anxiety in children, *AORN Journal* 84:5, 2006.
Fina D: The spiritual needs of patients and their families, *AORN Journal* 65:4, 1995.
McKennis A: Caring for the Islamic patient, *AORN Journal* 69:6, 1999.
National Center for Cultural Competence and the Center for Child and Human Development: A definition of linguistic competence. Accessed November 12, 2007, at http://gucchd.georgetown.edu/nccc.
National Center for Cultural Competence and the Center for Child and Human Development: Cultural competence: definition and conceptual framework. Accessed November 11, 2007, at http://gucchd.georgetown.edu/nccc.
Wood B: Caring for a limited-English-proficient patient, *AORN Journal* 75:2, 2002.

Death and Dying

CHAPTER OUTLINE

LEARNING OBJECTIVES

After studying this chapter the reader will be able to:

- Define the end of life
- Define death
- Describe Kübler-Ross's stages of dying
- Discuss other models used to describe the end of life period
- Discuss ways to provide comfort and support to patients in the dying period
- Understand the conflicts and stress families face during the dying period
- Discuss significant ethical issues surrounding death and dying
- Define cultural competence as it applies to the dying patient

- Define the criteria for death
- Discuss the physical changes in the body immediately after death
- Describe postmortem care
- Give examples of a coroner's case
- Define the criteria for organ procurement
- List organizations that provide education and services for organ and tissue donation
- Discuss how health care workers can obtain support for stressful events in their workplace
- Identify one's own plan for self-care in times of stress

TERMINOLOGY

Coroner's case: A patient death that requires investigation by the coroner, as well as an autopsy on the deceased.

Cultural competence: The ability to provide support and care to individuals of cultures and belief systems different from one's own.

Determination of death: A formal medical process to determine brain death.

DNAR: "do not attempt resuscitation," emphasizes the patient's desire to refuse intervention to resuscitate.

DNR: "Do not resuscitate." An official request to refrain from certain types of resuscitation, usually cardiopulmonary resuscitation.

End of life: A period within which death is expected, usually days to months.

Heartbeating cadaver: A cadaver maintained on cardiopulmonary support to provide tissue perfusion. This is done to maintain viability in organs for donation.

Kübler-Ross, Elisabeth: A Swiss psychiatrist who proposed a theory of developmental or psychological stages of the dying experience.

Living will: A legal document signed by the patient stating the conditions and limitations of medical assistance in the event of near death or a prognosis of death.

Livor mortis: A red and purple discoloration of the face that appears soon after death.

Non-heartbeating cadaver: A cadaver in which perfusion at and after death was not possible. Only certain tissues may be procured for donation.

Postmortem care: Physical care of the body to prepare it for viewing by the family and for mortuary procedures.

Required request law: A law requiring medical personnel to request organ procurement from a deceased's family.

Rigor mortis: The natural stiffening of the body that starts approximately 15 minutes after death and lasts about 24 hours.

Self-determination: The right of an individual to determine the direction and path of his or her life.

INTRODUCTION

Death in the operating room is a relatively rare event. Training in death has only recently returned to the curriculum of health care workers. All allied health personnel benefit from structured study on death, with the main focus on the psychosocial and procedural aspects.

This chapter is not intended to provide a course in death and dying. It is the basis for further study and exploration. This chapter discusses social, personal, ethical, legal, and medical perspectives on death. An understanding of the process of death and the events triggered by it can aid the surgical technologist in providing compassionate care to patients and their families. Knowledge and understanding also contribute to the health professional's beliefs and values.

The procedural aspects of death and the protocols that must be followed may seem "clinical" in nature; however, they are necessary to ensure dignity, order, and professionalism.

DEFINING THE END OF LIFE

Death and the end of life can be defined from many perspectives. The study and experience of different perspectives assists health professionals in their support of the dying patient and family.

> From a medical point of view, the **end of life** is that period when death is expected. Most clinicians pronounce the patient's entry into a dying state when death is expected within days, weeks, or months. The dying period is marked by inability to provide or the cessation of attempts to prolong life. However, this does not mean that comfort care is not provided in the dying period. It simply means that death cannot be avoided.

MODELS OF DEATH AND DYING

News that oneself or a loved one has begun the dying process triggers a cascade of emotional and psychological events. In the past few decades, a number of models have been presented that explain these events and processes. The best-known model was developed in the 1960s by Swiss psychiatrist **Elisabeth Kübler-Ross,** who described stages of death. In her model, the stages of death are not discrete, nor are they predictable in all people of all cultures. The Kübler-Ross's model proposes the following stages of grief and dying:

- **Denial:** The patient denies that he or she is dying. This is described by mental health professionals as a natural response to shocking events. Denial is a defense mechanism that forestalls the full impact of the fact of death until the mind is ready to accept it.
- **Anger:** Some patients express anger. Feelings of anger may be projected onto the family, oneself, health workers, or God. Some patients feel great anger and remorse that they did not heed warnings to change lifestyle habits they knew

were harmful. Others express anger at those who care for them or become very demanding in their care. Patients may express anger at themselves by refusing treatment or nutrition. These coping strategies may be an attempt to gain control over the environment.

- **Bargaining:** Kübler-Ross describes this stage as a way of postponing death. The patient may make an inner attempt to bargain with God or another spiritual entity, such as, "I just want to experience one pain-free day with my family" or "If I pray daily maybe God will allow me to live."
- **Depression:** True clinical depression may occur during the dying process. In recent years there has been a trend away from accepting depression as a natural result of dying and to treat it clinically.
- **Acceptance:** In Kübler-Ross's theory, death is "accepted." The idea and interpretation of death are no longer a source of psychological conflict.

Critics of Kübler-Ross's model believe that the stage theory is too constricting and does not allow for individualism in the experience of death. However, the stages model provided a framework for psychologists and social workers to look at the process of dying in a way that had not been previously studied.

Many modern models have been developed since Kübler-Ross conducted her research. These appreciate individuals according to their situation, personality, culture, and life experiences. For example, *William McDougall,* a well-known social psychologist, emphasized the need to integrate the dying process into existing life experiences. Rather than focusing on particular tasks or psychological stages, he advocated maintaining a sense of self-awareness in relation to the environment. Social psychologist, *Charles Corr* encouraged the dying to try different individual strategies and coping mechanisms based on their uniqueness as individuals and was a strong critic of the stage theory of death.

SUPPORT AND COMFORT FOR THE DYING AND BEREAVED

PATIENT

Perioperative caregivers may have only brief encounters with the dying patient in the surgical environment, whereas contact between patients and palliative care specialists is frequent and the relationships can last weeks or months. Perioperative staff members should always be aware that no matter how brief their contact with the dying patient, all encounters provide an opportunity to support and care for the patient in the dying process.

Communication with the dying patient requires keen listening and observation skills. It is important to recognize and acknowledge the fact of death and what this means to the patient in that moment and time. As a surgical technologist (ST), you should focus on what the patient is experiencing in the operating room or holding area. Observe facial expressions and gestures. Be alert to any changes in mood or signs of anxiety and fear related to death and isolation. Avoid communication that attempts to minimize, rationalize, or deny death. However, this does not imply blunt or insensitive communication. Focus on immediate physical and emotional comfort and acknowledgement, and above all, listen to the patient. Listening is sometimes the most effective source of comfort (but not always the easiest). A response may not be needed and should not be forced. Respect the patient's individuality and uniqueness in the present. Use the patient's verbal and physical cues as a guideline rather than making assumptions about what the patient feels or needs.

Never imply that a surgical procedure may "cure" the patient, but offer the possibility of a good outcome. Perhaps the patient is having surgery to reduce the size of a tumor or for treatment of intractable pain. These procedures offer hope for a longer survival period or one that is physically tolerable.

FAMILY

Families and friends react to dying and death in many different ways. Not only must they cope with the emotional and psychological impact of death, they also must make many significant decisions. They have a central role in the dying patient's emotional environment, and in sudden death they often need the assistance and guidance of health professionals.

The family's reactions of grief and sadness may be accompanied by bouts of anger and frustration with the health system, each other, and even the dying family member. Death triggers large and sometimes unmanageable emotions, and these cannot always be contained in a ways considered socially acceptable. This may be disconcerting to the family itself as they participate in the death and observe their own reactions as a family unit. The wise health professional recognizes when tensions are mounting and provides validation for these strong emotions. At the same time, the health professional can guide family members toward coping strategies to help defuse the tension and add order to the experience.

Families usually face many complex events associated with death and dying. The death may impose a financial burden. The dying patient may have children or other family members who rely on the individual for support, and these responsibilities must be shifted to other family members. Difficult decisions may need to be made about palliative care or "do not resuscitate" status. The administrative requirements, such as signing release forms or attending to the details of funeral arrangements, often seem too clinical or cold in the midst of grieving. Professionals who routinely care for the dying provide ongoing support in many areas. This includes not only management of the patient's medical needs, but also emotional support and even referral for counseling outside the medical and nursing environment.

SUDDEN UNEXPECTED DEATH

When death is sudden and unexpected, family and friends have many needs. In the clinical environment, these immediate needs are addressed by nurses, physicians, and spiritual counselors. Early reactions often focus on information about the cause and details of death. The need for cloistered privacy usually is very strong in the initial stages of shock and grief.

The surgical technologist should refrain from providing information to family or friends about the patient's medical condition. This is the responsibility of the physicians and nurses, and any discussions must be deferred to them. The surgical technologist may offer acknowledgement of the loss. The ST may also facilitate communication between the family and other professionals, such as showing the way to the consultation area and making sure the environment is appropriate.

ETHICAL CONSIDERATIONS IN DEATH AND DYING

The ethics of care and decision making in death and dying are highly personal, and there are many conflicting viewpoints. Beliefs and culture influence the decisions people make about how they want to die or how they would like others to go through the dying process. These beliefs are not universal. This means that whenever possible, an individual's personal wishes for his or her own death should be documented and validated by the individual and family.

SELF-DETERMINATION

Self-determination is the right of every individual to make decisions about how he or she lives and dies. Advanced care planning provides an accepted method for individuals to define their needs and wishes about death and dying. Patients may refuse treatment at any point in the dying process. They may select which palliative measures are performed and which are withheld. Decisions can then be communicated and made official for health care providers. Ethical issues arise when the patient is not competent to communicate. Decisions about end of life care fall to the family when the patient is not able to communicate his or her wishes. In these cases, health care workers help provide information about choices, as well as ongoing support through the decision process. Ethical decisions that cannot be resolved by the family and health care professionals may be brought before the hospital ethics committee for review.

RIGHT TO DIE

An individual may believe that he or she has a "right to die" and may refuse treatment to fulfill this right. However, *not treating a dying patient* is a completely different process from *treating with intent to harm.* Assisted suicide is perceived by many as intent to harm and on that basis is rejected. **Assisted suicide** is intentional harm to a person, at their request, to promote or cause death. The arguments for and against assisted suicide continue in many states and countries. The Netherlands allows assisted suicide, as does Oregon, Washington, and Montana. The process involves stringent preconditions and extensive review by an ethics committee.

ADVANCE DIRECTIVES

"Do not resuscitate" (**DNR**) and "do not attempt resuscitation" (**DNAR**) orders express the patient's decision to decline lifesaving efforts. In some cases the family makes this decision for the patient who is incompetent. The request not to resuscitate is made official when the patient signs a DNR order, which is charted in the patient's medical record. Exacting forms that define precisely the procedures that can and cannot be performed during resuscitation have been designed to alleviate ambiguity. However, ethical conflicts arise in spite of protocol. These usually occur when no DNR status has been stated and the decision is left for the family. The definition of "resuscitation" may also cause ambiguity. Active measures to prolong life are ethically different from those that do not halt the progression of death.

The individual's DNR status must be verified throughout the period of patient care. In most facilities, the DNR status must be renewed with each hospital admission. Health care providers may not realize that the patient has redefined his or her wishes at some point during illness. Admission to the surgical unit always includes verification of the DNR status.

CONFLICTS IN PALLIATIVE CARE

Palliative care is the medical and supportive care provided to the dying patient. Numerous types of surgical intervention may be included as a component of palliative care, such as debulking of a tumor or debridement of a pressure wound. Institution of some biomedical devices, such as a gastric feeding tube or renal dialysis access, require anesthesia in the interventional radiology department or operating room. Medical interventions for the dying patient include extreme measures, such as respiratory support ("artificial respiration"), intravenous feeding, dialysis, drugs to maintain and regulate failed metabolic processes, and many others.

The ethics of palliative care involve reasoned arguments about the definition of particular interventions. Many patients have signed a **living will,** which specifies the exact nature of palliative care that they accept. In the absence of a living will, clinical decisions sometimes are made by consensus of the patient (when able), the family, and care providers. Most people intend to do the "right thing." They try to resolve the conflicts about quality of life. However, families may have trouble deciding when to prolong life by supportive measures and when to discontinue them based on the suffering they might cause. These decisions are extremely difficult and often fraught with emotion and conflict within the family.

An ethical discussion that often arises is whether withdrawal of care constitutes suffering. Intravenous (IV) maintenance (hydration) and feeding often are the most sensitive areas for families to resolve. In these cases the health professional makes every attempt to inform the family about the effects of withdrawing care without interfering with their right to decide.

Health care workers often face personal conflict about the decisions made by their patients or the families of patients. They may not agree with the decisions, but they are obliged to honor them. In extreme cases of ethical conflict, the health professional may ask to be excused from participation in the care of the patient. Although this resolves the conflict temporarily, it does not offer long-term relief from an environment that frequently challenges beliefs and values. At some point in their career, health professionals usually need to define their own ethics and accept that others have differing perspectives.

ORGAN DONATION

Organ and tissue donation arise as an ethical issue when the patient has not left a clear directive before death. When no verifiable permission has been granted by the patient, the family may act as a surrogate for the patient.

Many cultures and faiths forbid organ removal after death, and these cases usually are straightforward for the family and patient. However, individuals often leave the question unresolved at the time of death. If no decision has been made by the patient, the attending physician must, *by law,* ask the patient and family to consider organ donation. In cases of sudden death without clear directives, conflicting views may be held by family members about organ donation. The ethical problem is whether the family can and should make such a decision for the deceased. Some families may feel very strongly opposed to organ donation, whereas others feel that it is a way of providing life.

CULTURAL RESPONSES TO DEATH AND DYING

SPIRITUAL AND RELIGIOUS CONCEPTS

Death, as perceived across cultures, often is defined through spiritual values and beliefs. Meaning in life and death often are linked to spiritual hope. The rituals and practices that people of different cultures observe are vital to the fulfillment of their duty to the dying person. In the United States, great efforts have been made to honor and respect the beliefs of others, but there is still a long way to go. Health care workers may question the validity of a belief or an expression of a patient's faith, often comparing it to their own. By definition, spiritual beliefs are valid for the believer and do not need approval or justification by others.

Support and care across cultures is called **cultural competence.** It is learned through experience and active learning. It begins with acceptance and respect. In many cultures, death is considered a natural phenomenon, a possible conclusion of serious illness and not a battle with the cause. Although grief and other deep emotions are present in all families at the time of death, these feelings often are mitigated by ritual and ceremony, which comfort as well as heal the living. In many cultures they also are believed to comfort the dead.

Handling of the body, especially its preparation for viewing by the family, may require special knowledge about the practices of certain cultures. As long as these practices do not conflict with health and safety standards, they should be carried out with dignity and respect.

DEATH IN THE CLINICAL SETTING

DETERMINATION OF DEATH

When death occurs in surgery, the surgeon and anesthesia care provider must verify that death has occurred; this is called **determination of death.** Death is determined by specific medical criteria, which have legal implications (Box 3-1). To determine brain death, specific medical assessment tests may be carried out on the patient, such as an electroencephalogram (EEG), administration of painful stimuli, and testing of cranial reflexes.

When death has been determined, the operating room supervisor communicates with other key individuals to prepare the morgue (or coroner in some cases) or the supervisor of the postanesthesia care unit (PACU). The deceased may be transported to the PACU for postmortem care. Arrangements are made for the family to meet with the surgeon or a designee in a quiet area near the surgical department or PACU.

The surgical wound is closed appropriately and dressed. Drapes are removed from the patient (if they were not removed during resuscitation), and instruments and supplies are prepared as they would be at the close of any case. The patient may then be transported to the PACU or another location in the surgical department for postmortem care.

POSTMORTEM CARE

Postmortem care prepares the body for viewing by the family and assists in further handling procedures carried out by the morgue and mortuary. The exact protocol for postmortem care is carefully defined by every health facility. All staff

members who perform postmortem care must be completely familiar with the protocol, and there should be no ambiguity about the process. The protocol for coroner's cases is different, and this procedure also is clearly documented in each health facility. General care of the body is based on the process of death.

NATURAL CHANGES IN THE BODY AFTER DEATH

Immediately after death, the body begins to cool. All sphincter muscles, including those controlling feces and urine, immediately lose tone. The eyes remain open, and the jaw drops down. Dependent areas of the body (those under pressure from body weight or gravity) begin to collect fluid, and the areas around the ears and cheeks may turn purple or red (a condition called **livor mortis**). The pooling of blood in these regions cannot be reversed in the embalming process. The sacrum and other pressure areas fill with fluid, possibly resulting in tissue rupture. **Rigor mortis,** the natural stiffening of the body, begins approximately 15 minutes after death and peaks at 8 to 10 hours. The exact time depends on the tissues and environmental temperature. At 18 hours the process regresses, and the body usually is relaxed after 24 hours. Rigor mortis begins at the head (eyelids) and progresses to the feet. When relaxation begins, it follows the reverse order of progression.

GENERAL POSTMORTEM PROCEDURES

All health care facilities have a postmortem kit, which contains the supplies needed to perform aftercare. During the aftercare procedure, the body is handled gently and with respect at all times. Postmortem care that conflicts with the patient's religious affiliation is not performed. In some facilities, with a death during surgery, the body must remain on the operating table, intact, until a decision is made about a coroner's investigation.

General procedures for postmortem care are as follows:
1. The head of the bed is raised to 30 degrees.
2. The eyelids are closed and held gently shut until they remain in place.
3. The jaw is closed and supported with a rolled towel. This may be difficult with an airway in place. A jaw strap sometimes is used to secure the jaw. Cloth adhesive tape should not be used to secure the jaw. The family will be viewing the body, and the face should retain a natural composure as much as possible.
4. Pads are placed under the patient to absorb urine and feces. A perineal pad may be positioned to prevent soiling of linens. A folded towel is placed beneath the scrotum to elevate the testicles. This prevents accumulation of fluid and distension of the scrotum. As mentioned above, fluid accumulates in areas of the body where there is any pressure—the scrotum swells and the skin may rupture. "Elevating" the scrotum prevents body fluid from draining into the scrotum because of gravity.

Box 3-1

Medical Assessment Criteria for Determining Death

1. Complete and irreversible cessation of the cardiovascular system
2. Irreversible respiratory failure that is not a result of drugs or hypothermia
3. Absence of any response to external stimuli
4. Cessation of cranial nerve reflexes
5. Cessation of all brain activity

5. All catheters, IV lines, tubes, and other devices are *left in place* for coroner's cases or according to hospital policy. These should be capped or occluded securely with tape and gauze to prevent leakage.

6. Wounds from venipuncture sites or other invasive procedures should be dressed with a single layer of gauze and surgical tape. Cloth adhesive tape should not be used on the skin, which may tear when the tape is removed. Every attempt is made to maintain the integrity of the body during postmortem care.

7. Any foreign objects or debris imbedded in the patient must be protected from dislodgement during postmortem care.

8. If the death is not a coroner's case, the body can be cleaned or washed. In medical settings, the family may want to perform this ritual themselves. In coroner's cases the body is not cleansed.

9. The patient's hair is combed for a presentable appearance, and a clean pillow is placed under the patient's head. All soiled sheets, including draw sheets, are exchanged for clean ones.

10. If the patient is to be viewed by the family, the body may be transferred to another location. The body should be transported in a closed stretcher or in a manner that is discrete and does not expose the body to others in the environment.

11. Required documentation is completed by the licensed nurse assigned to the case. All patient records remain with the patient until transport to the morgue. The patient's belongings are identified and collected. In coroner's cases, these may be transferred to the coroner. Otherwise, they are returned to the family with appropriate documentation to identify the transfer.

CORONER'S CASES

The circumstances of the patient's death determine whether the coroner must investigate the death; this process includes mandatory autopsy, and these cases are called **coroner's cases.** Most states have similar criteria for establishing coroner's cases, and the criteria may include the following circumstances of death:

- Death in the operating room or emergency department
- Unwitnessed death
- Death after admission from another facility
- Death in which criminal activity is suspected (the deceased may have been the perpetrator or the victim)
- Suicide
- Death of an incarcerated individual
- Death as a result of an infectious disease that might pose a public health risk

Death in the workplace. Other criteria may also apply, depending on the state law. Coroner's cases require that the conditions of the body remain intact for examination and investigation. In the medical environment, all implanted or invasive devices are left in place. The patient's property may also be transferred to the coroner rather than returned to the

family. Meticulous care and identification of specimens is always required, regardless of whether the specimens become part of the investigation. After a death in surgery, any specimens produced during surgery become the property of the coroner. They must be transferred directly from the operating room, as specified by hospital protocol, using universal precautions.

ORGAN AND TISSUE PROCUREMENT

Organ procurement is the donation of tissue or whole organs from a deceased person for transplantation into another individual. Once the decision has been made for organ procurement, exacting clinical protocols are followed to ensure the vitality of the organs.

Permission for Procurement

A person can make the decision to donate tissue or whole organs before the issue arises. In many states, this permission may be verified on an individual's driver's license or other identification card. Some states have a **required request law,** which requires medical professionals and other caregivers to ask the family for permission to procure organs from the deceased.

Protocols

The process of procurement is administered through tissue banks and organ procurement agencies, which locate donors, register recipients, and organize procurement. Many organizations are involved in the process (Box 3-2), which requires a high level of coordination and data exchange.

Donors are registered in different regions of the country, and the data are exchanged with procurement organizations. The protocols for medical procurement, care of tissue, and identification of tissue are formulated by the American Association of Tissue Banks, a nonprofit scientific organization that accredits tissue banks and procurement organizations to ensure professional standards of practice.

Organs are collected and stored by regional organ banks and provided to facilities as needed. Services are available on call 24 hours a day. Data are constantly exchanged between tissue banks and the organ procurement registries to match donor organs with compatible recipients.

Organ procurement takes place as soon as possible after death because the vitality of some tissues is time dependent.

Box 3-2

Organ Procurement and Tissue Bank Organizations

American Society of Transplant Surgeons (http://www.asts.org)
The Organ Procurement and Transplantation Network (http://www.optn.org)
United Network for Organ Sharing (http://www.unos.org)
American Association of Tissue Banks (http://www.aatb.org)

<u>Box 3-3</u>

Criteria for Organ Procurement in a Heartbeating Donor

- Systolic blood pressure: >90 mm Hg
- Central venous pressure: 5 to 10 mm Hg
- Urine output, minimum: 100 mL/hr
- Core body temperature: 98.6°F (37°C)
- Donor maintained on intravenous fluids and 100% oxygen

Modified from Phillips N: *Berry and Kohn's operating room technique*, ed 11, St Louis, 2007, Mosby.

Actual procurement takes place at the hospital or tissue bank organization. When procurement occurs at the host hospital, a transplant coordinator from the regional tissue bank arrives on site to ensure that medical, administrative, and supportive services are carried out according to set standards. The procurement team travels to the hospital as soon as possible after the death of a donor when time-sensitive tissue is to be procured.

Medical Criteria for Tissue Procurement

Different types of tissue require specific medical maintenance to remain viable after death. Donor cadavers generally are divided into two categories, heartbeating cadavers and non-heartbeating cadavers.

Heartbeating Cadaver

A **heartbeating cadaver** is one in which tissue perfusion can be maintained during and immediately after death to preserve the life of the tissue. Cardiopulmonary support provides intact circulation to organs suitable for procurement. The availability of cardiopulmonary support depends on the exact location of death; it usually is restricted to the emergency department, operating room, or critical care unit, where equipment, supplies, and trained personnel are immediately available. The physiological parameters for procurement include renal output, vascular pressure, temperature, and perfusion. The criteria for these parameters are listed in Box 3-3.

Nonheartbeating Cadaver

Tissues from a **nonheartbeating cadaver** are restricted to those that do not need perfusion to sustain viability for later transplantation. These include the cornea, blood vessels, heart valves, bone, and skin.

EMOTIONAL NEEDS OF THE HEALTH PROFESSIONAL

The emotional and psychological events triggered by the sudden death of a patient vary in health care workers. The reactions and coping skills available to these professionals often are influenced by the following factors:

- Previous experience with death
- Support available in the environment
- The health care professional's beliefs and values
- Knowledge about the process of death
- The health care professional's emotional well-being

The types of emotions or even severe psychological events that health care workers experience may be similar to those of the dying patient. Shock and denial are common in sudden death, especially when the patient is young or the death was violent.

For many health care workers, care of the dying is extremely rewarding and leads to important knowledge about one's own values and beliefs. The ability to provide comfort to both the patient and the family often results in the discovery of a special ability to nurture. This quality is the reason many health care workers begin a career in patient care.

However, some health professionals may experience crisis in connection with the death of a patient or in the care of the dying. Unresolved emotions related to previous loss or conflicts about beliefs and values may lead to depression or other severe psychological reactions. This is different from normal feelings of sadness, loss, and even frustration, which health professionals experience at various stages when caring for a dying patient. When these feelings arise, they can affect the quality of the health care worker's life and interfere with the individual's ability to cope with stress in the workplace.

A structured response may be required to help health care workers cope with death. This may involve planned "debriefing" periods, or spontaneous expressions of support and acknowledgement by individual team members. Health care workers often can benefit from coping skills that other professionals have found helpful:

1. Often it is helpful for staff who were involved in the patient's care or death to discuss the details of the death, going over exactly what happened and why. This is not to "medicalize" the death, but rather to discern the limitations of medical care and the fact that medical professionals cannot control all situations. It helps people understand that human intervention has limits, especially in the face of inevitable death.

2. Acknowledgement of one's feelings is helpful for many. Sometimes it is important to express the sadness, shock, and even anger that professionals feel after the death of a patient. It allows others to understand the feelings of their colleagues and to show acknowledgement and comfort. However, many people are not comfortable displaying their feelings or even discussing them, and this must be respected. No one should be coaxed into expressing that which is private and confidential.

3. Distraction provides a healthy break from severe stress. The effects of a tragic death in the operating room can linger for weeks, and this can have a serious effect on team morale and individual coping ability. Sometimes it is good to "lighten the conversation" or plan activities that do not remind people of the death. This does not diminish the meaning or significance of the death; it simply provides time to step away from it.

4. The health care worker must attend to self-care. At some point in their career, all health professionals must reflect on whether the stress of work is balanced by healthy coping mechanisms.

CHAPTER SUMMARY

- From a medical point of view, the dying patient is one in whom death is expected. Death may be expected within days, weeks, or months.
- The Kübler-Ross model of death has five stages: denial, anger, bargaining, depression, and acceptance.
- Many other models of death and dying have been developed since Kübler-Ross's work was published. These focus on other dimensions of death, such as the need for individual coping strategies (Corr) and the need to integrate the dying process into existing life experiences (McDougall).
- Care of the dying patient includes the family and other important people in the patient's environment.
- Ethical issues surrounding death include palliative care, the right to die, advance directives, and organ donation. Many more ethical issues also are involved, some extremely complex. In some cases, no satisfactory resolution may be possible for these types of ethical dilemmas.
- Death in the clinical setting triggers a series of professional responses for those involved in the care of the patient.
- Postmortem care is the preparation of the body of the deceased patient for viewing by family members.
- Postmortem care follows strict protocols established by the health care facility.
- Organ and tissue procurement may be performed after the death of a patient. The criteria for organ donation are previously established, and no organs are removed until the criteria have been met.

REVIEW QUESTIONS

1. Define the end of life from a medical perspective.
2. What are the five stages of death as defined by Kübler-Ross?
3. Name several administrative responsibilities of the family when death occurs in the clinical setting.
4. How can clinicians help families accomplish these administrative tasks while coping with the grief and shock of death?
5. What is self-determination? How does it apply to death and dying?
6. How can a patient express his or her "right to die?" How can this be carried out if the patient is unable to direct medical intervention?
7. Is there a difference between treating a dying patient for comfort measures and treating with intent to prolong life? Explain.
8. What are the functions of a tissue registry?
9. How does a person plan to become an organ donor?
10. How can health professionals honor cultural practices and beliefs in caring for the dying and the dead?
11. What is the purpose of postmortem care?
12. What is a coroner's case?
13. What is rigor mortis?
14. What specimens may be collected from a nonheartbeating cadaver?
15. What kinds of self-care are appropriate for you in times of stress? Why is it important to know this?

BIBLIOGRAPHY

American Academy of Hospice and Palliative Medicine: General educational materials. Accessed January 28, 2008, at http://www.aahpm.org/cgi-bin/wkcgi/browse?category=articlesion=CC.

Centers for Disease Control and Prevention, National Center for Health Statistics: Physicians' handbook on medical certification of death, 2003 edition. Accessed January 28, 2008, at www.gov/nchs/vital-certs-rev.htm.

Kuebler K, Heidrich D, Esper P: *Palliative and end of life care*, ed 2, St Louis, 2007, WB Saunders/Elsevier,

Porth C: *Pathophysiology concepts of altered health states*, ed 6, Philadelphia, 2002, Lippincott Williams & Wilkins.

Thibodeau G, Patton K: *Anatomy and physiology*, ed 6, St Louis, 2007, Mosby/Saunders.

Law and Ethics

CHAPTER OUTLINE

LEARNING OBJECTIVES

After studying this chapter the reader will be able to:
- Discuss the relationship between ethics and law
- Discuss the importance of terminology in the study of ethics and law
- Describe sources of the law
- Describe common hospital policies
- List common areas of negligence in the operating room

- Define criminal liability
- Describe and give examples of an incident report
- Describe informed consent
- Describe the advance directive and the living will
- Discuss why documentation is important
- Explain an ethical dilemma
- Describe several ethical conflicts

TERMINOLOGY

Abandonment: A health professional's failure to provide care to a patient, especially when there is an implied contract to do so. Examples include leaving the operating room during a surgical case without transferring care to another person, and leaving a patient on a stretcher alone in the hallway.

Administrative law: A law created by an agency or a department of the government.

Advance directive: A document in which a person gives instructions about his or her medical care in the event that the individual cannot speak for himself or herself. Examples are a living will and a medical power of attorney.

Cognitive impairment: A physiological condition in which a person is unable to carry out normal cognitive tasks, such as rational decision making.

Common law: Binding decisions made by a court judge and based on the precedent of a similar case.

Constitutional law: The supreme law of the nation in the United States.

Court trial: A trial in which a judge determines the factual evidence and makes the final judgment.

Damages: Money awarded in a civil lawsuit to compensate the injured party.

Defamation: A derogatory statement concerning another person's skill, character, or reputation.

Delegation: The assignment of one's duties to another person. In medicine, the person who delegates a duty retains accountability for the action of the person to whom it is delegated.

Deposition: The testimony of a witness given under oath and transcribed by a court reporter during the pretrial phase of a civil lawsuit.

Dilemma: A situation or personal conflict which arises from a need to made a decision and none of the choices are acceptable.

Ethical dilemmas: Situations in which ethical choices involve conflicting values.

Ethics: Standards of behavior that are accepted within groups.

Hospital policy: A set of rules or regulations that hospital employees are required to follow. They are created to protect patients and employees from harm and to ensure smooth operation of the hospital.

Incident report: A written description of any event that caused harm or presented the risk of harm to a patient or staff in the course of normal health care. For example, injury to patient or staff requires an incident report, regardless of the cause. A retained item such as a sponge, needle, or instrument in the surgical wound requires incident reporting, even if the item is subsequently found.

31

Informed consent: A process and a legal document that states the patient's surgical procedure and the risks, consequences, and benefits of that procedure. It must be signed by the patient or the patient's representative before surgery can proceed. Also known as a patient operative consent form.

Insurance: A contract in which the insurance company agrees to defend the policy holder if that individual is sued for acts covered by the policy and to pay any damages up to the policy limit.

Jury trial: A trial in which a case is presented to a selected jury, and the facts and final judgment are determined by the jury.

Laws: Standards that apply to all people in a given society.

Liable: Legally responsible and accountable.

Libel: Defamation in writing.

Living will: A legal document that states the patient's wish to refuse or limit care if the patient becomes incompetent. Living wills are used mainly for cases of terminal illness.

Malpractice: Negligence committed by a professional. Malpractice also may be committed if a person deliberately acts outside of his or her scope of practice or while impaired.

Medical ethics: A branch of ethics concerned with the practice of medicine.

Medical power of attorney: A legal document signed by a person who is giving another individual the power to make health care decisions for the first person if he or she becomes incompetent, unconscious, or unable to make decisions for himself or herself.

Medical practice acts: State laws that define the practice of medicine.

Negligence: Negligence can occur in two ways: it can be a failure to do something that a reasonable person, guided by the ordinary considerations that regulate human affairs, would do; or, it can be the act of doing something that a reasonable and prudent person would not do.

Nurse practice acts: State laws that define the practice of nursing.

Operative report: A patient record of the surgery, which is maintained and submitted by the attending circulating nurse.

Perjury: The crime of intentionally lying or falsifying information during court testimony after a person has sworn to tell the truth.

Professional ethics: Ethical behavior established by authoritative peers of a particular profession, such as medicine or law.

Professional license: Governmental permission to perform specified actions.

Punitive: Actions intended to punish a person who has violated the law.

Retained object: An item that is inadvertently left inside the patient during surgery.

Safe Medical Device Act: A federal regulation that requires the reporting of any incident causing death or injury that is suspected to be the result of a medical device.

Sentinel event: An unexpected incident resulting in serious physical injury, psychological harm, or death. The risk of injury or harm is also considered a sentinel event.

Sexual harassment: Sexual coercion, sexual innuendoes, or unwanted sexual comments, gestures, or touch.

Slander: Spoken defamation.

Standard of conduct: A set of rules or guidelines an organization writes for its members. The rules pertain to how people behave and are based on the principles that the organization values, such as honesty, professionalism, compassion, and integrity.

Statutes: Laws passed by legislative bodies.

Subpoena: A court order requiring its recipient to appear and testify at a trial or deposition. Medical records also can be the subject of subpoenas.

Summons: A court-issued document that is received by a person being sued, notifying the person that he or she is a defendant in the lawsuit.

Time out: A mandated procedure for ensuring that surgery is performed on the correct site and side. Time out is a pause before the start of surgery, before the incision is made, when all members of the team verify the correct side and site.

Tort: A wrong, independent of contract law violations, perpetrated by one person against another person or another person's property. Any act of negligence or fraud compensable by money damages. Torts may be intentional or negligent in nature.

INTRODUCTION

Health professionals in all settings are guided in their practice by society's rules and laws. The law generally is very clear about how we deliver care to others and what our responsibilities are to the public. Professional ethics are guiding principles of correct behavior. All health professionals agree to follow certain ethical standards established by their profession when they provide services to the public. This is different from ethical decision making, which involves difficult choices about one's beliefs and values.

This chapter discusses important legal issues about which perioperative professionals must become knowledgeable to provide health services to the public. The chapter also discusses ethical behavior in the health care setting and the professional standards expected of health care workers.

LAW AND THE SURGICAL TECHNOLOGIST

DEFINING LAW

Laws are society's standards, enacted and enforced by governments to protect all individuals and groups from harm. The consequences of violations of the law sometimes are **punitive** (i.e., involve punishment). Most people are familiar with the common laws of their country or state, especially those that govern day-to-day living and associating with others. However, many other laws are less well known and require expert knowledge to interpret. Particular professions have legal standards that are easily accessed and learned and that apply to circumstances these professionals encounter in their work.

❖ *Every health professional must be familiar with the laws that pertain to his or her practice.*

Ethics may influence the creation of laws, but ethical standards are not enforceable by government. Laws, however, *are* enforceable by government. That is the main difference between a profession's ethical standards and the law.

SOURCES OF LAW

In the United States, the laws that regulate society arise from a number of sources. The following are the types of laws most applicable to this discussion.

- **Constitutional law.** The U.S. Constitution is the supreme source of law in the nation; no other law may violate the provisions of the Constitution. Similarly, each state has a constitution that is considered the supreme law for that state.
- **Statutes.** Statutes are laws passed by legislative bodies. Bills passed by state legislatures and signed into law by the governor are called *statutes.*
- **Administrative law.** Administrative laws are created by agencies and departments of the government. Examples of administrative laws are the rules established by the Environmental Protection Agency (EPA) for the handling of medical waste and by the Drug Enforcement Administration (DEA) for the dispensing of prescription drugs. Other sources of administrative law that affect health care workers include the Department of Health and Human Services (DHHS) and the Occupational Safety and Health Administration (OSHA).
- **Judicial or common law.** When conflict arises between two parties, the courts may become involved to resolve the dispute. The rulings issued by courts have the effect of law and are binding (legal). Common law is based on precedence, which is set by previous cases.
- **Professional practice acts.** Each state has established laws that govern the actions of those licensed in a given profession. When a state board of practice establishes standards of practice, the board can take disciplinary action against a member who violates a standard. For example, if a professional nurse or physician practices under the influence of drugs or alcohol, the state board may revoke or suspend the person's **professional license,** declare the offense to other professionals, or require rehabilitation. In addition, because practicing under the influence of drugs or alcohol is illegal, the person also may face criminal charges.

LAWS, REGULATIONS, AND STANDARDS AFFECTING HEALTH PROFESSIONALS

Whether a legal action or a disciplinary action is taken against a health professional depends on whether the person has broken a law or violated a standard of practice. As explained previously, the two may occur simultaneously. If the health care worker is licensed (given the right to practice within specified boundaries by the government), each state sets precise legal limitations.

❖ *If a professional is not specifically regulated by medical or nursing practice acts, the individual's actions are judged according to the laws of civil or criminal law, just as are those of any other person in society.*

The legal boundaries for the surgical technologist are defined by *what is not permitted* rather than by *what is permitted.* A surgical technologist is not a doctor and therefore cannot practice medicine as defined by the law. A surgical technologist is not a licensed nurse and therefore cannot practice nursing. A few states now require surgical technologists to be registered (listed in public records) and many duties are performed under the direct supervision of a licensed medical or nursing professional. However, the surgical technologist remains directly responsible and may be held liable for any act of negligence or criminal wrongdoing, which includes practicing as a licensed nurse or medical doctor as defined by state law.

FEDERAL REGULATIONS

A number of federal regulations apply to health care personnel. Those issued by the DHHS prescribe standards for hospitals receiving funds under Medicare. OSHA issues and enforces standards that protect employees and patients against risks in the environment. These include hazards such as those caused by noxious chemicals and electrical devices and risks associated with blood-borne diseases. The EPA regulates the use of chemicals for disinfection and sterilization. The Food and Drug Administration (FDA) has established laws that protect the public from medical devices known to be defective, unsafe, hazardous, or prone to malfunction. An example of an FDA law is the **Safe Medical Device Act,** which requires hospitals to report any incident in which a medical device is believed to be the cause of an injury or death.

STATE LAW: MEDICAL AND NURSE PRACTICE ACTS

Under the U.S. Constitution, each state has the power to regulate the practice of medicine and professional nursing. These state laws are called **medical practice acts** and **nurse practice acts,** and they differ from state to state. They require a person to obtain a license before practicing medicine or nursing. For example, physicians may diagnose and treat disease, cut and suture tissue, prescribe drugs, and pronounce death. Nurses may administer medications prescribed by a physician. Because of the variation among states, each person must become familiar with the laws of the state in which he or she works.

HEALTH CARE POLICY AND PROCEDURE

Accredited hospitals and other health care facilities are required to provide orientation training for their employees and to supply printed documents that detail the required policies and procedures. New employees (or students) must become familiar with and understand the responsibilities and procedures of their job. Policies and protocols are updated constantly, and workers must keep aware of any changes.

> ❖ Forgetting to read about policy or protocol changes does not protect an employee from legal action in case of negligence.

Hospital policy is explained in the hospital policy manual, which describes the general administrative and logistical operations of the hospital. It includes an organizational chart that clarifies the chain of command and information on other topics, such as rules about employee identification, privileges, and salary procedures.

The operating room procedure manual and other protocol manuals describe safe practices and policies, such as infection control, aseptic technique, disinfection and sterilization methods, room turnover procedures, proper use of equipment, and chemical safety information.

STANDARDS OF CONDUCT

A **standard of conduct,** also called a *code of conduct,* is a set of rules an organization writes for its members. The rules pertain to how people behave and are based on the principles that the organization values, such as honesty, professionalism, compassion, integrity, and so on. These rules are not laws, and there is no *legal* consequence for violating them unless a standard coincides with an existing law. For example, honoring the patient's privacy is a standard of conduct established by all health professions. The consequences of violating this standard may be legal action by the patient or the family. However, the standard itself is not a legal document. Box 4-1 presents the *Standard of Practice* of the Association of Surgical Technologists.

DELEGATION

Delegation is the transfer of responsibility for a task from one person to another. This is a frequent occurrence in all health care settings, especially where licensed personnel work directly

---

Box 4-1

Standards of Practice of the Association of Surgical Technologists

Standard I
Teamwork is essential for perioperative patient care and is contingent on interpersonal skills.

Communication is critical to the attainment of expected outcomes of care. All team members should work together for the common good of the patient. For the benefit of the patient and the delivery of quality care, interpersonal skills are demonstrated in all interactions with the health care team, the patient and family, superiors, and peers. Personal integrity and surgical conscience are integrated into every aspect of professional behavior.

Standard II
Preoperative planning and preparation for surgical intervention are individualized to meet the needs of each patient and his or her surgeon.

The surgical technologist collaborates with the professional registered nurse in the collection of data for use in the preparation of equipment and supplies needed for the surgical procedure. The implementation of patient care identified in the plan of care is performed under the supervision of a professional registered nurse.

Standard III
The preparation of the perioperative environment and all supplies and equipment will ensure environmental safety for patients and personnel.

Application of the plan of care includes wearing appropriate attire, anticipating the needs of the patient and perioperative team, maintaining a safe work area, observing aseptic technique, and following all policies and procedures of the institution.

Standard IV
Application of basic and current knowledge is necessary for a proficient performance of assigned functions.

The surgical technologist should maintain a current knowledge base of procedures, equipment and supplies, emergency protocol for various situations, and changes in scientific technology pertinent to his or her performance description objectives. It is the responsibility of the surgical technologist to augment his or her knowledge base by studying recent literature, attending in-service and continuing education programs, and pursuing new learning experiences.

Standard V
Each patient's right to privacy, dignity, safety, and comfort is respected and protected. Each member of the operating room team has a moral and ethical duty to uphold strict observance of the patient's rights.

The surgical technologist, like all members of the health care team, is expected to perform as a patient advocate in all situations. This is an accountability issue and should be part of each aspect of patient care.

Standard VI
Every patient is entitled to the same application of aseptic technique within the physical facilities.

Implementation of the individualized plan of care for every patient includes the application of aseptic or sterile technique at all times by all members of the health care team. All patients are given the same dedication in their care.

Modified from the Association of Surgical Technologists.

with allied health professionals. Surgical technologists are valued members of the perioperative team, and they have responsibilities and duties specific to their training and skill. Many of the activities they perform in the work environment are delegated to them by another person. The student encounters delegation daily. Professionals who delegate tasks occasionally may request performance of a task that the delegee cannot or should not carry out. This presents both an ethical and a legal situation.

Because of the current situation in health care, which is one of staff shortages and expanding roles for allied health professionals, the guidelines for delegation are reviewed in this chapter. Specific conditions allow a person to delegate tasks to another individual:

- The delegee must be *legally permitted* to perform the task. For example, a licensed nurse cannot delegate drug administration to the surgical technologist, because it is illegal for personnel to administer drugs unless they are licensed to do so. A surgical technolgist is not licensed to give drugs in any state.
- The delegee must have received the proper training to perform the task safely, *without harm* to the patient. For example, a licensed nurse may not delegate urinary catheterization to a person who has not been previously trained to perform this procedure, even if the nurse is present and can guide the delegee through the task.
- The delegee must be competent to perform the task. The individual must admit with honesty and clarity whether he or she is competent. The delegator has a responsibility to ensure that the delegee has sufficient knowledge and experience to complete the task safely. For example, has the delegee been trained to perform the task? Has the delegee's trainer or mentor stated *in writing* that the delegee is capable of performing the task safely? Written verification of competence may be required to protect the patient, delegator, and delegee. Allied health personnel may not perform tasks defined as nursing or medical practice, such as making an incision or administering drugs. Each state has different practice acts, therefore the surgical technologist must become knowledgeable about the acts in his or her state.

LEGAL DOCTRINES

A variety of legal doctrines (a set of rules or conclusions drawn from many similar cases) have been developed to ensure accountability and responsibility for the safety of the patient. In legal language and documents, these doctrines are sometimes referred to in Latin translation. The concept of the doctrine and its significance in health care practice are of greater importance than the Latin terms which are used only in legal documents and proceedings by legal professionals.

- **An employer is responsible for the actions of an employee** (Latin: *respondeat superior*). This means that the employer (e.g., the hospital or other health care facility) can be sued if an employee acts negligently in his or her work. In this case, the employer has done nothing wrong but is nevertheless held legally responsible.
- **Certain cases of negligence are so evident that there can be no defense, or no further information is needed to prove the negligence** (Latin: *res ipsa loquitur*). In other words, "the thing speaks for itself." An example is leaving an instrument or a sponge in the patient.
- **Do no harm** (Latin: *Primum non nocere*). In all medical practice and in many other professions in which the public is served, professionals have a legal and ethical responsibility to refrain from any actions that would harm the person they serve. An example of this concept is the medical professional who knows he or she does not have adequate skill or training to perform a task safely but proceeds anyway, regardless of the potential risk.
- **Doctrine of detrimental reliance.** This doctrine specifies that in certain cases, a surgeon may rely on the professionalism of the scrub and circulator and therefore may deflect responsibility for an injury.

NOTE: In the past, perioperative staff members (called "borrowed servants") worked directly under the surgeon, who was held accountable for all activities in surgery. *This doctrine no longer holds true.* Hospitals now are held accountable for the actions of their employees, and all health care workers are accountable for their own actions.

ACTIONS OF CIVIL LIABILITY (TORTS)

A **tort** is a civil wrong, an act committed against a person or a person's property. A criminal act can result in a fine or imprisonment, but a civil wrong can result in a lawsuit in which money is awarded to the injured party. The person or organization that would be responsible for paying the award is said to be **liable.** The two types of torts are intentional torts and unintentional torts.

❖ An intentional tort *is a wrong purposefully and knowingly committed against a person.*

❖ An unintentional tort *is a wrong committed inadvertently, without intent to harm.*

Negligence (Unintentional Tort)

Negligence is an unintentional tort, or civil wrong. Negligence torts are the most common example of tort liability in the health care setting. Negligence is defined as "the commission of an act that a prudent person would not have done or the omission of a duty that a prudent person would have fulfilled, resulting in injury or harm to another person."[1] In other words, the negligent person fails to observe or act in a situation the individual should have known about and acted on.

Four elements of negligence must be proven:

- A duty to the patient existed. (A duty to the patient is initiated the moment the patient receives treatment or care from a hospital or physician).

- The duty was breached when a failure to meet the standard of care occurred.
- The breach of duty caused injury to the patient.
- The breach of duty resulted in damage to the patient.

A person who proves that negligence occurred may be awarded compensation, also called **damages.** This usually is financial compensation for future medical expenses, lost wages, or suffering.

In some cases a person may not be able to prove each of the four elements. In these situations the courts rely on the doctrine of *res ipsa loquitur* ("the thing speaks for itself"). This doctrine recognizes that the negligence is so obvious that no other proof of responsibility is needed. Examples include leaving a sponge or other object inside the patient or administering an incorrect medication. Other common acts of negligence in the perioperative environment are listed and described in the following sections.

In many situations in the surgical setting, negligence can result in injury to patients or coworkers. These injuries can lead to lawsuits against the perioperative staff member as well as the hospital. As is any employer, the hospital is liable for the negligent acts of its employees. The activities that carry the highest risk of harm are discussed in this chapter.

The following are the best guidelines for reducing or preventing the risk of harm to others:

- Be aware of what you do not know. Ask questions. Ask for help when you are unsure about the process of a task or its consequences.
- Be conscious of what you are doing. Not consciously thinking is one of the major causes of accidents in the operating room. Not responding to situations in which the potential for harm exists is an act of negligence.
- Come to work mentally and physically prepared for extreme situations. These occur unexpectedly and frequently in the operating room.

Retained Objects

A **retained object,** such as an instrument or a sponge, is one that is unintentionally left in the patient as a result of surgery. A retained object is a foreign substance, and the body reacts as it would to any foreign body, with inflammation and tissue destruction. A retained instrument can migrate through tissue, injuring solid or hollow organs and causing infection or hemorrhage. Delayed healing and unresolved pain are potential consequences of any retained object.

Accountability for a retained object lies with the entire operating team. The scrub and the circulator are responsible for the surgical counts; however, the physician is the one who actually places items inside the patient, therefore he or she also may be legally responsible for an item being left in the patient.

Court decisions have held the scrub, the circulator, and the surgeon equally liable. The courts also have held that the surgeon relied on the information given to him or her by the staff and therefore not liable. Surgical item counts must be completed according to hospital policy, and

---

Box 4-2
Surgical Counts

- Surgical counts are performed during any surgery in which an item can be lost in the patient.
- A count is performed by two people. The law does not specify the qualifications of those who perform the count (licensed or unlicensed) or the manner in which it is performed. However, the Association of periOperating Room Nurses (AORN) recommends that a registered nurse and a surgical technologist participate. One person must be in the scrub role. This is a standard that most institutions follow.
- Counts are performed at the beginning of surgery, at the closure of a hollow organ, at the closure of a body cavity such as the thoracic cavity or peritoneum, and at the closure of the skin.
- If at any other time there is suspicion of a retained item, a count should be performed.
- A count is performed whenever a change is made in the personnel performing the scrub and circulating roles, such as during a change of shift.
- In accord with the standard of practice, the circulating registered nurse identifies the scrub and circulator on the patient's operative record.

---

extra precautions may be taken according to individual circumstances.

The procedure for counts is described in Chapter 16. To reinforce understanding of this critical task, the reader should study Box 4-2 carefully.

Burns

Burns occur in the operating room as a result of misuse or negligent operation of electrosurgical equipment, heating blankets, hot solutions, hot instruments, lasers, or chemicals. Every person who works with these devices and agents is responsible for learning about the risks and adhering to safe practices. The following are examples of burn injuries caused by negligence:

- During laser surgery of the upper respiratory tract, special precautions for a laser-safe endotracheal tube are neglected. The endotracheal tube bursts into flames, causing third-degree burns in the patient's throat.
- Standard safety precautions for electrosurgery are neglected, and the patient suffers serious electrical burns.
- A warm airflow pad that covers the patient's body is connected improperly. The patient suffers massive burns that are not discovered until the end of surgery when the drapes are removed.
- An improperly placed dispersive electrosurgical pad allows current to flow to electrocardiograph leads, resulting in serious burns under the leads.
- Alcohol used during patient preparation pools under the drapes. When the electrosurgical equipment unit is activated, the drapes ignite and the patient catches fire.

- A stainless steel retractor is removed from the autoclave and immediately placed in the patient. The abdominal contents are burned by the hot instrument.
- Skin prep solutions (antiseptics) are allowed to pool under the patient. After the procedure, the drapes are removed to reveal the patient's blistered skin.
- Irrigation solutions are kept in warmers with excessively high temperatures. The cavity in which the irrigation solution is used suffers tissue damage from the intense heat of the solution.
- A hot ultrasound coagulation/dissecting instrument is placed on the patient's skin, causing a second-degree burn.

Falls

Falls can cause serious injury to the patient. The following are examples of circumstances in which a fall may result:

- The side rails on a stretcher are not kept raised, or a safety strap is not secured on the operating room table.
- Children are left unattended, enabling them to crawl out of cribs or beds.
- A patient left unattended or improperly restrained emerges from general anesthesia and struggles and thrashes.
- An insufficient number of staff members are available to transfer a patient to and from the operating table. A sedated or disoriented patient climbs over the side rails or becomes entangled between the rails.
- Unsafe transfer techniques are used to move a patient to and from a wheelchair.

Improper Positioning

The patient can be seriously and permanently injured as a result of improper positioning. Only personnel specifically trained and competent to position the patient should assist in this task. Overextension of limbs, pressure on bony prominences, loss of circulation as a result of improper padding, and restricted ventilation are some consequences of improper positioning. An unconscious or sedated patient cannot speak for himself or herself. Fractures, sprains, bruising, and damage to soft connective tissue can occur when such a patient is moved. The surgeon, anesthesiologist, nurse anesthetist, surgical assistant, and circulator should work collaboratively while positioning the patient to ensure safety.

Mistaken Patient Identity or Operative Site

No excuse is possible for mistaken identity or operation on the wrong side. Surgery on the wrong site, wrong side, or wrong patient is considered a **sentinel event.** To prevent such negligence, the registered nurse checks and rechecks the patient's identification card, wrist band, chart, and preoperative record. In addition, the patient is asked to describe what he or she understands the surgery will entail and on which side it is to be performed. If any discrepancy is found between the records and the patient's report, surgery is delayed until absolute surgical site verification (SSV) is ensured. Staff members should *never* rely on the surgical schedule for accuracy in this matter.

The Joint Commission, the Association of periOperative Nurses (AORN), American College of Surgeons, and AST require a **time out** immediately before the procedure starts or the first incision is made. Time out is a procedure, or set of procedures, to provide for final verification of the patient's identity, surgical procedure, and correct location of the incision. Both the AST and AORN have established guidelines for time out procedures. Guidelines among organizations may vary slightly in wording but are consistent in their actual practice.

Some hospitals require the surgeon to sign his or her name on the patient's skin at the operative site when an operative side applies (e.g., for limbs, eyes, and ears) to prevent surgery on the incorrect side; the patient may also be required to mark the operative site.

Specimen Handling

Specimens removed from the patient require careful and attentive handling. If the specimen is removed to confirm or rule out malignancy, loss or lack of proper labeling can have disastrous consequences for the patient, including misdiagnosis or delay in appropriate treatment. All specimens must be identified by the hospital pathology department. Some are forensic evidence that will be used to prove innocence or guilt in a criminal case. One of the responsibilities of the surgical technologist is to handle specimens properly and deliver them off the surgical field. The surgical team must identify, label, and ensure delivery of specimens to the pathology department or other area specified by hospital policy. This procedure is described in Chapter 16.

Medications

The surgical technologist is not licensed to administer any drug. However, the ST does accept drugs from the circulator. These must then be properly labeled and passed to the surgeon. If a medication is labeled improperly (or not labeled at all), the risk of injury to the patient increases. Accepting and passing the wrong medication to the surgeon can injure the patient and constitutes serious negligence. The scrub should always state the medication name and strength when passing drugs or solutions to the surgeon.

Abandonment

Abandoning or neglecting a patient who requires professional care and for whom the health professional has accepted the duty of care is a serious act of negligence. On a very basic level, abandonment results when the health professional stops caring for a patient without making provisions for another qualified person to assume the responsibility. Examples of abandonment are:

- Leaving a patient unattended in the operating room.
- a staff member leaves the operating room at the change of shift once the patient is on the operating table and no relief is available.
- A patient is being transported to the operating room by stretcher and is left unattended in a hallway.
- A staff member agrees to work overtime, then leaves without notifying anyone.

- A staff member refuses to work overtime when the hospital has a mandatory overtime policy.
- A health professional delegates care of the patient to a colleague who is unqualified to provide safe care.

Severe injury and even death may occur as a result of patient abandonment. Falls, cardiopulmonary arrest, and respiratory obstruction are just a few examples of the consequences of abandonment.

Failure to Communicate

Failure of a medical staff member to communicate a patient's complaint to the appropriate person (either because of forgetfulness or because the patient's communication is ignored) is considered negligence. Failure to communicate can result in serious injury. For example, the patient has had his leg casted and complains of extreme pain in his foot. The communication is not reported. Later, the patient requires amputation of the foot as a result of loss of blood supply to the area. In this case, the surgical technologist must report the patient's complaints to the licensed nurse or medical doctor, who will make further assessment and take action.

Loss of or Damage to the Patient's Property

Patients sometimes arrive in surgery with dentures, jewelry, hearing aids, or glasses. Loss of or damage to these items can be very traumatic for the patient. Any personal property must be properly labeled with the patient's name and hospital number and sent either to the hospital security department or to another depository according to hospital policy.

Differentiating Incompetence and Negligence

Negligence is a legal term that implies potential or actual harm to another. *Incompetence* is inability or refusal to perform one's job. It is important not to confuse these terms. An incompetent person may commit acts of negligence. However, negligence is not always the result of incompetence. A documentation error may be the result of incompetence, but it is not an act of negligence unless harm occurs as a result of the error. Likewise, an error in aseptic technique is not legal grounds for a civil case on the basis of negligence unless it can be proven that the patient suffered injury as a direct result of the error.

Intentional Torts

Invasion of Privacy

The patient has a right to both physical and social privacy. One of the most common offenses against the patient is invasion of privacy. Discussions about patients in public areas of the hospital are common. These are a violation of ethical and legal codes. Vivid descriptions of the patient's surgery or disease, including the names of the attending physicians, are commonly heard in cafeterias, hallways, and elevators. Family or friends overhearing these discussions can be devastated by their content. Any conversation about a patient must take place only within the therapeutic environment and never in public.

Box 4-3

Health Privacy Act Identifiers that May not Be Shared

Individual identifiers include but are not limited to the following:
- Name and address
- Birth date
- Social Security number
- Photographs
- Medical record numbers
- Fax numbers
- Electronic e-mail addresses
- Health plan beneficiary numbers
- Account numbers
- Certificate/license numbers
- Vehicle identifiers and serial numbers, including license plate numbers

The patient's operative record and all other medical records are permanent legal documents. They may not be altered or changed. A subpoena can be served for their use in a court of law, and they are considered evidence in the event of negligence or criminal action. The patient has a right to the information contained in his or her record, but the public does not. Records must be protected from public viewing at all times.

The Health Insurance Portability and Accountability Act of 1996 (HIPAA) protects patients' medical records and other health information through its Privacy Rule. The goal of the Privacy Rule is to ensure that the individual's health information is properly protected while the individual seeks or receives health care. Identifiable health information is any information relating to the individual's past, present, or future physical or mental health or condition and information about payments for health care. The Privacy Rule applies to any transmission of information through any medium, including electronic, paper, or oral means. Box 4-3 specifies information that cannot be shared.

Defamation

Defamation is a derogatory statement made by one person about another. If the statement is made verbally, it is **slander.** If the statement is written, it is **libel.** Medical personnel sometimes witness practices or acts that they consider incompetent or dangerous to the patient. Failure to report incompetence (or impairment, such as intoxication) to the appropriate person is negligence. However, discussing the suspected incompetence in public is defamatory. The appropriate response to any unusual or dangerous occurrence in the operating room is to inform that person's supervisor verbally and in an incident report. Although claims of defamation usually are made by a health care worker against a colleague or against the institution, a patient or the patient's family also can claim defamation by health care workers.

Two defenses can be made against a claim of defamation. The first is truth. In this defense, although a certain communication may be damaging to an individual's reputation, the statement is factual. The second defense is privilege. Health care workers are required to communicate certain information to ensure safe and effective care. If the communication is conducted in a private setting and is related to the care of the patient, the conversation is privileged.

Civil Assault

Civil assault is the threat or attempt to strike or harm another, regardless of whether the threat is carried out, provided the intended victim is aware of the danger. Any treatment given to a patient against his wishes may be considered assault. This is a punishable civil crime, and the victim may sue for mental distress as well as damages resulting from the assault.

Civil Battery

Civil battery is the actual unlawful touching or striking of a person, even if the injury is slight. Touching or striking a patient in any inappropriate way is battery. The injured party may file suit for damages as a result of the battery.

False Imprisonment

False imprisonment is the act of depriving a person of freedom of movement by holding him or her in a confined space or by physical restraint. A patient who is not a danger to himself or herself or to others and who is wrongfully restrained may be a victim of false imprisonment.

CRIMINAL LIABILITY

Civil liability is not the only risk in the operating room setting. Criminal liability also can arise, such as when a person's actions exceed the individual's scope of practice and when theft occurs.

Actions Exceeding the Scope of Practice

A person who fraudulently poses as a nurse or physician and proceeds to perform duties associated with that profession commits a criminal offense. However, the question arises: If an unlicensed person is delegated a task that is defined as practicing medicine or nursing, does he or she commit a crime in performing the task? The fact that a licensed nurse or doctor grants permission to perform a task to an unlicensed person does not give the unlicensed individual legal status. This means that if the act is in violation of the law, it does not matter who delegates the task; it remains a violation. Some states may allow the delegation of certain duties to unlicensed personnel, and others specifically forbid it. Hospital policy usually is very clear on this matter. When in doubt, the surgical technologist should seek the advice of the operating room supervisor or the hospital's legal staff. If a lawsuit should arise, the surgical technologist who asked for legal advice is in a more defensible position than one who proceeded blindly.

Any discussion concerning the surgical technologist's scope of practice ultimately becomes an ethical one. Because the surgical technologist often is eager to increase his or her expertise and because surgeons may offer the surgical technologist the opportunity to perform tasks that exceed the scope of practice, engaging in such activities may seem permissible and harmless. The fact that the task seems harmless, however, does not negate the legal boundary or the safety factors that define it. The professional chooses an ethical path that coincides with both patient safety and legality.

Theft

Theft is the willful taking of another's property with the intention of keeping it. In the operating room, as in any workplace, theft of supplies or equipment is a crime punishable by law.

LEGAL DOCUMENTS

Documentation is a requirement of all medical practice. It is both a method of communication among staff members and a record of all the patient's interactions with the medical system. Medical records are protected by law. Losing or misplacing a record or part of a record is a serious event. Remember that *all patient records and reports are legal documents.* Documentation commonly encountered in the perioperative setting includes the operative report and informed consent.

Operative Report

The **operative report** is completed by the registered nurse circulator. It includes a complete patient assessment, care plan, and technical information about the equipment and devices used during the procedure. A record of the sponge, sharps, and instrument counts are included in this document, along with details about specimens and medications. The names of all perioperative personnel who participated in the procedure are listed, and those who participated in the counts must sign at the close of surgery. Figure 4-1 shows an example of an operative report.

Informed Consent

A patient's operative consent form, or **informed consent,** is a legal document the patient must sign before surgery (Figure 4-2). The purpose of the consent is to include patients in decisions about their health care. It gives patients an opportunity to ask questions and provide feedback on their understanding of a procedure. The main elements of the consent are:

- The name and type of surgery, which are communicated using words and language the patient understands
- The risks, benefits, and possible outcomes of the procedure
- Alternatives to the procedure
- An assessment of the patient's understanding
- The patient's acceptance of the procedure

The patient has the right to be informed about the consequences and risks of the procedure, but the physician must also be cautious about overstating the risks, especially those that are statistically unlikely. It is neither a casual process nor one performed in haste.

The informed consent is not just a form that is signed before surgery. It is a process. It involves tactful, skilled com-

Operating Room
OPERATION REPORT (Long Form)   Page 1 of 2

Date:___/___/___ OR Room #:_____ Patient Type: ☐Inpatient ☐Outpatient   To OR via: ☐Stretcher ☐Bed ☐Wheelchair ☐AMB (with escort)

Procedure Type: ☐Elective ☐Emergency Class ☐1 ☐2____ ☐3 ☐Return to OR   A.S.A. (Physical status) ☐1 ☐2 ☐3 ☐4 ☐5   Wound Classification ☐1 ☐2 ☐3 ☐4

Patient Time in:_____ Anesthesia Induct Time:_____ Procedure Start Time:_____ Procedure Stop Time:_____ Patient Time Out:_____ Delay Code:_____ Delay Time:_____

☐ Allergies verified; Comments:_____

☐ Interdisciplinary Admission Data Base/Outpatient Preoperative Record (local anesthesia) reviewed.

☐ Implemented standard plan of care for the operative patient.

Exception(s) noted: Intervention(s)

_____   _____

_____   _____

_____   _____

                                        RN Initials:_____

ANESTHESIA TYPE: ☐GEN ☐SPINAL ☐EPIDURAL ☐M.A.C. ☐LOCAL ☐BLOCK (type):_____

☐OTHER_____

Preoperative Diagnosis:	Attending Surgeon:
	Attending Surgeon:
	Attending Surgeon:
	Resident:
Procedure:	Resident:
	Assistant: ☐M.S. ☐P-A ☐S-A ☐RNFA
	Assistant: ☐M.S. ☐P-A ☐S-A ☐RNFA
	Assistant: ☐M.S. ☐P-A ☐S-A ☐RNFA
	Anesthesiologist:
	Anesthetist:
	Perfusionist:
Postoperative Diagnosis:	Autotransfusionist:
	Cell Saver ☐Yes ☐No

Circulating Nurse:			Scrubperson		
Relief by:	Time in:	out:	Relief by:	Time in:	out:
Relief by:	Time in:	out:	Relief by:	Time in:	out:
Relief by:	Time in:	out:	Relief by:	Time in:	out:
Relief by:	Time in:	out:	Relief by:	Time in:	out:

Others/Observers:_____

Comments:_____

_____

X - RAYS: ☐Portable ☐Fluoro ☐Self Image ☐Yes ☐No **LASERS:** Type:_____ Total Time:_____ ☐Yes ☐No

By:_____

A

Figure 4-1 Sample operative report. *(From Rothrock JC: Alexander's care of the patient in surgery, ed 13, St Louis, 2007, Mosby.)*

Operating Room
OPERATION REPORT (Long Form)
Page 2 of 2

POSITION: ☐ Supine ☐ Prone ☐ Lithotomy ☐ Sitting ☐ Lateral ☐ R↑ ☐ L↑

ARMS Side Board Arm Holder Chest ☐ Other_____
Right ☐ ☐ ☐ ☐ Positioned by:_____
Left ☐ ☐ ☐ ☐ Comments: _____

Pre-op Skin condition: ☐ Intact _____
Post-op Skin condition: ☐ Intact _____

POSITIONING AIDS/DEVICES: Location

☐ Safety Strap_____ ☐ Vac Pac ☐ Donut ☐ Fracture Table ☐ Mayfield Headrest
☐ Tape _____ ☐ Stirrups ☐ Axillary Roll ☐ Andrews Bed ☐ Hall Relton Frame
☐ Blankets _____ ☐ Lami Rolls ☐ Gel Pad ☐ Stryker Frame ☐ McGuire Positioner
☐ Pillow(s) _____ ☐ Foam Headrest ☐ Other _____
☐ Sandbag(s) _____ ☐ Eggcrate Comments: _____

RN Initials

PREP: ☐ Betadine ☐ Iodine____% ☐ Alcohol ☐ Duraprep ☐ Other:_____ ☐ None

EQUIPMENT	MEDICATIONS

ESU ☐ Bipolar Setting: _____ Serial/I.D.#_____ ☐ Yes ☐ No

OTHER THAN THOSE GIVEN BY ANESTHESIA ☐ None

☐ Monopolar Coag _____ Cut_____ Serial/I.D.#_____

Dosage Route Time Given by

☐ Argon Beam Setting:_____ Serial/I.D.#_____
Dispersive Pad
Location: _____ Applied by:_____

_____

TOURNIQUET: Cuff Location_____ ☐ Yes ☐ No

Pressure:_____Time up:_____Time down:_____
Pressure:_____Time up:_____Time down:_____

IRRIGATION:_____

Applied by: _____ Serial/I.D. #_____

Amount in: _____ Estimated amount out: _____

COMPRESSION BOOTS: ☐ Yes ☐ No Pressure: _____

IRRIGATION:_____

Applied by: _____ Serial/I.D. #_____

Amount in: _____ Estimated amount out: _____

URINARY CATHETER	

To O.R. with catheter ☐ Yes ☐ No Inserted in O.R. by:_____

RN Initials: ☐ None

| | IMPLANTS/EXPLANTS |

Type/Size: _____ Amount: _____ mL Color:_____

☐ Yes See Implant/Explant Record ☐ None

Removed in O.R. by:_____ Time: _____

SPECIAL COMMENTS: _____

| PACKING/TUBES/DRAINS | |

Type: _____ Size: _____ ☐ None

_____

Location: _____ Amount of Packing:_____

_____

Comments: _____

_____

SPECIMENS	FAMILY COMMUNICATION DURING PROCEDURE (If applicable)

Examined and Disposed Per Dr._____
& Type of spec to Lab: ☐ None

Status discussed with _____
Name/Relation

_____ Tissue _____ Culture_____ FB _____ Fluid _____ Frozen Section

RN Signature Time

☐ Skin/Bone Freezer, describe: _____

Comments: _____ ☐ N/A

☐ Explant, describe:_____

| DISCHARGE VIA: |

Comments: _____

☐ Stretcher ☐ Patient Bed ☐ Crib ☐ Wheelchair ☐ Other _____

Verbal orders for intraoperative interventions given by: _____
Physician Signature Print Name/ID# Time Date

RN Initials & Signature Print Name Time Date

RN Initials & Signature Print Name Time Date

B

Figure 4-1, cont'd.

GENERAL REQUEST AND CONSENT

FOR OFFICE USE ONLY:

Patient Name: _____

Date of Birth: _____

Date of Procedure: _____

I _____ request and give consent to _____
            (Type or print patient name)   (Type or print Doctor or Practitioner Name(s))

to perform the following procedure(s) _____
                                          (Please list site and side if appropriate)

_____

The benefits, risks, complications, and alternatives to the above procedure(s) have been explained to me.

I understand that the procedure(s) will be performed at Christiana Care by and under supervision of my doctor or practitioner. My doctor or practitioner may use the services of other doctors or practitioners, or members of the resident staff as he or she deems necessary or advisable.

I authorize my doctor or practitioner and his or her associates and assistants to perform such additional procedures, which in their judgment are necessary and appropriate to carry out my diagnosis or treatment.

I authorize the hospital to retain, preserve and use for scientific, teaching or transplant purposes, or to make other dispositions of, at their convenience, any specimens, tissues, or parts taken from my body during the course of this operation.

I consent to observers in the operating room in accordance with hospital policy. I consent to photography or video taping of my surgical procedure for educational purposes, provided my identity remains anonymous and confidential.

I agree to being given blood or blood products as deemed advisable during the course of my procedure. The risks, benefits, and alternatives to receiving blood or blood products have been explained to me.

I consent to the administration of sedation or analgesia during my procedure. The risks, benefits, and alternatives to receiving sedation or analgesia have been explained to me.

If anesthesia is required, I consent to the administration of anesthesia by members of the Department of Anesthesiology. I also consent to the use of non-invasive and invasive monitoring techniques as deemed necessary. I understand that anesthesia involves risks that are in addition to those resulting from the operation itself including, but not limited to, dental injury, hoarseness, vocal cord injury, infection, nerve injury, corneal abrasion, seizures, heart attack, stroke and even death.

Please initial one of the following statements (females only):

_____ To the best of my knowledge I am not pregnant.   _____ I believe I am pregnant.

I certify that I have read and understand the above consent statements. In addition, I have been offered the opportunity to ask my doctor or practitioner any questions I have regarding the procedure(s) to be performed and they have been answered to my satisfaction. I acknowledge that I have been given no guarantee or assurance as to the results that may be obtained from the procedure(s).

_____   _____
Signature of Patient or Decision Maker   Date and Time   Doctor or Practitioner Signature   Date and Time

_____   _____
Relationship to Patient if Decision Maker   Doctor ID # or Print Name

_____   _____
Witness Signature   Date and Time   Practitioner Print Name/Title

_____
Witness Print Name

Telephone Consent: _____
            Name of person obtained from/Relationship to Patient

_____   _____
Witness(s') Signature(s)   Date and Time   Witness(s') Signature(s)   Date and Time

_____   _____
Witness(s') Print Name(s)   Witness(s') Print Name(s)

Figure 4-2   Sample informed consent document. *(From Rothrock JC: Alexander's care of the patient in surgery, ed 13, St Louis, 2007, Mosby.)*

munication between the physician and the patient. Communication begins long before the day of surgery (unless it is an emergency). It is the physician's responsibility to verbally explain the contents of the informed consent form and to obtain the patient's signature. Without this signed document, surgery cannot proceed. All informed consent forms must be witnessed by a person other than the physician providing the care.

Conditions of Signing

For surgery to proceed, the informed consent must be signed under specific conditions. It must be signed voluntarily by the patient. There can be no coercion or manipulation from the surgeon or other staff members. Also, the patient must be competent to make the decision. Patients who have taken medication that might impair their judgment or ability to make rational decisions must be evaluated on an individual basis. In such cases the physician would evaluate whether the patient understands the situation and the risks associated with the decision and is able to communicate an understanding of the information.

In some cases the patient is not competent to consent. **Cognitive impairment**, in which the patient is unable to form rational conclusions and cannot act in their own best interest may require someone else to sign the permit. Cognitive impairment may be caused by prescribed medications, substance abuse, or organic disease.

❖ *States have different laws regarding informed consent.*

In an emergency situation, when the patient is incompetent or unconscious and has no representative, the decision to act in beneficence may override other ethical considerations. This is a decision made by the physicians on duty, along with others involved in the case.

If the patient is a minor, the parent or guardian signs the consent. If there is no guardian, the physician, state, and hospital policy determine the protocol in the best interest of the child.

Other types of procedures also require informed consent. These include any invasive procedure (e.g., placing a central venous catheter or other vascular access device) and the administration of anesthesia. In the case of anesthesia, the nature of the medications and risks are detailed just as they are on the surgical informed consent.

A specific consent is needed to administer blood or blood cell products. Other consent forms are used for patients participating in experimental treatments or procedures and for patients undergoing elective sterilization.

In some specific cases the patient may not sign the surgical consent form, such as when the patient is a minor or is mentally incompetent. Other special cases determine who can sign the surgical consent form (Box 4-4).

Who Can Witness the Consent

The informed consent form is signed by the physician, patient, and a witness. By law, any adult can witness the patient's signature. However, hospital policy determines who can act as a witness in the perioperative environment.

Box 4-4

Special Considerations in Obtaining Informed Consent

1. If the patient is a minor, the parent or legal guardian may sign.
2. If the patient is illiterate, he or she makes an X, which is followed by the witness's signature and the words "patient's mark."
3. If the patient is mentally incompetent or incapacitated, a responsible guardian, agency representative, or court representative may sign.
4. In the case of an emancipated minor,* a responsible relative or a spouse may sign.
5. In an emergency, consent for immediate lifesaving treatment is not necessary. Verbal consent by telephone is permitted, but only if two registered nurses obtain the verbal permission. Written consent must then be obtained later.

*Surgical technologists must be sure to research the definition of an emancipated minor for the states in which they practice.

The witness to the consent can be a legal guardian, spouse, agency representative, or other authorized person who can attest to the identity of the patient, verify that the consent was signed without any coercion, and confirm that the patient was not mentally impaired at the time of the signing. The attending surgeon may not witness the consent because of conflict of interest.

Incident Report
Purpose

An incident report or unusual occurrence report is a document submitted to the operating room supervisor or other designated manager whenever an event occurs that is unusual or dangerous or requires further action. Remember that the purpose of the report is not to make a judgment about an event, only to report it. The incident report discloses all the events and people involved in the incident. The main reasons for the report are for quality assurance or risk reduction and to provide details in case legal action is taken by any of the individuals involved.

Events Requiring an Incident Report

An incident report is required whenever an event occurs that has resulted or might result in death, injury, or harm. The JCAHO defines such an occurrence as a sentinel event. *Harm* includes psychological as well as physical injury.

An incident report must be filed after events involving either patients or employees. Box 4-5 lists events that require an incident report. Other events require reporting according to hospital policy. If unsure whether an incident requires formal reporting, the surgical technologist should seek advice from a senior staff member.

Writing the Incident Report

Incident reports are completed in writing on the hospital's designated form. These forms include a place to list the personnel involved and the date, location, and time of the incident.

Box 4-5

Events that Require an Incident Report

- Surgery performed on the wrong side
- Failure to obtain informed consent
- Treatment or a procedure initiated on the wrong patient
- Medication error
- Cardiac or respiratory arrest
- Retention of an object after surgery *even if the object is subsequently retrieved*
- Incorrect count and steps taken to resolve the count
- Suspected intoxication of personnel
- Any injury to a patient while that person is in the care of the perioperative staff
- Equipment failure resulting in injury
- Suspected malpractice
- Extreme inappropriate behavior by physicians or other staff members
- Bullying
- Sexual harassment
- Battery of a patient (includes inappropriate touching or a procedure for which informed consent was not obtained)
- Any violation of the patient's rights by another
- Loss of patient property
- Death of a patient

NOTE: Other events may require reporting according to hospital policy.

A section is included in which the incident must be described by the person making the report in his or her own words. The statement must include *who* was involved, *where* the incident occurred, *when* it took place, and *how* it happened.

These guidelines can be followed in writing the narrative part of the report:

1. **Write and submit the form as soon as possible after the event.** If you are uncertain whether an incident report is needed, ask for help.
2. **State only the facts and do not give your opinion about the incident.** An example of a proper statement is, "Dr. X smelled strongly of alcohol. His speech was slurred" or "The needle count was found to be incorrect at the close of surgery. A radiograph was ordered, which did not reveal the needle, and the needle was not found outside the patient."
3. **Use professional and precise language whenever possible.** It is *more proper* to state, "Dr. X appeared agitated and angry. He denied us time for a sponge count and proceeded to throw surgical scissors off the sterile field onto the floor." Language such as the following should be *avoided*: "Dr. X was acting horrible. He wouldn't even take a sponge count, and he smashed the Metz across the room."
4. **Write in the first person.** For example, "When I arrived in operating room 4, I saw the patient lying on the floor" rather than "The patient was seen by the surgical tech (me) on the floor in room 4."
5. **Do not be intimidated by others who want to protect individuals.** In some circumstances, employees may

wish to protect others who were involved. Always use good ethical judgment, keep the safety of the patient in mind, and submit the incident report.

6. **Take your time in writing the report.** Try to write the report in a location where you are undisturbed by others. Fill out the form carefully and thoughtfully.
7. **Submit the incident report directly to the operating room supervisor or other designated personnel.** Do not leave the report where others can find it. Do not place it in the patient's chart.
8. **Remember that the report may be subpoenaed for legal action.** After an incident report is submitted to the risk management or legal department, an informal investigation may be conducted, or the hospital's **insurance** company will be notified. Further action is then taken if needed.

Advance Directive

An **advance directive** is a document in which a patient gives instructions about his or her medical care in the event the individual cannot speak for himself or herself because of incapacity. If the patient is incompetent or a minor, a guardian or family member may sign the advance directive. Different forms of advance directives can be used, and states have different regulations and standards for the implementation of directives. For example, an individual may refuse mechanical ventilation but accept medication. If the patient is considered to be in a persistent vegetative state, the guardian may request withdrawal from mechanical support systems. In most institutions, the advance directive must be reactivated with each separate hospital admission. The following sections explain the different types of advance directives.

Do Not Resuscitate Order

A "do not resuscitate" (DNR) order specifies that cardiopulmonary resuscitation must not be initiated in the event of cardiac or pulmonary arrest. When a patient has DNR status, this is clearly stated on the front of the patient's chart. Because of the effects of anesthetic agents on the cardiovascular and respiratory systems, some hospitals suspend a DNR order for the duration of the surgical procedure. The order must be rewritten when the patient is in the postanesthesia care unit (PACU).

Organ Donation

Patients have the right to refuse the removal of their organs for transplantation after their death. A number of religions and cultures forbid or limit certain types of organ transfer. With such patients, a written advance directive stating the refusal should be included in the patient's chart.

Refusal of Blood or Tissue Products

Patients may refuse blood or tissue products because of their faith or personal beliefs. Simply stating that one belongs to a certain faith does not automatically restrict medical intervention. If the patient is unable to communicate his or her wishes, lifesaving measures may be initiated. An advance directive is needed if the normal process of patient care, including transfusion, is to be interrupted.

Living Will

A **living will** is a legal document that specifically states the type of medical intervention or treatment the patient wants. Possible interventions include artificial feeding, transfusions, specific diagnostic tests, pulmonary maintenance on a ventilator, and the use of medications. Living wills can be created with help from the state bar association, state nursing association, state medical association, or hospital. A living will is not the same as a last will and testament, which is a legal document used for the distribution of a person's property after death.

Medical Power of Attorney

The patient may assign a specific person to act as his or her proxy with regard to medical treatment. After the **medical power of attorney** is prepared and signed, the proxy thereafter can speak on behalf of the patient regarding his or her medical treatment. The medical power of attorney does not give up legal authority in any area except medical treatment.

LEGAL ACTIONS

The average surgical technologist may never need a lawyer. However, every professional should be able to recognize when one is necessary and be able to select a competent one.

A lawyer is needed if **malpractice** is suspected and legal papers arrive. A certified surgical technologist (CST) who receives any legal document should show it to his or her lawyer or the hospital's lawyer immediately. Almost any lawyer will be able to explain the significance of the document, which usually will be a subpoena or a summons.

Subpoena

A **subpoena** is an order to appear as a witness to an incident. If a surgical technologist is required to testify about an incident at the hospital, the individual should check with the hospital administration before doing so. In some cases the hospital (or its insurance carrier) may provide a lawyer to be present during the testimony.

Two types of testimony might have to be given. The most common is called a **deposition.** This is testimony taken in a lawyer's office or in some other informal location. It is given under oath and transcribed by a court reporter. All lawyers involved in the case are allowed to question the witness. The witness may have a lawyer present and certainly will have one if he or she is also directly involved in the lawsuit. The deposition can be read to the jury during the trial if the witness is not available, or it can be read while the witness is testifying during the trial to show that the testimony has changed or to refresh the witness's memory.

The second type of testimony is that given in court during a trial. If required to testify at a trial, a surgical technologist should inform the hospital administration and consider consulting an attorney, depending on the seriousness of the case and the individual's degree of involvement in the suit. When

the CST testifies, it is imperative that he or she tell the truth, because the witness is under oath. Lying under oath is called **perjury,** which is a punishable crime.

A person who receives a subpoena must keep in mind that it is a court order requiring the individual's presence; disobeying the subpoena can result in criminal penalties.

Summons

A **summons** makes its recipient a party to a lawsuit; that is, if a person receives a summons, he or she is being sued. The person who was injured and is suing is called the *plaintiff.* The person being sued is the *defendant.* All summonses require action by the recipient within a limited time (usually 20 to 30 days). The papers should be taken to a lawyer or an insurance company immediately. Failure to do so could cause the defendant to lose the case without ever having had the chance to defend himself or herself.

Judgment

A claim for injury may be pursued in either a **court trial** or a **jury trial.** The trial determines whether the defendant is liable for the injury to the plaintiff and, if so, the extent of direct damages, indirect damages, and punitive damages. The judgment is the amount of money awarded to the plaintiff based on damages incurred.

ETHICS

What exactly is ethics? How is ethics related to the law? How does this affect our professional actions?

Ethics is a branch of philosophy that defines people's behavior in their relationships with others and their environment. The definition of ethics and whether morality is the same as ethics are the subject of many philosophical and scholarly debates. There is no correct answer in this debate. Morality, or morals, may be described as personal standards that often are influenced by culture, religion, and other traditions. Morality usually attempts to define what is right or wrong behavior. Ethics tends to be less focused on right and wrong and more intent on finding out what is *beneficial to humanity* in the long term or in looking at the specific circumstances of an act. In many ways, these concepts overlap. For example, most people agree that stealing another's property is wrong or immoral. However, ethics might argue that some situations allow stealing. For example, is it permissible to steal food to save a child from starvation?

For the purposes of this text, ethics is discussed as it applies to a health professional's conduct in the care of patients; that is, **medical ethics.** The focus is on standards of conduct that have been established by the health professions for their own members and that promote accountability and responsible, compassionate care of others.

❖ *Ethics refers to a standard of behavior created by specific groups of people to establish the conduct of its own members.*

One of the best-known ethical standards is, *"Do no harm."* This ethic was established by the medical profession but has been adapted by many others. This simple phrase has many deeper concepts, including the promise to every patient that no matter what treatment or advice is given, the patient will not suffer as a result. It is an implied contract between the patient and the health provider and the basis of trust in this relationship. Surgical technologists make this promise to their patients in every simple or complex task that involves safety or protection. They promise that no matter how difficult or stressful the surgery or how tired they are, their first priority is to protect that patient from injury and suffering. In other words, the patient comes first.

Conflict in ethical decision making arises when a standard of behavior creates a dilemma for the person making the decision. Perhaps the choice of actions conflicts with the rights of another person. For example, is it better to honor a patient's right to confidentiality or to reveal his confession to you before surgery that he committed a serious crime and only you know about it? In this case, the rights of society to protect itself against a criminal might be in conflict with the individual's right of confidentiality.

Some very important principles in society seem to be universal. Most people believe that murder, lying, and stealing are detrimental to individuals and society. Aside from these, however, ethical dilemmas always exist in society. Unless forced to adopt the views of others, people hold varied opinions about actions, and those opinions are governed by conscience. This is especially true when certain complex situations seem to pull people toward both ends of the ethical decision making spectrum. People can change their views as life and forceful events provide new insights. This often happens to caregivers, and it is a normal part of development and growth.

Professional ethics, such as those observed in medicine, nursing, and allied health, usually are very clear. The standards are defined by professionals who are highly regarded by their peers and who have the experience and authority to promote the standards. The standards are reviewed regularly and approved by members of the profession as a group. A health professional must agree to the standards of the profession before entering it. A professional who violates the standards may lose the right to remain a member of the profession. However, ethical standards are not laws, because they have no affiliation with government.

ETHICAL BEHAVIOR IN HEALTH CARE

Most people understand what is acceptable in a society and what is considered unethical. Professional ethics comprises the standards that society expects from those who provide services to them. Medical ethics defines the conduct of those in the health professions.

Ethical behavior in health care is based on a few very powerful directives for the health professional. These directives have far-reaching implications:

- Respect human individuality and uniqueness
- Do no harm
- Act with beneficence
- Act with justice
- Respect all confidences entrusted to you
- Act with faithfulness to the patient and others

- Act with honesty
- Respect the free will of the patient
- Give the patient's welfare priority over all else

These behaviors might be applied to any situation in life. In the care of patients, they have special meaning.

Respect Human Individuality and Uniqueness

Each person is different from all others. Each person has needs that are specific to his or her personality, medical condition, psychological state, emotions, social life, and culture. Respect for these qualities is demonstrated when health professionals treat the patient as a person with a name, a history, and a lifetime of experiences that probably are very different from their own. We must act without judgment or condemnation.

When we encounter a patient who acts or looks very different from what we consider "normal" or "mainstream," we sometimes feel off-guard or even offended. Our first impressions tell us that this person is different and therefore unpredictable or even threatening in some way. Health professionals learn to curb these feelings and transform them into therapeutic action. A person may behave outside the norm, but he or she is human, with all the needs and pain of any human being. It is these characteristics to which health professionals must respond, not the patient's lifestyle, appearance, or mannerisms.

Do No Harm

The health professional must maintain constant awareness of the potential for injury to the patient, others, and oneself. Almost every task in the surgical environment requires some form of protection from harm. Aseptic technique, sponge counts, and education about equipment are examples of protective measures.

Act with Beneficence

Beneficence implies empathy and commitment to healing. It requires health professionals to move beyond aspects of the patient's condition that offend their senses or make them emotionally uncomfortable and instead focus on the use of their professional and personal skills. Active care of a patient who has a purulent infection, shows self-neglect, or has a disease associated with a social stigma is an act of beneficence and compassion.

Act with Justice

All patients have the right to equal treatment regardless of age, physical attributes, mental state, ethnicity, or socioeconomic status. Advocating for justice may mean speaking out in the workplace when equal rights are violated. It also means monitoring and challenging our own beliefs and perhaps even our prejudices. Health professionals must be culturally and socially sensitive. To act without sensitivity is to act without justice.

Respect All Confidences Entrusted to You

Confidential information about the patient should not be shared with others outside the operating room. Confidence among coworkers is also an expected ethical behavior. Gossip is an insidious but common breach of confidentiality. It extracts enormous cost in emotional hurt and can affect the professional and personal lives of people in profound ways that we may never realize.

Act with Faithfulness

It is your responsibility to remain faithful to the patient as his or her advocate. At all times, you must respect the patient's personal and physical privacy and honor the patient's trust in you. It is important to have faith in the work you do and the people with whom you work.

Act with Honesty

If you make an error, it is crucial that you admit it. When you are unsure about a procedure, be sure to ask for help and accept that help without resentment or anger. Falsifying information or records is dishonest, as is embellishing or diminishing your actions or those of others.

Respect the Free Will of the Patient

All patients have the right to refuse care and to participate in their care. They have the right to receive information about their condition from their physicians and nurses and to ask for advocacy. Patients lose almost all physical freedom when they enter the hospital. Although not physically restrained (except in certain extreme circumstances), they lose mobility, the freedom to work and care for other family members, and the ability to participate in a normal life. Health care workers are expected to respect and respond to patients' freedom to make choices and express needs and concerns.

Give the Patient's Welfare Priority Over All Else

Surgical technologists are presented with many responsibilities and decisions during the course of a workday. Some decisions, such as what equipment to prepare for a case, or the ordering of supplies, seem to be straightforward, without ethical dilemma. Others situations such as reporting alleged malpractice committed by a colleage are laden with more serious ethical consequences. Most responsibilities and duties in the perioperative environment have a consequence (large or small) for the patient. The technologist has a duty of care to always act in favor of the patient's welfare. The implied contract between patient and care worker always favors outcomes that protect the patient from harm. During professional development, the surgical technologist learns to think "outside" immediate consequences when making decisions. They become increasingly aware of their patients' vulnerabilities. Patient protection and welfare is consciously or unconsciously factored into every action and task.

COMBINED ETHICAL AND LEGAL CONCERNS

Impairment

An impaired team member is a major threat to the safety of the patient and others in the environment. It is illegal to care

for others while under the impairment of drugs or alcohol. Health care workers have both a legal and an ethical responsibility to report suspected impairment of a coworker or, if needed, to seek treatment for themselves. Self-destructive behavior, such as drug or alcohol abuse, reveals not a weakness but an illness. In reporting these behaviors, team members protect not only everyone in the environment but also the abuser. Treatment programs are available to those who need help. The goal is to return the health care worker to a productive and satisfying role in the workplace and to enable the individual to resume a stable personal and social life.

Sexual Harassment

Sexual harassment is unwanted sexual coercion, lewd comments, innuendoes, or touching perpetrated by one person on another. Sexual harassment is identified when a person speaks or acts in a sexually aggressive manner that causes discomfort, embarrassment, humiliation, or shame. It is illegal and unethical. Over the past 20 years, sexual harassment increasingly has been condemned in the workplace. Incidents that used to be accepted as the norm in team relationships are no longer tolerated by institutions or health care workers themselves. No one in any profession is obliged to tolerate implied or actual physical or verbal sexual aggression. Because sexual harassment is defined differently by different individuals, it is best to document and report every instance of harassment as it occurs. The person who is harassed should retain an exact duplicate of the report. If the perpetrator is a superior, the report should be made above his or her administrative level or up the chain of command. Accepting sexual harassment is not an indicator of one's "toughness"; harassment is a violation of one's person and dignity, and it is punishable by law.

Refusal to Perform an Assigned Task

The surgical technologist has the right to abstain from participation in certain types of cases that violate his or her ethical, moral, or religious values (e.g., abortion or organ transplantation). The operating room must be informed of this when the surgical technologist is hired. It is not ethical suddenly to refuse to perform a task on moral grounds unless the case is one that could never have been anticipated by the staff member. When offered a position, the surgical technologist should submit, in writing, a list of cases in which he or she declines to participate.

Occasionally a team member refuses to work with another person based on that person's history of inappropriate behavior. The surgical technologist should report the behavior before the next time he or she may be working with this person. To suddenly refuse to participate in a case, or worse, to walk out in the middle of a case, could be interpreted as abandonment of the patient. If the reason for refusal is a personality clash, steps must be taken to resolve the problem before the surgical technologist is assigned to the case (see Chapter 6).

Any person must refuse to perform a task that is beyond the scope of his or her professional ability, skill, or training. If repeated requests to perform such tasks are made, the individual should submit a formal report to the operating room supervisor or the next person in the chain of command. However, if the task is in the person's job description, it is the individual's duty and obligation to learn to perform the task.

Staff Shortages

The shortage of health care personnel in recent years has resulted in greater risk for patients in nearly all health care settings. The staff-to-patient ratio is unsafe, and staff members and personnel often are asked to extend their shift to make up for the shortfall. Lack of attention, fatigue, hunger, and frustration all contribute to accidents and injury. This is both a legal problem and an ethical problem, and the solutions remain somewhat elusive.

ETHICAL DILEMMAS

A dilemma is personal conflict that arises from the need to make a decision based on choices that are not completely acceptable. A common example is the overloaded lifeboat. If everyone remains on the lifeboat, it will probably sink. To remove individuals and prevent the boat from sinking will result in the immediate death of those thrown overboard. Neither option is satisfactory from an ethical viewpoint. Society tries to resolve dilemmas in many areas of medical ethics through ethics committees, public debate, and even laws. Medical technology has exceeded our ability to cope with the many **ethical dilemmas** as they relate to health and society. There are no "answers" to these debates, but health professionals should be aware of them.

- **Right to die.** Should an individual have the right to die when and where he or she wishes? Should this include assisted suicide?
- **Stem cell research.** Is it ethical to use stem cells obtained from discarded human embryos for cell regeneration?
- **Human cloning.** Is it ethical to allow researchers to perform the replication of a human being?
- **Good Samaritan law.** Should a health professional be allowed to help someone in need of assistance outside the health care environment without threat of liability if things go wrong? (States allow this by law, but the issue is still debated.)
- **Abortion.** Is it ethical for a woman to terminate her pregnancy?
- **Refusal of treatment.** Can the family of an incapacitated individual decide to refuse treatment for that family member if they believe it will cause or prolong suffering?
- **Organ donation.** Is it ethical to remove vital organs from a patient who is brain dead but maintained on life support systems? Can the family make this decision if the patient cannot express his or her wishes? Is it ethical to donate a liver to a person who suffers from chronic alcoholism?

Many other ethical dilemmas occur in day-to-day clinical work, including the following:

- **Loyalty.** A loyalty dilemma requires that a person be loyal to one person while being disloyal to another. For example, you are asked to comment on an act of negligence committed by a coworker that you witnessed. Do you incriminate your coworker by telling the truth or try to defend her even though you know she was negligent?
- **Confidentiality.** Your patient informs you that she is pregnant, but she has not told her partner or the physician. She asks you not to tell anyone.
- **Spiritual values.** You have notified your employer that you decline to participate in abortion procedures. You are called in for an emergency. When you arrive at the hospital, you learn that you will serve as scrub on a case of an incomplete self-induced abortion. No one else is available to serve as scrub. The patient is hemorrhaging.
- **Honesty.** You have incorrectly reported the amount of a local anesthetic used during a procedure. The patient has a toxic reaction, but it is eventually resolved with a good outcome for the patient. No one knows that you miscalculated the dosage and caused the reaction. Do you report it anyway, knowing that it might cost you your job?

One method of resolving ethical conflict is to examine your own beliefs thoroughly and come to a resolution about how you will act in certain circumstances. Not every ethical dilemma is predictable, but surgical technologists frequently are confronted with ethical decisions both small and large. These issues deserve thoughtful consideration. Speaking with other health care professionals or those who have helped mentor you can help you define personal values and integrate them into your professional ethics.

PROFESSIONAL CODES OF ETHICS

Professional organizations, such as the Association of Surgical Technologists (AST), the American Nurses Association, the American Hospital Association, and the American Medical Association, have created codes of ethics that reflect expectations of those professionals as they make decisions involving ethical issues. By acting in accordance with these ethics, professional health care workers demonstrate their advocacy for human rights, patient protection, and the laws of society. In all situations, the health care worker is the patient's advocate; the health care worker is doing what the patient would do if he or she were able. The AST has adopted a Latin phrase to describe its ethos: *Aeger primo,* which means, "the patient first." The AST code of ethics is presented in Box 4-6.

PATIENTS' RIGHTS

Government agencies and established laws are created to protect patients. Professional organizations for health care workers establish and publish codes of ethics. These codes outline the behaviors expected of any member of the health profession. A health professional thus is expected to act in a certain way and within the ethical standards of the profession and the laws of the state. Health professionals have an unspoken contract to maintain a particular kind of relationship with their patients. The American Hospital Association has developed guidelines to help patients understand their rights in the hospital setting (Box 4-7).

Box 4-6

Code of Ethics of the Association of Surgical Technologists

1. To maintain the highest standards of professional conduct and patient care.
2. To hold in confidence, with respect to the patient's beliefs, all personal matters.
3. To respect and protect the patient's legal and moral rights to quality patient care.
4. To not knowingly cause injury or any injustice to those entrusted to our care.
5. To work with fellow technologists and other professional health groups to promote harmony and unity for better patient care.
6. To follow principles of asepsis.
7. To maintain a high degree of efficiency through continuing education.
8. To maintain and practice surgical technology willingly, with pride and dignity.
9. To report any unethical conduct or practice to the proper authority.
10. To adhere to the Code of Ethics at all times with all members of the health care team.

From the Association of Surgical Technologists.

Box 4-7

The Patient Care Partnership: Understanding Expectations, Rights, and Responsibilities

When you need hospital care, your doctor and the nurses and other professionals at our hospital are committed to working with you and your family to meet your health care needs. Our dedicated doctors and staff members serve the community in all its ethnic, religious, and economic diversity. Our goal is for you and your family to have the same care and attention we would want for our families and ourselves.

The following sections explain how you can expect to be treated during your hospital stay. They also cover what we will need from you to care for you better. If you have questions at any time, please ask them. Unasked or unanswered questions can add to the stress of being in the hospital. Your comfort and confidence in your care are very important to us.

What to Expect During Your Hospital Stay

- *High-quality hospital care.* Our first priority is to give you the care you need, when you need it, with skill, compassion, and respect. Tell your caregivers if you have concerns about your care or if you have pain. You have the right to know the identity of doctors, nurses, and others involved in your care, and you have the right to know when they are students, residents, or other trainees.
- *A clean and safe environment.* Our hospital works hard to keep you safe. We use special policies and procedures to avoid mistakes in your care and keep you free from abuse or neglect. If anything unexpected and significant happens during your hospital stay, you will be told what happened, and any resulting changes in your care will be discussed with you.
- *Involvement in your care.* You and your doctor often make decisions about your care before you go to the hospital. Other times, especially in emergencies, those decisions are made during your hospital stay. When decision making takes place, it should include discussing your medical condition and information about medically appropriate treatment choices. To make informed decisions with your doctor, you need to understand:
  - The benefits and risks of each treatment
  - Whether your treatment is experimental or part of a research study

- What you can reasonably expect from your treatment and any long-term effects it might have on your quality of life
- What you and your family will need to do after you leave the hospital
- The financial consequences of using uncovered services or out of network providers

Please tell your caregivers if you need more information about treatment choices.

- *Discussing your treatment plan.* When you enter the hospital, you sign a general consent to treatment. In some cases, such as surgery or experimental treatment, you may be asked to confirm in writing that you understand what is planned and agree to it. This process protects your right to consent to or refuse a treatment. Your doctor will explain the medical consequences of refusing recommended treatment. It also protects your right to decide whether you want to participate in a research study.
- *Getting information from you.* Your caregivers need complete and correct information about your health and coverage so that they can make good decisions about your care. That information includes:
  - Past illnesses, surgeries, or hospital stays
  - Past allergic reactions
  - Any medicines or dietary supplements (e.g., vitamins and herbs) you are taking
  - Any network or admission requirements under your health plan
- *Understanding your health care goals and values.* You may have health care goals and values or spiritual beliefs that are important to your well-being. They will be taken into account as much as possible throughout your hospital stay. Make sure your doctor, your family, and your care team know your wishes.
- *Understanding who should make decisions when you cannot.* If you have signed a health care power of attorney stating who should speak for you if you become unable to make health care decisions for yourself, or a "living will" or "advance directive" that states your wishes about end of life care, give copies to your doctor, your family, and your care

Continued

team. If you or your family need help making difficult decisions, counselors, chaplains, and others are available to help.

- *Protecting your privacy.* We respect the confidentiality of your relationship with your doctor and other caregivers, and the sensitive information about your health and health care that are part of that relationship. State and federal laws and hospital operating policies protect the privacy of your medical information. You will receive a Notice of Privacy Practices that describes the ways that we use, disclose, and safeguard patient information and explains how you can obtain a copy of information about your care from our records about your care.

- *Preparing you and your family for your departure from the hospital.* Your doctor works with hospital staff and professionals in your community. You and your family also play an important role in your care. The success of your treatment often depends on your efforts to follow medication, diet, and therapy plans. Your family may need to help care for you at home.

- *Helping you to identify sources of follow-up care and letting you know whether our hospital has a financial interest in any*

referrals. As long as you agree that we can share information about your care with them, we will coordinate our activities with your caregivers outside the hospital. You can also expect to receive information and, where possible, training about the self-care you will need when you go home.

- *Helping you with your bill and filing insurance claims.* Our staff will file claims for you with health care insurers or other programs, such as Medicare and Medicaid. They also will help your doctor with needed documentation. Hospital bills and insurance coverage often are confusing. If you have questions about your bill, contact our business office. If you need help understanding your insurance coverage or health plan, start with your insurance company or health benefits manager. If you do not have health coverage, we will try to help you and your family find financial help or make other arrangements. We need your help with collecting needed information and other requirements to obtain coverage or assistance.

While you are here, you will receive more detailed notices about some of the rights you have as a hospital patient and how to exercise them. We are always interested in improving. If you have questions, comments, or concerns, please contact _____.

CHAPTER SUMMARY

- Laws concerning the practice of medicine, nursing, and allied health have been established to protect the public.
- The surgical technologist's scope of practice is defined by state law.
- The medical and nurse practice acts of each state provide information about the roles and responsibilities of health care workers.
- Health care policy is established by professional organizations and by health care facilities.
- Delegation is an important legal and professional concept in medicine. It is the transfer of responsibility for a task from one person to another. The conditions of delegation must be determined to protect the patient from harm.
- Civil liability derives from an act committed against a person or property. Acts of negligence in health care are causes of civil liability.
- Negligence is "the commission of an act that a prudent person would not have done or the omission of a duty and a prudent person would have fulfilled, resulting in injury or harm to another person."[1]
- Negligence is the most common cause of patient injury and death in health care.
- Examples of negligence include patient burns, falls, medication errors, improper patient positioning, abandonment of a patient, and retained surgical objects. Failure to care for a surgical specimen

correctly and failure to communicate about a potentially dangerous situation are also considered negligence.
- Criminal liability involves breaking the law. Exceeding the scope of practice and theft of hospital or another's personal property are criminal actions.
- The patient's record is a legal document. Laws regarding the use of patient information are strictly enforced.
- Documentation in the perioperative environment is necessary to protect the patient.
- A sentinel event is one in which there is potential or actual injury or death in the work environment. An incident report must be completed for any sentinel event.
- A legal action may be brought against any health professional when a negligent act results in harm.
- Ethics is a branch of philosophy that defines people's behavior in relation to others and the environment.
- An ethical dilemma is a situation in which no desirable outcome exists no matter which ethical choice is made.
- Ethical behavior in health care is established by culture, society, and professional organizations.
- Professionals are expected to act in an ethical manner.
- Ethics in medicine involves issues such as confidentiality, honesty, respect for others, beneficence, and respect for the law.

REVIEW QUESTIONS

1. Define the relationship between accountability and delegation.
2. Who may delegate a task? Under what circumstances can a task be delegated?
3. What is sexual harassment? Why do you think people tolerate it in the workplace?
4. Negligence is the most common cause of lawsuits in medical practice. Define negligence and give three examples of negligent acts or behavior.
5. What are state practice acts?
6. The unlicensed medical professional is treated as a normal citizen when a lawsuit over patient injury arises. What source of law is applicable in this case?
7. What are the causes of negligence in the operating room?
8. What is informed consent? Why is it necessary? Who can witness informed consent?
9. How do you decide what ethical decisions to make?
10. What is the difference between the law and ethics?
11. What is an ethical dilemma?
12. Many bioethical dilemmas have arisen in our society, such as abortion, stem cell research, savior siblings, and organ donation. List at least five bioethical dilemmas that you find particularly difficult.

CASE STUDIES

Case 1

You are scrubbed on a case involving an exploratory laparotomy. The surgeon has revealed a large tumor involving the pancreas, liver, and mesentery. He calls in another assistant to help with retraction. The case becomes complex very quickly. The surgeon asks you to cauterize ("buzz") bleeders as he clamps them. What will you do?

Case 2

Your patient is a 50-year-old woman about to undergo breast biopsy with possible mastectomy. Your role is to act as assistant circulator to the registered nurse. The RN asks you to go to the holding area to see whether the patient has arrived. When you arrive at the holding area, the surgeon is there with the patient. As the surgeon looks over the chart, he notices that the patient has not signed the operative permit. He asks you to witness the patient's signing. What will you do?

Case 3

While scrubbed on a case involving surgical treatment of carpal tunnel syndrome, you complete the instrument, sponge, and needle count. You are missing a needle. You tell the surgeon that the count is incorrect. He replies, "Oh, don't worry. The needle can't be in the wound, it's too small. I would be able to see it. Let's close." What will you do?

Case 4

While in the locker room, you notice that one of your coworkers is emptying the pockets of her scrub suit. There are two vials of injectable medications. You cannot see what they are. She puts them in her purse and leaves. What do you do?

Case 5

You have been called into the office of the hospital's attorney to answer questions about a case 2 months earlier in which you served as scrubbed technologist. The case involves the retained needle in the patient undergoing carpal tunnel surgery (see case 3), who is suing the hospital and staff. Based on how you answered the question in case 3, what are your thoughts as you wait to see the hospital's attorney?

Case 6

You have been asked to help position an 80-year-old man for hip surgery. He is under general anesthesia and is intubated. After the surgery, the anesthesiologist discovers that the patient's right ulna is fractured. The surgeon says, "We'd better fix this ulna now." Think about the events in this procedure. Who is responsible for the fracture? Can the surgeon repair the ulna without a permit? What (if anything) is the appropriate action for you as a surgical technologist at this point? What will you do if you believe that you may have caused the fracture?

Case 7

You are scrubbed on a cholecystectomy case. You have been given sterile saline, Hypaque (a contrast medium used during radiography to observe strictures inside the ducts of the gallbladder), and thrombin (a coagulant). You put these in separate medicine containers on your back table. The surgeon asks you to prepare a syringe of 50% Hypaque and 50% saline. Instead, you hand her thrombin. Just as she begins to inject the bile duct, you realize that you made an error. What do you do? Who will be responsible for any injury to the patient? How could you have prevented this mistake?

REFERENCE

1. *Mosby's pocket dictionary of medical, nursing, and allied health*, ed 6, St Louis, 2009, Mosby.

BIBLIOGRAPHY

American Hospital Association: The patient care partnership: understanding expectations, rights, and responsibilities. Accessed November 1, 2007, at www.aha.org/aha/issues/Communicating-With-Patients.

Association of periOperative Registered Nurses (AORN): Position statement on correct site surgery. In *Standards, recommended practices and guidelines, 2007 edition*, Denver, 2007, AORN.

Association of Surgical Technologists (AST): Standards of practice. Accessed October 22, 2007, at http://www.ast.org.

Association of Surgical Technologists (AST): Code of ethics. Accessed November 2, 2007, at http://www.ast.org.

United States Department of Health and Human Services, Office for civil rights: Summary of the HIPPAA privacy rule. Accessed January 1, 2009 at http://www.hhs.gov/ocrprivacysummary.pdf

University of Washington School of Medicine: Informed consent: ethics in medicine. Accessed November 2, 2007, at http://depts.washington.edu/bioethx/.

CHAPTER 5

Introduction to the Health Care Facility

CHAPTER OUTLINE

LEARNING OBJECTIVES

After studying this chapter the reader will be able to:
- Identify operating room staff members and their duties
- Define hospital policy
- Describe the process of health care accreditation
- Describe the purpose of an organizational chart
- Define a chain of command
- State the importance of a job description
- List common hospital ancillary services and describe their functions

- Describe an organizational chart and explain its significance in an organization
- Discuss the purposes of the operating room design
- Describe safe traffic patterns in the operating room
- Differentiate restricted, semirestricted, and nonrestricted areas of the operating room
- Discuss environmental controls in the surgical suite and why they are important

TERMINOLOGY

Accreditation: The process by which a hospital is evaluated by an independent organization, which examines the hospital's practices, records, procedures, and outcomes.

Administration: Individuals who manage an institution, plan its activities, and provide oversight for day to day operations and employees. The administration is also a liaison between the facility and the community, government, and media.

Air exchange: The exchange of fresh air for air that has been recirculated in a closed area.

Back table: A large stainless steel table on which most of the sterile surgical supplies and instruments are placed for use during surgery. Before surgery, the back table is covered with a sterile drape and sterile instruments and other equipment are opened onto its surface. Supplies needed for immediate use are transferred to the Mayo stand.

Biomedical technologists: Professionals who specialize in the maintenance, repair, and safe operation of devices used in medicine, including surgical equipment.

Case cart system: Organizational method of preparing equipment and instruments for a specific surgery. Equipment is prepared by

the central services or supply department and sent to the operating room.

Central core: The restricted area of the operating room, where sterile supplies and flash sterilizers are located.

Certified Registered Nurse Anesthetist CRNA: A registered nurse trained and qualified to administer anesthesia.

Chain of command: A hierarchy of personnel positions that establishes both vertical and horizontal relationships between positions.

Contaminated: The condition of instruments, supplies, or items that have been exposed to a nonsterile item, particle, or surface through physical or airborne contact.

Decontamination area: A room or small department in which soiled instruments and equipment are cleaned of gross matter and decontaminated to remove microorganisms.

Efficiency: The economic use of time and energy to prevent unnecessary expenditure of work, materials, and time.

High-efficiency particulate air (HEPA) filters: Filters installed in the operating room ventilation system that remove 99.97% of particles equal to or larger than 0.3 micrometers (μm).

Integrated operating room: A type of structural and engineering design in which digital and computerized components such as cameras, monitors, and environmental controls can be controlled from a central location in the room. Components such as endoscopic control units and monitors are built into the room structure rather than as separate portable units.

Job description: A document which specifies duties, responsibilities, location, pay, and management structure of a job.

Job title: The name of a job, such as "Certified Surgical Technologist" or "Chief of Surgery."

Kick bucket: A stainless steel bucket which fits into a movable frame for positioning near the sterile field. The bucket is used primarily for discarding surgical sponges during a procedure.

Laminar airflow (LAF) system: A ventilation system that moves a contained volume of air in layers at a continuous velocity, with 800 to 900 air exchanges per hour.

Mayo stand: A stainless tray mounted on a floor stand, which is draped and placed within the immediate sterile field during surgery. Instruments and lightweight equipment are placed on the Mayo stand for immediate use. These are exchanged for others on the back table as required during the surgery.

Mission statement: A written declaration that defines the central goal of the health care institution and reflects the organization's ethical and moral beliefs in broad terms.

Operating table: A table or bed on which the patient is positioned for a surgical procedure. The operating table has many possible configurations, support structures, and accessories to facilitate positioning for access to the surgical site or focal area of the operation.

Organizational chart (organigram): A graphic depiction of an organization's chain of command that shows the lines of vertical (higher and lower) and horizontal (equal) administrative authority.

OSHA: Occupational Safety and Health Administration. The agency of the U.S. Department of Labor that establishes rules and standards to protect the safety of employees in the workplace.

Personnel policy: A policy that sets forth the health care facility's job descriptions, role delineations, requirements for employment, and rules of conduct for personnel.

Physician assistant (PA): A licensed medical professional who practices medicine under the direct supervision of a licensed medical doctor.

Policy manual: Operational guidelines, procedures, and protocols contained in written or electronic documents. Employees are required to follow the policies of the department in which they are employed and be familiar with procedures for emergency and general safety.

Postanesthesia care unit (PACU): The critical care area where patients are taken after surgery for monitoring, evaluation, and response to emergencies.

Restricted area: The area of the operating room where only personnel wearing surgical attire, including masks, shoe coverings, and head coverings, are allowed. Doors are kept closed, and the air pressure is greater than that in areas outside the restricted area.

Ring stand: A raised circular frame used to support one or two sterile stainless steel basins. Basins are filled with sterile water or saline for use in surgery.

Risk management: The process of tracking, evaluating, and studying accidents and incidents to protect patients and employees. Risk management produces change in policy or enforcement of policy if the risk reaches an unacceptable level.

Role confusion: Lack of clarity about one's job duties and requirements.

Satellite facilities: Community health care offices that are administered by a single institution but are located in communities in surrounding urban or rural areas. These facilities offer primary and preventive health care services in general medicine and other specialties.

Semirestricted area: A designated area in which only personnel wearing scrub suits and hair caps that enclose all facial hair are allowed.

The Joint Commission: The accrediting organization for hospitals and other health care facilities in the United States.

Traffic patterns: The movement of people and equipment into, out of, and within the operating room.

Transitional area: An area in which surgical personnel or visitors prepare to enter the semirestricted and restricted areas. Transitional areas include the locker rooms and changing rooms.

Unrestricted area: An area that people dressed in street clothes may enter.

INTRODUCTION

The services provided in the health care setting require specific facilities and a staff capable of delivering those services. Neither of these elements of health care can exist without the other. The facility itself must provide a safe environment for patients, staff members, and visitors. It also must *enable* the work of health care personnel in a way that encourages efficiency of time, movement (work), and space. This is done through the administrative and management process.

This chapter is an introduction to the perioperative environment and to the health care facility as a whole. It gives the rationale for operating room design and standards. It also provides important information about the professionals who work in the facility; specifically, what their roles are and where those roles fit into the larger organizational structure.

OPERATING ROOM ENVIRONMENT

PRINCIPLES OF OPERATING ROOM DESIGN

The surgical department is structured and engineered to provide a safe and efficient environment for patients and staff members. Many different designs can be used, but all must achieve the following objectives:

1. Infection control
2. Environmental safety
3. Efficient use of personnel, time, space, and resources

Infection Control

Infection control is a multidisciplinary process. It involves many different areas of expertise and practice. The physical design of the operating room is one focal area. It is based on two basic principles:

- Physical separation between the surgical environment and any source of contamination
- Containment of sources of infection

Clean and **contaminated** areas are physically separated when possible. For example, the cleaning and **decontamination area** is separated from the surgical suites by walls and corridors. The surgical department itself is separated from hospital corridors and units by doors that remain closed at all times.

When complete physical separation is impossible, contaminated objects are *contained*. Containment means confinement in a prescribed area or by a barrier. For example, the air in the surgical suite cannot be completely separated from the air outside the suite, therefore it is contained by keeping the doors closed and maintaining a higher air pressure inside the suite than outside. Nonporous materials are used for floors so that dirt, water, and body fluids remain contained on the surface, where they can be easily removed with disinfectant and water.

Environmental Safety

Many hazards can be found in the surgical environment. Some of these are obvious, but others are not. Environmental engineering in the operating room follows national medical engineering standards for electrical circuits, in-line gases, lighting, and other utilities. Strict safety standards ensure that patients and staff members are protected from extreme hazards and accidents such as fire, explosion, and electrocution. (Chapter 15 presents a more in-depth discussion of environmental safety in the operating room.)

Efficiency

Efficiency is the economic use of time and energy to save unnecessary work, material resources, and time. Efficient use of space influences the use of time and contributes to the safety of personnel. Work in the operating room is strenuous. Intelligent design can reduce physical stress by reducing movement and creating work systems that minimize strain. Time-saving practices are implemented to increase the number of patients served, but also to make the best use of people's skills and abilities. In an emergency, time sometimes is the most important factor in achieving a good outcome. Proper storage of sterile supplies and efficient use of space protects the sterility of the items and enables staff members to find what they need quickly and retrieve it safely. For example, equipment that is stacked too high for safe retrieval or equipment that obstructs hallways creates a risk of injury for both patients and employees.

PHYSICAL ENVIRONMENT

Floor Plans

Many different types of floor plans meet the goals of infection control, environmental safety, and efficiency. Figures 5-1 and 5-2 show two examples of floor plans. In Figure 5-1, the surgical suites are separated from the workroom by

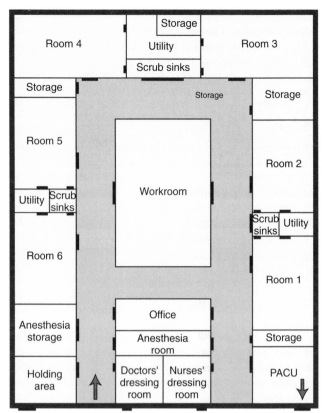

Figure 5-1 "Race track" style operating room floor plan. *(Modified from Phillips N: Berry and Kohn's operating room technique, ed 10, St Louis, 2004, Mosby.)*

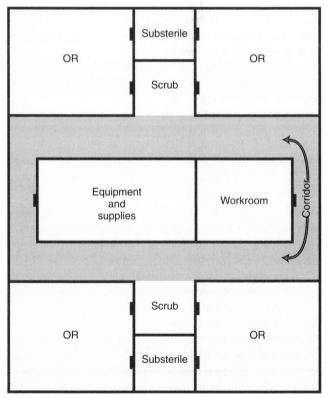

Figure 5-2 Operating room floor plan with a central core. *(Modified from Phillips N: Berry and Kohn's operating room technique, ed 10, St Louis, 2004, Mosby.)*

a corridor. The surgical suites are arranged around a continuous corridor. The transitional areas are located at one end so that traffic into the department can be controlled at one location. In Figure 5-2, the **central core** contains clean and sterile equipment and supplies. Contaminated instruments and equipment are processed outside the central core in another area. The primary design goal of the floor plan is to create a clear separation between soiled and clean equipment.

Traffic Patterns

The movement of people and equipment within and into the perioperative area is restricted. Traffic into the operating room is controlled by the specific location and lockout system of the entry doors. Personnel can enter the department only through monitored doors, and fire exits are equipped with alarms to prevent people from entering the department from the outside. **Traffic patterns** are designed to reduce the spread of disease by isolating the source.

Unrestricted Area

The **unrestricted area** is a monitored area where people entering the department may be directed to change into surgical attire, or they may remain in the unrestricted area. Personnel dressed in street clothes and portable equipment that has not been disinfected are confined to the unrestricted area. Family waiting areas and outer reception areas are unrestricted areas.

Semirestricted Area

Only personnel wearing surgical attire (a scrub suit and a hair cap that encloses facial hair) are allowed in the **semirestricted area.** The corridors between surgical rooms, the instrument and supply processing area, storage areas, and utility rooms are semirestricted areas.

Sterile or Restricted Area

Entry into a **restricted area** requires the highest level of precautions against contamination. Only personnel in scrub attire, including complete head, nose, and mouth covering, are permitted in these areas. Restricted locations include the surgical suites, procedure rooms, sterile corridor or substerile rooms where flash sterilizers are located, and sterile supply rooms.

Locker Room/Lounge Area

The locker room is a **transitional area** for those who need to change from street clothes to surgical attire. Clean scrub attire is located outside the locker room to protect it from contamination by fluids or soil inside the locker room. If the locker room leads directly into the lounge area, it is completely separated from the nonrestricted area. The areas are clearly delineated so that personnel dressed in street clothes do not frequent the lounge, offices, or other locations used by those who work in restricted zones. The lounge area often presents a problem for infection control, because personnel in street clothes may have easy access, and traffic control is limited or absent. It is very important that food and drink be limited to the lounge area and never taken into restricted areas.

SURGICAL SUITE

Equipment and Furniture

Equipment, furniture, and supplies in the surgical suite are stored in a standardized way that is familiar to all personnel. The purpose is to facilitate rapid setup and location of stored supplies. Every piece of equipment has a designated location; remember the wise old saying, *a place for everything and everything in its place.*

Many devices and equipment are standard to most surgical suites. Basic components needed during surgery include the operating table, instrument tables, ring stands for solutions, computer station, digital imaging equipment, and electrosurgical unit. All rooms contain an anesthesia machine and physiological monitoring equipment. Sterile supplies are stored in recessed cabinets or in substerile rooms just outside the suite. Suction and in-line gas and compressed air hoses are suspended from ceiling fixtures for safety and efficiency. Figure 5-3 shows a standard operating room with furniture and equipment in place.

The operating table is adjustable for height, degree of tilt in all directions, orientation in the room, articular breaks ("table breaks"), and length (Figure 5-4). This allows the patient to be positioned in any anatomical position to expose the surgical site fully and maintain safety. The surface is covered with a firm pad that may be removed for cleaning. (The operating table is discussed in more detail in Chapter 10.)

The back table is a large, stainless steel table on which all instruments and supplies except those in immediate use are placed (Figure 5-5). For some procedures, more than one back table may be needed. Just before surgery, a sterile pack (cover with towels and drapes enclosed) is opened onto the table. This provides a sterile surface on which instruments and sterile supplies are distributed. After gowning and

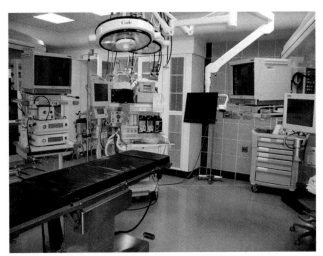

Figure 5-3 Operating room suite. *(Courtesy Allegheny General Hospital, Pittsburgh, Pa.)*

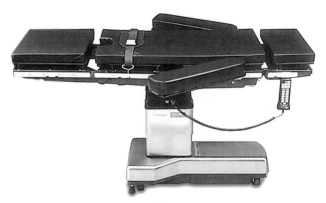

Figure 5-4 Operating table. *(Courtesy STERIS, Mentor, Ohio.)*

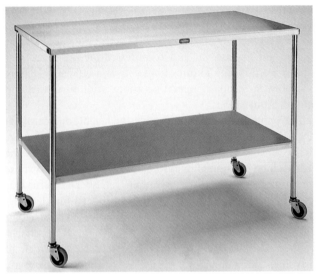

Figure 5-5 Back table. *(Courtesy Pedigo Products, Vancouver, Wash.)*

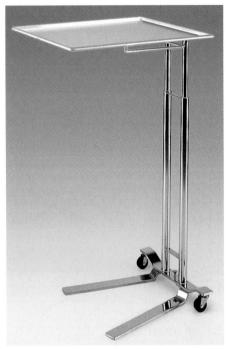

Figure 5-6 Mayo stand. *(Courtesy Pedigo Products, Vancouver, Wash.)*

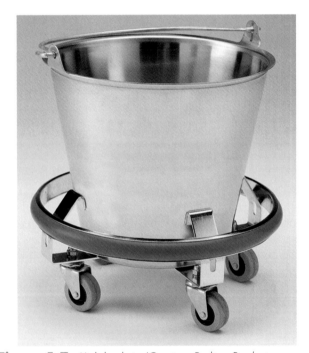

Figure 5-7 Kick bucket. *(Courtesy Pedigo Products, Vancouver, Wash.)*

gloving, the scrub arranges all the equipment in an orderly manner.

Other small tables are used for skin prep kits, power equipment, and extra sterile supplies that may be too heavy or bulky to place on the back table during surgery.

The Mayo stand is a smaller table with one open end that can be raised or lowered (Figure 5-6). It also is covered with a sterile drape and used for the placement of instruments and supplies that are immediately required during surgery. The table is placed over or alongside the patient for quick access to instruments. As the case progresses, new instruments or supplies are added and others removed.

The kick bucket is a stainless steel or plastic bucket on castors or wheels (Figure 5-7). It has a specific use and is not a "trash" receptacle. The kick bucket is designated for soiled surgical sponges and other lightweight, *nonsharp* items that must be discarded during surgery and accounted for. During surgery, it is placed in a strategic location near the surgical field so that the scrub can drop items directly into it for the circulator to retrieve.

The ring stand is used to contain one or two stainless steel basins (Figure 5-8). The ring stand is designed to support the lip of the basin, which has been previously wrapped and sterilized. Before surgery, the wrapped basin is placed in the ring stand and the wrapper opened up to expose the basin. Sterile water or saline is poured into the basin for use during surgery. The solutions are freshened as needed throughout surgery.

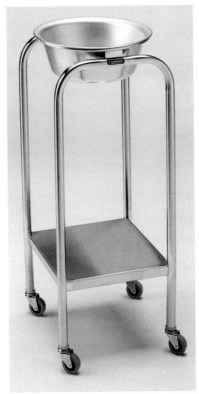

Figure 5-8   Single ring stand. *(Courtesy Pedigo Products, Vancouver, Wash.)*

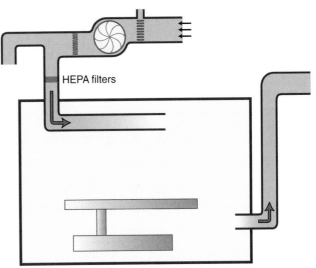

HEPA filters

Figure 5-9   Operating room air system. *(From Gruendemann BJ, Mangum SS: Infection prevention in surgical settings, Philadelphia, 2001, WB Saunders.)*

ENVIRONMENTAL CONTROLS

Airflow

Allowing airflow from unrestricted to restricted areas can increase the risk of infection. To reduce this risk, the air pressure in the surgical suite is maintained at a level 10% higher than the air pressure in adjacent semirestricted areas. The doors to the surgical suite must remain closed to maintain this positive pressure differential. Positive pressure forces air from the operating room into the hallways, preventing the potentially contaminated hallway air from entering the operating room.

Fresh filtered air enters the operating room ceiling vents and is combined with existing air in the room (Figure 5-9). The standard for **air exchange** is a minimum of 15 and a maximum of 20 filtered air exchanges per hour.

High-efficiency particulate air (HEPA) filters are installed in the operating room ventilation system and remove particles equal to or larger than 0.3 µm. HEPA filters must be changed regularly to maintain their efficiency. Bacteria and molds can easily colonize heating and cooling vents and dirty filters, creating a major source of infection, especially in burn units.

A **laminar airflow (LAF) system** moves a contained volume of air in layers at a continuous velocity. HEPA-filtered exchanges range from 400 to 600 exchanges per hour. The function of a LAF system is to move large volumes of air containing particles and microorganisms out of the operating room suite. A LAF system is very expen-

sive to implement and maintain. Infection control professionals currently debate the rate of surgical site infections (SSIs) when LAF systems are used compared with the rate when strict aseptic and surgical techniques are practiced meticulously.

Humidity

Air humidity is controlled to reduce the risk of infection and to minimize static electricity. When humidity is low, static electricity can create a fire hazard in the presence of flammable solutions and oxygen. High humidity may increase the risk of mold and bacterial growth on surfaces. The Joint Commission requires operating rooms to be maintained at 50% to 55% relative humidity.

Temperature

Temperature control is an important component of patient care and safety. The operating room is maintained at 68° to 73° F (20° to 23° C). This temperature range is less hospitable to the growth of microorganisms and maintains the temperature within the comfort range of patients and personnel. In extreme cases in which the patient's core temperature must be raised, such as for burn or pediatric patients, a warmer environment must be created to prevent hypothermia.

Lighting

Many different light sources are used in the operating room. Lighting in the operating room is produced by main overhead lights (room lighting) and by the surgical spotlights. The surgical lights usually are halogen lamps. These lights have a high color temperature (a measure of the hue that a light emits), which is very pale blue. Halogen provides extremely intense light that is less fatiguing to the eyes than other types of light of equal intensity. In addition, more of the energy emitted by halogen lighting is given off as light rather than as heat, making it safe to use near tissues.

SPECIAL PROCEDURE ROOM

Some types of surgical procedures require specialized rooms that contain the equipment and technology of that specialty. For example, transurethral (through the urethra) procedures of the genitourinary tract require continuous irrigation and a specialty operating table. A cystoscopy room is standard to all surgical departments. Other procedures, such as fluoroscopy-assisted surgery or cryosurgery, are performed in the interventional radiology or nuclear medicine department or the emergency department.

INTEGRATED OPERATING ROOM SYSTEMS

The integrated operating (OR) room provides centralized control of surgical devices and equipment through a sterile remote- or voice-activated system. This enables the surgeon to activate endoscopic controls, imaging components, operating lights, table adjustments, insufflators, environmental controls, and many other devices that previously were managed individually. Integrated systems allow the surgical team to view patient monitoring output, as well as diagnostic imaging, on the central monitor or "inside" the image seen by the endoscopic camera. A nonsterile work station in the system provides secondary control of equipment and a standard computer for intraoperative documentation and access to patient records. Integrated OR systems allow for advances in technology through software design that can be updated periodically.

OTHER WORKING AREAS

Surgical departments can vary widely in size, use of space, and types of work areas they contain. Regardless of the exact appropriation of space, every department strives to maintain the principles of asepsis—separating and confining contaminated areas to keep them apart from clean and sterile areas. The following are some examples of units within the surgical department.

Surgical Offices

A front office situated near the main entry doors serves as a central communication area for the department. General incoming calls may be received in and referred from this office or from a surgical switchboard area. Because of its location, the office also is a monitoring point for personnel entering the department. Other offices include those of the operating room supervisor, head nurse, anesthesia director, and other department heads.

Patient Holding Area

Hospitalized surgical patients are transported to the holding area before being taken into the operating room. Outpatients (i.e., those coming from outside the hospital) may be escorted to a changing area and then to the holding area. Patients

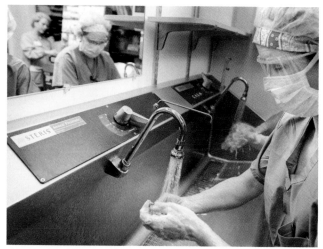

Figure 5-10 Scrub sink area. (© 2008 STERIS Corporation. All rights reserved.)

arrive via stretcher or wheelchair and await surgery. The holding area is a check-in point where the surgeon, anesthesiologist, and circulating nurse can confirm that all laboratory and preoperative documentation is in order, and the information on the preoperative checklist can be verified. If the surgery is an emergency procedure, the patient may be brought directly from the emergency department to the operating room suite without passing through the holding area.

Scrub Sink Areas

Scrub sinks are located outside the surgical suites so that personnel can proceed directly to surgery immediately after hand antisepsis (Figure 5-10). Some operating room designs include closed areas for the scrub sinks, and these are restricted (masks are required). Scrub sink areas contain antiseptic hand rub, masks, face shields, protective eyewear, brushes, and surgical soap. The area around the scrub sink is kept clean, and the floors are mopped frequently to prevent falls.

Substerile Room

The substerile room is directly adjacent to the operating room suite and is entered through a common door between the two rooms. This area may hold sterile supplies or a flash sterilizer. Some substerile areas are contiguous with other operating suites, which share access to the facilities and supplies. The area is restricted, requiring complete surgical attire, including a mask.

Sterile Instrument Room

Sterile wrapped supplies may be stored in designated restricted areas adjacent to the operating suites nearby. Specialty rooms, such as those used for orthopedics, genitourinary procedures, or cardiothoracic surgery, often have their own sterile supply rooms close by. Most hospitals now use a case cart system so that fewer instrument sets are stored in the operating room itself.

Equipment Storage Areas

Large equipment, such as the operating microscope, operating table attachments, and electrosurgical units, may be kept in special storerooms. Equipment must be arranged in a way that prevents damage during movement into and out of the room. Thousands of dollars of the operating room's yearly budget are spent on equipment repair as a result of careless handling. Many of these accidents occur when equipment is poorly stored in a space that is too small or in a manner that makes the equipment difficult to remove.

Utility Workroom and Decontamination Area

Soiled instruments and equipment are decontaminated and washed in a utility workroom or central processing area. Some operating rooms use a combination of systems, holding back certain specialty instruments for decontamination and sterilization in the utility workroom and sending the remainder to central processing. The workroom is located in an area convenient to the staff but well contained and away from all restricted areas to prevent cross-contamination of sterile and clean equipment and supplies.

When a **case cart system** is used, sterile supplies (e.g., wrapped instrument sets, single-use items, and drapes) are placed on a closed or open stainless steel cart by personnel in the central processing department. The case carts usually are prepared the night before and are sent to the operating room by the night shift personnel. As new cases are added to the schedule in the daytime, new case carts are assembled. After surgery, soiled instruments and equipment are carefully placed on a cart and returned to the utility workroom and/or the central processing decontamination area. The cart and instruments are decontaminated. The equipment then can be assembled in trays, wrapped, and resterilized.

Clean Processing Room

Any instruments that are not sent out of the department for decontamination and sterilization are brought to a clean processing room for assembly after decontamination. Items that are particularly delicate or that are used infrequently may be processed in this area. If an item must be reused in a later case and there is not enough time to send it to the central processing department, it may be cleaned and prepared for flash sterilization in the clean processing room.

Anesthesia Workroom

The anesthesia workroom contains clean respiratory equipment, anesthetic agents, and adjunctive drugs. Tubes, hoses, valves, and other equipment are stored in the workroom and organized neatly to avoid damage and to enable personnel to locate the items quickly in the event of an emergency. This semirestricted area also may have its own separate office.

Postanesthesia Care Unit

A patient emerging from anesthesia faces many physiological risks. These include airway obstruction, cardiac arrest, hemorrhage, neurological dysfunction, hypothermia, and pain.

Therefore patients are taken directly from surgery to the **postanesthesia care unit** (**PACU**). Critical care nurses in the PACU assist the patient in recovery from conscious sedation or general anesthesia. They assess, monitor, and document the patient's recovery from the time of arrival until the patient is discharged back to the hospital unit or home. (Chapter 12 presents a complete discussion of postanesthesia recovery.)

Surgery Waiting Area

The surgery waiting area for the patient's family and friends is located outside traffic areas leading into the operating room but near the department. This waiting area allows families to be close to the operating room in a relaxed environment.

HOSPITAL DEPARTMENTS AND FUNCTIONS

Team Approach to Patient Care

Perioperative staff members work in cooperation with many professionals and departments in the health facility. The operating room often seems to be an isolated environment, independent from other departments of the hospital. Physical barriers and procedures necessary to maintain strict asepsis seem to foster an atmosphere of isolation and independence. In fact, the operating room could not function without the collaborative efforts of departments outside the OR. The efforts of many departments and caring staff members contribute to a safe surgery and uneventful recovery. Perioperative staff members must communicate effectively with those outside the operating room and help facilitate a cohesive team approach. Knowledge about the roles of other departments and the activities they perform contributes to this team approach.

In many instances departments face multiple demands that may exceed their limits of available personnel and time. Patience, respect, and professionalism build good interdepartmental relationships and help reduce stress and improve patient care.

Departments in the health facility are distinguished by function (what they do) or by administration (the sector in which they are managed, such as nursing administrator, medical director, and so on). Every hospital has multiple departments and services. Box 5-1 lists the hospital departments found in most institutions.

Pathology

The pathology department receives all tissue samples and other specimens from surgery. A pathologist is a medical doctor who examines each specimen to determine the type of tissue, to identify disease within the tissue, and to create a permanent legal record. If the surgeon requires an immediate tissue evaluation, as in the case of a suspected malignancy, the pathologist is available to perform a frozen section analysis. The specimen is frozen with liquid nitrogen, and thin sections are removed for examination under the microscope. This examination immediately produces the information needed to determine the need for additional radical surgery. When a surgeon is excising a known malignancy, the pathologist also

Box 5-1

Hospital Departments

Patient Medical Services
- Diagnostic services
  Radiology
  Clinical laboratory/pathology
  Other diagnostic services (e.g., computed tomography, magnetic resonance imaging)
- Patient care units
  Cardiovascular
  Labor and delivery
  Medical/surgical
  Neonatal
  Neurological
  Orthopedic
  Pediatric
  Trauma
  Psychiatric
  Renal dialysis
- Intensive and critical care units (ICUs)
  Cardiac telemetry
  Cardiac (CICU)
  Medical (MICU)
  Neonatal (NICU)
  Neurological
  Operating room
  Postanesthesia care (PACU)
  Trauma (TICU)
  Pediatric (PICU)
- Anesthesia and pain management
- Blood bank
- Outpatient or ambulatory surgery
- Emergency department (ED or ER)
- Rehabilitation
- Physical therapy
- Outpatient medical clinics
- Nuclear medicine
- Food and nutrition services
  Dietitian
  Outpatient nutrition services

Psychosocial and Outreach Services
- Patient education
- Community health services

- Home health services
- Hospice
- Adult day care services
- Hospital chaplaincy
- Occupational therapy

Employee and Administrative Services
- Human resources
- Employee education
- Employee health services and insurance
- Accounting
- Patient accounts
- Reimbursement
- Managed care
- Auditor
- Payroll

Environmental Services
- Infection control
- Maintenance
- Bioengineering (clinical engineering)
- Housekeeping

Materials Management
- Central supply
- Distribution

Communications
- Switchboard
- Paging system
- Telecommunications
- Mobile radio communications
- Electronic communications

Safety
- Risk management
- Security

Records and Clerical Services
- Medical records
- Admissions

examines excised tissue to check tumor margins and ensure that all of the malignancy has been removed.

Nuclear Medicine and Interventional Radiology

Nuclear medicine involves the use of radioactive materials or radiopharmaceuticals to diagnose and treat disease. These special procedures are performed in a designated nuclear medicine department, which has the technical capability to perform a variety of different procedures following the strict regulations needed to ensure patient and staff safety.

Interventional radiology uses radiographic, magnetic resonance imaging (MRI), computed tomography (CT), ultra-sound, and other imaging techniques to guide instruments into vessels and organs. Surgical technologists may be required to assist in interventional radiology because sterile technique is required. Examples of interventional radiology procedures are angiography, angioplasty, and insertion of a gastrostomy tube, needle biopsy, and stereotactic procedures. (Chapter 20 presents a complete description of nuclear and interventional radiology.)

Infection Control

Infection control personnel are specialists in the prevention and control of nosocomial (hospital acquired) infections. The health care environment is a potential source for the spread of many types of infection. Whenever people are in physical proximity, especially people who are already ill or are debilitated by surgery, nutritional problems, stress, or trauma, the potential for infection is high. The infection control department develops policy based on the standards and recommendations of The Joint Commission, the Centers for Disease Control and Prevention (CDC), the Association for Professionals in Infection Control and Epidemiology (APIC), the Occupational Safety and Health Administration (**OSHA**), and the National Institute for Occupational Safety and Health (NIOSH).

The objectives of infection control are to reduce the incidence of nosocomial infections and prevent the transmission of infectious disease in hospitals. Policies affect nearly every department of the hospital. Important goals in infection control include educating staff members and patients, tracking policy compliance, and investigating the sources of infection. Infection control professionals also must keep current with the information in their field as new disease strains and types appear in the population.

Biomedical Engineering

Biomedical technologists (usually called biological engineers) are required to maintain the safety and operating condition of many of the hospital's medical devices, including those used in surgery. The complexity of sophisticated devices requires technologists who are specially trained in biomedical engineering. The biomedical engineering department may be located within the operating room or in a separate department. Technologists may be called to the operating room in the event of equipment failure during surgery. All biomedical devices must be routinely serviced by the department to ensure patient safety.

Materials Management

The Materials Management department of a health facility is the purchasing and logistics center for goods and supplies needed for the delivery of healthcare. It is also responsible for ordering new supplies, and for implementing tracking systems to maintain the supply chain.

Central Supply

Disposable items, linens, and equipment are distributed to hospital departments by the central supply department. Items usually are tracked by computer, and distribution is carefully managed to control hospital costs. In some hospitals this department may be responsible for receiving soiled equipment used in surgery. Wrapping and sterilization then are performed in separate areas of the department. Items may be purchased from this department or from a separate purchasing department.

Pharmacy

The pharmacy distributes medications to patient care units in the hospital. Medications and anesthetic agents used in the operating room are received from the pharmacy, either by regular delivery or by special requisition. Controlled substances are kept in locked storage on all units. Anesthetic agents usually are stored in the anesthesia department or pharmacy located in the surgical department.

Laboratory

Diagnostic tests are performed in the hospital laboratory, where clinical laboratory personnel examine and analyze body fluids, tissues, and cells. Laboratory personnel perform chemical, biological, hematological, immunological, microscopic, and bacteriological tests. They also type and cross-match blood specimens for the blood bank. The data and results obtained in the laboratory are returned to the physician to aid evaluation and treatment of the patient.

Blood Bank

The blood bank provides blood products for transfusion in the surgical, postanesthesia care, and medical units of the hospital. Because of the stringent protocols regulating blood product transfusion, strict methods are followed for handling, storage, transport, and identification of these products. The technologist may interact with blood bank personnel and should be familiar with the institution's policy regarding ordering and receiving blood products. Under most circumstances, blood may be transfused only after two licensed personnel together have verified all patient and blood identification information.

Risk Management Department

Because of the many environmental risks and the possibility for errors and omissions by personnel, surveillance is required to track the number and exact nature of adverse events in a given time period. The cause of each event is studied, and policies are enacted to prevent future incidents of the same type. For example, if the incidence of chemical burns among staff members were increasing, the risk management team would investigate the circumstances, time of day, personnel involved (e.g., housekeeping, nursing), and other important aspects to identify the cause. The team then would develop a plan to reduce the number of incidents. The team might change existing policy regulating the use of chemicals or give personnel intensive training. After the plan is implemented, an evaluation is performed to determine whether the measures taken actually did reduce the number of chemical burns. Incident reports (see Chapter 4) are very important to **risk management** because they contain the information needed to analyze incidents and develop a plan of intervention.

Switchboard/Paging Systems

The switchboard is the central communication point for the hospital. Calls are received from both inside and outside the hospital. Because of the volume of calls coming into and going out of the switchboard, every department posts a directory of numbers near central telephones so that calls can be made directly, without going through the switchboard.

Paging systems usually are set up by individuals. Hospital personnel can be reached through a private paging service or the hospital's own paging service. In a hospital paging system, the caller simply dials the desired party's number, followed by a specific in-hospital number. Before beginning surgery, the surgeon often leaves his or her pager in a convenient location in the surgical suite. When a call comes in, the circulator returns the call and either puts the caller on the room's speaker system or passes the caller's message to the surgeon.

Medical Records

The medical records department is responsible for receiving, maintaining, and transferring all patient records. Because patient records are considered legal documents, strict protocols determine when signatures are required, who may make entries, what must be included, and where the patient's documents are stored.

Maintenance

The maintenance department is responsible for environmental systems in the hospital. These systems include the hospital's power source (regular and emergency), ventilation, in-line gases, suction, electricity, water, light, heat, cooling, and humidity control. Standards for environmental control and safety are established by The Joint Commission and government agencies. The surgical technologist should never ignore or try to repair a system that malfunctions. Maintenance personnel are available at all times to respond to environmental emergencies.

Environmental Services

Environmental services personnel perform essential cleaning and decontamination services for all departments of the hospital. In the operating room, they maintain a clean environment and decontaminate the floors, furniture, and other surfaces between cases. They work with other team members to ensure rapid turnover from one case to the next.

PERSONNEL IN THE HEALTH CARE ENVIRONMENT

ADMINISTRATION AND POLICY

Most large health care organizations provide primary health care, inpatient and outpatient services, diagnosis, and outpatient rehabilitation services. Primary or secondary (preventive) medical care is provided in a fixed location, such as the community hospital. The community hospital, whether privately or publicly owned, brings together people with different professional skills to provide coordinated services. Larger hospitals or medical centers also operate **satellite facilities** in rural or urban areas away from the central facility. Satellite facilities deliver various types of care or treatments to patients. Services may include but are not limited to ambulatory surgery centers, clinics, urgent care centers, laboratory and radiology centers, physicians' offices, extended care centers, and rehabilitation facilities.

Surgery is performed in many different settings, including hospitals, community health centers, and freestanding clinics that may be privately owned or operated by nonprofit organization.

Ambulatory surgical centers perform minor surgery that does not require postoperative hospital recovery. Ambulatory surgery and outpatient surgery departments in hospitals also are becoming increasingly popular. In addition, some types of surgery are being performed in surgeons' offices.

Surgery that requires general anesthesia, conscious sedation, or complex local anesthesia is performed in a hospital facility, where perioperative services are coordinated with the services of other departments and the patient recovers in the hospital. This setting provides continuity of care and ensures that emergency services are immediately available. This chapter focuses on the hospital-based surgical department. However, the principles of administration, organization, and physical layout are similar for all settings.

ACCREDITATION

Accreditation, as it pertains to health care facilities, is the process by which a team of professionals evaluates a health care institution's practices and policies and the outcomes of patient care. The institution is awarded accreditation when these standards are met. Accreditation is a voluntary process, but government agencies and insurers use accreditation to determine whether an institution qualifies for patient care reimbursement. Accreditation implies a high standard of care and a commitment to public safety and welfare.

Health care facilities and institutions in the United States are accredited by The Joint Commission. To earn this accreditation, the institution must meet or exceed the high standards set by the commission. The Joint Commission bases its own standards on those of professional and governmental agencies. The Joint Commission is governed by a board of commissioners, which is made up of members of the American College of Physicians, the American Society of Internal Medicine, the American College of Surgeons, the American Dental Association, the American Hospital Association, and the American Medical Association, as well as nurses, ethicists, and other professionals. The Joint Commission standards apply to every area of the health care facility and focus on patient safety, protection, and quality care.

HEALTH CARE POLICY

The purpose of any policy is to create a standard that protects the patient, hospital personnel, and public from harm. Health care policies are formed with this goal in mind. Some are mandated by law, others by practice evaluation and outcome.

The Joint Commission requires that all hospital policies be available to staff members in written form. A health care facility may have many different policy manuals, each pertinent to a specific aspect of operations, activities, the hospital environment, or administrative issues.

All new employees are required to read and follow the policies applicable to their job descriptions and duties. Failure to comply with hospital policy may result in disciplinary action or termination of employment. Organizations that contribute to the knowledge and research used to create hospital policy are listed in Box 5-2.

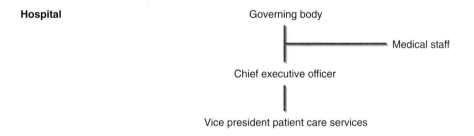

Box 5-2

Agencies and Organizations that Provide Research and Data Used to Develop Hospital Policy

Association for the Advancement of Medical Instrumentation (AAMI)
Association of periOperative Registered Nurses (AORN)
Association for Professionals in Infection Control and Epidemiology (APIC)
Centers for Disease Control and Prevention (CDC)*
Environmental Protection Agency (EPA)*
Food and Drug Administration (FDA)*
Joint Commission on Accreditation of Healthcare Organizations (The Joint Commission)
National Institute for Occupational Safety and Health (NIOSH)*
Occupational Safety and Health Administration (OSHA)*

*Government agency.

MANAGEMENT STRUCTURE

Hospital management and operational staff members usually are organized into separate bodies or groups of people whose joint functions and roles enable patient and community services. The board of directors or trustees usually is responsible for hiring the chief executive officer. It determines the hospital's administrative and development policies and mission and reviews the delivery of safe and ethical patient care.

The administrative sector designs and implements personnel procedures and policies and financial systems. The administration also communicates with the public and handles overall institutional issues, such as public relations and quality assurance.

The medical and other licensed professional staff deliver services according to the privileges granted them by license and state codes. Management within these sectors usually is organized by departments and profession. Medical staff members usually are managed by the chief or head physician of the department. Professional nurses are managed by the nursing department. Allied health staff members are managed by their own department heads, or they may be administered by the nursing department. The management structure can be horizontal (many people sharing the same level of management) or vertical (fewer people at the management level).

ORGANIZATIONAL CHART (ORGANIGRAM)

An **organizational chart (organigram)** is a graphic representation of the management chain of command (Figure 5-11).

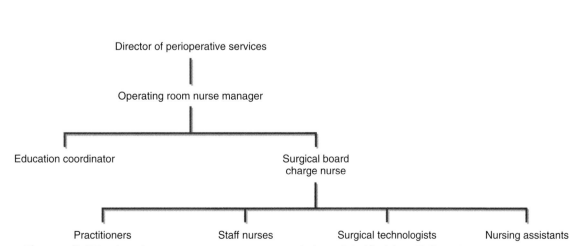

Figure 5-11 Sample operating room organizational chart. *(Modified from Phillips N: Berry and Kohn's operating room technique, ed 10, St Louis, 2004, Mosby.)*

The significance of the organizational chart is that it depicts each manager's areas of responsibility and accountability. It eliminates ambiguity about who is in charge of what and the level of responsibility.

It is important to note that there is no standard organizational system, and different hospitals use various titles for their administrative and management staff. The terms *supervisor, manager,* and *director* are interchangeable in the general sense. All staff members have a responsibility to understand the management structure of the institution and in particular their department (Figure 5-11).

CHAIN OF COMMAND

The **chain of command** defines the relationship between management and staff members. An employee reports (is responsible to) the person directly *upward* on the organizational chart. As stated previously, vertical alignment of positions indicates the authority that one position has over another. Horizontal alignment indicates equal authority. The fact that some positions are lower vertically than other positions does not necessarily mean that all the lower positions are under the authority of a given higher level person. For example, the chief medical engineer does not have administrative authority over the surgical technologist, even though that vertical position is higher.

Chain of command is important for several reasons. Management systems rely on the flow of information *from* specific people in particular positions *to* other specific positions. Certain information is critical to the outcome of work. For example, a safety warning about equipment is directed to all staff members who use that equipment. The direct link between the staff members and their immediate manager may be the most important source of that information. In another example, an incident in surgery must be reported to the individual positioned to act on the consequences of that incident. This includes not only immediate action on health and safety, but also the process of analysis and risk management. Certain people in the chain of command are responsible for these tasks. Following the chain of command puts the person (or position) previously designated as the most appropriate in charge of the response.

The types and volume of responsibility required of managers in today's hospitals are much greater than ever before. Chain of command defines the domains and specific areas of focus for each manager. It allows managers to focus their attention where it is intended. This creates a smoother running department and better patient outcomes.

Chain of command is important for resolution of policy and protocol questions. Each staff member has a line manager whose tasks include resolving issues or directing them to another appropriate source. For example, if a staff member experiences abusive treatment in the operating room, that staff member must present the situation to his or her line manager. The line manager must be made aware of staff relations in the department and is best placed to counsel the individual and refer the situation to other authority if necessary.

STAFF ROLES AND JOB DESCRIPTIONS

Personnel Policy

The responsibilities and functions of all employees in the surgical department are clearly defined in writing in the hospital manual covering its **personnel policy.** These policies are written to clarify job descriptions and to establish the accountability of each employee. They include topics such as employee safety, how to respond in emergency situations, insurance issues, and ethical conduct. These policies comply with state and federal laws and ensure that the hospital meets the minimum standards set by The Joint Commission. Policies must be strictly followed, because they define the scope of practice necessary for the safe and efficient operation of the department. Employees are required to read these policies and often must sign a form stating that they understand the policies in order for the hospital to enforce compliance.

Each member of the hospital staff has defined duties and responsibilities. These are often referred to as a job description. A job description for each position is necessary to ensure that every person knows what is expected of him or her. The job description is a management tool to ensure that all tasks have been assigned appropriately. It is equally important for the individual to know exactly what his or her role is. **Role confusion** is a common cause of conflict in the workplace. This occurs when delegation or assignments are not clear or when an employee is not sure who is responsible for what. Assumptions that *someone else* is responsible for completion of a task can lead to *no one* doing it. This presents risks for patient safety, because most tasks have *shared* responsibility. Staff members are required to read their job description at the time of hiring to prevent confusion and conflict later on. The job description includes a job title, which identifies the position by name. This is another method of clarifying roles and responsibilities.

Many different professional, allied health, and assistive personnel make up the modern perioperative team. Some roles overlap, whereas others are specific to a particular job according to professional standards, policy, training, and individual capability.

Licensed Professional Staff

Surgeon

The surgeon is the patient's primary physician in the operating room and is responsible for guiding the surgical team during the procedure. The surgeon operates under the prescribed policies of the hospital in which he or she works and is licensed under the medical practice acts in his or her state. The surgeon may be qualified as a medical doctor (MD), doctor of dental surgery (DDS), doctor of osteopathic medicine (DO), or doctor of podiatry (DPM).

Assistant Surgeon

The assistant surgeon, also called the *surgeon's assistant,* is a medical doctor licensed to perform and assist in surgery. The assistant provides direct care to the patient according to the delegation of the surgeon and the needs of the patient.

The assistant surgeon is qualified to deliver emergency care during a procedure, including assistance in the event of unexpected hemorrhage or patient injury. The assistant surgeon may also take charge of the surgical case in an emergency.

Anesthesia Care Provider

The anesthesiologist is either an MD or a DO and is a specialist in anesthesia and pain management. The anesthesiologist is responsible for the meticulous assessment, monitoring, and adjustment of the patient's physiological status during surgery.

The certified registered nurse anesthetist (CRNA) is a highly trained registered nurse who renders the same care as the anesthesiologist and may work under the supervision of an anesthesiologist in the operating room.

Perioperative Registered Nurse

The perioperative registered nurse holds a current license in nursing (RN) and also may have advanced certification in perioperative nursing (certified nurse–operating room [CNOR]). The perioperative nurse functions as a circulating nurse (circulator) or as a scrub. Additional training permits a registered nurse to become a registered nurse–first assistant (RNFA). The staff nurse performs his or her duties in accordance with laws regulating the practice of licensed personnel for the state in which the nurse is employed. The RN delegates tasks to allied health personnel in the perioperative environment.

Physician Assistant

A physician assistant (PA) is a medical professional who practices medicine under the supervision of a physician. A PA is required to pass a national certification examination and earn the title of a physician assistant–certified (PA-C). A PA in the operating room has received additional training in surgery. The PA may perform first-assistant tasks under the direct supervision of the surgeon and according to hospital policy.

Licensed Practical Nurse

The licensed practical nurse (LPN) (or licensed vocational nurse [LVN] in some states) has completed a 1- to 2-year program in a vocational or technical school. After completing a state-approved practical nursing program, an LPN or LVN becomes licensed after passing the National Council Licensure Examination for Licensed Practical Nurses (NCLEX-LPN), which is the national qualifying examination for LPNs. In the operating room, the LPN or LVN usually functions in the role of scrub.

Allied Health Personnel

Certified Surgical Technologist

Surgical technologists have a wide variety of roles within perioperative practice. Primarily they assist in surgical procedures under the supervision of the surgeons, anesthesiologists, and perioperative nurses. The certified surgical technologist (CST) prepares equipment and instruments before surgery, ensuring that all devices are safe and operative. Surgical technologists also assist in preparation of the patient immediately before surgery. They help position the patient for surgery, perform the antiseptic skin prep, and apply sterile drapes to protect the surgical site from contamination. They arrange the equipment and maintain it during surgery and hand instruments to the surgeons. They also are responsible for setting up and maintaining instruments during the procedure and for safely handling and transporting soiled instruments for reprocessing. The surgical technologist has expanded tasks according to the individual's education and experience. Career choices available to the certified surgical technologist were detailed in Chapter 1.

Certified Surgical Technologist–Certified First Assistant

The certified surgical technologist-certified first assistant (CST-CFA) is a certified surgical technologist who has completed an educational program for assisting the surgeon during a procedure. Certification requirements are established by National Board of Surgical Technology and Surgical Assisting (NBSTSA). The CST-CFA assists the surgeon with selected procedures by providing aid in exposure, hemostasis, and other technical functions. This assists the surgeon to carry out a safe procedure and provide the best results for the patient. The CST-CFA usually is hired by a specialist surgeon or health care facility to perform in a role specific to that specialty, such as ophthalmic surgery, ear, nose, and throat (ENT) surgery, or orthopedic surgery.

Certified Surgical Assistant or Nonphysician Surgical Assistant

The certified surgical assistant (CSA) or nonphysician surgical assistant is an allied health qualification achieved by certification through the National Surgical Assistant Association. Qualifications for certification include graduation from an accredited surgical assistance school, military training, or a foreign medical degree. Physician assistants and registered nurses may also apply for qualification, which is recognized by the Accreditation Review Council on Education in Surgical Technology and Surgical Assisting (ARC/STSA) and approved by the Commission on Accreditation of Allied Health Education Programs (CAAHEP). There are also other credentialed surgical assistants (i.e., SA-C).

Certified Anesthesia Technologist

The certified anesthesia technologist is a member of the anesthesia patient care team and department. Anesthesia technicians directly assist the anesthesiologist, residents, and nurse anesthetist. They prepare and maintain equipment and supplies needed for administration of anesthetics and calibrate monitoring devices used during surgery. They assist with laboratory tests and obtain blood products and pharmaceuticals. Depending on their expertise, they may also perform technical and support roles in procedures involving anesthesia.

Administrative and Educational Personnel

Health care managers or executives are needed to provide oversight and development of the facility's goals and operations.

Health Care Facility Management

The chief executive officer (CEO) of the health care facility is responsible for the overall operational planning and implementation of the facility's strategic plan. This role may be shared with the chief operations officer, who is expected to assume the role of CEO in that individual's absence. Additional roles of the CEO are ensuring that the facility complies with regulatory requirements and developing good communication among departments within the facility. The executive officer provides leadership within the facility and in the community.

Chief Operational Officer

The chief operational officer (COO) is responsible for oversight of the health facility with a particular focus on the functioning of the medical services, personnel, and fiscal areas. This individual works with all levels of operations, developing strategic plans for operation and implementing them. Operations covers a broad range of areas, including workforce recruitment and safety, information technology, communications, liaison with educational institutions, and research. The COO is a manger who troubleshoots problems in the actual day-to-day operations from a global perspective. The COO then coordinates with midlevel managers to develop solutions.

Director of Surgical Services/Operating Room Supervisor

The director of surgical services (also known in some areas as the operating room supervisor) is responsible for overseeing all clinical and professional activities in the department. He or she creates and implements policies about clinical and professional practices in the operating room using evidenced-based standards. The operating room supervisor may represent the department at supervisory meetings, where he or she helps coordinate activities in other departments with those of the operating room.

Perioperative Nurse Manager

A perioperative nurse manager may assist the operating room director with his or her duties or may have separate responsibilities. If the director is absent from the department, the nurse manager may assume the role of supervisor if necessary. The nurse manager is responsible for the day-to-day activities of the operating room, although the individual may or may not participate in surgical procedures. The nurse manager usually is an RN with a baccalaureate degree in science (BSN). Responsibilities may include ordering and management of devices and materials, environmental safety, education, infection control, staff scheduling, and resolving staffing problems. The nurse manager often is responsible for organizing triage and emergency responses in the OR.

Operating Room Educator

The operating room nurse educator usually is an RN with extensive operating room experience. This individual develops and implements educational programs, seminars, and in-services (informational training on new products or techniques) within the department. Not all surgical departments have a designated educator; some provide training on a more informal basis. The surgical technologist instructor is designated by the health facility to orient and teach newly recruited surgical technologists or those in a specialty.

Independent surgical technology instructors are affiliated with their educational institution, not with the health care institution in which students have internships. The instructor upholds the policies of the health care institution and supervises them in compliance with these standards. The students also interact with staff members who may delegate individual tasks in accordance with the goals and objectives of the educational program. Cooperation and good communication between the surgical technology instructor and operating room staff ensure that students complete their educational requirements while following the policies of the health care institution in which they are learning.

Ancillary Staff

Unit Secretary

The surgical unit secretary receives scheduling requests from the surgeons or their representatives. The secretary also must answer the telephone and relay messages within and out of the surgical department. In the event of emergency, the secretary must assist the manager in rescheduling any cases that have been canceled and notify all personnel involved in these cases. The unit secretary is under considerable strain to maintain an orderly schedule and satisfy the scheduling needs of many different surgeons. Consequently, the job requires a composed and efficient personality. The individual must be knowledgeable about medical and surgical terminology, have excellent communication skills, and be able to cheerfully but firmly cope with the many demands made during the workday.

Surgical Orderly or Aide

The surgical orderly participates in many types of patient care services, including transportation of the patient to and from the surgical department. The orderly also may participate in the safe clean-up of the surgical suite after procedures and the restocking of supplies. Orderlies often assist in the preparation of supplies and instruments for decontamination and sterilization. The work is demanding, because many members of the surgery department make many requests for their attention.

Central Sterile Processing Technician

The central processing or sterile processing technician is responsible for the safe management of equipment in preparation for and after its use in surgery and other care units. Technicians are knowledgeable about the process of sterilization and decontamination, asepsis, and standard precautions. They assemble instruments and safely process them according to hospital standards. They also keep hospital and operating room inventories of instruments and equipment and may be responsible for ordering supplies.

CHAPTER SUMMARY

- The operating room is designed and engineered to provide infection control; environmental safety; and efficient use of personnel, time, space, and resources.
- The layout of the surgical department is based primarily on the principles of infection control – confining and containing areas and sources of contamination.
- Traffic patterns in the surgical department contribute to infection control and are strictly enforced.
- Operating room equipment and furniture is managed in a way that promotes safety and efficiency.
- The physical environment of the OR such as lighting, air exchange, temperature, and humidity is strictly controlled. Standards for these elements are enforced by accreditation and safety organizations.
- Basic equipment and furniture needed for surgery are kept in each surgical suite. Special procedure rooms include supplies and equipment for surgical specialties such as genitourinary surgery, orthopedics, and plastic surgery.
- Designated areas of the surgical department include the surgical suites, sub sterile rooms, instrument storage areas, anesthesia workroom, and scrub sink areas. These are restricted areas.

- The health care facility has many different departments that interact with each other to provide patient care. Coordination among departments is essential for smooth teamwork.
- Perioperative personnel rely on departments such as interventional radiology, materials management, pharmacy, and the blood bank for the day-to-day activities in surgery.
- All health care facilities have a mission statement and community goals on which they base their policies, procedures, and activities.
- Hospital policies are established in consultation with accreditation and safety organizations. Every employee must be familiar with personnel, health, and safety policies. They are also required to understand the policies of the department they work in.
- An organizational chart establishes the relationships between management and staff. These are ranked by chain of command.
- All personnel are required to have a job description so that they know what is expected of them.
- The surgical department utilizes many different types of professional and nonprofessional staff. Everyone has a responsibility to coordinate their work with others and to become familiar with each other's roles in the work place.

REVIEW QUESTIONS

1. How is the floor plan of the operating room related to patient safety?
2. What is a restricted area in the operating room?
3. How does the environmental air pressure in the operating room relate to the spread of infection?
4. Why is the operating room maintained at 50% to 55% humidity?
5. What is an integrated operating room?
6. What is the purpose of hospital accreditation?
7. What types of problems might employees experience if they are not familiar with the policies of their employer?
8. An organizational chart outlines, in graphic form, the levels of responsibility within an organization. Why do you think it is important to delineate management responsibilities?
9. What is the purpose of a chain of command?
10. A job description should describe exactly what the employee's responsibilities and duties are. What might be the consequences of a vague or unclear job description?

BIBLIOGRAPHY

Association of periOperating Room Nurses (AORN): Position statement on allied health care providers and support personnel in the perioperative practice setting. In *Standards, recommended practices and guidelines, 2007 edition,* Denver, 2007, AORN.

Association of periOperating Room Nurses (AORN): Position statement on workplace safety. In *Standards, recommended practices and guidelines, 2007 edition,* Denver, 2007, AORN.

Association of periOperating Room Nurses (AORN): Recommended practices for traffic patterns in the perioperative practice setting. In *Standards, recommended practices and guidelines, 2007 edition,* Denver, 2007, AORN.

US Department of Labor, Occupational Safety and Health Administration: Surgical suite module. Accessed November 10, 2007, at http://www.osha.gov/SLTCetools/hospital/surgical/surgical.html.

Communication and Teamwork

CHAPTER OUTLINE

LEARNING OBJECTIVES

After studying this chapter the reader will be able to:

- Describe the meaning of content and tone in communication
- Demonstrate body language and describe its meaning
- Discuss the significance of touch in communication
- Role-play situations to demonstrate assertive behavior
- Describe the dimensions of assertive behavior
- Use active listening skills

- Discuss types of problem behavior and how to cope with them
- Define sexual harassment and discuss how to confront it
- Describe the qualities of good teamwork
- Describe how poor teamwork results in poor patient care
- Discuss how to approach problem behavior in the workplace
- Describe three approaches to solving conflicts and give examples

TERMINOLOGY

Aggression: The exertion of power over others through intimidation, loudness, sarcasm, or bullying.

Assertiveness: A quality in people with self-esteem; assertive behavior seeks to protect one's own rights while respecting those of others.

Body language: Communication through facial expressions, posture, and gestures.

Brainstorming: A method of contributing to group discussion in which people informally state their ideas as they occur.

Consensus: Agreement among members of a group.

Content: The substance or actual information contained in a message.

Delivery: The way in which a message is conveyed.

Facilitator: A group leader that coordinates the direction and flow of a group meeting without influencing the content of people's contributions. Similar to an **enabling** position in which people are encouraged to express ideas without fear of judgement.

Feedback: The response to a message; a component of effective communication.

Gossip: The telling and retelling of events of another's personal life, professional life, or physical condition.

Groupthink: In sociology and group behavior theory, the conformity of a group to one way of thinking and behaving. Groupthink creates two factions, those who agree (in-group) and those who disagree (out-group). This generates resentment and conflict in the workplace.

Horizontal abuse: Verbal abuse or sabotage among people of equal job or professional ranking.

Message: The idea, concept, thought, or feeling expressed during communication.

Norms: Behaviors that are accepted as part of the environment and culture of a group. Norms usually are established by custom and popular acceptance rather than by law, although the two may not be mutually exclusive.

Receiver: The person to whom a message is communicated by a sender.

Sender: The person who communicates a message to another.

Sexual harassment: An extreme abuse of power in which an individual uses sexualized language, gestures, or unwanted touch to coerce or intimate another person.

Therapeutic touch: The purposeful touching of another person to convey empathy, care, and tenderness.

Tone: The expression of emotion or opinion contained in the delivery of a message. It is not explicit but is implied by intonation, emphasis on certain words, or measured delivery of words. Tone also is established by nonverbal communication.

Values: Beliefs, customs, behaviors, and norms that a person defends and upholds.

Verbal abuse: Deliberate attempts to devalue, intimidate, bully, or embarrass another person using loud, vulgar, sexualized, or intimidating language.

Win-lose solution: In conflict resolution, a solution that leaves one party satisfied but the other party dissatisfied.

Win-win solution: In conflict resolution, a solution that allows both parties in a conflict to gain.

INTRODUCTION

Communication and teamwork are two of the most important components of patient care. Information must be passed accurately, and often very precisely, in the health care setting. The ability to communicate well is highly valued in professional settings. For some it is easy, whereas others require study and self-reflection to increase their communication skills.

Surgery is performed by *teams* of health professionals. Within the team, each person knows his or her tasks and roles and is guided by knowledge and experience. The surgical team may be composed of people who have worked together before, or new members may have been added. The ability to form a cohesive group quickly and efficiently is one of the challenges of surgery. Other teams in the perioperative setting are more permanent. Department committees, policy groups, and surgical specialty teams meet regularly to communicate policy, scheduling, and educational needs or for social functions. In all these situations, common objectives obtain. Hundreds of models are available to help people form teams, get along, be productive, and enjoy the process. No matter what model (if any) is used, the process requires active participation and willingness to work with others for the common goal.

COMMUNICATION

WHY STUDY COMMUNICATION?

Communication is a two-way process whereby one person (the **sender**) expresses ideas and feelings, and another person (the **receiver**) receives them, processes them, and gives feedback. In patient care, effective communication is important in understanding the patient's needs, feelings, and experiences. Clear communication among coworkers is equally important, because it produces cohesion and efficiency in the workplace. It gives personnel the information needed to establish priorities and act on them. It also helps solidify roles so that all individuals know what is expected of them. Clear communication clarifies relationships and helps establish professional and social boundaries. It increases teamwork and reinforces team goals. Good communication greatly increases the safety of the environment for the patient. Poor communication results in poor patient care, errors, conflict, and stress.

In the health care setting, the exchange of information is a primary responsibility of every staff member. We communicate information about patients to others involved in their care, and this triggers specific actions. Information about

equipment and safety is transmitted throughout the workday. Many messages need an immediate and specific response. In these and many other situations, effective communication can be critical in preventing accidents and injury.

Good communication is not accidental. It requires skill and practice. Everyone wants to be understood and to have his or her ideas and feelings respected. Even under the best of circumstances, however, communication can be difficult. Many health care workers are surprised to find that the greatest challenge in their work is not the work itself but the interactions and social climate of the workplace. This chapter is intended to increase the reader's understanding of communication skills and the way communication affects interpersonal relationships and team building.

Among the most important reasons to improve communication skills is maintaining respect, trust, and empathy among coworkers and management. The operating room environment often is rushed, tense, and even brusque. In this atmosphere, people sometimes feel a loss of control over their work. Long hours, insufficient breaks, low pay, and verbal abuse result in a loss of morale and may lead to burnout. This downward spiral can be avoided. When individuals are allowed to express their needs in the workplace and others are willing to listen and respond, conflicts and destabilizing events can be addressed or prevented.

ELEMENTS OF COMMUNICATION

In this chapter we discuss the five components of communication:

- The sender
- The receiver
- The message
- Feedback
- Methods of communication

Communication requires both a sender and a receiver. No communication takes place without both. The message is the concept, thought, idea, or feeling that is being expressed. It is the actual information conveyed in a communication. For example, "Please keep the doors closed." This **content** is simple information. Information can be perceived as negative ("You must work the next two weekends"), positive ("Everyone is getting raises next month"), or neutral ("Shut the door"). The message has an effect based on the content itself.

For communication to be considered effective, one additional item is required. This is known as feedback. **Feedback** is a response by the receiver that acknowledges the message that was sent. An example of this is a commercial on television. A company wants to sell a product or service. The company is the sender. The company creates a visual and audio display that appears during the intermission of your favorite television program. This is called the *message.* You, sitting in the comfort of your living room, are the receiver. The sender obtains feedback when you go out and inquire about the product or service. Feedback tells the company whether its advertisement (the message) was effective. Feedback in the health care setting is critical to patient safety. Feedback ensures that the message was conveyed and that the receiver understood the message.

The method used to communicate is almost as important as the content of the message. The **delivery** is the way the message is expressed; it includes verbal and nonverbal communication. We use deliberate methods to communicate, such as speaking and writing. We also communicate through facial expression, body movement, and tone of voice. Some of these actions are deliberate, and others are inadvertent, a result of our feelings and attitudes.

VERBAL COMMUNICATION

Verbal communication is communication that is spoken or written. Examples of spoken communication include telephone calls and face-to-face discussions. Written communication includes electronically transmitted messages and those written by hand. They can take the form of a policy or a document in the patient's chart.

In health care, the ability to convey information is critical to patient care, group morale, and team cohesion. The words that we select in day-to-day communication can have a powerful effect on the listener's reaction. When we speak thoughtlessly, without considering how the message is interpreted, we can cause conflict and harm. When we speak as we would like to be spoken to, we are more likely to produce an environment conducive to problem solving and collaboration.

Some situations in the operating room require communication of brief, accurate information with little or no dialogue. Even in these cases, it is important to use language and a tone that are respectful and polite. Box 6-1 lists important considerations for communicating verbally.

Tone is the environment of the message. It reflects the sender's emotions, such as respect for the receiver, or the sender's opinion about the message or attitude toward the receiver. Most people are familiar with the effect that tone has on the message. For example:

"Please! Keep—the—doors—closed!"
"Would you mind keeping those doors closed?!"
"Please keep the doors closed—thanks!"

In the first example, the sender emphasizes words by volume and by measured delivery. This conveys impatience and frustration. In the second example, the sender uses a bit of sarcasm to emphasize annoyance. In the third example, the sender simply expresses a need to keep the doors closed and shows appreciation for compliance.

The following sentence can be stated in many different ways to convey additional information about the message:

Box 6-1
Guidelines for Verbal Communication

1. Focus on the receiver.
2. Use concrete words. Avoid descriptions that are vague and require the listener to "fill in the blanks" or guess your meaning.
3. Do not assume how the receiver will respond. Allow the person the freedom to express personal views and opinions.
4. Do not judge the receiver or others in your dialogue; this engenders mistrust.
5. Avoid using strong emotional words; these trigger emotional reactions in others.
6. When speaking with someone, make eye contact with the person and be alert to cues that the individual is not listening or wants to terminate the conversation. Such cues include looking away or from side to side, fidgeting, and backing up.
7. On the telephone, do not carry on a background conversation while speaking to the person on the phone. It disrupts the phone conversation and prolongs it unnecessarily. If someone interrupts you while you are on the phone, ask that person to wait until you are finished.

"I'm scrubbing with you again today, Dr. X . . ." (neutral information)

The sender's tone might convey any of the following additional meanings:

". . . and I'd rather have a root canal done." (dread)
". . . and I'm really glad, because things go so smoothly in your rooms." (relief)
". . . and if you start yelling today, I'm going to report it." (hostility)

NONVERBAL COMMUNICATION

Body Language

The way we use posture, gestures, and expressions to convey ideas and messages is called body language. These cues can emphasize the message or convey a meaning that differs significantly from what was originally intended.

❖ *Even if a person does not want to express his or her true feelings about the message, those feelings probably will be conveyed by the individual's body language.*

One of the qualities of good communication is genuineness. Watch your own body language. Does it express what you feel? How do you think others read your body language? For example, you can request assistance from a colleague in many ways. Your words may sound polite, but your body language may convey impatience.

Another example is the manner in which we receive job assignments for the day. Not everyone can be assigned the cases he or she wants. When assignments are made, most supervisors try to match the skills of the personnel with the tasks required while also considering a complicated schedule and staffing problems. When you receive an assignment, do

Table 6-1

Body Language Observed in Western Culture

Element of Body Language	What It Demonstrates
Hands on hips	Authority or anger
Arms folded across the chest	Resentment or guarding
Eye contact	Attention and respect for the speaker, confidence
Eye rolling	Discontent, disagreement, or impatience
Lack of eye contact	Lack of social comfort (note that people of different cultural backgrounds may not hold eye contact with the speaker because of their culture or faith)
Eyes cast downward	Contemplation, embarrassment, or contrition
Backing up	Social distance that is too close or a desire to leave
Rigid posture	Restrained emotions or tension
Upright posture	Confidence or a sense of well-being
Hand brushed over the forehead or eyes	Exasperation, despair, or fatigue
One eyebrow raised	Doubt or mistrust
Both eyebrows raised	Surprise
Mouth covered by hand	Shock or sudden grief

you respect the need to consider these factors? What does your body language convey? If you were the supervisor, how would you react to the person who rolls his eyes, shakes his head, sighs, or turns away abruptly when given an assignment? Table 6-1 describes some common examples of body language observed in Western culture.

Touch

Touch can be both an expression of comfort and a way of controlling people. Except in social gestures, such as shaking hands, touch is almost never neutral. It is a powerful means of communication that can soothe and comfort. It also demonstrates dominance. People who want to show their power over others sometimes use touch in a condescending manner. For example, consider the team leader who lays his hand on a subordinate's shoulder and says, "I know you won't mind working overtime tonight since you had last weekend off." This person is saying, "You will work overtime tonight whether you mind it or not." Touch also is sometimes used in sexual harassment to overpower another person.

Touch is a very delicate issue for many people. Consider the following behaviors that occur in the workplace:

- Engaging in horseplay or jostling
- Making intimate gestures in view of others (jokingly or not)
- Surprising someone from behind by touching or grabbing them

To some people, these behaviors seem innocent and acceptable, whereas others find them repugnant and offensive. Very often, the person who finds the behaviors acceptable cannot understand why others will not "loosen up" and participate. People who lack respect for others' feelings, values, and experiences demonstrate this in many ways, and touch is one of them. Many people simply do not want to be touched.

❖ *No one has the absolute right to touch another person. It is a privilege earned by trust and limited by the boundaries of culture and social custom.*

Therapeutic touch is purposeful touch that conveys empathy, tenderness, and care. Therapeutic touch is one of the health professional's roles. For many people, it is a natural response to another's suffering. Training in therapeutic touch is directed toward the development and awareness of how touch can have a positive effect on patient outcome.

Silence and Stillness

Silence and stillness communicate powerful messages. Silence can mean contemplation, shock, inability to speak, disagreement, or concentration. Many people misinterpret silence and stillness as "dead space" that must be filled. They are uncomfortable with silence. However, allowing others to think carefully before speaking shows respect and self-confidence. Some people are naturally quiet and still, even in a busy environment. Individuals with this trait sometimes cause others discomfort because they behave differently from the norm. All people have a right to express their individual personalities unless they harm or disrespect the rights of others.

Sometimes a person who is uncomfortable with silence feels the need to provide a running dialogue (or monologue) to avoid silence. In the operating room, speaking can spread airborne contaminants. However, the modern operating room is far from silent. Even here, team members may keep up a constant dialogue.

CULTURAL DIFFERENCES

Culture reflects the **values,** social practices, and communication methods of a group of people. Important considerations in cross-cultural communication include but are not limited to:

- Acceptable social distance between people
- Gender value
- Preference for collective versus independent action
- Methods of coping with conflict and uncertainty
- Ways of expressing emotion
- Body language

Communication with people of different cultures requires respect for all human beings. Most people have heard others criticize newcomers to the United States with comments such as, "They should act like we do" or "They should learn the way we do things" or worse, "If they can't do it like we do, they should go back where they came from." These statements show the speakers' disdain for others who are different from them and a lack of knowledge about how cultural behavior or **norms** are formed. Social and interpersonal norms are imbued in people from the time they are born. Cultural beliefs are based on tradition and value systems that cannot be switched off and on. All people esteem their cultural values and deserve to have them respected by others.

QUALITIES OF GOOD COMMUNICATION

Listening (Receiving Skills)

People find it easy to talk with those who have good listening skills. Good listeners are often placed in management positions because of their ability to communicate ideas in a concise, accurate, and nonjudgmental way. People seek them out for advice because they know they will be heard fairly and with respect.

Listening requires active participation. Passive listening frequently leads to inaccurate interpretation or inability to respond to the information. Parts of the message may be lost because the listener is distracted or impatient to speak.

> ❖ *Many people begin to formulate a response before they have heard everything the sender has to say. Their thoughts are focused on what they want to say, and they fail to receive the message. Box 6-2 presents positive listening skills.*

Assertiveness

Assertiveness is the ability to express one's own needs and rights while respecting the needs and rights of others. It is not aggression or confrontation. However, **aggression** is the exertion of power over others by intimidation, loudness, or bullying; these traits ignore others' feelings or take advantage of another's vulnerabilities. The aggressive person puts his or her own needs and wants above those of everyone else. In contrast, the assertive person communicates self-worth without showing arrogance or "pulling rank."

> ❖ *The assertive person does not submit to the aggression of others, but rather states his or her needs clearly, without hesitation or self-effacement.*

You can convey assertiveness through nonverbal or verbal language. To show assertiveness using *body language*:

- Maintain good posture.
- Use eye contact when speaking and listening. In maintaining relaxed eye contact, shift your gaze on the other person from one eye to the other. A fixed stare can convey emotional intensity.
- Stand still and do not fidget or shift your weight; this conveys ambivalence.
- Place your arms at your sides; this communicates acceptance and genuineness.
- Curb annoying actions, such as knuckle cracking and foot tapping, which can be distracting.

To express assertiveness through *verbal language*:

- Do not interrupt people. Patience shows respect.
- State your question, request, information, or comment without hesitation.
- State your message without blame or criticism.

Box 6-2
Positive Listening Skills

1. Focus on the sender. Avoid listening to background noise or other conversations.
2. Avoid listening for what you want to hear; you may misinterpret the message.
3. Do not judge the sender. If you are preoccupied with personal details about the sender, you cannot interpret the message accurately.
4. Watch for nonverbal cues, such as facial expressions and body language. These help clarify the sender's attitude about the message and help you understand important aspects of the information.
5. Ask for clarification!
6. Rephrase the sender's content so that both of you know the message is understood. For example, "You mean that . . ."
7. If the sender begins to get sidetracked from the topic, redirect the conversation. Ask questions about the original issue or ask the sender to return to the topic.
8. If you find that your attention has drifted, ask the sender to repeat what was just said.
9. Do not assume background information unless you know it. If the message seems unreasonable, there may be circumstances of which you are unaware. Be open to the possibility that a much bigger picture is involved than the one you see.
10. If you find the sender's language or comments in bad taste or offensive, say so without judgment. For example, "I feel uncomfortable when you talk about Dr. X that way" or "I wish you wouldn't use that kind of language, it's offensive to me." When asking another to change his or her tone or language, be sure to state your own feelings about it. For example, "When you get angry with me in front of everyone, I feel very uncomfortable. Can we talk in your office instead?"

- State your own needs or feelings in a straightforward manner.
- Accept the consequences of your message. Remain calm and deliberate in your speech. Remain open to the responses.
- Remain engaged and attentive during conversation.
- If you are emotionally upset, take time to calm down before speaking (unless the patient or a coworker is in direct harm). Strong emotions cloud the ability to think and speak coherently.
- Never assume that, because the work environment is intense, your own intensity has no effect on others; it does.

Consider the following examples.

Example 1

Statement A: "I came to ask you for the weekend off. My brother's coming in from overseas. I really want to spend time with him before he leaves again."

Statement B: "Uh, oh, I was thinking about this weekend. I, well, I've been on call for the last two weekends. I mean, I know you are short staffed, but I was wondering if, you know, I could have this weekend off. I don't know, maybe it'll throw your schedule off. I just thought I'd ask."

Example 2

Statement A: "I want to report that Dr. X threw another bloody sponge across the room today. It hit the wall and barely missed the circulator. Please speak to him."

Statement B: "I was in a room with Dr. X. You know how he is. But, well, I think maybe someone might need to talk to him. Maybe he shouldn't throw sponges. I mean, he did it again today. I know he's chief of surgery, but, well, isn't it bad practice? I mean, couldn't someone get hepatitis or something?"

Statement C: "This operating room is so awful. I mean, to let someone like that get away with throwing bloody sponges all over the room. No wonder people get hepatitis. Why don't you do something? You make these policies, but no one ever does anything about them!"

These examples demonstrate several ways of communicating the same problem. In example 2, the sender is concerned about appropriateness and safety with regard to the behavior of Dr. X. In statement B of both examples, the sender is not confident about reporting. He or she has needs but is reluctant to express them directly. In statement A of both examples, the messages are polite, clear, and to the point. They state the problem clearly, show respect for the receiver, and deliver the message without hesitation. The receiver knows exactly what the request is and can make a decision. Statement C in example 2 communicates disrespect for the receiver and anger at the situation, without actually stating what the problem is or who is involved. This type of approach is aggressive, not assertive. And equally important, it does not provide information for problem solving.

Respect

Respect for others communicates the recognition of value, both our own and that of other people. It shows that although we may not agree with another's opinion or beliefs, we value that person's right to express and act on them, as long as the person does not cause harm to others.

People immediately sense when another person respects them. The person's actions and speech clearly show it.

❖ *We all know individuals who are always respectful and easy to talk to. We admire them because we can trust them.*

The respectful person:
- Does not judge others
- Does not gossip
- Does not reveal personal or confidential information about others
- Speaks directly and listens attentively to others
- Responds with empathy to others
- Does not interrupt
- Does not demand another's attention
- Values the views and ideas of others

- Does not use others to gain personal advantage
- Does not disparage another person to appear smarter, more skilled, or "better"

Respectful people are well liked because others feel accepted in their presence. This quality is developed from one's past experiences and one's own self-esteem. Sometimes people do not realize that their behavior shows a lack of respect. *They do not see the cues or have never been told that their communication is offensive or hurtful.* Others feel entitled to treat people in a disrespectful manner because they were treated this way at some time in their lives. This type of person is often self-centered and may be socially isolated. Such individuals seek out others who find their behavior acceptable and even validate their inappropriate behavior, often to avoid becoming a target themselves.

Clarity

Clarity means that the important aspects of the message are delivered without ambiguity or unnecessary information. Consider the following examples:

Example 1

"You know, I just went to sterilize Dr. X's curettes; you know, the ones he always wants on his total knee surgeries . . . and when I closed the door I hit "Start" and a little steam kept coming out from around the door and the buzzer never went off, and I tried to turn it off and I couldn't. These old sterilizers . . . I think the seal is broken; maybe someone should look at it. Can you call someone? I need those curettes and I don't have time."

Example 2

"Sterilizer number 3 is leaking steam around the door, it won't open, and Dr. X's curettes are inside. Would you mind calling engineering? I need to scrub."

When you report a problem, such as the one in the previous examples, give the right person the necessary information, as in example 2. In that example, the receiver knows exactly what and where the problem is. He or she also understands the level of urgency and can act on this information without further questioning.

❖ *Information in the perioperative setting often is communicated on a "need to know" basis. Economical communication is not the same as withholding information.*

Feedback

As mentioned previously, feedback is the response to the sender's message. Effective communication includes clear feedback. Poor communication results when a message is delivered but the receiver does not acknowledge understanding. In this case, feedback is missing. This may happen when the receiver is distracted, in a hurry, or reluctant to seek clarification.

Look for cues that the receiver understands the message. When the message is understood, the receiver should seek additional information or indicate the appropriate action. Just as the sender has a responsibility to clarify the message, the receiver should give direct, specific feedback. In health care, feedback is critical in discussions or reporting of safety issues. In the previous examples, a request is made to solve a problem with a flash sterilizer. The person who asks for help must not assume that the other person will follow through. He or she must determine whether the coworker really will be able to call engineering.

How do we give feedback? By repeating the message or reporting our response to the sender. Feedback gives the sender confidence that the receiver understands the importance of the message and will act on it. Without feedback, some ambiguity may exist about the receiver's ability or intention to take the information on board and respond appropriately. Consider the following examples.

Example 1
A: "I just talked to the ED, and there's a patient with a gunshot wound in the chest. I'm calling thoracic to see who's on call. Can you call the anesthetist on duty?"
B: "Well, okay, but I was just going to lunch."

Example 2
A: "Can you tell Dr. X that his 2 o'clock has been cancelled because the patient refused to sign the permit?"
B: "I'll do that right now. I just saw him going into the locker room. Do you want me to let him know that the patient is still in the holding area?"

In example 1, the sender has given an urgent message. The receiver does not convey assurance that the message is important. He or she may even wonder whether the requested task will be carried out. The person delivering the message does not need to know that the receiver was just going to lunch, and it is not relevant to the situation, which requires immediate attention.

Example 2 is a clear response to the request and includes clarification. There is no doubt about this person's understanding or willingness to follow through.

Appropriate Person, Time, and Place
Effective communication results when the delivery is appropriate to the situation.

❖ *Communication should take place with the right person at the right time in the right place.*

The chain of command must be respected in communication. Ask yourself, "Does this person need to know this?" If the message is urgent, do not delay. However, do not rush to someone with a problem that is not under that person's control or that the individual cannot resolve. Think about the consequences of your communication.

❖ *Remember that deliberately withholding information that could affect a person's work is considered sabotage.*

BARRIERS TO COMMUNICATION
Communication between individuals or groups can fail for many reasons. The following are some of the most common.

- **Perceptions.** Our perceptions of the environment may not coincide with those of others. We make assumptions about what we see, hear, and understand based on our perception of the situation. For example, one person may perceive an unemotional patient as "stoic," a strong, brave person facing illness. Another person may see the same patient as extremely anxious and fearful, speechless, and unable to express emotion because of the intensity of his or her emotions.
- **Bias.** Personal bias is our preexisting opinions about people because of their affiliations, culture, economic status, and even their diseases. Bias is an effective communication stopper because it does not allow new ideas or opinions to develop or to be revealed. The biased receiver already "knows" all he or she wants to know and is firmly rooted in a narrow point of view.
- **Lack of understanding.** Sometimes the receiver does not have sufficient knowledge to understand exactly what the sender is trying to communicate. This is why *clarification* is so important in communication. Both parties have a responsibility to ensure that the message is clear. If the communication requires action on the part of the receiver, the need for clarification is even more pressing.
- **Social and cultural influences.** How we perceive a problem, situation, or action depends on our social and cultural background. These affect the way we evaluate and comprehend what is being communicated. Communication in any form is integrated into what we already know and believe. In a sense, there is no "pure" communication, each of us has a unique point of view of ourselves and the environment.
- **Emotions.** How we feel at the time of communication can have a powerful effect on our ability to receive and send messages. Emotions can block communication through distraction or prejudice. Communication is extremely difficult when people are in a state of anger or resentment. These emotions not only distort the message, but also prevent concentration and mental imaging, which are necessary for good communication.
- **Environmental barriers.** Communication sometimes fails simply because the environment prevents reception. Hearing is a particular problem in the operating room. Masks can cause words to sound muffled, and background noises, such as suction, irrigation, power equipment, or even loud music, can distort communication.
- **Lack of a desire to communicate.** To be successful in sending and receiving information, a person must *want* to communicate. The desire to communicate creates greater attention, focus, and concentration, which are necessary for clarity and understanding.

STRESSORS IN THE PERIOPERATIVE ENVIRONMENT

Coping with problem behaviors in the workplace is always a challenge. Because the operating room is a unique environment that often involves an established hierarchy and intense work, problem behaviors frequently are accepted as the norm.

The following are some characteristics of operating room work that contribute to lack of communication and disrupt team cohesion.

- **The work is stressful.** The operating room requires its personnel to work at a high level of mental, physical, and emotional strength. Because of the demanding schedules, strong lines of authority, and wide diversity of behavior and personality types, excellent communication skills are vital.
- **Close teamwork is necessary.** This holds true even when team members have little knowledge of each other's work styles and personalities. It is especially true in a teaching hospital, where surgical residents and medical, nursing, and surgical technology students rotate through the department regularly. Even when communication is good among team members, working under intense conditions with new people can be challenging.
- **People and departments compete for time, space, materials, and personnel.** All operating rooms, whether in a large metropolitan area or in a small community, must meet the needs of the patients with fixed levels of staffing, equipment, and time. When the patient load requires more resources than are immediately available, the potential exists for conflict over available personnel, supplies, and space. Conflict arises when the needs of one person override those of the others.
- **The model for team relationships is in transition.** The social model for teams in the operating room traditionally has been authoritarian, hierarchical, and intended to put people "in their place." Many of these social traditions are no longer accepted by administrators and professional associations. Whenever a major change in a social structure occurs, a period of testing and adjustment also occurs.

Problem behaviors cause mistrust, frustration, and interpersonal conflict. The person with problem behaviors uses extreme defensive or aggressive tactics to achieve a level of social comfort. Supervisors cannot resolve every conflict that arises. Each person on the unit must make an effort to communicate effectively and assertively. When personal attempts to resolve conflict fail, then the issue must be referred to management.

When working with people with problem behaviors, one must remember to focus on the behavior, not the person. Difficult people relate poorly to each other, their environment, and themselves because they have not learned how to meet their own needs in socially acceptable ways. They have not learned to cope. This does not dismiss the frustration and even humiliation that others experience with them. However, attacking the person in an attempt to cope with the behavior is neither productive nor helpful. In fact, it usually increases defensive behavior and alienates the person even more.

VERBAL ABUSE

Verbal abuse is a significant problem in the operating room. Despite changing social norms and professional acknowledge-

ment of the problem at all levels, it persists. It is among the leading causes of burnout among team members. Verbal abuse has a negative effect on patient care, because it causes staff members to become tense, upset, and distracted, and the result is an increase in errors. Verbal abuse also reduces productivity and increases staff turnover.

What Is Verbal Abuse?

Verbal abuse is one of several types of sabotage in which the perpetrator overpowers an individual by demeaning the person and devaluing him or her. This is done through deliberate and often aggressive (and loud) criticism, public embarrassment, vulgar language, and personal attack. Sometimes verbal abuse involves sexual innuendos or insults.

Verbal abuse includes but is not limited to the following behaviors:

- Vulgar remarks directed toward staff members
- Violent public criticism and demeaning of another person
- Loud and abrasive comments or demands
- Comments intended to deliberately embarrass or hurt another person
- Sexual remarks directed toward staff members

Violent behavior may accompany verbal abuse. This includes throwing or deliberately destroying instruments and other items. Any staff member who threatens or throws a dangerous object at another person may be violating the law and certainly should be reported to the hospital administration.

Perpetuation of Verbal Abuse and Violence

No excuse is possible for verbal abuse. However, research has shown that circumstances and beliefs perpetuate it.

Verbal abuse by surgeons increases when they are allowed to show favoritism toward particular staff members. Others who are obliged to work with these surgeons on emergency calls or under other circumstances often are the targets of severe verbal abuse because they lack the "inside knowledge" of the select group. This type of treatment leads to conflict and resentment among staff members and increases the scope of the problem. People in the select group who feel secure in their positions sometimes use their power to belittle and criticize others, especially students or new employees. This behavior damages self-esteem and inhibits the newcomer's ability to fit into the group.

Verbal abuse sometimes is built into the operating room culture. An administration that does not address and act on the problem in a serious manner gives implied permission to continue the behavior. Victims who cannot seek sympathy from or action by those who can affect policy are left with little recourse. They may leave the job or suffer the abuse silently as their stress level increases. Administrative support is very important to changing operating room culture.

Rude, vulgar, and offensive behavior is *not a natural reaction to stress.* It is a choice made by those who perpetrate it.

The job stress experienced by surgeons and other operating room personnel is no greater than that of people in many other professions, such as firefighters, rescue workers, and police officers. Yet in these groups, one finds increased cohesion and support rather than abuse among coworkers. A culture of verbal abuse and passive aggression does not flow naturally from the environment; it comes from individuals who use their authority to hurt others.

Remember, as a student it is important to inform your instructors if you are the target of verbal abuse and to allow them to help resolve the situation.

Coping with Verbal Abuse

Assertive behavior is one of the most effective ways to counteract verbal abuse. The following guidelines describe specific coping behaviors.

1. **Remain calm.** To deescalate rising tension and disarm the abuser, you must prepare yourself to address the person. This often is very difficult, especially when the outburst is extremely demeaning and loud and includes foul language.

2. **Remind yourself of the following facts:**
   - "I have the right to confront this person."
   - "I have the right not to take this abuse."
   - "There is no acceptable excuse for this behavior."

3. **Make an assertive statement.** Do not engage in sarcasm or personal attack; this usually escalates the situation. Instead, state what you feel and what you want:
   "Dr. X, please don't speak to me like that. It is rude and demoralizing."
   "Dr. X, it is not necessary to scream at me. When you do that, I can't work."
   "Dr. X, if I make an error, tell me what the error is. It's not necessary to yell and curse at me."
   After you have made your statement, proceed with your work. If the abuser continues, it sometimes is helpful just to ignore the person. The abuser will soon realize that you are not listening. The important fact is that you have stated your rights and are in control of yourself. If the situation continues, restate your position calmly.

4. **"Sidestep" the behavior.** With this tactic, you simply change the direction of the communication. For example, in response to an aggressive remark about an instrument that is not working, you state, "I'll get a replacement for that instrument right now."

5. **Do not become aggressive.** When you act aggressively in the face of aggression, it escalates the conflict and may cause a major crisis. This creates a risk to the patient and is not acceptable. The patient must never bear the consequences of anyone's behavioral problems. If you cannot stop the behavior, wait until after surgery, then confront the abuser.

6. **Stand up for your coworkers.** If you are in a room where your coworker is being abused, defend the person. Your silence is approval of the abuser's behavior.

7. **If the abuse becomes violent (objects are thrown or threats are made), call for the supervisor.** Do not allow the abuse or other disruptive behavior to continue. Do not be afraid to request the presence of others who are in an administratively stronger position to stop the abuser.

8. **Challenge authorities who allow abuse to continue.** Seek justification for allowing abuse to continue and do not allow yourself to feel personal defeat in the face of the administration's complacency.

When an abusive situation has occurred, it is natural to want to tell the first person you see what has happened. However, pick the correct time and place. The operating room corridor is not the appropriate place to vent your feelings. Patients can overhear talk and become frightened and insecure. File a complaint with the operating room supervisor. You can do this face to face or in a written report, stating when the abuse occurred, what was said, and who was in the room. If you choose to meet with your supervisor, make an appointment. Do not burst into the supervisor's office demanding that the person "do something about Dr. X." If you need to vent your anger, avoid lashing out at others. This only spreads the effects of the abuse and multiplies the abuser's ability to demoralize people. If possible, take a break and write down your feelings. Vent your stress in physical activity or other appropriate ways.

If you work with the abuser again, continue to reinforce your position: that that person is the abuser, and you have the right to tell him or her to stop. Continue to file appropriate written reports of the abusive behavior.

HORIZONTAL ABUSE

As stated previously, horizontal abuse takes place among staff members of equal rank and position. This type of abuse may be completely ignored by management because they consider it a private problem involving personal conflict. In reality, it often is not a matter of personal conflict but a form of sabotage. Some examples of vertical abuse include the following behaviors:

- Failure to share information
- Demeaning a person in front of others
- Open or covert discrimination
- Mocking another person
- Taking the credit for another's work or accomplishments
- Directly sabotaging another's work
- Falsely reporting another to management or staff

The most effective management of this type of abuse is assertiveness and reporting in writing. Defend your colleagues by exposing the abuser. If you do not agree with what others are saying, let them know. *Silence shows agreement with the abuser.* Act as you would like others to act for you if you were the one being abused.

PROBLEM BEHAVIORS

Complaining

Legitimate complaints about conditions in the workplace are important and should be addressed. Legitimate complaints often lead to creative solutions that produce a safer and more efficient operating room. However, when people complain without the intention of seeking solutions, they erode morale and sometimes cause conflict. Chronic complaining can be contagious. When it becomes part of the workplace culture, it spreads discontent and feelings of helplessness or despair. Habitual complaining usually is not about occasional incidents. Habitual complainers usually are unhappy about many aspects of their lives. They do not look for solutions; they simply want everyone to know how they feel and seek out others to hear and validate their many complaints. It is helpful for people to share their feelings about incidents. By sharing their thoughts and emotions, they find support and empathy. Chronic complainers, however, have little regard for or knowledge about the unhappiness that they spread in the work environment. The following guidelines can be used in dealing with chronic complainers.

- Do not become a complainer yourself. Often we are tempted to jump in and agree with a complainer. This only perpetuates the problem. Offer a solution or suggest how the person might solve the problem. If the complainer rejects the solution immediately or gives more examples of how bad things are, you know that the individual is not interested in seeking solutions but simply wants to state and restate the negative aspects of work or of his or her personal life.
- Just listen. Sometimes silence has a powerful effect on the complainer. Listen without emotion and then simply leave. This is not a satisfying response to the complainer, and the person may stop.
- Confront the complainer. Complainers often dominate locker room conversation or complain in front of patients. If you are in the presence of a patient, simply say, "Not now . . ." or "This isn't the time . . ." Speak to the complainer in private and tell the person how you feel about the complaining and the effect it has on the team. Ask the person to curb the behavior. It is not necessary to speak harshly or unkindly. The individual does not complain out of maliciousness. The complainer is unhappy and does not know how to cope with this unhappiness.
- If possible, remove yourself from the situation. If other solutions do not work, simply do not stay with the complainer. Understand that listening to the complainer regularly is frustrating and tiring. Do not allow this person to increase your stress.

Gossip and Rumors

Gossip is the telling and retelling of events about another's personal life, professional life, or physical condition. It is insidious behavior that hurts people, erodes teamwork, and damages group ethics. Gossip is not the same as the normal sharing of news or events that occur in people's lives. It is communication about another person or event that is confidential or personal. The goal of gossip is to shock or evoke intrigue. As gossip spreads, the story may change slightly and facts may become blurred, so that the only importance of the story is its ability to entertain, at the expense of someone else.

A rumor is information for which the validity is in question. The damaging effect of a rumor is that, after the story begins to circulate, people assume that it is true and react as if the rumor were fact. If the rumor is unpleasant news, conflicts arise and people may become resentful, angry, or even fearful. Ironically, people who spread rumors often fail to validate the rumor. As with gossip, the value of the rumor lies in its effect on others during the telling and retelling, not in whether it is based on reality.

Adopt the following rules in coping with gossip and rumors:

- Do not perpetuate rumors or gossip about others. If you find yourself participating in rumors or gossip, ask yourself whether you would want others to discuss the details of your personal life or other private news in public.
- Call attention to the behavior. One very effective way to do this is to make a remark such as, "We shouldn't be talking about Dr. X. That's his personal business." (Note that it is important not to accuse the other person; that is, do not say, "You shouldn't . . .") You might also say, "It's not fair to talk about someone when he can't defend himself." The point is to reinforce to the gossiper that the behavior is damaging and that you are not going to participate.

Groupthink

Groupthink is collective behavior and thinking. It is based on peer pressure and occurs when members of a group are polarized in their opinions, ways of doing things, and means of expression. It produces two categories of people: those who are "in" and those who are "out." Whether the values of the group are positive or negative, people avoid becoming isolated and strive to become part of the "in" group. They change their own values to fit those of the "in" group. In this way, group culture is created and maintained.

Groupthink establishes unwritten, unspoken rules. Those who do not follow the rules may be criticized or ostracized by their peers. Standards of practice are deeply affected by groupthink. When the group sets high standards, groupthink is a positive force, but when aseptic technique and other practices slide, the people in the "out" group may be the only ones trying to uphold the high standard.

Groupthink usually is a negative force because it does not allow freedom of speech or action without the implied threat of isolation. A surgical technologist should be an independent and critical thinker, uphold high standards, and act in a professional manner in every situation.

Criticism

Criticism is a helpful tool in correcting work habits or raising awareness about harmful or unsafe situations. When offered appropriately, criticism is specific, nonjudgmental, and focused on the task, not on the person. When criticism is used to exercise power over others or boost one's own self-confidence, however, it can be very destructive. People who criticize usually are insecure in their own lives. They use criticism as a way to soothe the anxiety they experience as a result of self-dissatisfaction. Nevertheless, this does not give them the right to demoralize or demean others. Some critics are expert at finding vulnerabilities in their coworkers and using these to demonstrate their superiority. Staff members must not tolerate this behavior.

Habitually critical people often are defensive and may become resentful when confronted with their behavior. However, it is important to point out when their criticism is causing conflict. When confronting the critical person, you should do the following:

- State that you find the person's behavior distressing rather than helpful.
- Tell the person that if he or she wishes to discuss your work, you will do so in private. This formalizes the critical process and removes its ability to cause embarrassment in front of others.
- Ask the person to be specific about the problem. Respond with a request for clarification or simply state without emotion or further discussion your reason for behaving as you did.

Example 1
Person A: "The way you stacked these things, I can't find anything!"
Person B: "Tell me how you would like them arranged."
Person A: "I don't know, that's not my job."
Person B: "But I can't improve the situation unless you can identify the problem."

Example 2
Person A: "Why can't you ever loosen up in surgery? You're so serious."
Person B: "What bothers you about it?"
Person A: "You never laugh at any of my jokes."
Person B: "I just don't find that kind of humor amusing, and I'm usually pretty quiet during surgery."

In both of these examples, person B deflected person A's comments by being assertive or asking for clarification.

SEXUAL HARASSMENT

Definition
Despite increased awareness and the enactment of laws and policies regarding sexual harassment, it continues to be a problem in the operating room. Sexual harassment is an extreme abuse of power in which a person engages in the following types of behavior:

- Expects sexual favors in exchange for personal or professional gain (sexual coercion)
- Directs sexually explicit comments toward another
- Makes *any* unwanted sexual or casual physical contact with another person
- Directs vulgar or sexual innuendoes at another

The legal implications of and responses to sexual harassment were discussed in Chapter 4. Behavioral responses to aid in coping with this behavior are discussed in this chapter.

Box 6-3

Defenses Against Sexual Harassment

- If the institution does not have policies covering reporting and discipline, request that the process of developing such policies be initiated.
- Do not engage in sexual jokes or conversation yourself. Walk away from the scene or simply change the subject. If you are scrubbed and cannot leave, confront the person either at that time or later. If you are afraid to make the report, ask another person who was present to do it. Explain why.
- Inform your coworkers that you recognize a given behavior as sexual harassment. If they agree, ask them to participate in a confrontation. If you are not the subject of the harassment but are present, help others by confronting the perpetrator as your coworker's advocate, especially if the victim is so humiliated that he or she cannot respond.
- Report all incidents of sexual harassment, even if you are not the victim.
- Stand up for your rights. If you feel victimized, others probably do, too. Seek others out for support in taking appropriate action.
- If your supervisor does not respond to repeated reports, write a letter or speak to the person at the administrative level directly above the supervisor.

Coping with Sexual Harassment
Sexual harassment is illegal. However, because the victims are humiliated and embarrassed and often feel powerless to do anything, incidents go unreported and perpetrators continue the behavior. The perpetrator often considers sexual harassment to be innocent behavior. He or she may believe that acts of sexual harassment may be open to interpretation (unless the sexual content is blatant). Consequently, the victim may feel that there are no grounds on which to make an incident report. Any act that evokes humiliation, shame, or guilt should be reported. Documentation of an incident is the best way to elicit disciplinary action by those in a position to enforce the law.

Although it sometimes is difficult, the victim should confront the perpetrator when sexual harassment occurs and afterward submit a written report. For example:

"Don't touch me again. I don't like it, and I won't tolerate it."

"Don't use those kinds of sexual references around me. Your comments are inappropriate."

"My personal life is not open for discussion."

Box 6-3 presents specific defenses that personnel can use, in addition to confrontation, to prevent and stand up to sexual harassment.

TEAMWORK

TYPES OF TEAMS

A team is a group of people who come together to reach a common goal or set of goals. The surgical team is only one type of team that plans and implements patient care in the operating room. In some large hospitals, certain personnel work within a surgical specialty, such as cardiology or orthopedics. In this type of structure, surgical technologists work with their peers to design instrument sets, order equipment, and update the surgeons' procedural changes. The team may or may not have a team leader.

The surgical technologist also may participate in other types of interdepartmental teams to improve care or produce information for surveillance and monitoring. Within a team, different personalities, work styles, values, and cultures are brought together. The team must identify and prioritize the steps of the process to reach the desired goal of a positive outcome for patient treatment.

The surgical team includes the surgeons, anesthesia provider, assistants, surgical technologist, and registered nurse. They all work together on a single procedure. Communication usually is focused, task oriented, and at times intense.

A *group* does not have a common goal, but the people in the group share common professions, task requirements, or other characteristics. Group work and teamwork are very similar. Interpersonal relationships and the ability to resolve differences are equally important in a team and in a group. When people work on the same shift in the operating room, they form a group. An understanding is formed among them that they will help each other with certain tasks and try to resolve work-related obstacles.

CHARACTERISTICS OF GOOD TEAMWORK

Good teamwork is the result of healthy relationships within the team. This does not mean that conflicts do not arise. Conflict in groups is normal, because people have different ideas, problem-solving skills, values, and beliefs. The qualities of a good team reflect how conflict is managed. Individuals must retain valued traits, such as genuineness, self-assertion, and empathy, yet at the same time be willing to discuss, yield, and accept change.

Many different social and professional models of team building and collaboration have been devised. There is no "best" model for every situation. People work in teams for immediate (emergency) results, long-term project goals, creative output, and many other reasons. The dynamics of team interaction always include common social and psychological behavior. An earlier business model developed in the 1960s by Bruce Tuckman was based on four group processes: "forming, storming, norming, and performing." More modern models allow for greater integration of psychological, social, and cultural perception, more flexibility in the creative process, and an emphasis on conflict resolution.

Conflict cannot be managed unless people communicate about their problems. Discussion means that the group must admit that a problem exists. Identifying the problem requires sharing of experiences and interpretations of events without judgment. Members of successful groups do not accuse others of wrongdoing. They simply state the facts and relate the effect. Although people's perceptions of events, situations, or problems may be different, it is important to focus on the problem, not the people. Attacks on others in the group lead to defensive behavior, which is counterproductive to creating solutions.

Yielding

Yielding in teamwork does not mean giving up one's values or beliefs. It means accepting the fact that others have valid points of view and conceding when one has made incorrect assumptions or conclusions. People who are able to yield are open-minded and retain a sense of fairness during team interaction. A team member who tries to gain control of all decisions and conversations is unable to yield to other people's right to express their views. Such individuals cannot imagine any way but their way and make little or no attempt to broaden their thinking.

Change

The ability to accept change is crucial to good teamwork. Many people experience change as a positive event, but others face it with dread. One of the purposes of a team is to adjust to a changing environment, such as unfolding events during a surgical procedure, a change in instrumentation, or new responsibilities. When teams are confronted with change, they must adjust their ways of working to accommodate the change. Team members must identify new tasks or procedures and implement them with as little disruption as possible. This requires personal flexibility, one of the positive character traits identified in the successful surgical technologist.

Politeness

Politeness concerns the manner in which people speak to and behave toward each other. The attributes of acceptable behavior include respect, gratitude, and acceptance. The operating room culture does not always promote these attributes. This does not mean that they are unimportant. On the contrary, teams that honor and practice these qualities have a pleasant work atmosphere, are efficient, and show a high level of professionalism. They experience fewer conflicts, and team members show high self-esteem. Unfortunately, group thinking and aggressive behavior often overcome civility in the operating room. The most powerful way to instill civility in a group is to model it.

Polite behavior is not complicated or difficult. Saying, "Thank you" or "Please" makes people feel appreciated and respected. Offering to help another person even if you have not been asked and responding to requests for help without resentment create an atmosphere of cohesion and empathy among coworkers. Speaking with others in a calm manner without sarcasm promotes evenness and reduces stress.

Collaboration

Collaboration is working together for a common purpose. In the operating room, personnel contribute their skills, time, and energy to the care of the surgical patient. Collaboration requires that everyone solve problems and obstacles as a group. Cooperation and the ability to accept one another's individual personalities contribute to successful collaboration. Successful patient outcomes result when each team member recognizes the relationship of his or her own responsibilities to the tasks of the other members. Each person understands that his or her contribution is one of many and that problems or strengths in one area affect the entire collaborative effort.

TEAM CONFLICT

Interpersonal Conflict

Personality clashes, attempts to gain control of the group, and power plays are some causes of team conflict. When stress occurs between two or more people on a team, all team members feel the tension. Other members feel frustrated because they cannot solve the problem. Team cohesion disintegrates, and members worry about productivity, safety, and accountability. Resolving the conflict may require mediation if the individuals involved cannot resolve their differences. Particularly in health care, the overall goal (patient care) must not suffer because of individuals' inability to get along or resolve differences.

Conflict Between Team Goals and Personal Goals

On the surface, a team's goals might seem obvious. Although each person is aware of the final outcome (i.e., the surgery is completed), the manner in which each person contributes to the final outcome is affected by personal goals. For example, if a student is scrubbed with a surgical technologist, the role of the surgical technologist is to be a teacher (preceptor). The overall goal remains the same: completion of the surgery in a safe and efficient manner. The goals of the student, however, are to learn about the procedure and practice skills that will allow the student to work independently. The surgical technologist may not want to give up control of the case. The surgical technologist may be concerned that the surgeon will blame him or her if the surgery is slowed or errors are made. Perhaps the surgical technologist wants to show the student how much he or she knows rather than allow the student to participate actively. In such a case, the student becomes frustrated, because a conflict of goals has arisen. In this type of conflict, the needs of each person must be discussed. The most favorable outcome is for each person to recognize the overall priority of needs and to be willing to yield to these priorities.

Conflicting Priorities

Setting team priorities requires **consensus,** which is agreement on what the goals are and how they will be reached. Everyone may understand the goal, but people may disagree on how to reach it. For example, during surgery, the surgeon's goal is to work quickly without pauses in the flow of the procedure. The surgical technologist's goal is to remain ahead of the surgeon, anticipating what will happen next and what instruments and supplies will be needed, while at the same time providing what is needed in the present. To do this, the surgical technologist must use every moment to prepare as well as work in the present.

Consider a scenario in which the surgeon places used instruments out of the surgical technologist's reach. Suction devices, hemostats, and needle holders soon pile up at the opposite end of the work area from the surgical technologist. The surgeon has created a situation in which the surgical technologist cannot do the work. The surgical technologist reminds the surgeon of the need to return instruments. This causes interruption. The surgeon is frustrated, because he or she must periodically retrieve the instruments, and the surgical technologist must spend time requesting the instruments and sorting them. Cooperation is lacking. The solution, of course, is for the surgeon to place the used instruments within the surgical technologist's reach immediately after using them, but this is not the surgeon's main priority. In this case, it would be helpful for the surgical technologist to point out that the procedure would go more quickly and more smoothly if the used instruments were placed within reach. The surgeon may be unaware of this need or may not have thought about the effect of his or her work habits on achievement of the overall goal.

Role Confusion

Role confusion was discussed in Chapter 5. However, it is reemphasized here in the context of team conflict. It occurs when individuals are uncertain of what is expected of them. The following comments are common expressions of role confusion:

"That's not *my* job." (anger)

"I thought *you* were supposed to do that." (surprise and confusion)

"What am *I* supposed to do about that?" (anger)

"No one told *me* that was part of my job description." (distress and anger)

Most role confusion is a result of poor communication. Conflict occurs when one person assigns a task to another who does not have the knowledge or time to complete the task. In cases of delegation, the person who delegates the job is responsible for evaluating the outcome and assisting if help is needed.

When a task is transferred from one person to another with the same qualifications, the person completing the task must have both the freedom to work independently and the authority to carry out the task. You should never assign a task to someone else just to get rid of it. Learn whether that person is qualified, capable of doing the job, and has the time to do it. Always request a specific job description when beginning employment.

When working on a team, ask for clarification of what is expected of each person. Do not give up responsibility for a task after you have accepted it. If you cannot complete it, you must pass the task to someone else who agrees and is qualified to complete it.

Conflict Resolution

The goal of conflict resolution is to attempt to find a solution that is acceptable to all parties. This is called a **win-win solution.** The other type of resolution is a **win-lose solution,** in which one party is satisfied but the other is not. This is not a satisfactory resolution, because resentment and frustration will continue.

The goal of conflict resolution is to find a win-win solution. This requires behaviors such as a nonbiased approach, flexibility, willingness to yield, and the ability to focus on the problem, not the people. The following are some steps for resolving conflicts:

- When discussing the problem, try not to consider your personal opinion or bias about the situation. Consider the problem and the objective (e.g., to provide smoother turnaround between cases).
- Remain open-minded about solutions. Do not get stuck on a single fact or solution.
- Gather information about the problem before discussing it. Then assess the information and how it relates to the problem.
- View the problem as a team problem, not as *your* problem. Even interpersonal conflict is a team problem because it affects everyone.
- Brainstorm for solutions. Offer suggestions without deep analysis. Brainstorming allows people to suggest creative or different solutions without fear of judgment.
- Address any interpersonal conflicts in the team before other problems are solved. Tension in the team competes for energy needed for other types of problem solving.
- Formulate a plan for improvement that includes necessary behaviors and the rationale for changes.
- Try to reach a win-win solution. If such a solution is not reached, go back over the plan and evaluate whether concessions can be made to achieve a more satisfactory resolution.
- Seek mediation if the conflict cannot be resolved.

MANAGING TEAMS

Surgical technologists are increasingly becoming team managers. They may manage other technologists on a specialty team or serve as managers for projects or for situations requiring technical expertise. Few technologists have previous management training, therefore they must learn how to develop those skills by doing the job. Management practices have changed significantly in the past decade. Professional teams are more participatory in decision making, and a completely top-down approach is reserved for emergency situations in which the team leader must make decisions that have immediate and serious consequences.

Management styles were first popularized in the 1970s, when businesses began to seek methods of training managers for increased production. Early texts identified these styles based on the behavior of the manager and the context. The following styles were described:

- *Authoritarian* or *autocratic:* With this method, the manager makes most decisions with little or no input from the team.
- *Democratic:* This style allows team members to provide input in the decision-making process, and extensive discussion is pursued to support the final decisions.
- *Laissez-faire:* With this method, the manager allows the team to make the decisions based on loosely organized communication and little or no management.

The modern team leader is a facilitator or enabler. Managers are trained to develop the ideas of individual team members, clarify their common goals, and help set a course that will accomplish the objectives. Good management or team leading reflects particular qualities. An effective team leader will follow these rules:

Box 6-4

Guidelines for Serving as a Preceptor

1. If you are a student now, notice the problems you encounter. Think of the preceptors from whom you have learned the most and consider why you learned from them.
2. Develop a plan with the person for whom you are serving as preceptor. Discuss with the learner what each of you will do and how it will be done. For example, as the preceptor, you might start the case and then allow the learner to step in and complete it. You might also have the student perform certain tasks while you do others.
3. Never try to perform the same task at the same time as your student. For example, if the learner is passing instruments, allow your student time to think and act. Silently point to the correct instrument, but do not reach for it; this would result in hand collisions on the Mayo stand and frustration for everyone.
4. If the learner is struggling, try to help by coaching quietly in the background. If this is insufficient, ask the learner whether you should take over for awhile. This allows the student to regain composure.
5. Never make a learner feel inadequate or foolish; this will only intensify the person's lack of confidence. Encouragement is much more productive than criticism. If you cannot contain negativity, ask to be excused from preceptor duties.
6. Always introduce the learner to the surgical team before beginning the procedure. This allows the learner to feel like part of the team and encourages confidence.
7. Respect the learner as a person. Remember that the learning phase is only one aspect of this person's life. You have a privileged job in helping the student achieve goals. You are also in a position to hurt the student's confidence. This is especially true of adult learners, who may not be accustomed to steep learning curves.
8. If the surgeon becomes irritated or anxious because of the learner's lack of experience, support the learner. If the situation becomes critical, ask the learner to wait until the critical situation has passed. Then invite the student back into the case after assessing whether the surgeon is tolerant.

1. Listen to everyone with equal attention and respect.
2. Set realistic goals.
3. Keep the team focused and interested in the goals.
4. Be alert for friction among team members.
5. Remain unemotional in team interactions.
6. Enable every team member to participate in discussion and input.
7. Recognize that new ideas can be brought to the team in many ways; integrate them into the objectives.
8. Allow team members to make mistakes; allow them to be human.
9. Remember to encourage team members frequently; point out accomplishments.
10. Meetings should be short, well planned, and focused.
11. Allow others to speak more frequently than you do.
12. Do not become involved in department politics and do not criticize management.
13. Be generous with your knowledge and humble about your opinions.

THE SURGICAL TECHNOLOGIST PRECEPTOR

The experienced surgical technologist may be asked to become a preceptor to new employees or surgical technology students. In this role, the surgical technologist tutors the student and shares the duties of a scrubbed technologist. Those who enjoy teaching and sharing information find the role very satisfying. However, patience and a good sense of timing are important. A balance between allowing the student freedom and while preventing serious errors or frustration on the part of other team members is crucial to the preceptor role. Box 6-4 outlines important guidelines for serving as a preceptor.

CHAPTER SUMMARY

- Effective communication skills are extremely important in the health care professions. Patient safety and team work are based on the ability to deliver and receive information in all forms.
- The elements of communication are a sender, a receiver, the message, the means of communication, and feedback about the message.
- Verbal communication is written and spoken. Our choice of words and tone of voice often can alter the meaning of a message, resulting in positive or negative reactions in those with whom we are communicating.
- Communication is influenced by culture, attitude, point of view, emotions, and the desire (or lack of desire) to communicate.
- The qualities of good communication include focused listening, assertiveness, respect, and clarity.
- Stressors in the environment can block good communication and teamwork.
- Verbal abuse in the workplace deeply affects relationships and attitudes on a team.
- Verbal abuse used to be an accepted norm in the workplace. It is no longer acceptable behavior and requires action on the part of those involved, as well as management.
- Skills to manage verbal abuse are learned. Ample resources for these skills are available through human resource departments and in professional literature.
- Sexual harassment is not acceptable in today's workplace. All staff members can learn how to recognize and stop sexual harassment.
- Characteristics of good teamwork include yielding, the ability to change, politeness, and collaboration.
- Team conflict often arises when the goals of the team conflict with the priorities of individuals.
- Role confusion is an important source of team conflict. Clarification of everyone's role on the team is of utmost importance.
- Conflict resolution is a learned skill that can benefit all health care professionals.
- Important goals of team management are to enable the team to reach its objectives and to do this in a way that fosters appreciation for individual contributions.

REVIEW QUESTIONS

1. Give three examples of groupthink that you have observed.
2. Define sexual harassment. Give three examples of sexual harassment in the workplace.
3. What is the purpose of having teams?
4. What are the characteristics of good communication?
5. Why does communication sometimes fail?
6. What does it mean to withhold information deliberately?
7. What are some constructive ways to work with chronic complainers?
8. What would you do if you believed a coworker was spreading rumors about you?
9. What are the causes of cultural discrimination?
10. How do you distinguish between true verbal abuse and indiscriminate rude comments?

CASE STUDIES

Case 1

You have repeatedly been the victim of verbal abuse by one member of the surgical team. You avoid working with this person, as does almost everyone else. When you are assigned to work with her, you are tense and upset even before the case begins. How will you prepare yourself to work with this difficult person?

Case 2

In the situation described in the previous example, you have made repeated complaints to the operating room supervisor, who tells you that she cannot really do anything about it. What steps will you take next?

Case 3

You are among six surgical technologists on an orthopedics team in a large hospital. The team leader is aggressive and rude to you. You feel that his technical expertise is lacking and that he was made team leader because of his relationships with the sales representatives. How will you handle your working relationship with this person? How can you reduce your own stress?

Case 4

You are a new employee in a large hospital operating room. You have been assigned a preceptor with whom you have difficulty working. You are not learning much, because she won't let you do anything except observe. When you tell her you would like to do more, she declares, "You're not ready to do anything; just watch." After several weeks, the situation has not changed. What will you do?

Case 5

You are a student scrubbing in with your preceptor. When draping begins, you reach for the drapes and he pushes you out of the way, saying, "Dr. X likes me to do this." What will you do?

BIBLIOGRAPHY

Association of periOperative Registered Nurses (AORN): Position statement on workplace safety. In *Standards, recommended practices and guidelines, 2007 edition,* Denver, 2007, AORN.

Bevea S: Employee morale and patient safety, *AORN Journal* 80:6, 2004.

Buback D: Assertiveness training to prevent verbal abuse in the OR, *AORN Journal* 79:1, 2004.

Clancy C: Team STEPPS: optimizing teamwork in the perioperative setting, *AORN Journal* 86:18, 2007.

Dunn H: Horizontal violence among nurses in the operating room, *AORN Journal* 78:6, 2003.

Reina D, Rein M: *Trust and betrayal in the workplace,* San Francisco, 1999, Berrett-Koehler.

CHAPTER 7

Microbes and the Process of Infection

CHAPTER OUTLINE

LEARNING OBJECTIVES

After studying this chapter the reader will be able to:

- Discuss how disease is transmitted
- Describe the relationship between environment and infection
- Explain why the host-microbe relationship changes
- Explain the significance of spores in medicine
- List body fluids that transmit the human immunodeficiency virus (HIV)
- Describe some of the body's defense mechanisms
- List the ways a person acquires immunity to pathogenic organisms
- Describe blood-borne pathogens
- Explain the significance of multidrug-resistant organisms
- Describe different kinds of vaccines and how they protect against infection

TERMINOLOGY

Abscess: A localized accumulation of pus. An abcess may be any size and is usually the result of a bacterial infection. The abscessed tissue is usually inflamed and may be very painful.

Acquired immunity: Disease immunity established through cellular memory following exposure to the disease antigen.

Active immunity: Production of antibodies which combat a specific disease. Acquired by contracting the disease or by vaccination.

Aerobes: Organisms that favor an environment with oxygen. Strict aerobes cannot live without oxygen.

Aerosol droplet: A droplet of moisture small enough to remain suspended in the air; it can carry microorganisms within it.

Anaerobes: Organisms that prefer an oxygen-poor environment. Strict anaerobes cannot survive in the presence of oxygen.

Anaphylactic shock: A type I hypersensitive immune reaction that occurs in response to previous sensitization to a substance, usually a protein. Anaphylactic shock can be quickly fatal.

Antibiotic: A chemical agent used specifically for the treatment of bacterial infection.

Antibiotic resistant: A microorganism that is able to resist destruction by antimicrobial therapy.

Antibodies: Complex glycoproteins produced by the immune system that are formed in response to antigens. An antibody makes contact with an antigen to destroy or control it.

Antigens: Macromolecules (e.g., proteins, glycoproteins, lipoproteins, and polysaccharides) on the surface of cells that identify them as part of the organism ("self") or foreign ("nonself"). Antigens can trigger a response by the immune system, which seeks out and destroys the marked cell.

Antimicrobial therapy: Use of antimicrobial drugs to combat an infection.

Archaea: Primitive, single-celled prokaryotes.

Autoinfection: The spread of infection from one part of the body to another part.

Bacilli: Rod-shaped bacteria that occur in pairs, chains, or filaments.

Bacteriology: The study of bacteria.

Bacteriophage: A virus that invades bacterial cells and can replicate from within the cell.

Bacterium (sing); **bacteria** (pl): A unicellular microorganism with a rigid cell wall.

Binomial system: A method of classifying living organisms by their genus and species.

Bioburden: A measure of the number of bacterial colonies on a surface.

Capsule: With regard to cells, a surface layer on some cells that resists chemicals and the invasion of viruses; also called a slime layer.

Carrier: An individual who harbors disease microbes and is capable of transmitting the disease to others but may not show signs of the infection.

Cell theory: An early hypothesis in biology that stated that cells are the basic unit of all living things, cells are derived from other cells, and all living things are composed of cells.

Cell wall: A rigid structure surrounding certain types of cells.

Chromatin: A protein substance containing the genetic code of the cell.

Chromosomes: Double strands of specifically paired proteins that contain the genetic code of a cell.

Chronic infection: An infection that is unusually prolonged, usually months beyond the normal healing period.

Cocci: Round or spherical bacteria that occur in chains, pairs, or clusters.

Colony (Colonization): A group of microbes—usually refers to the normal growth pattern of bacteria.

Commensalism: The relationship between two organisms in which one uses the other for physiological needs but causes it no harm.

Community-acquired infection: Infectious disease acquired in the community rather than in a health care facility.

Contaminated: A surface, substance, or tissue that is not completely free of microorganisms.

Cross-contamination: The spread of infection from one person to another or from an object to a person.

Culture: The process of growing a microbe in a laboratory setting so that it can be studied and tested.

Culture and sensitivity: A test in which a specific sample of bacteria is grown in the laboratory in the presence of various antibacterial agents to test the bacteria's sensitivity to them.

Cystitis: Infection of the urinary bladder.

Cytoplasm: Substance contained within the cell which contains a fluid called cystosol, and functional "organs" of the cell.

Dehiscence: Separation of the tissue edges of a surgical wound; dehiscense may be partial or involve the full thickness of the wound.

Diaphragm: Mechanism for adjusting the amount of light entering the microscope.

Diffusion: Uniform dispersal of particles in a solution or across a membrane.

Direct transmission: The transfer of microbes from their source to a new host by direct physical contact with the microbes; for example, a water droplet containing respiratory virus is exhaled by one person and inhaled by another.

Droplet nuclei: Dried remnants of previously moist secretions containing microorganisms. Droplet nuclei are an important source of disease transmission.

Endocytosis: A process by which the cell engulfs large particles in the environment.

Endoplasmic reticulum: An extension of the nuclear membrane in the cell that facilitates the movement of protein out of the nucleus.

Endospore (spore): The dormant stage of some bacteria that allows them to survive without reproducing in extreme environmental conditions, including heat, cold, and exposure to many disinfectants. When conditions are favorable for reproduction, the spore again becomes active and produces bacterial colonies.

Endotoxins: Bacterial toxins that are associated with the outer membrane of certain gram-negative bacteria. Endotoxins are not secreted but are released when the cells are disrupted or broken down.

Entry site: In microbial transmission, the sites where microorganisms enter the body.

Eukaryote: The basic type of cell; it is surrounded by a membrane and contains complex organs for metabolism and reproduction.

Evisceration: The protrusion of an internal organ through a wound or surgical incision.

Exostosis: A process in which substances are removed from a cell.

Exotoxins: Toxic substances produced by microorganisms and excreted outside the bacterial cell. Exotoxins differ in the particular tissues of the host that they may affect.

Extensively drug resistant TB (XDR TB): A strain of tuberculosis which is resistant to first and second line drugs normally used to treat TB.

Facultative: The ability of some organisms to live with or without oxygen.

Fomite: An intermediate, inanimate source in the process of disease transmission. Any object, such as a contaminated surgical instrument or medical device, can become a fomite in disease transmission.

Golgi apparatus: An extension of the endomembrane of the cell that stores, modifies, and transports large molecules.

Gram staining: A method of differential staining of bacteria that separates them into one of two groups, gram positive (accepts the stain) or gram negative (is not stained). Each group has common characteristics that identify its members and aid in diagnosis and treatment.

Hemolysis: Breakdown or rupture of red blood cells.

Host: The organism that harbors or nourishes another organism (parasite).

Immunity: The body's ability to defend itself from "nonself" substances.

Infection: The state or condition in which the body or body tissues are invaded by pathogenic microorganisms that multiply and produce injurious effects.

Inflammation: The body's nonspecific reaction to injury or infection that causes redness, heat, swelling, and pain.

Innate immunity: Non-specific immunity present from birth; the body's normal physiologic reaction to injury.

Live attenuated vaccine: Vaccine containing live virus that has been modified physically or chemically to prevent the effects of the disease.

Lysogenesis: The process whereby viruses replicate their genetic material and then cause the host cell to rupture, releasing the genetic material and forming new virions.

Lysosome: An organelle capable of releasing enzymes to kill the cell.

Macro-parasite: Large parasites such as insects and worms.

Microbes or microorgansims: Microscopic organisms such as bacteria and viruses.

Microbiology: The study of microbes, or organisms that require a microscope for observation.

Micro-parasite: Parasitic microbes.

Mitochondrion (sing); mitochondria (pl): An organelle that synthesizes adenosine triphosphate (ATP) to provide cellular energy.

Molds: A type of fungi.

Mutualism: The relationship of two organisms of different species in which both benefit by the association.

Mycotic: Referring to fungi.

Necrosis: Tissue death.

Nonpathogenic: Refers to an organism that does not cause disease in a healthy individual. About 95% to 97% of all bacteria are nonpathogenic.

Nosocomial infection: Another term for hospital-acquired infection (HAI) or healthcare-acquired infection; an infection acquired as a result of being in a health care facility.

Nucleoid: Region of the prokaryotic cell where DNA is located but not enclosed.

Nucleolus: An organelle inside the nucleus that contains proteins necessary for cell reproduction.

Nucleus: The organ structure in the cell that contains the genetic material for replication and reproduction of the cell.

Opportunistic infection: Infection occurring in a weakened individual, usually by colonization of a bacterium that does not usually cause disease. The host may be debilitated by another disease or the immune system may be compromised.

Organelles: Functional organs within the cell which perform various metabolic processes.

Osmosis: The movement of liquid through a semi-permeable membrane according to the differences in the concentration of substances in the liquid.

Parasite (parasitism): An organism that lives on or within another organism and gains an advantage at the expense of that organism. Parasitology is the study of parasites.

Passive immunity: Protection against a disease by antibodies from another person or animal. Maternal antibodies are passed to the fetus from the mother's blood, an example of passive immunity.

Passive transport: Movement of substances or liquid by diffusion or osmosis.

Pathogen: A disease-causing (**pathogenic**) microorganism.

Pathogenicity: An organism's biological and chemical mechanisms that cause disease.

Pathology: The study of disease.

Phagocyte: Any cell capable of ingesting particulate matter and microorganisms.

Phagocytosis: A defensive mechanism in which a cell engulfs a substance or another cell.

Pili: A rodlike attachment extending from the cell membrane that is capable of attaching to another cell to transfer genetic material.

Plasmid: Circular molecule of DNA located in the prokaryotic cell.

Prion: An infectious protein substance that is resistant to common sterilization methods.

Prokaryotes: Cellular organisms that lack a true nucleus or nuclear membrane. Prokaryotes include only bacteria and the Archaea, a smaller primitive group of single-cell organisms.

Resident microorganisms: The microorganisms that normally live in certain tissues of the body; also called normal flora.

Ribosomes: The site of protein synthesis for reproduction in the cell.

Spirochetes: Curved or spiral-shaped bacteria.

Spore: The highly resistant dormant stage of some bacteria. Spores can live in extreme environmental conditions, sometimes indefinitely; also called an endospore.

Stage: Area of the microscope where the slide is placed.

Staining: The process of coloring microbial specimens so that they can be seen with the optical microscope.

Standard Precautions: Guidelines recommended by the Centers for Disease Control and Prevention (CDC) to reduce the risk of transmission of blood-borne and other pathogens.

Sterile: Completely free of all microorganisms.

Strict aerobe: A microorganism that requires oxygen to live and grow.

Strict anaerobe: An organism that must live in the absence of oxygen to survive.

Suppurative: Having developed pus and fluid.

Symbiosis: The environmental relationship between two or more organisms in which each benefits from the other.

Vaccination: Injection of a small amount of disease antigen in order to stimulate the immune system to produce antibodies against the disease.

Vacuoles: Cellular compartments formed by the "pinching off" of the endomembrane.

Vector: A living intermediate carrier of microorganisms from one host to another. An example is the transmission of the bubonic plague. The vector is a flea, and the bacterium is transmitted to the human through a bite from an infected flea.

Vesicle: Cell organelle which stores substances for transport and waste.

Virion: A complete virus particle.

Virology: The study of viruses.

Virulence: The degree to which a microorganism is capable of causing disease.

Virus particle: A genetic element containing either deoxyribonucleic acid (DNA) or ribonucleic acid (RNA) that replicates in cells but is characterized by an extracellular state. It is parasitic in that it is entirely dependent on nutrients inside cells for its metabolic and reproductive needs. Viruses are different from other microbes in that they cannot reproduce their genetic material but must produce within a living host.

Yeast: Type of fungi.

INTRODUCTION

Microbiology is the study of microscopic animals and plants (i.e., those that require a microscope for observation). These organisms are called microbes or microorganisms. In the operating room, we are particularly concerned with preventing infections caused by bacteria and viruses transmitted by instruments, equipment, and personnel. To understand how disease is transmitted and prevented, we first need to study the organisms themselves and the diseases they cause. This chapter in particular (as well as other chapters) explains the relationship between microbes and **infection.** Box 7-1 presents a short summary of important events in the history of microbiology.

Microbiology is a highly complex field with many subspecialties. *Medical microbiology* is the study of infectious diseases caused by microorganisms. Subspecialties of medical microbiology are concerned with specific species (e.g., **virology, bacteriology,** and parasitology). **Pathology** is the study of disease mechanisms, diagnosis, and treatment. Nonmedical microbiology includes the study of microbios in the environment or those used in commercial products. *Plant microbiology* is an important field of study for understanding habitats in the environment and preservation of species. The study of microbial diseases in plants focuses on the development and protection of food crops.

Important Events in the History of Microbiology

1677: Anton van Leeuwenhoek develops the light microscope and observes "little animals" under magnification.
1796: Edward Jenner develops the first smallpox vaccination.
1850: Ignaz Semmelweis discovers the association between hand washing and a decrease in puerperal infection.
1861: Louis Pasteur disproves the theory of spontaneous generation and develops the germ theory of infection.
1867: Joseph Lister first practices surgery using antiseptic practices.
1876: Robert Koch offers the first proof of the germ theory using *Bacillus anthracis*.
1882: Robert Koch develops the Koch postulates. Paul Ehrlich develops the acid-fast stain.
1884: Christian Gram develops the Gram stain.
1885: Louis Pasteur develops the first rabies vaccine.
1892: Dimitri Iosifovich Ivanovski discovers the virus.
1900: Walter Reed proves that mosquitoes carry yellow fever.
1910: Paul Ehrlich discovers a cure for syphilis.
1928: Alexander Fleming discovers penicillin.
1995: The first microbe genome sequence (for *Haemophilus influenzae*) is published.

OVERVIEW OF ORGANISMS AND CELLS

CLASSIFICATION OF ORGANISMS

A system for classifying organisms enables scientists to identify and study living things. One of the earliest systems was developed approximately 300 years ago by Carol Linnaeus, and his system is called the *Linnean system*. Linnaeus greatly clarified the system of nomenclature and ranking of organisms. The Linnean system classifies living things as either plant or animal according to evolutionary descent. Since Linnaeus' work, taxonomy has become much more sophisticated, and new systems have been developed. A commonly used system in biology has seven categories or classifications, listed here from smallest to largest:

* Genus
* Family
* Order
* Class
* Phylum
* Kingdom
* Domain

CLASSIFICATION OF MICROBES

Microbes belong to a variety of different groups, both prokaryotic and eukaryotic (terms discussed later). Classification by certain characteristics within each group allows them to be identified. The important microbes in human disease are:

* Bacteria
* Viruses
* Prions
* Fungi
* Protozoa
* Rickettsiae

BINOMIAL SYSTEM

The binomial system, which was also developed by Linnaeus, is a method of naming organisms. Each organism is named specifically according to its genus and species, which are Latin or Greek words. For example, human beings are classified as genus: *Homo* and species: *sapiens.* Any scientific discussion should include the binomial name of a disease organism to differentiate it from others that cause the same disease. For example, the disease typhoid is caused by the bacterium *Salmonella typhi.* The bacterium *Salmonella enterica* has many different strains, each with its own name. When the scientific name of an organism (genus and species) is typed, the genus is capitalized *(Salmonella)* and both the genus and species are italicized *(Salmonella enterica);* when the scientific name is written, the capitalization stays the same and the name (both parts) is underlined.

THE CELL

Cell Theory

The **cell theory** was developed in the 1600s, shortly after the development of the light microscope. This theory stated that:
1. The cell is the fundamental unit of all living things.
2. All living things are composed of cells.
3. All cells are derived from other cells.
The cell theory formed the basis of modern biology.

Types of Cells

The cell is the basic unit of a living organism. Cellular organisms are divided into two types, prokaryotes and eukaryotes, each descended from different groups. Figure 7-1 shows both types of cells.

Characteristics of the Eukaryote

Plants, animals, and many types of single-celled organisms are composed of many types of cells that are basic in structure but have variations. The basic type of cell is called a **eukaryote.** All cells that make up the human body are eukaryotic cells. Different tissues are composed of variations of the eukaryote. For example, a muscle cell has features that distinguish it from a nerve cell (neuron). However, both are eukaryotes. The cells of a fish or a fungus are also eukaryotic cells.

❖ *The eukaryote is the basic cell that makes up multicellular organisms and some types of single-celled organisms. There are many different kinds of eukaryotes, but all have the same basic structure.*

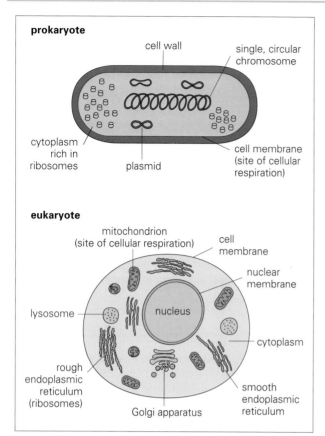

prokaryote

cell wall

single, circular
chromosome

cytoplasm
rich in
ribosomes

plasmid

cell membrane
(site of cellular
respiration)

eukaryote

mitochondrion
(site of cellular respiration)

cell
membrane

nuclear
membrane

lysosome

nucleus

cytoplasm

rough
endoplasmic
reticulum
(ribosomes)

Golgi apparatus

smooth
endoplasmic
reticulum

Figure 7-1   Eukaryote and prokaryote cells. Only bacteria
and the Archaea groups are prokaryotes. *(From Goering R,
Dockrell H, Wakelin D et al: Mim's medical microbiology,
ed 4, St Louis, 2008, Mosby.)*

A eukaryotic cell is surrounded by a double-layered membrane. Plant cells also have a cell wall that is lacking in other types of eukaryotic cells. The inside of the cell contains cytoplasm. Cytoplasm is composed of a semiclear liquid, called *cytosol,* and small organs, called organelles, which perform the cell's metabolic functions.

A eukaryotic cell has many types of organelles (Figure 7-2). The **nucleus** is the largest organelle. It is surrounded by a membrane and contains the cell's deoxyribonucleic acid (DNA), which enables the cell to replicate. The DNA is contained within the cell's **chromatin,** a protein substance that contains the genetic code for the cell. During reproduction, the chromatin forms double strands called **chromosomes.** The nuclear membrane forms a complex set of interconnected folds called the **endoplasmic reticulum,** which facilitates the movement of protein out of the nucleus.

The nucleus also contains a **nucleolus,** which has proteins and ribonucleic acid (RNA) necessary for cell reproduction. RNA transfers the cell's genetic information from the DNA in the nucleus to the ribosomes along the folds of the endoplasmic reticulum. These small organelles are the site of protein synthesis for cell reproduction.

The cell has a complex network of membranes that form compartments for the organelles. This system is called the

endomembrane system. The endomembrane can "pinch off" to form new closed compartments as needed; these are called **vacuoles.** The vacuoles do not communicate with the organelles but remain separated. They have many different functions depending on the type of cell. They may store molecules or transfer wastes out of the cell. They also wall off any harmful substances within the cell. Smaller sacs that are very similar to the vacuoles are called vesicles. Like vacuoles, they store substances and transport waste. The **Golgi apparatus** is another extension of the endomembrane. This organelle is composed of layered sacs, the function of which is to store and modify large molecules and transport them inside the cell.

The **mitochondria** are composed of a double outer membrane and numerous inner compartments formed by the folds of inner membranes. Mitochondria are responsible mainly for synthesizing a chemical called *adenosine triphosphate (ATP);* this process provides energy for the cell. Other important functions include calcium storage and regulation of cell death.

Characteristics of the Prokaryote

A **prokaryote** is one of a group of single-celled microbes; this group includes only bacteria and a smaller, primitive group of single-celled organisms called Archaea. In medicine, we are concerned with the bacteria, because they cause disease and far outnumber the Archaea.

❖   *A prokaryote is a type of single-celled organism. This group of cells includes only bacteria and the Archaea.*

A prokaryotic cell does not develop into a complex organism with tissue differentiation. The primary structural difference between a prokaryote and a eukaryote is the absence of a distinct nucleus in the prokaryote. The genetic material for the cell is coiled into an area called the nucleoid. This structure contains chromosomes, but DNA may also lie outside this region in a small circular molecule called a plasmid. The only true organelle of the prokaryote is the ribosome, which synthesizes protein.

All prokaryotes are surrounded by a cell membrane, and some have a rigid **cell wall.** The cell wall is very important in the classification of bacteria. A long filament extends from the surface of the cell. This structure may occur as a single strand *(flagellum)* or in small "tufts" *(flagella).* The flagella provide a means of motility for the prokaryotic cell. **Pili** are another type of surface extension on bacterial cells. A single *pilus* attaches to another bacterium as a means of infusing its cytoplasm and genetic material. Some bacteria can attach their pili to human tissue and can alter the body's immune response to the bacteria. Some bacteria have a **capsule,** or *slime layer.* This protects the cell from drying and also provides resistance to chemicals and invasion by viruses.

Cell Transport and Absorption

Cells absorb molecules and other substances across the cell membrane and synthesize others from substances available within the cell. The movement of substances occurs either by passive transport or active transport.

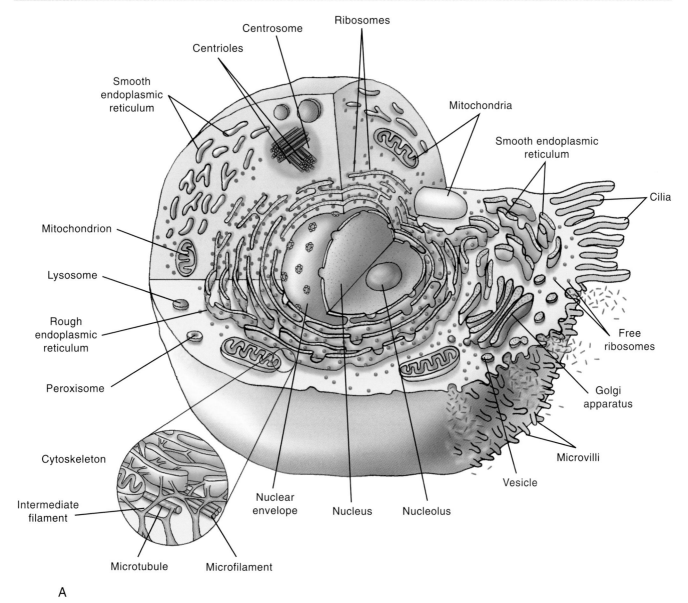

Centrosome
Centrioles
Ribosomes
Smooth endoplasmic reticulum
Mitochondria
Smooth endoplasmic reticulum
Cilia
Mitochondrion
Lysosome
Rough endoplasmic reticulum
Peroxisome
Free ribosomes
Golgi apparatus
Cytoskeleton
Microvilli
Vesicle
Intermediate filament
Nuclear envelope
Nucleus
Nucleolus
Microtubule
Microfilament

A

Figure 7-2 Eukaryote demonstrating organelles, which are units of metabolic function within the cell. *(From Thibodeau G, Patton K:* Anatomy and physiology, *ed 6, St Louis, 2007, Mosby.)*

Continued

Passive Transport

Diffusion of particles is the uniform dispersal of particles in a solution or across a membrane as a result of spontaneous movement (Figure 7-3).

Osmosis is the movement of liquid through a semipermeable membrane according to differences in the concentration of substances on either side. Because the membrane allows only certain substances to cross, the osmotic pressure depends on the nondiffusible particles on each side. Water moves from the side with fewer particles to the side with more particles. This results in dilution of the more concentrated side. Water continues to move until the concentration and water pressure are equal on both sides of the membrane (Figure 7-4).

Active Transport

The metabolic or functional requirements of a cell may require movement of substances, resulting in unequal distribution between the outside and inside of the cell. For example, the inside of the cell requires a higher concentration of potassium ions than is available in the extracellular fluid. The cell must maintain a lower concentration of sodium inside than outside. The electrical charges of the ions prevent the proper ratio of positive to negative ions inside the cell. Therefore they must be "pumped" across the membrane using energy generated from the cell. Sodium is moved out of the cell and potassium is moved into it by means of the sodium-potassium pump. This is one form of active transport. At the cellular and molecular levels, the cell doesn't actually "filter" substances. Sub-

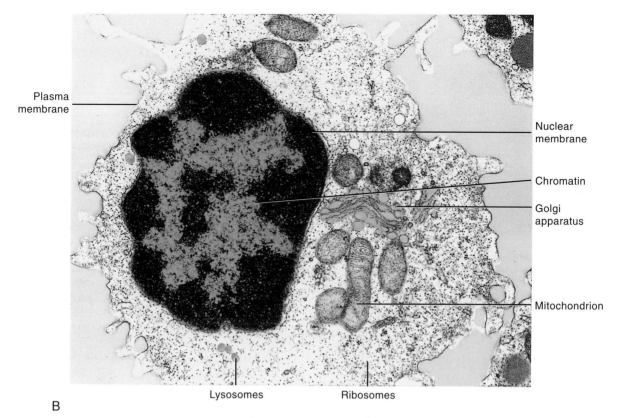

Plasma membrane

Nuclear membrane

Chromatin

Golgi apparatus

Mitochondrion

Lysosomes

Ribosomes

B

Figure 7-2, cont'd.

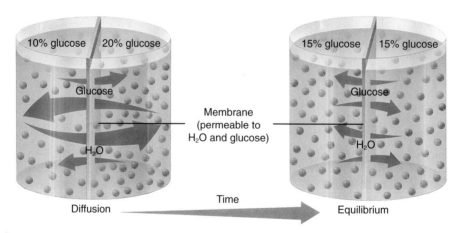

10% glucose   20% glucose

Glucose

H₂O

Diffusion

15% glucose   15% glucose

Glucose

H₂O

Equilibrium

Membrane (permeable to H₂O and glucose)

Time

Figure 7-3 Diffusion across a membrane. The container on the left shows two separate concentrations of glucose. The membrane allows glucose to pass through until the two sides are equal in concentration. *(From Thibodeau G, Patton K:* Anatomy and physiology, *ed 6, St Louis, 2007, Mosby.)*

stances are actively brought into the cell because of the properties of the molecules that make up the cell membranes.

Endocytosis is a process in which the cell engulfs large particles from outside the cell. Two types of endocytosis occur.

In *pinocytosis*, the cell takes in water and small particles by surrounding them with a membrane-covered blister or vesicle. The material is completely enclosed by the membrane and moved to the interior of the cell, where it transported to the needed location in a vesicle, or it is released from the cell.

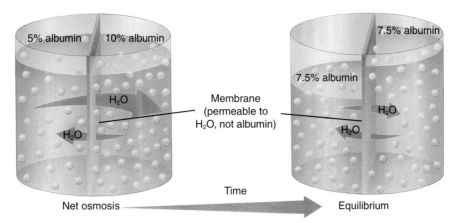

Figure 7-4 The process of osmosis, which is the passage of water through a *selectively permeable* membrane. On the left, the container holds two concentrations of albumin. On the right, the membrane has allowed water, but not albumin, to pass through, creating equilibrium. *(From Thibodeau G, Patton K: Anatomy and physiology, ed 6, St Louis, 2007, Mosby.)*

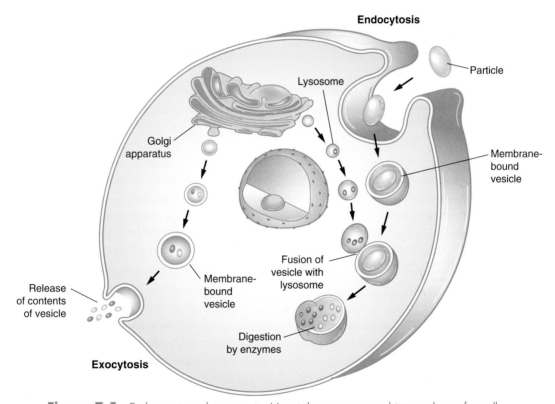

Figure 7-5 Endocytosis and exocytosis. Materials are transported into and out of a cell by means of a vesicle. Fusion of the vesicle with the lysosome causes the material to break down. The contents of the vesicle are released by exocytosis. *(From Thibodeau G, Patton K: Anatomy and physiology, ed 6, St Louis, 2007, Mosby.)*

In **phagocytosis,** large particles such as microbes are engulfed and digested by the cell. In this process, the particle is surrounded by a membrane that fuses with another cell organelle called the **lysosome.** Enzymes in the lysosome degrade and destroy the microbe cell. The contents of the lysosome are released from the cell through **exocytosis** (Figure 7-5).

MICROBE-HOST RELATIONSHIPS

Biological advances in the past decade have led to a new understanding of how microorganisms interact with the human body to cause disease. The traditional model described organisms as beneficial, neutral, or harmful. We now under-

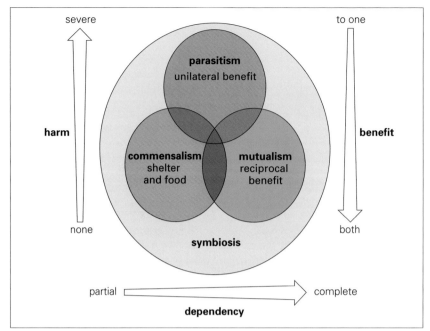

Figure 7-6 Schematic drawing of symbiotic relationships. This modern model of relationships among living things is flexible and more realistic with regard to the natural world. *(From Goering R, Dockrell H, Wakelin D et al: Mim's medical microbiology, ed 4, St Louis, 2008, Mosby.)*

stand that the microbe-**host** relationship changes according to specific conditions in the environment or in the microbe. Certain microbes cause disease when conditions are favorable for them. When conditions are favorable to the host, disease is more likely to be resisted. These variable conditions include:

- The number of microbes in the body (the *dose*)
- The physiological environment in the body (e.g., pH, temperature, amount of moisture, pressure, or presence of chemicals or immune proteins)
- The location of entry into the body (the *portal of entry*)
- The strength of the body's immune system, which determines the body's ability to recognize and destroy harmful organisms
- The disease-producing potential of the bacteria
- The number of pathogenic microorganisms that penetrate the body
- The pathogen's ability to adhere to the target tissue and secrete enzymes that destroy the target cells
- The pathogen's ability to evade the body's defense system by chemical or physical means or by mutation

The process by which organisms of two different species live together is called **symbiosis.** If neither organism is harmed, the association is called *commensalism;* **commensalism** if the association benefits both, it is called mutualism; and if one is harmed and the other benefits, it is called parasitism (Figure 7-6).

Commensalism

In **commensalism,** one organism uses another to meet its physiological needs but causes no harm to the host. For example, the human intestinal tract has many different types of bacteria, such as *Escherichia coli,* that are essential for

metabolism. The bacteria survive in balance with the body as long as they remain in the intestine. However, if *E. coli* enters the sterile tissues of the body, such as when the bowel is perforated by trauma or disease, the result can be deadly. When *E. coli* bacteria are in the bloodstream, they destroy vital organs and can cause death very quickly. This is an example of how a change in the environment of a bacterium changes its relationship with the host from commensal to parasitic.

Mutualism

In mutualism, both organisms benefit from the relationship. For example, *Staphylococcus aureus* inhabits normal healthy skin. These bacteria benefit from their environment, and they protect the skin from other invading organisms. However, the stress of disease, a break in the skin, and other conditions cause the bacteria to multiply rapidly and create infection. In this case, a mutualistic relationship turns parasitic.

Parasitism

A **parasite** is an organism that lives on or within another organism (the host) and gains an advantage at the expense of that organism. Infectious disease is the result of a parasitic relationship between the host and the invading organism. Any organism that causes infectious disease is pathogenic. Microparasites include the bacteria, viruses, protozoa, and fungi. Macroparasites are the larger organisms, which include arthropods (insects) and helminths (worms). Microparasites can overwhelm their host, and many have the potential to cause death. Macroparasites cause disease but do not usually remain in the host once they have reproduced.

Only about 3% to 5% of all microorganisms are pathogenic. However, **nonpathogenic** microbes (those that do not

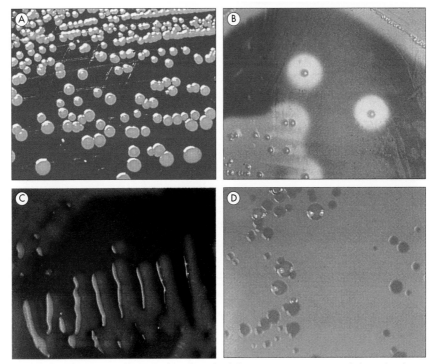

Figure 7-7 Bacteria colonies cultured in the laboratory using a Petri dish and culture media. *(From Goering R, Dockrell H, Wakelin D et al: Mim's medical microbiology, ed 4, St Louis, 2008, Mosby.)*

usually cause disease) that live in and on the body can become pathogenic under certain conditions. When this occurs, the microorganism is described as opportunistic. An opportunistic infection is one that occurs when the host is weakened in some way and its usual defenses are inadequate to prevent the parasite from causing disease.

Tools for Studying and Identifying Microbes

The study of microbes in medicine includes their identification and sensitivity to antimicrobial drugs. This requires special laboratory procedures and tools. Most basic laboratory procedures focus on the bacteria, because this group of microbes causes most infectious diseases, and accurate identification often is critical for treatment and prevention.

Culture

For identification of a particular microbe, a minimum number of colonies or individual microbes often is required to have a representative sample for study. Bacterial culturing is the most common type. After a sample of tissue or fluid is obtained from the patient or other source, a very small amount of the sample is applied to a special plate or test tube that contains a medium conducive to microbial growth. Many different types of culture media are used to grow colonies of bacteria. After the bacteria are inoculated into the culture medium, the plate or test tube is placed in a warm culturing oven for several days to a week to allow the bacteria to proliferate. Samples of the newly cultured microbes are then ready for testing and identification. Figure 7-7 shows bacterial colonies growing on culture media.

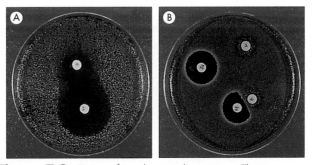

Figure 7-8 Testing for culture and sensitivity. This is a common method of determining which antibiotics are effective against a specific bacterium or fungus. Various types of antibiotic agents impregnated on paper are positioned in the culture medium, which has been inoculated with the microorganism. Note the areas of no colonization around some of the squares. *(From Goering R, Dockrell H, Wakelin D et al: Mim's medical microbiology, ed 4, St Louis, 2008, Mosby.)*

Bacteria are routinely tested for their sensitivity to antimicrobials. This is done by inoculating a culture plate with the microbe and placing small paper discs impregnated with various antibacterial agents on the sample. The procedure is called **culture and sensitivity.** The antimicrobial agents that prevent microbial growth show no cultures in that region of the culture plate. The microbe is said to be *sensitive* to that chemical. The antimicrobial discs that are *not* effective in halting microbial growth show a proliferation of colonies in the region of that agent (Figure 7-8).

Staining

Staining is a procedure used to prepare a microbial specimen for examination under the microscope. A large variety of colored stains are available to perform specific tests. Staining takes place after the microbe has been applied to a glass slide. Many staining techniques require multiple steps, which include several "baths" with different stains and meticulous care of the specimen. Bacteria commonly require staining, but fungi also may be stained for microscope viewing.

Gram Stain

Gram staining is routinely performed to differentiate bacteria into two primary classifications. The bacterial cell wall contains a layer of sugars and amino acids. In some bacteria, this wall is very thin, whereas in others it is thick. Gram staining reveals the thicker wall, and these bacteria are said to be gram positive. The bacteria with the thinner wall do not absorb the stain and are categorized as gram negative. The Gram staining procedure requires two dyes: crystal violet as the primary stain and safranin as the counterstain. Under the microscope, gram-positive bacteria appear dark purple, and gram-negative bacteria are pink (Figure 7-9).

Acid-Fast Stain

The acid-fast staining technique is used primarily for identification of *Mycobacteria* organisms, especially *Mycobacterium tuberculosis*. In this procedure, the bacteria are exposed to an acidic stain, which is retained by the cell wall. The Ziehl-Neelsen test is most commonly used. This test uses the stain carbofuschin or methylene blue, which colors the cell wall pink, leaving a blue background that is identified under the microscope. Another form of acid staining uses a fluorescent stain, which requires fluorescent microscopy for identification.

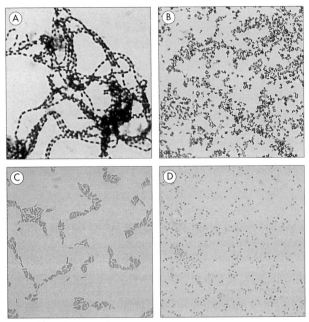

Figure 7-9 Gram staining. This technique is used to differentiate between gram-positive and gram-negative bacterial types for identification. *(From Goering R, Dockrell H, Wakelin D et al: Mim's medical microbiology, ed 4, St Louis, 2008, Mosby.)*

Biochemical Testing

Identification of the shape and size of bacteria is insufficient to establish the exact species. Tests that analyze the cell's biochemical activity are performed to differentiate bacteria. All metabolic functions are mediated by enzymes, which act on a substrate or base substance. Different biochemical tests reveal the substrates involved in metabolism and the end products. This information is used to identify specific bacteria or other microbes.

Microscopy

The Microscope and its Use

The laboratory microscope is one of the most important tools used to identify and study microbes. The microscope magnifies specimens for identification of shape, size, staining properties, and other important properties. Below is a discussion on the use of the microscope. The two main types of microscopes are the *optical microscope* and the *scanning probe microscope*. The optical microscope uses a series of lenses to focus light on the object being viewed. The light waves provide contrast, which can be enhanced by stains and other substances. The electron microscope is a type of optical microscope that uses electrons rather than light waves to provide contrast.

The scanning probe microscope uses a physical probe that tracks the contours and surfaces of the object and creates an image based on the findings. This type of microscope can view the object at a molecular level and is used in extremely fine examinations for industrial, biochemical, and medical purposes.

The optical microscope is commonly used in medical microbiology for routine identification and study of tissue, cells, and microorganisms. The simple optical microscope is pictured in Figure 7-10. Many different types of optical microscopes use an exterior or interior light source to illuminate the subject.

Parts of a Microscope

A microscope has one or two eyepieces, a series of lenses, a light source, focus adjustment, and a strong base that stabilizes the microscope. Modern microscopes use an electric light source contained inside the body or located at the bottom under the stage, where the specimen slide is placed for viewing. The following parts make up the microscope.

1. **Ocular (eyepiece):** One or two oculars are located at the top of the microscope. The viewer looks into the eyepieces, through which the image of the object is viewed. The eyepieces are directly in line with the series of lenses that focus the light and bring the image into clear view. A monocular microscope has only one eyepiece, and a binocular microscope has an eyepiece for each eye. Binocular microscopes allow adjustment of each eyepiece to accommodate the viewer's visual acuity and the distance between each eye. The eyepiece lenses are located near the top of the eyepiece.

2. **Tube:** The tube, or viewing tube, connects the eyepiece to the objective lens, which is located directly over the stage.

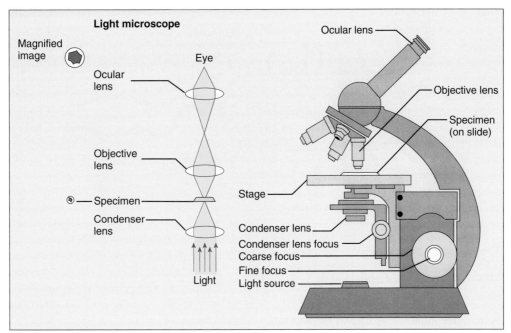

Figure 7-10 Light microscope showing the lens system and parts. *(From Erlandsen SL, Magney JE: Color atlas of histology, Figure 3-22 [p 27], St Louis, 1992, Mosby.)*

3. **Arm:** The arm connects the viewing tube to the base and balances the microscope. It also is used for carrying the microscope; one hand is placed on the base and the other around the arm.

4. **Objective lens:** This set of lenses is located at the bottom of the tube. The lens powers, or magnification, differ among microscopes. The common laboratory microscope has 10×, 40×, and 100× lenses. These are in line with the eyepiece lens, which is usually 10×. Thus the collective magnification is 10 times the power of the objective lens. Objective lenses are color coded for easy identification.

5. **Focus adjustment knobs:** Two focus adjustment knobs are located near the arm. These provide fine and coarse focus by moving the serial lenses vertically. Because the focus adjustment moves the objective lenses directly over the subject, the danger exists of direct contact (and damage) to the objective lens. Some microscopes have a rack stop to prevent this.

6. **Rack stop:** This is a vertical adjustment that prevents direct contact between the objective lens and the specimen. The rack stop is common on student microscopes to prevent damage to the objective lens (and slide).

7. **Nosepiece:** This is a round fitting for the objective lenses. The nosepiece revolves to place one of the objective lenses directly over the subject being viewed.

8. **Stage:** This is the flat area just under the objective lenses where the specimen slide is placed. The stage can be moved with knobs so that the specimen can be scanned from side to side or up and down. The slide is secured on the stage by a clip mechanism.

9. **Illuminator (light source):** Intense, evenly distributed light is needed to view the specimen. This is provided by the light source, which is located under the base of the microscope directly under the condenser. Tungsten or quartz halogen light bulbs are commonly used in the laboratory microscope.

10. **Condenser:** This mechanism is located under the stage and contains two sets of lenses that focus light on the subject. The condenser has a diaphragm, or iris, that can be adjusted to allow more or less light into the viewing area. The condenser is operated with a diaphragm lever located just under the stage.

How to Use a Microscope

Using a microscope properly requires "hands on" instruction and practice. The microscope itself is a delicate and expensive instrument with numerous components. In addition, the specimen itself requires preparation. If the slide is prepared improperly, the specimen will be damaged or obscured.

Guidelines for caring for the microscope include the following:

1. Always carry the microscope by the arm and the base, using both hands.

2. Use only laboratory-grade, lint-free lens paper to clean the objective lenses. The lenses are very delicate and can be easily scratched with coarse paper. Lint from cleaning materials can obscure the lenses.

3. Provide a clutter-free surface for the microscope during use.

4. Always store the microscope with the objective lenses in their highest position to prevent damage.

5. Never attempt to insert a slide with the objective lenses lowered.

6. Store the microscope in a dust-free environment with a cover.

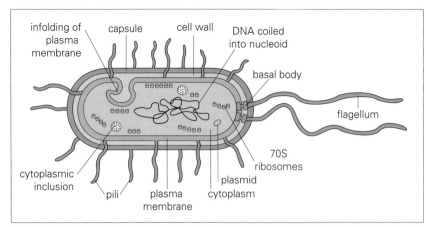

Figure 7-11 Generalized bacterial cell. Note both the cell wall and the plasma membrane, which differentiate the prokaryote from most eukaryotic cells. A wide variation in morphology is seen among bacteria types. *(From Goering R, Dockrell H, Wakelin D et al: Mim's medical microbiology, ed 4, St Louis, 2008, Mosby.)*

The microscope requires some setting up and adjustments in the illumination system before use. Once these are accomplished, a simple specimen can be used to practice with the microscope. Below are the steps to prepare a simple specimen for viewing under the microscope.

1. Prepare the specimen using a glass slide and cover slip. (Slides that have been commercially prepared beforehand are best for learning in the beginning.)
2. Make sure the lowest power objective is in position over the stage. It should be placed in its closest position over the specimen.
3. Position the slide specimen on the stage and secure the spring clip. The stage should be centered under the objective.
4. Observe the specimen through the eyepiece. Slowly raise the objective using the coarse adjustment knob. Use the fine focus adjustment to clarify the image.
5. Use the condenser diaphragm to adjust the amount of light, which is critical for a clear view.
6. View the specimen on the next highest power by turning the nosepiece. Do not move the specimen.
7. Use the fine focus adjustment to clarify the image.
8. Immersion oil is required to view images with the red-coded objective lens. This further focuses the light.

MICROORGANISMS AND DISEASE

BACTERIA

Bacteria are prokaryotic organisms. They represent a very large population of microbes in the environment and affect animals, humans, and plants. Most live without harm to other organisms. However, a few species cause serious disease. Bacteria that cause infection are called *pyogenic*. This group includes streptococcal, staphylococcal, meningococcal, pneumococcal, and gonococcal organisms, and the coliform (intestinal) bacilli. These organisms typically cause suppuration (pus) and tissue destruction that can lead to systemic involvement and ultimately death.

Structure

Bacteria represent the largest variety of infectious microorganisms and cause the greatest number of postoperative infections and other hospital-acquired infections (HAIs). Bacteria exist in a variety of shapes, sizes, and forms, which are created by the cell wall. Bacteria can exist singly or in groups, called colonies. Figure 7-11 shows a generalized bacterium.

Identification of specific bacteria is an important goal in the diagnosis of infectious diseases. Many tests can be performed on bacterial cells to identify their exact classification and disease potential. Other tests are performed to determine the organisms' susceptibility to antibacterial drugs.

Bacteria are partially classified according to their shape (Figure 7-12). This can be determined by staining the bacteria and observing them under the microscope. Bacteria take the following shapes:

- Rod-shaped bacteria are **bacilli,** which occur singly or in pairs, chains, or filaments. Rods can be slightly curved or straight.
- Curved or spiral-shaped bacteria are **spirochetes,** which may be coiled or loosely curved.
- Spherical bacteria are **cocci,** which occur singly (micrococci), in chains (streptococci), in pairs (diplococci), or in clusters (staphylococci).
- Other shapes sometimes seen are square and tetrahedral, but these are less common.

Motility

Bacteria move using a number of different kinds of mechanisms. The flagella and pili described previously are the most common methods. The flagella rotate and propel the cell in different directions. Pili also create motility by anchoring to a surface and retracting, which allows the pili to move the cell along. Some bacteria move by using the host's cytoskeleton, a network of filaments within the cytoplasm.

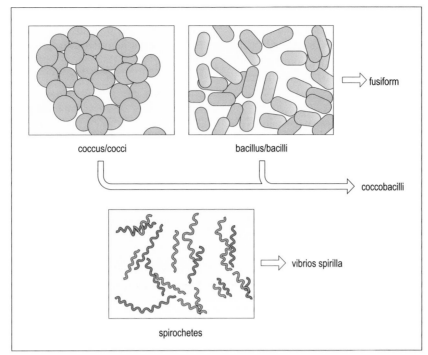

Figure 7-12 The three basic shapes of bacteria. *(From Goering R, Dockrell H, Wakelin D et al: Mim's medical microbiology, ed 4, St Louis, 2008, Mosby.)*

Environmental and Nutrient Requirements

Important environmental parameters for all microorganisms include temperature, oxygen, pH, moisture, and atmospheric pressure. Bacteria are found everywhere in the natural world, living under a wide variety of conditions. Those that infect human beings require moderate conditions.

Bacteria that produce spores can live in temperature ranges of −4° to 194°F (−20° to 90°C). Oxygen requirements for bacteria vary widely. Some require oxygen to live and grow (strict **aerobes**). Others cannot live in the presence of oxygen; these are called strict **anaerobes.** Anaerobes are important in the process of infection, because they can proliferate in deep traumatic or surgical wounds. **Facultative bacteria** can live with or without oxygen.

Bacteria have evolved to withstand extremes of the pH spectrum. For example, the normal pH of blood is 7.35 to 7.45. *Helicobacter pylori* can invade the gastric mucosa and reproduce at a pH of 2. The normal pH in the body prevents most pathogenic organisms from proliferating, but a change in pH can destroy the normal "resident" bacteria and allow pathogens to invade the body.

Bacteria that are significant in infectious disease prefer a moist environment. One method of destroying bacteria is *desiccation* (drying). Resistance to drying makes bacteria such as mycobacteria, which cause tuberculosis, a public health problem, because the bacteria can spread through dried sputum.

Bacteria obtain nutrient substances from their immediate environment. Some bacteria can synthesize many nutrients from substances available within the cell. Others require a more complex variety of organic compounds, which they take in from their environment. Most bacteria require basic elemental nutrients:

- Carbon
- Oxygen
- Nitrogen
- Hydrogen
- Phosphorus
- Sulfur
- Potassium

Reproduction

Bacterial cells reproduce by asexual fission into two new cells. In this process, the genetic material is replicated and moves to separate areas of the cell. A septal membrane develops, splitting the mother cell into two halves, which separate into daughter cells.

Some bacteria are capable of producing a vegetative reproductive form called an **endospore** (commonly referred to as a **spore**). This is a dormant phase in the reproductive cycle in which the bacteria form a thick, multilayered protein wall around their genetic material. The wall resists extreme environmental conditions such as boiling, drying, chemical destruction, and high pressure. When environmental conditions are favorable, the spore becomes active and growth (**colonization**) begins. Two important spore-forming bacteria are *Clostridium tetani* (tetanus) and *Bacillus anthracis* (anthrax).

Bacterial Growth

Bacteria grow at a rate that corresponds to their environment and nutritional status. A favorable environment, one that meets the bacteria's essential requirements, results in more rapid growth than an environment in which the bacteria has to compete for resources. In the laboratory, bacteria can be provided with essential environmental and nutritive requirements. In this way, their growth patterns can be studied.

Bacteria show four characteristic phases of growth:

1. **Lag phase:** This period occurs immediately after the growth medium is inoculated with the sample bacteria. During this phase, the bacteria do not divide, but they may be processing or synthesizing components of the growth medium in preparation for cell division. This is a period of increased metabolism for the bacteria as they adjust to the environment.
2. **Exponential (log) phase:** This phase is characterized by active and sometimes rapid cell division. The rate usually is constant, depending on the growth medium. This rate often is referred to as the *doubling time* or *generation time* of the bacteria.
3. **Stationary phase:** In this phase, the bacteria have used up their available nutrition in the growth medium and the amount of space available for growth. The by-products of reproduction have accumulated, and these inhibit further growth. During this phase, cell division stops.
4. **Death phase:** In the restricted culture medium, the death phase follows the stationary phase. The bacteria can no longer survive, and the colony dies out, usually at the same rate as the growth phase.

Pathogenicity

Bacteria cause disease by gaining entry into the host and colonizing tissue. Bacteria have many different mechanisms for adhering to host cells and evading the immune system. They can overcome and destroy the body's defensive white blood cells. Some are capable of hemolysis, the destruction of red blood cells. One of the most potent pathogenic mechanisms of bacteria is the toxins released by the bacterial cell.

Endotoxins are chemicals contained within the cell wall of bacteria. When the bacterial cell ruptures, endotoxins are released into the bloodstream and spread to different organ systems. The toxic effects of these substances include fever, diarrhea, shock, extreme weakness, and sometimes death.

Exotoxins are proteins produced as a result of bacterial metabolism. Exotoxins break down surrounding tissue, which allows the **pathogen** to spread and colonize freely. Exotoxins enter specific body cells and disrupt the cell's chemical and physical structure. For example, *Clostridium botulinum* produces a highly concentrated toxin that damages the nerve-muscle mechanism and causes paralysis in the host. Exotoxins released by bacteria and other microbes are listed in Table 7-1.

Important Bacterial Pathogens
Gram-Positive Cocci

Gram-positive cocci are responsible for about one third of all bacterial infections in human beings. Many are responsible for surgical site infections. They produce pus, and some are resistant to antibiotic therapy.

The streptococci are further classified by their ability to reduce the levels of iron in hemoglobin, through hemolysis. Two groups of hemolytic streptococci are the *alpha-hemolytic* streptococci and the *beta-hemolytic* streptococci.

Staphylococcus aureus

Staphylococcus aureus is the most widespread cause of surgical site infections. It normally resides in healthy skin, but when transmitted to the surgical wound by direct or indirect contact, it can cause an infection. From 30% to 70% of people are skin carriers of *S. aureus*. When confined to the surgical wound itself, it produces copious amounts of pus, which spreads and erodes tissues. The organism also causes endocarditis (infection of the lining of the heart) when it colonizes heart valves. Invasion of the bone causes osteomyelitis.

Staphylococcus epidermis

Staphylococcus epidermidis is a normal resident of the skin. However, it can cause infection in other parts of the body when spread by medical devices such as catheters, prosthetic valves, and orthopedic implants.

Streptococcus pyogenes

Many HAIs are caused by *Streptococcus pyogenes* (a group A beta-hemolytic streptococcus). This potentially lethal pathogen causes surgical site infection; it spreads via the lymphatic system to other sites in the body, causing anaerobic infection and tissue death (necrosis). Burn patients are particularly vulnerable to streptococcal infection. Surgical site infection is most commonly caused by **direct transmission** from a contaminated surface.

Streptococcus pneumoniae

Streptococcus pneumoniae, is the primary cause of pneumonia and otitis media (middle ear infection). The pathogen is spread mainly through the respiratory tract. It colonizes the nose and nasopharynx and then spreads to the lungs and middle ear. The bacteria are coated with a thick capsule and cell wall, which prevent its destruction by the body's white blood cells. Because of this resistance mechanism, respiratory disease caused by *S. pneumonia* can be fatal in children and the elderly.

Gram-Negative Rods and Cocci (Aerobic)
Pseudomonas aeruginosa

Pseudomonas aeruginosa is found in the normal gastrointestinal tract and in sewage, dirt, and water. It has emerged as an increasingly important pathogen in hospitalized patients. It can infect nearly all body systems. *P. aeruginosa* infection is especially prevalent in burn patients who lack healthy skin as a barrier against the airborn bacteria. *P. aeruginosa* can cause septicemia (systemic vascular infection), osteomyelitis, urinary tract infection, and endocarditis. It is highly resistant to antimicrobial agents.

Neisseria gonorrhoeae

Gonorrhea is a sexually transmitted disease spread from person to person by direct contact with *N. gonorrhoeae*. The infection usually remains localized in the reproductive tract

Table 7-1
Bacterial Toxins and Diseases

Bacteria	Exotoxin	Tissue Damaged	Mechanism	Disease
Clostridium tetani	Tetanospasmin	Neurons	Spastic paralysis	Tetanus
Clostridium perfringens	Alpha-toxin	Erythrocytes, platelets, leukocytes, endothelium	Cell lysis	Gas gangrene
Clostridium botulinum	Neurotoxin	Nerve-muscle junction	Flaccid paralysis	Botulism
Corynebacterium diphtheriae	Diphtheria toxin	Throat, heart, peripheral nerve	Inhibits protein synthesis	Diphtheria
Shigella dysenteriae	Enterotoxin	Intestinal mucosa	Fluid loss from intestinal cells	Dysentery
Escherichia coli	Enterotoxin	Intestinal epithelium	Fluid loss from intestinal cells	Gastroenteritis
Vibrio cholerae	Enterotoxin	Intestinal epithelium	Fluid loss from intestinal cells	Cholera
Staphylococcus aureus	Alpha-toxin	Red and white cells (via cytokines)	Hemolysis	Abscesses
	Hemolysin	Red and white cells (via cytokines)	Hemolysis	Abscesses
	Leukocidin	Leukocytes	Destroys leukocytes	Abscesses
	Enterotoxin	Intestinal cells	Induces vomiting, diarrhea	Food poisoning
	TSST1	—	Release of cytotoxins	Toxic shock syndrome
	Epidermolytic	Epidermis	Cell lysis	Scalded skin syndrome
Streptococcus pyogenes	Streptolysin O and S	Red and white cells	Hemolysis	Hemolysis, pyogenic lesion
	Erythrogenic	Skin capillaries	Inflammation	Scarlet fever
Bacillus anthracis	Cytotoxin	Lung	Pulmonary edema	Anthrax
Bordetella pertussis	Pertussis toxin	Trachea	Destruction of epithelium	Whooping cough
Legionella pneumophila	Numerous	Neutrophils	Cell lysis	Legionnaire's disease
Listeria monocytogenes	Hemolysin	Leukocytes, monocytes	Cell lysis	Listeriosis
Pseudomonas aeruginosa	Exotoxin A	Cell lysis	Cell lysis	Various infections

but may become systemic. The bacteria can cause blindness in the newborn of an infected mother; however, this can be prevented by instilling antibiotic into the newborn's eyes. If the disease is not treated, it may lead to sterility and endocarditis.

Neisseria meningitidis

Bacterial meningitis is a highly contagious infection of the meninges which cover the brain and spinal cord. Two forms of the disease are caused by *Neisseria meningitidis*, one that is transient and resolves spontaneously and a more serious form that can result in seizures, respiratory arrest and coma.

Bordetella pertussis

Bordetella pertussis is a bacterium that causes whooping cough, a life-threatening disease in children. Vaccination against *B. pertussis* has reduced the mortality rate significantly. Before the vaccine was developed, whooping cough was a major killer of children.

Enteric bacteria

The enteric bacteria are also gram-negative rods; however, they are facultative anaerobes and can grow in an oxygen-poor environment. This group of pathogens inhabits the intestinal tract of human beings in both a disease state and as resident (normal) bacteria.

Escherichia coli

E. coli organisms are resident bacteria of the gastrointestinal tract. Postoperative infection caused by this bacterium occurs when the organisms are transmitted via a contaminated object such as a urinary endoscope or catheter. Direct transmission occurs when the gastrointestinal tract is perforated and bowel contents spill into the sterile peritoneal cavity. *E. coli* is the most common cause of urinary tract infections. In the bloodstream, *E. coli* can spread to other organs and cause severe tissue destruction or death.

Salmonella enterica

S. enterica is a common cause of food poisoning (acute gastroenteritis). The bacterial infection is spread from person to person by contaminated food and fecal contact. The disease causes diarrhea, vomiting, and fever, which usually resolve without treatment.

Salmonella typhi

As mentioned previously, the bacteria *S. typhi* causes the disease typhoid. The infection is spread via contaminated water and food. In communities where sewage treatment is lacking, the bacteria can contaminate local drinking water and cause widespread infection. Bacterial colonies can persist in the intestine long after antibiotic treatment, and a disease carrier may continue to infect others while showing no symptoms.

When ingested, the bacteria penetrate the intestinal wall and enter the mesenteric lymph nodes. They release a powerful endotoxin that enters the bloodstream and causes septicemia, cardiovascular infection, and death. Several types of typhoid vaccine are available, but the vaccine usually is given only to individuals at risk, such as those traveling or working in an area where sanitation is poor.

Spore-Forming Bacteria

The spore-forming bacteria are significant because of their ability to resist destruction. They are extremely important in the health care setting. In the perioperative setting, any process of sterilization is defined by its ability to destroy not only all microbes but also bacterial spores.

Clostridium perfringens

Clostridium perfringens is an anaerobic bacteria that causes rapid tissue death in deep wounds deprived of oxygen. This is a relatively rare infection, but it does occur in health care settings. Historically, it has been a common infection of deep, penetrating, combat wounds. In true gas gangrene, the tissue is destroyed by the toxins of the *C. perfringens* bacilli. *C. novyi* bacilli, another type of clostridia, invade the necrotic tissue and release toxic gases Systemic absorption of these gases is fatal. The disease is transmitted directly from a contaminated source to an open or penetrating wound.

Clostridium tetani

Clostridium tetani is the causative bacteria of tetanus, a disease of the nervous system. *C. tetani* bacterium is an anaerobic organism commonly found in soil and intestinal tract of humans and other mammals. The toxins released by the bacilli travel along the peripheral nerve pathways, eventually reaching the central nervous system. Severe muscle spasm, convulsions, and eventual paralysis of the respiratory system lead to death from asphyxia. Transmission is through direct contact with the bacilli usually through an open or penetrating wound.

Clostridium difficile

Clostridium difficile is a spore-forming bacterium that cause severe diarrhea. It is easily spread among patients who are immunocompromised, and the infection can be rapidly fatal. Strict attention to asepsis, especially hand washing, is needed to control its spread in the health care setting.

Mycobacterial Infections

As mentioned previously, the bacillus *Mycobacterium tuberculosis* causes the disease tuberculosis (TB). The human strain of the bacterium causes dense nodules or tubercles to form in localized areas of the body, including the lungs, liver, spleen, and bone marrow. Lung involvement occurs in all cases.

Tuberculosis is a serious concern in areas where people live or work in crowded conditions. Multidrug-resistant strains of

M. tuberculosis are increasingly common throughout the world. TB kills about 3 million people and infects about 9 million every year worldwide. The organism primarily causes respiratory disease, but it also can infect other areas of the body, including vital organs. The infection is spread by inhalation of the bacteria in droplets or dust containing dried mycobacteria. The infection can be introduced into the body via medical equipment such as respiratory diagnostic equipment or anesthesia equipment.

After the bacteria have entered the respiratory system, they are engulfed by white blood cell components. The mycobacteria that are not destroyed by the body become encased in granular "tubercles," which remain in the lungs. These become calcified and fibrotic. If the infected person's immune system becomes weakened, the bacteria can again become active.

Rickettsiae

Rickettsiae are a type of bacteria carried by specific species of ticks, mites, and fleas. The insect transmits the bacteria to its host through a skin bite. Once the bacteria enter the host's body, they move through the bloodstream and attach to the inner lining of the blood vessels (endothelium). The cell then ingests the bacteria. Once inside the cell, the bacteria destroy it by releasing enzymes and continue to multiply and enter other host cells. Rickettsiae are identified by staining, using the same techniques as those for bacteria in general.

Diseases caused by Rickettsiae include typhus, Q fever, and Rocky Mountain spotted fever. Rickettsial disease can persist in the body for long periods. Prevention of disease involves avoiding exposure to ticks, fleas, and mites that carry the bacteria.

Important bacterial diseases are listed in Table 7-2.

VIRUSES

A **virus** is a nonliving infectious agent that ranges in size from 10 to 300 nm. A virus is not a cell. It is referred to as a virus particle. A complete virus particle is called a virion. These agents cause some of the most lethal infections known. Although they can be extremely pathogenic, they are unable to metabolize outside the host cell. While inside the host's cells, they are unable to infect another individual. Viruses are transmitted by inhalation, in food or water, and by direct transmission from an infected host via blood or body fluids. Some viruses may also be transmitted by insects. Viruses are found throughout the living environment and cause disease in many different organisms.

Classification

Viruses are classified by a number of complex systems and categories, such as by morphology (shape and structure), chemical composition, and method of replication.

Morphology

A virion consists of a double or single strand of either DNA or RNA. This genetic material is surrounded by a protein coating (capsid). The total structure is called a nucleocapsid. Depending on the type of virus, the nucleocapsid can take on

Table 7-2

Important Bacterial Infections

7-2A: GRAM-POSITIVE COCCI

Organism	Major Infection	Less Common Infection	Vaccine Preventable
Staphylococci			
S. epidermidis	Bacteremia in immuno-compromised individuals	Most often associated with indwelling devices	No
S. saprophyticus	Urinary tract infections	—	No
S. aureus	Boils, impetigo, wound infections, osteomyelitis, septicemia	Pneumonia, endocarditis, toxic shock syndrome, food poisoning	No
Streptococci			
Beta-Hemolytic			
S. pyogenes (group A)	Tonsillitis, impetigo, cellulitis, scarlet fever (rheumatic fever, glomerulonephritis)	Puerperal sepsis, erysipelas, septicemia	No
Alpha-Hemolytic			
S. pneumoniae	Pneumonia, otitis media	Meningitis, septicemia	Yes (some serotypes)
S. viridans	Dental caries	Subacute bacterial endocarditis	No
Group D Streptococci			
S. faecalis (enterococci) (Enterococcus faecalis)	Urinary tract infections, wound infections, intraabdominal abscess	Bacteremia, endocarditis	No

7-2B: GRAM-NEGATIVE COCCI AND COCCOBACILLI

Organism	Major Infection	Less Common Infection	Vaccine Preventable
Neisseria			
N. meningitidis	Meningitis, septicemia	Arthritis	Yes (serogroups A/C)
N. gonorrhoeae	Gonorrhea, pelvic inflammatory disease	Arthritis, conjunctivitis	No

7-2C: AEROBIC GRAM-POSITIVE BACILLI

Organism	Major Infection	Less Common Infection	Vaccine Preventable
Spore Forming			
Bacillus			
B. anthracis	Anthrax	—	Yes
Non–Spore Forming			
Listeria			
L. monocytogenes	Neonatal sepsis, meningitis	Septicemia in immunocompromised individuals	No
Corynebacterium			
C. diphtheriae	Diphtheria	Skin infections	Yes
C. urealyticum	Cystitis	—	No
C. jeikeium	Infection associated with prosthetic devices and intravenous or cerebrospinal fluid (CSF) catheters		No

Modified from Hart T, Shears P: *Color atlas of medical microbiology*, London, 2000, Mosby.

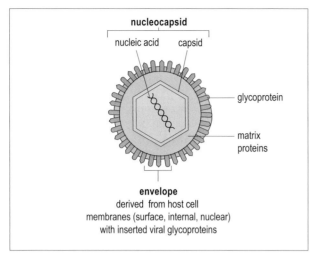

Figure 7-13 Construction of the virus, showing the envelope and nucleocapsid. *(From Goering R, Dockrell H, Wakelin D et al: Mim's medical microbiology, ed 4, St Louis, 2008, Mosby.)*

many different complex geometric shapes. Some virions are enclosed in a membrane, or envelope, derived from the host cell (Figure 7-13). A virion has no organelles.

Replication and Transmission

Although viruses contain genetic material, they cannot replicate without a host cell. To replicate, they inject their DNA or RNA into another cell and dissolve its genetic material. The virus uses the host cell's physiological mechanisms to replicate its own genetic material. The virus then synthesizes new capsids, assembles new virions, and ruptures the cell to release them. The cycle of replication and lysis (bursting) of the host cell is called **lysogenesis.**

Some types of viruses remain inside the host cell in latent form. In this state the virus is not infective, but it continues to replicate. Under certain favorable conditions, the virus begins to replicate more actively and produces disease symptoms, perhaps years later. Examples of viruses that follow this cycle are the herpes simplex virus and the poliovirus.

A virus that invades bacterial cells is called a **bacteriophage** (Figure 7-14). Bacteriophages are widely dispersed throughout living organisms and may display a parasitic, commensal, or symbiotic relationship with their bacterial host. Bacteriophages

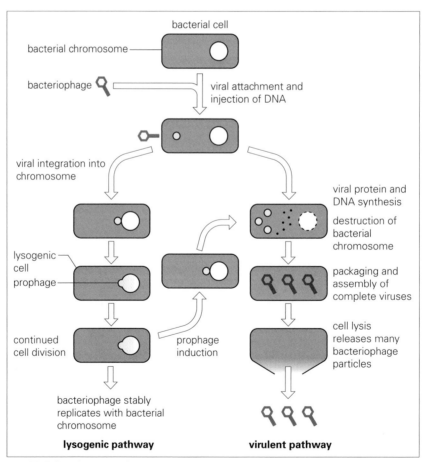

Figure 7-14 Life cycle of the viral bacteriophage. The bacteriophage is a viral bacterium that can survive outside or inside the bacterium and reproduce using the bacterial cell. *(From Goering R, Dockrell H, Wakelin D et al: Mim's medical microbiology, ed 4, St Louis, 2008, Mosby.)*

can replicate and spread through lysogenesis or remain inside the bacterial cell. Alteration of the bacteria's genetic code can provide beneficial as well as harmful results. Modification of genetic material can cause antibiotic resistance in bacteria. Bacteriophages are currently being tested for use in medicine and food production as a way to destroy harmful bacteria.

Viruses are also capable of transforming normal cells into cancerous cells, which lose their original functional and metabolic characteristics through genetic changes. These cells divide rapidly and develop into tumor tissue. Specific cancer-inducing viruses include the hepatitis A virus and certain types of the human papilloma virus.

Pathogenicity

Pathogenicity is defined less clearly in viruses than in bacteria. We know some of the mechanisms that create and sustain viral disease in certain strains. These include the following:

- **The ability to enter a healthy cell:** The virus enters the host cell by attaching to its membrane or wall, where it is absorbed by phagocytosis.
- **The ability to develop:** The virus is able to redirect the cell's genetic material to viral replication rather than cell reproduction.
- **The ability to resist the host's defense mechanisms:** The virus may be recognized by the body's immune system, which attacks its own cell, killing it.
- **Cell transformation:** The virus's ability to mutate the cell can result in the formation of cancer growth in some cells.
- **The ability to synthesize substances not normally produced by the host cell.**
- **The ability to initiate structural changes in the host cell:** These changes lead to cell death or to abnormalities that alter the cell's functions.

Pathogenic Viruses

Human Immunodeficiency Virus/Acquired Immunodeficiency Syndrome

Infection with the human immunodeficiency virus (HIV) is pandemic (a worldwide epidemic). Approximately 39 million cases of HIV have been reported worldwide (Joint United Nations Committee on HIV/AIDS and the Work Health Organization [UNAIDS/WHO], 2006). The global effect of acquired immunodeficiency syndrome (AIDS) has changed practices and procedures in health care dramatically.

HIV is transmitted via blood-to-blood contact, sexual contact, and contact with certain body fluids. The body fluids known to transmit HIV are:

- Blood
- Semen
- Vaginal secretions
- Breast milk
- Cerebrospinal fluid
- Synovial fluid
- Amniotic fluid
- Any body fluid containing blood

HIV may be transmitted when the body fluids of an infected person are deposited on the mucous membranes or into the vascular system of another person. Sexual contact and use of contaminated needles are primary modes of transmission in the general public. The risk of transmission during sexual contact increases when partners also are infected with another sexually transmitted disease. HIV can be transmitted to the fetus in utero and to the infant who receives breast milk from an infected mother. A neonate also may be infected during delivery.

Casual contact with an infected person does not transmit the virus. Although HIV has been found in saliva, tears, and sweat, the number of pathogens found in these body fluids has been very small. Contact with these fluids has not been shown to result in the transmission of HIV. Occupational risk to health care workers is highest in needlestick and other sharps injuries. There is little evidence of a risk of transmission from an infected health care worker to a patient.

A person infected with HIV may be show no symptoms yet still transmit the disease to others. This is because early in the disease process, the body's immune system is able to attack the virus. As long as such individuals are not tested, they may continue to transmit the disease to others without realizing that they are infected. Weeks after the initial infection, mild illness occurs, followed by increasingly serious disease manifestations. Years may pass before symptoms of AIDS begin to appear. The conversion from HIV infection to AIDS-related complex to AIDS is poorly understood. HIV infection is confirmed by the presence of specific antibodies.

AIDS is not a separate disease organism but a syndrome that results from infection with the HIV virus. Patients with AIDS lack normal immune response, and certain diseases are common in these individuals. A true diagnosis of AIDS is made when the presence of one or more of these diseases is confirmed (Box 7-2). Currently, AIDS has no cure. However, the disease now can be controlled with drug therapy.

Extensive information about AIDS and its treatment can be found on Web sites for the Centers for Disease Control and Prevention (CDC) and the United Nations Committee on HIV/AIDS.[1]

Viral Hepatitis

Viral hepatitis is a disease of the liver that is caused by one of five significant viruses. The hepatitis B, C, and D viruses are blood-borne pathogens, which are transmitted when blood from an infected person enters the body of another person (a transmission similar to that for HIV). Hepatitis A and hepatitis E are transmitted through contaminated food or water.

The hepatitis A virus (HAV) is transmitted by ingestion and by close contact with an infected person. Fecal and oral routes are the common modes of transmission. This virus cannot be cultured, but hepatitis can be diagnosed through a serological test that shows the presence of antibodies to HAV. Hepatitis A is rarely fatal, and one infection results in permanent immunity to the disease.

Infection with the hepatitis B virus (HBV) causes chronic hepatitis, cirrhosis, massive liver necrosis, and death. Like HIV, HBV is transmitted through blood and body fluids. The virus is 100 more times infective than HIV. It can be spread through sexual contact and is found in most body secretions.

Box 7-2

Opportunistic Infections and Tumors in Acquired Immunodeficiency Syndrome (AIDS)

Viruses
Disseminated cytomegalovirus (lungs, retina, brain)
Herpes simplex virus (lungs, gastrointestinal tract, central nervous system [CNS], skin)
JC papovavirus (brain: progressive multifocal leukoencephalopathy)
Epstein-Barr virus (EBV)

Bacteria*
Mycobacteria (e.g., *Mycoplasma avium, Mycobacterium tuberculosis:* disseminated, extrapulmonary)
Salmonella (recurrent, disseminated; septicemia)

Protozoa
Toxoplasma gondii (disseminated, including the CNS)
Cryptosporidium (gastrointestinal tract: chronic diarrhea)
Isospora (gastrointestinal tract: diarrhea persisting longer than 1 month)

Fungi
Pneumocystis carinii (lungs: pneumonia)
Candida albicans (esophagus, lung)
Cryptococcus neoformans (CNS)
Histoplasma capsulatum (disseminated, extrapulmonary)
Coccidioides (disseminated, extrapulmonary)

Tumors
Kaposi sarcoma†
B-cell lymphoma (e.g., brain; some are EBV induced)

Other
Wasting disease (cause unknown)
Human immunodeficiency virus (HIV) encephalopathy (AIDS dementia complex)

Data from Goering R, Dockrell H, ZuckermanM, Wakelin D, Roitt I, Mims C Chiodini P: *Mims'Medical microbiology,* ed 2, London, 1998, Mosby.
*Also pyogenic bacteria (e.g., *Haemophilus, Streptococcus, Pneumococcus* spp.), which cause septicemia, pneumonia, meningitis, osteomyelitis, arthritis, abscesses, and other diseases; multiple or recurrent infections, especially in children.
†Associated with human herpes virus 8, an independently transmitted agent; 300 times more common in AIDS than in other immunodeficiency conditions.

Infected mothers also pass it to infants in 70% to 90% of births. Infected infants have a 90% chance of becoming chronic (long term) carriers.

The incubation period of HBV is 10 to 12 weeks, during which time the virus can be detected through serological testing. The disease causes general weakness, arthralgia, myalgia, and severe anorexia. Fever and upper abdominal pain also may be present. Some patients develop cirrhosis and liver cancer as a complication of the disease. There is no cure for the disease so only the symptoms are treated. However, a safe, effective vaccine is available, and all health care workers and those coming in contact with blood products or body fluids should be vaccinated.

Hepatitis C virus (HCV) is transmitted by blood transfusions and blood products. The virus also is found in saliva, urine, and semen. Health care workers, those who receive blood transfusions, intravenous drug abusers, organ transplant recipients, and hemodialysis patients are at high risk for the disease. The symptoms are similar to but milder than those of hepatitis B. About 50% of patients develop chronic hepatitis and cirrhosis and may require liver transplantation. The highest rates of infection are found in transfusion recipients and intravenous drug abusers. HCV is a causal agent of liver cancer.

Hepatitis D virus (HDV) is associated with HBV as a coinfection. It is a blood-borne virus that is acquired as a secondary infection with HBV or as a result of HBV. When the two infections occur together, they result in more rapid liver destruction and more severe clinical manifestations than HBV alone.

Hepatitis E is caused by a the hepatitis E virus. It causes serious acute liver disease and is transmitted by contaminated water. The disease is does not develop into chronic form.

Human Papilloma Virus

The human papilloma virus (HPV) is a potentially cancer-producing virus that occurs in about 15% of the population. Approximately 40 types of HPV exist, although only a few of them are oncogenic. The virus is found throughout the animal population but is species specific. It is transmitted through sexual contact and therefore is a significant public health concern. Both men and women can be affected. Chronic HPV infection is likely to develop into cervical cancer in women and noninvasive penile and anal cancer in men. The virus types are divided into two groups: high risk and low risk (for cancer association). Some of the low risk types cause genital warts (condylomata), which can be removed. However, the virus may persist in the body after removal of the lesions.

HPV may cause no symptoms and can lie dormant for many years. Predictors for HPV in women include:
- Women under 25 years of age
- Multiple sex partners
- Early onset of sexual activity (younger than 16 years old)
- Male partner with a history of multiple partners

Predictors in men include multiple partners. Disease rates are higher in the males having sex with males (MSM) population.

A vaccine for HPV is available for girls and young women. No evidence supports the effectiveness of the vaccine for men. A routine Papanicolaou (PAP) test is one of the best methods of preventing cervical cancer in women. The PAP test detects changes in the cervical endothelium caused by the HPV virus. Information on HPV from the CDC can be found at http://www.cdc.gov/STD/Hpv/hpv-clinicians-brochure.htm.

PRIONS

The **prion** (a proteinaceous infectious particle) is a unique pathogenic substance. It is a protein particle that contains no nucleic acid. It is believed to be a modified form of normal cellular protein that arises through mutation. It then is transmitted by ingestion or direct contact, especially during medical or surgical procedures. Prions are resistant to all forms of disinfection and sterilization normally used in the medical setting. They cannot be cultured in the laboratory, and the immune system does not react to them. Only a few prion diseases affect human beings. The most important is Creutzfeldt-Jakob disease (CJD) and newly emergent variant CJD, which are always fatal.

CJD is a rare transmissible disease of the nervous system that is progressive and always fatal. The virus cannot be killed by ordinary sterilization processes, and the disease has no cure. The disease may have an incubation period of up to 20 years. Although CJD is not contagious, it is transmissible. The mechanism of transmission currently is unknown. CJD represents a threat in the health care setting, because it is known to be transmitted by contaminated electrodes during neurosurgical stereotactic surgery, corneal grafts, and direct contact with neurosurgical instruments that have been used on patients with CJD. For these reasons, current infection control standards require the use of disposable instruments for these types of surgical procedures or specialized decontamination procedures. Protocols for CJD have been established to help prevent transmission.

FUNGI

Fungi are found worldwide on living organic substances, in water, and in soil. More than 70,000 species of fungi exist, but only 300 are pathogenic. They are composed of eukaryotes classified into two groups, molds and yeasts.

Characteristics

Yeasts are unicellular, and molds are multicellular. Like the bacterial endospore, fungal spores are resistant to heat, cold, and drying. They have a cell wall and obtain their nutrients through absorption. Fungi are distinct from plants and animals. They occur as a single cell or as filaments called hyphae. These occur as a complex mass called a mycelium. The mycelium is divided into compartments, each containing a nucleus. Many fungi are visible without a microscope, and colonies may be grown in the laboratory for identification and drug sensitivity testing.

Identification

Fungi can be identified in the laboratory by direct observation of their form after culture. A specimen of the fungus is allowed to grow in a suitable medium and then observed for the shape, pattern, and color of the fungal colony. Further testing can be done by staining the cells and observing them under the microscope.

Reproduction

Fungi are capable of sexual or asexual reproduction, depending on the species and environment. Sexual reproduction takes place in the mycelium, which contains the sex cells needed for meiosis (reproductive cell division). Spores are released through sexual reproduction, and these may go on to produce a new colony. Fragmentation of the mycelium may also initiate the growth of a new colony.

Transmission to Humans

Fungal diseases occur as superficial or deep mycoses. Superficial fungi, which affect the skin, hair, nails, mouth, and vagina, are transmitted by direct contact with the source and cause mild disease symptoms. The yeast *Candida albicans* normally is established in the oral cavity of the newborn and persists as a commensalate organism throughout life. At times of immune stress or disease, oral *Candida* can proliferate. Deep fungi enter the body through the respiratory tract or through breaks in the skin or mucous membranes. Medical devices, such as catheters and intravenous cannulas, also can infect a health individual. In the health care setting, fungi can survive in the heating and cooling ducts of the ventilation system, releasing spores into the environment from which patients and workers can become infected.

Pathogenicity

Deep or disseminated fungal infections can be fatal. Patients who are immunosuppressed or who are weakened by metabolic disorders, infectious diseases, or trauma are at high risk for serious **mycotic** (fungal) disease. Healthy individuals are rarely infected with deep mycosis. Pathogenic fungi are described in Table 7-3.

Table 7-3
Medically Important Fungal Infections

Type of Fungus	Location	Disease	Causative Organism
Superficial	Keratin layer of skin, hair shaft	Tinea nigra, pityriasis versicolor	*Trichosporon Malassezia Eosinophilia*
Cutaneous	Epidermis, hair, nails	Tinea (ringworm)	*Microsporum Trichophyton Epidermophyton*
Systemic	Internal organs	Coccidiomycosis	*Cryptococcus*
		Histoplasmosis	*Candida*
		Blastomycosis	*Aspergillus*
		Paracoccidioidomycosis	*Pneumocystis*

Modified from Goering R, Dockrell H, Zuckerman M et al: *Mim's medical microbiology*, Philadelphia, 2007, Mosby/Elsevier.

Pathogenic Fungi
Aspergillus fumigatus

Aspergillus fumigatus is a significant fungal pathogen. It is an opportunistic infection in immunosuppressed patients. This fungus invades the body through the lungs and blood vessels and can cause vascular thrombosis and partial blockage of the airways. In a severely compromised patient, invasive *Aspergillus* infection often is fatal.

Candida albicans

Candida albicans is a common cause of opportunistic infection. It is a normal resident of the mouth, vagina, and intestine. However, it can proliferate in individuals who are immunosuppressed or weakened by disease and in patients taking antibiotics. When localized in the oral cavity or vagina, the infection usually can be treated successfully with antifungal drugs. Systemic or disseminated infection can spread to any location in the body, including the heart, kidneys, and other vital organs.

Pneumocystis carinii

Pneumocystis carinii infection is widespread in the general population but usually produces only mild symptoms. *P. carinii* pneumonia (PCP) is a common respiratory disease among patients with AIDS. Patients who are immunosuppressed, including those receiving immunosuppressive drugs for organ transplantation, are at high risk for the disease. The infection is difficult to diagnose because the symptoms are nonspecific and the fungus cannot be isolated from the patient's sputum through normal methods.

Cutaneous Mycoses

Superficial fungal infections invade the superficial layers of the skin. The filaments of the fungus spread into dead (keratinized) skin, hair, and nails. These cause irritation and oozing and may encourage the development of a superficial bacterial infection.

PROTOZOA

Characteristics

Protozoa are a group of single-cell eukaryotic organisms. Protozoa are free living in a variety of freshwater and marine habitats. Approximately 65,000 different species have been identified (compared to 4,500 species of bacteria). A large number of protozoa are parasitic in animals, including human beings. Most have complex life cycles with intermediate hosts that facilitate their transmission and reproduction. Single-celled protozoa reproduce by binary fission. They can infect any tissue or organ of the body. The organisms usually enter through an insect bite or by ingestion. Once in the body, they selectively reproduce in particular anatomical structures, such as the intestine, skin, blood, liver, or central nervous system. Protozoa feed on a wide variety of substances in the environment, including algae and bacteria. These are absorbed through the cell membrane.

The structure of protozoa varies widely by species, which allows identification by microscopic examination. Most protozoa have a well-defined shape and cell membrane, or envelope. They range in size from 1 to 300 μm. Many have an outer layer, called an *ectoplasm,* that contains the organelles used for feeding, locomotion, and defense. The cytoplasm contains organelles usually found in eukaryotic cells (described previously).

Mobility

Protozoa move through their watery environment by a variety of mechanisms. These are used to classify the protozoa. *Ciliates* are protozoa that move by multiple projections (cilia), which extend as hairlike fibers around the periphery of the ectoplasm. The cilia move in waves, providing locomotion. *Flagellates* have a single flagellum ("tail") or multiple flagella, which propel them in different directions. *Amoebae* move by using a pseudopod (false foot), which extends and pulls the cell along. Amoebae are attracted or repelled by concentration gradients in their environment, and they feed by absorption through the pseudopod.

Pathogenicity

Protozoa cause a wide variety of diseases in animals and human beings. These diseases often are characterized by destruction of the host cells by ingestion. Protozoa are able to resist or avoid many of the body's defenses by changing the antigens on their surface or by ingesting the immune complement of the cell, thereby disabling it. Widespread cell destruction results in the disease characteristics of different protozoal species and of the tissue they invade.

Gastrointestinal disease is characterized by simple diarrhea or dysentery. Protozoa feed on the mucosa and red blood cells of the host. This can result in severe dehydration, anemia, perforation of the intestine, and proliferation in other organs.

Protozoal diseases of the central nervous system (CNS) can result in severe destruction of nerve cell tissue or blood vessels. This leads to encephalitis and death. Malaria is the most significant protozoal disease of the CNS and a major killer of children in Africa and Asia. Protozoa that infect blood and organs destroy blood cells and tissue, including the liver, kidneys, heart, and lymph system. Important pathogenic protozoa are described in Table 7-4.

ALGAE

Algae are eukaryotes that belong to the plant kingdom; they include sponges and seaweed. They are classified as microbes but have no pathogenic effect on human beings. Structurally they vary widely, from single-cell organisms to colonies and large plants that can reach several hundred feet in length. They occur in freshwater and saltwater sources globally. Widespread commercial harvesting of algae for food products, manufacturing, and agriculture threatens these species, which are important in the food chain and in the ecology of wetlands and water-borne animals.

PROCESS OF INFECTION

REQUIREMENTS FOR INFECTION

Not every contact with a pathogen results in infection. Certain conditions must be favorable for the pathogen to gain entry into the body and proliferate:

Table 7-4

Important Protozoal Parasites

Anatomical Location	Species	Disease	Method of Transmission
Intestine	Entamoeba histolytica	Amebiasis	Ingestion of parasite cysts in water or food
	Giardia intestinalis	Giardiasis	
	Cryptosporidium spp.	Cryptosporidiosis	
	Microsporidia	Microsporidiosis	
Urogenital tract	Trichomonas vaginalis	Trichomoniasis	Sexual contact
	Trypanosoma spp.	Trypanosomiasis	Reduviid bug
		Sleeping sickness	Tsetse fly
		Chagas disease	
	Leishmania spp.	Visceral leishmaniasis (kala-azar)	Sand fly
		Cutaneous leishmaniasis	
Blood and tissue	Plasmodium spp. (P. vivax, P. ovale, P. malariae)	Malaria	Anopheles mosquito
	Toxoplasma gondii	Toxoplasmosis	Ingestion of cysts in raw meat; contact with infected cat feces

Modified from Goering R, Dockrell H, Zuckerman M et al: *Mim's medical microbiology*, Philadelphia, 2007, Mosby/Elsevier.

1. **The microbe must have an entry site and an exit site.** Microbes often are environmentally suited to a specific body system, and their entry site and exit site are often the same.
2. **Microbes must be present in sufficient numbers.** The number of invading microbes is called the *dose.* An infection or disease can be established only if a sufficient number of disease organisms is present. The number of microbe colonies on a surface is referred to as the **bioburden.**
3. **The environment must be well suited to the pathogen.** Once the pathogen gains entry into the body, the conditions for nutrition, oxygen needs (or lack of oxygen), pH, and temperature must be conducive to establishment of the infection.
4. **The host must be unable to overcome the harmful mechanisms of the pathogen.** Infection develops only if the host's natural or artificial immunity cannot prevent microbial proliferation.

METHODS OF TRANSMISSION

Diseases can be transmitted through a number of different pathways (Figure 7-15).

Direct Contact

Microorganisms are transferred from a host through direct contact or an intermediate source. The source can be nonliving (**fomite**) or living (**vector**). In the operating room, only sterile supplies and instruments are used. **Sterile** means completely free of all microorganisms.

A nonsterile (**contaminated**) surgical instrument can become a fomite by transmitting microorganisms into sterile tissue. Instruments and medical devices can harbor pathogenic bacteria encased in dried blood and body tissue that was not removed during the cleaning process. Other common fomites in the hospital are bed linens, wound dressings, and contaminated urinary catheters. Insects or rodents (vectors) carry pathogens from one surface to another or between hosts. Food attracts vectors and therefore is not permitted in the operating room.

Airborne Transmission

Water droplets carry organisms from one surface to another. They can also enter the body directly through the respiratory tract or another entry site. Water droplets are forcefully expelled during talking, coughing, or sneezing. Another example of contamination by water droplets occurs in the processing of instruments and equipment in the surgical department. Cleaning always takes place away from restricted and semirestricted areas to prevent contamination by droplets released from contaminated wash water.

Airborne transmission also occurs via **droplet nuclei** (dried remnants of previously moist secretions containing microorganisms). Droplet nuclei or aerosole droplets can remain suspended in the air because of their small size (usually 1 to 5 μm). They are infective for long periods and transmit disease when individuals breathe in the particles. Aerosole droplets can settle on surfaces and transmit disease by direct contact.

Transmission by Body Fluids

Blood-borne pathogens are a risk to hospitalized patients and health care personnel who may acquire disease through contact with blood and body fluids. Strict protocols for isolating and handling medical waste, body fluids, specimens, and soiled equipment in the hospital environment have been established to prevent infection. These protocols are called **Standard Precautions.** Exposure to blood-borne pathogens in the workplace requires immediate attention. The CDC has established guidelines for the management of exposure based

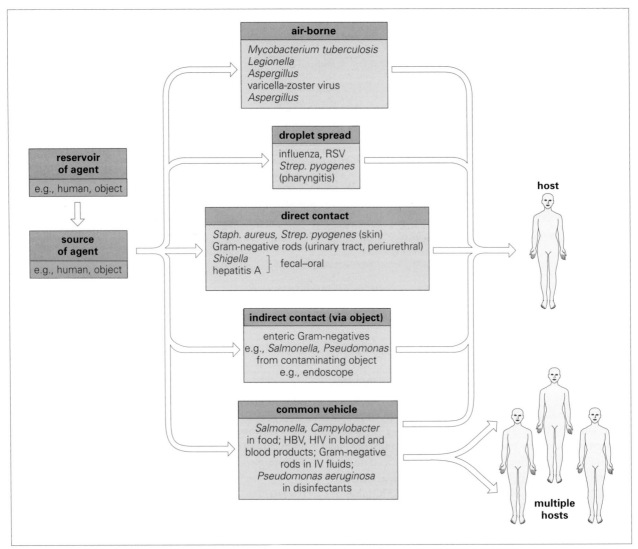

Figure 7-15 *Methods of disease transmission. Microorganisms leave or gain entry into the body through one of these routes and may colonize unless the body is able to overcome and destroy the microbes. (From Goering R, Dockrell H, Wakelin D et al: Mim's medical microbiology, ed 4, St Louis, 2008, Mosby.)*

on the type of pathogen and the nature of the exposure. Immediate care is available to all health care workers.

Oral Transmission (Ingestion)

Oral transmission occurs when a pathogen is ingested in food or through fecal-oral transmission. Fecal-oral transmission occurs when the infectious agent is shed by the infected host and acquired by the susceptible host through the ingestion of contaminated material. Poor hygiene among patients and hospital staff contributes to the spread of pathogens in this way. Frequent hand washing in the health care setting is very important to the prevention of oral disease transmission.

PORTAL OF ENTRY

To proliferate and cause disease, infectious organisms must gain entry to the body. The following are common means of entry.

- *Urogenital infection* almost always results from an outside source, usually the urethral orifice. The female urogenital tract is especially vulnerable to infection, because it is very short. Bacteria enter the urethral orifice and proliferate in the bladder, causing cystitis (infection of the bladder). The most common cause of urinary tract infection in females is *E. coli*, which is present in the large intestine and shed with feces.
- *Skin penetration* can result in local, regional, or systemic infection. The skin normally is a very efficient barrier against bacterial infection. However, when the skin is broken, bacteria can invade less protected tissues and cause local infection. If not resolved, a local infection can enter the vascular system and cause systemic disease.
- *Sexually transmitted diseases (STDs)* are spread when the mucous membrane of an infected person comes in contact with the mucous membrane of an uninfected person,

usually during sexual contact. The intact mucous membrane can help defend the body against disease transmission by secreting mucus, which cleanses the membrane. However, sexually transmitted diseases are prevented only with the use of condoms or abstinence.

- *Mother to infant transmission,* or vertical transmission, occurs from one generation to another prenatally or perinatally through breast milk.

PHASES OF DISEASE

The course of an infection follows distinct phases or patterns.

1. **Incubation:** In this phase the pathogens actively replicate, but the host shows no symptoms. This may be a short period (hours), or it may continue for days or even months. The incubation period is affected by the physical status of host, the port of entry, and the number of infectious organisms present in the body.
2. **Prodromal phase:** In this phase symptoms begin to appear. They may be very mild or vague at the start of the infection or may include certain clinically important signs of the disease.
3. **Acute phase:** In this phase the organism is at its most potent, and symptoms are very apparent. Cellular damage and destruction of tissue are characteristic of many diseases at this stage.
4. **Convalescence:** During this phase proliferation of the infectious organism slows and symptoms subside. Tissue begins to heal, and the body starts to regain strength and normal function.

These stages apply to diseases that resolve with treatment or by natural course. However, not all diseases resolve. A **chronic infection** may develop in some individuals. Weeks or months may be required for resolution, when all the disease organisms are eliminated from the body. Also, a person may harbor disease organisms but show no signs or symptoms; this person is referred to as a **carrier.**

CONTROL OF INFECTION

Prevention

The most important reason for studying certain aspects of microbiology is *disease prevention.* No other area of health care has a greater impact on populations, including patients undergoing surgery. Important methods of disease prevention in the health care facility include the following:

- Hand washing
- Learning and practicing Standard Precautions
- Learning and practicing aseptic technique
- Good personal hygiene practices
- Strict sanitation in the facility (cleaning, disinfection)
- Proper use of antiseptics and chemical disinfectants
- Isolation of infected patients according to standard guidelines

Community-acquired infection is prevented by public health education, immunization, rapid diagnosis of communicable disease, and reporting of specific diseases to state public health agencies.

Hand washing is the most important and effective method of disease prevention in the health care facility and in the community.

Treatment

The treatment of a patient with drugs to eradicate or minimize the effects of disease caused by microorganisms is called antimicrobial therapy. **Antibiotics** are used in bacterial and fungal infections.

Antibacterial agents are classified according to the way they destroy bacteria. The main mechanisms are:

- Inhibition of cell wall synthesis
- Interference with genetic replication (protein synthesis)
- Inhibition of metabolic pathways in the microbe

HOSPITAL-ACQUIRED INFECTION

A hospital-acquired infection (HAI), also called a **nosocomial infection,** is an infection acquired while the patient is in a health care institution. In the United States, about 2 million patients a year develop infections, including surgical site infections, as a result of hospitalization. Seventy percent of the bacteria that cause these infections are resistant to at least one of the drugs commonly used to treat that infection. The spread of a hospital-acquired infection from person to person is called **cross-contamination.** Introduction of an infection into a part of the body from another part of the body is called *self-infection* or **autoinfection.** The most common HAI is urinary tract infection, usually in patients who have been catheterized.

SURGICAL SITE INFECTION

Surgical site infection is the second most frequent type of HAI in U.S. hospitals. About 60% to 70% of surgical site infections are confined to the incision, and the remaining spread to distant or adjacent sites. Physiological complications of surgical site infections include the following:

- Tissue destruction or necrosis
- Wound dehiscence (splitting apart of deep and superficial wound edges)
- **Evisceration** (protrusion of visceral contents outside the body through the ruptured incision)
- Incisional hernia (protrusion of tissue through a weakened area of the abdominal wall at the site of a previous incision)
- Septic thrombophlebitis
- Single or multiple organ failure
- Recurring pain
- Increased metabolic requirements that result in malnutrition and bacteremia (circulatory involvement)
- Disfigurement
- Loss of function

Surgical site infection begins when a pathogenic or nonpathogenic microorganism colonizes sterile tissues. Some wound infections are minor, involving only the skin, whereas others occur in deep tissue or body cavities. The infection may remain localized or spread throughout the body. The patient's general condition at the time of surgery is a predictor of risk. Certain surgical patients have a high physiological risk of infection (Box 7-3).

The severity of the infection is influenced by the type, **virulence,** and number of invading bacteria, as well as the organisms' sensitivity to antibiotic treatment. Surgical wounds are classified according to the risk of contamination and infection at the time of the surgery.

PROCESS OF INFECTION

A small area of infection sometimes develops at the wound site. If the area is localized, it is referred to as an abscess and usually is easily treated. However a surgical site infection that spreads and becomes systemic can cause serious disease or death. In moderate to severe infection, the patient's temperature becomes elevated soon after surgery. The patient may experience pain at the incisional site or deep within the wound.

Exudate (an accumulation of pus, drainage, dead cells, and serum) may appear around the incision. The wound then is described as **suppurative.** The site becomes extremely tender or painful. If the infection is localized, antimicrobial therapy may be initiated and the infection eradicated. Deep infections, however, may lead to widespread areas of tissue necrosis, accumulation of pus, and breakdown of the sutured tissue layers. Infection can result in the breakdown of the surgical repair that was the focus of the surgery. As suture materials degrade in the presence of bacteria, the wound may split open, a condition known as **dehiscence.**

A large accumulation of pus leads to the spread of infection into adjacent tissues. An uncontrolled infection in a body cavity results in inflammation of the lining of that cavity (e.g., peritonitis in the abdomen). This can be rapidly fatal as vital organs are infected and become unable to function.

Treatment of Surgical Site Infection

A superficial surgical site infection usually is treated at the first signs. A **culture** specimen is taken. This is a sample of the wound exudate that is incubated and allowed to proliferate for testing. Antibiotic treatment may be initiated immediately. The wound is observed for further signs of infection and the patient monitored closely. Deep infection may not be diagnosed until days after the surgery. Antibiotic treatment is started immediately. If the symptoms do not resolve, the wound may be incised again and pus and necrotic, devitalized tissue removed. This procedure is called an *incision and drainage* (I & D). More extensive treatment includes intravenous (IV) antibiotic therapy and continued drainage. If the infection remains localized, the prognosis for resolution is good. However, systemic infection can result when bacteria migrate into the vascular system, causing septicemia.

When infection is present, the wound cannot be sutured, because infected tissues cannot withstand the tension of sutures and bacterial toxins rapidly break most suture material. Instead, the wound is packed with gauze dressings and allowed to heal from the bottom to the exterior.

MULTIDRUG-RESISTANT ORGANISMS

Important Concepts

Certain strains of pathogens have evolved to be partly or completely resistant to the most powerful antimicrobial agents available. Certain strains of bacteria are of grave concern, because they are easily transmitted, colonize rapidly, and can be lethal. The symptoms of these infections are the same as with the original, nonresistant strains. However, treatment becomes problematic, because resistance leads to spread of the infection and severe debilitation and/or death.

Treatment with antimicrobial agents destroys some pathogens, but the more resistant microbes survive and are transmitted to other hosts. The resistance is passed to succeeding

---

Box 7-3

Physiological Risks for Surgical Site Infection

- *Age:* The immune system of an elderly patient is less responsive than that of a younger patient. Tissues heal more slowly, and innate body defenses are less effective. Elderly patients are often undernourished.
- *Undernourishment or malnourishment:* Essential proteins required for tissue healing and body defenses against infection often are missing in the diet of these patients. Low body fat predisposes the patient to lowered body temperature, which increases physiological stress.
- *Diabetes mellitus:* The diabetic patient is at extremely high risk of infection because of problems with the circulatory system, which must be properly functioning to have a healthy immune system. Poor peripheral and visceral circulation prevents the flow of nutrients and oxygen to traumatized tissue, which increases the overgrowth of both resident and disease-producing microorganisms.
- *Substance or alcohol abuse:* These patients are often malnourished. Liver damage related to substance abuse and alcohol abuse leads to poor conversion of glycogen to glucose, which is necessary for cellular metabolism. Immune function often is depressed.
- *Immune suppression:* Patients with acquired immunodeficiency syndrome (AIDS) or other immune diseases, those undergoing cancer therapy, and those who have been prescribed high doses of corticosteroids have impaired immune function.
- *Long preoperative stay in the hospital:* A prolonged preoperative stay allows the body to incubate and colonize bacteria and other microorganisms commonly found in the hospital environment, especially antibiotic-resistant forms
- *Surgical wound classification:* Contaminated wounds, are associated with a higher risk of infection in the postoperative patient.
- *Long operative procedure:* Long procedures put the patient at higher risk for exposure to airborne pathogens and direct contact with contaminated medical devices and instruments.

generations of microbes through simple replication or via plasmid exchange, which carries the genes of the resistant strain to other microbes. Resistance occurs when the antibiotic used only partly destroys the pathogen or when antibiotic treatment is stopped before the microbes are destroyed.

Natural selection of resistant strains has been hastened by a combination of microbe strength and the indiscriminant and improper use of antibiotics. **Antibiotic-resistant** bacterial infection is a primary focus of public and clinical health researchers. Unfortunately, as new and more powerful drugs are developed, resistant strains also develop. The incidence of multidrug-resistant organisms (MDROs) in the United States has increased steadily in the past few decades.

Strict isolation protocols are used for patients with an MDRO. The surgical technologist must be knowledgeable about these protocols, which are established by the health institution in which they work. In addition to following all protocols, all health care workers must carefully practice hand washing procedures. These are discussed in detail in the next chapter.

Methicillin-Resistant *Staphylococcus aureus*

Methicillin-resistant *Staphylococcus aureus* (MRSA) is a virulent form of staphylococcus that is transmitted mainly by direct contact with the hands, equipment, and supplies. Health care workers who carry the bacteria in their respiratory system may become carriers of the disease. They do not become ill but can transmit the pathogens to others in their environment. MRSA can occur in surgical incisions, burns, and on devices such as urinary catheters, chest tubes and other common devices used in the health care setting.

Recently MRSA has been discovered in the community, outside the health care setting. The infection can be fatal and is particularly serious in debilitated patients. Vancomycin traditionally has been used to treat MRSA. However, a new strain has developed—vancomycin-resistant *Staphylococcus aureus*.

Vancomycin-Resistant and Vancomycin-Intermediate Resistant *Staphylococcus aureus*

Infection with vancomycin-resistant *S. aureus* (VRSA) was first diagnosed in the United States in 1997. Since then, the infection has increased steadily, and a new strain has also emerged, vancomycin-intermediate resistant *S. aureus* (VISA). These strains can be treated with other antibiotics. However, the infection can be fatal in severely debilitated patients.

Vancomycin-Resistant Enterococci

Vancomycin-resistant enterococci (VRE) infection is transmitted by direct contact or through intermediate sources, including furniture, equipment, and the hands of health care workers. Enterococci inhabit the intestine and female genital tract of healthy individuals. However, patients previously treated with vancomycin, surgical patients, and those who are debilitated or have a suppressed immune system are at particular risk for VRE infection. The bacteria are transmitted through contact with stool, urine, or blood and by the hands of health care workers. The bacteria cause urinary tract infection, septicemia (blood infection), and wound infection.

Multidrug-Resistant Tuberculosis

Multidrug-resistant tuberculosis (MDR TB) has emerged in the past few decades as a serious public health risk worldwide, including in the United States. It also is a risk for all health care workers. Transmission is the same as for nonresistant TB. However, MDR TB continues to increase in virulence and is fatal without treatment. A newer strain, called extensively drug resistant TB (XDR TB), is rare but has a greater risk of mortality. This strain is resistant to both the first- and second-line drugs normally used to treat TB. All strains of TB are transmitted by airborne particles and droplets, direct contact with inanimate objects, and direct contact with an infected individual.

IMMUNITY

GENERAL TYPES OF IMMUNITY

The immune system defends the body against harmful substances, including disease microorganisms. **Immunity** is the body's ability to accept substances that are part of the body ("self") and eliminate those that are not ("nonself"). The study of immunity and the immune system often is difficult, because it involves many terms and complex concepts.

The body has two general types of immunity, innate immunity and acquired immunity.

Innate immunity (also called *nonspecific immunity*) exists from the time of birth. This type of protection is not targeted at a specific substance but occurs as a physiological reaction whenever an injury occurs or any kind of foreign substance enters the body.

Acquired immunity, is conferred through exposure to a specific substance or microbe called an *antigen*. When exposure occurs, the immune system develops *antibodies*, which are specific proteins that trigger the immune system to launch its defenses.

MECHANISMS OF INNATE IMMUNITY

Chemical and Mechanical Body Defenses

The body has many different chemical and mechanical defenses against infection.

- **Intact skin,** including the mucous membranes, serves as an excellent barrier against the transmission and spread of infection. The normal flora of the skin, fatty acids derived from perspiration, excretions of sebaceous glands, and the rapid growth of keratin prevent bacterial entry into deeper tissues. Specific skin tissues are specialized in their ability to defend the body against infection. For example, skin appendages such as the eyelashes and nasal and ear hair prevent contamination by dust and droplets.
- **The respiratory system** has many different defense mechanisms. Microscopic cilia that line the respiratory tract continually sweep particles from the surface of the tract. The

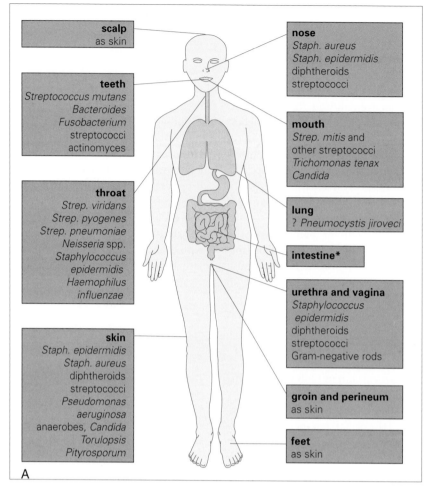

Figure 7-16 A, Normal body flora (resident bacteria). Normal flora protect the body against infection by competing successfully for resources (e.g., nutrition, moisture). They are well adapted to the body and also aid in body functions, such as digestion. **B,** Normal flora of the gastrointestinal system and their frequency. *(From Goering R, Dockrell H, Wakelin D et al: Mim's medical microbiology, ed 4, St Louis, 2008, Mosby.)*

action of the cilia moves material toward the mouth and nose and prevents them from settling in the lower respiratory tract. Mucus in the respiratory system traps particles and bacteria, which are forced out through the cough reflex.

- **Bacteriostatic chemicals in saliva, low pH in the stomach, and resident flora in the intestine prevent infection.** Gastrointestinal transmission occurs by ingestion (eating or drinking food or water contaminated with infectious microorganisms). We ingest many different types of foreign material and bacteria each day. Despite the body's defenses, virulent disease organisms can quickly invade the tissues of the intestine and proliferate.

- **Normal (resident) flora.** Shortly after birth, an infant's body begins to acquire a wide variety of bacterial colonies that live in symbiosis with the host in certain tissues of the body. These are called *normal* or *resident flora.* Resident flora, or **resident microorganisms,** are found in areas of the body that communicate with or are exposed to the outside environment (Figure 7-16). All other tissues in the body are normally sterile. Throughout a person's life,

the number and type of microorganisms in the resident population grow and recede according to environmental exposure. Important functions of resident flora are:

- To prevent invading organisms from colonizing by dominating the "ecological niche" provided by the host tissue
- To maintain the pH of the skin and mucous membranes to prevent the growth of harmful microorganisms
- To produce fatty acids on the skin to serve as a barrier against bacteria.

- The **inflammatory response** is the body's innate immune response to injury. The four classic signs of **inflammation** are:
  - Heat
  - Redness
  - Swelling
  - Pain

Almost immediately after tissue injury, blood vessels temporarily constrict at the site of injury. Constriction of capillaries helps reduce bleeding and restricts the movement of any microbial toxins present. This is rapidly fol-

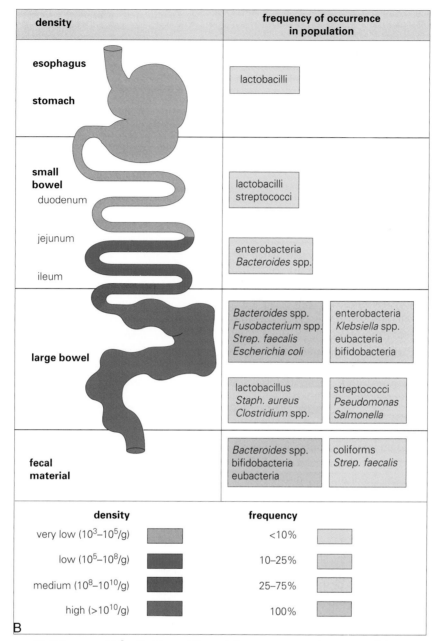

density		frequency of occurrence in population	
esophagus **stomach**		lactobacilli	

small bowel
  duodenum
 	
  jejunum
 	
  ileum
		lactobacilli
		streptococci
		
		enterobacteria
		Bacteroides spp.	

large bowel		*Bacteroides* spp. *Fusobacterium* spp. *Strep. faecalis* *Escherichia coli*	enterobacteria *Klebsiella* spp. eubacteria bifidobacteria
		lactobacillus *Staph. aureus* *Clostridium* spp.	streptococci *Pseudomonas* *Salmonella*
fecal material		*Bacteroides* spp. bifidobacteria eubacteria	coliforms *Strep. faecalis*

density		frequency	
very low (10^3–10^5/g)		<10%	
low (10^5–10^8/g)		10–25%	
medium (10^8–10^{10}/g)		25–75%	
high (>10^{10}/g)		100%	

B

Figure 7-16, cont'd B, Normal flora of the gastrointestinal system and their frequency. *(From Goering R, Dockrell H, Wakelin D et al: Mim's medical microbiology, ed 4, St Louis, 2008, Mosby.)*

lowed by localized arterial and venous dilation. As a result the injured area becomes red and warm. Local capillaries become more permeable, which allows plasma to escape into the surrounding tissue. The plasma dilutes any toxins in these tissues and also increases the thickness (viscosity) of the local blood supply and encourages clotting. These processes result in swelling, pain, and impaired function of the affected part.

• **Cellular response.** When microorganisms invade the body, specialized leukocytes rush to the site and surround and engulf them. Phagocytosis is an immune response triggered by the process of inflammation. Once the microorganism is inside the leukocyte, the leukocyte's lysosomes fuse with the microorganism and digest it. Nonliving remnants of the microorganism are then released from the leukocyte. Two types of **phagocyte** are involved in this process. *Neutrophils* are carried to the site of infection within 90 minutes. Within about 5 to 48 hours, *macrophages* arrive and continue to engulf and digest large amounts of bacteria. The neutrophil has a shorter life span than the macrophage but is quicker to respond.

As part of the immune process, regional lymph nodes collect cellular debris and act as centers for more intensive phagocytic activity. Pus at the site of an infection is composed of dead cells, lymphocytes, and living and dead pathogens.

Acquired Immunity

Acquired immunity is triggered by exposure to a specific potentially harmful substance, such as a disease microorganism. This protein substance is referred to an *antigen.* When exposed to an antigen, the body forms antibodies, which attach to the cells and remain there temporarily or throughout life.

❖ Antigens are non-self substances that trigger the immune system to launch defense.

❖ Antibodies are self substances that provide protection to the body.

Active Immunity

Active immunity develops when the body is stimulated to form its own antibodies against specific disease antigens. This type of immunity usually is permanent. The best immunity is formed from a live antigen. Active immunity can occur after vaccination or exposure to the disease. In this process, T and B lymphocytes are activated to bring about the production of antibodies (proteins that remain in the immune system memory). When the body is exposed to the disease pathogen again, the antibodies are activated and quickly destroy the organisms. Immunity can last for years or a lifetime.

A person can develop active immunity in two ways:
1. By getting the disease
2. By vaccination which is an injection containing a small amount of disease antigen. The antigen is modified to prevent the recipient from developing the disease, but it is effective in stimulating the formation of antibodies.

Passive Immunity

Passive immunity develops when the body receives the specific disease antibodies from an outside source. This eliminates the need for the body to synthesize them. Passive immunity, which is temporary, occurs when:
1. The fetus receives antibodies in utero from the mother's immune system or breast milk (natural immunity).
2. A person receives a specific antibody for a specific antigen, created in horse or human tissue. The antibody usually is given by injection. Tetanus antitoxin is an example of an injectable antibody.

VACCINES

Vaccination provides a form of acquired immunity. Vaccines are modified forms of disease organisms that create immunological memory in the body. They produce the same immunological response as the disease itself, without the risks involved in the disease process. Vaccination provides artificial immunity against specific organisms.

Vaccines are classified into two main types and their subtypes:
1. Live attenuated vaccines
   * Viruses
   * Bacteria
2. Inactivated vaccines
   * Whole
   * Fractional

Live attenuated vaccines contain modified disease organisms, either viruses or bacteria. Modification of the organism prevents the recipient of the vaccine experiencing the effects of the disease, but immunity is still conferred. Examples of attenuated vaccines licensed in the United States are polio, measles, mumps, varicella, and rubella.

Inactivated vaccines contain whole viruses or bacteria, or fractional components of the organisms. Protein-based fractional vaccines are called toxoids. These are inactivated bacterial toxins.

HYPERSENSITIVITY

Immune response to a substance is referred to as hypersensitivity. Hypersensitivity occurs only in individuals who have previous exposure and sensitivity to the substance. A hypersensitivity reaction may be mild, producing a rash, mild respiratory distress leading to asthma, or gastrointestinal symptoms. The reaction can be immediate or delayed up to 12 hours after exposure. A severe immediate reaction is referred to as **anaphylactic shock,** which can be quickly fatal.

ALLERGY

True allergy is hypersensitivity to a substance in the environment, a process that is mediated by the immune system. A substance that causes a hypersensitivity reaction is called an allergen. Allergens gain entry into the body by many routes, including those used for medication. Inhalation of pollens and pollutants is another way in which people experience allergy. In the operating room, the greatest concern is whether the patient is allergic to drugs or other substances (e.g., latex) in the perioperative environment.

Immediate and Delayed Reaction

As mentioned previously, the two types of allergic reactions, are immediate reactions and delayed reactions. Delayed reactions are more common with simple compounds, inorganic chemicals, and metals. These reactions are mediated by T lymphocytes. Immediate reactions are mediated by antibodies. Allergic reactions are divided into four categories:
* *Type I:* These reactions are characterized by inflammation of tissues, which is caused by the release of *histamine* in the body. This causes increased permeability of blood vessels and constriction of bronchioles, leading to difficulty breathing. The most extreme form of sensitivity is anaphylactic shock, which can lead to death. (The symptoms and treatment of anaphylactic shock are described in Chapter 12.)
* *Type II:* A type II reaction is called a *cytotoxic reaction.* It is the result of interaction between two antibodies and cell surface antigens. It causes the onset of powerful immune defense mechanisms, which can result in injury or death.

Mismatched blood transfusion and hemolytic disease in newborns are type II reactions.

- *Type III:* Type III reactions are caused by antigen-antibody complexes, which produce tissue damage when they trigger an immune response. An example of a type III reaction is allergy to antibiotics. Symptoms include itching, rash, severe tissue swelling, and fever. This usually resolves in several days.
- *Type IV:* Type IV reactions are cell-mediated reactions (not related to antibodies) that occur 24 to 72 hours after exposure to the agent. An example of this delayed hypersensitivity is a positive reaction to the tuberculin skin test, in which a small amount of killed *M. tuberculosis* is injected.

Autoimmunity

In certain diseases, the body does not recognize "self." Consequently, it mounts a mild to severe immune response to its own tissues, causing fever, swelling, and tissue destruction. Examples of autoimmune diseases are rheumatoid arthritis, systemic lupus erythematosus, and ulcerative colitis.

CHAPTER SUMMARY

- Microbiology is the study of microorganisms and their relationship to the environment.
- The Linnean system of classification is used in biology to distinguish specific groups of organisms.
- Living cellular organisms are divided into two groups, eukaryotes and prokaryotes.
- Bacteria belong to the prokaryote class of cells.
- Microbes are identified by their morphology, staining tendencies, and reactions to biochemical tests. Gram staining is a basic test performed for differentiation.
- Chemical tests can be performed on bacteria only if they are grown in a laboratory environment (culturing). After culturing, the bacteria are tested for sensitivity to antimicrobial drugs (culture and sensitivity).
- Microbes are classified by types according to the Linnean system. The major groups are bacteria, viruses, fungi, protozoa, Rickettsiae, and prions.
- Cells contain various types of organelles, which aid in the cell's metabolism.
- Substances move into the cell mainly by diffusion, osmosis, active transport, and pinocytosis.
- The relationship between a microbe and its host depends on the environment, the condition of the host, and the condition of the microbe.
- The biological relationship between organisms living together is called *symbiosis.* If neither organism is harmed, the association is called *commensalism;* if the association benefits both, it is *mutualism;* and if one is harmed and the other benefits, it is *parasitism.*
- Bacteria are the most important group of microbes in medicine, because they cause most diseases.
- Bacteria vary in their environmental and physiological needs. These include nutrition, oxygen requirements, pH, and temperature. Oxygen requirements are particularly important in wound management. Aerobic bacteria require oxygen, and anaerobic bacteria do not. Anaerobic bacteria produce powerful toxins that can be fatal in the host.

- Bacterial toxins are produced by living bacteria as products of metabolism (exotoxin), or the toxins are released after the bacteria die (endotoxin).
- Specific types of bacteria live normally in human tissues. These are called *resident flora,* and they aid in digestion and defense against disease.
- Prions and viruses are nonliving but able to cause disease.
- Creutzfeldt-Jakob disease and variant CJD are fatal, transmissible diseases of the nervous system. They are important in surgery because although rare, the prion responsible for the diseases cannot be destroyed by normal sterilization methods.
- Hepatitis and HIV/AIDS are the most important infectious diseases caused by viruses. The hepatitis B virus and HIV are blood-borne microbes transmitted through contact with body fluids.
- Disease transmission occurs only when certain conditions are met. These include a method of transmission, a portal of entry into the body, a sufficient dose of microbes, a suitable environment for microbe reproduction, and insufficient resistance in the host.
- Infectious disease is transmitted by direct contact, airborne droplets, oral transmission, and ingestion of microbes.
- Urinary catheterization causes the greatest number of hospital-acquired infections in the United States. Surgical site infection is the second most frequent HAI.
- Multidrug-resistant organisms have evolved because of the overuse and misuse of antimicrobial agents worldwide.
- The immune system defends the body against infection by innate immunity and acquired immunity. Innate immunity is present at birth, and acquired immunity is conferred by previous exposure to the disease-causing organism, either naturally or by immunization.
- Hypersensitivity to a substance in the environment is also mediated by the immune system and can result in serious illness or death.

REVIEW QUESTIONS

1. How is the environment of a pathogen related to the disease it causes?

2. In what ways are viral and bacterial diseases transmitted?

3. List the body fluids that can transmit HIV.

4. What particular protection does the bacterial spore provide in prolonging the life of bacteria?

5. Why are antibiotics not effective against viral infections?

6. What is a resident bacterium? What protection does it provide?

7. How do viruses replicate?

8. How is hepatitis B transmitted?

9. What characteristics make CJD such a risk?

10. Define these terms: *antibody, antigen, passive immunity,* and *active immunity.*

11. What is the most important method of preventing disease transmission in the health care setting?

REFERENCE

1. Joint United Nations Committee on HIV/AIDS and the Work Health Organization (UNAIDS/WHO): AIDS epidemic update 2006. Accessed November 9, 2007, at http://data.unaids.org/pub/EPIReport/2006/2006_EpiUpdate_en.pdf.

BIBLIOGRAPHY

American Social Health Association: Fact sheet on HPV. Accessed November 10, 2007, at http://www.ashastd.org/pdfs/HPV-factsheet.pdf.

Atkinson W, Hamborsky J, McIntyre L, Wolfe S, editors: *Epidemiology and prevention of vaccine-preventable diseases,* ed 10, Washington, DC, 2007, Public Health Foundation. Accessed November 13, 2007, at http://www.cdc.gov/vaccines/pubs/pinkbook/default/htm.

Centers for Disease Control and Prevention: Guideline for hand hygiene in health-care settings: recommendations of the Healthcare Infection Control Practices Advisory Committee and the HICPAC/SHEA/APIC/IDSA Hand Hygiene Task Force, *Morbidity and Mortality Weekly Report* No RR-16, 2002.

Centers for Disease Control and Prevention: Prion diseases: about prion diseases. Accessed November 10, 2007, at http://www.cdc.gov/incidoc/dvrd/prions.

Centers for Disease Control and Prevention: Healthcare-associated infections (HAIs). Accessed November 9, 2007, at http://www. gov/ncicoc/dhqp/healthDis.html.

Centers for Disease Control and Prevention: Human papillomavirus: HPV information for clinicians. Accessed November 12, 2007, at http://www.cdc.gov/std/Hpv/hpv-clinicans-brochure.htm.

Control Practices Advisory Committee: 2007 Guidelines for isolation precautions: preventing transmission of infectious agents in healthcare settings. Accessed May 25, 2008, at http://www.cdc.gov/ncidod/dhqp/pdf/isolation2007.pdf.

Edwards J, Peterson K, Ndrus M et al: National Healthcare Safety Network report: data summary for 2006. Accessed Nov 7, 2007, at http://www.cdc.gov/ncidod/dhqp/nhsn_members.html.

Goering R, Dockrell H, Zuckerman M et al: *Mim's medical microbiology,* St Louis, 2008, Mosby.

Klevens M, Morrison M, Nadle J et al: Invasive methicillin-resistant *Staphylococcus aureus* infections in the United States, *Journal of the American Medical Association* 298:15, 2007.

Siegel JD, Rhinehart E, Jackson M, Chiarello L, and the Healthcare Infection

Seigel J, Rhinehart E, Jackson M et al: Management of multi drug–resistant organisms in healthcare settings, 2006. Accessed November 5, 2007, at http://www.cdc.gov/ncidod/dhqp/ar.html.

Decontamination, Sterilization, and Disinfection

CHAPTER OUTLINE

LEARNING OBJECTIVES

After studying this chapter the reader will be able to:

- Correctly use terms related to disinfection and sterilization
- Distinguish between the process of sterilization and other processes that render objects clean
- Define a prion and access information about Creutzfeldt-Jakob disease (CJD)
- Describe special processing required for instruments exposed to CJD
- Explain the Spaulding system of classification
- Describe the steps of reprocessing from the point of use to sterilization

- Describe the different methods of sterilization used in the operating room
- Explain the rationale for proper loading of the steam sterilizer
- Explain the principles of gas sterilization
- Describe the environmental concerns associated with the use of a gas sterilizer
- Distinguish between disinfection and sterilization
- Recognize the hazards associated with the use of chemical disinfectants
- Describe terminal decontamination of the operating room environment and equipment

TERMINOLOGY

AAMI: Association for the Advancement of Medical Instrumentation. The AAMI is an authoritative source of standards for sterilization and disinfection.

Antisepsis: A process that greatly reduces the number of microorganisms on skin or other tissue.

Autoclave: A small steam sterilizer used in low volume clinical settings.

Bactericidal: Able to kill bacteria.

Bacteriostatic: Chemical agent capable of inhibiting the growth of bacteria.

Biofilm: A matrix of extracellular polymers produced by microorganisms. These substances bind the microorganisms tightly to a living or nonliving surface, making them highly resistant to anti-

microbial action. Biotin increases the risk of disease transmission on internal medicine devices such as catheters and endoscopic instruments.

Biological indicator: A quality control mechanism used in the process of sterilization. It consists of a closed system containing harmless, spore-forming bacteria that can be rapidly cultured after the sterilization process.

Case cart system: A method of receiving clean and sterile equipment and preparing it for transportation to a central decontamination area. All equipment is contained within a covered movable storage cart.

Cavitation: A process in which air bubbles are imploded (burst inward), releasing particles of soil or tissue debris.

Central Service department: The area of the hospital where medical devices and equipment are processed; also called *Central Surgical Supply*, the *Surgical Processing department*, and the *Central Processing department*.

Central Service Technician: A skilled professional who specializes in processing and maintenance of medical devices used in the health care facility.

Chemical monitor: A method of testing a sterilization parameter. Chemical strips sensitive to physical conditions, such as temperature, are placed with the item being sterilized and change color when the parameter is reached; sometimes called a chemical indicator.

Chemical sterilization: A process that uses chemical agents to achieve sterilization.

–cidal: A suffix indicating death. For example, bactericidal means "able to kill bacteria."

Cleaning: A process that removes organic or inorganic soil or debris using detergent and mechanical or hand washing.

Cobalt-60 radiation: A method of sterilizing prepackaged equipment using ionizing radiation.

Contaminate: To render nonsterile and unacceptable for use in critical areas of the body.

Decontamination: A process in which recently used and soiled medical devices, including instruments, are rendered safe for personnel to handle.

Detergent: A chemical that breaks down organic debris by emulsification (separation into small particles) to aid in cleaning.

Disinfection: Destruction of microorganisms by heat or chemical means. Spores usually are not destroyed by disinfection.

Enzymatic cleaner: A specific chemical used in detergents and cleaners to penetrate and break down biological debris, such as blood and tissue.

Ethylene oxide: A highly flammable, toxic gas that is capable of sterilizing an object.

Event-related sterility: A wrapped sterile item may become contaminated by environmental conditions or events, such as a puncture in the wrapper. Event-related sterility refers to sterility based on the absence of such events. The shelf life of a sterilized pack is event related, not time related.

Evidence based practice: Methods and procedures proven to be valid by rigorous testing and professional research.

Exposure time: This is the amount of time goods are held at a specific time, temperature, and pressure during a sterilization process. Exposure time varies with the size of the load, type of materials being sterilized, and type of sterilizer. Exposure time is sometimes called the **hold** time.

Fungicidal: Able to kill fungi.

Gas plasma sterilization: A process that uses the form of matter known as plasma (e.g., hydrogen peroxide plasma) to sterilize an item. Also referred to as plasma sterilization.

Germicidal: Able to kill germs.

Gravity displacement sterilizer: A type of sterilizer that removes air by gravity.

High level disinfection (HLD): A process that reduces the bioburden to an absolute minimum.

High vacuum sterilizer: A type of steam sterilizer that removes air in the chamber by vacuum and refills the chapter with pressurized steam. Also known as a prevacuum sterilizer.

Inanimate: Nonliving.

Indicator: A device used in the sterilization process to verify that a parameter of the process (e.g., temperature) has been achieved.

Indicators are not used to verify that an item is sterile, only that a parameter has been achieved.

Just-in-time sterilization: Items to be sterilized shortly before surgery must be processed so they are ready as close to the time of surgery as possible. This is referred to as just-in-time sterilization.

Material Safety Data Sheet (MSDS): A government mandated requirement for all chemicals used in the workplace. The MSDS describes the formulation, safe use, precautions, and emergency response. The MSDS must be available for each chemical an employee is required to handle in their work.

Medical devices: Any equipment, instrument, implant, material, or apparatus used for the diagnosis, treatment, or monitoring of patients.

Noncritical items: Items that are not required to be sterile because they do not penetrate intact tissues. Patient care items such as a blood pressure cuff and a stethoscope are noncritical.

Nonwoven: A fabric or material that is bonded together as opposed to a process of interweaving individual threads.

Peracetic acid: A chemical used in the sterilization of critical items.

Personal protective equipment (PPE): Approved attire worn during the reprocessing of medical devices and the cleaning of patient areas. PPE protects the wearer from contamination by microorganisms.

Prion (proteinaceous infectious particle): A unique pathogenic substance which contains no nucleic acid. The prion is transmitted by direct contact or ingestion and is resistant to all forms of disinfection and sterilization normally used in the health care setting.

Process challenge monitoring: A sealed, harmless bacteriological sample is included in a load of goods to be sterilized. The sample is recovered following the sterilization process and cultured to test for viability. This process is also called a biological monitoring.

Reprocessing: Activities or tasks that prepare used medical devices for use on another patient; these activities include cleaning, disinfection, decontamination, and sterilization.

Reusable: A designation used by manufacturers to indicate that a medical device can be reprocessed for use on more than one patient.

Sanitation: A method that reduces the number of bacteria in the environment to a safe level.

Sharps: Any objects used in health care that are capable of penetrating the skin, causing injury.

Shelf life: The length of time a wrapped item remains sterile after it has been subjected to a sterilization process.

Single-use items: Instruments and devices intended for use on one patient only; sometimes called disposable items.

Spaulding system: A system used to determine the level of microbial destruction required for medical devices and supplies based on the risk of infection associated with the area of the body where the device is used. Categories include critical, semi-critical, and non-critical.

Sporicidal: Able to kill spores.

Sterilization: A process by which all microorganisms, including spores, are destroyed.

Terminal decontamination: Thorough cleaning and disinfection of supplies or an environment such as the operating room suite after patient use. Specific protocols and procedures are used during terminal decontamination.

Ultrasonic cleaner: Equipment that cleans instruments using ultrasonic waves.

Viricidal: Able to kill viruses.

Washer-sterilizer/disinfector: Equipment that washes and decontaminates instruments after an operative procedure.

Woven wrappers: Also called linen or cloth wrappers, these are fabric cloths used to wrap clean, disinfected supplies in preparation for a sterilization process.

INTRODUCTION

This chapter is about preventing the transmission of disease by instruments and other **medical devices** in the perioperative environment. The concepts and practices in this chapter bring together the science of microbiology and the recommended practices of reprocessing: decontamination, disinfection, and sterilization. Medical devices must be reprocessed after use to render them safe for use on the next patient. The steps of this process and the underlying rationales are basic to the education of surgical technologists.

In the previous chapter, discussed the ways in which disease is transmitted. In the community, people avoid infection through hygiene practices and healthy lifestyle behaviors. In the health care setting, the transmission of disease by means of equipment, instruments, personnel, and other patients is a significant risk. The hospital or clinic is a congested setting in which pathogens have ample opportunity to thrive. The purpose of decontamination, disinfection, and sterilization is to control the spread of disease by reducing the number of microbes and preventing their proliferation on the equipment used in patient care.

PRINCIPLES OF DECONTAMINATION, STERILIZATION, AND DISINFECTION

BASIC TERMS

Before studying the material in this chapter, the reader should become familiar with basic terminology related to the processes discussed. Ongoing research and new technology often produce new terms. The surgical technologist should strive to learn updated terms because they accurately describe current technology and have been validated by standards agencies. The following are very basic definitions.

- An antiseptic is a chemical used to remove microorganisms on skin or other tissue. This process is referred to as antisepsis. Surgical hand rubs and soaps contain an antiseptic. The patient's skin is cleaned with an antiseptic just before surgery to reduce the number of microorganisms. Some chemicals have dual-purpose qualities (i.e., they may be used on tissue and objects). However, if a chemical is labeled a *disinfectant,* it is intended for **inanimate** surfaces only.
- Bacteriostatic refers to an agent that inhibits bacterial colonization but does not destroy bacteria.
- As discussed in Chapter 7, **bioburden** is the number and type of live bacterial colonies on a surface before it is sterilized. For example, an endoscope used in gastrointestinal procedures will contain a high bioburden and require meticulous cleaning and high level disinfection after use. Contaminated refers to any surface or tissue that has come in contact with a *potential* or actual source of microorganisms. A sterile

item is considered contaminated even if the surface it touches is clean. Only sterile surfaces may touch other sterile surfaces in order to remain uncontaminated.

- **Cleaning** is the removal of blood, body fluids, dirt, and organic debris, usually with **detergents** and mechanical action.
- **Decontamination** is a process in which instruments and supplies are first cleaned and then processed through chemical or mechanical means so that they are safe for handling. The decontamination process must kill all pathogens.
- **Disinfection** is a process that removes most but not all microbes on inanimate surfaces. A disinfectant is a chemical used to destroy microorganisms on *inanimate or nonliving surfaces only*. Most disinfectants are not safe for use on tissues. Some disinfectants are formulated for use on surgical equipment, whereas others are used for environmental cleaning. There are three types of disinfection: high, medium, and low level.
- **High-level disinfection** is the destruction of all microorganisms including mycobacteria, but not forms (e.g., high levels of bacterial spores). **Medium-level disinfection** is effective against mycobacteria and most viruses. **Low-level disinfection** destroys most viruses and bacteria. The type of disinfection process used on a medical device depends on where it is used in the body—e.g., a critical, semi-critical, or non-critical area (see Table 8-1).
- **Reprocessing** refers to all the steps necessary to render soiled medical devices safe for use on the next patient.
- **Sterilization** is a process that results in the complete destruction of all viable forms of life on an object. An object is either sterile or not sterile. There are no "levels" of sterility.

Application of Terms

The terms just defined are used every day in the health care environment, especially in the operating room. Before and after a surgical case, the floors, walls, and tables are *cleaned* using a detergent. The floor is wet-vacuumed to loosen all soil and debris and remove it completely. Perioperative staff put on *clean* scrub attire, which is freshly laundered at the start of each working day. Clean scrub attire is put on at the start of every work day and changed whenever it becomes soiled or wet. Instruments are cleaned thoroughly before disinfection.

Instruments are *disinfected* after use so that they can be safely handled by staff members. This reduces the bioburden, so that instrument trays and other equipment can be *sterilized* for a surgical case.

Before surgery begins, the surgical technologist (ST) dons *sterile* gloves and gown. The ST then proceeds to arrange the sterile instruments and supplies. Sterile supplies and instruments are prevented from touching *contaminated* surfaces or objects. Touching a contaminated object will **con-**

taminate the sterile object, which then must not be used in surgery.

At the close of the case, the used instruments are removed from perioperative environment for extensive cleaning and decontamination. After this process, the instruments can be safely handled with bare hands.

STANDARDS AND REGULATIONS

Standards for sterilization and disinfection of instruments, devices, and equipment in the perioperative environment are established by the following authoritative sources.

- *The Association for the Advancement of Medical Instrumentation (AAMI).* The **AAMI** provides recommended practices and technical information for the U.S. medical professions. Standards are developed with the support of the Food and Drug Administration (FDA). The AAMI's Web site is http://www.aami.org.
- *The Association of Surgical Technologists.* The AST is the professional organization of surgical technologists. The AST Web site is http://www.ast.org.
- *The Association of periOperative Registered Nurses (AORN).* AORN is the professional association for perioperative nurses. Its Web site is http://www.aorn.org.
- *The Centers for Disease Control and Prevention (CDC).* The CDC is a federal agency that provides research and protocols in all areas of public health. The Web site is http://www.cdc.gov.
- *The Joint Commission.* The Joint Commission is the accreditation agency for all health care organizations in the United States. It oversees compliance with environmental and patient safety regulations.

Standards are established to maintain evidenced-based practice. Evidenced-based practice constitutes the practices and processes that are based on sound research and professionally conducted studies. The standards also establish accepted definitions of terms used in the processes. These definitions further clarify the biological and technical basis of the standards.

In recent years, infection control has become one of the most important areas of patient and staff safety. Concerns about multidrug-resistant organisms, disease caused by prions, and blood-borne pathogens have led to new standards and increasingly strict protocols. The role of the surgical technologist in infection control is to implement the specified procedure correctly and safely according to protocol.

Standards and regulations are implemented through the policies of the health care provider. Management teams in infectious control and in the Central Service (CS) and surgical departments develop ways to implement the standards and monitor the outcomes. The actual tasks are performed by perioperative and CS staff. These tasks are set out in the health care facility's procedures manual.

SELECTING A REPROCESSING METHOD
Spaulding Method

The decision to sterilize, disinfect, or merely clean equipment used in the health care environment is based on cat-

egories established by the **Spaulding system**. The system assigns a risk category (i.e., critical risk, semicritical risk, and noncritical risk) that is *specific to the regions of the body in which the device is to be used* (Table 8-1). Instruments and patient care equipment are processed according to their level of risk.

Critical Risk
Critical risk is assigned to sterile body tissues, including the vascular system. Nearly all body tissues are sterile. Exceptions are the external orifices (openings) of the body, such as the urethra, anus, vagina, ear, nose, and mouth, which are covered by mucous membranes. All other tissue is considered critical because contamination, even by microbes with relatively low or no pathogenicity, can lead to serious infection.

Semicritical Risk
Mucous membranes and nonintact skin are semicritical areas. Mucous membranes are not sterile. In the past, less attention has been given to high level disinfection or even sterilization of endoscopes that enter the mucous membranes. However, there is a trend toward sterilization to prevent any cross-contamination among patients.

Noncritical Risk
Intact skin is considered noncritical. Medical devices that touch *only the skin* are assigned to the noncritical category. The skin has many innate defenses against infection. However, the hands are the most common method of disease transmission in the health care environment.

BEST PRACTICE FOR REPROCESSING

Reprocessing is one of the primary activities in the health care facility. The following form the basis of safe reprocessing:

1. Soiled instruments and other surgical equipment are reprocessed in a designated area of the facility. This area is separated from the surgical suites and the patient care areas to prevent cross-contamination.
2. Staff members are fully trained in the standards and approved methods of reprocessing.
3. Staff members understand the rationale used in reprocessing.
4. The health care facility provides written policies and procedures based on the accepted standards of professional and accrediting organizations.
5. Evidence-based methods for quality control are used to validate and monitor the efficacy of the reprocessing methods.

Quality Control Monitoring

Procedures and methods for reprocessing medical devices must be monitored to ensure patient safety. The outcome of the process should be a statistically acceptable rate of hospital-acquired infection. Quality control includes monitoring the

<u>Table 8-1</u>

Summary of Disinfection and Sterilization Processes (Spaulding System)

Definition	Items and Devices	Processes Used*	Products Used
Critical Items Enter vascular systems or sterile tissues, or have blood flowing through them	Surgical instruments Implants Needles Catheters (vascular and urinary) Laparoscopes and arthroscopes (if sterilization is not feasible, these should receive at least high level disinfection) Endoscopy accessories (e.g., biopsy forceps, cytology brushes) Some dental instruments (e.g., scalers, burrs, forceps, scalpels)	***Sterilization*** Heat (steam, dry) Chemical gas, vapor, plasma Radiation Peracetic acid with hydrogen peroxide NOTE: Longer exposure times are required for sterilization than for disinfection.	*Liquid chemicals, sporicidal sterilants* Aldehydes (e.g., glutaraldehyde) Hydrogen peroxide Peracetic acid
Semicritical Items Come in contact with mucous membranes or nonintact skin	Gastrointestinal endoscopes Laryngoscopes Bronchoscopes Endotracheal tubes Respiratory therapy and anesthesia equipment Dialyzers Diaphragm-fitting rings Cryosurgical probes Some dental instruments (e.g., amalgam, condensers, air/water syringes) Hydrotherapy tanks (if used for patients with intact skin) Tonometers (5-min immersion recommended) Thermometers (alcohols preferred)	***High-level disinfection*** 20-min minimum required; 12 min for orthophthalaldehyde (Cidex OPA) *NOTE:* Sterilization may be preferred.	*Wet pasteurization agents or liquid chemicals* Aldehydes (e.g., glutaraldehyde) Cidex OPA Hydrogen peroxide Peracetic acid Peracetic acid with hydrogen peroxide Chlorines (sodium hypochlorite, 1000 ppm, 1:50 dilution)
		Intermediate level disinfection ≤10-min immersion NOTE: With label claim for tuberculocidal activity.	Alcohols (70% to 90%) Iodophors Phenolics Chlorines
Noncritical Items Come in contact with intact skin (not mucous membranes)	Stethoscopes Blood pressure and tourniquet cuffs Electrocardiogram leads Bedpans Linens Environmental surfaces (e.g., tabletops, bedside stands, furniture, floors)	***Intermediate level disinfection*** NOTE: Required if contamination is heavy and with significant blood contamination. *Low level disinfection* NOTE: Adequate for most noncritical items and surfaces.	Alcohols (70% to 90%) Iodophors Phenolics Chlorines Alcohols (70% to 90%) Iodophors Phenolics Chlorines (sodium hypochlorite, 100 ppm, 1:500 dilution) Quaternary ammonium compounds ("quats")

From Gruendemann BJ, Mangum SS: *Infection prevention in surgical settings*, Philadelphia, 2001, WB Saunders.
ppm, Parts permillion.
*Using products approved by the Environmental Protection Agency (EPA) and the Food and Drug Administration (FDA) and following the manufacturer's instructions.

technologies used in reprocessing, as well as the *human* factor. The two are equally important.

Technology-Based Parameters

- The parameters of the sterilization or disinfection method, such as a maximum temperature, pressure, or chemical concentration are verified by printable data generated by the system itself or by external testing methods.
- All batches of goods processed together in a single load are identified by batch number and date; these data are maintained to allow tracking of items for monitoring or in case of an adverse event related to system or equipment failure.
- Sterilization and disinfection systems undergo regular maintenance and inspection by bioengineering professionals.

Human (Personnel) Resources

- Central Service and perioperative personnel are involved in the coordination of roles and responsibilities that directly affect their safety.
- Personnel are provided with the tools and methods needed to meet the objectives of their work. They understand how to operate disinfection and sterilization equipment that is within their area of responsibility.
- Personnel document the procedures and results of specific reprocessing activities.
- Accurate records of responsibilities and tasks are maintained for the purpose of tracking adverse events related to sterilization and disinfection.
- Staff members are offered and encouraged to participate in ongoing training as new technologies and evidence-based practices are introduced.

Reprocessing of Disposable Devices

Single-use, or disposable, medical devices and products have come into extremely widespread use in the past two decades. The debate over environmental damage, use of shrinking natural resources, and waste is a separate issue and should be an ongoing discussion. The trend favoring disposables is unlikely to change as long as patients and medical professionals create a demand for such products.

The increased acceptance of single-use products has created a need for regulations and recommendations covering reprocessing of these items. **Single-use items** manufactured under FDA approval have a high level of safety. However, many items opened for surgery are never used and eventually are discarded as waste. To cut costs and retrieve the expense of these items, some institutions reprocess the items. Commercial reprocessing services are available for instruments and equipment *approved for reprocessing* by the manufacturer. However, unless the manufacturer sanctions reprocessing, the safety of any device intended for single use may be compromised. The health care facility is liable for any patient injury that occurs as a result of malfunction of a reprocessed single-use item that is not approved for multiple use.

COORDINATING THE ROLES OF CENTRAL SERVICE AND PERIOPERATIVE PERSONNEL

In most facilities, high volume processing takes place in the health facility's **Central Service department.** The personnel responsible for this are the Central Service (CS) technicians. This is a skilled, certified profession that requires expertise in the science and practice of materials management, decontamination, and sterilization.

Nearly all instruments and equipment used in surgery are transferred to Central Service for reprocessing. A high level of coordination is required between perioperative personnel and the CS staff to ensure a smooth turnover of supplies. Central Service must make sure that equipment is safe and ready for scheduled surgery and that thousands of instruments are organized and processed according to strict standards. Perioperative staff members are under pressure to deliver equipment fully intact with no pieces missing, ready for immediate use in the surgical field. This collaboration works when staff members from the departments understand and respect each other's roles. A bond of trust exists as well. The CS staff must handle extremely sharp and potentially dangerous equipment that arrives directly from the operating room. The surgical technologist and circulating nurse have a responsibility to prepare equipment for processing in a way that protects CS personnel from injury. CS staff members must appreciate the need for instrument trays to be complete and ready for use in time for the scheduled procedure.

Personnel in both departments also must understand the critical nature of their work—disease prevention and patient safety.

CYCLE OF REPROCESSING

All equipment used in providing patient care is potentially contaminated with pathogenic microorganisms and must be reprocessed for safe use on the next patient. Reprocessing is a step-by-step procedure that follows an exact protocol, which starts at the point of use (Figure 8-1). In this protocol, the equipment is:

1. Maintained in a clean and orderly way at the point of use. Transferred to the processing area in a way that protects it so as to prevent contamination of the environment or personnel
2. Decontaminated for safe handling
3. Prepared for sterilization or disinfection
4. Subjected to a sterilization or disinfection process, with simultaneous monitoring and validation of the process
5. Stored so as to maintain its state of sterilization or disinfection

These steps are consistent whether an item is to be disinfected or sterilized. Sterilized items must be wrapped or protected from contact with nonsterile surfaces during the preparation phase because the packs must be handled and stored after the process is complete.

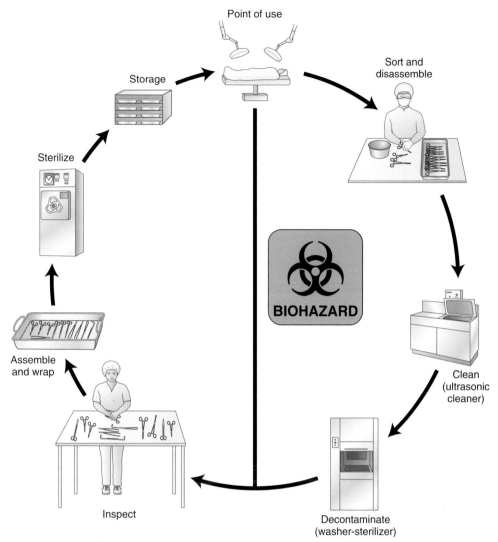

Figure 8-1 Cycle of reprocessing, starting at the point of use.

CLEANING AND DECONTAMINATION

CLEANING AT THE POINT OF USE

The preparation of equipment and instruments for patient use begins at the point of use. In the perioperative environment, this means during surgery and immediately afterward. During surgery, instruments and equipment exposed to blood and body tissue are periodically wiped free of blood and debris to prevent caking and drying. This prevents the instrument from becoming difficult to operate and also prevents dried blood and tissue from being reintroduced into the surgical wound. A sponge moistened with water can be used for this purpose, or instruments may be placed in a basin of water. Suction tips should be periodically flushed with water. Saline is never used for cleaning or soaking instruments, because it causes pitting, rusting, and corrosion.

Equipment that is not immersible should also be wiped down periodically. This includes digital or electronic cameras, light cables, pneumatic drills, and other power equipment.

At the close of surgery, sharp instruments are separated out to prevent injury. Other instruments usually are placed in a separate basin with the heaviest ones on the bottom and lighter ones on top. The water used to soak the instruments is suctioned off before the equipment is transported out of the surgical suite; this prevents spills and contamination of the transport cart. The equipment is placed on a covered or closed transportation cart for transfer to the decontamination area.

DECONTAMINATION

Many surgical departments use a case cart system to collect and transport instruments and equipment for a surgical procedure (Figure 8-2). Sterile instruments and supplies are loaded onto the cart before surgery and transported to the surgical suite. Immediately after surgery, instrument trays, basins, and any other soiled equipment are placed on the cart, which has closed shelving units. All water must be suctioned from basins before transport. The covered cart then is transferred to the decontamination area for processing. If the

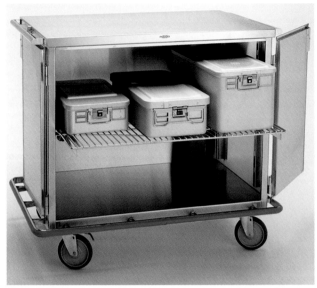

Figure 8-2 Case cart used to transport sterile packs to the surgical suite and return them to the decontamination area after surgery. A closed cart system is recommended. *(Courtesy Pedigo Products, Vancouver, Wash.)*

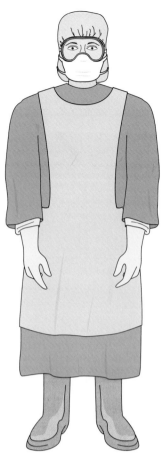

Figure 8-3 Personal protective attire (PPE). All personnel working in the decontamination area are required to wear a face shield or goggles, mask, cap, waterproof gown, and protective shoes.

health care facility has a cart decontamination system, basins and trays can be placed directly on the shelves at the point of use before transport to the decontamination area. If no such system is available, all soiled items must be contained in leak-proof bags to prevent gross contamination of the cart, and the cart is thoroughly hand cleaned with disinfectant before reuse. Instruments and equipment are transported directly to the decontamination area by the scrubbed technologist or nurse. The decontamination area may be adjacent to the surgical department or outpatient facility.

Decontamination Attire

All staff members who work in the decontamination area must wear **personal protective equipment (PPE)** in compliance with government regulations (Figure 8-3). PPE includes:

- Protective eyewear (i.e., goggles with side shields)
- Face mask
- Gloves approved for contact with chemical disinfectants (surgical or patient care gloves are not permitted)
- Full protective body suit or gown with waterproof apron and sleeves
- Waterproof shoes and covers

Sorting

The first phase of reprocessing is sorting. Items are removed from the transport cart and grouped together by category:

- Nonimmersible equipment or instruments
- Instruments with sharp edges or points
- Small gaskets, screws, pins, and other small parts
- Heavy instruments
- Delicate instruments
- Heat- and pressure-sensitive instruments
- Instrument containers

- Basins and cups
- Tubing, suction tips, or other instruments with a lumen
- Instruments or equipment requiring repair or replacement

As mentioned previously, instruments and equipment must be cleaned before they are disinfected or sterilized. Dried blood, body fluids, and tissue debris trap microorganisms and become contaminants. This debris can also cause instrument damage and malfunction. Cleaning is performed by hand, ultrasonic cleaner, and automated washer.

Hand Cleaning

After the instruments have been sorted, selected instruments are soaked and hand cleaned using cold water and enzymatic detergent. The instruments are placed in a large basin of water and submerged during cleaning to prevent the release of contaminated airborne droplets (aerosol effect).

Areas that are difficult to clean must be scrubbed with a small brush. Particular attention is paid to hemostats and other clamps, orthopedic rasps, and other instruments that contain bits of trapped soft tissue or bone. Items with a lumen (e.g., short tubing) are cleaned with a soft, narrow brush. Suction tips are cleared with a *stylet,* a fine wire that can be passed through the instrument to push out soil.

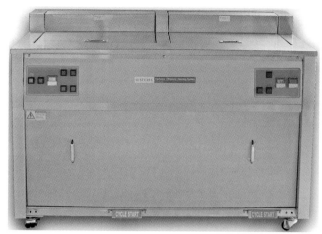

Figure 8-4 Ultrasonic cleaners remove tissue and other debris from instruments through a process called *cavitation*. (© 2008 STERIS Corporation. All rights reserved.)

Equipment and specialty instruments that are not immersible, such as those with lenses or electronic parts, are cleaned according to the manufacturer's written specifications.

Ultrasonic Cleaner

The **ultrasonic cleaner** removes debris from instruments by a process called **cavitation.** High-frequency sound waves are generated through a water bath. Cavitation causes tiny air spaces trapped within debris to implode inwardly (explode inwardly), and this releases the debris from the surface of the instrument. The ultrasonic cleaner has one or more recessed cavities that are filled with a special **enzymatic cleaner** intended for use in the system (Figure 8-4). Ultrasound may also be incorporated into the automated washer-sterilizer/disinfector. Only instruments that are free of gross debris are processed in the ultrasonic cleaner. Many instruments are damaged by ultrasound energy. Manufacturers of medical devices are careful to state whether the item can be cleaned by ultrasound. Ultrasound alone does *not* decontaminate or sterilize instruments. If a stand-alone ultrasonic system is used during the cleaning process, instruments must be decontaminated before handling.

DECONTAMINATION

Washer-Sterilizer/Disinfector

The washer-sterilizer or washer-disinfector is used to process all instruments that can tolerate water turbulence and high pressure steam. Instruments are opened and hinges extended to their widest adjustment. The instruments are then placed on metal trays and loaded into the washer chamber (Figure 8-5).

Steel basins, bowls, and containers are also processed in an automatic washer. These are not placed in with instruments but handled separately to prevent damage to instruments and ensure complete contact with water and steam.

Washer-sterilizer/disinfectors are available in several different designs. They include cleaning by immersion in a water

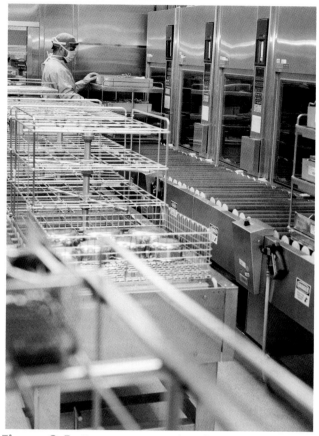

Figure 8-5 Processing area and washer-sterilizer or decontaminator used to process soiled instruments and equipment so that personnel can handle them for assembly, wrapping, and storage. (© 2008 STERIS Corporation. All rights reserved.)

bath with air injection or direct water spray wash. Newer systems include an ultrasonic phase. In the final stage, the instruments are sterilized by steam under pressure. At the conclusion of this process, the instruments can be handled by personnel.

Lubrication

Instruments are lubricated to ensure smooth mechanical action. This process is used on stainless steel instruments and other selected equipment according to the manufacturer's recommendations. Only lubricants approved for use on medical devices is used. Oils are not used for lubrication, because the sterilization process may not penetrate oil. Steel instruments may be dipped in a combined lubricating and protective "milk" as the final stage in cleaning and decontamination. The product is white when wet but dries as an invisible film.

PROCESSING IN THE CLEAN WORK AREA

After terminal decontamination, instruments are taken to the clean assembly area for sorting, inspection, and assembly (Figure 8-6). The clean processing area is separated from the

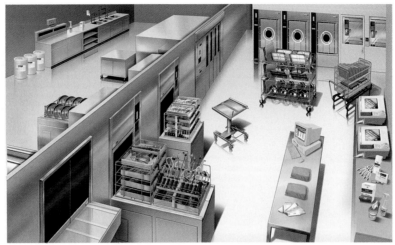

Figure 8-6 Clean processing area. This area is used for sorting, inspecting, tracking, and wrapping instruments. (© 2008 STERIS Corporation. All rights reserved.)

decontamination area to prevent cross-contamination. The clean processing area includes a workroom with ample table space for sorting instruments and assembling instrument "sets." Attire in the clean assembly area includes a clean scrub suit with long sleeves and a surgical cap.

Large-volume sterilizers are located adjacent to the clean work area for easy transfer of instruments once they have been arranged in sets and wrapped for a specific sterilization process.

NOTE: Instruments and equipment designated for semi-critical and noncritical use (e.g., endoscopes and endoscopic instruments) may be processed and stored in another location near the point of use. These instruments often are processed by perioperative staff members within that department. (Chapter 21 presents a complete discussion of the processing of fiberoptic endoscopes.)

INSTRUMENT INSPECTION

Before instruments are assembled and wrapped for sterilization, they are inspected for soil, stains, proper function, and structural soundness.

The shanks of instruments such as hemostats, needle holders, and scissors should be straight. The instrument should be opened and shut several times. If the hinge is stiff during opening and closing, it can be treated with an approved instrument lubricant. While examining the instrument, the inspector should consider the following: Do the ratchets mesh properly? Does the instrument stay shut after it is closed? With time, hemostats and needle holders may spring open unexpectedly. To determine whether an instrument is "sprung" (i.e., will not stay closed), the inspector should perform this test: Close the jaws and lock the ratchets in place. Then rap the edge of the finger rings gently on a firm surface. An instrument that is sprung will pop open when bumped.

Cutting instruments such as scissors, curettes, osteotomes, rongeurs, and shears should be examined for pitting along the cutting edge. Sharp instruments should be inspected to ensure

that the blade surfaces meet smoothly and properly. Forceps must be tested for spring. When the tips are compressed and then released, they should immediately return to the open position. The tips of forceps should close freely and meet precisely in alignment.

Microsurgical instruments are very expensive to purchase, repair, and replace. These instruments should never be mixed with heavier ones. The tips of microsurgical instruments should be inspected under magnification to ensure that the sharp points are smooth, sharp, and in proper alignment. Any instrument found to be malfunctioning should not be packaged and sterilized; rather, it should be sent for repair.

Inspection of lensed instruments is very important. Chapter 21 presents a complete description of this process.

INSTRUMENT SET ASSEMBLY

After inspection, the instruments are ready for assembly and wrapping. Lists of all instruments and equipment usually are maintained in a computer database or hard copy file. Materials management systems allow CS personnel to track both individual instruments and instrument sets. Standardized trays are assembled to so that staff members know what is included in an instrument tray at the point of use. Lists are printed out so that they can be checked at the time of clean instrument tray assembly and wrapping.

Finger ring instruments are opened (unlocked) and strung together with an instrument stringer or in racks designed to hold the instruments in an open position during the sterilization process (Figure 8-7). When assembling instrument sets, make sure any sharp or pointed items are turned downward to prevent injury or glove puncture when the pack is opened and sorted.

Instruments that have movable parts intended for disassembly must be disassembled before sterilization. Any instrument that was not disassembled before disinfection may not be clean and should be returned for disinfection.

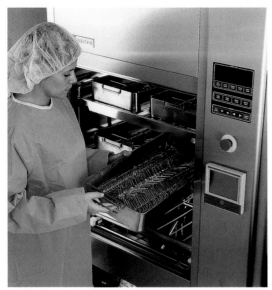

Figure 8-7 Instrument tray ready for wrapping. Instruments must be secured to prevent damage but are opened to allow the sterilant to flow to all surfaces. (© 2008 STERIS Corporation. All rights reserved.)

Instrument trays have a perforated bottom so that steam can circulate up through the tray and adequately cover all surfaces of the instruments. Make sure no instrument tips are caught in the perforations, where they could be damaged. A towel may be placed on the bottom of the tray to prevent damage to the instrument tips during the sterilization process. Heavy instruments are placed on the bottom of the tray, and the others are packed or nested so that they cannot shift and damage each other during processing.

For items with a lumen, a small amount of sterile, deionized (distilled) water should be flushed through the item immediately before sterilization. This water vaporizes during sterilization and forces air out of the lumen. Any air that is left in the lumen may prevent sterilization of its inner surface.

NOTE: Instrument trays should not contain separate items wrapped in "peel pouch" packages. Air can become trapped inside the pouches and prevent steam from reaching all surfaces of the items inside.

Power-driven surgical instruments (e.g., drills and saws) should be disassembled before steam sterilization. Hoses can be coiled loosely during packaging, and all delicate switches and parts should be protected during preparation. Before sterilization, power-driven instruments should be lubricated according to the manufacturer's specifications. Finally, before processing, make sure that all switches and control devices are in the safety position.

WRAPPING EQUIPMENT FOR STERILIZATION

Rationale
All items to be sterilized by pressurized steam, ethylene oxide, or gas plasma methods must be wrapped according to

approved methods. The purpose of wrapping an item before sterilization is to protect it from contamination after the sterilization process.

Qualities of a Wrapping System
A quality wrapping system accomplishes the following:
- Allows the sterilant to penetrate the wrapper and reach of all parts of the device
- Allows complete dissipation of the sterilant when the process is finished
- Contains no toxic ingredients or nonfast dyes
- Does not create lint
- Resists destruction by the sterilizing process (e.g., melting, delamination, blistering, and alteration of the chemical structure of an item)
- Permits complete enclosure of the package contents
- Produces a package strong enough to withstand storage and handling
- Is convenient to work with (i.e., pliable and easy to handle)
- Facilitates a method of opening and distributing the device that prevents contamination at the point of use
- Is cost-effective
- Matches the method of sterilization to be used

Wrapping Materials
Two broad categories of wrappers are woven and nonwoven paper or polymer material. Polypropylene pouches are also used to wrap items for sterilization (see below).

Reusable Woven Wrappers
Two types of woven materials are used to wrap medical devices. Cloth (often called muslin or linen wrappers) and "fabric" manufactured from chemical polymers.

Reusable cloth wrappers are made from high quality cotton or a combination of cotton and polyester. Cloth wrappers are sufficiently dense to protect goods from contamination, yet porous enough to allow penetration of steam or gas. The thread count (number of threads per square inch) must be at least 140 for an effective wrapper. Two double-thickness muslin wrappers or the equivalent (one double-thickness wrapper of 280-count muslin) are used to wrap items (Association of periOperative Registered Nurses, Recommended practices, 2007).

Before use, all cloth wrappers must be laundered and the lint must be removed. The rationale for fresh laundering is to ensure a minimum level of moisture in the cloth, which prevents superheating during sterilization. Wrappers are inspected on a light table for any pin holes or tears in the cloth, which must be repaired before use for sterilization processes.

Single-Use Nonwoven Materials
Disposable **nonwoven** wrappers are intended for one-time use only. These materials are manufactured from spun, heat-bonded fibers such as polypropylene. Nonwoven fabrics must

be used in accordance with their thickness. Lightweight fabrics require the same treatment as muslin (i.e., four thicknesses for complete protection). Heavier fabrics may be used according to the manufacturer's specifications. These are valuable for wrapping heavy instruments and flat-surfaced items such as basins and trays or heavy linen packs.

Paper derived from cellulose is *not* used for wrapping items for sterilization because paper recoils when the package is opened, making it difficult to distribute the goods inside aseptically. Also, paper is not compatible with many sterilization processes.

Wrapping Methods Using Flat Sheets

When goods are wrapped in cloth or synthetic material, the most common method is the envelope technique (Figure 8-8).

Items may be single wrapped or double wrapped, according to the specifications of the *wrapper* and in accordance with standard protocols for wrapping.

Peel Pouch

Combination synthetic and paper wrappers, commonly called *sterilization pouches* or *peel pouches,* are available in various compositions and styles (Figure 8-9). Pouches are made of a number of different synthetic materials that meet the standards for the sterilization process. The item is placed inside the pouch, which is closed with a self-sealing strip or heat sealed.

Peel pouch wrapping must be performed according to accepted standards to ensure that the item is sterile at the point of delivery:

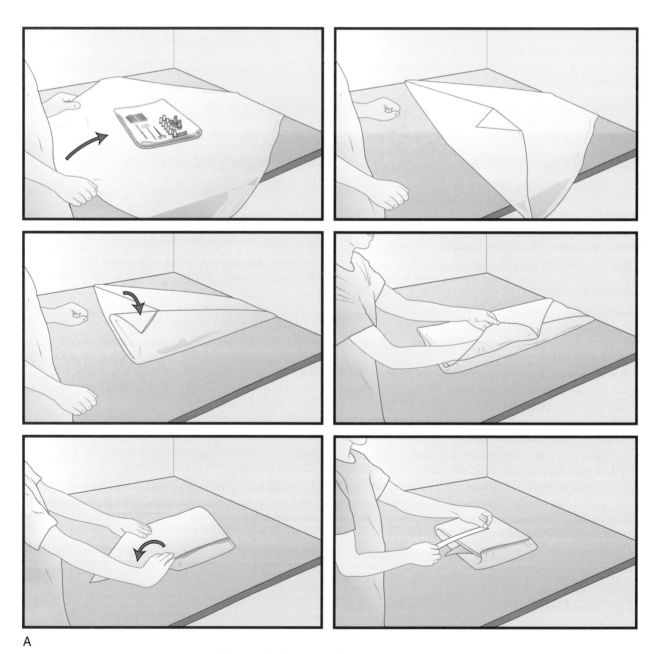

A

Figure 8-8   A, Envelope-style wrapping.

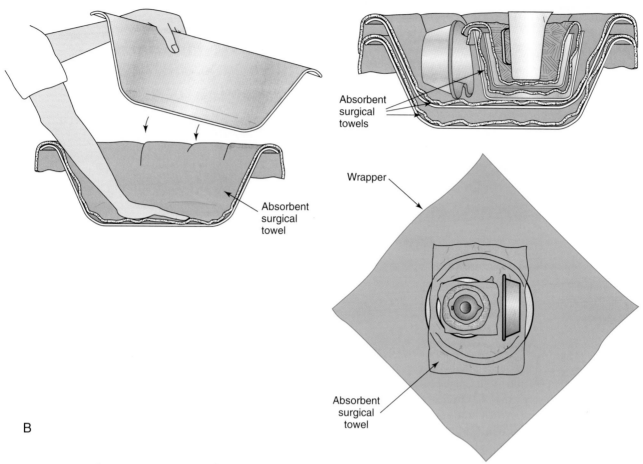

Figure 8-8, cont'd   B, Method of wrapping basins and cups for steam sterilization. Note the absorbent towel placed between objects to distribute steam evenly through the pack.

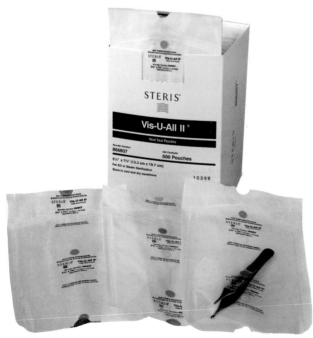

Figure 8-9 Peel pouch wrapping system used for lightweight items. (© 2008 STERIS Corporation. All rights reserved.)

- Items wrapped in peel pouches must not be placed inside an instrument tray. The sterilant may not penetrate the pouch.
- Double pouches are unnecessary and may prevent sterilization of the item.
- The item in the pouch should clear the seal by at least 1 inch (2.5 cm).
- Peel pouches are intended only for lightweight instruments and devices. Using this system for heavy items (e.g., bone rongeurs, rasps, and multiple instruments) usually leads to tearing and loss of integrity of the pouch.
- Air should be evacuated from the pouch before it is sealed. Otherwise, the package may rupture during sterilization.
- When a mechanical heat-sealing device is used, the seal should be checked very carefully to ensure that no air pockets have formed along the seal.

Sterilization Containers

Manufactured containers also are used to hold equipment for sterilization (Figure 8-10). These are convenient and safe for both gas and conventional steam sterilization. Sterilization

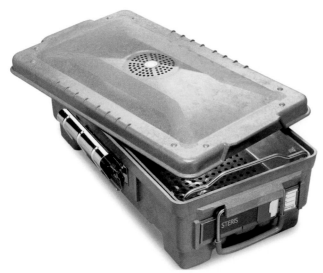

Figure 8-10 Closed sterilization container.

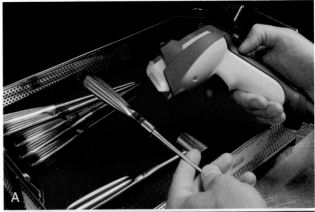

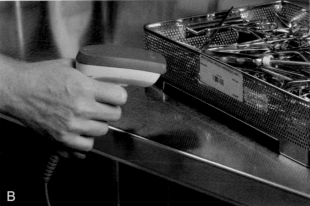

Figure 8-11 **A,** Scanning system for tracking instruments. **B,** Tracking codes are recorded in a central database, which can be used to verify the location and status of equipment. (© 2008 STERIS Corporation. All rights reserved.)

containers incorporate disposable filters into the construction of the container, and these must remain in place after sterilization to maintain the sterility of the enclosed items. A tamper-proof seal is used to verify that the cover of the container was not removed before use. When sterilization containers are used, the manufacturer's recommendations must be followed. Some containers are suitable only for a single method, whereas others are suitable for a number of different sterilization methods.

Equipment Tracking

Regardless of the type of packaging or wrapping system used, each package must be properly labeled. The date of processing, name of the item and a lot control number must be included on the label. The lot control number is used to identify items that have been included in a sterilization load that may have yielded a positive biological or mechanical control test. Any information written by hand on the outside of a wrapped package usually is placed on the sealing tape, the main purpose of which is to verify the parameters of the sterilization process (discussed in following sections).

A variety of computer-based technologies allow for accurate management of surgical supplies and equipment. Some programs track surgical instruments by bar code scanning, which allows the CS department to track specific instrument sets and identify their location at any given time (Figure 8-11). These programs identify instrument sets that have been used a certain number of times and automatically advise CS personnel to take a routine action, such as holding an instrument set for sharpening of scissors or replacing certain reusable items.

To improve the management of single-use items, special cabinets and carts have been designed to allow personnel to obtain items through a computerized system. Items are stored in the cabinet and retrieved by pushing the button associated with that item. A computer printout in a central inventory office tells the supply or stock personnel to replace that item. These systems may be connected to the hospital billing system. In this way, equipment charges are automatically assigned to individual patients.

METHODS OF STERILIZATION

Instruments and equipment used in critical areas of the body must be sterile before use. This means the instruments must be completely free of all forms of microorganisms. Common methods of sterilization include:

- High temperature steam
- Ethylene oxide gas
- Gas plasma sterilization
- Peracetic acid processing
- Dry heat
- Ionizing radiation (used in commercial manufacturing of sterile goods)

SELECTING A METHOD

In the past, surgical nurses and technologists have been confronted with decisions about which sterilization method to use for items such as wooden tongue depressors, petroleum-based gauze, liquid in glass bottles, and dry powders. These products are now less expensively and more safely sterilized by the manufacturer.

The selection criteria for the modern perioperative environment have changed with advances in technology and economics and with the increased focus on patient and personnel safety. Because steam sterilization is the most efficient method of sterilization, this is the first choice whenever possible. However, many delicate items, or those that have a complex structure may require alternative methods.

The enormous variety of instruments and equipment used in surgery does not fit easily into a generalized protocol for selecting a sterilization method. This complexity of methods also means that the manufacturer's recommendations must be followed exactly. And these methods can change quickly when new models are marketed. For example, some endoscopic instruments must be hand cleaned and gas sterilized, whereas others, even those with digital imaging capability, can be safely sterilized by high pressure steam. The current line of robotic instruments (discussed in Chapter 21 is disassembled, cleaned, decontaminated, and sterilized in an exact manner. These instruments can be steam sterilized, but only according to the manufacturer's detailed instructions. Charts and reference guides are available for most equipment, and these should be readily available in the processing area for staff members to consult.

Safety and Economic Considerations

- All devices used in the health care setting, including surgery, are sold or leased by manufacturers with instructions and recommendations for their care, including methods of reprocessing. These devices include a wide range of digital, electronic, electric, pneumatic, and lensed instruments and equipment.
- Patient safety cannot be ensured unless devices are handled according to the manufacturer's recommendations. Manufacturers are liable for any injury caused by their products as long as the products are used according to exact specifications. This includes the method of reprocessing. Consequently, reprocessing methods are specified exactly.
- Specific categories of devices, such as stainless steel (or other alloy) instruments, are processed according to standards established by professional organizations, such as the AAMI.
- The structure of a device and its composition help determine the method of reprocessing. The complexity and variety of manufactured materials are greater than in the past. Parameters for reprocessing are established according to the *exact type of material* used in the manufacture of the device, including plastics and elastomers such as such as silicone, polypropylene copolymer, ethylene-propylene rubber, and others. Compatible reprocessing methods for these materials are widely referenced and easily available.
- Speed of delivery is an important consideration in the selection of a method. A need for rapid turnover disqualifies many items for gas sterilization. Manufacturers are well aware of this constraint, and newer models of digital and electronic equipment are being developed for quicker turnover.

PROCESS-RELATED PARAMETERS OF STERILIZATION

A method of sterilization is effective only when certain conditions are met. Microbial destruction depends on the process itself and on the burden, virulence, and resistance of the microorganisms.

- **Time:** Items must be exposed to the process long enough to destroy microorganisms.
- **Saturation and surface exposure:** All parts of the item must be exposed to the sterilization process.
- **Temperature:** Some processes depend on the temperature at which the items are exposed.
- **Quality of the sterilant, air, and water:** The agent must be pure, as must the air and water used in conjunction with it. Chemical or elemental residue in water can reduce the efficacy of the process.
- **Presence of moisture:** Humidity is necessary in most sterilization processes.
- **Method of packing (where applicable) and loading the sterilizer:** This is related to saturation and exposure. Items must be loaded in a manner that allows the sterilant to penetrate all surfaces. The choice of packaging materials must be suitable for the process.

QUALITY ASSURANCE IN STERILIZATION PRACTICES

Several methods are used to determine whether the parameters of sterilization have been met. Subjecting items to the process of sterilization does not ensure that the items are sterile, only that the parameters such as heat and pressure have been reached. Objective testing or monitoring is needed to verify both the mechanical process and the outcome.

Modern sterilizers have microprocessors that supply a printout of the parameters of each phase of the sterilization process. These quality assurance methods provide valuable information and the means to detect a malfunction. Everyone involved in steam sterilization, including surgical technologists and perioperative nurses, must understand the information provided by these printouts. A malfunction is detected from the information, and the causes of load rejection must be investigated to ensure patient safety. Data for loads include the atmospheric and barometric pressures during all phases of the sterilization process, temperatures at all phases, steam quality, and vacuum levels. The most effective method of learning to operate the sterilization system properly is direct instruction by the manufacturer's clinical representative.

Chemical Monitor

A chemical monitor is a paper strip or specially treated tape that changes color when exposed to a specific temperature, pressure, and humidity (Figure 8-12). The pellet form of this **indicator** is contained in a glass vial. Chemical monitors are available for both steam and ethylene oxide sterilization. The chemical responds to high temperature, pressure, and humidity but does not register exposure time, which is critical to the

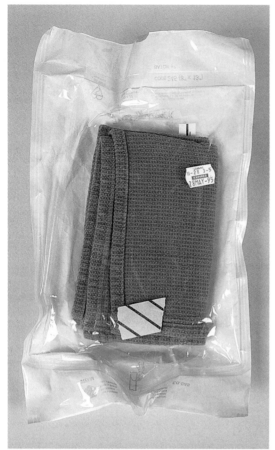

Figure 8-12 Chemical monitor. The striped monitor changes color when exposed to specific parameters used in the sterilization process. *(From Elkin MK, Perry AG, Potter PA: Nursing interventions and clinical skills, ed 3, St Louis, 2004, Mosby.)*

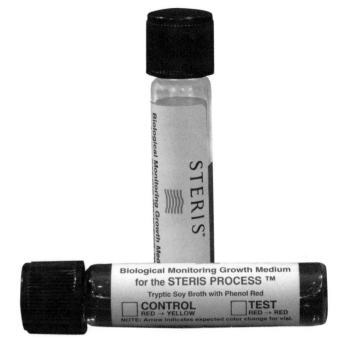

Figure 8-13 Biological indicators (BIs) contain harmless, spore-forming bacteria that can be quickly cultured after the sterilization process to monitor the load. (© 2008 STERIS Corporation. All rights reserved.)

sterilization process. A chemical monitor should be placed inside and outside all packs to be sterilized.

Biological Monitoring

Biological monitoring is the most reliable method of determining sterilization parameters. The sterility of an item cannot be *guaranteed*, because errors can prevent some items in a load from being exposed to the process. The load might be too compact, or air pockets may be present in the sterilization chamber. However, a bacterial sample can be exposed to the sterilization process and tested for viability. This is called process challenge monitoring or biological monitoring. The bacteria used during biological monitoring can differ according to the sterilization process:

- Steam sterilization: *Geobacillus stearothermophilus*
- Dry heat and ethylene oxide sterilization: *Bacillus subtilis*
- Hydrogen peroxide gas plasma: *Bacillus subtilis*
- Peracetic acid: According to the manufacturer's specifications
- Flash or high-speed steam sterilizer: *Geobacillus stearothermophilus* enzyme (fluorescence testing)

The test bacteria are encased in a self-contained unit that usually is placed in the most challenging area of the load; that is, near the outlet drain of the chamber (steam sterilizer). For ethylene oxide monitoring, the biological test pack is positioned in the center of the load. After the sterilization process, the bacterial spores are cultured. The growth of bacteria in the test culture indicates that the sterilization process probably was ineffective. If no bacteria grow, all items in the load are presumed to be sterilized.

Biological controls should be administered at least once weekly in all sterilizers and daily if possible. Biological monitors are always used when an artificial implant or prosthesis is sterilized. If any **biological indicator** shows a positive result, all items included in that load must be retrieved and resterilized. If the items have already been used in surgery, the physician must be notified so that the patient can be monitored or given prophylactic treatment.

Figure 8-13 illustrates a sample of biological monitors.

Rapid biological monitoring uses an enzyme that binds to spores. After the sterilization process, the level of enzyme is measured. This corresponds with destruction of the bacterial spores. The monitoring system is used for both high-pressure steam and ethylene oxide (EO) sterilization. Results can be obtained in 1 to 4 hours, depending on the sterilization process.

Air Detection Testing

To test and monitor the efficiency of the **high-vacuum sterilizer,** a test called the daily air removal test (DART) is performed. Commercially available Bowie-Dick tests also are available. High-vacuum sterilizers are monitored to detect air in the chamber during the exposure phase. In these tests, a special package of properly wrapped towels is taped with heat-sensitive chemical monitor tape and stacked to a height of 10 or 11 inches (25 to 27.5 cm). The package is then placed by itself in the sterilization chamber and run for the appropriate time. An unsatisfactory DART indicates a failure in the vacuum pump system or a defect in the gasket of the sterilizer door. Unsatisfactory results must be reported to the biomedical engineering staff, so that they can inspect the vacuum system and door seals.

STEAM STERILIZATION

Mechanism and Process

Steam sterilization is the most widely used, effective, and efficient method of sterilization in the health care setting. Normal atmospheric steam is not hot enough to achieve complete destruction of microbes and spores. Steam under pressure can reach the temperature necessary to destroy microbes. A high pressure steam sterilizer has a central chamber where goods are placed and a mechanism for creating extremely high pressure. Steam is pumped into the chamber, and as the pressure increases, so does the temperature. The items in this sealed environment are exposed to the temperature and pressure needed for sterilization.

Steam under pressure coagulates the nucleic acids and protein that make up the cell's genetic and enzymatic material. Pressurized steam also destroys the cell's resilient outer wall and bacterial spores.

Selection of Items for Steam Sterilization

Surgical instruments, steel basins, and cloth are routinely sterilized with steam. However, other equipment may not tolerate the high pressure and exposure to water. Some items are impenetrable to steam.

Items that should not be sterilized by steam include those made of rubber or wood and those containing materials that could melt. The appropriate processing method should always be verified with the manufacturer. This is particularly true of power-driven instruments and those that have an optical system, internal computer, or microprocessor. Some synthetic materials, such as Silastic, Teflon, polyethylene, polypropylene, and other complex polymers, are also sensitive to steam sterilization.

Temperature, Pressure, and Time Requirements

Steam sterilization is achieved at 250°F (121°C) or 270°F (132°C), depending on the items being sterilized (some items require a higher temperature than others). The laws of physics tell us that to raise the temperature of steam, we must also raise the pressure in the closed sterilization chamber:

- To achieve 250°F (121°C), the required pressure is 15 pounds per square inch (psi).
- To achieve 270°F (132°C), the required pressure is 27 psi.

The **exposure time** is actual amount of time the load is held at the designated temperature and pressure. This depends on the type of steam sterilizer, the size of the load, the temperature, and the type of materials or supplies being processed.

Moisture Concentration (Steam Quality)

Effective steam sterilization requires a specific concentration of moisture. If too little moisture is present, items become superheated and eventually can be damaged. Too much moisture leaves items wet after removal from the chamber; this can result in contamination of the item. The amount of moisture in the steam is referred to as the *steam quality*. Water is converted to steam at 212°F (100°C). At this temperature, steam is ineffective for sterilization. Steam that contains more than 97% water is necessary for sterilization to take place.

Water Quality

Although the water used during steam sterilization is filtered, contaminants are still present. These usually consist of minerals that are too small to be trapped by filters. These minerals are deposited on the surfaces of sterilized items and on the internal surfaces of the sterilizers. The presence of orange, white, brown, or black spots on sterilized items may indicate the presence of excess minerals in the water supply. As these minerals become deposited in the box locks of surgical instruments, they can impair the function of these instruments.

Gravity Displacement Steam Sterilizer

The **gravity displacement sterilizer** (also called a *downward displacement sterilizer*) operates on the principle that air is heavier than steam (Figure 8-14). The sterilizer has an inner chamber, where goods are loaded, and an outer, jacket-type chamber, which forcefully injects steam into the inner chamber. Any air in the inner chamber blocks the passage of pressurized steam to the goods and prevents sterilization. All the air must be removed from the inner chamber, because all surfaces of the items must be exposed to the pressurized steam to ensure sterilization. The sterilizer is constructed in such a way that air is pushed downward by gravity (hence the name *gravity displacement sterilizer*) and is replaced by steam. Small gravity steam sterilizers are often used in clinics or dental offices. These are called autoclaves. Large hospital steam sterilizers are commonly referred to as autoclaves.

The air exits the chamber through a temperature-sensitive valve. As the amount of steam builds up in the chamber, the temperature increases, and when the sterilization temperature is reached, the valve closes. Careful loading of items in this type of sterilizer is critical, because if the load is too dense or improperly positioned, air may become trapped in pockets. Items in these air pockets are not sterilized, because the steam cannot displace the air, which acts as an insulator.

Prevacuum Steam Sterilizer

A prevacuum steam sterilizer *pulls* air from the chamber with vacuum force and replaces it with steam. The chamber pres-

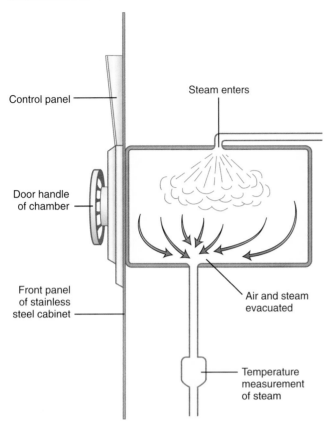

Figure 8-14 Prevacuum steam sterilizer. (Redrawn from Phillips N: Berry and Kohn's operating room technique, ed 10, St Louis, 2004, Mosby.)

sure and temperature are held for a specified period. The steam is removed through a filter, and the chamber pressure is reduced to normal (atmospheric) temperature. A cool cycle reduces the temperature to a level at which personnel may safely handle the sterilized goods. In some systems the air is removed by pulsed steam. This process is not affected by air leaks that may occur through the valves and around the door seal.

Loading and Operation of a Large Steam Sterilizer

Large steam sterilizers are used for bulk processing of hospital equipment, including surgical instruments. They usually are located in the Central Service department. Smaller sterilizers, called *flash sterilizers,* are located in the surgery department (see the following section). Bulk sterilization requires special loading techniques.

Because steam sterilization depends on direct contact of steam with all surfaces of the items, the sterilizer must be loaded so that the steam penetrates each pack. Instrument pans with mesh or wire bottoms are placed flat on the sterilizer shelf.

Linen packs, because of their density, require special attention. Linen packs are best sterilized by placing the packs on their sides. Packs and instrument trays should be placed so that they do not touch, or touch only loosely, and small items

should be placed crosswise over each other. Heavy packs should be placed at the periphery of the load, where steam enters the chamber. Basins, jars, cups, or other containers should be placed on their sides with the lids slightly ajar so that the air can flow out of them and steam can enter. Any item with a smooth surface on which water can collect and drip during the cooling phase of the sterilization cycle should be placed at the bottom of the load. Figure 8-15 shows the proper methods of loading a gravity displacement sterilizer.

Modern steam sterilizers are programmed by microprocessor. Parameters such as temperature, time, and pressure are preprogrammed for specific types of leads. The sterilizer passes through its phases automatically. Information about each load is stored in memory, and hard copies are maintained for quality assurance. The total time necessary to expose goods to pressurized steam and sterilize them depends on the density of the goods and the temperature in the sterilizer. The minimum temperature and time standards for metal and nonporous equipment are listed in Table 8-2.

These exposure times and temperatures do not reflect the entire time needed to include all phases of the sterilization process. These minimum standards apply only to the amount of time necessary for the pressurized steam to contact all surfaces of the load. Total exposure time includes the warm-up phase, holding phase (sometimes called the *kill time*), a factor of safety time, and an exhaust phase. Some sterilizers also include a drying phase. Because these times may vary from load to load, depending on the items to be sterilized, the operator should always check the specifications of the item's manufacturer, not the sterilizer's manufacturer, for recommended sterilization times and temperatures. Many items, especially heavy instruments and power-driven orthopedic tools, require longer periods of sterilization and cooling.

To assist in the removal of moisture and to prevent "wet packs," the sterilizer operator may use a dry cycle as part of the steam sterilization process. Regardless of whether a dry cycle is used, items that have been steam sterilized should be allowed to remain in the sterilizer chamber for 15 to 30 minutes after the cycle to prevent the formation of condensate.

Flash Sterilizer

A flash sterilizer is used in the operating room and in other areas of the hospital to sterilize unwrapped items quickly. A flasher sterilizer usually is located just outside the operating suite, in the substerile area. This type of sterilizer is used *only when no alternative is available* (AORN, *Standards, recommended practices, and guidelines,* 2007). Items are sterilized just before use; this is called just in time processing. Ideally, items to be flash sterilized should be in a covered metal tray. However, some flash sterilizers can be used with a drying cycle that is suitable for items wrapped in a single layer of woven material.

Recommended Practices for Flash Sterilization

1. Implants should never be flashed sterilized before use. If an implant must be sterilized in an emergency, a rapid readout biological indicator must be used.

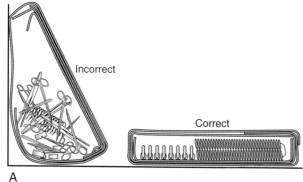

A

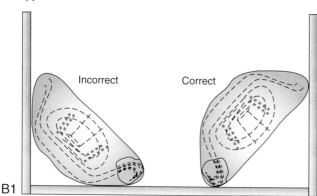

B1

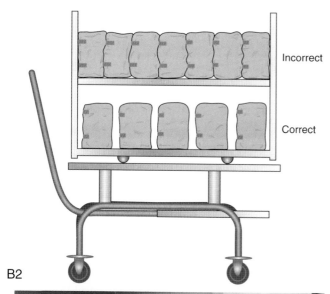

B2

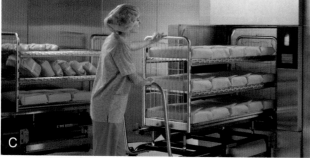

C

Figure 8-15   A, Proper method of placing instrument trays in a steam sterilizer. **B,** Proper method of loading basins and packs for steam sterilization. **C,** Loading trays into a steam sterilizer. *(Redrawn from STERIS Corp., Mentor, Ohio.)*

2. The manufacturer's specifications for exposure time and temperature must be followed.

3. If a covered sterilization container is used to flash sterilize instruments, parameter values specified by the manufacturers of the container *and* the instrument are consulted.

4. Power-driven equipment and cords are never flash sterilized without first verifying the manufacturer's recommendations.

5. Flash sterilizers must be located in an area where unwrapped sterile items can be transported directly from the sterilizer to the sterile field.

6. Items for flash sterilization are never wrapped unless this is permitted by the manufacturer's specifications.

7. Sterilization monitors must be used with every load.

8. Sterilization containers with tamper proof seals may be used for flash sterilization. Always follow manufacturer's instructions for use.

Table 8-3 presents the parameters for flash sterilization.

Removing Items from the Flash Sterilizer

To remove items from in the sterilizer chamber, the circulator dons sterile gloves and grasps the edges of the tray using sterile transfer handles. The tray is offered to the scrub who removes the sterile items from the tray with care to prevent contamination of her or his gown or gloves. The tray should not be transferred to the sterile field, and the scrub should not leave the sterile field or the room to retrieve the item from the sterilizer as this is considered poor aseptic technique

Precautions and Hazards

Most modern flash sterilizers have an alarm and lockout system that prevents personnel from opening the chamber door until it is safe to do so. In spite of safety features, accidents can occur in older models that do not have lockout systems.

The operator should be particularly careful when opening or closing the door. It is held in the lock position by a pressure-sensitive valve that prevents the door from being opened when the chamber is under pressure. Because a tremendous amount of pressure is exerted on the door by the steam in the chamber, the valve is designed to withstand very high temperatures and force from within. If the valve malfunctions for any reason, the operator may be able to open the door while the chamber is partly pressurized with steam. If this happens, the operator will be exposed to a rapid burst of hot steam when the door is opened.

The operator should always check the pressure level on the control panel before opening the door. If the pressure has not dropped to atmospheric level (0) at the completion of the sterilization cycle, the operator should wait for it to do so. If the pressure remains elevated, the operator should not attempt to open the door, nor should he or she attempt to resolve the malfunction. Rather, the malfunction should be reported so that trained personnel can be called for assistance.

Occasionally the operator may fail to close the door all the way. This usually is caused by misalignment of the spokelike locks mounted on the front of the door on older models.

Table 8-2

Minimum Exposure Time Standards for Steam Sterilization after Effective Steam Penetration and Heat Transfer

Materials	GRAVITY DISPLACEMENT		PREVACUUM
	250°F (121°C)	270°F (132°C)	270°F (132°C)
Basin sets—wrapped	20 min	NA (not applicable)	4 min
Basins, glassware, and utensils—unwrapped	15 min	Not recommended	3 min
Instruments, with or without other items—wrapped as set in double-thickness wrappers	30 min	NA	4 min
Instruments—unwrapped but with other items, including towel in bottom of tray or covering them	20 min	10 min	4 min
Instruments—completely unwrapped	15 min	3 min	3 min
Drape packs	30 min*	NA	4 min
Maximum size: 12 × 12 × 20 inches (30 × 30 × 50 cm)			
Maximum weight: 12 pounds (5.5 kg)			
Fabrics, single items—wrapped	30 min*	NA	4 min
Rubber and thermoplastics, including small items and gloves but excluding tubing—wrapped	20 min*	Not applicable	4 min
Tubing—wrapped	30 min	NA	4 min
Tubing—unwrapped	20 min	NA	4 min
Sponges and dressings—wrapped	30 min	NA	4 min
Solutions—flasked	(Slow exhaust)	NA	Automatic selector determines correct temperature and exposure period for solutions.
75-mL flask	20 min		
250-mL flask	25 min		
500-mL flask	30 min		
1000-mL flask	35 min		
1500-mL flask	45 min		
2000-mL flask	45 min		

From Phillips N: *Berry and Kohn's operating room technique*, ed 10, St Louis, 2004, Mosby.
*Fabrics and rubber deteriorate more quickly with repeated sterilization for prolonged periods in gravity displacement sterilizers.

Table 8-3

Time-Temperature Parameters for Flash Steam Sterilization

Type of Sterilizer	Load Configuration	Temperature °F (°C)	Time
Gravity displacement	Metal or nonporous items only (no lumens)	270°-275°F (132°-135°C)	3 min
	Metal items with lumens and porous items (e.g., rubber, plastic) sterilized together	270°-275°F (132°-135°C)	10 min
Prevacuum	Metal or nonporous items only (no lumens)	270°-275°F (132°-135°C)	3 min
	Metal items with lumens and porous items sterilized together	270°-275°F (132°–135°C)	4 min or manufacturer's instructions
Pulsing gravity	All loads	Manufacturer's instructions	Manufacturer's instructions
Abbreviated prevacuum	All loads	Manufacturer's instructions	Manufacturer's instructions

From Rothrock JC, editor: *Alexander's care of the patient in surgery*, ed 12, St Louis, 2003, Mosby.

When this happens, a constant flow of steam escapes from around the edges of the door. Most models have a steam shutoff valve close to the floor, below the sterilizer. The valve can be turned to the "off" position only if it can be approached without risk of injury. Steam should then be allowed to dissipate from the sterilizer until it is safe to open the door completely. The operator should not attempt to reach the valve unless the area around it is completely cool and free of steam.

ETHYLENE OXIDE STERILIZATION

Mechanism and Process

Ethylene oxide is used to sterilize objects that cannot tolerate the heat, moisture, and pressure of steam sterilization. It can be used for delicate instruments, including microsurgical instruments and those with optical systems. It is highly penetrating, which makes it ideal for complex instruments with delicate inner components.

EO is a highly flammable liquid that, when blended with inert gas, produces effective sterilization by destroying the deoxyribonucleic acid (DNA) and protein structure of microorganisms. Ethylene oxide is used in 100% pure form, blended with carbon dioxide gas, or mixed with hydrochlorofluorocarbons.

Ethylene oxide kills microorganisms and their spores by interfering with the metabolic and reproductive processes of the cell. The process is intensified with both heat and moisture. The EO sterilizer operates at a low temperature. The temperature of the gas directly affects the penetration of items in the chamber. Operating temperatures range from 85° to 100° F (29° to 388° C) for a "cold" cycle and 130° to 145° F (54° to 63° C) for a "warm" cycle.

Humidity is required to make spores more resistant to the EO gas. The preferred moisture content for EO sterilization is 25% to 80%. The length of exposure depends on the type and density of material to be sterilized, temperature, humidity, and concentration of the gas.

Precautions and Hazards

A number of environmental and safety hazards are associated with ethylene oxide. Exposure to the gas can cause burns to skin and mucous membranes. Prolonged occupational exposure to EO gas is known to cause respiratory damage. EO is a stable compound with a long half-life. Its advantage as a penetrating sterilant also poses hazards. It is difficult to remove, and the level of EO residue is not the same in different materials. In addition, it reacts with many different substances, causing them to disintegrate or creating other toxic compounds, such as ethylene glycol and ethylene chlorohydrins. These chemicals also are difficult to remove from the environment.

To prevent injury from EO exposure, the Occupational Safety and Health Administration (OSHA) requires air sampling in areas likely to contain high concentrations of ethylene oxide. The level of ethylene oxide must not exceed 0.5 ppm in any area. Personal dosimeter badges measure ethylene oxide exposure. Air samples should be taken regularly in the sterilization area. Other safety precautions include the installation of an exhaust system that vents the gas to the outside of the building through an exhaust vent located above the chamber door. Six to 10 exchanges of fresh air per hour are delivered to the sterilization area.

Observing the following precautions reduces occupational and patient risk:

- After the sterilization process is finished, keep the sterilizer door opened slightly for about 15 minutes.
- Make sure goods transported from the sterilizer to the aerator (discussed later) remain on a transport cart.
- Always wear protective gloves when handling unaerated items.
- Never retrieve an instrument from the aerator before completion of the approved aeration period. Do not ask anyone else to do this, even if a surgeon requests it.
- Always pull the transport cart rather than pushing it. Pushing the cart places personnel in back of the air flowing from the unaerated items.
- Follow the manufacturer's exact specifications for aeration.

Preparation of Items for Gas Sterilization

All items to be gas sterilized must be clean and dry. Any water left on equipment bonds with EO gas and produces a toxic residue, which can cause burns or a toxic reaction in those who come in contact with it. Any organic material or soil exposed to ethylene oxide also may produce toxic residues, therefore all items processed for EO gas must be completely clean. Items are loaded in the sterilizer loosely so that the gas is free to circulate over every surface.

Every attempt should be made to load items that have similar aeration requirements. Some items must not be gas sterilized. These include acrylics and some pharmaceutical items.

Because ethylene oxide does not penetrate glass, solutions in a glass vial or bottle cannot be sterilized by this method. Any instruments with fittings or parts should be disassembled before ethylene oxide sterilization to facilitate exposure to the gas.

Wrapping techniques for EO sterilization are the same as for high pressure steam sterilization. However, some materials are not suitable for ethylene oxide processing. These include wrappers made of natural fiber combined with nylon and rayon, polyester, and polyvinyl chloride. Double-wrapped peel pouches are not suitable for some ethylene oxide sterilizers. The manufacturer's recommendations should always be followed.

Loading and Sterilization

The ethylene oxide sterilizer is loaded in such a way that gas can penetrate all surfaces of the packages. Packages must not touch the bottom or top of the chamber and must be placed loosely on their sides. The EO sterilizer is preprogrammed for exposure time, temperature, and aeration parameters. The sterilizer is operated from the control panel by trained CS technologists.

<u>Table 8-4</u>

Minimum Aeration Times after Ethylene Oxide Sterilization at Different Temperatures

Materials	AMBIENT ROOM AIR 65°-72°F (18°-22°C)	MECHANICAL AERATOR 122°F (50°C)	140°F (60°C)
Metal and glass			
Unwrapped	May be used immediately		
Wrapped	2 hr	2 hr	2 hr
Rubber for external use—not sealed in plastic	24 hr	8 hr	5 hr
Polyethylene and polypropylene for external use—not sealed in plastic	48 hr	12 hr	8 hr
Plastics except polyvinyl chloride items—not sealed in plastic	96 hr (4 days)	12 hr	8 hr
Polyvinyl chloride	168 hr (7 days)	12 hr	8 hr
Plastic and rubber items—those sealed in plastic and/or those that will come in contact with body tissues	168 hr (7 days)	12 hr	8 hr
Internal pacemaker	504 hr (21 days)	32 hr	24 hr

From Phillips N: *Berry and Kohn's operating room technique*, ed 10, St Louis, 2004, Mosby.

Aeration

Unlike with steam sterilization, items sterilized with ethylene oxide require aeration to dissipate any residual gas remaining on the items. The manufacturer's recommendations for aeration are critical to the safety of both the patient and the hospital personnel handling equipment that has been gas sterilized. Aeration takes place in a special aeration chamber or by room air, provided that safety precautions are followed. In many newer models, aeration takes place within the sterilizer chamber through the addition of an aerator that evacuates the gas from the chamber and flushes the chamber with room air. The aeration time for an object depends on its porosity and size (Table 8-4). Aeration can require to 12 hours for some items.

GAS PLASMA STERILIZATION

Mechanism and Process

Gas plasma sterilization is used on items that are heat and moisture sensitive. The time required for gas plasma sterilization is much shorter than that required for EO sterilization. Gas plasma is made up of ionized gases. During the sterilization process, hydrogen peroxide is exposed to a vacuum. This creates a vapor, which is forced into the central chamber where goods have been loaded. Radiofrequency energy is transmitted through the vapor, which excites the hydrogen peroxide molecules. This action destroys microorganisms by interfering with the cell membrane, genetic material, and cell enzymes.

The gas plasma sterilization cycle has four phases:
1. **Vacuum phase:** Air is evacuated from the chamber to reduce the pressure.
2. **Injection phase:** Liquid hydrogen peroxide is injected into the central chamber, where it is vaporized.
3. **Diffusion phase:** Hydrogen peroxide vapor disperses throughout the load.
4. **Plasma phase:** Radiofrequency energy breaks apart the hydrogen peroxide vapor, creating a plasma cloud containing free radicals and ultraviolet (UV) light. The compounds recombine into oxygen and water and are dissipated from the chamber. This completes the cycle.

The exposure time depends on the type and size of the load but ranges from 30 to 60 minutes. No toxic chemicals are created by this process, and aeration time is not necessary. After the sterilization cycle, hydrogen peroxide gas is converted to its molecular components, water, and oxygen.

Cloth and cellulose products cannot be processed by gas plasma sterilization. Only specific nonwoven wrapping materials can be used (e.g., Tyvek/Mylar wrappers). Materials compatible with gas plasma sterilization are listed in Box 8-1.

Preparation of materials for gas plasma sterilization is the same as for EO sterilization. Items are decontaminated as usual, dried, assembled, and wrapped according to the manufacturer's specifications. Quality control indicators to verify sterilization parameters are used just as with other sterilization procedures (see later discussion).

LIQUID PERACETIC ACID STERILIZATION

Mechanism and Process

Peracetic acid is a liquid chemical made up of 35% peracetic acid, hydrogen, and water. This system is an alternative to cold sterilization processing, commonly performed with a glutaraldehyde solution. During the sterilization process, peracetic acid inactivates many cell systems through a chemical process called *oxidation*. As the peracetic acid decomposes after the sterilization process, it converts to acetic acid (vinegar) and oxygen. Peracetic acid does not leave a chemical residue, but it must be rinsed thoroughly from instruments.

Materials Compatible with Gas Plasma Sterilization

Metals
- Stainless steel 300 series
- Aluminum 6000 series
- Titanium

Nonmetals
- Glass
- Silica
- Ceramic

Plastics and Elastomers
- Acrylonitrile-butadiene-styrene (ABS)
- Chlorinated polyvinyl chloride (CPVC)
- Ethylene-propylene rubber (EPDM)
- Polycarbonate (PC)
- Polyetherketone (PEEK)
- Polyethermidide (Ultem)
- Polyethersulfone (PES)
- Polyethylene
- Polymethyl methacrylate (PMMA)
- Polymethylpentene (PMP)
- Polyphenylene oxide (Noryl, PPO)
- Polypropylene (LDPP, HDPP)
- Polypropylene copolymer (PPCO)
- Polysulfone (PSF)
- Polyvinyl chloride (PVC)
- Polyvinylidene fluoride (PVDF)
- Teflon (PTFE, PFA, FEP)
- Tefzel (ETFE)
- Most silicones and fluorinated silicones

From Johnson & Johnson: Material compatibility for STERRAD system.

Peracetic acid is used in a closed commercial processing system manufactured by the STERIS Corp. (Mentor, Ohio).

Cobalt-60 Radiation Sterilization

Most equipment available prepackaged from a manufacturer has been sterilized by ionizing radiation (**cobalt-60 radiation**), which destroys all microorganisms. Items such as **sharps,** sutures, sponges, and disposable drapes are just a few of the many types of presterilized products available.

Also included are anhydrous materials such as powders and petroleum goods. These products traditionally have been sterilized by dry heat in the hospital setting. However, the current trend is away from dry heat sterilization because of its inconvenience and because these substances now are available as single-use items, packaged in one-dose containers to prevent cross-contamination. Items intended for single use, whether supplies for use in the surgical field or other substances meant to be used only once, must never be resterilized by conventional methods (steam sterilization, ethylene oxide, or chemical sterilization) without the manufacturer's express recommendation to do so. The item might change in composition or deteriorate and could become a hazard to the patient or personnel.

INSTRUMENTS EXPOSED TO CREUTZFELDT-JAKOB DISEASE (CJD) PRIONS

Creutzfeldt-Jakob disease (CJD) and variant CJD are fatal diseases caused by prions. A prion is a protein particle that is not a cell and is not related to bacteria or viruses. These prions are highly infective in central nervous system tissue, and they are a special concern in the processing of instruments and equipment. Prions are not destroyed by normal means of mechanical or **chemical sterilization.** Specific procedures are necessary to control and destroy the prion on medical devices in the clinical setting (Table 8-5 presents general guidelines). Perioperative staff members can update their knowledge of the recommended procedures by consulting the CDC Web site (http://www.cdc.gov) and the AORN Web site (http://www.aorn.org).

STORAGE AND HANDLING OF STERILE GOODS

After an item has been processed and sterilized, consideration must be given to how the item can be kept sterile. Time-related sterility measures (based on the length of time since sterilization) are not considered valid. **Event-related sterility** or terminal sterilization is the accepted standard.

> ❖ *Event-related sterility or terminal sterilization is based on the principle that sterilized items are assumed sterile between uses unless environmental conditions or events interfere with the integrity of the package.*

Guidelines for Storage

Items should be stored according to the following guidelines:

- Sterile items should be stored in areas that are separate from those used to store clean nonsterile items.
- Sterile items must never be stored near sinks or other areas where they can be exposed to water.
- Sterile items should be stored in critical areas or in the sterile core when possible. They should be placed in a draft-free area away from vents and windows. The area must be dust and lint free.
- Closed cabinets are preferred to open storage areas.
- If items are stored in open bins, the bins or drawers should be shallow to prevent excess handling of the items.
- Mesh or basket containers are preferable over those with a solid surface where dust and bacteria can collect.
- Packages should be placed loosely on shelves to prevent crushing, tearing, or damage to items and wrappers.
- Heavy items must never be stacked on top of lighter ones. Stacking heavy instrument trays poses a risk that wrappers will be torn as the top tray is removed.
- Seldom-used items can be wrapped in protective dust covers.
- Wrappers should be inspected for damage and expiration before they are opened for use.

Table 8-5

Care of Items Exposed to Creutzfeldt-Jakob Disease (CJD) Prions

Tissue Infectivity	Item/Device (Spaulding Classification System)	Cleanable	Heat/Moisture Stable	Disposition
High infectivity	Critical/semicritical instruments and devices	If easily cleaned	If yes	1. Thoroughly clean with antiseptic detergent 2. Process at 272°F (134°C) immersed in water in prevacuum sterilizer for 18 min (extended cycle) or 3. Process instruments immersed in water at 250°F (121°C) in gravity sterilizer for 20 min; 60 min if not immersed in water or 4. Immerse in 1 N NaOH (1 normal sodium hydroxide) for 60 min at room temperature. After 60 min, remove items from NaOH, rinse, and steam sterilize at 250°F (121°C) in gravity sterilizer for 30 min. 5. After processing as selected from 1-4, prepare instruments in the usual fashion and sterilize for future use.
			If no	Discard

	Critical/semicritical instruments and devices	If difficult to clean	If yes	1. Discard or
				2. Decontaminate initially by:
				  a. Autoclaving at 272°F (134°C) in prevacuum sterilizer for 18 min or
				  b. Autoclaving at 250°F (121°C) in gravity sterilizer for 60 min or
				  c. Immersing in 1 N NaOH for 60 min at room temperature. After 60 min, remove items from NaOH, rinse, and steam sterilize at 250°F (121°C) in gravity sterilizer for 30 min.
				3. After initial decontamination as above, thoroughly clean, wrap, and sterilize by conventional methods for future use.

			If no	Discard
	Critical/semicritical instruments and devices Noncritical instruments and devices	If impossible to clean	NA	Discard
	Noncritical instruments and devices	If cleanable	NA	1. Clean according to routine procedures. 2. Disinfect with 1:10 dilution of sodium hypochlorite or 1 N NaOH, depending on which solution would be least damaging to the items. 3. Continue processing according to routine procedures.
		Noncleanable	NA	Discard
	Environmental surfaces	NA	NA	1. Cover surface with disposable, impermeable material. 2. Incinerate material after use. 3. Disinfect surface with 1:10 dilution of sodium hypochlorite (bleach). 4. Wipe entire surface using routine facility decontamination procedures for surface decontamination.
Medium/low/no infectivity	Critical/semicritical/noncritical instruments and devices	Cleanable	NA	1. Clean, disinfect, or sterilize according to routine procedures.
		Noncleanable	NA	Discard
	Environmental surfaces	NA	NA	1. Cover surface with disposable, impermeable material. 2. Dispose of material according to facility policy. 3. Disinfect surface with OSHA-recommended agent for decontamination of blood-contaminated surfaces (e.g., 1:10 or 1:100 dilution of sodium hypochlorite).

Data from Favaro MS, Bond WW: Chemical disinfection of medical and surgical materials. In Block SS, editor: *Disinfection, sterilization, and preservation*, ed 5, Philadelphia, 2001, Lippincott Williams & Wilkins; New clues on how to inactivate prions, *OR Manager* 20:23, 2004; Rutala WA, Weber DJ: Creutzfeldt-Jakob disease: recommendations for disinfection and sterilization, *Clinical Infectious Diseases* 32:1348, 2001; World Health Organization, Department of Communicable Disease Surveillance and Response: *WHO infection control guidelines for transmissible spongiform encephalopathies*. Accessed at www.who.int/site-search/data-who-hq-live/search.shtml.

NA, Not applicable; *OSHA*, Occupational Safety and Health Administration.

- Items commercially prepared and sterilized by manufacturers may be considered sterile indefinitely as long as the wrapper is intact. An expiration date printed on the package shows the maximum time the manufacturer can guarantee product stability and sterility.

DISINFECTION

TERMS RELATED TO DISINFECTION

Disinfection is the destruction of some but not all types of microorganisms. Common terms used to describe chemicals and the process of disinfection help distinguish chemicals and also clarify their action.

The suffix **-cidal** means to kill. A **bactericidal** chemical is one that kills bacteria, and a **viricidal** chemical kills viruses. A **sporicidal** chemical destroys bacterial spores, and a **fungicidal** agent is one that kills fungi. The term *germicide* ("germ killing," or **germicidal**) is commonly used by the general public but not in medicine. *Germ* is the lay term for infectious microorganism.

As previously discussed, the *bioburden* is the number of reproducing bacterial colonies on a contaminated surface. **Biofilm** is a matrix of extracellular polymers formed by some types of bacteria. This substance forms an adhesive, which enables the microorganisms to remain attached to their host. Biofilm must be penetrated for the microbes to be removed or destroyed.

USE OF CHEMICAL DISINFECTANTS

Disinfectants commonly used in patient care are categorized by chemical type (Table 8-6). The selection of a disinfectant is based on the result required. Some disinfectants are effective at destroying a limited number of microorganisms; others are very effective at killing all organisms, including bacterial spores. Some are extremely corrosive, whereas others are relatively harmless to common materials found in the hospital. Factors that affect a disinfectant's activity (or "-cidal" ability) include the following:

1. *Concentration of the solution:* Every chemical disinfectant is used at a prescribed dilution. Chemicals may require premixing with water. This must be done with a measuring device.
2. *The bioburden on the object:* As the bioburden increases, the effectiveness of the disinfectant may decrease.
3. *Water hardness and pH:* The mineral content and pH of the water used for dilution may alter the action of the chemical.
4. *Presence or absence of organic matter on the item:* Nearly all disinfectants are weakened in the presence of organic material such as blood, sputum, or tissue residue. Therefore items to be disinfected must undergo cleaning (removal of organic debris and soil) and thorough drying before the disinfection process.

Precautions and Hazards

Many disinfectants are unsafe for use on human tissue, including skin. This means that employees must be extremely cautious when handling them. Warnings and instructions for use must be strictly followed. Do not be misled by the mild odor of some disinfectants. Many chemicals do not emit noxious fumes. This is not an indication of any lack of toxicity to skin or the respiratory system.

Every health care facility is required by law to provide employees with information about hazards in their work environment. This includes specific training and information about the chemicals they handle. Every chemical used in the workplace has a corresponding Material Safety Data Sheet (MSDS), as mandated by OSHA. The MSDS describes the chemical, potential hazards, and what to do if the chemical comes in contact with the skin or is splashed into the eyes. The MSDS for each chemical is easily accessed and should be read by all who work in the perioperative environment. (A more complete discussion of chemical safety is presented in Chapter 15.)

Safety Guidelines for Disinfectants

- All disinfectants should be stored in well-ventilated rooms, and their containers should be kept covered.
- All personnel handling disinfectants must wear personal protective equipment.
- The dilution ratio of a liquid chemical should never be changed except by hospital protocol.
- A measuring device designated for mixing liquid disinfectants with water should always be used. Personnel should not rely on haphazard techniques or guesswork when preparing solutions.
- Two disinfectants should never be mixed; this could create toxic fumes or unstable and dangerous compounds.
- Liquid chemicals should be disposed of as directed by hospital policy and the chemical's label instructions. Some chemicals are unsafe for disposal through standard sewage systems.
- An unlabeled bottle or container should never be used and should be discarded. Personnel should always be aware of what chemical is being used and its specific purpose.

HIGH LEVEL DISINFECTION

High level disinfection (HLD) is a process in which most but not all microorganisms are killed with a liquid disinfectant. HLD does not usually destroy bacterial spores, therefore it is used only for instruments that will be used in semicritical areas of the body (i.e., nonintact skin and mucous membranes). Instruments and other items that are semicritical include:

- Anesthesia equipment
- Gastrointestinal endoscopes
- Bronchoscopes
- Respiratory therapy equipment

HLD is used for flexible and rigid endoscopes that are used in noncritical areas of the body. Processing takes place in a special area of the operating room adjacent to or near the point of use, such as the endoscopy department or cystoscopy suite.

The process uses a commercial reprocessing unit, or the instrument is simply soaked in a large basin or tray. Before any instrument is disinfected, it must be thoroughly cleaned

Table 8-6

Properties of Disinfectants

Chemical	Level of Disinfection	Kills Spores	Kills HIV	Kills M. Tuberculosis	Kills HBV	Uses	Risk
Isopropyl alcohol (70% to 90%)	Intermediate (some semicritical and noncritical items)	No	Yes	Yes	Yes	Limited; no longer used as a general disinfectant.	Flammable; can damage lensed instruments.
Phenolic detergent compounds	Low	No	Yes	Yes	No	Environmental cleaning only.	Highly toxic.
Glutaraldehyde (2%)	High (critical items)	Yes	Yes	Yes	Yes	Endoscopes, respiratory equipment, anesthesia equipment, immersible items. Long shelf life. Disinfectant active for long periods when used properly.	Vapor causes eye, skin, and nasal irritation. Improperly rinsed endoscopes can cause tissue damage.
Stabilized hydrogen peroxide (6%)	High (critical items)	Yes	Yes	Yes	Yes	Must contact all surfaces when used as a sterilant.	Can cause tissue irritation.
Formalin (37% formaldehyde)	High	Yes	Yes	Yes	Yes	Currently used for specimen preservation.	Highly noxious fumes; carcinogenic.
Iodophor (free iodine in a detergent-disinfectant solution)	Intermediate to low, depending on concentration	No	Yes	Yes	Yes	As a disinfectant, limited to use in cleaning hydrotherapy tanks and thermometers, environmental cleaning.	May cause reaction in sensitive individuals.
Quaternary ammonium detergent	Low (noncritical items)	No	Yes	No	No	Limited effectiveness; used for low level environmental disinfection.	May cause reaction in sensitive individuals.
Sodium hypochlorite (5%, 500 ppm)	Low (noncritical items)	No	Yes	No	Yes	1 : 100 ppm for spot disinfection and blood spills; environmental cleaning.	Fumes can irritate skin and mucous membranes.

HBV, Hepatitis B virus; *HIV*, human immunodeficiency virus.

to remove all traces of blood, tissue, and body fluids. Cleaning proceeds in a systematic fashion so that no areas are overlooked.

A complete discussion of the techniques used in the reprocessing of endoscopes can be found in Chapter 21. Important guidelines are listed in Box 8-2.

CHEMICAL DISINFECTANTS FOR MEDICAL DEVICES

The chemicals most commonly used in high level disinfection are glutaraldehyde and orthophthaldehyde (commercially prepared as Cidex and Cidex OPA).

Glutaraldehyde

Glutaraldehyde is a high level disinfectant that is sporicidal, bactericidal, and viricidal. It is tuberculocidal in 20 minutes. This disinfectant is weakened considerably by unintentional dilution, which occurs if instruments are wet when placed in the immersion tank. Glutaraldehyde is also weakened by the presence of organic matter. When glutaraldehyde solutions are mixed and kept for repetitive use, the solution must be completely renewed after 14 days because it is ineffective after that time. In addition, during its time in use, the solution must be evaluated often with test strips to ensure that the proper concentration is maintained (2% glutaraldehyde).

Important Guidelines for Processing Endoscopes

Manual Cleaning

- Always wear PPE when reprocessing instruments in a chemical solution.
- Always leak test any flexible endoscope before cleaning.
- Submerge the instrument in detergent solution and clean all surfaces with a clean cloth.
- Use a suction pump and syringe to flush detergent through the instrument channels and ports.
- A soft brush can be used to clean channels.
- After cleaning the instrument completely, rinse it in deionized water to remove all traces of detergent.
- Inspect the instrument for any soil or debris missed during cleaning. If any debris remains, repeat the cleaning process, including all channels, valves, and stopcocks.
- Remove all water from the instrument channels and exterior. Low level compressed air may be used to dry channels, valves, and stopcocks.

High Level Disinfection

- Processing should be done just before use.
- If an automatic reprocessor is used, following the manufacturer's guidelines exactly.
- Make sure the instrument is completely dry before submerging it in disinfectant.
- For manual processing of items in a tray or basin, make sure all channels are filled with solution.
- Cover the tray and start timing.
- Do not add any instruments or change the dilution after processing has begun.
- When timing is complete, remove the item and rinse thoroughly according to operating room policy at least three times to remove all traces of disinfectant.

Occupational hazards of glutaraldehyde most commonly arise when the solution is kept in open immersion baths in a poorly ventilated work area. The safe levels of formaldehyde or glutaraldehyde in the air are under 0.2 ppm. Any amount over that causes irritation of the eyes and nasal passages. Glutaraldehyde is toxic to tissue; items that have been disinfected or sterilized in glutaraldehyde must be completely rinsed with sterile, distilled water before they are used on a patient.

Orthophthaldehyde

Orthophthaldehyde 0.55% (Cidex OPA) is a non–glutaraldehyde-based, high level disinfectant that can be used for immiscible medical devices. Instruments and equipment are thoroughly cleaned, dried, and placed in the solution for 12 minutes. The items must be thoroughly rinsed with water three times. Items not properly rinsed will stain the skin of the handler or the patient. Orthophthaldehyde has a **shelf life** of 14 days; daily testing is required to ensure that the concentration of the disinfectant is at the required level.

LOW LEVEL DISINFECTION: NONCRITICAL AREAS

Low level disinfection is performed on equipment that comes in contact with skin but not mucous membranes or any other tissue. The process of low-level disinfection kills most, but not all, bacteria and viruses. This category of disinfection is performed on patient care items, transport devices, and furniture, such as:

- Operating room table and accessories
- Furniture in the surgical suite
- Floors and walls
- Intravenous (IV) stands
- Stretchers
- Blood pressure cuffs
- Stethoscopes

Low level disinfection is performed as part of routine decontamination of the operating room and in all patient care settings.

ENVIRONMENTAL DISINFECTANTS

Environmental disinfectants are used for routine low level disinfection and terminal decontamination.

Phenolics

Phenol (carbolic acid) is formulated as a detergent for hospital cleaning. It is not sporicidal, but it is tuberculocidal, fungicidal, viricidal, and bactericidal. Because scant information is available on the specific effects of phenol on microorganisms, its use is restricted to disinfection of **noncritical items.** It is extremely important to follow the manufacturer's instructions for dilution and mixing, because phenolic mixtures can be very toxic. Phenol has a very noxious odor and causes skin lesions and respiratory irritation in some individuals.

Quaternary Ammonium Compounds

Quaternary ammonium compounds, or "quats," are fungicidal and bactericidal but not effective at killing spores. This group of disinfectants is less effective in hard water, which can limit their use in some regions. Benzalkonium chloride and dimethyl benzyl ammonium chloride have been widely used as disinfectants.

Hypochlorite

Hypochlorite is sporicidal, tuberculocidal, and effective against the human immunodeficiency virus (HIV). The CDC recommends this product for use in spot cleaning of blood spills, because it is very fast acting. However, it is deactivated in the presence of organic material, therefore the area must be cleaned before hypochlorite is applied. The chemicals in the hypochlorite family are not used on instruments, because they are corrosive. However, they are widely used for environmental cleaning, because they are effective and inexpensive. Sodium hypochlorite, for example, is common household bleach. Hypochlorite must be diluted properly to prevent respiratory irritation and skin burns.

Alcohol

Alcohol is a commonly used disinfectant that is composed of two components: ethyl alcohol and isopropyl alcohol. Both are water soluble (mix easily in water). Alcohol is not sporicidal, but it is bactericidal, tuberculocidal, and viricidal. It is effective against *Cytomegalovirus spp.* and HIV. Alcohol's optimum disinfection ability occurs at a 60% to 70% dilution. Alcohol must never be used on surgical instruments, because it is not sporicidal and is very corrosive to stainless steel.

Alcohol greatly reduces the number of bacteria on skin when used as a surgical hand rub. However, it also removes fatty acids from the skin and has a drying effect when used routinely.

Because it is highly flammable and volatile, alcohol must never be used around electrocautery instruments or lasers. It must be stored in a cool, well-ventilated area. Skin preparation solutions that contain alcohol must be allowed to dry completely before draping.

Hydrogen Peroxide

As previously mentioned, hydrogen peroxide is a potent sterilizing agent when used in high concentration. It is not used for environmental cleaning, because it is unstable and corrosive.

ENVIRONMENTAL CLEANING

The perioperative environment is cleaned with disinfectants to reduce the bioburden to a safe minimum. Cleaning should be the responsibility of everyone in the department. In certain settings, the responsibility belongs to specific personnel assigned by the nurse manager or by the job description given to them by the hospital. The duties and tasks associated with sanitation and decontamination must never be taken lightly.

Disinfection or **sanitation** is the process by which surfaces, materials, and equipment are cleaned with specific substances (disinfectants) that render them safe for their intended use. Any item that is soiled with organic matter such as blood, tissue, or any body fluids is considered contaminated. The process that renders the surface or item safe is decontamination. The disinfection or sanitation process may achieve the same result as decontamination. One must assume that all items are contaminated and clean all items properly. *Cleaning* refers to the process by which any type of soil, including organic material, is removed. This is accomplished with detergent, water, and mechanical action. Cleaning precedes all disinfection processes. The purpose of sanitation and disinfection is to prevent cross-contamination between patients and between patients and personnel.

ROUTINE DECONTAMINATION OF THE SURGICAL SUITE

Before the Workday

The recommended practice before the first case of the day is damp dusting of surgical lights, furniture, and fixed equipment in the operating suite. A clean, lint-free cloth and a hospital-grade chemical disinfectant are used.

During Surgery

The principles of Standard Precautions apply to all surgical procedures, and all cases are considered contaminated and treated accordingly. During surgery, the circulator and his or her assistants are responsible for ensuring that the environment in the surgical suite is kept as disease free as possible. They do this by confining and containing all potential contaminants. The following activities, which are part of the Standard Precautions, must be performed to prevent cross-contamination with blood-borne pathogens.

- Any blood spills or contamination by other organic material should be removed promptly with a hospital-grade disinfectant. Household bleach should not be used for this purpose because of its potential to damage certain equipment and instruments.
- All articles used and discarded in the course of surgery must be placed in leak-proof containers. This prevents spilling of contaminated liquid onto other surfaces.
- Any contaminated or suspect item must be handled in a manner that protects personnel from contamination. Non-scrubbed personnel must wear PPE. This includes gloves, a cover gown, a face shield or mask, and protective eyewear. An instrument can be used to transfer contaminated articles to a waste or other receptacle (this is called the *no-touch method*).
- Tissue specimens, blood, and all other body fluids must be placed in a leak-proof container for transport out of the department. The outside of any specimen container that is passed off the surgical field to the circulator must be cleaned with a hospital-grade disinfectant.
- Because paper products are difficult or impossible to decontaminate, every effort should be made to keep patients' charts, laboratory slips, radiograph reports and radiographs, and any paper documentation free of contamination.
- Contaminated sponges must be collected in a kick bucket in which a plastic bag or liner has been previously placed. Sponges must not be lined up on the floor for counting. Sponges should be counted and immediately placed in plastic bags representing increment numbers such as five or 10 sponges.
- Instruments that fall off the surgical field must be retrieved by the circulator (with gloves protecting the hands) and placed in a basin containing a noncorrosive disinfectant. In this way, organic debris on the instrument is prevented from drying and becoming airborne. If the instrument is needed to continue surgery, it may be cleaned in the decontamination room and flash sterilized.
- During surgery, the scrubbed surgical technologist should periodically wipe blood and tissue from instruments. Those that are difficult to clean (e.g., orthopedic rasps, drill bits, and suction tips) should be kept moist at all times to prevent blood, tissue, and body fluids from drying on the surface.
- Small-bore cannulas and suction-tip lumens should be flushed frequently to prevent interior buildup of debris. If a suction tip becomes completely occluded, a metal stylet should be used to remove the debris before flushing. When blood and tissue are allowed to dry on an instrument, they

stick to the surface and may pass intact through subsequent phases of processing, including vigorous mechanical washing.

- Any organic debris or residue that remains is a potential source of pathogenic microorganisms, even if the item has been through the sterilization or disinfection process. A basin of sterile water should be available during surgery to aid in keeping instruments clean. Instruments should never be soaked in saline, because it causes the metal to corrode.

Terminal Decontamination

The process of terminal decontamination follows every surgical case. This is the thorough cleaning and disinfection of all equipment and soiled surfaces in the operating room. It follows the removal of instruments and contaminated, disposable items used during surgery.

The goal of terminal decontamination is to prevent disease transmission. A systematic routine is followed to ensure that no step in decontamination is missed. Rapid turnover of patients is important in a busy operating room. However, environmental safety takes priority over scheduling. After a surgical procedure, duties are shared between the scrub person, who handles equipment and instruments directly related to the performance of the surgery, and the personnel responsible for case cleanup. These can be housekeeping personnel, scrub persons, circulators, or surgical aides. Regardless of the type of personnel participating in the cleanup, all should be attired in PPE.

During decontamination, an approved disinfectant is used to clean surfaces and fixtures. High level disinfectants are not used in terminal disinfection.

The steps in the procedure are described below:

1. After surgery, the scrub prepares equipment and instruments for transport out of the surgical suite. Any instrument exposed to the sterile field must be processed whether it appears soiled or not. All instruments are placed in leak-proof containers and placed into a closed cart for transport to the decontamination area.
2. All disposable sharp instruments (e.g., knife blades, sutures, trocars) are placed in a designated sharps container in a manner that prevents injury to the personnel who next handle the container. If other personnel are responsible for cleaning up the back table, the scrub person should verbally communicate the presence of sharps on the table and visually identify them to the other personnel.
3. All disposable anesthesia equipment is removed in closed bags.
4. Suctioned blood and body fluids may be treated with a hypochlorite solidifier and then placed in leak-proof biohazard bags or containers.
5. Soiled linens and/or single-use drapes are gathered from the outer edges inward to contain contaminants. Linen is placed in waterproof biohazard bags in such a way as to prevent the soiled areas from touching bare skin. Open bags should not be compacted, because this releases contaminated particles into the air.

6. All disposable items contaminated with blood must be placed in waterproof bags or containers and clearly labeled as biohazardous waste. If any items are likely to leak blood or body fluids, they must be removed from the operating room in a closed container system.
7. All soiled equipment that is routinely kept in the operating suite is removed to the decontamination area or safe disposal area.

After instruments, supplies and contaminated equipment have been removed from the surgical suite, the walls, floors, furniture, and fixtures are cleaned.

- Floors are cleaned with disinfectant and may be wet vacuumed. A 3- to 4-foot area (about 1 to 1.2 m) around the sterile field is considered efficient for routine decontamination between cases.
- The pads of the operating table are removed to expose the undersurface of the table. All surfaces of the table and pads are cleaned, with particular attention to hinges, pivotal points, and castors.
- The operating table is moved aside for cleaning underneath and to check for any items that may have dropped to the floor during surgery.
- All soiled operating room equipment is cleaned with disinfectant.
- Walls, doors, surgical lights, and ceilings are spot cleaned if they are soiled with blood, tissue, or body fluids. Additional attention is given to supply cabinet doors, especially the latches and handles.
- All contaminated items used during the cleaning process are removed from the room.

After decontamination, all furniture is repositioned, and clean linen is placed on the operating table. Clean covers are also placed over table accessories. Clean liner bags are placed in kick buckets and linen frames.

CHAPTER SUMMARY

- All instruments and equipment used in critical areas of the body are sterilized before use. Sterilization is the complete destruction of all viable forms of life on an object.
- An object is either sterile or not sterile; there are no "levels" of sterility.
- The Spaulding system is used to determine a method of processing medical and surgical equipment. The system assigns a risk category *specific to regions of the body in which that device is to be used.*
- Critical risk is assigned to sterile tissues, including the vascular system.
- Mucous membranes and nonintact skin are semicritical areas.
- Intact skin is considered noncritical.
- Disposable items are not reprocessed unless this is approved by the manufacturer.
- Surgical personnel coordinate disinfection, decontamination, and sterilization processes with the

Central Service department, where bulk sterilization takes place.

- The cycle of sterile reprocessing begins at the point of use and includes cleaning, decontamination, sterilization, assembly, and storage.
- A case cart system is the preferred method of transferring contaminated surgical instruments and supplies to the decontamination area.
- The purpose of decontaminating instruments after use is to render them safe to handle.
- Instruments and equipment are decontaminated in a designated area away from clean and sterile equipment to prevent cross-contamination.
- Equipment for sterilization is wrapped in a specific way that prevents contamination during storage and allows the equipment to be distributed safely to the sterile field.
- The sterilization process is monitored by chemical and biological methods to ensure patient safety.
- Biological monitoring during sterilization is performed by exposing the load to a harmless bacterial spore, which is then recovered and cultured.
- Steam under pressure is the most common and economical method of sterilizing surgical equipment.
- The flash sterilizer is used to rapidly sterilize clean decontaminated equipment on a "just in time" basis. This method is used only when no other method is available. Implants are not flashed sterilized except in an emergency and must be monitored with a biological control system.
- Other methods of sterilization include ethylene oxide gas, gas plasma, liquid peracetic acid, and ionizing radiation (commercial use only).
- All equipment used on a patient must be cleaned and decontaminated before sterilization.
- Disinfection is performed on equipment used in semicritical areas of the body. High level disinfectants are capable of destroying bacteria and their spores.
- Low level disinfection is used for environmental cleaning.
- Terminal decontamination of the operating room is performed after each case according to established methods and protocols.

REVIEW QUESTIONS

1. What is the *bioburden*?
2. What three conditions are necessary for any sterilization or disinfection process to be effective?
3. Why are instruments processed in the washer-sterilizer?
4. What is the purpose of wrapping instruments for steam sterilization?
5. What disinfectant is approved for cleaning blood spills in the surgical suite?
6. Why doesn't a control monitor determine that sterilized goods are sterile?
7. What is DART?
8. Describe each of the three levels of the Spaulding classification system.
9. What is "just in time" processing?
10. What is terminal disinfection?
11. Why are sterile packages given a lot number?

CASE STUDIES

Case 1

While scrubbed, you open a basin set and find a small amount of water pooled in the bottom of the basin. What are the possible causes of this? What will you do?

Case 2

During the setup for a case, you notice one of the indicator strips in a pan of instruments on your back table has not changed color. What should you do?

Case 3

You are employed in a small community hospital. In your first week, you are scrubbed on a laparotomy case. The circulator opens a single-use electrosurgery pencil that has been resterilized with EO in the hospital's Central Service department. What will you do?

Case 4

You are the afternoon shift relief scrub on a plastic surgery case. About an hour into the case on which you have relieved, you happen to notice the chemical sterilization monitor at the bottom of the instrument tray, which is on the sterile back table. The monitor has not changed color. The surgeon is using instruments from this tray. What do you do?

Case 5

You are about to scrub on an orthopedic case in which a stainless steel implant will be inserted into the patient's hip. The surgeon wants to see the implant before surgery. He opens the package and examines it with bare hands. He then instructs you to flash sterilize the implant. What will you do? Who is responsible? What are the risks associated with flash sterilization of implants?

Case 6

You have been assigned to work in the gastrointestinal laboratory for the day. You will use gastrointestinal endoscopes. When you arrive in the laboratory, you notice that the endoscope to be used first is soaking in disinfectant solution that has expired (has been held beyond the date approved for disinfection). The physician tells you that he will use the endoscope anyway. What is your response?

Case 7

While opening sterile goods for a case, you find a basin set that has been wrapped in one double thickness wrapper. You are able to open the basin set using sterile technique. Is it sterile?

BIBLIOGRAPHY

Association of periOperative Registered Nurses (AORN): Recommended practices for environmental cleaning in the surgical practice setting. In *Standards, recommended practices and guidelines, 2007 edition,* Denver, 2007, AORN.

Association of periOperative Registered Nurses (AORN): Recommended practices for sterilization in the perioperative practice setting. In *Standards, recommended practices and guidelines, 2007 edition,* Denver, 2007, AORN.

Association of periOperative Registered Nurses (AORN): Sterilization in the perioperative practice setting. In *Standards, recommended practices and guidelines, 2007 edition,* Denver, 2007, AORN.

Association of Surgical Technologists (AST): Aseptic technique in *Standards of Practice,* available at http://www.ast.org/educators/standards_table_of_contents.aspx. Accessed March 19, 2009.

Carlo A: The new era of flash sterilization, *AORN Journal* 86:1, 2007.

Comprehensive guide to steam sterilization and sterility assurance in health care facilities. ANSI/AAMI ST79: 2006.

International Association of Healthcare Central Service Materiel Management: *Enhancing cooperation between the central service and operating room departments* Accessed May 20, 2008, at http://www.iahcsmm.org/.

Medical Device and Diagnostic Industry: Global sterilization: making the standards standard. Accessed November 13, 2007, at www.devicelink.com/mddi/archive/05/03/008.html.

Spry C: Care and handling of basic surgical instruments. *AORN Journal* 86(Suppl 1): 77-81, 2007.

US Department of Labor: Hazard communication: foundation of workplace chemical safety programs. Accessed November 13, 2007, at http://www.osha.org.

CHAPTER 9

Aseptic Technique

CHAPTER OUTLINE

LEARNING OBJECTIVES

After studying this chapter the reader will be able to:
- Describe evidence-based practice
- Clearly define the terms *sterile, nonsterile,* and *asepsis*
- Explain surgical conscience
- Explain the concept of barriers
- Practice the rules of aseptic technique
- Explain the relationship between personal hygiene and aseptic technique

- Perform the surgical hand scrub correctly
- Demonstrate aseptic technique by donning gown and gloves
- Don sterile gloves using proper open gloving technique
- Remove gown and gloves using aseptic technique
- Remove contaminated gloves from another person
- Discuss reasons personnel might not follow the rules of asepsis

TERMINOLOGY

Airborne contamination: An incident of contamination in which microorganisms carried in the air by moisture droplets or dust particles make contact with a sterile surface.

Antiseptics: Chemical agents approved for use on the skin that inhibit the growth and reproduction of microorganisms. Antiseptics are used to cleanse and paint the surgical site to reduce the number of microorganisms to an absolute minimum.

Asepsis: The absence of pathogenic microorganisms on an animate surface or on body tissue. Literally, *asepsis* means "without infection." In surgery, asepsis is a state of minimal or zero pathogens. Asepsis is the goal of many surgical practices.

Aseptic technique: Methods or practices in health care that reduce infection.

Centers for Disease Control and Prevention (CDC): The U.S. government agency that researches public health issues and educates the lay public and professionals about disease transmission, origin, and prevention.

Chemical barrier: The barrier formed by the action of an antiseptic; it not only reduces the number of microorganisms on a surface, but also prevents recolonization (regrowth) for a limited period.

Closed gloving: A technique of gloving in which the bare hand does not come in contact with the outside of the glove. The sterile glove is protected from the nonsterile hand by the cuff of a surgical gown.

Contamination: The consequence of physical contact between a sterile surface and a nonsterile surface in surgery. Contamination also can result from airborne dust, moisture droplets, or fluids that act as a vehicle for transporting contaminants from a nonsterile surface to a sterile one.

Containment and confinement: A foundation concept of aseptic technique which sterile and non sterile surfaces are separated by physical barriers or distance (space).

Double gloving: Wearing two pairs of gloves, one over the other to reduce the risk of contamination as a result of glove failure or puncture.

Gross contamination: Contamination of a large area of tissue by a highly infective source.

Hand antisepsis: A technique for removing transient flora from the hands using alcohol-based hand rub or surgical hand scrub.

Hand washing: A specific technique used to remove debris and dead cells from the hands. Hand washing with an antiseptic also reduces the number of microorganisms on the skin.

Latex allergy: Sensitivity to latex, which can cause itching, rhinitis, conjunctivitis, and anaphylactic shock leading to death. Personnel and patients with latex allergy must not come in contact with any articles that contain latex.

Nonsterile personnel: In surgery, team members who remain outside the boundary of the sterile field and do not come in direct contact with sterile equipment, sterile areas, or the surgical wound. The circulator, anesthesia care provider, and radiographic technician are examples of nonsterile team members.

Open gloving: A gloving technique in which the bare skin does not touch any part of the outside of the glove. Open gloving generally is used when a health care worker does not wear a sterile gown.

Pathogenic: Having the potential to cause disease.

Physical barrier: In surgery, a barrier that separates a sterile surface from a nonsterile surface. Examples are sterile surgical gloves, gowns, and drapes. A physical barrier, such as a clean surgical cap, also can prevent a bacteria-laden surface, such as the hair, from shedding microorganisms.

Resident flora: Microorganisms that are normally present in specific tissues. Resident flora are necessary to the regular function of these tissues or structures. Also called *normal flora*.

Scrub: The scrubbed surgical technologist or nurse assisting in surgery. Also refers to the surgical hand scrub performed before surgery and if the hands are contaminated with body fluids.

Scrubbed personnel: In surgery, members of the surgical team who work within the sterile field. Also called *sterile personnel*.

Sharps: Any objects that can penetrate the skin and have the potential to cause injury and infection, including but not limited to needles, scalpels, broken glass, broken capillary tubes, and exposed ends of dental wires.

Standard Precautions: Protocols and guidelines established by the CDC to prevent the transmission of microorganisms in the health care environment. All aseptic technique practices are based on Standard Precautions.

Sterile field: An area that includes the draped patient, all sterile tables, and sterile equipment in the immediate area of the patient. The patient is considered the center of the sterile field.

Sterile item: Any item that has been subjected to a process that renders it free of all microbial life, including spores.

Sterility: A state in which an inanimate or animate substance harbors absolutely no viable microorganisms.

Strike-through contamination: An event in which fluid from a nonsterile surface or air penetrates the protective wrapper of a sterile item, potentially contaminating the item.

Surfactant: A surface agent such as soap that lowers surface tension, allowing greater permeability.

Surgical conscience: In surgery, the ethical motivation to practice excellent aseptic technique to protect the patient from infection. Surgical conscience implies that the professional practices excellent technique regardless of whether others are observing.

Surgical hand rub: The systematic application of antiseptic foam or cream on the hands before gowning and gloving for a sterile procedure. The surgical hand rub may be used as an alternative to the traditional hand scrub under certain conditions.

Surgical hand scrub: A specific technique for washing the hands before donning a surgical gown and gloves before surgery. The scrub is performed with timed or counted strokes using detergent-based antiseptic. The surgical hand scrub is designed to remove dirt, oils, and transient microorganisms and reduce the number of resident microorganisms.

Surgical site infection (SSI): Postoperative infection of the surgical wound, most commonly caused by the normal bacteria found on the patient's skin or shed from the skin or hair of surgical team members. The goal of surgical skin preparation is to prevent postoperative wound infection.

Topical antiseptics: Agents applied to skin or mucous membranes that temporarily reduce or prevent the growth of microorganisms.

Transient flora: Microorganisms that do not normally reside in the tissue of an individual. Transient microorganisms are acquired through skin contact with an animate or inanimate source colonized by microbes. Transient flora may be removed by routine methods of skin cleaning (see Hand washing and Surgical hand scrub).

INTRODUCTION

Aseptic technique is a set of practices and methods that prevent the transmission of disease in the health care setting. In the operating room, these practices are the foundation of *sterile technique,* which is used to prevent microbial contamination of the surgical wound.

When students first begin to learn aseptic technique, with its many rules and precautions, they often feel awkward and afraid of making errors. This is a normal reaction to a completely new way of performing what previously was a simple task, such as pouring liquid from a bottle or putting on gloves. It is important to understand that the learning process always feels uncomfortable, especially when others are watching. However, the learning environment is where mistakes are made and corrected. There is no easy way to assimilate new ways of doing things, except by practice and error.

Repeated practice develops the confidence necessary for learning.

EVIDENCE-BASED PRACTICE

Evidence-based practice (EBP) is both a way of way of thinking and a way of carrying out professional duties. It depends on the scientific method of proof and evidence (in the form of quantitative data) to decide *how* and *why* a certain process or policy is adopted in health care. Evidence-based practice is a way of using critical thinking skills to achieve objectives.

The study and practice of disease transmission (including aseptic technique) have undergone expansive growth in past decade. As a result of this research, we have a set of evidence-based practices that provide a high level of patient care.

Evidence-based practice is now the gold standard of professionalism in the health sciences and biotechnology. As surgical technologists take on more demanding roles in clinical practice and biotechnology, it becomes imperative for them to learn how to "think" and use EBP.

EVIDENCE-BASED PRACTICE IN PRACTICE

EBP does not rely on *past* practices to define *current* ones. It relies on science and evidence rather than opinion or tradition. It abolishes the "sacred cows" of procedure and practice that were assumed to be adequate in the past; these are no longer valid, because scientific investigation and discovery have superseded the old practices. Perhaps they never were valid, or they seemed to work at the time. EBP does not consider this; it considers only best practices based on current study and proof.

Evidence-based practices are rooted in the following questions:

- Why is this technique used in this situation?
- What is the rationale (logical, reasoned basis) behind a particular practice or procedure?
- Is this the "best" (e.g., beneficial, scientifically based, most effective) way to accomplish this? What is the evidence that this works?

EBP is used to provide rationales for all the standards and recommendations made by professional organizations in disease transmission, biotechnology, patient safety, and advances in surgical practice. Throughout this text, you will see sections titled Standards and Recommendations. These sections list the professional bodies that have been established as authoritative sources of information for that area of practice. No professional organization would attempt to set a standard without first carrying out the scientific studies and research required to support that standard. When we follow a directive in the operating room, we always have the right to ask, "What is the rationale for this, and what is it based on?" If there is no evidence-based rationale, the practice may not be valid.

EXAMPLES OF EVIDENCE-BASED PRACTICE

The following are just a few examples of evidence-based practice.

1. **Double gloving.** In the past, double gloving (wearing two pairs of stterile surgical gloves) was practiced only in orthopedic cases in which heavy cutting instruments were used. Glove splitting and tearing are common in traditional orthopedic surgery. The current practice is for all **scrubbed personnel** to double glove, regardless of the type of surgery. This is based on numerous studies arising from the perceived risk of infection with the human immunodeficiency virus (HIV) in surgery. These studies have demonstrated a reduced risk of skin contact with blood and body fluids when double gloving is practiced.

2. **Surgical hand scrub.** Historically, the **surgical hand scrub** was a symbol of excellent aseptic technique. A full 10-minute scrub using a stiff brush and strong antiseptic was considered the only method adequate for preparing the hands before each and every surgical procedure. Raw skin and dermatitis were common among surgeons and **scrub** personnel. Studies now have shown that vigorous scrubbing actually breaks down the skin, reducing its natural barrier against microorganisms and inviting infection. The **surgical hand rub,** using an effective antiseptic, has been shown to be at least as effective as the hand scrub, as long as visible dirt is removed. In the past, the hand rub would not have been acceptable because of professional opinion and the highly regarded tradition of the 10-minute hand and arm scrub.

3. **Annotated research.** All professional journals and textbooks have an ethical responsibility to publish information that is based on research and evidence. Recommendations for techniques and standards must be backed up by a reference to the evidence. This may be in the form of a bibliography or a list of references. Information also may be validated with a *citation.* This is a note following the information that states the source of the information and usually refers to a person or organization that is established as an authority.

LEARNING TO USE EVIDENCE-BASED PRACTICE

Students should begin to incorporate evidence-based practice into their profession from the day they being learning. Curiosity and academic inquiry should lead to a desire to validate the learning. As a student, you have a right to look for references following an article you read. You also have the right to look up these references and determine whether they are authoritative or merely opinion.

The Internet provides a vast amount of information for students to learn about their chosen profession. However, students should seek evidence that the Web site is authoritative and presents evidence-based information. Just because something is in print does not mean it is true. If no references follow an article or a book chapter and none are cited in the text material, this might mean that the author bypassed this standard. Students should always check the dates of a reference. A reference that is 8 or 10 years old probably is not valid for today's technology and medical practices. If it is worth practicing and learning, it is worth getting right. A good source of Web sites for exploring evidence-based practice is http://healthlinks.washington.edu/ebp/ebptools.html.

STANDARDS AND RECOMMENDATIONS

All practices that prevent the transmission of infectious disease in the health care setting flow from standards established by the **Centers for Disease Control and Prevention (CDC).** These practices are called **Standard Precautions.** Aseptic technique is among the behaviors and protocols specified in the Standard Precautions. Standard Precautions evolved from a previous policy called *Universal Precautions,* which were oroginally established to prevent the spread of HIV and acquired immunodeficiency syndrome (AIDS).

CDC guidelines are interpreted by professional associations whose members are committed to patient and staff safety in health care settings. These interpretations are referred to as *recommendations, best practice standards,* or *statements of practice.* Professional consensus on the control of disease transmission has been established for most procedures used in the perioperative environment. The following agencies contribute to and enforce interpretation of these practices.

- **Association of periOperative Registered Nurses (AORN):** The professional organization for operating room nurses that sets standards and recommends procedures for operating room practice.
- **The Association of Surgical Technologists (AST):** The AST establishes Recommended Standards of Practice, which apply to the duties and responsibilities of the surgical technologist. These standards and guidelines are approved by the association's board of directors and include recommended practices in safety, aseptic technique, sterilization, and disinfection.
- **Association for Professionals in Infection Control and Epidemiology (APIC):** This professional organization performs research and recommends standards and procedures in the area of infection control.
- **Occupational Safety and Health Administration (OSHA):** OSHA is a federal agency that sets standards for safe environmental conditions for workers in all fields, including health care.
- **The Joint Commission:** The Joint Commission is the official private agency that accredits health care facilities according to approved standards for outcomes, procedures, and safe environmental conditions in the health care institution.
- **The Association for the Advancement of Medical Instrumentation (AAMI):** This organization sets standards for sterilization and disinfection in the health care setting. It also influences methods of aseptic technique.

IMPORTANT DEFINITIONS

Aseptic technique is:
- A method of "doing and thinking" that is used during the entire surgical process
- A method of performing tasks that reduces the risk of infection for patients and staff members

- A method based on the central principle that microorganisms transmit disease from objects, surfaces, air, and dust to patients and personnel
- A method that results in the *containment, confinement, reduction, or elimination of microorganisms* to prevent them from coming in contact with the sterile field

The concepts and activities described in this chapter form the foundation of surgical technique. Developing good aseptic technique takes time and practice, and everyone makes mistakes. Minor breaks in aseptic technique usually can be corrected *as long as they are reported.*

Aseptic technique requires constant self-monitoring. All surgical personnel should observe their own practices and ask, "Are my practices consistent with my professional and ethical responsibility? Are my standards consistent with what I would want for myself or my family?"

ASEPSIS

Literally defined, **asepsis** means *without infection.* Asepsis is the goal, whereas **aseptic technique** comprises the methods used to achieve that goal. A few examples of practices that promote and maintain asepsis are:
- The surgical hand scrub and rub
- Patient skin preparation
- Air filtering in the surgical suite
- Sterilization of surgical instruments
- Proper surgical attire
- Use of sterile gowns, gloves, and drapes
- Separation of soiled instruments from clean instruments during processing
- Strict environmental cleaning between surgical cases
- Air filtering, control of traffic patterns, and creation of restricted areas to confine microorganisms
- Protection of the surgical wound with sterile dressings
- Draining of the wound to remove a medium (blood and serum) for bacterial growth in the body

STERILITY

When an object is sterile, it is completely free of all viable microorganisms, including bacterial spores.

❖ *The term sterile is absolute. An item either is sterile, or it is not sterile.*

The process of sterilization is detailed and exact. After an item has been sterilized, its **sterility** is maintained by aseptic technique. Items exposed (opened) to the surgical field are considered surgically clean after they have been exposed to the air or to a patient's tissues and must be resterilized before being used on another patient. In the health care setting, all nonsterile surfaces are considered potentially contaminated with **pathogenic** microorganisms.

CONTAMINATION

A contaminated object is an object or body tissue that is not sterile or that has come in contact with a nonsterile object or surface. Recall from Chapter 7 that microorganisms are spread by direct contact, moisture, dust, and droplet nuclei. These are sources of **contamination.**

Gross contamination is the contamination of the surgical wound or sterile site by a highly infective source. An example is the spilling of bowel contents into the peritoneal cavity during surgery. Gross contamination can lead to systemic infection because of the number and type of microorganisms that enter the body. Even in cases of gross contamination, aseptic technique is maintained, because wound contamination with one type or strain of microorganism does not eliminate the pathogenic potential of others in the environment.

SURGICAL CONSCIENCE

Aseptic technique is based on surgical conscience; that is, the ethical and professional motivation that regulates a professional's behaviors regarding disease transmission. All members of the surgical team are jointly responsible for reporting and responding to breaks in aseptic technique so that steps can be taken to mitigate the risk of infection. In the case of gross contamination, this may mean starting the patient on intravenous antibiotics. If a glove or drape is contaminated, the appropriate action is to change the glove or redrape. If fluids are contaminated, they are discarded and new sterile basins and fluids are obtained.

Admitting and reporting any break in technique demonstrate a high level of professional maturity and surgical conscience. Aseptic technique is closely associated with the health professional's motivation to protect the patient.

CONCEPT OF BARRIERS

The principles of aseptic technique are based on the concept and practice of placing a barrier between a source of contamination and a sterile surface. To better understand and practice aseptic technique, consider the concept of containment and confinement. Sterile objects are contained by a physical barrier or confined to a specified area to prevent contact with nonsterile objects.

A **physical barrier** prevents a nonsterile surface from touching a sterile surface. For example, sterile drapes are a barrier between the patient and all sterile items. A physical barrier is one that contains (encloses) or separates a source of contamination.

Hair caps and masks are examples of barriers that contain sources of contamination. Back table covers and Mayo stand covers all separate contaminated areas from surgically clean areas. A **chemical barrier** is produced by the residual effect of **antiseptics** used during patient skin preparation.

Distance is another type of barrier. As the distance between a sterile surface and a nonsterile surface increases, the risk of contamination decreases. When you are learning aseptic technique, visualize an imaginary space around sterile objects and the sterile field. This space is perceived, first consciously and then unconsciously, as "off limits" to nonsterile objects and personnel. Over time, surgical personnel develop a sense of

intrusion when nonsterile objects are too close to the field. Generally, **nonsterile** items and **personnel** must remain at least 12 inches (30 cm) from a sterile field.

HEALTH AND HYGIENE

Perioperative personnel should be free of any contagious illness or open infection that might be transmitted to the patient and others in the surgical environment. Bacterial shedding from the nasopharynx and skin is a particular risk. Evidence indicates that open sores, cuts, or small skin wounds harbor bacteria, which are spread in the course of handling surgical equipment. Research also demonstrates that bacteria in open hand sores are resistant to elimination through hand washing. Surgical personnel should maintain good personal hygiene. Hand washing is particularly important.

JEWELRY

Jewelry of any kind is a potential source of pathogens. Surgical personnel must remove all rings, bracelets, and wristwatches before entering the restricted areas of the surgical department. Microorganisms proliferate freely under rings and bracelets and may resist destruction during hand washing. Necklaces and earrings that are not confined under scrub attire pose a risk of falling onto the surgical field or even into the surgical wound. Exposed necklaces or earrings may become contaminated with blood or other aerosolized particles that can spread infection. The recommended standard is to remove all jewelry or *completely confine it* inside scrub clothes. Body piercing is considered jewelry and ideally should be confined or removed. A draining or inflamed pierced track is considered an open infection (see previous discussion).

SCRUB SUIT

The scrub suit is worn by both sterile and nonsterile surgical personnel. The suit is designed to prevent the release of skin particles and hair into the environment and to protect the wearer from contact with soil and body fluids. Perspiration and normal exudate from sebaceous glands in the skin contain large colonies of bacteria, which are released with friction and movement. The scrub suit helps prevent the release of these substances into the surgical environment. The process used to launder surgical scrub suits in the hospital is vigorous and effective at lowering bacterial counts.

The scrub suit consists of a shirt and pants (Figure 9-1). It is made of lint-free material and should fit closely to the body. The suit should not be so tight as to produce chafing, which increases the release of skin and hair particles laden with bacteria. The top should be secured at the waist, tucked into the pants, or fit close to the body to prevent contact with sterile surfaces.[1] The drawstring ties should be tucked into the pants.

A clean scrub suit is donned whenever personnel enter the restricted or semirestricted area of the operating room, and the suit must be changed if it is contaminated by blood or body fluids.

In some facilities, surgical personnel are required to wear a cover gown or laboratory coat over the scrub suit whenever they leave the department to protect the scrub suit from microbial contamination. This is a policy decision of the individual institution.

When a scrub suit has been soiled by blood or body fluids, surgical personnel must remove it in such a way as to prevent skin contact with the soiled area. Grossly soiled scrub suits must be placed in a biohazard laundry receptacle so that they do not spread contaminants.

NONSTERILE COVER JACKET

Long-sleeved cover jackets are worn by nonsterile personnel to prevent contamination of the surgical field from bacterial shedding from the arms. OSHA recommends that jackets be buttoned or snapped closed during use. Previously worn jackets should never be kept in lockers and then reused; this presents a source of contamination rather than a barrier. Ideally, jackets should be freshly laundered by the health care facility. When this is not possible, home laundering must follow safe parameters for microbial destruction, including exposure to high heat and detergent. Operating room policy dictates whether this is permissible in a particular institution.

HEAD CAP

Head caps or hoods are worn to reduce contamination of the surgical field by loose hair and dander from the scalp. Surgical site infections have been traced to *Staphylococcus aureus* and group A streptococci from the hair or scalp of surgical personnel. Caps are meant to contain all hair and to cover the scalp line and sideburns completely (Figure 9-2). Males with facial hair should wear a cap that is specifically designed to cover this hair. The cap is put on before the scrub suit to prevent shedding of hair onto the clean scrub top.

Most faculties use disposable caps. They are inexpensive and readily available in the operating room. The use of cloth (home laundered) caps is not recommended, but their use is governed by the policy of the individual institution or state. Cloth caps that are reused day after day are a source of contamination rather than a barrier against disease transmission.

PROTECTIVE EYEWEAR AND FACE SHIELD

All surgical team members must wear impervious protective eyewear or face shields during all procedures and whenever there is a risk that blood, body fluids, or particles of tissue could splash on the face. When power equipment is used, bone chips, liquefied tissue, and other debris splatter into the air and onto personnel. Eyewear must cover the eye area from the brow to the top of the surgical mask and must extend over the temples. This protects the eyes from the front and sides. Impervious face shields offer increased protection (Figure 9-3).

A variety of goggles and face shields are available. The professional's choice should be based on visual clarity, expense, and comfort. Personnel are less likely to comply with regulations requiring eyewear and face shields when the equipment is uncomfortable or causes glare or visual distortion.

MASK

Masks are worn to protect the intraoperative environment from contamination by aerosol droplets generated by the mouth, oropharynx, nose, and nasopharynx. Talking, coughing, and sneezing forcefully spread droplets onto the sterile field and surrounding environment. When used properly, masks block droplets and filter air. They also protect the wearer's nose and mouth from contact with particles of tissue and body fluids, especially during drilling, sawing, cutting, and tissue liquefaction. Masks should be worn at all times by all surgical personnel in restricted areas and in locations where sterile instruments and supplies are stored or processed.

Masks are made of lint-free synthetic material that is woven loosely enough to allow the breath to pass through effectively but tightly enough to filter 99% of particles of 5 μm or larger.

To protect the patient and the wearer, masks must be worn properly:

- The mask must cover both the nose and the mouth. Any pliable insert over the nose bridge of the mask should be molded over the nose to fit snugly.
- Ties must be secured at the crown of the head and around the neck. Crossing the ties at the back of the head allows the sides of the mask to tent, which causes the breath to bypass the mask and escape from the sides.
- Double masking is not recommended. When two masks are worn, the open spaces of the material are doubled, requiring the wearer to exert more respiratory force during inhalation and exhalation. This causes air to be forced in and out of the sides and defeats the filtering process.
- The wearer must remove and dispose of the mask immediately upon leaving any restricted or semirestricted area. Even after a short time, bacterial colonization increases to a very high level on the inside surface of the mask. Masks are to be changed between surgical procedures. When masks are worn around the neck, they present a significant source of contamination.
- To remove the mask properly, the wearer should untie the top strings, then the bottom strings, without handling the portion that covers the face. The mask should be discarded in the proper waste receptacle and the hands washed thoroughly. Fresh masks are to be worn for each surgical procedure.
- Masks should either be left on or left off; they should never be worn around the neck with the ties dangling.
- Specialized masks are worn during laser procedures. These masks are designed to filter out particles that are smaller than those filtered by standard surgical masks;

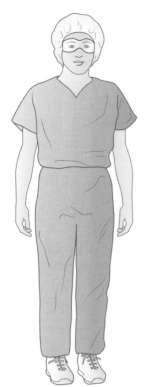

Figure 9-1 Correct attire for perioperative personnel working in restricted areas.

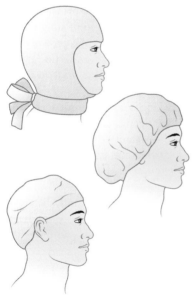

Figure 9-2 Approved head covers. All hair must be completely covered.

these smaller particles are created when cells are destroyed by laser energy.

SHOES AND SHOE COVERS

Perioperative personnel should wear shoes that are comfortable and easy to keep clean and that protect the wearer

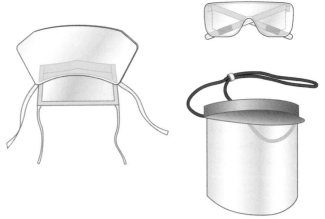

Figure 9-3 Protective eyewear required for surgical personnel.

against foot injury. Shoe covers protect shoes from contamination by blood and body fluids and should be worn when splashes or spills can reasonably be expected to occur. No evidence indicates that the use of shoe covers reduces the risk of **surgical site infection (SSI);** the primary purpose of shoe covers is to facilitate sanitation. If shoe covers are worn, they should be changed daily or when they become torn, wet, or soiled. They must be changed or removed before the staff member leaves the department. If gross contamination or pooling of blood, body fluids, or other liquids is possible, such as during some orthopedic or obstetrical cases, impervious shoe covers that extend to the knee should be worn.

HAND HYGIENE

PURPOSE

Hand hygiene is the most important tool for preventing the transmission of microorganisms in the health care setting. Hands are a significant cause of hospital-acquired infection. Organic debris, soil, and microorganisms can exist on the hands without any visual evidence. As personnel move from one task to another, touching patients and equipment, they transmit microbes.

Hand hygiene is the most effective way to reduce disease transmission in the health care setting. Two types of hand hygiene are practiced in the operating room and other health care settings: hand washing and hand antisepsis.

FINGERNAILS

The subungual area (the area under the fingernails) hosts a greater number of bacterial colonies than any other area of the hand. This area requires specific cleaning during normal hand washing, as well as during the surgical hand scrub. Nail tips must be level with the tip of the finger. Long nails easily puncture gloves and make handling of equipment more difficult. Scrubbed personnel sometimes wear gloves that are too large to protect long, manicured nails. Gloves that are too large for the hand can become caught in equipment. Long nails can scratch or dig into the patient's skin during transfer and positioning.

Nail polish itself has not been proven to be a source of bacteria; however, if the polish has chips or is flaking, it can be a site of bacterial growth. Nail polish often is worn over artificial or long nails, both of which are unacceptable in the operating room. AST recommends that nail polish should not be worn by surgical personnel.

Artificial nails harbor pathogenic bacteria (particularly gram-negative bacteria) and fungi (e.g., *Candida* and *Pseudomonas* organisms) between the real and synthetic nails, especially when the artificial nail is chipped or cracked. Bacterial counts remain high even after hand scrubbing of artificial nails with antiseptic solution. Therefore, artificial nails should not be worn by surgical personnel.

HAND WASHING

Hand washing is an event related practice (performed before and after a specific task or event). It requires a specific method with individual steps. To be effective, hand washing must be done with adequate friction, for an adequate time, and with an effective washing agent.

Liquid soap is used in the health care setting. When used properly, soap is effective at removing soil and debris. However, it has little or no antimicrobial activity. The effectiveness of soap depends on friction to remove organic and inorganic matter from the skin.

Antiseptic detergents (**topical antiseptics**) are used for hand washing and the surgical scrub (Table 9-1). They reduce the number of bacterial colonies, and some provide barrier protection that inhibits the growth of bacteria over time. This action is produced when the antiseptic binds chemically with the superficial layer of the skin. Detergents are among the most destructive agents routinely used on skin. Increased amounts of **surfactant** (an agent that lowers the surface tension of a liquid) cause more rapid and extensive skin damage. Damaged skin is more resistant to antimicrobial action and harbors greater numbers of microbes. Detergent antiseptics that contain skin emollients are available to prevent the breakdown of skin.

Table 9-1
Surgical Hand Scrub Agents

Agent	Residual Protection	BACTERICIDAL ACTIVITY Gram-Negative Organisms	Gram-Positive Organisms	Toxicity	Comments
Povidone iodine (iodophors)	Minimal	Moderately good	Moderately good	Possible irritation, allergy, and toxicity. Can be absorbed through skin.	Commonly used. Effective against mycobacteria, fungi, and viruses. Effective in the presence of organic substances. Must be rinsed thoroughly from skin. *Caution:* Care must be taken not to allow iodophor detergents to splash into the eyes.
Chlorhexidine gluconate (alcohol-detergent based)	Good with repeated use	Good	Good	Nonirritating to skin. Highly ototoxic; causes severe eye damage on contact with cornea.	Not absorbed by the skin. Not effective in the presence of organic debris except in a detergent base.
Alcohol-based skin cleaners	None	Excellent	Excellent	Damaging to mucous membranes and eyes. Nontoxic on skin. Can be very drying.	Contain skin emollients to prevent drying. If used as a surgical hand cleaner, should be preceded by thorough mechanical cleaning.
Triclosan	Moderate with repeated use	Inhibits growth	Inhibits growth	Nontoxic on skin. Absorbed through skin.	Not fungicidal. Viricidal activity unknown. Effective against *Mycobacterium tuberculosis*. Least effective of surgical hand scrubs. Use only when personnel cannot use other skin scrub agents.

When to Wash the Hands

Hand washing should be performed at the following times:

- Whenever hands are visibly soiled
- Before the surgical scrub and at the conclusion of a surgical case
- Before contact with sterile packages
- Before and after any contact with a patient
- Between contacts with potentially contaminated areas of the same patient
- Immediately after contact with blood or body fluids, regardless of whether gloves were worn at the time of contact
- Before and after eating
- After personal hygiene care
- After toileting
- Before the beginning and at the end of the workday

Hand Washing Procedure

First, all jewelry should be removed from the hands and fingers. The process then goes as follows:

1. Wet the hands thoroughly under running water.
2. Apply soap to the hands and wrists.
3. Rub the hands together vigorously, including the backs of the hands, interdigital spaces, and wrists. To ensure that the spaces between the fingers are adequately washed, spread the fingers and weave the two hands together, rubbing continuously.
4. Continue the hand scrub for at least 15 seconds, increasing the time after gross contact with known pathogenic surfaces, blood, or body fluids.
5. Rinse all soap from the hands.
6. Dry the hands by blotting them with a towel.
7. Use the towel to turn off the water faucet.

HAND ANTISEPSIS

Hand antisepsis is the application of an approved antiseptic to all surfaces of the hands and fingers.

Ethyl or isopropyl alcohol combined with skin emollients is now available in the form of foams and creams for use in health care settings. When used correctly, these products destroy both gram-positive and gram-negative bacteria at high levels.

An alcohol-based hand rub can take the place of hand washing and is more effective. However, this procedure should be used only when no soil is visible on the hands. Operating protocol should always be followed in the use of hand rubs.

SURGICAL HAND SCRUB/RUB

SURGICAL SCRUB

The purpose of the surgical scrub is to reduce the number of resident (normal) and transient (those transmitted by direct contact from a contaminated source) microorganisms on the skin to an absolute minimum. The surgical scrub does not sterilize the skin. Living tissue cannot be sterilized; however, the use of certain antiseptics along with the standardized scrub technique reduces the number of microbes on the skin and can provide continuous antimicrobial action. This is important, because bacteria proliferate quickly in the moist environment between the skin and a glove.

If nondisposable brushes are used, they must be sterile. During the scrub, avoid harsh friction with the brush. Repeated skin irritation with a scrub brush encourages colonization of both resident and transient bacteria on the hands and arms.

Sterile members of the surgical team perform the surgical scrub:

1. Immediately before donning sterile gown and gloves
2. After direct exposure (skin contact) with blood or body fluids

NOTE: Before beginning the surgical scrub, the surgical technologist or scrub nurse opens the sterile gown, towel, and gloves onto a small table on which no other sterile supplies have been opened. Never don gown and gloves directly from the back table or Mayo stand, and do not allow anyone else entering the sterile field to do so. This is done to prevent the contamination of sterile instruments, table covers, and other equipment by water dripping from the hands and arms onto the sterile items.

Government and professional organizations have researched the amount of time required for an effective surgical scrub. A timed scrub or counted stroke method may be used, and a 2- to 3-minute scrub is effective. However, the length of time for the surgical scrub is an individual institutional policy. The length of the scrub should be the same for both the initial surgical scrub and all scrubs that follow during the day. Manufacturers of antiseptic agents recommend a specific scrub time for a particular agent. These recommendations should be followed.

TECHNIQUE

The surgical scrub is performed with disposable sterile scrub sponges; a sponge-brush combination; or a sterile, nondisposable brush as mentioned above. The disposable scrub sponge is impregnated with antiseptic and prewrapped.

The steps for performing a surgical scrub are as follows (Figure 9-4):

1. Prepare for the surgical scrub by ensuring that the scrub suit top is tucked into the scrub pants or is sufficiently snug so that it remains dry. Remember to adjust the surgical mask and protective face shield or eyewear before starting the scrub.
2. Perform routine hand washing and include the forearms, according to institutional policy, using antiseptic soap. Rinse the hands and arms thoroughly.
3. Unwrap a sterile scrub brush packet and remove the nail cleaner. Hold the brush in one hand while carefully cleaning the subungual area on each finger, using a nail cleaner under running water. Discard the nail cleaner.
4. Moisten the sponge with antiseptic soap, create a lather, and begin with the nails. Keep the surfaces of the fingers, hands, and arms in mind as you begin the scrub. If using the counted method, scrub the nails with 30 strokes.

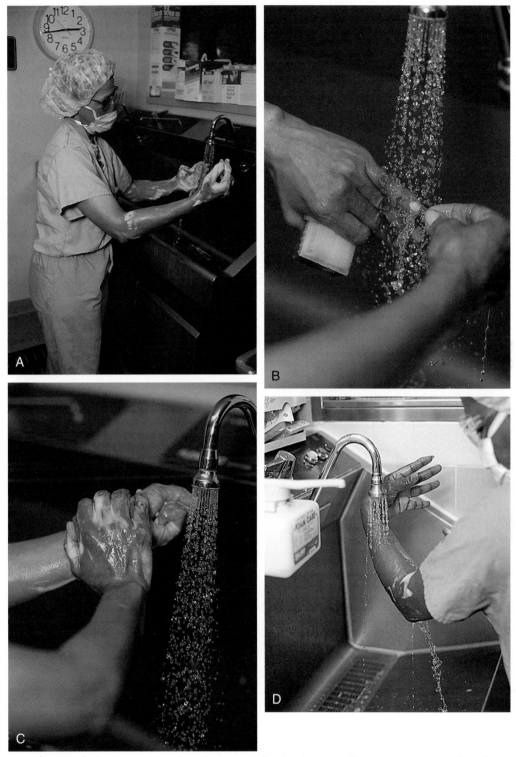

Figure 9-4 Surgical hand scrub. See text for details. *(From Perry AG, Potter PA: Clinical nursing skills and techniques, ed 5, St Louis, 2004, Mosby.)*

5. Scrub each side of each finger and the hand separately. Each finger has four sides. Scrub each side individually, first on one hand and then on the other.

6. Proceed to the arm (20 strokes on each of four surfaces) and then to the other without returning to previously scrubbed areas. Extend the scrub to 2 inches (5 cm) above the elbow.

7. Do not allow the scrubbed hand or arm to contact any part of the sink, faucet, or scrub suit. Avoid splashing water on the scrub suit. Donning a sterile gown over a wet scrub suit is not acceptable because of the danger of **strike-through contamination.**

8. Keep the hands higher than the elbows at all times. When the scrub is complete, rinse the hands and arms

by passing first the hand and then the arm under running water. Keep the elbows flexed. Do not move the arms back and forth through the water. Try to remove all residual soap, because it can harbor debris and also make gloving more difficult.

9. Proceed to the operating room. Enter by pushing the door open with your back, keeping the elbows flexed. Proceed to drying, gowning, and gloving. Make sure to dry the hands well, because gloves are difficult to put on moist skin, and moist environments are a breeding ground for bacteria.

SURGICAL HAND RUB

An approved, alcohol-based rub designated for use in preparation for surgery can be used before sterile gloves are donned. Because the application of hand rub products does not remove debris, the hands—including the subungual area—and arms must be thoroughly washed and dried before the product is applied. Many studies have demonstrated that, when appropriate amounts of the product are applied to the hands and arms and friction is used to completely moisten all surfaces, an alcohol-based surgical hand rub is as effective as a standard surgical scrub. When scrubbing with these products, consult the manufacturer's instructions about recommended use.

GOWNING AND GLOVING

DRYING YOUR HANDS

The following is the proper technique for drying the hands and arms (Figure 9-5):

1. After entering the operating room from the scrub sink area, proceed to the gowning and gloving table.

2. Remove the towel by grasping only the edge and lift it up and away from the sterile gown and gloves. Do not hesitate, because water may drip from the hands onto the sterile gown and gloves, which would contaminate them.

3. Allow the towel to unfold so that the long edge hangs down between your two hands. Bend forward slightly at the waist so the sterile towel does not touch the scrub suit. Use one end of the towel for one hand and arm and the other end for the other hand and arm.

4. Blot the skin, working from hand to wrist to arm, without moving back over a previously dried area.

5. Keep the towel out in front of you where you can see it. After drying one hand and arm with one end of the towel, begin drying the other hand by placing the wet hand at the other end of the towel while confining it to its own side.

6. Dry the second hand and arm using the same blotting technique. When you are finished, drop the towel into a nearby receptacle. Proceed immediately to gowning.

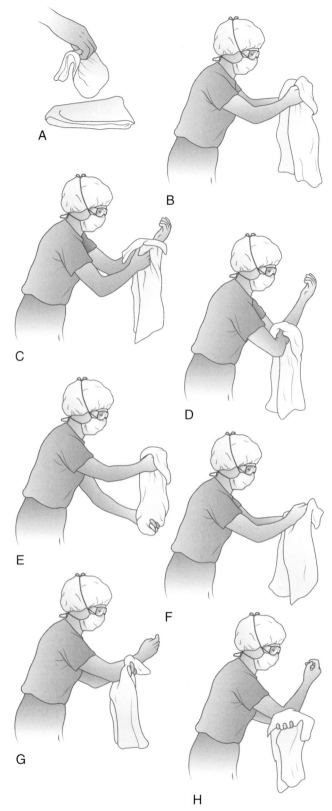

Figure 9-5 Procedure for drying the hands after the surgical scrub.

GOWNING YOURSELF

Surgical gowns are worn by all sterile personnel. The gown is donned immediately before the start of surgery and may be changed during surgery if it is penetrated by blood or other fluids. Many types of surgical gowns are available, but the most common type wraps around the body and is designed to cover both the front and back of the wearer. However, the back is considered nonsterile because it cannot be observed by the wearer.

Most disposable gowns are water resistant. For gowns used in orthopedics, obstetrics, and other specialties in which copious amounts of blood or irrigation fluids end up on and around the sterile field, a waterproof or reinforced shield is laminated to the front of the gown.

The surgical technologist or scrub nurse dons a sterile gown immediately after drying the hands. When gowning, consider the gown as having two surfaces: an inside surface that will contact the nonsterile scrub suit and bare skin of the hands and arms, and an outside surface that will be considered sterile only from the waist to the axillary line and from the hands to the elbows.

Surgical gowns are folded inside out before packaging. This allows scrubbed personnel to grasp the presenting surface of the gown with bare hands to put it on, because that surface will be the nonsterile side. Care must be taken not to grasp the gown at the neckline, because the sterile (outer) section of the gown may become contaminated.

Gowning should be performed according to the following guidelines (Figure 9-6):

1. After drying the hands and arms, grasp the gown just below the neckline and lift it up and away from the table, without touching anything else with bare hands. Remember, the inside surface of the gown faces outward.
2. Step away from the table and allow the gown to unfold. Do not touch the (outside) surface facing away from you.
3. Being careful not to lower the gown, look for the armholes and place your hands and arms inside the sleeves. Advance your hands, pushing them through horizontally from your shoulders, not above your head, to within about 1 inch (2.5 cm) of the knitted cuff edge. At this time the circulator may secure the neck and inside ties and assist in securing the back wrap. Glove immediately, using the closed technique.

GLOVING YOURSELF

Many types of surgical gloves are commercially available. The common considerations in choosing gloves are the glove material (**latex allergy** is a major concern), tensile strength, thickness, and economy. Tactile sensation is important, especially in surgical specialties that require the use of fine instruments and in which delicate tissues are encountered. Thicker gloves are more appropriate for repeated contact with heavy instruments or if copious bleeding is likely, such as during orthopedic surgery.

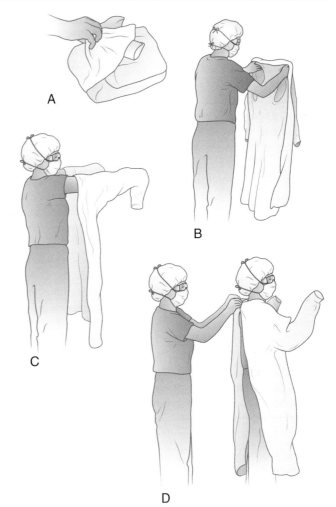

Figure 9-6 Procedure for gowning oneself.

DOUBLE GLOVING

Double gloving (wearing two pairs of surgical gloves) has been demonstrated to reduce the risk of glove failure, which increases with increased surgical time and increased handling of tissues and supplies. Glove punctures are associated with the transmission of blood-borne pathogens to health care workers and microbial contamination of the surgical site. The CDC and AORN now recommend double gloving on all invasive procedures. No set rule governs glove sizes when double gloving. The outer glove can be one size larger or smaller or the same size.

CLOSED GLOVING

Closed gloving is performed after gowning. It is the most effective method for preventing contact between the skin and the outside of the sterile glove. When you are learning the closed gloving technique, think of the glove as having two surfaces or planes, the inside and the outside. Before the gloves are touched, the entire glove is sterile, inside and outside. As soon as gloving is initiated, however, the *inside* surface is considered nonsterile.

The technique for gloving is among the most difficult skills for students to learn. One of the best ways is to have an experienced person glove while you are also gloving in a practice session or "dry run." Follow each step as the other person gloves. The experienced person must move slowly so that the student can follow these actions. The actions will need to be repeated in order to firmly establish correct technique. Always stand next to (not across) from the demonstrator to avoid confusion about which way the hand and glove are oriented. Take your time when learning to glove. It is better to be methodical and slow at first. Speed and efficiency will follow with practice.

Use the following technique to perform closed gloving. In this description the left hand is gloved first, but the right hand can be gloved first (Figure 9-7):

1. Begin closed gloving after donning a sterile gown. Do not allow your fingers to protrude outside the knitted cuff of the gown. You will maneuver sterile gloves onto your hands with your hands hidden from view under the gown's cuffs.

2. The glove wrapper is folded so that the side edges come together at the middle. The gloves are oriented in the wrapper with the fingers up and the cuffed (wrist) part at the bottom edge of the wrapper. The upper and lower edges of the wrapper are folded inward. To open the wrapper, grasp the two center edges and open them outward to expose the gloves. To keep the edges from closing up again, evert them slightly; this will remove some of the memory in the folds.

3. Position the left hand with the palm facing upward, as if you are about to receive an object in your hand. Pick up the glove with your right hand shielded by the gown and place the glove, palm to palm and cuff to cuff, over the left hand. The glove is oriented correctly if the fingers point to your wrist.

4. Working inside the gown cuff, grasp the under edge of the glove cuff between your left thumb and fingers. Using your protected right hand, grasp the upper edge of the glove cuff. The palm of the glove should still be oriented to your palm. If it is not, you will have difficulty sliding the hand into the glove, a common problem at this point. To correct misalignment of the glove, grasp it at the cuff and realign it correctly, *palm to palm.*

5. Keep the hidden fingers within 1 inch (2.5 cm) of the outside edge of the knitted cuff, and make sure your thumb is well inside the seam of the cuff. This prevents another common obstacle, which occurs when the left hand slips back into the gown sleeve.

6. Pull the glove on. Grasp the left glove cuff and advance your left hand into the glove.

7. Repeat with the other hand. After gloving, check both hands for any sign of punctures or tears. If a defect is apparent, the circulater removes the glove and gloving is repeated on that hand.

OPEN GLOVING

Open gloving is used during sterile procedures that do not require a sterile gown, such as preoperative skin preparation

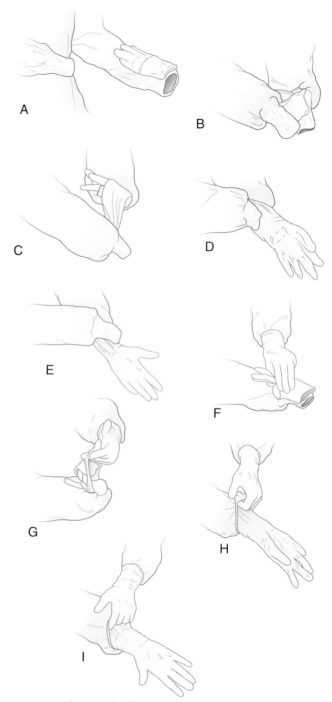

Figure 9-7   Closed gloving technique.

of the patient, assisting in minor skin procedures, catheterization, and when a scrubbed member changes a glove without changing his or her gown. The hands are not usually scrubbed before open gloving, although they should always be clean.

When gloving, consider the two surfaces of the glove, the outside and the inside. The glove has a cuff that exposes the *inside* of the glove. This inner surface is considered the nonsterile surface, even though it is sterile until touched with the bare hand. The outside remains sterile. The wrapper is considered sterile to within 1 inch (2.5 cm) of the edges.

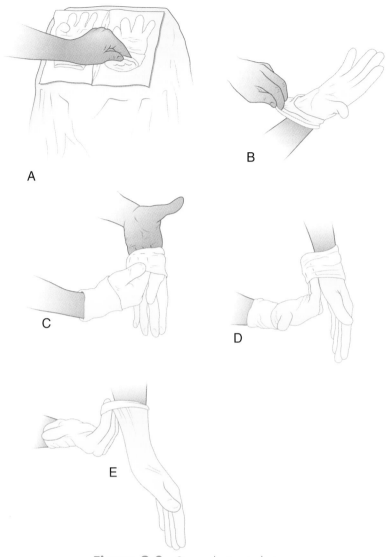

Figure 9-8 Open gloving technique.

The following are the steps in the technique for open gloving (Figure 9-8). In this description, the right hand is gloved first.

1. Open the outer, nonsterile wrapper and deliver the inner, sterile, wrapped gloves onto a clean, dry surface.
2. Grasp the edges of the glove wrapper with bare hands and expose the gloves. Before releasing the glove wrapper, make sure that it will stay open. The palms of the gloves should be facing upward, thumbs to the outside.
3. Using your left hand, grasp the upper folded lip of the right glove cuff. Do not touch the wrapper underneath or the outside of the glove. Pick up the glove and slide your right hand into it, keeping your hand palm up, oriented to the palm of the glove. Leave the cuff turned down until you glove the other hand.
4. To glove the left hand, slide the fingers of your sterile, gloved hand under the cuff. This positions your gloved hand (sterile) in contact with the outside (sterile) surface of the other glove. Keep the palm up as you slide your bare hand into the glove. You may unroll the cuff carefully, but do not allow the gloved hand to touch any bare skin.

When learning to glove, students sometimes experience difficulty removing the glove from the open sterile wrapper. Very thin or short-cuffed gloves are difficult to put on without contaminating the sterile side of the glove or the glove wrapper. Remember that as long as you do not touch the sterile surface with your nonsterile fingers, you have not contaminated either one.

GOWNING AND GLOVING OTHER TEAM MEMBERS

After the surgical technologist has set up sterile supplies and instruments, the other members of the surgical team enter from the scrub sink area. Gowning and gloving of the other team members precede all other activities and are as much a social tradition as a necessary part of the surgical routine. During gowning and gloving, the surgeon greets the scrub, circulator, and anesthesiologist and may introduce other members of the team. This time allows formal acknowledgment of the team members and what is to be done before the actual start of surgery. The surgeon also may clarify the need for special instruments or equipment at this time. Interaction among team members during the process of gowning and gloving often sets the tone for the entire surgery.

When the sterile team members enter the operating room, the scrub hands a towel to the surgical team leader (lead surgeon) and then to the other members of the team.

Gowning Other Team Members

The following technique is used to gown other team members (Figure 9-9):

1. When the team member reaches out for a towel for drying, pass the sterile towel over the team member's hand so that the long edge of the towel falls between the person's two hands.
2. Grasp the folded gown, step away from any nonsterile surface, and allow the gown to unfold. Cuff your gloved hands from contamination by placing your hands below the neckline and shoulders (away from the top edge) of the gown so that the outside of the gown (the part of the gown that will remain sterile) faces you. Position the gown so that the person you are gowning can easily insert his or her hands into the armholes as shown.
3. After the team member has stepped forward and placed his or her arms into the sleeves, pull the gown over the elbows toward the shoulders and then step back and away and grasp the gloves.
4. Glove the team member (see the next section).
5. The circulator secures the neck closure and ties located on the inside (nonsterile) surface of the gown.
6. After the team member is gloved, grasp one of the sterile outside ties of the gown while the wearer turns toward the wrap that encircles the front of the gown. Hand the tie to the wearer to be secured in front.

Gloving a Gowned Team Member

The following technique is used to glove a gowned team member (Figure 9-10):

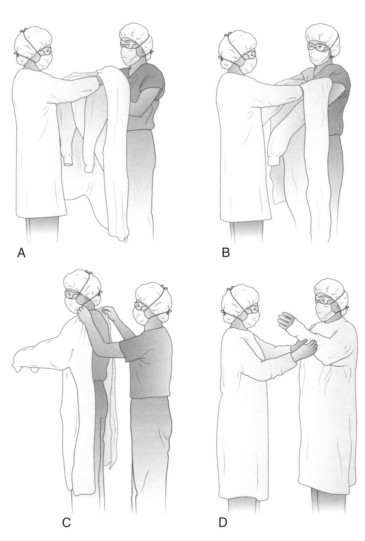

A

B

C

D

Figure 9-9 Gowning another person.

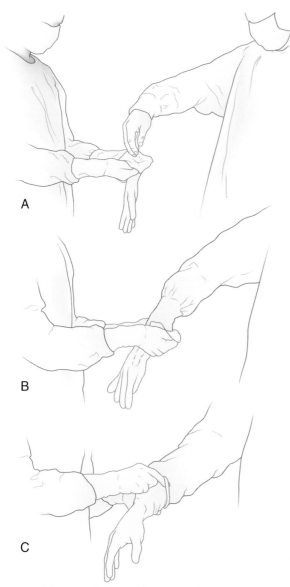

Figure 9-10 Gloving another person.

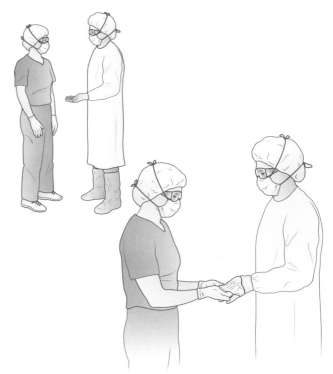

Figure 9-11 Circulator removing a contaminated glove. Note that the circulator does not touch the scrub's glove with bare hands.

1. Open the glove wrapper and place the gloves and wrapper near you on the sterile table.
2. Grasp the glove under the cuff and spread the opening with your thumbs held well away from the glove or tucked securely under the cuff.
3. Orient the glove so that the palm of the glove faces the person you are gloving. Offer the right glove first, then the left.
4. Make sure the sterile team member inserts his or her hand into the glove by pointing all fingers downward. Allow the cuff edge to recoil gently. Repeat the process with the other glove.

REPLACING A CONTAMINATED GLOVE

The following technique is used to remove a contaminated glove during surgery:

1. The team member presents the contaminated hand to the circulator palm upward or removes the glove aseptically (Figure 9-11).
2. The circulator, wearing nonsterile gloves, grasps the contaminated glove below the wrist and removes it.
3. Remember that the cuff of the gown is no longer considered sterile after the glove is removed. It must not come in contact with the outer surface of the sterile replacement glove.
4. The scrub regloves the team member as described previously.
5. If the scrub contaminates a glove, he or she may replace his or her own outer glove using open technique or may place a second sterile glove over the contaminated one until it is convenient to replace it.

REMOVING STERILE ATTIRE

When removing sterile attire, always remove the gown first and then gloves (Figure 9-12):

1. Grasp the gown at the shoulders, releasing or breaking the ties or snaps, and pull the sleeves downward. This rolls the gown inside out as it slides over your gloved hands.
2. Roll the gown so that the contaminated outside surface faces inward.
3. Dispose of the gown in a biohazard bag.

The gloves should be removed after the gown (Figure 9-13):

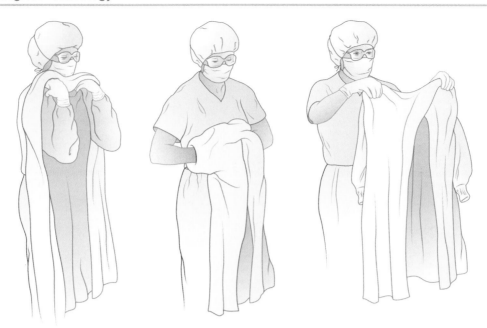

Figure 9-12 Removing the gown using aseptic technique. Note that the gown is immediately turned inside out to contain the contaminated side.

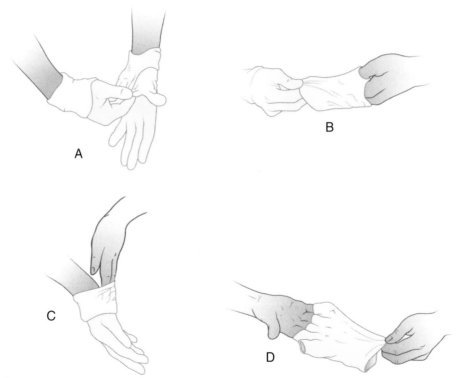

Figure 9-13 **A** to **D,** Procedure for removing contaminated gloves. Note that the bare hand does not touch the outside of the glove.

1. Grasp one glove at the outer wrist, using the opposite gloved hand.
2. Pull the glove off. It will turn inside out as you remove it.
3. Place your bare fingers inside the cuff of the opposite hand and roll this glove off your hand.
4. Dispose of both gloves in a biohazard receptacle without touching the contaminated outside of the gloves.

❖ *Remember*—glove to glove, hand to hand *when removing a soiled glove.*

OPENING A CASE

Opening a case means to prepare the surgical suite for a procedure and open sterile items. All equipment and furniture are arranged, and sterile supplies are brought into the room.

Depending on the complexity of the surgery, the amount of equipment to be prepared, and the degree of emergency, the scrub and circulator open the case about 15 to 20 minutes before the start of surgery. In extremely large cases, more time may be needed to allow for opening supplies and setting up the case.

After the case is opened, the sterile items should be monitored constantly. The ideal technique is to have someone physically in the room to observe the sterile setup and verify that nothing is contaminated.

❖ *Covering the setup with a sterile drape is not recommended because of the risk of contamination when the cover is removed. Leaving a room vacant and posting a sign on the door advising staff members that the case is open also is not an acceptable practice.*

LARGE PACKS

Large packs are included in almost all surgical setups. These include linen or nonwoven gowns, towels, sponges, and other items. Preassembled case packs can be custom designed by the institution to include surgical supplies routinely used during specific types of surgery. Some commonly preassembled packs include abdominal, orthopedic, and minor surgery packs. The large case pack is the first to be opened.

Before opening any sterile pack, always check the integrity of the outside of the package and the external chemical indicators for verification of exposure to the sterilization process. Any packages with tears, holes, or water marks are contaminated and should be removed from the room for reprocessing and replaced with new packs.

The large pack is opened on the back table, because that is the center of the scrub's work area. After the large pack is unwrapped, instruments, suture packs, and other sterile items are opened onto the draped surface and later organized and set up in logical order.

The following technique is used to open the large pack on the back table (Figure 9-14):

1. Center the pack on the table and orient it so that the long ends of the outside drape line up with the long end of the table.
2. If the pack is very large and has been square wrapped, the recommended practice is to move around the package rather than reaching across it. In this case, grasp the folded edge of the top fold with both hands and pull the edges toward you.
3. Move to the other side of the table and repeat this process on the opposite top fold. Allow 1 inch (2.5 cm) of margin between the edge of the drape and

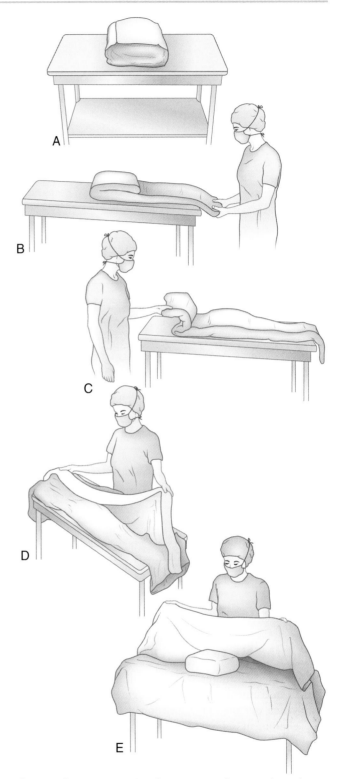

Figure 9-14 Procedure for opening a linen pack on the back table. The linen pack usually is opened first to provide a sterile surface on which other items can be distributed.

your nonsterile hand. Remember not to lean over the table while opening the pack. Keep a safe distance away.

4. Do not readjust the table drape after it has been opened.

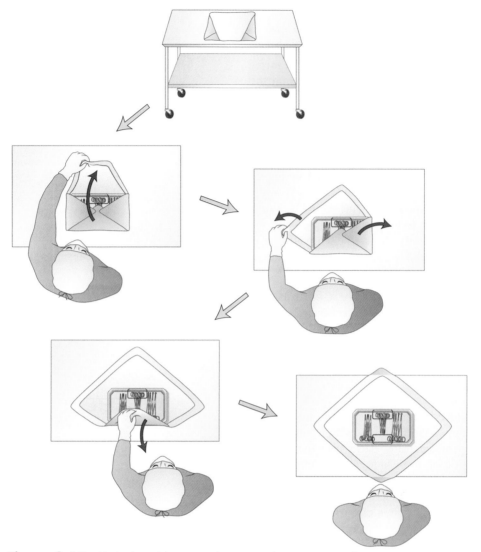

Figure 9-15 Method used by nonsterile personnel to open a small instrument tray on a table. Note the order in which each flap is folded back to prevent contamination by the hand and arm.

INSTRUMENT TRAYS

The following technique is used by nonsterile personnel to open an instrument tray properly (Figure 9-15):

1. When opening large instrument trays or other heavy equipment, set the tray on a small table and then open in place.
2. Orient the item so that the flap farthest from the body is grasped first. The flap is opened away from the body and gently pulled down.
3. Open each side flap. Open the flap closest to the body last, pulling it toward you. This prevents the nonsterile arm from reaching across the sterile surface inside the pack.
4. Drape small tables in the same manner. Place the drape on the table. Grasp only the edges of the drape and unfold the top corner or edge of the drape away from you. After the first flap has been pulled back, subsequent flaps must be opened in such a way that the nonsterile

arm and hand do not reach across the sterile surface. Move around the table if necessary, always bringing the edge of the drape toward you.
5. As sterile items are opened, use more tables if necessary.
6. Do not stack heavy sterile instruments precariously high or in such a way that they might be dropped.
7. Avoid holding a heavy instrument tray in one hand and removing the wrapper with the other. This puts excessive strain on the wrist, and you may drop the tray. Put the tray on a nonsterile table before opening the wrapper.

BASINS

Basin sets are placed on a ring stand and opened in the same manner as large instrument trays. Open the flap farthest away from you first, then the side flaps. Do not reach over the basin.

It is better technique to move around the sterile package and pull flaps toward you.

If water is found in a basin when the sterile wrapper is opened, the basin is considered contaminated. This is caused by a problem in steam sterilization, and the Central Service department must be notified. The load in which the basin was sterilized will be located, and those items will be removed from service.

INTRAOPERATIVE TECHNIQUES

DELIVERING STERILE GOODS

When items are opened during the setup and the scrub is sterile, the circulator opens these items and delivers them aseptically. Envelope-wrapped trays or other small items are opened by grasping the top flap and pulling it back, away from the person doing the opening, and under the item. Side flaps are opened next, followed by the near flap. The scrub may take the item directly (Figure 9-16), or the circulator may carefully set the item on a sterile surface without allowing contamination of the object (e.g., tray, instrument) or the sterile surface.

PEEL POUCHES

Items wrapped in sealed pouches are delivered directly to the scrub (Figure 9-17, A). Suture packets also may be flipped onto the field (Figure 9-17, B). This is done by opening the peel pouch halfway and then quickly popping the wrapper open the rest of the way to propel the contents out of the package and onto the sterile field. Extreme care must be taken when flipping items onto the field to avoid reaching over the sterile field or flipping the item past the sterile field and onto the floor.

When opening peel pouch wrappers, do not allow the item to slide out of the package; this contaminates it. Instead, peel the wrapper back far enough to permit the item to drop out cleanly, away from the exposed edges of the wrapper.

SHARPS

Scalpel blades and other **sharps** should be passed directly to the scrub or unwrapped in an open area where they are easily seen. Blades, trocars, and other sharps are not to be opened into instrument trays, because the sharps can be hidden by other instruments. Items should never be opened so that

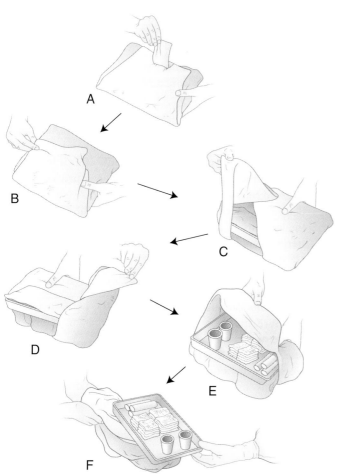

Figure 9-16 Procedure for distributing wrapped items. Note that the nonsterile (outside) of the wrapper does not touch the sterile inner surfaces.

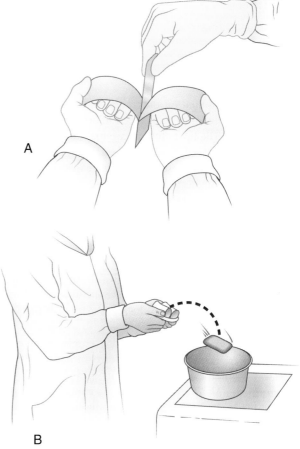

Figure 9-17 **A,** Distributing suture contained in a peel pouch wrapper. **B,** Suture packs may be flipped onto the sterile field. *(Redrawn from Phillips N: Berry and Kohn's operating room technique, ed 10, St Louis, 2004, Mosby.)*

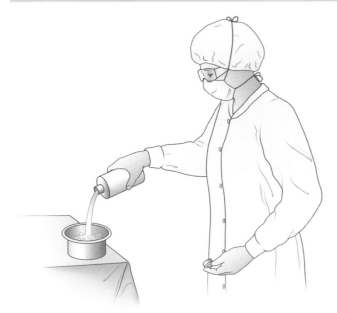

Figure 9-18 Distributing sterile liquids to a sterile container. Note that the bottle is not suspended directly over the sterile bowl. *(Redrawn from Phillips N: Berry and Kohn's operating room technique, ed 10, St Louis, 2004, Mosby.)*

sharps are hidden from plain view. If a sharp item is accidentally covered during opening, warn the scrub of its location to prevent injury during the setup.

SOLUTIONS

Solutions are distributed on the sterile field so that the fluid does not come in contact with the side of the bottle or any area below the sterile lip. Solutions are manufactured so that the cap can be removed aseptically, preserving the lip of the container. (Chapter 14 presents a complete discussion of the delivery of liquid medications to the sterile field.)

The recommended practice for distributing solutions is as follows:

1. The lip of a solution bottle is considered sterile only if it is covered with a sterile top that extends over the edge of the container.
2. The recommended method of distributing a solution is to pour the solution directly into a container set close to the edge of the table or held in the hand of the scrub (Figure 9-18).
3. When pouring sterile liquids, empty the entire container and move the down-turned container away from the sterile field. This prevents any liquid from running over the edge of the container and contaminating the field. After the bottle has been opened and its contents poured, the lip of the bottle is no longer considered sterile. Do not recap the sterile solution bottle.
4. It is poor practice to remove the cap of a medicine vial using an instrument and then pour out the contents. The lip of the vial is potentially contaminated by the

instrument. (Chapter 14 presents a complete discussion of the sterile distribution of drugs.)

CONTAMINATION DURING SURGERY

When an item or surface becomes contaminated during surgery, it must be isolated or removed from the sterile field. Contamination events must be treated on a case by case basis. Instruments and other small items can be passed off to the circulator. The scrub may need to change gloves if *any* possibility exists that the gloved hand touched the contaminated item.

When draped equipment or the sterile field becomes contaminated, all items in the area of the contamination must be passed off to the circulator. The contaminated surface is then contained with a nonpermeable drape. If the boundaries of the contamination are not clear, a wide area of containment or covering is necessary.

MAINTAINING THE STERILE FIELD

The **sterile field** is the physical area of which the center is the operative site and all sterile surfaces around it. It may also be restricted to particular sterile surfaces, such as when the sterile field is created and the patient has not yet been draped nor has sterile equipment been moved into place. The following practices pertain to any situation in which a sterile field exists.

1. **Sterile surfaces contact only sterile surfaces; nonsterile surfaces contact only nonsterile surfaces.**
   Contamination of a sterile surface occurs when a nonsterile surface touches a sterile surface (e.g., the circulator's bare hand accidentally touches the surgical technologist while delivering sterile items to sterile personnel).
2. **A sterile item is considered sterile only after it has been processed using methods that have been proven effective and that yield measurable results.**
   Before any sterile item is distributed to the sterile field, the integrity of the wrapper and the reading of chemical sterility indicators must be verified. Biological indicators are used to verify the correct functioning of a sterilizing system. Although an item has been through the process of sterilization, it might not be sterile. Many conditions and events can alter the sterility of the item, including puncture holes or tears in the wrapper, moisture, or failure of the sterilizer system.
3. **Sterile drapes, gowns, gloves, and table covers are barriers between a nonsterile surface and a sterile surface.**
   Materials used as barriers against contamination are chosen for their density, strength, ability to resist moisture, and ease of use. Materials that do not meet minimum standards for patient safety should not be used.
4. **The edge of any sterile drape, wrapper, or covering is considered nonsterile.**
   When a sterile item is opened, the edge of its wrapper must not touch the item. Maintaining a wide margin between the sterile item and the edge prevents possible

contamination of the item as it is delivered to the field. A 1-inch (2.5-cm) margin from the perimeter of a sterile wrapper is considered not sterile. When sterile items are opened and distributed, the nonsterile hand is protected under the wrapper. A specific technique is used to open and distribute sterile goods.

5. **Sterile liquids in bottles with an edge (lip) that is protected with a sealed sterile cap may be delivered directly from the bottle into a sterile container on the field.**

Medication vials often are sealed with aluminum caps. When the metal cap is pried open, the edge of the vial is considered contaminated, because the top cannot be removed without dragging the nonsterile cap across the lip of the vial. When you begin to pour sterile solution into a container, do not stop pouring until the container is empty. Pull the container away from the sterile field so that no residual liquid can drip down the nonsterile side of the container into the sterile receptacle below. Never recap a sterile fluid container.

6. **If any doubt exists about the sterility of an item, consider it contaminated.**

Before opening the wrapper of any sterile item, inspect it for signs of contamination. Tears, holes, wear marks, or water spots on any wrapper are signs of questionable sterility. When in doubt, do not use the item.

7. **The draped patient is the center of the sterile field during surgery.**

Other draped items and sterile personnel form the periphery of the field. Sterile drapes create a barrier between a nonsterile surface and the working area of the sterile field. For example, the operating microscope, ring basin, and back table are draped. Equipment that is not draped must remain outside the sterile field, with at least 12 inches (30 cm) allowed between the sterile and nonsterile surfaces.

8. **Sterile gowns are considered sterile only in front from midchest to table level.**

Sterile personnel should not drop their forearms or hands below waist level nor raise them above the axillary line. The axilla itself is considered nonsterile even though protected by a gown because of the large population of bacteria in the axillary region.

Sterile personnel must pass other sterile personnel back to back or front to front. Even though wraparound gowns are used in most surgical settings, the sterility of the back cannot be guaranteed because the person wearing it cannot observe it. Sterile personnel never turn their back to the sterile field.

9. **Sterile tables are considered sterile only at table height.**

The top of a sterile table is the only surface considered sterile. Suture ends must not hang over the table edge. Table drapes must not be repositioned once they have been placed, because this changes the level of the sterile area. Tubing, cords, and hoses that are secured to the patient drape must not be pulled up to create additional slack. This brings the nonsterile portion of the tubing up

to the sterile field. The scrub is responsible for measuring and allowing for necessary slack before securing these items in place when they are first brought onto the sterile field.

10. **Sterile personnel remain within the immediate area of the sterile field.**

Scrubbed personnel must not move away from the sterile field. Sterile personnel are sometimes required to move around the periphery of the field to perform their tasks. However, moving outside the immediate sterile area compromises aseptic technique. Sterile personnel should not leave the room to retrieve items from another area, even if that area is restricted (e.g., the sterile core where supplies are flash sterilized).

11. **Nonsterile team members never lean over or reach over a sterile surface to distribute sterile goods to the field. They do not pass between two sterile surfaces.**

When sterile packages are opened, the opener must hand items to personnel or deposit them on sterile surfaces in such a way as to avoid reaching over previously opened goods. Many commercially prepared surgical items are packaged so that they can be flipped onto the sterile field from a safe distance. If the wrapper does not permit this technique to be used, nonsterile personnel must pass the item directly to scrubbed personnel.

12. **Movement is kept to a minimum during surgery.**

Team members should move around the operating suite as little as possible. This applies to both scrubbed and nonsterile personnel. Traffic into and out of the surgical suite creates air currents that sweep contaminated particles into the operating room. Doors to the operating room suite should remain closed when sterile supplies are opened and when surgery is in progress.

13. **Drapes and linens should be handled as little as possible and with a minimum of movement.**

This prevents the release of lint and dust particles, which create a vehicle for transmission of airborne bacteria. When draping a surface, always unfold the drapes; never shake a drape to loosen or unfold it. At the close of surgery, fold or roll soiled drapes toward the center, taking care to contain the contaminants. Never drag a drape from a surface and bundle it up against your body, even if you are wearing protective attire. This spreads contaminated particles into the environment.

14. **Talking is kept to a minimum during surgery.**

The mouth is a major reservoir for bacteria. Talking forces the breath into the air and immediate environment. Masks worn to prevent the release of bacteria-laden moisture are not 100% effective and when improperly worn provide little protection against the dissemination of aerosol droplets containing microorganisms.

15. **Moisture carries bacteria from a nonsterile surface to a sterile surface.**

When water comes in contact with a sterile drape or gown, it can cause strike-through contamination. This occurs when moisture from either side of the drape serves as a vehicle for bacteria to infiltrate the drape from the nonsterile surface. Most disposable drapes are tightly woven to prevent strike-through. With continuous contact, blood and fluids can penetrate gowns and drapes. Woven (reusable) drapes are treated with a chemical that resists moisture, but they are not completely impervious.

16. **The sterile field is created as close as possible to the time of surgery and is monitored throughout the procedure.**

    When sterile supplies have been opened, the sterile setup is vulnerable to contamination. The longer a sterile setup remains exposed, the greater the risk of contamination, which is event-related rather than time-related.

Sterile supplies should be opened as close to the time of surgery as possible. In reality, however, cases often are delayed or even canceled. Currently no data are available to suggest that leaving a sterile setup exposed increases the risk of a surgical site infection. After a room is opened, it must be constantly monitored for contamination. Most health care institutions have their own internal policies regarding unused setups.

REALITY VERSUS STANDARDS

As surgical personnel develop experience, they clarify their own practices and compare them with those of the people around them. Even after acquiring excellent technique, people may consciously (or unconsciously) disregard certain practices because of lack of peer or administrative support, professional motivation, or simple apathy. Even when the numbers of serious surgical infections is small, the increased suffering for the patient and family, costs, extended hospital stay, lost workdays, and inability to meet one's personal goals create long-lasting effects in that person's life.

Standards vary slightly according to the practice setting and the policies of individual institutions. Surgical personnel can and should discuss the aseptic technique practices of their team, department, or institution as long as they have *evidence* to demonstrate that these practices are below the normal safety standard. Always remember, however, that criticism of those in your internship facility will not be welcomed.

CHAPTER SUMMARY

- Evidence-based practice is a way of making decisions and acting on proven methods. It uses rational decision making rather than opinion or past practice. Methods derived through evidence-based practice can be traced to accepted authority (peer review) and the highest level of professional inquiry.
- Professional surgical technologists are engaged in health care practices that use evidence-based knowledge and methods. The modern surgical technologist must be familiar with evidence-based thinking and acting.
- Aseptic technique is a method of preventing contamination of instruments, supplies, and equipment used in critical and semicritical areas of the body.
- Aseptic technique is based on a set of principles that must be learned and practiced until they are intuitive.
- The basis of aseptic technique is the concept of barriers between contaminated and sterile surfaces. Sterile objects or surfaces are contained or confined to prevent contact with nonsterile objects.
- A contaminated surface is one that has potentially or actually come in contact with a nonsterile object.

- The domains of aseptic technique include surgical attire, hand hygiene, gowning and gloving, surgical drapes, and techniques for handling sterile equipment.
- Perioperative personnel are required to wear scrub suit attire that has been freshly laundered and not previously worn.
- A surgical cap is worn to cover all hair, which is a primary source of surgical wound contamination.
- During surgery, a sterile gown and gloves are worn as barriers between nonsterile skin and clothing and the surgical wound and sterile equipment.
- The sterile field is the area covered by sterile drapes. It includes scrubbed personnel who are gowned and gloved. The draped patient is the center of the sterile field.
- The rules of asepsis include methods of moving around the sterile field, the distribution of sterile supplies and equipment, and methods of preserving sterility.
- Surgical conscience is the practice of aseptic technique, reporting when sterility has been broken, and taking measures to re-establish sterility when necessary. In cases of gross contamination of the surgical wound, medical therapy may be initiated to prevent infection.

REVIEW QUESTIONS

1. What is the purpose of aseptic technique?
2. What established standards are used for setting aseptic technique protocols?
3. Why are artificial nails prohibited in most surgical settings?
4. What antiseptic is used in the surgical hand rub?
5. Transient flora are found on the uppermost layer of the skin. Where are resident flora found?

6. While putting on sterile gloves, you touch the glove wrapper with your finger. Is the wrapper still sterile?
7. What is the sterile field?
8. During surgery, a team member contaminates his gowned arm. A sterile sleeve sometimes is used to cover the area of contamination. What concept of aseptic technique is put into practice in this situation?
9. What do you think is the best way to correct contamination of an entire instrument tray during surgery?

10. How does surgical technique relate to aseptic technique?

CASE STUDIES

Case 1

After you have performed the hand scrub, you enter the surgery suite and proceed to the area where your gown and gloves are located. As you are removing the towel, you notice that some water from your hand has dripped onto your sterile gown. What will you do?

Case 2

During surgery, you notice that the surgeon has a hole in his glove. You notify him of this. He replies, "Don't worry about it." How will you respond?

Case 3

When you arrive in surgery, you note that someone has placed your wrapped sterile instruments next to the heating vent. You notice moisture on the outside of the pack. What should you do?

Case 4

During surgery, you are moving a heavy instrument tray from one area of the sterile table to another. As you pick up the tray, the corner of the instrument tray accidentally rips the sterile sheet covering the entire back table. What will you do?

Case 5

The surgeon has just spoken abruptly to you about how you hand her sutures. A minute later, you rip your glove on the suture, and the surgeon must wait while you remove your contaminated glove and put on a sterile one. The surgeon is visibly irritated. What would you say to the surgeon, if anything, while changing your glove?

Case 6

When you open your sterile basins while setting up a case, you notice moisture on the inside of one of the basins. What is the significance of this?

Case 7

After gowning, you are donning your sterile gloves when you puncture the glove, creating a large hole. What should you do? What is the proper technique for correcting this problem?

Case 8

After gowning the surgeon, you notice a large tear in the sleeve of the surgeon's gown. What should you do? What is the proper technique for correcting this problem?

REFERENCE

1. Association Association of periOperative Registered Nurses (AORN): Recommended practices for surgical attire in *Standards, recommended practices and guidelines,* 2007 edition, Denver, 2007, AORN.
2. Association of Surgical Technologists (AST): Aseptic technique in *Standards of Practice,* available at http://www.ast.org/educators/standards_table_of_contents.aspx. Accessed March 19, 2009.

BIBLIOGRAPHY

Association of periOperative Registered Nurses (AORN): *Standards, recommended practices and guidelines,* 2007 edition, Denver, 2007, AORN.

Centers for Disease Control and Prevention: Airborne precautions. Retrieved November 15, 2007, at http://www.cdc.gov/ncidod/dhaq/gl_isolation_droplet.html.

Centers for Disease Control and Prevention: Contact precautions. Retrieved November 15, 2007, at http://www.cdc.gov/ncidod/dhaq/gl_isolation_html.

Centers for Disease Control and Prevention: Droplet precautions. Retrieved November 15, 2007, at http://www.cdc.gov/ncidod/dhaq/gl_isolation_droplet.html.

Centers for Disease Control and Prevention: Hand hygiene in health care settings. http://www.cdc.gov/Handhygiene/ Retrieved January 6, 2009.

Paulson D: Hand scrub products: performance requirements versus clinical relevance, *AORN Journal* 80:2, 2004.

Sehulster L, Chinn R, Arduino M et al: Recommendations from CDC and the Health Care Infection Control Practices Advisory Committee (HICPAC), Chicago, 2004, American Society for Health Care Engineering/American Hospital Association.

Seigel JD, Rhinehart E, Jackson M et al and the Health Care Infection Control Practices Advisory Committee: 2007 Guideline for isolation, precaution, and preventing transmission of infectious agents in health care settings: June, 2007. Retrieved November 15, 2007 at http://www.cdc.gov/ncidod/dhqp/pdf/isolation2007.pdf.

Weinstein R: Controlling antimicrobial resistance in hospitals: infection control and use of antibiotics. Retrieved November 15, 2007, at www.cdc.gov/ncidod/eid/vol7no2/weinstein.htm.

CHAPTER 10

Transporting, Transferring, and Positioning the Surgical Patient

CHAPTER OUTLINE

LEARNING OBJECTIVES

After studying this chapter and laboratory practice, the reader will be able to:

- Use safe body mechanics during patient transportation, transferring, and positioning
- Describe the responsibilities of the surgical technologist in patient transport and transfer
- Use the correct procedure to identify a patient
- Demonstrate how to assist a patient from a bed to a wheelchair
- Identify how to ease a patient to the ground in the event of a fall
- Describe how to transport a patient safely by stretcher
- Demonstrate the transfer of a patient from a bed to a stretcher
- Identify the proper transport for a pediatric patient
- Demonstrate the transfer of a patient from a stretcher to the operating table

- Describe the use of common operating table accessories
- Demonstrate the transfer of a semiconscious patient from the operating table to a stretcher
- Describe the consequences of nerve and blood vessel compression
- Describe the principles of safe positioning
- Describe how to prevent shear injury
- Describe the stages of decubitus ulcers and how to prevent them
- Participate in commonly used methods of patient positioning
- Describe compartment syndrome and how to prevent it
- Describe how to do the following when positioning a patient:
  - Prevent brachial plexus injury
  - Prevent ulnar nerve injury
  - Prevent injury to the face, ear, and eye during positioning
  - Prevent injury to the breasts and genitalia in prone position

TERMINOLOGY

Abduction: Movement of a joint or body part away from the body.

Compartment syndrome: Severe swelling and tissue injury caused by constriction of the blood and lymph. Compartment syndrome can progress to tissue necrosis.

Compression injury: Tissue injury caused by continuous pressure over an area

Dependent areas of the body: Areas of the body subject to pressure from gravity and weight. For example, the sacrum is a dependent area when a person is in the supine position.

Embolism: A clot of blood, air, organic material, or a foreign body that moves freely in the vascular system. An embolus travels from larger to smaller vessels until it cannot pass through a vessel. At that level, it interrupts the flow of blood and may result in severe disease or death.

Fasciotomy: A surgical treatment for compartment syndrome in which the fascia is incised to release severe tissue swelling.

Footboard: Operating table attachment which braces the patient's weight when the table is tilted toward the feet.

Fowler position: The sitting position, which is used for cranial, facial, and some reconstructive breast procedures.

Headrest: Operating table attachment used to support and provide peripheral access to the head.

Hyperextension: Extension of a joint beyond its normal anatomical range.

Hyperflexion: Flexion of a joint beyond its normal anatomical range.

Hypotension: Decreased blood pressure.

Ischemia: Loss of blood supply to a body part either by compression or as a result of a blockage in the blood vessels. Prolonged ischemia causes tissue death from lack of oxygen to the tissue.

Jackknife (Kraske) position: A type of prone position in which the patient lies on the abdomen with the hips flexed into an inverted V.

Knee-chest position: A familiar term that describes the patient position used for administration of spinal anesthetics and for access to the rectum in patient (nursing) care. The patient lies in the lateral position with the knees drawn toward the abdomen and the spine flexed outward.

Lateral (Sims) position: The position in which the patient lies on his or her side on the operating table or bed.

Lithotomy position: The position used for vaginal, perineal, and occasionally rectal surgery. The patient's legs are positioned on stirrups.

Log roll: A technique for moving the patient in which a bed sheet or draw sheet is used to roll the patient onto his or her side.

Necrosis: Tissue death.

Neuropathy: Permanent or temporary nerve injury that results in numbness or loss of function of a part of the body.

Prone position: The position in which the front of the body is in contact with the operating table.

Range of motion: The normal anatomical movement of an extremity.

Reverse Trendelenburg position: The position in which a prone or supine patient is tilted with the feet down.

Semi-Fowler position: A semisitting position, which is used for surgery on the neck and thyroid.

Shear injury: Tissue injury or necrosis that results when two tissue planes are forcefully pulled in opposite directions. Shearing usually occurs when the body is pulled or slides by gravity across a high-friction surface, such as a bed sheet. Shearing can lead to a decubitus ulcer.

Stirrups: Operating table attachment used to elevate the legs in lithotomy position.

Supine position: The position in which the patient lies on the back, facing upward.

Table break: The hinged joint between sections of the operating table that can be flexed in any direction.

Thoracic outlet syndrome: A group of disorders attributed to compression of the subclavian vessels and nerves. Such compression can cause permanent injury to the arm and shoulder.

Thromboembolus: A blood clot that breaks loose and enters the systemic circulation, causing obstruction or occlusion of a blood vessel. Also referred to as a *thrombus*.

Toboggan (also called a sled): Operating table attachment that secures the patient's arm at the side of the body.

Traction injury: A nerve injury caused by stretching or compression of the nerve.

Transfer board: A thin Plexiglas, fiberglass, or roller board that is placed under the patient to move the person from the operating table to the stretcher or bed.

Trendelenburg position: The position in which a prone or supine patient is tilted with the head down.

Ventilation: The physical act of taking air into the lungs by inflation and releasing carbon dioxide from the lungs by deflation.

INTRODUCTION

In the perioperative setting, patients must be transferred to and from a variety of conveyances, including stretchers, beds, wheelchairs, and the operating table. The transportation and positioning of patients are among the responsibilities that create the most risk for patients and health care workers alike. Patients may be unsteady, semiconscious, or unconscious and unable to use protective mechanisms that normally would prevent falls or other injuries. Diagnostic and operating room tables are narrow. Transfer vehicles, such as stretchers and wheelchairs, can slip unexpectedly. Perioperative work is physically demanding, and staff members may be tired or even themselves injured from the continual strain on the legs, back, and hips. Perioperative staff members, including surgical technologists, are responsible for the safe transfer of patients and protection against injury during surgery. Surgical technologists must be aware of the risks and dangers associated with positioning the patient for surgery. All staff members need to protect their own health by using approved methods for patient movement and handling. This chapter provides an introduction to hands-on technique necessary to ensure the safety of patients and staff members.

TRANSPORTING AND TRANSFERRING THE PATIENT

BODY MECHANICS

Health care workers are at high risk for back injury and other types of musculoskeletal injury while caring for, moving, and transferring patients. Workers are injured because these tasks are unpredictable. A weak or sedated patient lacks muscle tone, which results in flaccid limbs and general unwieldiness. The adult human body is asymmetrical and heavy, and unlike a large inanimate object, the human body cannot be held close to the health care worker's center of gravity when moved.

Moving a patient always poses the risk of an accident. The patient can fall, equipment can become entangled during transfer, or a weak patient may pull the health care worker off balance. A sudden shift of weight may be required to prevent injury to the patient or health care worker. Hospital rooms are small and crowded, which may necessitate some twisting motions. These motions put the health care worker off balance, which increases the risk of back injury.

Injuries are reduced when health care providers use proper body mechanics and patient transfer devices. Chapter 15 presents a complete discussion of body mechanics. The following guidelines can help prevent injuries:

- Always make sure you have sufficient help when moving a patient.
- Know your limits and do not exceed them.
- Be prepared for possible weight shifts.
- Maintain the spine in a neutral position whenever possible.
- Avoid twisting the spine, especially while lifting or bending.
- Position yourself as close to the patient as possible; this greatly reduces the spinal load.
- Keep your feet well apart to provide a wide base of support.
- When performing horizontal moves, such as transferring the patient from one surface to another, *do not bend the knees.*
- For vertical moves (up or down), *do bend the knees.*
- Avoid awkward positions that reduce your base of support.
- Never try to lift or maneuver the patient while reaching forward, away from your center of gravity. If necessary, place one knee on the stretcher to bring the patient closer to your center of gravity.
- Use abdominal, arm, and leg muscles when lifting the patient. The abdominal muscles can support the trunk much more efficiently than the lower back muscles.

PRINCIPLES OF SAFE PATIENT TRANSPORT AND TRANSFER

Many risks are associated with patient transport and transfer. A weak, disoriented, or pediatric patient may attempt to climb out of the stretcher or climb out of the crib and become entangled in side rails or climb over them and fall. Catheters, tubing, and other medical devices can cause tissue trauma or injury if pulled out of the body. The patient can sustain a shear injury (see the section on positioning injuries later in the chapter) if dragged across a high-friction surface such as bed linens or a draw sheet. Changes in posture can result in severe **hypotension** (low blood pressure) or elevated cerebral pressure. Even when transfers are done slowly and deliberately, accidents can occur.

Transport and transfer injuries occur more often in the following circumstances:

- There aren't enough people to help with the move.
- Personnel assisting in the transfer or transport do not have a plan.
- Personnel are rushed.
- The patient is disoriented or combative.

The following principles apply to all types of patient transport and transfer:

- *Know the risks.* To keep the patient safe, you must understand exactly what the risks are and how to prevent injury.
- *Protect the patient's personal dignity at all times.* The patient has a right to be protected from exposure and embarrassment. Many patients fear that their personal rights, such as a right to modesty, are forfeited upon admission to a health care facility. Try to avoid passing through crowded areas while transporting the patient. This is not always possible, but it is desirable. Use a patient elevator instead of visitor elevators during transportation.
- *Perform all patient movement deliberately and carefully.* You must have a plan before you begin. Prepare for the unexpected. Think ahead.
- When a patient is transferred, one person should be in charge of the move and guide the others. Because of the risks involved in patient movement, coordination is absolutely necessary. This requires one person to guide the action of others so that all are working together during each step.
- *Know your equipment.* Before moving any patient, know how to operate patient care equipment. Never use a mechanical lifting or transfer system without assistance.
- *Think about what you are doing while you are doing it.* As you move the patient, maintain your focus on the task at hand. Do not allow yourself to become distracted. Think ahead and be prepared for each step of the process.
- *Protect the patient from hypothermia.* The patient should be adequately covered with blankets. Corridors can be very cold and drafty. A patient that has become cold during transport is at higher risk for hypothermia during surgery.
- *Use approved protocol for patient identification at all times.* Check the name and number on the wrist or ankle band, identification card, permits, and chart.
- *Explain the process to the patient before and during the transfer.* This may relieve the patient's anxiety and make the person more relaxed during the transfer.
- Expect the unexpected.

PATIENT IDENTIFICATION

Patient identification is a critical issue in health care. The health care assistant is responsible for identifying the patient according to a standard policy. No patient should be transported and no procedure should be initiated until the protocol for identification has been completed, even if the patient is known to the health care assistant.

All patients are identified in at least three ways. The patient's wrist or ankle band is imprinted with the patient's name and hospital number and the physician's name. If a card system is used, the patient's identification card is used to stamp all paperwork and matches the patient's identification bracelet. This card must be firmly attached to the chart during transport and must remain with the chart until the patient returns to his or her hospital unit. The patient's chart must accompany the patient whenever the individual is transported from the unit.

Appropriate verification of the patient's identity proceeds as follows:

1. Examine the patient's identification band. Compare both the name and the number with those on the patient's chart.
2. Ask the patient to state his or her full name. Do not call the patient by name before asking the patient to state his or her name.
3. Ask the patient to tell you what procedure he or she is undergoing and to point to the side on which the surgery will take place.

Example 1

Incorrect: *"Good morning Mr. X, I'm here to take you to surgery."*
Correct: *"Good morning, my name is _____. I'm here to take you to surgery. Can you say your full name for me?"*

Example 2

Incorrect: *"So, Dr. X is planning to fix your arm today."*
Correct: *"What surgery will you be having today?"*

> ❖ *If the patient's name, hospital identification number, surgery, and surgical site do not match the chart or operative documents, you must report this to the unit charge nurse. Do not transport the patient if patient information does not match the chart. Call the operating room to let personnel know about the delay and the reason.*

> ❖ *If the patient has no identification band, you must report this to the unit charge nurse or nurse manager. Under routine circumstances an identification band must be obtained before the patient leaves the unit.*

ASSISTING THE AMBULATORY PATIENT

Transferring a Patient from a Bed to a Wheelchair

Transfer of a patient from a bed to a wheelchair is performed in distinct steps. First, help the patient to a sitting position, then to a standing position, and finally back to a sitting position in the wheelchair. Explain these steps to the patient before beginning the transfer. During the transfer, reinforce your instructions and prepare the patient for each step. This increases the patient's confidence and reduces fear. Remember that weak or elderly patients often are afraid of falling. Seek help when transferring a patient who is at high risk of falling (i.e., a patient who is heavy, unstable, or encumbered with medical devices).

Before beginning the transfer, familiarize yourself with the patient's equipment. Make certain that the wheelchair's brakes and steering mechanism are functioning properly. Do not transport a patient in a wheelchair that has no foot supports or other safety attachments. The wheelchair must fit the patient's size and weight.

Check the patient's identification as described previously. Free up any tubes or lines and make certain there is enough slack between the patient and the wheelchair to prevent entanglement or restriction during the transfer.

> ❖ *Transfer equipment first, then the patient.*

Assisting a Patient from a Lying to a Sitting Position

Whenever you are responsible for transporting the patient, be aware of the location of the call bell in case you need assistance or emergency help.

To help a patient move from a lying position to a sitting position, follow these steps:
1. Verify the identity of the patient before taking any actions. Bring the wheelchair to the side of the bed so that it is lined up with the bed. Lock the wheels. Make sure the wheels on the bed also are locked, and lower the bed to its lowest position.
2. If the patient is weak on one side, place the wheelchair on the opposite side of the bed. Raise the head of the bed slowly.
3. If the patient reports dizziness or any other changes, seek nursing help before proceeding. Dizziness may be caused by rapid hypotension that results in cardiac arrhythmia or a sudden loss of blood to the brain. The patient should be immediately returned to a supine position.
4. To assist the patient into a sitting position, support the patient under the shoulders and thighs if necessary.
5. Pull the patient's legs gently over the side of the bed to a sitting position. Allow the patient to remain in the sitting position for a few moments. Do not proceed if the patient shows or reports any physical or mental changes.

Assisting a Patient from a Sitting to a Standing Position

To help a patient move from a sitting position to a standing position, follow these steps:
1. Standing directly in front of the patient, place your hands around the patient's torso and under the arms to support the shoulder blades.
2. Slightly bend your forward leg while placing your opposite foot in a bracing position (Figure 10-1, *A*).
3. Slowly rock back and raise the patient to a standing position (Figure 10-1, *B*).

Assisting a Patient from a Standing Position to a Wheelchair and Transporting the Patient

To help a patient move from a standing position to a sitting position in a wheelchair and then to transport the patient, follow these steps:
1. Taking one small step at a time, rotate your entire body as the patient does the same until the patient's back is lined up with the wheelchair.
2. Slowly lower the patient into the wheelchair. Spread your feet so that they are approximately shoulder width apart. Use your abdominal muscles to support your

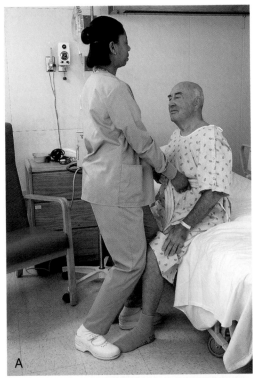

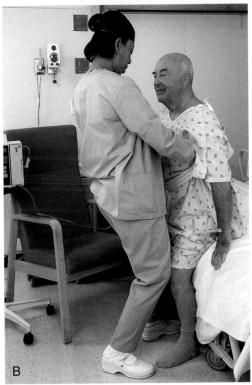

Figure 10-1 Lifting the patient to a standing position. *(From Potter PA, Perry AG: Basic nursing: essentials for practice, ed 7, St Louis, 2009, Mosby.)*

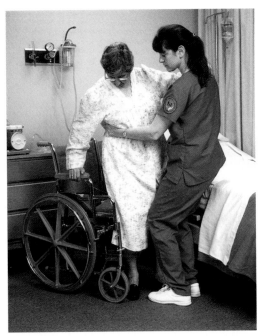

Figure 10-2 Lowering the patient into a wheelchair. *(From Harkreader H, Hogan MA: Fundamentals of nursing, ed 2, St Louis, 2004, WB Saunders.)*

4. Place the patient's feet on the footrests and cover the patient with a blanket or sheet. Secure the safety strap.
5. Make sure that you have the patient's chart and medical records.
6. Proceed to your destination. When entering an elevator or doorway, pull the wheelchair rather than pushing it ahead as this protects the patient's head. Secure doorways in the open position before passing through them. Make sure you have the patient's chart before leaving the area.

Transferring a Patient from a Wheelchair to a Bed or the Operating Table

To transfer a patient from a wheelchair to a bed or operating table, follow these steps:

1. Place the table or bed at its lowest height.
2. Reverse the steps used to transfer the patient to the wheelchair. Place the wheelchair in line with the bed and lock the wheels.
3. If the patient can put weight on the hands, ask the patient to push down. At the same time, lift the patient by placing your arms under the person's arms and securing your hands over the patient's shoulder blades.
4. Place your bracing foot back and rotated slightly outward.
5. As you lift the patient up, rock back on your bracing foot and, step by step, rotate your body with the patient's until the person is positioned to sit on the edge of the operating table or bed.
6. Remember to keep your spine and the patient's back in alignment while turning. Ease the patient down to a sitting position on the operating table or bed.

back as you lower the patient. Do not allow the patient's weight to pull your torso downward.

3. Bend your knees, use the larger thigh muscles, and use your abdominal muscles to support your upper body. Lower the patient when your spine and body are in alignment with the patient and wheelchair (Figure 10-2).

7. One person should support the patient's back and head while another assists in bringing the legs to a horizontal position on the operating table or bed. A third assistant should stand at the opposite side of the operating table or bed to prevent the patient from falling.

8. Ease the patient to a lying position. Place a blanket or sheet over the patient and secure the safety strap immediately.

Assisting a Falling Patient

In the ambulatory care setting, patients walk or are transported by wheelchair from the holding area to the surgical area, and the surgical technologist may be responsible for assisting them. There is always a risk that the patient may fall during ambulation. The patient may suddenly experience a drop in blood pressure or become light-headed. Always anticipate the possibility of a fall, even when the patient is mobile and seems able to walk without assistance.

Patient falls can be dangerous for both the patient and the health care worker. The weight of the falling person can cause you to lose your own balance, which can result in a twisting injury or fracture. Patients who feel unsteady or insecure may take hold of the health care worker and pull them off balance, causing injury to both the health worker and the patient.

Guidelines for Assisting an Ambulatory Patient

1. Position yourself slightly behind the patient's shoulder while helping the person walk. This places you in a position to support the patient if the individual becomes weak or falls. If the patient seems unsteady, use a wheelchair.

2. To assist the falling patient, do *not try to support the patient's weight*. Instead, ease the patient to the floor while protecting the person's head (Figure 10-3). Spread your feet to create a wide base of support. Bend your knees and use your thigh muscles for support.

3. Follow the patient's movements with your own body to prevent the patient from dropping.

4. Immediately call out for assistance while remaining with the patient.

5. Do not abandon the patient under any circumstances.

ASSISTING THE INPATIENT

Transferring a Mobile Patient from a Bed to a Stretcher

Inpatients usually are transferred to the operating room by stretcher using the following steps:

1. Before bringing the stretcher into the patient's room, notify the unit clerk or nurse in charge that you have arrived to transport the patient to surgery. Collect the patient's chart and any other documents required. Do this before entering the patient's room. .

2. Knock on the patient's door or prepare the patient of your arrival before entering. Avoid simply entering the patient's room with the stretcher and announcing that you are taking the individual to surgery.

3. After introducing yourself, verify the patient's identity.

4. Arrange the furniture to make adequate space for the stretcher. Patient rooms and cubicles often are very

small. It is easier to make a path for the stretcher before entering with it.

5. Lower the bed rails on the side where the stretcher is located.

6. Align the stretcher with the bed and lock the wheels on both the bed and the stretcher. Under no circumstances should you move a patient to an unlocked stretcher. Align the bed to the height of the stretcher.

7. Identify and free up all tubing, drainage bags, or other devices that can restrain the patient or become dislodged during the transfer. Drainage collecting units (such as urinary or chest units) must remain lower than the patient's body at all times, and intravenous (IV) lines should be higher than the patient's body.

8. Guide the patient slowly across the bed to the stretcher. Be mindful of the bed sheets and prevent them from wrapping under the patient.

9. Proceed from step 3 in the following section (Moving a Conscious Patient with Limited Mobility).

Moving a Conscious Patient with Limited Mobility

A patient with limited mobility is transferred manually to the stretcher (Figure 10-4, *A*) using a draw sheet, which is a folded bedsheet or thick torso pad placed under the patient. This move requires at least three people. If the patient is unable to support the head, one person must guide the head and neck together, making sure that the cervical spine is in neutral position during the move, while two people assist from each side of the patient.

To move a patient with limited mobility, follow these steps:

1. Lower the bed rails on the stretcher side.

2. Align the stretcher with the bed and lock the wheels. Under no circumstances should a patient be moved to an unlocked stretcher. Align the bed to the height of the stretcher (Figure 10-4, *B*).

3. Make sure all tubing and medical devices have been freed.

4. Transfer medical equipment and devices first, then transfer the patient.

5. Roll the sides of the draw sheet toward the patient and grasp it firmly with both hands (Figure 10-4, *C*).

6. On the count of three, all assistants move the patient horizontally to the stretcher in two lifts. The first lift moves the patient to the edge of the bed. The person on the bed side may kneel on the bed and then proceed to a second lift to the stretcher. Moving a patient in one step could lead to injury due to the long reach over the bed.

7. Cover the patient and raise the side rails.

8. Place a pillow under the patient's head unless directed otherwise. Some patients must be transported flat.

9. Apply the safety strap midway between the knees and hips on top of the blanket or sheet. Allow two fingers' breadth between the strap and the patient. Do not place the safety strap over the patient's bare skin.

10. If the patient is cooperative, have the patient place the hands over the abdomen, with the elbows away from the side rails. The patient's feet must not protrude over the edge of the stretcher.

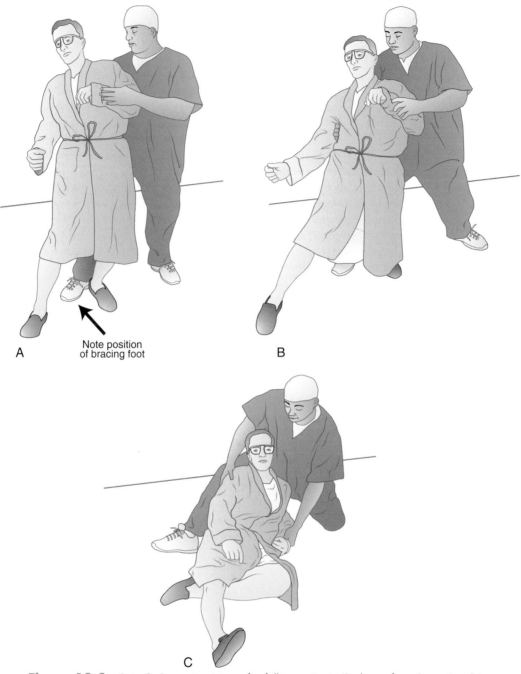

A   Note position of bracing foot

B

C

Figure 10-3 **A** to **C,** Preventing injury of a falling patient. *(Redrawn from Sorrentino SA: Mosby's textbook for nursing assistants, ed 7, St Louis, 2008, Mosby.)*

11. Notify the charge nurse that you are leaving the unit so this can be documented. Never remove a patient from a ward without notifying a staff member.

12. Proceed directly to your destination. If the patient is going to the operating room holding area, wait for the attending nurse to accept the patient before you leave. Do not leave the patient unattended at any time.

Transporting a Patient by Stretcher

Use the following guidelines when transporting a patient by stretcher:

1. When transporting the patient by stretcher, stand at the patient's head and push the stretcher forward. Look ahead as you move. Try to anticipate obstructions, sudden hallway traffic, and corners. Use ceiling mirrors when approaching corners.

2. When rounding blind corners, be careful of oncoming traffic. Check first before proceeding. Stopping a rolling stretcher is difficult, especially when the patient is heavy and medical devices are attached to the frame. If two people are available for transport, one person pushes from the head of the stretcher and the other guides the stretcher from the foot.

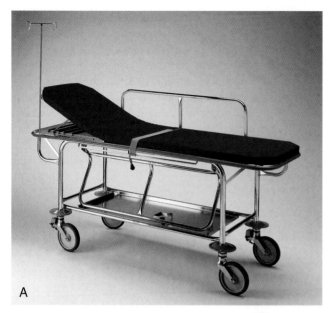

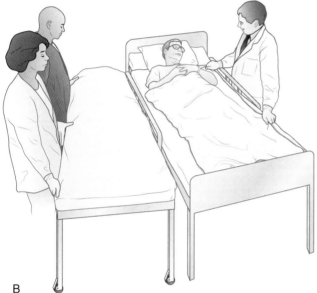

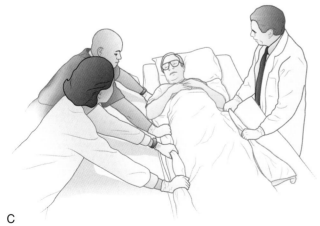

Figure 10-4 **A,** Standard stretcher. **B,** Aligning the bed with the stretcher. **C,** Moving a conscious patient with a draw sheet. (**A** courtesy Pedigo Products, Vancouver, Wash; **B** and **C** redrawn from Sorrentino SA: Mosby's textbook for nursing assistants, ed 7, St Louis, 2008, Mosby.)

3. Be sure to tell the conscious patient to keep the hands and arms within the stretcher rails. Patients often try to "help" during transport, which exposes them to the risk of injury.

Anticipation prevents accidents. Stretcher rails do not protect the patient from injury. The patient can easily bruise or even fracture an elbow, fingers, or wrist on walls or doorways. The transporter is responsible for protecting the patient from these injuries. Keep an eye on the patient and remind the individual to keep the hands and arms well within the boundaries of the side rails.

Ramps, doors, and elevators must be negotiated using carefully. Unless the patient is required to remain flat, raise the head of the stretcher so that the patient can see where he or she is going. Always warn the patient of bumps or other unfamiliar movements that will be encountered, such as entering or exiting an elevator.

Ramps

When rolling the stretcher down a ramp, do not rely on your strength to hold the stretcher against gravity. Ask for assistance. One person should stabilize the foot of the stretcher while the second is at the head. Traveling up the ramp also requires two people: one to push, the other to pull.

Doors

Remember the following when transporting a patient through doors:

- When passing through manually operated doors, open the doors first and secure them open. Do not push the foot of the stretcher forward against the closed doors, which would allow the doors to slam against the stretcher. This is unacceptable patient care.
- Stand at the patient's head and push the patient through the open doors or pull the patient through from the head of the stretcher.

Elevators

When transporting a patient on an elevator:

1. Use the patient elevator. Do not transport the patient in an elevator full of visitors.
2. When the elevator doors open, lock the doors open.
3. Standing at the patient's head, pull the stretcher head-first into the elevator.
4. Do not unlock the doors until you are certain that the foot of the stretcher has cleared the threshold.
5. Locate the emergency alarm and know how to use it.

Emergency During Transport

The patient may suffer sudden hypotension, cardiac arrest, seizure, or another emergency during transport. The effects of moving the patient from bed to stretcher can cause vascular or fluid shifts that may not manifest symptoms immediately.

If an emergency occurs during transport:

- Maintain verbal contact with the patient. If the person reports dizziness or lightheadedness or if you suspect a problem, call for help immediately.
- If you are in the corridor, shout for help.

• If you are in an elevator, activate the emergency alarm system, which is clearly marked.

Transferring a Conscious Patient from a Stretcher to an Operating Table

The patient is transported to the operating room shortly before the start of the procedure. The circulator and anesthesia care provider should be present to receive the patient and assist in the transfer to the operating table. At least two and preferably three people should be present during the transfer of a mobile and alert patient. As the stretcher is lined up next to the operating table, one person must stand on the opposite side so that the patient does not move too far and fall. The second person stands alongside the stretcher to brace it against the operating table. A third person should stand at the head of the table. Make certain that the brakes on the stretcher and the operating table are locked before beginning the transfer.

To transfer a conscious patient from a stretcher to an operating table, follow these steps:

1. Align the head of the stretcher with the head of the operating table. Lock the wheels of the stretcher and the operating room table.
2. Free up IV lines and other tubing. Transfer medical equipment and devices first, then transfer the patient.
3. Ask the patient to slide slowly onto the operating table, taking the top sheet along.
4. Open the back of the patient's gown to allow placement of cardiac leads or other monitoring devices.
5. Center the patient on the table and apply the safety strap immediately. Apply the safety strap midway between the knees and hips on top of the blanket or sheet. Allow two fingers' breadth between the strap and the patient. Do not place the safety strap directly over the patient's bare skin. The patient should always be secured on the operating table except during transfer.

Transferring an Immobile or Unconscious Patient from a Stretcher to an Operating Table

At least four people are required to transfer an immobile or unconscious patient from the operating table to the stretcher. More than four are needed if the patient is very obese or requires turning from prone to supine position. If other restrictions apply, such as spinal injury or special orthopedic considerations, extra personnel should be available to help. Teamwork is absolutely essential, with the anesthesia provider taking the lead.

Several methods can be used to manually transfer an unconscious patient from the stretcher to an operating table. For example, a Plexiglas **transfer board** or patient roller can be used. The patient is transferred to the board or patient roller, which is then pulled from one bed to the other. In addition to preventing shear injury, these aids reduce the vertical exertion required to move the patient and protect those doing the moving.

To use a transfer device, follow these steps:

1. Align the stretcher with the operating table and make sure the wheels are locked on both the stretcher and the operating table. Never move a patient onto an operating table with wheels that do not lock. The patient may fall to the floor between the stretcher and the table.
2. Before beginning the move, always tell the patient what you are going to do. Begin by freeing up all tubing and monitoring leads to allow slack during the move. To free up tubing and leads, follow the attachment at the patient's body to the source, making sure that nothing is pinched or tangled.
3. Transfer drainage tubes, IV bags, and other attached medical equipment items first and then move the patient.
4. One assistant, usually the anesthesia care provider, guides and directs the move. This person remains at the patient's head to protect the airway and prevent cervical injury.
5. Another person should assist with the patient's feet while two others assist at each side of the patient.
6. To use a transfer board, the movers must **log roll** the patient (Figure 10-5, A). Two or three people stand at

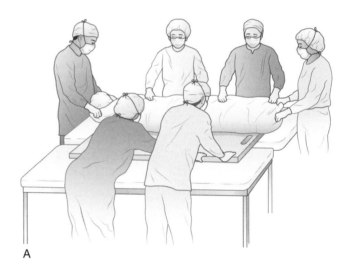

A

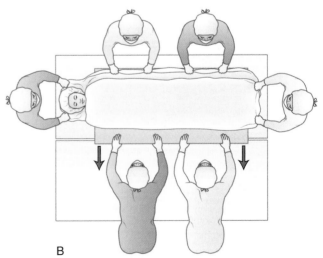

B

Figure 10-5 **A,** Log rolling the patient to slide the transfer board into position. **B,** Pulling the transfer board and patient in one or two coordinated moves.

the patient's side and grasp the opposite edge of the bed sheet or draw sheet.

7. The edge of the draw sheet is pulled toward the assistants to log roll the patient into a side-lying position with the front of the patient's body facing the assistants.

8. The anesthesia care provider protects the patient's neck and airway. The transfer board is placed to the back side of the patient, and those supporting the patient gently ease the person back into supine position on the board.

9. By grasping the board and pulling it across the stretcher, personnel can easily transfer the patient to the table (Figure 10-5, *B*). NOTE: If patient is semiconscious, another health care worker should help carry the patient's feet and lower legs across to the stretcher.

10. Make sure IV lines and drainage bags are all secured before unlocking the stretcher wheels to remove the stretcher from the room.

11. The transfer of patients in traction is directed by the surgeon and anesthesia care provider with strict attention to alignment and tension on the traction device.

12. To ensure patient safety, extra staff members may be needed to accompany patients requiring transport with a mechanical ventilator.

13. Whether the patient is conscious or unconscious, the same precautions are used when the individual is moved from the operating room table to the stretcher after surgery.

TRANSPORTING PEDIATRIC PATIENTS

Children are transported to the operating room by stretcher, crib, or bassinet. The crib must always be equipped with a Plexiglas cover during transportation. However, this may not prevent a small toddler from climbing between the top rail of the side bars and the crib cover.

All safety and procedural considerations apply to children as well as to adults. Young children are capable of climbing out of cribs with amazing speed and agility.

❖ *Never leave a child unattended or unobserved.*

Remember the following when transporting a child:

- Caregivers may accompany the child to the holding area, and in many hospitals a parent or other caregiver is permitted to stay in the operating suite during induction of anesthesia.
- Most young children, especially toddlers and preschoolers, suffer extreme anxiety when separated from their caregivers. Talk with the child during transport and explain what the child sees and hears in simple, nonthreatening terms. Children from 5 to 9 years old are curious about their environment. Preteens want to take part in their care. Teenagers are likely to seem unconcerned but appreciate explanations of the environment.

- Always allow caregivers to soothe the child during transport. As you talk with the child, remember that children understand the meanings of words in their most literal sense.
- Do not treat the child like a small adult. Provide a calm, supportive presence, showing respect for the child at all times. Children are quick to understand when they are being falsely reassured.
- Refrain from saying, "Oh, don't be afraid; this won't take long." A child who is afraid will not be reassured by being told to calm down. A more comforting approach would be to evaluate the child's understanding of what is happening and to clarify his or her perception in simple, concrete terms. .
- The child's developmental age is critical to communication. The trip between the safety of the hospital room or holding area and the operating room can either cause great distress or provide a means for the child to integrate the experience of surgery into the hospital stay. The child arriving in surgery may be frightened and difficult to treat or anesthetize. Your calming presence during transport can help prepare the child before arrival.

POSITIONING THE SURGICAL PATIENT

RATIONALE

Patients are placed in specific surgical positions for the following reasons:

- To reduce adverse physiological effects and mechanical injury to an irreducible minimum.
- To allow optimum access to the operative site.
- To permit optimum access for the anesthesia care provider. This includes venous, arterial, and respiratory access and access to monitoring sites.
- To give the surgeon unobstructed access to the operative site. The need for physiological stability, protection from injury, and access to the surgical site all affect positioning decisions.

The following elements are important in the safe positioning of patients:

- **Knowledge of anatomy, physiology, and the individual patient's specific medical condition.** Positioning is not a regimented routine. Each patient is unique and has specific considerations, such as age, joint mobility, and disease. Because of the high risk of serious and permanent injury, the surgical team must be guided and directed in the positioning process. The anesthesia care provider, surgeon, and circulator draw this direction from their knowledge of the patient's status.
- **Planning.** Planning promotes an organized and efficient effort by everyone involved. All necessary equipment must be assembled ahead of time. Padding, pillows, positioning devices, table accessories, and transfer devices must be on hand before positioning begins. Adequate personnel must be available to complete the task safely.

- **Teamwork.** Teamwork is needed to create smooth, step-by-step coordination. Coordinated activities complement each other.

DUTIES OF THE SURGICAL TECHNOLOGIST

Surgical technologists have specific responsibilities during patient positioning of They must:

- Understand common positions and the surgeries for which these positions are used
- Know ahead of time the position that will be used for each assigned surgical procedure
- Proactively prevent accident and injury during positioning
- Question any aspect of the patient's position that appears to have risk potential
- Remain alert and focused on patient safety
- Communicate clearly with other members of the team.

GENERAL OPERATING TABLE

The general operating table is used for most surgical procedures (Figure 10-6, *A*). It can be configured into many positions and accommodates accessories for different types of surgery (Figure 10-6, *B* to *E*). The frame is stainless steel and attaches to a hydraulic lift. Weight restrictions for operating tables vary. Extremely large or heavy patients require a table that is specifically designed to safely accommodate excess weight and girth.

Table Features

Table pads are covered with washable material. The pads are removable for cleaning. The top of the table can be rotated, flexed, or disassembled. Some table tops are radiolucent to allow intraoperative x-rays. A handheld remote control unit is used to operate the hydraulic components to change the angle and height. The headboard and footboard can be flexed or removed. The base is centered on the frame or may be offset to accommodate radiographic and C-arm fluoroscopy equipment. The kidney rest can be elevated to raise the flank and offer wide exposure. A perineal cutout allows unrestricted access when the patient is in the lithotomy position.

Table Attachments

The standard arm board is used when the patient's arms are outstretched (Figure 10-7, *A*). At least one arm is abducted during surgery to accommodate access to IV and monitoring sites. The arm is secured by means of a padded strap, semirigid brace, or rigid cradle.

The toboggan (Figure 10-7, *B*) (also called a *sled*) is a stainless steel or Plexiglas attachment that slides under the patient and holds the arm at the person's side.

Shoulder braces are fixed to the head of the table to prevent the patient from sliding downward when he or she is in the Trendelenburg position.

Stirrups are used to elevate and abduct the legs for access to the perineal area. The type of stirrups used depends on the

procedure, the surgeon's preference, and the patient's physiological tolerance for the position (see the section on the lithotomy position). Figure 10-9 show three types of low lithotomy stirrups used for endoscopic, gynecological, genitourinary, and obstetrical procedures.

The headrest is attached to the operating table and stabilizes the head and neck during a craniotomy or when the patient is in the Fowler (sitting) position. The horseshoe rest is a padded, U-shaped attachment that supports the forehead when the patient is in the prone position. Other attachments, such as the Gardner and Mayfield headrests, penetrate the skull with sterile pins and hold the head in precise position (see the section on the prone position).

The chest or back brace **is** a padded, elevated frame which elevates the upper thorax. It is used when the patient is in the prone position to create access to the spine and back. Several types of patient braces have been designed to overcome the many risks of prone positioning. Most frames have two raised lateral pieces attached to a base that rests on the operating table. Other styles have lateral crosspieces that extend at right angles to the long axis of the body. All frame styles must be checked carefully to ensure that they fit the patient and do not impinge on nerves and blood vessels.

The footboard attaches at a right angle to the foot of the operating table. It prevents the patient from sliding downward when the table is tilted into a foot-down (reverse Trendelenburg) position.

Padding is used to distribute the weight of the body, especially where vulnerable areas contact the operating table or table pad. Gel, foam, and deflatable "beanbag" pads are available to conform to the patient's anatomy. When these are not available, pillows, towels, and rolled blankets are used. However, the rough surfaces of linen pads can cause patient injury. In an older person who has fragile skin, indentations can lead to skin breakdown and sloughing. Improperly placed padding causes skin and deep tissue injury and creates pressure in areas subject to **compression injury.** Remember that the purpose of padding is weight distribution, not just cushioning.

PATIENT INJURIES AND POSITIONING

Principles of Safe Positioning

Positioning injuries usually are the result of pressure on neurovascular structures. These injuries are related to the failure of a mechanical accessory, inattention to detail, haste in meeting the demands of a full (or unreasonable) schedule, and lack of adequate help. A shortage of personnel must never be allowed to interfere with patient safety.

Injury awareness is the first step in prevention. When workers participate in patient positioning, it is not just desirable but necessary that they have specific knowledge of anatomy, range of motion, risks of pulmonary compromise, and effects of intravascular fluid shifts. Positioning is not a "cookbook" process. Although each position requires the body to assume a certain posture, the positioning team must have specific information about the patient's individual needs and medical condition. This information requires medical

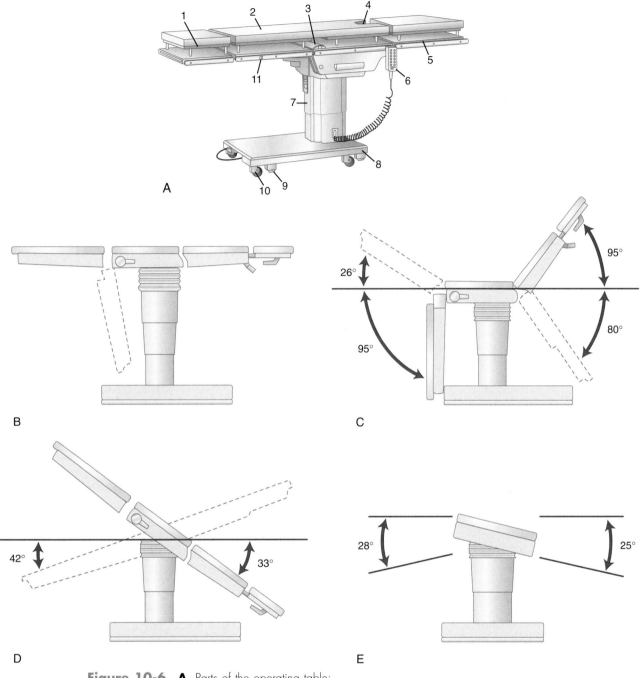

Figure 10-6   A, Parts of the operating table:
1. Removable head section
2. Table pad (mattress)
3. Kidney elevator
4. Perineal cutout
5. Radiolucent top and removable head section
6. Hand control unit
7. Hydraulic lift cylinder
8. Table base
9. Floor locks
10. Locking swivel casters
11. Side rail locking system

B to **E,** Positions of the operating table. *(Modified from Martin JT, Warner MA: Positioning in anesthesia and surgery, ed 3, Philadelphia, 1997, WB Saunders.)*

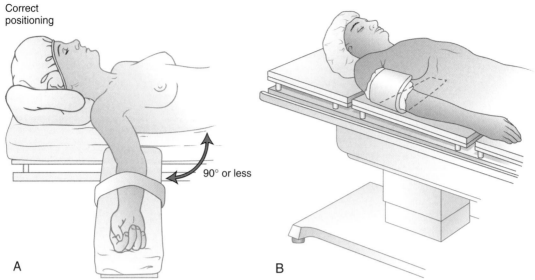

Correct
positioning

90° or less

A

B

Figure 10-7 A, Arm board. **B,** Toboggan arm holder. (**A** *redrawn from Phillips N: Berry and Kohn's operating room technique, ed 10, St Louis, 2004, Mosby;* **B** *redrawn from Martin JT, Warner MA: Positioning in anesthesia and surgery, ed 3, Philadelphia, 1997, WB Saunders.)*

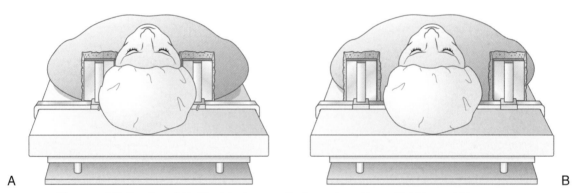

A

B

Figure 10-8 A and **B,** Shoulder braces. *(Redrawn from Martin JT, Warner MA: Positioning in anesthesia and surgery, ed 3, Philadelphia, 1997, WB Saunders.)*

and nursing assessment skills and is provided by the anesthesia care provider, surgeon, and circulator.

The following guidelines apply to all positioning procedures:

- All equipment needed for positioning must be assembled and prepared for use before the patient is brought into the room.
- Adequate personnel must be available to assist before positioning begins. Do not risk the patient's safety because of a crowded surgical schedule.
- Before positioning begins, all team members should be familiar with the position, and each person must understand his or her role in positioning.
- The patient should not be moved except on the instruction of the person directing the move. Everyone must be aware of the motion direction, movement process, and resting point of the body. Positioning is a collaborative task. Although everyone involved is respon-

sible for the patient's safety, one person—usually the surgeon, anesthesia care provider, or surgical assistant—guides and directs the others. This ensures that movements are coordinated which reduces injury to both the patient and team members. In general, the anesthesia care provider must give permission before any change is made in a patient's position because these can cause physiological alteration such as a drop in blood pressure.

- Always check equipment before using it. Tighten the locking devices of all weight-bearing accessories.
- Make sure the table is locked securely in position and do not assume that any accessory equipment is in working order.
- Move slowly when positioning the patient.
- Always move the body within its normal range of motion. This requires knowledge of joint types and anatomy.

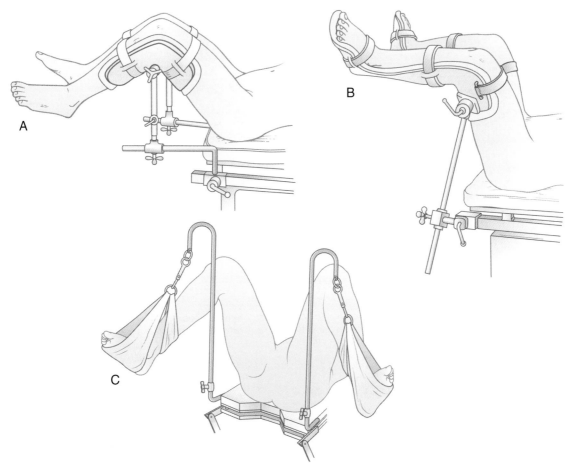

Figure 10-9   A, Crutch stirrups. **B,** Multipurpose stirrups. **C,** Sling stirrups. *(Modified from Phillips N: Berry and Kohn's operating room technique, ed 11, St Louis, 2007, Mosby.)*

- When positioning an unconscious, sedated, or weak patient, make certain that you have complete control of the part you are moving before you begin.
- Before moving the patient, make sure all tubing, leads, and other medical devices are untangled. Move devices first, then the patient.

Nerve and Vascular Injury

Nerves are injured when they lose their blood supply, are stretched, or compressed. During general anesthesia, central nervous system depressants and muscle relaxants are administered, and muscles lose their normal tone. This allows the joints to assume exaggerated positions that the patient normally would not be able to tolerate. **Hyperextension** (greater than normal extension) and **hyperflexion** (greater than normal flexion) can result in a nerve injury called a **traction injury** (or stretching injury).

Continuous pressure on the nerve or its blood supply can cause **necrosis** (tissue death) within 2 hours. Nerve damage can result in loss of mobility or sensation.

Compression of vessels restricts the blood supply to the tissue, a condition called **ischemia.** Loss of oxygen to the tissue causes necrosis. Pressure injuries may not be readily apparent, because underlying tissues, such as muscle and fascia, are more susceptible to damage than skin (Box 10-1).

Box 10-1

Classification of Pressure Damage and Stages of Pressure Ulcers

The National Pressure Ulcer Advisory Panel has developed a ranking system for evaluating the extent of damage caused by pressure. Pressure damage is a risk for surgical patients and for bed-bound, debilitated, and elderly patients.

Stage I: Nonblanchable erythema of intact skin, the heralding lesion of skin ulceration. NOTE: Reactive hyperemia normally can be expected for one half to three fourths as long as the time that pressure occludes blood flow to the area.

Stage II: Partial-thickness skin loss involving the epidermis and/or dermis. A superficial ulcer evolves and develops clinically as an abrasion, a blister, or a shallow crater.

Stage III: Full-thickness skin loss, involving damage to or necrosis of subcutaneous tissue, that may extend down to but not through underlying fascia. The ulcer presents clinically as a deep crater with or without undermining of adjacent tissue.

Stage IV: Full-thickness skin loss with extensive destruction, tissue necrosis, or damage to muscle, bone, or supporting structures (e.g., the tendon of a joint capsule). NOTE: Undermining and sinus tracts also may be associated with stage IV pressure ulcers.

Modified from Martin JT, Warner MA: *Positioning in anesthesia and surgery,* ed 3, Philadelphia, 1997, WB Saunders.

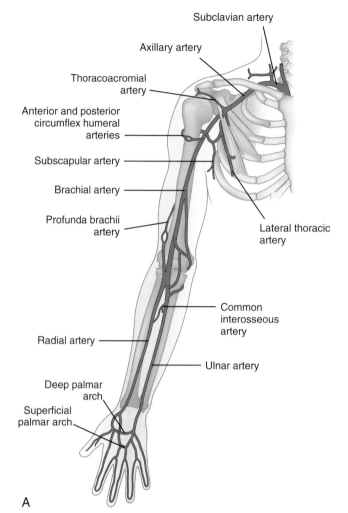

Subclavian artery

Axillary artery

Thoracoacromial
artery

Anterior and posterior
circumflex humeral
arteries

Subscapular artery

Brachial artery

Profunda brachii
artery

Lateral thoracic
artery

Common
interosseous
artery

Radial artery

Ulnar artery

Deep palmar
arch

Superficial
palmar arch

A

Figure 10-10   A, Arteries and nerves of the upper limb (dorsal view).

Ischemia is time and weight related. To prevent ischemia and necrosis, all bony prominences and **dependent areas of the body** (areas of the body under gravitational force) must be adequately padded and the weight distributed over a large area. Figure 10-10 shows the large blood vessels and nerves of the upper and lower limbs.

Locations of Common Nerve and Vessel Injuries

Nerve and vessel injuries often occur at the following locations:

- The ulnar nerve where it passes through the condylar groove of the elbow. Here the nerve is covered only by skin and subcutaneous fat and is subject to compression (pressure) injury when the elbow is tightly flexed or when the nerve is under direct pressure from the edge of the operating table.
- The ulnar nerve where it passes through the condylar groove and then at the cubital tunnel. Injury in this area is the second most common cause of postoperative **neuropathy** (temporary or permanent nerve injury).
- The common peroneal and tibial nerve and vessels where they pass through the popliteal fossa at the back of the knee.

- The brachial plexus, which is a complex anatomical area where the branches of nerve roots from C5 to T1 or T2 merge (Figure 10-11). The brachial plexus is vulnerable to injury because the nerves and blood vessels lie close to bony structures and are subject to direct compression. Injury in this area can be caused by shoulder braces, arm boards, and wrist supports.
- The lumbosacral nerve roots at the base of the spine.

Prevention of Compression Injury

The following guidelines can help prevent compression injury:

- Padding can distribute weight over a larger surface area, or it can impinge on a vulnerable space. Make sure that in preventing one type of injury, you do not cause another. Rolled blankets must be used with caution, because uneven folds in the outer covering may cause skin or compression injury, especially in older or debilitated patients. Axillary rolls must never be placed *in the axilla*, because this increases pressure on the axillary nerve and vessels. The axillary roll actually is positioned slightly inferior to the axilla when the patient is in the lateral position.

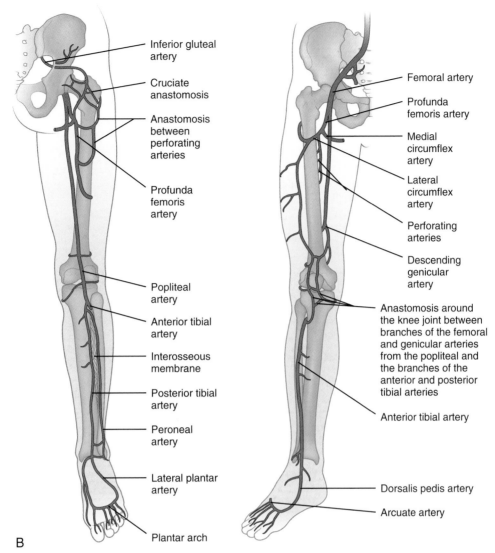

B

Figure 10-10, cont'd   B, Arteries and nerves of the upper limb (ventral view).

Continued

- Pressure on the "downside" shoulder of a patient in the lateral position is removed by shifting the upper arm and shoulder slightly forward and placing a foam or gel pad under the flank area. This prevents retroclavicular compression and nerve injury (Figure 10-12).
- All linens and padding must be smooth. Wrinkles can deform the skin and cause the tissue to break down.
- Arm abduction must be limited to less than 90 degrees or less than the angle the patient can tolerate awake.
- If shoulder braces must be used, they should be liberally padded and positioned at the acromion rather than at the base of the neck or clavicle. Pressure close to the cervical spine can damage peripheral nerves and muscle. When the braces are placed wide apart, pressure over the shoulders can cause enough compression to force the clavicle into the first rib and damage the subclavicular vessels and brachial nerve plexus.
- Keep the cervical spine and head in neutral position.

Shear Injury and Pressure Ulcers

Shear injury is associated with pressure injury. It occurs when two parallel tissue planes are forced in opposite directions. The most common cause of shear injury is sliding the patient across a high-friction surface. Shearing also is associated with particular positions, particularly the Trendelenburg and reverse Trendelenburg positions.

Shearing causes blood clots and tissue death. Tissue damage that begins as a shear injury can easily progress to a pressure ulcer. Pressure ulcers occur in dependent areas of the body. The skin and underlying tissues slough as a result of compression and loss of blood supply. Any pressure on the ulcer causes continued breakdown until the bone is exposed. Exposed tissues become infected and can be very resistant to healing. In extreme cases, skin grafts are required to close the defect. Pressure ulcers are classified by stage and progress rapidly from mild to severe.

Continuous compression or extreme flexion can result in vessel compression and severe swelling below the area of

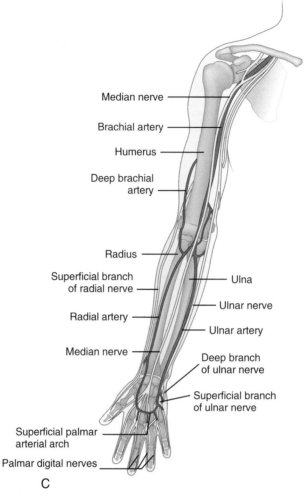

C

Figure 10-10, cont'd C, Arteries of the lower limb.

compression. This is called **compartment syndrome.** In this situation blood cannot return to the heart but pools in the extremity. As the surrounding tissues become more and more swollen, the risk arises of complete loss of blood supply to the whole limb and even distant organs. Treatment of compartment syndrome requires an emergency procedure called a *fasciotomy* to relieve the pressure on deep tissues. In a **fasciotomy,** deep incisions are made in the long axis of the limb to open the tissues and relieve pressure.

Skeletal Injury

Skeletal injury occurs when the joint is manipulated out of a neutral position or is stressed beyond a tolerable load. Sudden dislocation can occur when the limb of a sedated or anesthetized patient is allowed to drop over the table edge. This can happen when positioning is hurried or too few personnel are used to maintain safety during positioning. Skeletal injury also can occur when the patient is not restrained properly. Do not position the patient unless adequate help is available.

Safe joint manipulation requires a knowledge of the joint capacity, including its type and range of motion, and specific knowledge of the patient's condition. To avoid exceeding normal ranges of motion, one must know what those ranges are. Avoid skeletal injury by referring to the range-of-motion illustrations shown in Figure 10-13. Remember that the unconscious body can be manipulated into positions that would not be tolerable to a conscious patient, and this must be avoided.

Determine whether the patient has any skeletal conditions, such as a previous injury, joint implants, or arthritic disease. Remember that every patient is unique.

NORMAL RANGE OF MOTION

The joints of the human body allow a specific type of movement, or **range of motion.** For example, the elbow joint is hinged; that is, it can move freely in only one direction. Its movement is described by the angle created by the upper and lower arm. The movement of this joint is called *extension* or *flexion.* As the elbow is bent closer to the body, the angle becomes smaller. This is called *flexion.* As the arm straightens, the angle becomes wider or larger. This is called *extension.* Some joints, such as the ball-and-socket joint in the hip, allow rotation of a body part inward and outward. Such inward and outward rotation is called *internal* and *external rotation.*

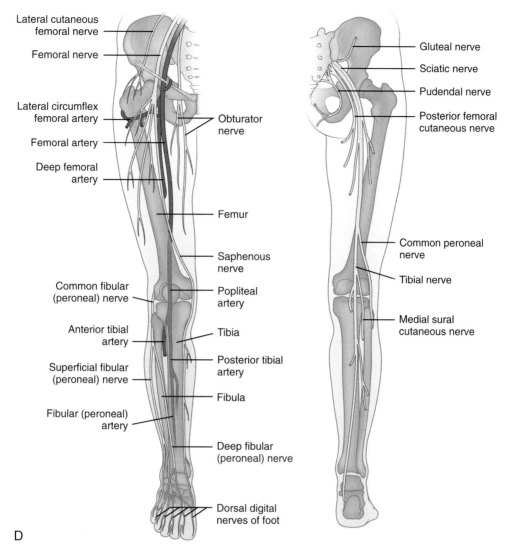

D

Figure 10-10, cont'd D, Nerves and arteries of the lower limb. *(Redrawn from Jacob S: Atlas of human anatomy, St Louis, 2002, Churchill Livingstone.)*

When the patient is positioned, it is critical not to exceed the limits of a joint. Most joint movements are described in degrees of movement. For example, in the positioning of the patient's arm on an arm board, it is critical to restrict **abduction** to less than 90 degrees. This means that the angle between the side of the patient's body and the arm is less than 90 degrees. Figure 10-13 shows directions of motion and the proper terms to describe them.

OTHER INJURIES AND ACCIDENTS

Embolism

A **thromboembolus** (or thrombus) is a blood clot that circulates in the vascular system and lodges in a vessel, causing obstruction or occlusion. Circulating blood normally does not form clots. When blood is allowed to slow or pool, however, as can occur during surgery, clots form in the

lower extremities and migrate through the systemic circulation. A circulating thrombus can lodge anywhere in the body. When it blocks blood supply to the lungs, brain, or heart, these vital tissues are deprived of oxygen and the tissue dies.

Antiembolism stockings or a sequential compression device (SCD) is placed on patients' legs before long procedures or on patients predisposed to clot formation. The SCD wraps around the leg, much like a large blood pressure cuff, and sequentially fills with air and then deflates. During the inflation phase, the cuffs push venous blood toward the heart, and during deflation, the vessels refill. This reduces the risk of blood pooling (stasis) and thrombus formation.

Respiratory Compromise

Positioning can affect the patient's **ventilation** (ability to fill the lungs with air). Patients in the prone position and steep

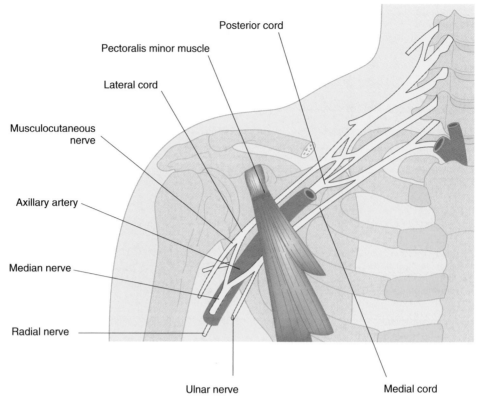

Posterior cord

Pectoralis minor muscle

Lateral cord

Musculocutaneous
nerve

Axillary artery

Median nerve

Radial nerve

Ulnar nerve

Medial cord

Figure 10-11 Brachial plexus. *(From Jacob S: Atlas of human anatomy, St Louis, 2002, Churchill Livingstone.)*

Trendelenburg position are particularly vulnerable to ventilation problems. Both gravity and the position of the chest wall determine the amount of gas that enters the lungs. The prone position must allow expansion of the thorax. Different types of open braces have been developed to raise the thorax from the operating table (see the section on the prone position). This increases ventilatory capacity by taking pressure off the thorax.

Falls

Although patients do not often fall from the operating table, this is a devastating occurrence. Falls can result in major fractures and serious injury to the head and soft tissue. To prevent a patient fall, study and follow these guidelines:

- Never leave a patient unattended, not for any reason or any length of time.
- When transferring the patient between the stretcher and the operating table, lock both the table and the stretcher firmly in place.
- Make sure that at least one person is standing at the receiving side of the operating table or stretcher to prevent the patient from moving too far over the edge.
- Do not position or move the patient without adequate help. Administrative support may be necessary to establish strict safety standards.
- Do not rush while moving an unconscious patient. Likewise, allow a conscious patient to move slowly during any move from one surface to another.

- As soon as the patient has moved to the operating table, secure the safety strap halfway between the knees and hips (as described earlier).
- Position a morbidly obese patient on a specialty table built to hold extreme weight and size. Know the limits of the standard surgical table. A very heavy patient can tilt the tabletop to one side, which may cause the patient to roll off the table and onto the floor.

CONDITIONS THAT INCREASE THE RISK OF INJURY

Physical examinations by the anesthesia care provider and physician reveal pre-existing conditions that affect positioning, including the initial positioning and the repositioning that takes place during the procedure (intraoperatively). Workers assisting in positioning may not be aware of these conditions. Therefore those who have assessed the patient medically must guide the team. Box 10-2 describes physical conditions that affect patient positioning.

SURGICAL POSITIONS

Supine Position

The **supine position,** or dorsal recumbent position, is used for procedures of the abdomen, thorax, and face and in

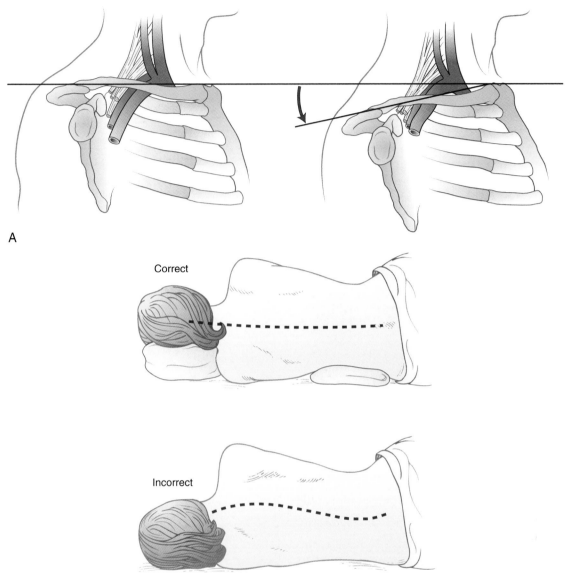

A

Correct

Incorrect

Figure 10-12   A, Potential injury to the retroclavicular space related to compression of the clavicle. **B,** Note the position of the padding to level the spine and prevent compression of the clavicle. (**A** *redrawn from Martin JT, Warner MA: Positioning in anesthesia and surgery, ed 3, Philadelphia, 1997, WB Saunders;* **B** *redrawn from Phillips N: Berry and Kohn's operating room technique, ed 11, St Louis, 2007, Mosby.*)

Box 10-2

Patient Conditions that Influence Positioning

- Pre-existing nerve compression syndrome
- Neuropathy (nerve disorder)
- Diabetes mellitus
- Osteoarthritis (progressive arthritic disease)
- Venous stasis (pooling of blood as a result of inactivity or cardiovascular disease)
- Pre-existing decubitus ulcer (pressure sore)
- Previous traumatic injury
- Alcohol abuse
- Vitamin deficiencies
- Malnutrition
- Renal disease
- Hypothyroidism
- Previous joint fractures
- Rheumatoid arthritis
- Corticosteroid use
- Contractures (scar tissue that restricts joint movement)
- Poor skin turgor (lack of skin and tissue firmness)
- Peripheral edema (intracellular fluid swelling in the legs and arms)
- Reduced range of motion
- Weakness in the extremities

Modified from Martin JT, Warner MA: *Positioning in anesthesia and surgery,* ed 3, Philadelphia, 1997, WB Saunders.

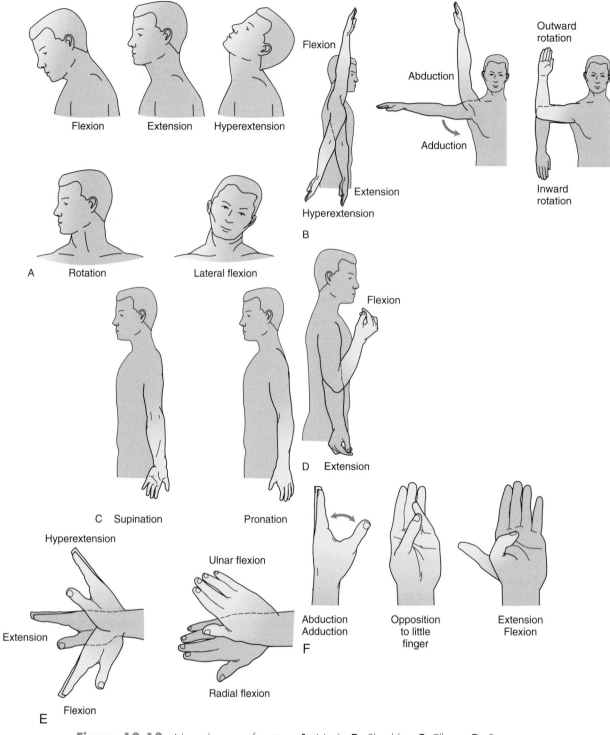

Figure 10-13 Normal range of motion. **A,** Neck. **B,** Shoulder. **C,** Elbow. **D,** Forearm. **E,** Wrist. **F,** Thumb. **G,** Fingers. **H,** Hip. **I,** Knee. **J,** Ankle. **K,** Foot. *(From Sorrentino SA: Mosby's textbook for nursing assistants, ed 7, St Louis, 2008, Mosby.)*

orthopedic and vascular surgery (Figure 10-14). The patient is positioned with the head and spine in alignment. When an arm board or toboggan is not used, the arm is placed in a natural position at the patient's side, and the draw sheet is tucked smoothly underneath. The patient's feet must not extend over the edge of the table, and the legs must not be crossed one over the other.

The patient's weight is distributed over the occipital bone, back, sacrum, heels, and posterior legs. Patients with spinal or pelvic malformation or total joint prostheses may require special padding to support irregular curvatures and prevent hyperextension. A foam or gel pad is used to support the head. The safety strap is placed midway between the knees and thighs.

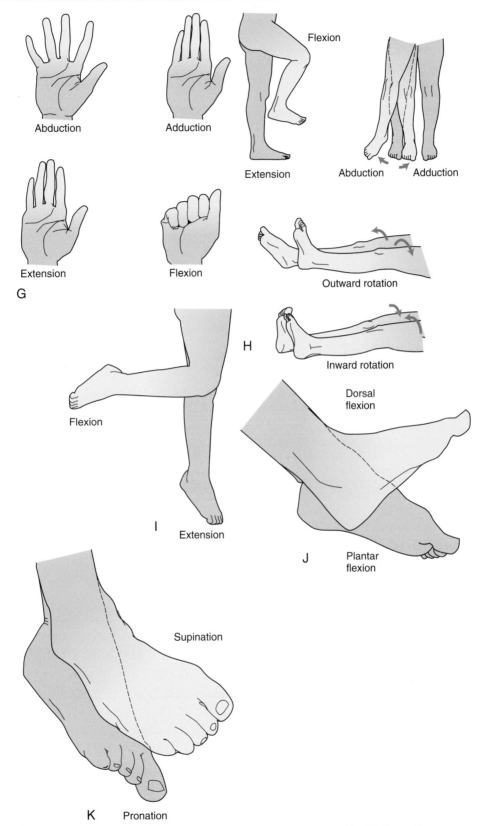

Figure 10-13, cont'd G, Fingers. **H,** Hip. **I,** Knee. **J,** Ankle. **K,** Foot. *(From Sorrentino SA: Mosby's textbook for nursing assistants, ed 7, St Louis, 2008, Mosby.)*

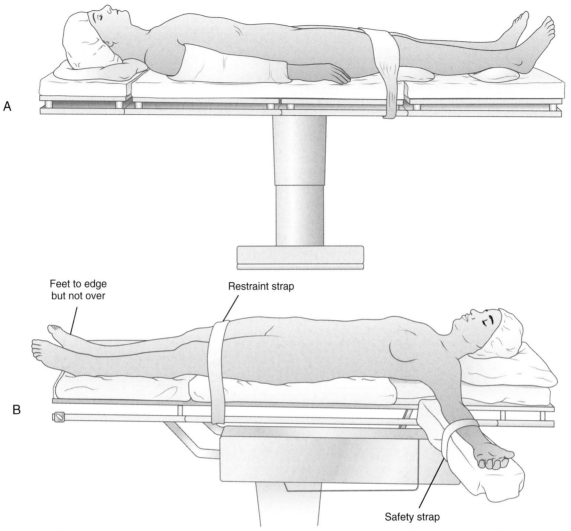

Figure 10-14 Supine position. **A,** With the arms tucked. **B,** With the arms positioned on arm boards and the safety strap applied. (**A** redrawn from Phillips N: Berry and Kohn's operating room technique, ed 11, St Louis, 2007, Mosby; **B** from original artwork by Sandra McMahon.)

Labels on figure: Feet to edge but not over; Restraint strap; Safety strap

Safety Precautions

1. Keep the cervical spine and head in neutral alignment.
2. Distribute weight evenly over the ulnar nerve area; remember that padding may not be sufficient to prevent nerve damage and may even compress the nerve and cause injury.
3. Protect the brachial plexus. Arm boards must not be abducted more than 90 degrees.
4. Prevent decubitus ulcer formation at the lumbosacral area in elderly or debilitated patients. Place a soft, pliable surface under this dependent area.
5. Protect the popliteal fossa from impingement. Do not place pillows directly under the knee joint. Pillows or rolls are placed just proximal to this area. Distribute weight over the area.
6. Separate the patient's feet so that they do not touch each other. Padding under the heels may be advised.
7. Avoid the use of knee crutches (leg holders) during extended orthopedic surgery. Compartment syndrome and severe vascular damage can result.

8. Place an SCD or antiembolism stockings on the patient's legs to prevent an **embolism.**
9. Make sure the patient's legs are not crossed, as this puts pressure on the peroneal nerve and blood vessels of the posterior leg.

Trendelenburg Position

The **Trendelenburg position** is a variation of the supine position in which the operating table is tilted head down (Figure 10-15). This position permits greater access to the lower abdominal cavity and pelvic structures by allowing gravity to retract organs such as the small intestine, proximal large bowel, and omentum toward the head. The position is commonly used during lower gastrointestinal surgery and pelvic surgery. It can cause hypertension, respiratory restriction, and increased intracranial pressure.

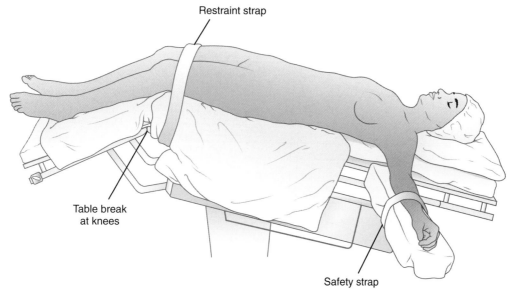

Figure 10-15 Trendelenburg position. *(From original artwork by Sandra McMahon.)*

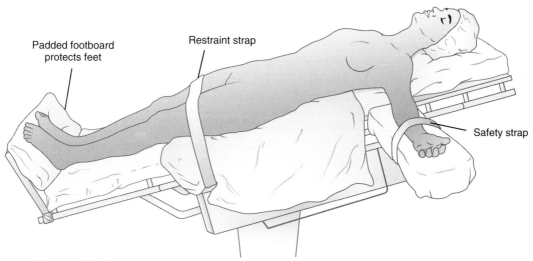

Figure 10-16 Reverse Trendelenburg position. *(From original artwork by Sandra McMahon.)*

Safety Precautions

1. Distribute the weight of the elbow and upper arm evenly in the area of the ulnar nerve.
2. Protect the brachial plexus. Arm boards must not be abducted more than 90 degrees.
3. Keep the Mayo stand from coming into contact with the patient's body if it is positioned over the patient's legs during surgery. If the patient's position is altered in any way, always check the Mayo stand to make sure it is not touching the patient.
4. Anticipate the onset of severe hypertension or respiratory depression during intraoperative positioning from level supine to Trendelenburg position. Surgery may be halted until the patient's condition is stabilized.

5. When the patient is returned to the supine position from the Trendelenburg position after surgery, move the patient very slowly, because returning the patient to the supine position too quickly may result in hypotension.

Reverse Trendelenburg Position

The **reverse Trendelenburg position,** or foot-down position (Figure 10-16), is used when the surgeon requires unobstructed access to the upper peritoneal cavity and lower esophagus. When the operating table is tilted toward the patient's feet, gravity drops the viscera into the lower cavity, which allows a clear view of the diaphragm, cardiac sphincter, and esophagus.

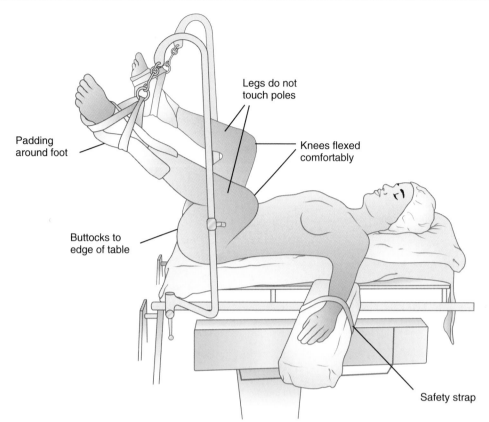

Legs do not
touch poles

Knees flexed
comfortably

Padding
around foot

Buttocks to
edge of table

Safety strap

Figure 10-17 Lithotomy position using sling stirrups. *(From original artwork by Sandra McMahon.)*

During intraoperative positioning to the reverse Trendelenburg position, all instruments lying on the surgical field must be secured by a magnetic pad or pocket holders. Special care must be taken to ensure that endoscopes and all accessories are removed to prevent them from sliding to the floor. All tubing should be well secured at the beginning of surgery. The Mayo stand may be moved to accommodate the shift in the patient's position.

Safety Precautions
1. Follow all safety precautions applicable to the supine position.
2. Prevent the patient's body from sliding toward the floor, which can cause a shear injury. Use a footboard if necessary, but use soft padding or protective foam boots to prevent nerve and vascular compression.
3. Make sure that the weight of each leg is distributed over a wide area at the popliteal fossa if the patient will be placed in reverse the Trendelenburg–lithotomy position. Do not rely on padding alone to protect the patient from compartment syndrome or nerve or vessel damage. Use of a low conforming stirrup with moldable gel or foam inserts helps prevent impingement on the back of the knee.

Lithotomy Position
The **lithotomy position** is a variation of the supine position. The patient's thighs are abducted, and both the knees and hips are flexed. The feet are suspended in stirrups, or the legs rest on low leg braces. The lithotomy position is used for gynecological, obstetrical, and genitourinary procedures (Figure 10-17). Incorrectly implemented, lithotomy position can cause severe tissue injury; therefore it is critical that protocol be followed. Attention to pressure points is very important. Patients with limited range of motion in the hip, spine, or knee joints are at particular risk. Respect the patient's dignity by placing a cover sheet over the perineum during positioning.

Safety Precautions
1. Before anesthesia induction, the patient receiving a general anesthetic is positioned with the sacrum at the lower **table break.** An extension (or the head portion of the operating table) is fitted to the lower end of the table to support the patient's legs. The offside stirrup or leg brace is secured to the table. The remaining stirrup is attached after the patient is moved to the operating table. Both legs must be elevated simultaneously by two people.
2. When the patient is unconscious and sufficiently relaxed, the anesthesia care provider announces when it is safe to elevate the legs. The lower portion of the table is flexed downward, or the end section is removed.
3. Raising both legs at the same time keeps the body in alignment and prevents twisting of the lumbar spine.
4. If the patient's arms are tucked at the sides, care must be taken to ensure that the patient's fingers do not become impinged as the lower table portion is flexed or raised.

5. When the legs are placed in stirrups, the knees must be flexed first, keeping them in midline position; then the thighs are abducted while the knees are kept flexed after the anesthesidogist gives permission.

6. The femoral vessels are at risk of compression during lithotomy when the angle of hip flexion is severe. (When femoral vessels are compressed, blood supply to the lower legs and abdominal viscera can be reduced significantly.)

7. Sudden shifts in blood pressure and spinal injury can occur as the legs are positioned in, or removed from, stirrups. To prevent this, the maneuver must be performed very slowly.

8. When attaching the stirrups and securing the patient's position, make sure the locking device is tight and that no portion of the patient's legs rests against the vertical extensions (Figure 10-18).

9. Protect the peroneal nerve when stirrups are used. Do not place the stirrup sling directly over the Achilles tendon. Distribute the weight of the leg between both slings on the stirrup.

10. Two people are required to lower the legs after surgery. Release the feet from the stirrups or leg rests, slowly bring the knees together on the midline, and gradually extend the hips and knees. Coordination between the two people lowering the legs prevents lumbar torsion.

11. Slow manipulation is necessary to allow blood to flow back into the limbs gradually. If the legs are lowered too quickly, a sudden shift of blood to the lower extremities and a sudden drop in blood pressure can occur.

Low Lithotomy Position

Low lithotomy position is maintained by stirrups or knee crutches that allow the surgeon access to the perineum and pelvic structures. Many endoscopic abdominal surgeries also require low lithotomy position.

A cystoscopy or urology table is used during endoscopic procedures involving the genitourinary tract (Figure 10-19). The patient is positioned in the low lithotomy position. Because copious amounts of fluid are used during urological procedures, the table contains a drain path that exits the end of the table and passes directly into the floor drainage system. The table also is constructed to accommodate video and fluoroscopy imaging processes. Patients often are awake during positioning for urological procedures.

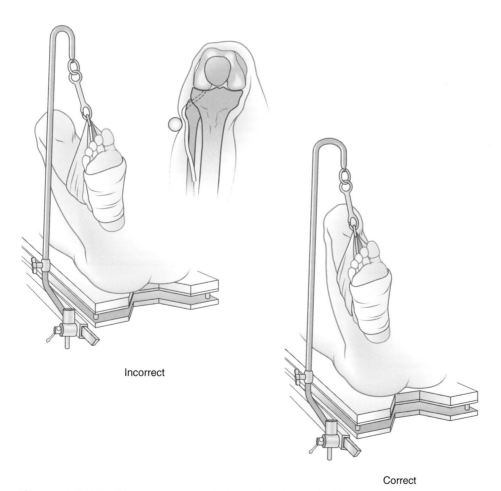

Incorrect

Correct

Figure 10-18 Lithotomy injuries. *(Redrawn from Martin JT, Warner MA: Positioning in anesthesia and surgery, ed 3, Philadelphia, 1997, WB Saunders.)*

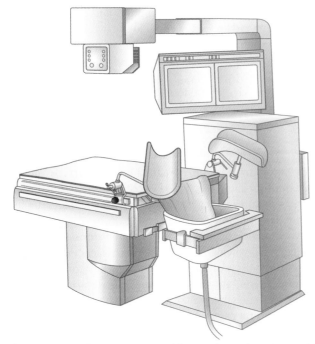

Figure 10-19 Cystoscopy table. *(Redrawn from Martin JT, Warner MA: Positioning in anesthesia and surgery, ed 3, Philadelphia, 1997, WB Saunders.)*

Safety Precautions

1. Follow all precautions described for the standard lithotomy position.
2. Using knee rests in the low lithotomy position can risk compartment syndrome of the lower leg because the popliteal artery and vein lie close to the surface and rest directly on the table attachments. The angle of the knee and distribution of weight in the popliteal fossa must be carefully planned.
3. The patient's arms must be maintained on arm boards, with precautions taken to protect the ulnar nerve and cubital tunnel. If the patient receives only a local anesthetic, the arms can be placed on the patient's abdomen.

Positioning on the Orthopedic Table

The orthopedic or fracture table allows the patient to be positioned for hip and other orthopedic procedures of the lower extremities. The orthopedic table or fracture table allows circumferential access to the patient's leg while producing horizontal traction during surgery (Figure 10-20). The patient rests with the injured leg restrained in a bootlike device. The leg may be rotated, pulled into traction, or released as the surgery requires. The unaffected leg rests on an elevated leg holder. The open structure of the table allows intraoperative fluoroscopy and radiography.

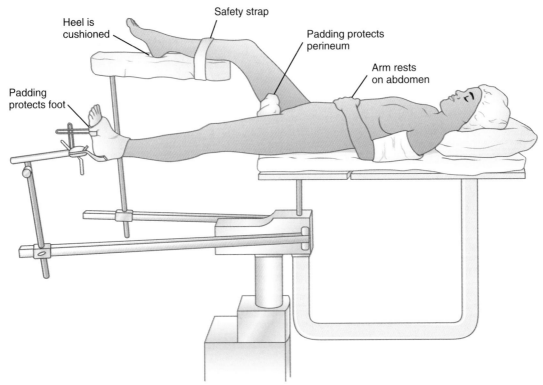

Figure 10-20 Patient positioned on an orthopedic table. An arm board and padding accessories are used to protect nerves and blood vessels. *(From original artwork by Sandra McMahon.)*

Many different types of attachments are available, depending on the complexity and needs of the surgery. At least four people are required to position the patient on the orthopedic table.

Safety Guidelines

1. When moving the patient from the stretcher to the orthopedic table, maintain the spine and head in neutral position at all times.
2. The center post of the orthopedic table must be removed before the patient is moved. The post is repositioned, and the patient's genitalia are protected with padding during positioning.
3. Pressure points on the sacrum, heels, and unaffected lower leg must be adequately padded, and weight must be distributed. The extended leg is held by a boot or a combination of boot and straps.
4. The perineal area and genital structures must not rest against the center post.
5. Traction on the affected leg is adjusted by the surgeon who directs the positioning team.
6. Because of its design, this table is used for patients with fractures of the hip. Moving and transfer of the injured patient must be carried out slowly and carefully to prevent further injury.

Sitting (Fowler) Position

The sitting position, or **Fowler position,** occasionally is used for facial, cranial, or reconstructive breast surgery (Figure 10-21). Use of the position requires experienced personnel who are familiar with the protocol and who practice it frequently enough to prevent accidents. When this position is used, the general operating table is flexed to allow a Fowler position or **semi-Fowler position.** The head may be secured by a craniotomy headrest or stabilized with a doughnut-shaped gel or foam pad.

Lateral (Sims) Position

The **lateral (Sims) position** is used for procedures involving the renal system and for cardiothoracic surgery (Figure 10-22). When the lateral position is described, the side named is the side lying on the table. For example, in the left lateral position, the left side lies on the table. The opposite side is the operative or "up" side.

When general anesthesia is used, the patient is anesthetized in the supine position and maneuvered into the lateral position after intubation. At least four people are needed for this maneuver (Figure 10-23).

1. Abduct the down-side arm so that it does not become compressed under the trunk. To put the patient in a left lateral position, the assistants stand at the patient's right.
2. The assistant at the hips places his or her right hand under the pelvis and the left hand on the iliac crest. At the same time, the assistant at the shoulders reaches around the back of the patient's neck (never around the front, because this would compress the patient's airway) and grasps the patient's shoulder.

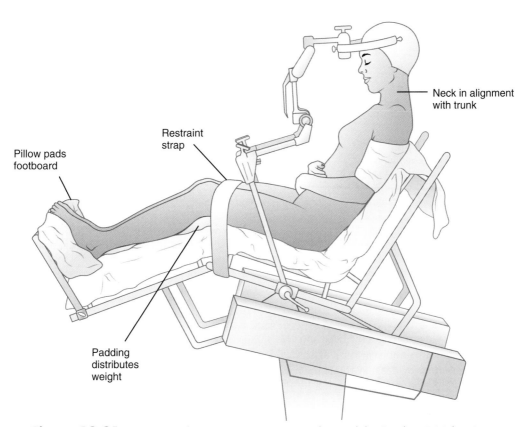

Pillow pads footboard

Restraint strap

Padding distributes weight

Neck in alignment with trunk

Figure 10-21 Sitting (Fowler) position. *(From original artwork by Sandra McMahon.)*

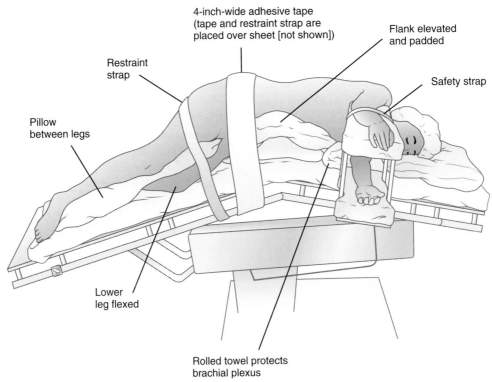

Figure 10-22 Lateral (Sims) position. *(From original artwork by Sandra McMahon.)*

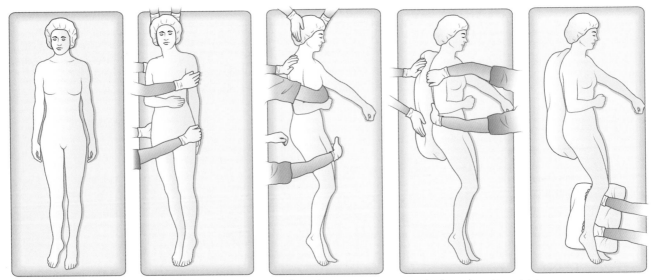

Figure 10-23 Turning the patient from the supine position to the lateral position. Note the correct placement of staff members to protect the joints from injury during the transfer.

3. The anesthesia care provider manages the head and cervical spine. If the patient does not have a risk of cervical injury, the anesthesia care provider may rotate the head in advance of the body. The move is directed by the anesthesia care provider.

4. At the count of three, the assistants simultaneously pull the down-side hip and shoulder while pushing the up-side hip and shoulder. This effectively turns the patient while maintaining alignment.

5. Flex the lower leg and place padding between the legs. The upper leg remains extended.

6. Protect the brachial plexus with padding. The arms may be extended on double arm boards, or the down-side arm, which is the most vulnerable, may be placed in

front of the body. An overhead arm sling also may be used.

7. In addition, use flank padding and a head stabilizer.

Use of the flexed lateral position may require stabilization of the hips and/or shoulders with wide tape. The tape is placed on top of the top sheet, not on the patient's skin. It is secured to the table frame on both sides and passes over the pelvic rim or the shoulder. The tape is meant to stabilize, not to secure the patient's entire weight. Excess compression by the tape can cause tissue damage. The safety strap is placed midway between the thighs and knees. Flexing the middle table break widens the operative exposure. The kidney elevator, located under the table pad, is used to lift the flank region but must be used with caution. It can cause excessive pressure on the deep blood vessels of the abdomen, and its use may result in vascular injury or hypotension.

Safety Precautions

1. During the move from supine to lateral position, the patient's shoulders and pelvis must be moved in the same plane without any torsion.
2. The anesthetized patient must be moved as one unit; that is, the head, neck, spine, pelvis, and legs all must be moved together to prevent twisting injury to joints.
3. The down side of the face should rest on an open horseshoe pad or pillow to protect the facial nerves, ear, and eye from compression.
4. When the patient is turned from supine to lateral, the head and neck must be kept in alignment at all times.
5. The patient's arms should be protected by extending them on double arm boards or positioning them with the up-side arm flexed at an angle of 90 degrees or less and the down-side arm lying close to the torso. The down-side arm can be flexed (no more than 90 degrees). The weight of the upper torso must be distributed evenly with padding.
6. When the patient is in a flexed lateral position, the angle of flexion and padding must be meticulously checked to avoid pressure damage to vessels and nerves in the flank.
7. Padding always should be placed between the legs so that it extends the full length of the leg. The up-side ankle must not rest directly on the down-side leg.

Prone Position

A number of variations of the **prone position** are used to allow access to the spine, cranium, and perianal region. This position can compromise physiological and structural mechanisms in the body, and its use requires extreme caution. The pressure exerted on the abdomen restricts normal ventilation, and the cervical spine may be forced into a position that would be intolerable to the patient if the person were conscious. There is risk to the nerves, eyes, genitalia, breasts, and spine. In the prone position, the patient's upper body rests on a raised padded frame or elongated pads placed on each side of the patient's thorax.

When a patient is to be placed in the prone position, the person is anesthetized in the supine position on the stretcher. After intubation the patient is repositioned on the operating table into the prone position. Four to six people are required to turn the patient. If the patient is turned on the operating table (Figure 10-24), two people lift and pull the patient close to them and then slowly rotate the body onto the arms of the other two helpers. The spine is maintained in alignment, and the head is controlled by the anesthesia care provider. The female patient's breasts should be placed between the chest rests (Figure 10-25). Check that the breasts are free of any unnecessary pressure from the chest rests. If the patient is a male, the genitalia must be assessed for pressure that could cause injury.

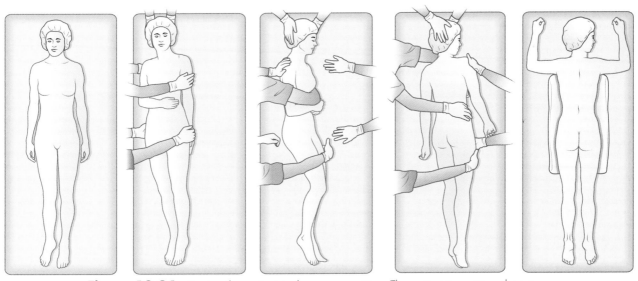

Figure 10-24 Turning the patient to the prone position. The patient is positioned on a padded mold for respiratory clearance.

To turn the patient into the prone position (pronation), follow these steps:

1. Align the stretcher with the operating table.
2. If the patient is to be catheterized, perform catheterization before turning the patient.
3. When the anesthesia care provider is ready, he or she will temporarily disconnect the patient's ventilation circuit.
4. Two people positioned on the receiving side of the table reach across, while those on the other side slowly lift and rotate the patient's body onto the arms of the receiving personnel. The head is controlled by the anesthesia care provider and the feet by another helper.
5. The patient's shoulders are anatomically rotated and placed on arm boards.
6. Reconnect the airway, and make adjustments in the position.
7. Place the arms on arm boards with the elbows flexed.

A laminectomy brace is used to elevate the trunk and allow expansion of the lungs during spinal or back surgery. The patient is turned from the stretcher directly onto the padded lift or brace (Figure 10-26).

Surgery of the posterior spine or cranium often is performed with the patient in prone position and the head supported by a headrest. The head is secured by sterile tongs that attach to the head brace (Figure 10-27).

Jackknife (Kraske) Position

The **jackknife (Kraske) position** is a modification of the prone position (Figure 10-28). The lower table break is flexed downward to achieve a simultaneous head-down and foot-down posture. This position may be used for anorectal surgery. The lower legs are elevated and rest on pads to distribute the weight.

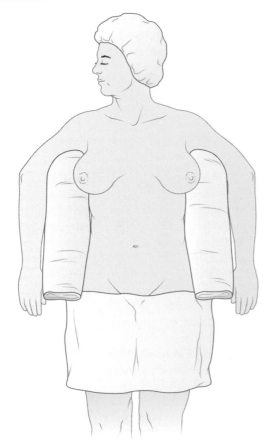

Figure 10-25 Correct position of the breasts in the prone position (as seen from below).

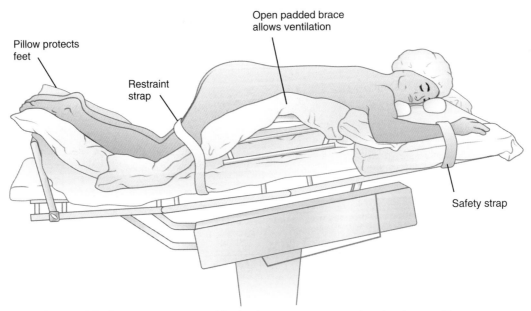

Open padded brace allows ventilation

Pillow protects feet

Restraint strap

Safety strap

Figure 10-26 Patient positioned for back surgery on a raised pad or brace. *(From original artwork by Sandra McMahon.)*

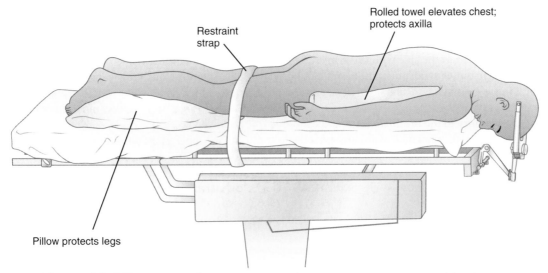

Figure 10-27 Positioning for a craniotomy in the prone position using a rigid head stabilizer. *(From original artwork by Sandra McMahon.)*

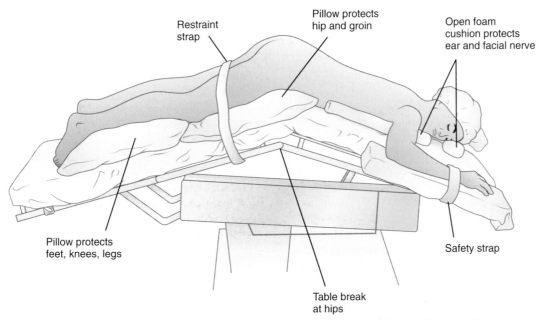

Figure 10-28 Jackknife (Kraske) position. *(From original artwork by Sandra McMahon.)*

Safety Precautions

1. The spine must be kept in a neutral position at all times during positioning.
2. There must be sufficient clearance to allow deep lung inflation. When a brace is used, the two sides of the brace should not impinge on the abdomen.
3. Corneal abrasion can result from compression on the globe of the eye and can cause blindness. This can be prevented through the use of a hollow headrest.
4. A female patient's breasts must be protected. A patient with heavy breasts is likely to be unstable on the operating table because of the lack of firm support in the upper thorax.
5. Forcing the breasts laterally during positioning can cause bleeding and tearing of deep tissue at the breast margins.
6. Particular care must be given to positioning patients who have had a mastectomy or radiation treatment to the chest wall, because the skin and underlying tissues are tender and may be painful.
7. The male genitalia must be protected from compression. When a brace is used, the genitalia must be clear of any part of the frame. Pads placed across the thighs must not entrap the scrotum and penis.

8. If the patient has an intestinal stoma, this area must be completely free of contact with the brace or padding.
9. Pressure on the subclavian artery and brachial plexus when the head is turned to the side with the arms raised can lead to **thoracic outlet syndrome.** The result can be permanent injury, causing pain and loss of sensation along the ulnar nerve.
10. The risk of severe injury to the brachial plexus and cervical spine arises when the patient's arms are extended above the head. To prevent brachial plexus injury, the upper arms should be placed at an angle of 90 degrees or less to the trunk with the forearms parallel to the trunk.
11. When the patient's head is rotated to the side, the risk of a traction and compression injury to the brachial plexus is increased. Many patients cannot tolerate this degree of cervical rotation. Preoperative evaluation must include an assessment of this area to prevent temporary or permanent injury.
12. A wide area around the ulnar nerve must be amply padded.
13. In the knee-chest position, ventilation is a primary concern. Lateral padding of the chest is required in this position, even during short procedures performed with the patient under local anesthesia.

CHAPTER SUMMARY

- Whenever patients are transported or transferred, a risk of injury exists. Health care personnel are required to understand and practice safe moving techniques to prevent injury to their patients and themselves.
- Most injuries occur because of insufficient training in patient handling, insufficient help, and pressure to accomplish tasks quickly.
- Certain patients are at particular risk during handling. Sedated, weak, anxious, and resistant patients may be difficult to balance and guide during moving and handling.
- The conscious patient must always be alerted before any moving or handling begins. Communication during movement is equally important.
- The foundation of safe moving and handling is establishing a wide base of support and maintaining it throughout the move. Accidents occur when balance is shifted to an unstable base.
- When moving patients who have attached monitoring or medical devices, move the equipment first, then the patient.
- Use common sense when moving and handling patients. If it feels unsafe, it probably is.
- Never abandon a patient during transportation—not for any reason or for any length of time.
- The surgical patient is positioned in a specific way to provide the best exposure to the surgical site while maintaining safety.
- The anesthesia care provider or surgeon directs the team during patient positioning.
- Positioning is performed by trained personnel only.
- The greatest risks to patient safety during positioning are dislocation or avulsion of a limb and falls.
- Transferal of an unconscious patient requires at least four people and a transfer board or other device so that the patient is not dragged across the bed or stretcher.
- During positioning, vulnerable nerves and blood vessels are protected from injury.
- Spinal alignment and movement of joints within anatomically correct range are of primary importance during positioning.
- The patient's airway and ventilatory function are preserved throughout the positioning process.
- Nerve damage resulting from improper positioning can cause permanent paralysis. Damage to blood vessels can cause ischemia and tissue death.
- The supine position is used for procedures of the abdomen, limbs, face, neck, and thorax. The supine position also is used for vascular, ear, and eye surgery.
- A modified sitting position is used for breast reconstruction and plastic surgery of the face.
- The lithotomy position provides access to the perineum for gynecological and genitourinary surgery.
- The lateral position is used for procedures of the thorax and renal structures.
- The prone position and its modifications are used for back surgery and rectal procedures. Some craniotomy procedures are also performed with the patient in the prone position and the head fixed in a brace or headrest.

REVIEW QUESTIONS

1. What is a shear injury?
2. How can you best protect yourself from injury if a patient you are escorting begins to fall and leans into you?
3. Describe the proper method for identifying a patient.
4. What are the exact anatomical risks when moving a patient from a stretcher into prone position?
5. What are the anatomical risks in the lithotomy position?
6. Why is a sequential compression device used on patients during surgery?
7. What is *respiratory compromise*?
8. Why are patients more prone to skeletal injury when under general anesthesia or unconscious sedation?
9. What is *thoracic outlet syndrom*?
10. What are the physiological risks of Trendelenburg position?

CASE STUDIES

Case 1

You are asked to bring a patient from the medical unit to surgery. When you arrive on the unit, the patient is not in his room or in the hallway. What will you do?

Case 2

You are transporting a patient from the medical unit to the operating room. You discover that the patient elevator is out of order. What will you do?

Case 3

While turning the patient into the lateral position, you suddenly realize the patient is falling off the table in your direction. What will you do? What precautions can be taken to prevent falls?

Case 4

You are assigned to act as circulator in a procedure in which the patient is placed in the lithotomy position. The patient emerges quickly from anesthesia, and she begins to struggle. Her legs are still elevated in stirrups. What are the risks to the patient in this situation? What will you do?

Case 5

You are scrubbed on a laparotomy case. A number of medical students have been brought in to observe. One of the medical students is scrubbed and is holding a retractor. You notice the student has placed his elbow on the patient's shoulder, and he is resting his weight on the patient. The surgeon has said nothing. What will you do?

BIBLIOGRAPHY

Association of Surgical Technologists (AST): Aseptic technique in *Standards of Practice*, available at http://www.ast.org/educators/ standards_table_of_contents.aspx. Accessed March 19, 2009.

Porth C: *Pathophysiology: concepts of altered health states,* ed 6, Philadelphia, 2002, Lippincott & Williams.

CHAPTER 11

Surgical Skin Preparation and Draping

CHAPTER OUTLINE

LEARNING OBJECTIVES

After studying this chapter the reader will be able to:
- Describe urinary catheterization and the rationale for the method used
- Explain the risks of urinary catheterization
- List the characteristics of common surgical prep solutions

- Describe the fundamental steps in a surgical skin prep
- Explain the rationale for the surgical skin prep
- Identify necessary precautions to prevent injury associated with the skin prep
- Describe the protocols for hair removal

TERMINOLOGY

Antiseptics: Chemical agents approved for use on the skin that inhibit the growth and reproduction of microorganisms.

Autograft: A tissue graft taken from the patient. Autograft sites are usually prepped at the same time as the primary operative site.

Barrier drape: A drape intended to separate a contaminated area from the incision site. For example, a barrier drape is placed across the perineum between the vagina and anus during gynecological procedures.

Debridement: The removal of devitalized tissue, debris, and foreign objects from a wound. Debridement is performed on trauma injuries, burns, and infected wounds either before surgery or as part of the surgical procedure.

Decompression: The removal of air or fluid from an organ.

Desiccation: Tissue drying. Alcohol is a desiccating skin prep solution. It destroys tissue protein and therefore is never used around the eyes or on mucous membranes.

Drapes: Sterile materials, including towels and sheets, that are placed around the prepared incision site to create a sterile field.

Fenestrated drape: A sterile body sheet with a hole or "window" (**fenestration**) that exposes the incision site. The fenestrated drape is positioned after other drapes and towels have been placed in keeping with the procedure. Fenestrated drapes are differentiated by type (e.g., laparotomy, thyroid, kidney, eye, ear, and extremity drapes).

Half sheet: Also called a body sheet, a large rectangular drape used to increase the size of the surgical site. It has many general uses whenever a plain, sterile sheet is required.

Head drape: A turban-style drape created with two surgical towels that covers the patient's head and eyes. The ability to prepare and place this drape is a valuable draping skill.

Impervious: Waterproof.

Incise drape: A plastic, self-adhesive drape that is positioned over the incision site after the surgical skin prep. The incise drape creates a sterile surface over the skin. The incision is made directly through the incise drape and skin.

Prep: The use of antiseptic solutions to clean the skin, reduce the microbial count, and prevent unnecessary contamination of an area for a sterile invasive procedure (e.g., skin incision) or a sterile noninvasive procedure (e.g., urinary catheterization).

Residual activity: The "–cidal" activity of an antiseptic or a disinfectant that continues after the solution has dried.

Retention catheter: A urinary catheter with an inflatable balloon that is used to drain the bladder continuously during surgery. It is inserted before the surgical skin prep. Also called an *indwelling* or a *Foley catheter*.

Single stage prep: Also called a "paint prep." The skin prep is performed using only antiseptic solution which is painted on the skin at the operative site.

Sterile field: An area that includes the draped patient, all sterile tables, and sterile equipment in the immediate area of the patient. The patient is considered the center of the sterile field.

Straight catheter: A urinary nonretaining catheter used to drain the bladder.

Surgical site infection (SSI): Postoperative infection of the surgical wound, most commonly caused by the normal bacteria found on the patient's skin or shed from the skin or hair of members of the surgical team.

Top drape: The uppermost drape in a layered draping routine. This may also be referred to as a **procedure drape**, because the design

of the drape, size, and orientation of the fenestration are specific to certain procedures such as thoracotomy, or laparotomy.

Towel drape: Small sterile towel, the approximate size of a hand towel. These have many uses in surgery. The surgical towel is used to enclose or frame the incision site. A "sticky" towel drape is a proprietary item which is made of plastic and has one self adherent edge. These can be used in place of a sterile towel for draping the wound site, especially around the face or ear.

Two-stage skin prep: Surgical skin prep which includes a scrub prep and application of antiseptic solution to the surgical site.

INTRODUCTION

Bacteria colonize all layers of the skin, including its appendages (i.e., sweat and sebaceous glands and hair follicles). Before surgery the skin must be cleansed with an antiseptic solution to reduce the number of transient and normal microorganisms to an absolute minimum. After skin **prep**, the patient is covered with sterile **drapes** that expose only the surgical site and create the center of the **sterile field**. Skin prep begins before the patient arrives in surgery. At least 1 day before surgery, the patient may be required to bathe with antiseptic soap. This allows thorough cleaning of the hair and skin.

The day of surgery, the patient is brought into the holding area and admitted to the department. (The procedure for ensuring that all preoperative orders have been completed is explained in Chapter 15.) The patient usually is required to wear clean hospital attire, which contributes to overall asepsis. Outpatients preparing for superficial procedures may have fewer restrictions. When admission is completed, the patient is brought to the surgical suite and transferred to the operating bed. Anesthesia preps are begun, and if general anesthesia is planned, the patient is induced and intubated. At this stage the patient is ready for skin prep and draping, which take place immediately before the start of surgery.

URINARY CATHETERIZATION

DESCRIPTION

Urinary catheterization is performed before surgery to empty the bladder and provide continuous urinary drainage throughout the procedure. This is necessary for certain procedures and circumstances:

- Continuous drainage prevents distension of the bladder during lengthy procedures.
- Surgery of the lower abdominal and pelvic cavity requires **decompression** (collapse) of the bladder to protect it from injury during procedures.
- Catheterization allows easy measurement of urine and thus assessment of renal output.

The most common method of continuous drainage is a Foley urinary catheter (Figure 11-1, *A*). This is a **retention catheter**, which has a small inflatable balloon at the tip. After the cath-

eter is inserted into the bladder, the balloon is inflated to keep the catheter in place. A **straight catheter** is used when continuous urinary drainage is unnecessary (Figure 11-1, *B*). Catheterization often is performed immediately before the surgical skin prep.

SUPPLIES

Prepackaged sterile catheter kits contain most of the supplies needed for catheterization. The correct catheter is selected based on assessment of the patient's age, size, and gender. A size 14 to 16 French (Fr) Foley catheter generally is appropriate for a female patient; males usually require a 16 or 18 Fr catheter. Pediatric patients require considerably smaller sizes, and this should be assessed by qualified personnel. The patient's allergy status must be verified before catheterization, because latex allergy is a risk of this procedure.

The standard catheter balloon inflates to 10 mL. When the catheter is in place, a Luer-Lock syringe is used to fill the balloon with 10 mL of sterile water. A valve prevents backflow and deflation of the balloon. The distal tip of the catheter is connected directly to the drainage tube, or a plastic connector is used. This tube is fitted to the drainage bag, which has

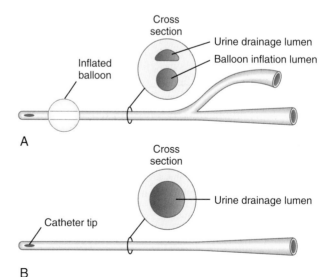

Figure 11-1 A, Foley catheter with balloon tip. **B,** Straight catheter.

graduated markers for measuring the amount of urine. After the catheter has been inserted and connected to the drainage device, the collection unit must not be raised above the level of the patient, because this would cause urine to drain back into the bladder.

The supplies for catheterization must be gathered, checked, and opened before the patient is positioned. A small catheterization table is prepared and moved into place immediately before the procedure.

The following supplies are needed for catheterization:
- Containers for the antiseptic or saline
- A Foley catheter
- Gauze prep sponges
- Antiseptic solution
- Sterile lubricant
- Sterile gloves
- A 10-mL syringe prefilled with water
- A perineal drape
- Forceps
- Cotton balls
- Drainage tubing and a urine collection unit

PROCEDURE

Catheterization is performed only after the anesthesia care provider has indicated that it is safe. If the operative procedure requires the lithotomy position, the patient is positioned using the correct technique. A female patient is positioned with the knees slightly flexed and the hips externally rotated. A male patient is placed in the supine position for catheterization.

The sterile technique required for catheterization entails keeping one hand sterile and the other nonsterile. The hand used to insert the catheter and perform the skin prep is referred to here as the *insertion hand*. The *assisting hand* is used to stabilize the genitalia and expose the urethral meatus. The assisting hand does not contact sterile supplies, including the catheter itself. The insertion hand remains sterile and is used to cleanse the area and guide the catheter into place.

If the insertion hand becomes contaminated, the procedure must be stopped and the contaminated glove changed. If the catheter becomes contaminated, a fresh sterile catheter must be obtained.

The following guidelines describe the step-by-step procedure for prep and insertion of a Foley catheter. Although catheterization is a sterile procedure, only the insertion hand remains sterile throughout. The catheterization kit is prepared by adding antiseptic solution, sterile lubricant, and the correct size catheter. Step-by-step illustrations for catheterization are presented in Figures 11-2 (female) and 11-3 (male).

1. Arrange the patient in the proper position. Then put on sterile gloves using the open gloving technique (see Chapter 9.
2. Place the prep sponges in the antiseptic.
3. The balloon may be tested before insertion. However, some manufacturers discourage this, because it can weaken the balloon and lead to rupture after insertion. Follow the facility's and the manufacturer's recommendations. To test the balloon, inject 5 mL of sterile water

from the prep syringe into the Luer-Lock tip of the catheter and observe for leakage. Withdraw the water back into the syringe and put it aside.
4. If the sterile lubricant is provided in a sealed pouch, open the pouch and place a small amount of lubricant in a sterile area of the prep tray or on the tip of the catheter. Position the catheter so that it can be easily grasped with one hand.
5. If the patient is already in the lithotomy position, tuck a **barrier drape** under the buttocks with the tails of the drape directed toward a prepositioned kick bucket.
6. If the patient is in the supine position, place a fenestrated barrier drape over the genitalia.
7. *Female prep:* With the *assisting hand*, spread the labia, using the thumb and forefinger to form a C. Then, use the *insertion* (sterile) *hand* to cleanse the genitalia. Grasp the prep sponge with the sterile forceps. Cleanse the meatus and internal labia by drawing the cotton prep sponge downward from the superior apex of the labia majora to the anus. Drop this sponge into the kick bucket. Do not allow the sponge to touch the area just prepped. Repeat this process several times.
8. *Male prep:* With the *assisting hand*, retract the foreskin and stabilize the penis just below the glans. Use the *insertion hand* to cleanse the penis. Grasp the prep sponge with the sterile forceps and, starting with the urethral meatus, draw it in a circular direction, widening the circle to include the outer portions of the glans. Do not draw the sponge back over the area just prepped. Discard the sponge and repeat this process several times.
9. Maintaining traction on the genitalia, grasp the insertion end of the catheter and lubricate the tip (if this was not done in step 4).
10. Guide the tip of the catheter into the urethra with slow, steady pressure. *Do not force the catheter into the urethra.* It should slide easily into place with little resistance. When the tip of the catheter reaches the bladder, urine will begin to flow through the tubing. (With males, replace the foreskin into its normal position.) If blood returns through the urethra at any time during insertion, gently retract the catheter and request a medical assessment immediately.
11. Connect the distal end of the catheter to the sterile tubing and urine collection unit.
12. Make sure no tension is placed on the catheter tubing once it is in place. This can traumatize the bladder neck and may result in dragging of the inflated balloon through the narrow proximal urethra. Some institutions require that tape or a special strap be placed on the patient's thigh to secure the tubing.
13. Remove your gloves. Lower the drainage unit to allow gravity drainage. When urine stops flowing, secure the drainage unit to the operating bed and measure the baseline amount. Document this amount according to policy.

RISKS OF CATHETERIZATION

Catheterization is a routine procedure performed by (circulating) perioperative personnel. Recently the trend has been

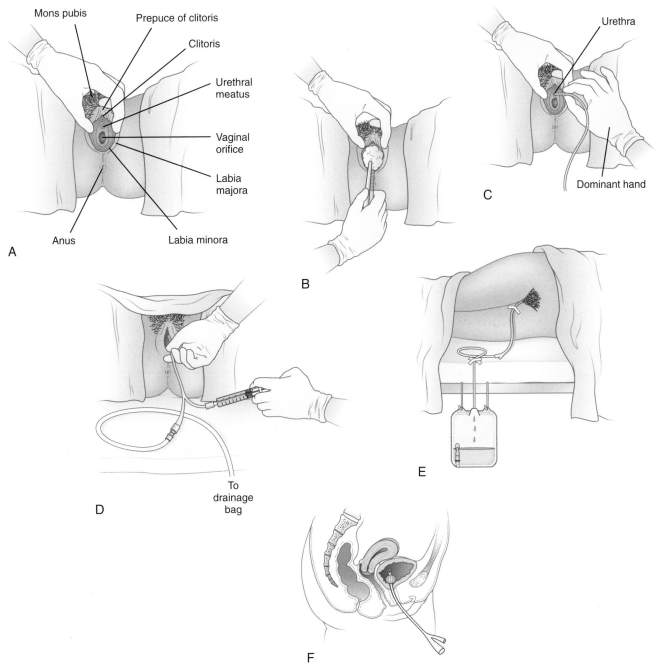

Figure 11-2 Urinary catheterization of the female. **A,** Exposure of the urethra using the assisting hand. **B,** Cleansing of the labia using the no-touch technique. **C,** Insertion of the catheter. **D,** Inflation of the balloon tip. **E,** Attachment of the drainage bag. **F,** Anatomical position of the catheter.

to reduce the number of catheterizations of hospitalized patients because of the risks involved. *Urinary catheterization is the most common cause of hospital-acquired infections in the United States.* Two primary risks are associated with catheterization: infection and trauma to the genitourinary tract.

Urinary catheterization is a sterile procedure. The urinary bladder and proximal urethra are sterile, and contaminants introduced by catheterization increase the risk of urinary tract infection. Because of its proximity to the rectum (especially in female patients), the urinary meatus can be easily contaminated with *Escherichia coli*, which may be introduced into the

urinary system during catheterization. Urinary tract infection can progress to systemic infection, with serious consequences. Strict aseptic technique is required to perform catheterization safely.

Catheterization can cause trauma to the urethra and bladder. Repeated attempts at catheterization can produce mucosal abrasions that cause pain and increase the risk of infection. Damage to the urethra and sphincter muscle can result in prolonged urinary retention and inability to urinate. In elderly males, enlargement of the prostate gland may contribute to difficulty in catheterization.

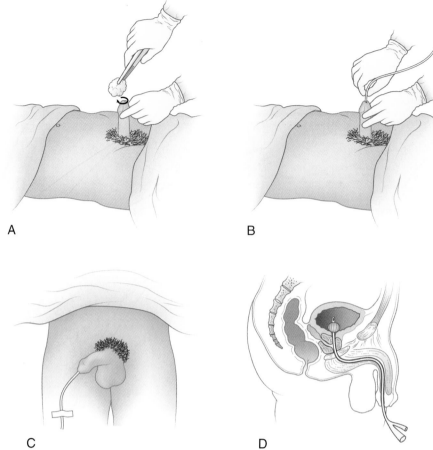

Figure 11-3 Urinary catheterization of the male. **A,** The assisting hand stabilizes the penis and draws back the foreskin. The insertion hand is used to cleanse the urethral meatus and glans. **B,** Insertion of the catheter. The assisting hand replaces the foreskin. **C, D** The catheter is secured to the leg. Anatomical position of the catheter.

❖ *Only trained personnel who have demonstrated technical proficiency should catheterize a patient. The anesthetized patient cannot respond during painful and injurious catheterization.*

THE SURGICAL SKIN PREP

The skin is the body's primary defense against infection. A surgical incision creates a portal of entry for microorganisms. Healthy skin has colonies of microorganisms (normal flora), which compete with and usually overcome foreign or transient bacteria (bioburden). When normal or transient floras are introduced into the surgical wound, they can cause a **surgical site infection (SSI)**.

The surgical skin prep is performed immediately before the start of surgery, after the patient has been positioned and anesthetized. The surgical site and a wide area around the site are cleansed and painted with antiseptic solution. Skin cannot be sterilized, but the number of bacteria can be reduced significantly with antiseptic cleansing or a coating of antiseptic on the skin.

Hair removal may be part of the skin prep, before skin cleansing or performed prior to surgery in the holding area or other location near the operating room.

HAIR REMOVAL

Hair generally is not removed from the surgical site unless the surgeon orders it. If hair is removed, the following guidelines should be followed:

- Hair removal requires an order from the physician, and the exact procedure used follows operating room policy.
- Hair should be removed as close to the time of surgery as possible. If the skin is to be shaved, this should be done immediately before surgery.
- Hair is removed with a razor, electric clippers, or a chemical depilatory.
- Shaving the hair results in injury to the skin that may not be visible. Small skin abrasions create a site for bacterial colonization and become a source of surgical site infection. Studies have shown that the incidence of surgical site infection increases when the skin is shaved. If shaving is necessary, shave in the direction of hair growth no more than 30 minutes before surgery.
- Hair should be removed in an area away from the location where surgery is performed.
- Any shaving equipment that comes in contact with the patient is discarded in a biohazard container.

- If a depilatory is used, the patient first must be tested for sensitivity to the agent. This sensitivity test takes a minimum of 12 hours.
- Cranial procedures often are performed with minimal hair removal. However, in some cases that require removal of a great deal of hair, it is returned to the patient after surgery. The surgeon usually removes the hair in these cases.
- Eyebrows are never shaved, because they may fail to regrow or may grow abnormally after surgery.

RECOMMENDED GUIDELINES FOR THE PREP

Supplies

Supplies for the basic skin prep are available in disposable kits or may be assembled on site. They include the following:

- Sterile gloves
- Towels
- Gauze or foam prep sponges
- Sponge forceps
- Antiseptic paint prep
- Antiseptic scrub soap (if a scrub prep is performed)
- Sterile water
- Several small basins
- Cotton-tipped applicators as needed (for abdominal prep)

PREPPING AGENTS

Only antiseptic agents approved for use on skin may be used for the prep. Five **antiseptics** are commonly used for the surgical skin prep:

- Alcohol
- Chlorhexidine gluconate
- Iodophor
- Triclosan
- Parachlorometaxylenol

Alcohol

Alcohol solution contains isopropyl alcohol. At 70% concentration, isopropyl alcohol is 95% effective against both gram-negative and gram-positive bacteria, mycobacteria, fungi, and viruses. It is not completely effective against bacterial spores. Isopropyl alcohol is extremely flammable and volatile. It can be a source of fire in an oxygen-rich environment when laser and electrosurgery are used. All traces of alcohol must be completely dry on the skin before drapes are applied.

Alcohol destroys microorganisms through **desiccation** (drying out) of the cell proteins. For this reason, alcohol is never used on mucous membranes or the eyes or in any open wound. Alcohol prep solutions are available in liquid or gel form and are combined with other antiseptics.

Chlorhexidine Gluconate

Chlorhexidine gluconate (CHG) is a broad-spectrum antiseptic that has better microbicidal action than povidone-

iodine. This antiseptic provides **residual activity**, which means that it continues to kill microorganisms after application. It is not absorbed by the skin. A disadvantage of CHG is that it is not effective in the presence of soap and organic debris such as skin oils, blood, and body fluids. If it is used for preoperative bathing, the patient first must bathe normally, and chlorhexidine solution then is used as a final wash after all traces of soap have been removed from the skin and hair.

CHG has been linked to hearing loss when accidentally introduced into the middle ear, therefore it must never be used during prep of the ear or face. It is not recommended for use on large, open wounds, such as burns.

Iodophor

Iodine alone is irritating to tissue, but when combined with povidone (a synthetic dispersing agent), it becomes iodophor, a commonly used antiseptic. Iodophor is combined with detergent and used for the surgical hand scrub. It is effective against gram-positive bacteria but weaker against gram-negative organisms, mycobacteria, fungi, and viruses. It has some residual activity and retains its microbicidal action in the presence of organic substances.

Iodophor is absorbed through the skin and may cause toxicity. After use it must be rinsed from the skin. Although it normally is nonirritating to tissue, first-degree and second-degree chemical burns can result from improper prep technique or if the patient is sensitive to iodine. Detergent forms are not used on mucous membranes or near the eyes. Iodophor sometimes is commercially formulated with 70% alcohol as a prep solution. Gel and spray preps also are available.

Triclosan

Triclosan 1% solution is an antiseptic commonly found in deodorants, antibacterial soaps, and other proprietary cosmetics. Its use in surgery is limited, because its full microbicidal effect occurs only with repeated application. It is safe for ophthalmic use and for use on the face.

Parachlorometaxylenol

Parachlorometaxylenol (PCMX) has limited use in surgery. It is nontoxic and can be used in the area of the eyes and ears. It has limited bactericidal, tuberculocidal, viricidal, and fungicidal properties.

GUIDELINES

Before the surgical skin prep is started, all supplies are gathered and placed on a small prep table near the patient. The skin prep is a sterile procedure. Sterile gloves are worn, and supplies are sterile. Manufactured sterile prep trays are available that contain all or most of the supplies needed to perform the skin prep. Many different types of commercial prep systems are available, some with sponges on handles or other devices. The rationale and procedure for the prep remain the same, regardless of the system.

The skin prep follows a prescribed protocol. Before the prep is started, the prep kit is positioned on a small table and the outer wrapper is opened using sterile technique. The sterile outside wrapper is folded down over the table, and a sterile field is created. Prep solutions such as antiseptic scrub soap and paint prep are poured into a basin, and all other supplies are placed on the table.

When more than one procedure is planned during the same surgery, the circulator must prepare each site separately, using a different prep setup for each site. This can occur in cases of multiple trauma or in grafting procedures when the graft is taken from the patient's own tissues. Two people may prep simultaneously if enough staff members are available.

Do not use radiographically detectable surgical sponges to perform the patient. prepSurgical sponges are reserved for surgery and must never be used for the patient prep. They may be confused with the surgical sponges and count. Used prep sponges are discarded according to facility policy to keep them away from the surgical field and out of the incision. In some facilities the kick bucket is used to collect prep sponges which are then collected and bagged before surgery begins to keep them separated from surgical sponges.

It is common practice to identify the surgical side and site by marking it. This is done by applying indelible ink on the skin site. Before the prep is started, the operative site should be cross-checked with the patient's chart to confirm that these marks agree with information in the medical chart, the preoperative checklist, and the patient's knowledge.

Natural skin excretions act as a water-repellant barrier. While these provide protection to the tissue, they can also prevent the prep solution from reaching deeply imbedded soil and bacteria. Special pre-prep solutions containing alcohol are available to remove skin oils. These are used only in patients who have particularly oily skin. The basic principles of the skin prep are based on the rules of aseptic technique, However, the details of the prep may vary somewhat, depending on the location of the surgical site.

There are two methods of prepping. One method uses an antiseptic soap solution followed by a coating of antiseptic **two-stage skin prep**. The other method uses antiseptic solution alone (**single stage prep**). The type of prep used depends on the surgeon's preference.

During procedures performed using regional anesthesia, it is important to respect the patient's modesty and provide a brief explanation of the procedure before starting the prep.

PROCEDURE FOR THE SKIN PREP

Before starting the skin prep, the surgical technologist should perform a mental check of patient safety considerations. These are listed in Box 11-1.

1. The prep site must be assessed before the prep begins. Any lesion or disruption in the skin must be documented in the patient's chart.
2. If the prep area is grossly contaminated with dirt, debris, industrial chemicals, or other foreign material, the site is cleansed as a separate procedure before the surgical skin prep.
3. Prepare the prep supplies on small table near the patient. If a scrub prep to planned, antiseptic scrub soap, such as

---

Box 11-1

Checklist for Starting the Skin Prep

- **Prepare the patient.** Have you checked the patient's record for allergies? Has the patient been positioned properly? Has the surgical site been verified? Has all jewelry been removed? Has the anesthesia care provider given permission to start the prep? Are the surgeons present and available to start surgery?
- **Prepare the supplies.** Note what items are not included in the prep kit. Are sterile gloves available? Have the prep solutions been poured? Is the prep table positioned close to the patient? Is a receptacle at hand for soiled prep sponges? Do you have adequate light on the prep area?
- **Prepare yourself.** Do you have a plan? Do you know the exact boundaries of the prep area? Is your clothing contained so that it does not touch the prep area? (A loose warm-up jacket or baggy sleeves may drag across the prep area.)

Betadine soap, is added to sterile water in a small basin. The ratio of water to antiseptic soap is determined by facility policy and the manufacturer's recommendation. Do not alter the ratio. A small amount of paint prep solution is poured into a separate basin. This is painted on the skin following a scrub prep.

4. Don sterile gloves using the open gloving technique.
5. Place two or more sterile towels on either side of the patient to catch any prep solution that might pool. When placing the towels, make a wide cuff in the towel to protect your gloved hands from contamination.
6. Dip a prep sponge in the antiseptic solution and squeeze out any excess. Use one sponge at a time to perform the prep.
7. The prep is performed in a circular pattern starting at the incision site and moving outward. As the area of the prep is extended outward, do not bring the sponge back to an area already prepped. A new prep sponge is used to widen the circle as needed or to repeat the pattern. As each sponge reaches the periphery of the prep boundary, it is discarded.
8. Any area that is highly colonized with microorganisms (i.e., a contaminated area), such as a colostomy, skin ulcers, or a foreign body, is prepped with fresh sponges *after* the surrounding area has been prepped.
9. After the scrub prep, use a towel to blot the soap from the skin.
10. *Two-stage prep:* Antiseptic paint prep solution is applied to the surgical site after the scrub prep. Dip fresh sponges into the paint solution and squeeze out the excess. Beginning with the incision site, apply paint prep in a circular motion from the center to the periphery. Apply the paint prep solution without allowing the sponge to return to an area previously prepped. When the periphery is reached, discard the sponge.
11. Allow the paint prep solution to air-dry. This enhances its bacteriocidal effect.

12. Document the skin prep in the patient's chart, including the skin assessment, prep area, solutions, and the name of the person who performed the prep.

❖ *Note: DuraPrep Surgical Solution is commonly used for patient prep in the United States. This solution contains iodine povacrylex and isopropyl alcohol. The solution is self-contained in an applicator, which is applied to the surgical site using standard technique. The solution must be allowed to dry before drapes are applied.*

RISKS ASSOCIATED WITH THE SURGICAL PREP

Chemical Burns

Chemical burns result when prep solutions are allowed to pool under the patient. Pressure and contact with the chemical over time can result in severe blistering and skin loss. To prevent burns, the prep area should be framed with sterile surgery towels that can absorb the excess solution at the periphery of the prep area. Towels must be tucked between the operating table and the patient to catch any runoff solution. Towels are removed after the prep. The circulator must check the entire site for pooling or dampness before drapes are applied.

Fire

Alcohol and alcohol-based prep solutions are volatile and flammable. When alcohol solution or volatile fumes come in contact with heat sources, they can easily cause a fire on or inside the patient. Approximately 100 surgical fires occur each year in the United States. These fires result in about 20 serious injuries and two deaths annually.[1]

In the presence of concentrated oxygen or in an oxygen-enriched environment such as the operating room, the risk is even greater. Ignition can occur during electrosurgery or laser surgery. Closed cavities, such as the throat, are particularly at risk because they are small, contained areas. Prevention of alcohol-related fires requires vigilance and proactive measures on the part of all members of the surgical team. To prevent a fire arising from a prep solution, make sure the prep area, towels, linens, and operating bed are dry before applying sterile drapes. All team members are responsible for making sure that the surgical site and bed linen is dry before draping begins.

Thermal Burns

Prep solutions must never be warmed in a microwave unit or autoclave. Heating in this manner is uncontrolled, and the exact temperature is unknown, creating a risk of thermal burns. When iodine is heated in a closed container, it combines with free oxygen, causing the iodine to be lost from the solution, which reduces its concentration.

SPECIFIC PREP SITES

Special procedures and precautions are needed for particular surgical sites. Some of these procedures and precautions require supplies that are not included in a routine prep kit.

Eye

Special Supplies
- Adhesive barrier drape
- Lint-free cotton balls
- Small basins with warm saline solution and prep solution
- Towels
- Bulb syringe
  Note: Eye prep solutions must be diluted according to the surgeon's orders.

Procedure
1. Explain the procedure to the conscious patient. Advise the patient not to touch the face during and after the prep.
2. Turn the patient's head slightly toward the operative side.
3. Start the prep at the eyelid. Prep in a circular pattern around the eye to within 1 inch (2.5 cm) of the hairline, including the nose, cheek, and jaw on the affected side. If the procedure includes both eyes, prep both sides of the face.
4. Prevent prep solutions from entering the patient's ear. Iodophor and chlorhexidine solutions can damage the inner ear. Although the tympanic membrane separates the external auditory canal from the middle ear, solutions may enter through a rupture or tear in the membrane. Place a cotton ball at the ear canal opening or an adhesive barrier drape along the side of the face to prevent solution from draining into the ear.
5. Discard each sponge after reaching the periphery of the prep area.
6. Repeat the prep at least three times, using fresh sponges each time.
7. Rinse the prepped area using warm saline and cotton balls. Discard each used cotton ball and obtain a fresh one. Rinse the area at least twice.
8. Use a bulb syringe and small basin to flush the conjunctiva. Using one finger, pull the conjunctival sac slightly downward while flushing with normal saline solution or a solution ordered by the surgeon.

Ear

Special Supplies
- Mild prep solution (e.g., triclosan or PCMX)
- Normal saline
- Small plastic drape with adhesive edge
- Cotton-tipped applicators

Procedure
1. Use a sterile plastic drape to exclude the eye on the affected side.
2. Do not use alcohol, iodophor, or chlorhexidine prep solutions around the ear. Follow the surgeon's written order for the correct prep solution.
3. Cleanse and rinse the folds of the pinna (external ear) with cotton-tipped applicators.
4. Extend the prep area with sponges to the edge of the hairline, face, and jaw.

Face

Apply only nonalcohol solutions to the face. Triclosan is a mild antiseptic commonly used in this area. The hair contains a high concentration of bacteria and is still considered a contaminated area.

Special Supplies

- Nonalcohol prep solution (e.g., triclosan)
- Warm normal saline
- Cotton swabs
- Cotton-tipped applicators
- Towels
- Comb and water-soluble hair gel (nonsterile supplies)

Procedure

1. Apply gel to the hair if necessary before combing it back away from the face. Use clips if necessary to hold the hair away from the face and ears.
2. Place a towel on each side of the neck to prevent the bed linen from becoming soaked.
3. Prep the face from the neck or chin upward to the hairline. The ears may be included in the face prep.
4. Use cotton-tipped applicators to cleanse the folds of the pinna. Do not allow prep solution to drain into the ear canal.
5. Prep the face from the incision area outward. Prep the incision site again with fresh sponges. No prep sponge that touches the hairline should be brought back over the skin. Rinse the skin with cotton swabs dipped in warm normal saline solution.

Neck

The neck and throat area is prepared for thyroid surgery, tracheotomy, carotid artery surgery, lymph node biopsy, or radical dissection of the mandible, shoulder plexus, and mediastinum. If radical dissection is anticipated or scheduled, the prep area extends from the chin to the nipple line or waist and around the side of the body to the operating table on each side (Figure 11-4).

Procedure

1. Turn the patient's gown down to several inches below the prep area.
2. Place sterile towels at the periphery of the prep site.
3. Begin the prep at the incision site, applying prep solution in a circular motion to the periphery of the site.

Breast and Thorax

The boundaries of the prep area for breast and thoracic procedures depend on the extent of the surgery and the patient's position. The prep area for radical breast or thoracic surgery extends from the chin to the umbilicus and includes the lateral thorax on each side.

When the surgery involves removal of a mass without the possibility of more extensive surgery, the breast is prepped from the clavicle to the midthorax and from the midline, including the sides of the thorax to the operating table on the affected side. The prep area is extended into

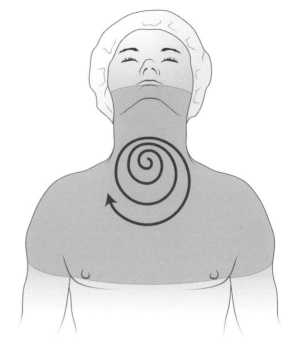

Figure 11-4 Skin prep for neck and throat procedures. *(Modified from Phillips N: Berry and Kohn's operating room technique, ed 10, St Louis, 2004, Mosby.)*

the axilla for lesions in the upper lateral quadrant of the breast.

Surgery that includes both biopsy of a mass and the possibility of mastectomy requires a much wider prep area. A radical mastectomy requires a prep boundary that encompasses the neck, shoulder of the affected side, thorax to the operating table surface, and midpelvic region (Figure 11-5).

Tissue that is suspected of being cancerous must be prepared gently. The area should be painted with as little friction and pressure as possible to prevent tumor cells from migrating into surrounding tissue. Skin prep for surgery of the thoracic cavity uses a bilateral extension of the boundaries for radical breast surgery.

Procedure

1. Square the prep boundary with sterile towels.
2. If the umbilicus is included in the prep, clean it with cotton-tipped applicators.
3. Prep the operative area, starting at the incision site.
4. If the shoulder is included in the prep, an assistant should abduct the arm so that solution can be applied circumferentially.

Shoulder

The shoulder prep includes the neck, shoulder, upper arm, and scapula on the affected side (Figure 11-6). One assistant is required to elevate the patient's arm. The subscapular and midback area also may be elevated on a pad.

Procedure

1. Remove the patient's gown to the umbilicus.
2. Place sterile prep towels at the periphery of the prep area.

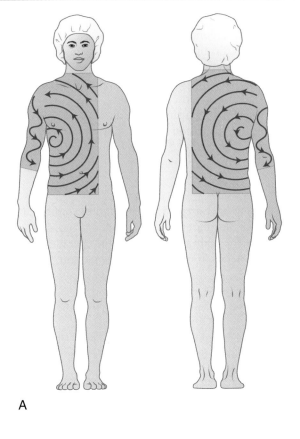

A

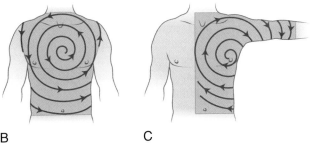

B   C

Figure 11-5 Skin prep for the breast and thorax. *(Modified from Phillips N: Berry and Kohn's operating room technique, ed 10, St Louis, 2004, Mosby.)*

3. Place an **impervious** sheet between the operating table and the subscapular area.
4. Have a gloved assistant elevate the arm.
5. The hand may be excluded from the prep. Some surgeons wrap the hand in an occlusive drape after the prep.
6. Do not pull the patient's shoulder laterally to expose the scapular area. This can cause injury. Seek guidance from the surgeon about the exact nature of the injury or repair to prevent damage.
7. Begin the prep at the incisional site and extend it to the periphery.

Arm

Depending on the incision site, the arm is prepped in total or in one section. If a nerve block anesthesia will be performed, the entire arm usually is prepped. The hand is normally laden with transient and resident bacteria. It may be prepped but then excluded from the operative site by an occlusive drape.

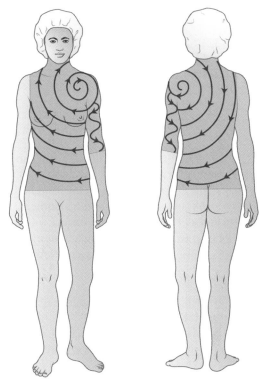

Figure 11-6 Shoulder prep. *(Modified from Phillips N: Berry and Kohn's operating room technique, ed 10, St Louis, 2004, Mosby.)*

If the operative site is on the upper arm, the prep extends several inches above the elbow.

In all cases, the arm or hand is prepped circumferentially. An assistant supports the arm and hand while another person performs the prep. If a pneumatic tourniquet is in use, is it important to prevent prep solutions from becoming trapped between the tourniquet and the patient' skin.

Procedure

1. Elevate the arm carefully, keeping it in anatomical alignment.
2. Place an impervious sheet under the arm, covering the operating table and the patient's torso.
3. Place sterile towels at the periphery of the prep site and under the shoulder. Towels are not required for hand prep.
4. Begin the prep at the incision site and move to the periphery.
5. When the prepped area is dry, remove the impervious sheet.
6. Continue to elevate the arm during draping.

Hand

Large colonies of resident and nonresident bacteria are present on the hand. The subungual area (under the nails) may contain debris and nonresident bacteria, requiring more thorough cleansing. The routine hand prep begins at the fingernails. A brush can be used to cleanse the subungual area. After the hand is cleaned, prep solution is applied as usual, beginning at the incision site and moving outward and circumferentially. The upper boundary is a few inches above the elbow unless.

Special Supplies
- Nail cleaner
- Scrub brush
- Impervious sheet
- Sterile gloves

Procedure
1. Elevate the hand carefully, keeping it in anatomical alignment.
2. Place an impervious sheet under the arm and hand.
3. Clean the subungual areas with a nail cleaner or brush.
4. Beginning at the incisional area, prep the hand in the usual manner, moving outward. Include the interdigital spaces, fingertips, and all four sides of each finger.
5. Extend the prep to the arm, covering all sides.
6. Blot excess antiseptic soap and paint with antiseptic solution.
7. Remove the impervious drape.
8. Support the hand until draping begins and the surgeon takes control of it.

NOTE: If there is extensive trauma to the hand involving a crushing or tearing injury, the surgeon may perform the prep.

Abdomen
The abdominal prep extends from the nipple line to midthigh and both sides of the body to the operating table (Figure 11-7). If a pelvic laparoscopy is planned, a vaginal prep may be included, and two separate preps are necessary.

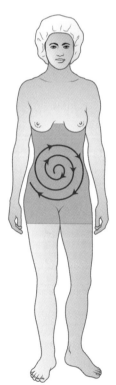

Figure 11-7 Abdominal prep. (Redrawn from Phillips N: Berry and Kohn's operating room technique, ed 10, St Louis, 2004, Mosby.)

Procedure
1. Square the abdomen with sterile towels. The upper towel is placed at the nipple line and the lower towel at the pubis.
2. Begin the prep at the umbilicus. Cleanse the umbilicus using cotton-tipped applicators dipped in prep solution to remove detritus (loose, dead skin).
3. Prep the abdomen using antiseptic soap or prep solution, starting at the incision site and moving to the periphery.
4. If soap solution is used, blot dry and apply prepping solution. Allow the prep solution to dry before applying drapes.

Flank or Back
The flank and back areas are prepped in the same manner as the abdomen, starting at the incision site and moving outward. The sides of the body are prepped to the operating table. The back prep extends from the neck to the sacrum.

Procedure
1. Remove the patient's gown and the cover sheet to the iliac crest.
2. Square the periphery of the prep site with sterile towels.
3. Begin at the incision area and apply prep solution in a circular pattern, continuing to the periphery. Complete this pattern at least twice, beginning again at the incision site and working outward to the surface of the operating table.

Vagina and External Genitalia
The vaginal prep is performed with the patient in the lithotomy position. After the patient has been placed in lithotomy position, the lower table break is flexed downward. Before beginning the prep, place the kick bucket at the foot of the table to receive used sponges.

An impervious drape is placed under the buttocks to prevent prep solution from seeping between the coccyx and the table. If a single impervious sheet is used, place the tail of the sheet in the kick bucket to drain excess prep solution. Place a prep towel above the pubis.

The vaginal prep is performed in two stages. The pelvis, labia, perineum, anus, and thighs are prepped first as one stage, and the vagina is prepped separately (Figure 11-8). Sponge forceps are used to prep the vaginal vault. The rationale for the two-step procedure is to ensure that bacteria from the external genitalia and perineum are not introduced into the vagina.

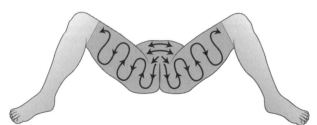

Figure 11-8 Vaginal prep. (Redrawn from Phillips N: Berry and Kohn's operating room technique, ed 10, St Louis, 2004, Mosby.)

NOTE: For combined abdominal-vaginal procedures, such as pelvic laparoscopy, the vaginal prep is done first, followed by the abdominal prep.

Procedure

1. Start the pelvic prep at the pubis, using back-and-forth strokes. This area is prepped to the level of the iliac crest.
2. Apply prep solution at the labia majora, using downward strokes only and including the perineum and anus. Discard the sponge after the anus is prepped. Do not return to the area previously prepped.
3. Using clean sponges, prep the inner aspects of the thighs. Start at the labia majora and move laterally, using back-and-forth strokes. Discard the sponge as it reaches the periphery.
4. Prep the vaginal vault last. Use sponges mounted on forceps and ample prep solution to reach the folds of the vaginal rugae. Discard the sponge and repeat.
5. Use a dry-mounted sponge to blot excess fluid from the vaginal vault and remaining prep area.

Perianal Prep

The perianal prep is performed with the patient in the prone position with a midpelvis break in the operating table. Because the anus is a contaminated area, the surrounding area is prepped first and the anus last. The anus is exposed by separating the buttocks with wide adhesive tape.

Procedure

1. Remove the patient's gown and the cover sheet to expose the lower trunk. Keep the patient's legs and upper body covered.
2. Begin the prep outside the anal mucosa and extend the prep area outward about 12 inches (30 cm) in all directions.
3. Prep the outer anus. In some institutions, the anal prep is omitted.

NOTE: For abdominoperineal resection, the patient is placed in the lithotomy position. The technique requires separate abdominal and perineal preps.

Leg and Foot

The leg prep is similar to that of the arm. The prep extends from the ankle to the groin (Figure 11-9). The limb must be elevated by an assistant or placed in a vertical leg holder attached to the operating table. Use a leg holder with extreme caution, because it can cause serious injuries. If the leg holder is not strong enough to support the leg of a heavy patient, it can rotate or slip, causing injury. For knee surgery, the entire leg is prepped and the foot is wrapped in a separate drape. If a pneumatic tourniquet is in place, prevent prep solutions from seeping under the tourniquet cuff.

Hip surgery requires a circumferential prep from the midcalf to the iliac crest, excluding the groin (Figure 11-10).

Procedure

1. Remove the patient's blanket to the level of the groin, keeping the upper body covered.

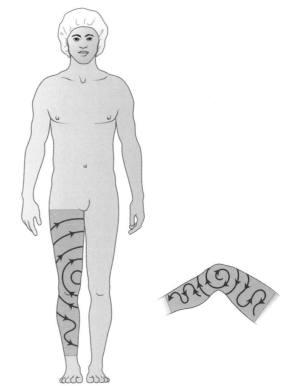

Figure 11-9 Leg prep. (Redrawn from Phillips N: Berry and Kohn's operating room technique, ed 10, St Louis, 2004, Mosby.)

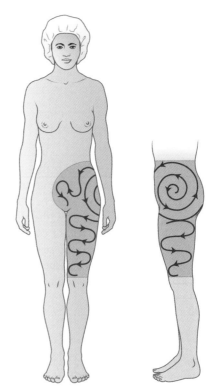

Figure 11-10 Hip prep. (Redrawn from Phillips N: Berry and Kohn's operating room technique, ed 10, St Louis, 2004, Mosby.)

2. Place a towel between the groin and the fold of the upper leg.
3. Elevate the leg.
4. Place an impervious sheet over the operating table and patient's nonoperative leg.
5. If the foot is to be included in the prep, scrub it as you would a hand. Remember that because the leg is elevated, the prep must begin at the highest level and move to the lowest level.
6. If the foot is excluded from the prep, perform wide skin prep around the operative site.

Prep for Trauma Cases

Trauma patients who have a penetrating and open fracture (i.e., a foreign object protruding from the wound) usually are prepped by the surgeon. The entire site is contaminated, and small pieces of bone and foreign material must be washed from the wound. A pressurized water system may be used to clean the wound. This requires specialized drapes with drain pockets to collect and drain runoff solution. During the cleansing process, the surgeon removes all foreign material and trims away devitalized tissue. This is called **debridement**. Preliminary debridement takes place in the emergency department or in some cases in a separate treatment room to prevent gross contamination of the surgical environment. All tissue and foreign material are retained as specimens. After debridement, the wound can be prepped and draped.

Autograft Prep

A tissue autograft is a graft that is removed from one site on the patient and grafted to another site. This requires two separate preps. Clear prep solutions are used on the donor site, especially for skin grafts. This is necessary to maintain a clear view of the vascular bed of the graft. It is important to maintain an aseptic barrier between the donor and recipient sites when grafting is performed in a contaminated or open wound.

DRAPING THE SURGICAL SITE

RATIONALE

Draping is performed immediately after the skin prep. The purpose of draping is to provide a wide sterile area around the surgical site. Drapes act as a barrier surface between nonsterile objects and the sterile field. They allow the sterile team to work in relative freedom without risk of contaminating the wound. Once the patient is draped, the center of the sterile field is defined. Draped tables and equipment are moved into position close to the patient, and scrubbed team members work within the sterile area.

PRINCIPLES

Draping of a surgical patient is one of the more difficult skills for surgical technologists and perioperative nurses to master. The principles of draping are not difficult to understand. However, the actual handling of drapes while maintaining strict aseptic technique sometimes is problematic for students.

To make the process more difficult, there are many variations on basic draping materials based on slightly different designs. However, all drapes and all draping procedures are based on the same principles. Understanding the principles can help clarify the practice.

Drapes are large sheets of impervious material or bonded fabric designed to fit the contours of the body and provide a large sterile surface that is both a barrier against the nonsurgical areas of the patient's body underneath (except for the relatively small area called the *wound* or *surgical site*) and a large sterile surface on which to work (the top side of the drape).

Drapes are available in all sizes and configurations. The draping routine for a surgical procedure is a *process*. Drapes are applied in layers, in a specific order around and over the surgical site using aseptic technique.

DRAPING FABRICS AND MATERIALS

Drapes are made of woven material (cotton or cotton/synthetic blend) or nonwoven material (bonded synthetics). Sterile drapes must create a moisture barrier between the patient and the sterile field.

Nonwoven drapes are disposable, single use items. They are impervious to moisture and breathable, to prevent the patient from becoming hyperthermic. Many different types of nonwoven draping materials are available for specific uses and types of surgery. Woven drapes are reinforced around the fenestration and chemically treated for moisture resistance to prevent strike-through contamination. They are more pliable and easier to handle than nonwoven drapes but require laundering and repair. Self adhering, transparent plastic drapes provide an impervious barrier over an incision site and the incision can be made through the drape (see technique below).

Woven drapes are made of sewn cotton and synthetic fabric. This type of drape has become much less common than in the past, as synthetic single-use materials have become more popular. Woven materials require reprocessing, which may be more costly than single-use materials. However, the environmental impact may be less. Woven drapes must be carefully inspected for tears, holes, and fraying, which may become sources of contamination. Because the fabric is not waterproof, extra precautions, such as increased layers, are needed to prevent penetration with irrigation solutions and blood during surgery.

TECHNIQUES USED IN DRAPING

1. Layering begins with a plain sheet, half sheet or body sheet. In upper body surgery, this is used to cover the patient's legs and lower torso. The plain sheet may also be called a half sheet or cover sheet, depending on regional differences.
2. Surgical towels made of heavy, absorbent cloth are used to make a frame around the incision site. Towels are folded along one edge before they are positioned on the patient. *Framing* the incision means providing an opening in the drapes for the incision. The open area inside the frame is

called the fenestration. The fenestration can be square, oblong, or oval if a disposable **fenestrated drape** is used.

3. Plastic drapes and towels are used to cover the patient's skin and in many different applications. The towel drape, also called a *sticky drape*, is a sheet of smooth plastic or bonded draping material with one adhesive edge. The towel drape is commonly used to exclude an area from the prep. For example, during the skin prep for eye surgery, a towel drape can be applied to prevent prep solution from draining into the patient's ear on the affected side. The drape is then removed when the prep is complete. A towel drape usually is applied across the perineum to exclude the anus from the vagina during gynecological surgery.

4. The plastic **incise drape** (Figure 11-11) is commonly placed over the entire surgical site on top of the towels and any bottom sheets and towels that form the fenestration. The sterile incise drape is coated with adhesive on one side and may be impregnated with antiseptic. The drape is packaged with a paper backing on the adhesive side. The whole drape, including paper backing, is then folded lengthwise and contained in a plastic sleeve wrapping. During draping, the paper backing is peeled away while the drape is applied. This is done in a way that prevents the drape from tangling and sticking to itself. The surgical technologist and surgeon usually apply the drape together.

5. The last drape to be applied is the top drape, also called a *procedure or specialty drape*. Drapes are fan-folded to be compact and allow convenient unfolding over the patient. The folded drape must be positioned over the surgical site

correctly before it is unfolded. It cannot be shifted once it is positioned, therefore it must be correct the first time. The fenestration is centered over the incision site, and the drape is unfolded over the patient's body. Many different specialty drapes are available (Figure 11-12). Printed directions are located on the edge of the fenestration for correct orientation.

ASEPTIC TECHNIQUE DURING DRAPING

The rules of asepsis are followed throughout all draping procedures. When draping, visualize the drape as having two surfaces or sides. One side is in direct contact with the patient and other nonsterile surfaces. The other side can contact only other sterile surfaces, such as the gloved hand or sterile instruments. This principle follows the rules of asepsis.

The following guidelines support the principles of asepsis and safety during draping:

- Handle drapes with as little movement as possible. This reduces the risk of contamination and prevents release of airborne particles that can become vehicles for bacteria.
- When placing a drape, do not touch the patient's body or any other nonsterile surface. Remain a safe distance from the patient to avoid contamination of your gown.
- After a drape has been placed, do not shift or move the drape. To protect the gloved hand during draping with flat sheets, grasp the edge of the sterile sheet and roll your hand inward. This forms a cuff. Position the drape and release the edge of the cuff, keeping your hands on the sterile side of the drape or towel.
- Use only nonpenetrating towel clamps for securing drapes. A hole in a drape creates a passageway for bacteria to contaminate the sterile field. When drapes are stapled to the patient's skin, the stapled area should be covered by an impervious (plastic) drape.
- After a drape has been placed, any portion that falls below the edge of the operating table is considered contaminated. If an area of the drape is suspected of being contaminated, the area may be covered with another impervious drape.
- After a drape has been placed, the edges are considered nonsterile.
- Do not reach over the prepped surgical site to place a towel or drape. Instead, move around the table to position yourself.
- Strike-through contamination occurs when a drape becomes soaked during surgery and solution penetrates to a nonsterile surface. Whenever possible, use only impervious drapes.
- Drapes fitted with a pocket reservoir and drainage system are used for cases in which extensive fluids or bleeding may cause strike-through contamination.
- Aluminum-coated drapes are used whenever laser surgery is planned. These deflect laser energy and prevent ignition in an oxygen-rich environment, especially in head and neck surgery.

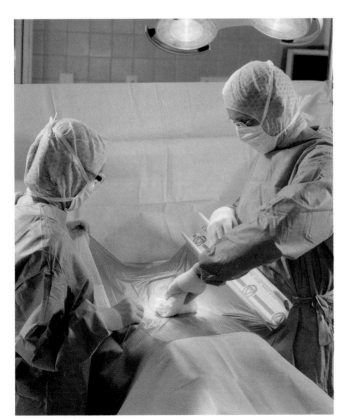

Figure 11-11 Incise drape. *(Courtesy 3M.)*

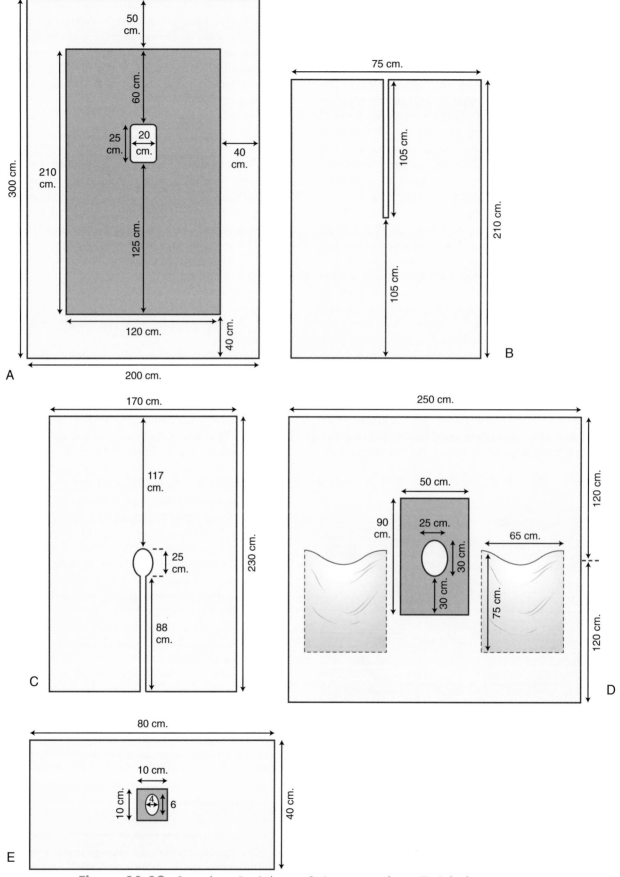

Figure 11-12 Specialty or "top" drapes. **A,** Laparotomy drape. **B,** Split sheet. **C,** Craniotomy drape. **D,** Lithotomy drape (leggings for draping stirrups included). **E,** Eye or ear drape.

- Plan ahead for draping. Verify the surgeon's procedure at the start of the case and stack drapes on the back table in reverse order of application. Have extra sterile towels and sheets available.

DRAPING THE SURGICAL SITE

Abdomen

The procedure for draping the abdomen can be used to drape many other surgical sites (Figure 11-13):

1. Place a plain sheet over the patient's legs.
2. Place four towels (folded cloth, disposable nonwoven material) in a square to frame the operative site. These may be held in place with nonpenetrating towel clamps.
3. A plastic (adhesive) incise drape may be applied over the towels. Two people are required to perform this step. One person holds one end of the drape while the other pulls the paper backing away.
4. Smooth the plastic drape over the contours of the patient's skin.
5. Center a fenestrated body drape over the incision site and unfold it to provide a sterile field.

Lithotomy (Perineal) Draping

Lithotomy, or perineal, draping is used for gynecological surgery, transperineal surgery of the prostate, and combined abdominal-perineal resection of the colon (Figure 11-14). In most cases the anus is excluded from the surgical site with a barrier drape. An impervious drape is tucked under the patient's buttocks to begin draping. The bottom edge of this drape may be placed in the kick bucket to collect runoff fluids. Alternatively, a drainage bag drape may for this purpose.

1. For gynecological surgery, a barrier is necessary between the anus and the vulva. Apply an adhesive towel across the perineum midway between the vulva and anus.
2. Use leggings to cover the patient's legs in stirrups (or the perineal drape may have inserts that extend over the stirrups and the patient's legs).
3. Center a fenestrated body sheet over the perineal area and extend it upward over the patient's abdomen and upper body. Secure the top to the anesthesia screen.

Leg

When draping the leg, the foot is excluded from the surgical site by wrapping it in a towel and then covering it with a tube drape (tube stockinet). The limb must be held up and away from the operating table while the stockinet is applied. With the limb suspended, a sterile, impervious sheet is placed directly beneath the limb.

1. A towel is wrapped around the pneumatic tourniquet. (Note: Chapter 17 contains a complete discussion of the pneumatic tourniquet which is applied above (proximal to) the surgical wound site in limb surgery)
2. Place rolled stockinet over the foot or hand and unroll it to cover the limb.
3. Secure a split drape around the proximal (upper) part of the limb.
4. Apply a fenestrated drape to complete the surgical field.

Hand or Arm

Hand procedures are performed with the surgeon and assistant seated.

1. After the skin prep, suspend the hand and forearm while the first drape is placed on the surgical arm board.
2. Use a towel to wrap the proximal arm and cover the pneumatic tourniquet.
3. A tube stockinet may be used to cover the arm.

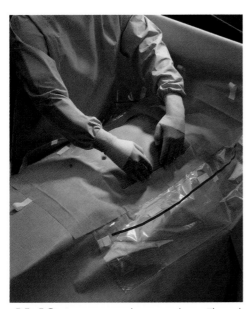

Figure 11-13 Laparotomy drape in place. The edges are reinforced and adhesive. After application, the edges are pressed in place. An incise drape may be placed over the top of the opening. (© Kimberly-Clark Worldwide, Inc. Used with permission.)

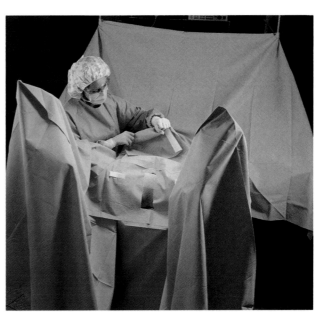

Figure 11-14 Lithotomy draping. (© Kimberly-Clark Worldwide, Inc. Used with permission.)

4. Position a split sheet with the tails draped toward the patient's hand.
5. Place the arm through a fenestrated sheet and complete the sterile field (Figure 11-15).

Shoulder

The shoulder is draped with the patient in semisitting (Fowler) position. The arm is suspended away from the body with the hand and lower arm excluded from the surgical site. The arm is draped free so that it can be manipulated during surgery (Figure 11-16).

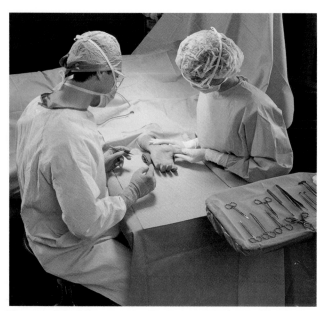

Figure 11-15 Completed draping for the hand and upper arm. The surgeon and assistant or surgical technologist are seated during hand surgery. *(© Kimberly-Clark Worldwide, Inc. Used with permission.)*

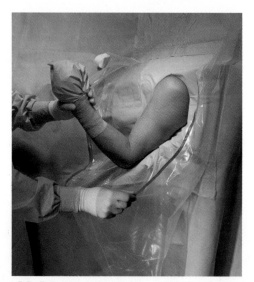

Figure 11-16 Shoulder draping. Note that the arm is draped free for manipulation during surgery. *(© Kimberly-Clark Worldwide, Inc. Used with permission.)*

1. Place an impervious drape between the upper torso, shoulder, and operating table.
2. Position a body or half sheet over the torso.
3. The hand and lower arm may be occluded with towels and stockinet applied over the arm. This may be secured with an impervious drape.
4. Use towels to frame the shoulder and cover them with an incise drape.
5. Apply a split drape.
6. Place the arm and shoulder through a fenestrated sheet.

Head Drape

The **head drape** occasionally is used for nose and throat procedures to maintain a sterile barrier between the face and the head. The head drape is created with two towels or plain draping sheets. The head is slightly elevated, and both towels are placed under the patient's head as shown in Figure 11-17. Each corner of the uppermost towel is brought to the center over the hairline and secured with a nonpenetrating towel clamp.

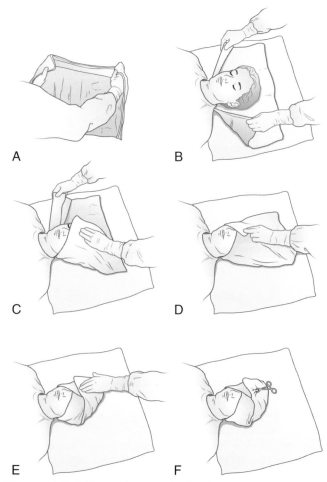

A   B

C   D

E   F

Figure 11-17 Application of a head drape, which is used to protect the eyes during nasal and oromaxillofacial surgery.

Craniotomy

Draping for a cranial procedure is similar to that for other routines that require a large body sheet with a fenestration. Cranial access usually is obtained with the patient in the prone position using a Mayfield headrest. This allows the anesthesia care provider access to the patient's airway while providing access to the skull.

1. Position a body sheet at the neck and extend it to the legs.
2. Apply surgical draping towels to square the incision site. These may be secured to the scalp with skin staples.
3. An incise drape may be positioned on the scalp.
4. Center a large, fenestrated procedure drape over the incision site and open it to cover the patient fully.

HOW TO DRAPE LARGE EQUIPMENT

Large equipment, such as the operating microscope, C-arm, and robotic equipment used within the sterile field, is draped before surgery. Most equipment drapes are designed to fit with cutouts and ample material to allow smooth draping. Adhesive strips and drape openings are imprinted with arrows and directions. The circulator assists during equipment draping by grasping the periphery of the drape and pulling it into place (the edge of a sterile drape is not considered sterile).

When the operating microscope is to be used right away during a case, it is draped before the patient prep. If it will not be used for an hour or more after the case begins, it can be draped during the procedure.

The single-use microscope drape is a continuous plastic sleeve that is fan folded for easy application. The drape has "pockets" that cover the protruding parts of the scope. The scrub starts the draping. The circulator assists by pulling the drape down by holding the bottom portion, which will be outside the sterile field after the drape is in place. The ocular portions and optics of the microscope are not covered. The drape is secured over the lenses with sterile caps. After the drape is in place, it is loosely bound to the body of the microscope with adherent tapes that are an integral part of the drape itself.

REMOVING DRAPES

At the close of a procedure, all instruments and equipment are removed from the tope drape, including the sterile sections of power cords, air hoses, and other devices that might become tangled in drapes as they are removed. One member of the sterile team holds any dressings in place while the drapes are slowly removed. When removing drapes, pull them away from the patient, starting at the patient's head, and proceeding to the feet.

Remove one layer at a time. Be sure not to dislodge any wound drains. Drapes should be contained with as little movement as possible, with the ends wrapped or rolled toward the inside, to confine blood and body fluids in the middle of the drape. The drapes are placed in a designated biohazard bag. No drapes are removed from the room until the final sponge, needle, and instrument count has been verified.

CHAPTER SUMMARY

- Urinary catheterization is performed before surgery to empty the bladder and provide continuous urinary drainage throughout the procedure.
- Urinary catheterization is a sterile procedure that follows the rules of asepsis and Standard Precautions.
- Catheterization increases the risk of urinary tract infection and is performed by trained personnel only.
- The patient skin prep is performed to reduce transient and normal microbes to an absolute minimum.
- The skin prep is performed immediately before the start of surgery, after the patient has been positioned.
- Only antiseptic agents approved for use on skin are used for the surgical prep.
- Alcohol prep solutions increase the risk of fire in an oxygen-rich environment. Prep solutions must be completely dry before drapes are applied.
- The skin prep may include a scrub prep of the skin or only a paint prep using antiseptic solution.
- Hair is not removed from the surgical site unless ordered by the surgeon
- If skin is to be shaved, it is done immediately before surgery to prevent infection at the site.
- The skin prep is performed according to an exact protocol and procedure, depending on the surgical site and whether gross contamination is present.
- Sterile drapes are applied to the surgical site so that only the surgical site is exposed. The surgical site is the center of the sterile field.
- Draping routines are established by individual surgeons and health care facilities and are based on the rules of asepsis.
- Draping materials are made of woven cloth, plastic, or laminated synthetic sheeting. Drapes are supplied as single-use or nondisposable items.
- Draping routines include towels, draping sheets, and a procedure drape, which exposes the surgical site.
- Surgical equipment used within the sterile field (e.g., the fluoroscopy C-arm) is draped before use.

REVIEW QUESTIONS

1. Describe the risks of urinary catheterization.
2. Why is continuous urinary drainage required during surgery?
3. Explain how to maintain sterility while inserting the catheter.
4. Explain the rationale for the surgical skin prep.
5. Why are plain (not radiographically detectable) sponges used for the skin prep?
6. During the skin prep for a contaminated region, the area of highest contamination is prepped last. Why is this?

7. What is the rationale for surgical draping?

8. What is the purpose of aluminum-coated drapes?

9. What parts of a drape are considered nonsterile after the drape is in place?

10. What techniques are used to prevent contamination of the gloved hand while draping the patient?

REFERENCE

1. Association of periOperative Registered Nurses (AORN): Fire safety in perioperative settings, *AORN Journal* Vol 86, Supplement 1, Page 2141-S145, 2007.

BIBLIOGRAPHY

Association of periOperative Registered Nurses (AORN): Recommended practices for hand antisepsis/hand-scrubs. In *Standards, recommended practices and guidelines*, Denver, 2007, AORN.

Association of periOperative Registered Nurses (AORN): Recommended practices for skin preparation of patients. In *Standards, recommended practices and guidelines*, Denver, 2007, AORN.

Boyce J, Pittet D: Guidelines for hand hygiene in health-care settings, *Morbidity and Mortality Weekly Report* 51:16, 2002. Available online at http://www.cdc.gov.

Healthcare Infection Control Practice Advisory Committee: Recommendations from the CDC guideline for hand hygiene in healthcare settings. Available online at http://solutions.3m.com.

CHAPTER 12

Anesthesia, Anesthetics, and Physiological Monitoring

CHAPTER OUTLINE

LEARNING OBJECTIVES

After studying this chapter the reader will be able to:
- Explain terms used to describe important anesthesia concepts
- Explain the basic physiology of neurotransmission
- Describe basic anesthesia equipment
- Explain the rationale and parameters of physiological monitoring during anesthesia
- Describe the components of an anesthesia evaluation
- Explain the preoperative preparation of the patient for anesthesia
- Define general anesthesia and describe induction, maintenance, and emergence

- Describe the methods used in conscious sedation
- Recognize the names of general anesthetic agents
- List the classes of drugs used as adjuncts during general anesthesia
- Define the role of the surgical technologist during the use of regional anesthesia
- Define common types of regional anesthesia
- Recognize the names of regional anesthetic drugs
- Describe important anesthetic and physiological emergencies

TERMINOLOGY

Agonist: A drug that potentiates the release or uptake (or both) of a particular neurotransmitter.

Airway: The anatomical passageway or artificial tube through which the patient breathes.

Amnesia: The loss of recall of events or sensations.

Analgesia: The absence of pain, produced by specific drugs.

Anaphylaxis: A life-threatening allergic reaction to a drug or substance.

Anesthesia: The absence of sensory awareness or medically induced unconsciousness.

Anesthesia care provider (ACP): A professional who is licensed to administer anesthetic agents and manage the patient throughout the period of anesthesia.

Anesthesia machine: A biotechnical device used to deliver anesthetic gases or volatile liquids and provide physiological monitoring.

Anesthesia technician: An allied health professional trained to assist the anesthesia care provider.

Anesthesiologist: A physician specialist in the administration of anesthetics and pain management.

Anesthetic: A drug that reduces or blocks sensation or induces unconsciousness.

Antagonist: A drug that counteracts the effects of another agent or physiological process.

Antegrade amnesia: In anesthesia, the patient's inability to recall events that occur after the administration of specific drugs. After the drug is metabolized and cleared from the body, normal recall returns.

Anxiolytic: A drug that reduces anxiety.

Apnea: A period of cessation of breathing.

Balanced anesthesia: A somewhat outdated term used to describe the use of multiple drugs to produce sedation, analgesia, amnesia, and muscle relaxation during general anesthesia.

Bier block: Regional anesthesia in which the anesthetic agent is injected into a vein.

Bispectral index system (BIS): A monitoring method used to determine the patient's level of consciousness and prevent intraoperative awareness.

Bolus injection: A single dose of medication administered all at one time.

Breathing bag: The reservoir breathing apparatus of the anesthesia machine. Gases are titrated and shunted into the breathing bag, which is connected to the patient's airway.

Bronchospasm: An involuntary smooth muscle spasm of the bronchi.

Certified registered nurse anesthetist (CRNA): A registered nurse trained and licensed to administer anesthetic agents.

Coma: The deepest state of unconsciousness, in which most brain activity ceases.

Consciousness: Neurological status in which a patient is able to sense environmental stimuli such as sight, sound, touch, pressure, pain, heat, and cold.

Controlled hypothermia: Deliberate lowering of the patient's core body temperature during general anesthesia.

Cricoid pressure: Direct manual pressure on the cricoid cartilage to prevent aspiration and facilitate intubation.

Cyanosis: A blue or dusky hue of the skin that results from inadequate perfusion of tissue.

Delirium: A state of confusion and disorientation.

Emergence: The stage in general anesthesia in which the anesthetic agent is withdrawn and the patient regains consciousness.

Endotracheal tube: An artificial airway (tube) that is inserted into the patient's trachea to maintain patency.

Esmarch bandage: A rolled bandage made of rubber or latex that is used to exsanguinate blood from a limb.

Extubation: Withdrawal of an artificial airway.

Gas scavenging: The capture and safe removal of extraneous anesthetic gases from the anesthesia machine.

General anesthesia: Anesthesia associated with a state of unconsciousness. General anesthesia is not a fixed state of unconsciousness, but rather ranges along a continuum from semiresponsiveness to profound unresponsiveness.

Homeostasis: A state of balance in physiological functions.

Hypertonic: A physiological solution which has greater solute concentration than plasma.

Hypothermia: A subnormal body temperature.

Hypotonic: Physiological solution with a solute concentration lower than plasma.

Induction: Initiation of general anesthesia with a drug that causes unconsciousness.

Infusion: Gradual administration of a drug over a specified period.

Intraoperative awareness (IOA): A rare condition in which a patient undergoing general anesthesia is able to feel pain and other noxious stimuli but unable to respond.

Intraoperative cell salvage: A method of collecting blood at the surgical site and immediately reusing it by infusing it back to the patient during surgery.

Intravascular volume: Fluid volume within the blood vessels.

Intubation: The process of inserting an invasive artificial airway.

Isotonic: Physiologic solution that is equal in solute concentration with plasma.

Laryngeal mask airway (LMA): An airway consisting of a tube and small mask that is fitted internally over the patient's larynx.

Laryngoscope: A lighted instrument used to assist endotracheal intubation.

Malignant hyperthermia: A rare state of hypermetabolism that occurs in association with inhalation anesthetics and neuromuscular blocking agents. In extreme cases, the condition causes hyperpyrexia, seizures, and cardiac arrhythmia.

Monitored anesthesia care (MAC): Monitoring of vital functions during regional anesthesia to ensure the patient's safety and comfort.

Nasopharyngeal airway: Artificial airway between the nostril and the nasopharynx; used in semiconscious patients or when an oral airway is contraindicated.

Neuromuscular blocking agent: A drug that blocks nerve conduction in striated muscle tissue.

Neurotransmitter: Biochemical that carries nerve transmission from one neuron to another.

Nondepolarizing neuromuscular blocking agent: Agent that binds to the muscle's cholinergic receptor to increase muscle paralysis.

Oropharyngeal airway: Artificial airway that is inserted over the tongue into the larynx; used in patients in which endotracheal intubation is difficult or contraindicated.

Parasympathetic nervous system: Part of the autonomic nervous system that is responsible for energy conservation and rest, including relaxation of muscle groups, dilation of blood vessels, and decreased blood pressure.

Perfusion: Circulation of blood to specific tissue, organ, system, or the whole body is called perfusion. Perfusion is necessary to maintain life in the cells.

Physiological monitoring: Assessment of the patient's vital metabolic functions.

Pneumatic tourniquet: An air-filled tourniquet used to prevent blood flow to an extremity during surgery.

Polarizing neuromuscular blocking agents: Drugs used to cause muscle paralysis by stimulating involuntary muscles followed by fatigue.

Postanesthesia recovery unit (PACU): The critical care area in which patients recover from the sedation of general anesthesia.

Preoperative medication: One or more drugs administered before surgery to prevent complications related to the surgical procedure or anesthesia.

Protective reflexes: Nervous system responses to harmful environmental stimuli, such as pain, obstruction of the airway, and extreme temperature. Coughing, blinking, shivering, and withdrawal (from pain) are protective reflexes.

Pulmonary embolism (PE): An obstruction in a pulmonary vessel caused by a blood clot, air bubble, or foreign body caused sudden pain and possible pulmonary arrest.

Pulse oximeter: A monitoring device that measures the patient's hemoglobin oxygen saturation by means of spectrometry.

Regional block: Anesthesia in a specific area of the body, achieved by injection of an anesthetic around a major nerve or group of nerves.

Sedation: An arousable state in which an individual is unaware of sensory stimuli. Depression of the central nervous system.

Sedative: A drug that induces a range of unconscious states. The effects are dose dependent. At low doses, sedatives cause some drowsiness. Increasing the dose causes central nervous system depression, ending in loss of consciousness.

Sensation: The ability to feel stimuli in the environment (e.g., pain, heat, touch, visual stimuli, and sound).

Sympathetic nervous system: Part of the autonomic nervous system responsible for "fight or flight" response to danger and stress. Physiologic reactions include diversion of blood to essential organs, increased heart rate, and blood pressure.

Synapse: The synapse is the small space in which the neurotransmitter passes from one nerve cell to another.

Topical anesthesia: Anesthesia of superficial nerves of the skin or mucous membranes.

Unconsciousness: A neurological state in which the person is unable to respond to external stimuli. Unconsciousness can be induced with drugs or may be caused by trauma or disease.

Ventilation: The physical act of taking air into the lungs by inflation and releasing carbon dioxide from the lungs by deflation.

INTRODUCTION

Anesthesia means *without sensation*. The goal of *surgical anesthesia* is to allow the patient to tolerate surgery and maintain the body in a balanced physiological state, called **homeostasis**. Anesthesia is achieved by altering the patient's level of consciousness, by interrupting nerve pathways that transmit sensation, or a combination of the two.

❖ *Modern anesthesia is characterized by an alteration in the patient's sensory awareness and consciousness.*

IMPORTANT ANESTHESIA CONCEPTS

1. **Sensation** is the awareness of stimuli. Most people are familiar with the "five senses" (hearing, sight, smell, taste, and touch). The nervous system is capable of many other sensations, including temperature (heat and cold), pressure, and pain. Sensory awareness is a complex biochemical process involving specialized nerves, electrical activity, and chemical transmitters.

2. **Analgesia** is loss of pain sensation. Specialized "pain" nerves transmit signals from the source of injury to the brain. Analgesic drugs interrupt these pain nerve pathways.

3. **Consciousness** is a state of awareness in which a person is able to *sense the environment and respond to it*. In a fully conscious person, all autonomic and sensory functions are intact and the patient is "awake."

4. **Sedation** is a *state of consciousness* described along a continuum. At one end a person is fully aware of the surroundings. At the other end is unconsciousness, in which the patient is not aware of the environment and cannot respond to external stimuli such as pain or temperature.

5. **Central nervous system depression** refers to diminished mental, sensory, and physical capacity. It is another way of expressing sedation.

6. **Unconsciousness** is severe depression of the central nervous system (CNS) resulting in the *inability to respond to external stimuli*. Deep unconsciousness, such as that achieved during general anesthesia, results in the absence of **protective mechanisms**, such as swallowing, coughing, blinking, and shivering. General (surgical) anesthesia produces reversible unconsciousness.

7. **Coma** is the deepest state of unconsciousness, in which most brain activity ceases.

8. **Amnesia** is the loss of recall (memory) of events that occur while the drug is present in the patient's system. Drugs that produce amnesia often are given during anesthesia. For example, the drug diazepam is given intravenously during diagnostic procedures such as a colonoscopy.

ANESTHESIA PRINCIPLES AND PERSONNEL

PHYSIOLOGY OF THE CENTRAL NERVOUS SYSTEM

A knowledge of nerve transmission is basic to an understanding of how anesthetics and other CNS drugs work. The following basic description of how stimuli are transmitted provides useful background for the study of anesthesia.

The transmission of nerve impulses (signals) is a complex biochemical process. In simple terms, impulses are chemical and electrical. Chemicals that carry impulses from nerve cell to nerve cell are called *neurotransmitters*. The biochemical work of the neurotransmitter is to transport the signal from one nerve cell to the next until the signal reaches the target tissue.

Each nerve cell (neuron) is separated from an adjacent nerve cell by a synapse (also called the *synaptic cleft*). The synapse is the small space in which the neurotransmitter passes from one nerve cell to another. For the neurotransmitter to transport a signal, it must be released from the presynaptic neuron (the neuron before the synapse) and received by the next neuron in line (the postsynaptic neuron).

The neurotransmitter is contained in small vesicles (cell sacs). The receptor for a particular neurotransmitter is a specific molecule in the postsynaptic neuron (Figure 12-1).

Nerve Transmission

The body has many different types of neurotransmitters, each carrying a different type of impulse. About 30 known neurotransmitters occur in specific tissues of the body.

One type of neurotransmitter can be blocked without affecting the others. For example, the neurotransmitter for motor control can be blocked by a muscle-paralyzing agent while the neurotransmitter for pain remains unaffected. This would result in the ability to feel pain but the inability to withdraw from the agent causing it. Likewise, sedation or loss of consciousness can be achieved without reducing the sensation of pain.

One method of blocking neurotransmission is to administer a drug that has an affinity for the postsynaptic receptor. A limited number of receptors are available for the neurotransmitter molecule. When the drug attaches to the receptor site,

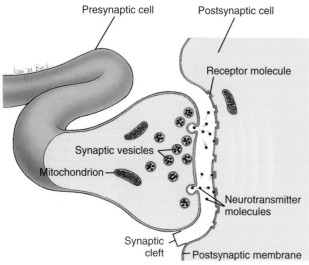

Figure 12-1   Neuron junction and neurotransmitter molecules. *(From Thibodeau GA, Patton KT: Anatomy and physiology, ed 6, St Louis, 2007, Mosby.)*

the neurotransmitter cannot continue on its path, because no unbound receptors are available. The neurotransmitter remains in the space between the two neurons (the synapse) and eventually is reabsorbed by the presynaptic cell or broken down by enzymes in the synapse. The path of transmission is broken. A drug that works in this manner is called a *competitive* **antagonist**. Certain drugs can increase the availability of postsynaptic receptors and the movement of neurotransmitters. If a drug potentates the release or uptake (or both) of a particular neurotransmitter, it is called an *agonist*.

Autonomic Nervous System

Stimuli in the autonomic nervous system produce specific involuntary responses in body organs and tissues. These responses occur in smooth muscle tissue, including cardiac smooth muscle and glands. Examples of autonomic responses are changes in heartbeat, the release of glandular secretions (e.g., insulin in the pancreas), and intestinal contractions (peristalsis).

Two types of responses can occur in the autonomic nervous system: sympathetic and parasympathetic (Figure 12-2). These are often called "fight or flight" responses. Sympathetic and parasympathetic responses generally produce opposing effects, such as increasing or decreasing the heart rate and decreasing or increasing bronchiole dilation.

Somatic Nervous System

The somatic nervous system is under direct voluntary control. Neurotransmitters of the somatic nervous system conduct impulses to the striated muscles of the body. This results in voluntary (consciously controlled) muscle activity that produces movement. Paralysis occurs when nerve impulses are interrupted. A neuromuscular blocking agent is used during surgery to relax or paralyze muscles for easier intubation and tissue manipulation. (Neuromuscular blocking agents are discussed later in the chapter.)

ANESTHESIA PERSONNEL

Anesthesia Care Provider

The **anesthesia care provider** (**ACP**) is trained to administer **anesthetic** agents, perform physiological monitoring, and respond to anesthetic and surgical emergencies. An **anesthesiologist** is a medical doctor with specialist training in anesthesia (MDA). The **certified registered nurse anesthetist** (**CRNA**) is licensed to deliver anesthesia after achieving a master of science degree in nursing and obtaining certification. Specialty areas in the field of anesthesia care include chronic pain management and clinical anesthesia specialties, such as obstetrical, cardiac, pediatric, and ambulatory anesthesia.

Role of the Anesthesia Care Provider

The primary role of the ACP is to provide an adequate level of anesthesia while assessing and managing the patient's physiological responses to the surgery and anesthesia. The tasks of the ACP include the following:

- Protect and manage the patient's vital functions during surgery.
- Manage the patient's level of consciousness and ability to sense pain.
- Provide an adequate level of muscle relaxation during general anesthesia.
- Provide sedation as needed during regional anesthesia.
- Communicate with the surgeon about the patient's responses to intraoperative stimuli. This includes information on homodynamic changes, fluid and electrolyte balance, level of muscle relaxation, and level of consciousness.
- Report and respond to any surgical or anesthetic emergency.
- Provide psychological support to the patient throughout perioperative experience.

To perform these tasks effectively, the ACP must collaborate and communicate with the surgeon. The surgeon gives information to the ACP about the patient's physical responses during surgery, such as level of muscle relaxation and movement. The ACP communicates information to the surgeon about the physiological assessment of intravascular pressure, oxygen saturation, cardiovascular status, and other physiological parameters. All work together to maintain an appropriate anesthetic level and homeostasis.

The ACP monitors the patient from the time the individual enters the surgical suite until the person is discharged from the hospital. Intraoperative care begins when the patient arrives in surgery and continues through the duration of the procedure and into the next phase, postoperative care. This begins when the patient is transported to the postanesthetic care unit and continues until discharge. The ACP is available to respond to medical problems related to the anesthesia, including management of postoperative pain.

Anesthesia Technician

The **anesthesia technician** is an allied health professional trained to assist the ACP in nonmedical tasks. These include

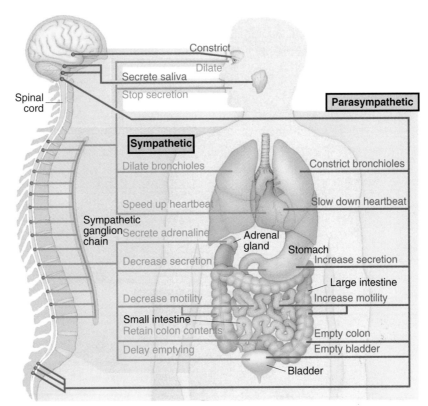

Figure 12-2 Sympathetic and parasympathetic nervous systems: the "fight or flight" system. (*From Thibodeau GA, Patton KT: Structure and function of the body, ed 11, St Louis, 2000, Mosby.*)

maintaining anesthesia and physiological monitoring equipment, preparing drugs and supplies, and providing nonmedical assistance during routine anesthesia delivery. To obtain certification as an anesthesia technician, a person must graduate from an approved 2- or 4-year college or university program and pass a certification examination.

PREOPERATIVE EVALUATION

Before surgery, the ACP or other qualified personnel (e.g., nurse practitioner, physician assistant) perform an assessment of the patient. This takes place 1 to 3 days before the date of surgery. In an emergency, the assessment is performed just before the procedure and may be done in the patient holding area. Patients coming in for day surgery or for minor procedures for which regional (local) anesthesia will be used may not require an in-depth assessment because the risks are fewer and less complex.

The purpose of the assessment is to determine the patient's specific needs and risk factors for anesthesia. The decision on the type of anesthesia to be used (general, sedation, regional) may be made at this time. During the preoperative evaluation, patients have the opportunity to discuss specific concerns about their physical or psychological well-being as it relates to the anesthesia and postoperative care. Patient education

during the assessment often resolves many fears and misconceptions about the effects of anesthesia and pain control.

Specific information about the patient's physical status is needed to ensure safe delivery of anesthesia. The preoperative assessment is modified according to the type of surgery and known risks to a particular patient. For example, if the patient is diagnosed with a metabolic or other systemic disease, the assessment may require specific investigations. Figure 12-3 shows an example of a preanesthesia questionnaire.

Physical Status and Anesthesia Classification

Most patients will have had a recent physical examination and assessment before the anesthesia evaluation. In the outpatient setting, the anesthesia evaluation may be done at the same time as the preoperative examination. The evaluation includes a current or past history of systemic disorders, such as:

- Cardiovascular abnormalities
- Respiratory disease
- Metabolic diseases of the kidney or liver
- Neurological conditions

Systemic disease may alter the action of drugs. Many anesthetics and adjunct agents are toxic to the kidneys and liver or are metabolized or excreted by these organs. A patient with liver or kidney disease may have problems with medication clearance. This results in sustained medication action or decreased tolerance. Certain disease states can also increase the patient's risk for cardiopulmonary arrest, especially during general anesthesia. In patients with certain disease conditions, the normal dose may require adjustment and additional complex monitoring may be needed during surgery. If general rather than regional anesthesia is planned, greater focus is placed on systemic disease.

The American Society of Anesthesiologists (ASA) has developed an assessment system that classifies patients according to their risk of anesthesia-related complications (Box 12-1). This system was developed to identify an individual's level of risk. The system currently is being challenged by medical authorities as an inadequate method of establishing risk, especially compared with other means available.

Current Medications and Allergies

The patient's current medications include over-the-counter medications and herbal remedies. Drugs and agents the

Addressograph

Breath Sounds

- A - Absent ☐
- C - Clear ☐
- D - Decreased ☐
- R - Rales ☐
- RH - Rhonchi ☐
- W - Wheezes ☐
- SNN - See Nurses Notes ☐

P.S.S. VITAL SIGNS BP____ P ____ R ____ T ____ SaO_2 ____ (presedative room air)

VITAL SIGNS BP____ P ____ R ____ T ____ SaO_2 ____ (presedative room air)

DATE:________ TIME:________

PRE-ANESTHETIC EVALUATION

PRIMARY PHYSICIAN/SURGEON:

PRE-OP DIAGNOSIS:

SCHEDULED OPERATION:

MEDICATIONS:

CIGARETTES: ☐ QUIT SMOKING ________
ETOH:
DRUG ABUSE: ________

REMARKS / FAMILY HEALTH HISTORY:

CARDIOVASCULAR: ☐ ASHD ☐ CHF ☐ H.V.D. ☐ ANGINA ☐ ORTHOPNEA ☐ VALVULAR DISEASE ☐ PREV. M.I. ☐ EDEMA ☐ MVP ☐ ARRHYTHMIA ☐ CYANOSIS ☐ OTHER ☐ THROMBOEMBOLISM ☐ PVD ☐ NEG

RESPIRATORY: ☐ PNEUMONIA ☐ COPD ☐ TRACHEOSTOMY ☐ URI ☐ COUGH ☐ ASTHMA ☐ SOB AT REST ☐ BRONCHITIS ☐ OTHER ☐ SOB W/EXERTION ☐ WHEEZING ☐ NEG

NEUROLOGIC: ☐ SYNCOPE ☐ TIA ☐ LOW BACK PAIN ☐ SEIZURES ☐ COMATOSE ☐ OTHER ☐ CVA ☐ NEUROPATHY ☐ NEG

ENDOCRINE/METABOLIC/RENAL/ HEPATIC: ☐ CIRRHOSIS ☐ DIABETES ☐ ANEMIA ☐ HEPATITIS ☐ HYPOGLYCEMIA ☐ BLEEDING ☐ JAUNDICE ☐ OTHER ☐ SICKLE CELL ☐ CRF ☐ NEG

OTHER: ☐ HIATAL HERNIA ☐ FULL STOMACH ☐ PREGNANCY ☐ H/O MH-FAM ☐ PSYCHIATRIC ☐ NEG

PREVIOUS SURGERIES:
☐ NONE

PREVIOUS ANESTHETIC COMPLICATIONS:
☐ NO KNOWN FAMILY HISTORY OF ANESTHESIA COMPLICATIONS
☐ NONE

REASSESSED IMMEDIATELY PREOP ☐
COMMENTS:

NPO since ________

P.E. AIRWAY MALLAMPATI CLASS 1 2 3 4

ROM: NECK:
TEETH: ☐ DENTURES ☐ CAPS ☐ LOOSE TEETH ☐ CHIPS ☐ RAGGED DENTAL EDGE ☐ PERMANENT BRIDGE
LUNGS:
HEART:
NEURO:

LABS: HGB: ____ ECG ☐ NORMAL ☐ ABNORMAL
HCT: ____ CXR ☐ NORMAL ☐ ABNORMAL
Na+: ____ SMA ☐
K+: ____ CREATININE ____
FBS: ____ PT ____
DOS: ____ PTT ____
PREG TEST: ☐ NEGATIVE ☐ POSITIVE

ASA CLASSIFICATION
1 2 3 4 5 6 E

PROPOSED ANESTHESIA
☐ REGIONAL
☐ IV ☐ EPIDURAL
☐ SPINAL ☐ OTHER
☐ GENERAL
☐ LOCAL W/ SEDATION
☐ LOC/GENERAL
☐ RAPID SEQUENCE INDUCTION

PROPOSED MONITORING
☐ A-LINE
☐ CVP
☐ SWAN

☐ PATIENT CONFUSED, UNABLE TO INTERVIEW
☐ PATIENT RELATIVE INTERVIEWED
☐ RELATIVE UNAVAILABLE
☐ MINOR - MOTHER OR FATHER INTERVIEWED

RISKS/BENEFITS: ☐ DISCUSSED AND UNDERSTOOD
☐ ALL QUESTIONS ANSWERED

SIGNATURE ________

Figure 12-3 Example of a preanesthesia evaluation form. *(Courtesy St. Joseph's Mercy of Macomb, Clinton Township, Mich.)*

Box 12-1

Classification of Patients by Risk of Anesthesia-Related Complications (American Society of Anesthesiologists [ASA])

ASA 1	The patient is normal and healthy.
ASA 2	The patient has mild systemic disease that does not limit the individual's activities (e.g., controlled hypertension or controlled diabetes without systemic sequelae).
ASA 3	The patient has moderate or severe systemic disease that does limit the individual's activities (e.g., stable angina or diabetes with systemic sequelae).
ASA 4	The patient has severe systemic disease that is a constant potential threat to life (e.g., severe congestive heart failure, end-stage renal failure).
ASA 5	The patient is morbid and is at substantial risk of death within 24 hours, with or without intervention.
E	Emergency status; any patient undergoing an emergency procedure is identified by adding "E" to the underlying ASA status (1-5). Therefore, a fundamentally healthy patient undergoing an emergency procedure would be classified as E-1.

Modified from Hata T et al: *Guidelines, education, and testing for procedural sedation and analgesia*, Iowa City, 1992-2003, University of Iowa.

patient takes routinely may interfere with, block, or increase the effect of drugs used during surgery. In some cases patients must withdraw their regular medication to prevent adverse effects. Known allergies are very important, and these should be clearly documented according to facility protocol. The patient also is asked about illegal or illicit use of drugs and alcohol and about tobacco use.

Previous History of Anesthesia

A history of having undergone general anesthesia or conscious sedation is important, especially if the patient experienced any adverse reaction during the procedure. Adverse reactions may have been the result of sensitivity to the anesthetic agents, metabolic problems, or disease. Patients who have previously experienced complications are at high risk for subsequent reactions, which might be life-threatening. The ACP attempts to determine the cause of the complications and plan the anesthesia accordingly.

Airway and Dental Status

Any abnormality of the **airway** or potential obstruction can create an anesthesia emergency. General anesthesia requires complete assessment of the airway to evaluate conditions that might lead to an airway obstruction or make intubation difficult. Dentures are removed before surgery to prevent them from becoming dislodged. Loose teeth or crowns may break loose and become an airway obstruction. Jewelry implanted in the tongue, lips, cheeks, or teeth also create a risk. These can easily become a tracheal or bronchial obstruction, especially during placement of an artificial airway, which requires

manipulation of structures in the mouth, pharynx, and larynx. Even during local or conductive anesthesia, a patient may need emergency resuscitation, requiring placement of an artificial airway.

Some patients have an anomalous or "difficult" airway. These patients are difficult to resuscitate during general anesthesia, cardiac arrest, aspiration, and other airway emergencies because they are difficult to intubate by normal means. During the preoperative evaluation, the ACP assesses the patient's airway to determine the level of risk.

Musculoskeletal Assessment

Impaired mobility, skeletal injuries, and other structural problems might lead to patient injury during positioning. The ACP therefore documents any joint replacements, previous skeletal injury, disease, and areas of nerve damage. This information is available in the patient's chart, and the ACP may provide specific information to other perioperative team members before patient positioning. During regional or monitored sedation anesthesia, the patient is not positioned while unconscious. However, any mobility problems must be considered regardless of the patient's level of consciousness.

Psychological Assessment

Many patients fear anesthesia and pain more than the surgery itself. Many people are concerned that they will have inadequate medication for pain or that they will become addicted to pain medication. Misinformation from various media sources and lack of knowledge about the pharmacology of analgesics often contribute to these fears. The ACP or perioperative nurse can answer the patient's questions about the action and duration of postoperative medication, which frequently allays the patient's fears.

Social Assessment

The patient's emotional and social well-being are important to recovery. The ACP inquires about the patient's family and friends and whether the patient will have a caregiver or helper after surgery. This affects not only the physical care of the patient, but also the psychological support available in the postoperative period. Patients who are fearful or anxious about their surgery and the possible consequences for work, family, and social environment may have a higher threshold for sedation and antianxiety medication.

Selection of Anesthesia

After the patient evaluation, an appropriate type and method of anesthesia are selected. This is a cooperative and informed decision made by the ACP, the surgeon, and the patient. The decision is based on the following:

- The patient's current physical status
- The presence or history of metabolic disease
- The patient's psychological status
- The type of surgery, including positioning requirements
- The length of the procedure
- Any past history of adverse reactions to anesthetics and drug allergies

The patient's safety and well-being are always the primary considerations in the selection of the method of anesthesia. The medical and surgical goals are to provide the appropriate level of anesthesia without compromising the patient's safety. This means that not only the patient's physical condition and past history are considered, but also the requirements of the surgical procedures. For example, some procedures may be performed with a **regional block** without unconsciousness. Patients generally are more relaxed and experience less stress when monitored sedation is provided. Many orthopedic surgeries are in this category. Other surgeries, such as those of the abdomen and thorax, require general anesthesia and invasive monitoring. The surgeon may participate in the decision based on his or her knowledge of the time required for surgery and the extent of the procedure.

Patients participate in their own anesthesia care by expressing preferences. However, these must be informed choices based on safety and environmental considerations. The ACP helps the patient choose among the "best choices." This is especially important for patients who have moderate or high risk factors to consider. Patients differ in their desire to be awake during the procedure, fully sedated, or only partly conscious. All patients have the right to be fully informed of the risks and benefits of various types of anesthesia to help determine the course of their treatment.

Preoperative Testing

Diagnostic testing to determine the patient's risk level has been routine for many decades. In current practice (in the United States), fewer tests are performed than previously. Institutions vary in their requirements for preoperative testing, and the rationale for ordering tests generally is based on the patient's history and physical examination findings. In these cases, the tests are intended to confirm or elaborate upon a finding rather than to discover an abnormality.

PREOPERATIVE PREPARATION OF THE PATIENT

Admission Documentation and Preoperative Checklist

Every precaution is taken to ensure the patient's safety in the perioperative period. When the patient arrives in surgery, a checklist is used to ensure that all preoperative procedures have been completed. The admission procedure is extremely important to the patient's emotional well-being. Reassurance and physical comfort are critical in this first encounter.

In the ambulatory setting, patient teaching is done before the day of surgery and the patient is made aware of special precautions and procedures. Inpatients are prepared in the ward. Routine preoperative care is provided plus any specific needs required because of the patient's individual physical or emotional status. Hospitals and other surgical facilities have individual check-in protocols. However, specific details are always verified:

1. **Patient identity** is meticulously checked. The health care provider asks the patient his or her name and verifies this with the patient's identification band, the surgery schedule, and the medical records at hand.
2. **Correct procedure, side, and site** are validated with the patient, the medical record, the surgical schedule, and the consent form. Preoperative procedures may have included skin markings on the operative side. These are matched with all other information available.
3. **Surgical and anesthesia consent forms** must be signed according to facility protocol. (Details on legal aspects of the consent were described in Chapter 4.)
4. **Resuscitation orders** and any other legal documents are checked.
5. **Patient allergies** must be noted on all medical records, and the patient is asked about allergies again in the holding area.
6. **Preoperative medications** are documented in the patient's medical and preoperative records. Any medication ordered but not yet given may be administered in the holding area as directed by the surgeon or ACP.
7. **Prostheses,** including dentures and hearing aids, must be removed before surgery whenever possible. In the event a prosthesis is removed in the holding area, extreme care is taken to protect it from loss or misidentification.
8. **Jewelry** is removed before induction of general anesthesia or any procedure in which electrosurgery is used. Any jewelry removed in the holding area is placed in a container, labeled, and placed in a secure location until it can be safely returned to the patient. A wedding ring may be taped in place.
9. **Any medical records** accompanying the patient are noted. Diagnostic results accompanying the patient, such as radiographs or other imaging studies, are clearly labeled.

Any **preoperative medication** is administered the night before surgery or in the perioperative holding area. Historically, preoperative drugs were given routinely while the patient was awaiting surgery on the hospital ward. In the past, patients were heavily sedated, and most arrived in the operating room disoriented and difficult to rouse. These sedatives also prolonged their anesthesia recovery, caused **delirium**, cardiovascular risks, and produced many unpleasant side effects. The purposes of premedication are to:
- Reduce anxiety
- Enable a smooth induction
- Reduce gastric acidity and volume
- Reduce the amount of general anesthetic used

The current practice in anesthesiology is selective preoperative medication for patients with specific risks or conditions that can be mitigated by drugs. For example, a patient at high risk for aspiration of stomach contents is given drugs to reduce the pH of gastric secretions and to reduce gastric volume. Patients who are extremely anxious before surgery may be given a light sedative. *Antibiotic prophylaxis* is the preoperative administration of antibiotics for patients at high risk for postoperative infection.

Preoperative fasting is required to minimize aspiration (inhalation) of gastric contents during general anesthesia. In the past, all liquids and food were withheld after midnight the day of surgery. However, this rigid parameter is no longer considered standard practice. Strict fasting in pediatric and geriatric patients may lead to dehydration, headache, and irritability, especially when surgery is delayed. A safer and more realistic fasting period is now determined by the type of surgery and the patient's age and condition. Clear fluids generally are now acceptable 2 to 3 hours before surgery within a 7- to 8-hour fasting period.

Arrival in the Surgical Suite

After being admitted to the surgical department, the patient is brought to the operating suite. The person usually is transferred to the operating bed but in selected cases may be anesthetized on the stretcher. Warmth and other comfort measures are very important at this time. The anesthesia personnel and circulator ensure that the patient is comfortable on the operating bed and that safety straps have been applied. An intravenous (IV) line is established as soon as possible to provide a method of drug administration. An IV line is necessary both for general anesthesia and for regional anesthesia.

PHYSIOLOGICAL MONITORING DURING SURGERY

PURPOSE AND RATIONALE

In a state of well-being, the body responds readily to stimuli to maintain life. Many complex biochemical, physical, and metabolic processes control the balance between stimuli and responses. Examples are *shivering* (uncontrollable muscle tremor) when the body's temperature drops and *vasoconstriction* (constriction of blood vessels) when blood pressure falls. This maintenance of physiological balance is called *homeostasis*.

During surgery, the ACP and registered nurse assess and control the body's normal responses to noxious (harmful or painful) stimuli. Physiological monitoring provides the basis on which personnel assess homeostasis and respond to the patient's needs.

Physiological monitoring is assessment of the patient's vital metabolic functions. All anesthetics (regional, general, or sedative) require physiological monitoring. Not all monitoring requires an ACP, but standards for safe care must be followed by licensed perioperative personnel. A surgical technologist may be asked to measure the patient's vital signs if he or she has not received anesthetic drugs. Assessment and interpretation requires that a licensed clinical nurse and a licensed nurse *must be present in the room at all times* with the patient receiving an anesthetic or adjunct drugs.

Monitoring is necessary because anesthetic drugs, position changes, and the trauma of surgery itself alter and in some cases prevent normal body functions. Protective reflexes (e.g., respiration, gagging, swallowing, and withdrawal from pain) are suppressed during general anesthesia. Rapid physiological changes can occur during positioning (e.g., tilting the patient's body or placing the legs in stirrups). Many types of anesthetic agents cause changes in the blood pressure and heart rate. Sedating and analgesic drugs can depress respiratory function. The complexity and type of monitoring depends on the patient's physical condition, the known risks, and the anticipated complications.

MONITORING PROCESS

The standards for monitoring patients in the United States are set by the ASA. The routine parameters that must be monitored include the following:

- **Oxygenation:** The oxygen levels in the inspired gas and blood are measured.
- **Ventilation:** The exchange of oxygen for carbon dioxide through the lungs is verified by blood tests.
- **Perfusion:** The circulatory system must be monitored continually to ensure that blood reaches all vital tissues of the body.
- **Body temperature:** The patient's core temperature must be assessed and maintained within a range compatible with normal homeostasis.
- **Neuromuscular response:** This parameter is monitored in selected cases when neuromuscular blocking agents are used.
- **Fluid balance:** Electrolyte and fluid balance are continually monitored, especially during lengthy cases or in very ill patients.

Oxygenation

Oxygenation is the ratio of oxygen present in inspired gas and the amount available to tissues through the circulating blood. Devices used for monitoring oxygenation are:

- **Oxygen analyzer:** This device is a mechanism of the machine used to deliver general anesthesia. The analyzer measures the amount of oxygen delivered and triggers an alarm when the percent is too low.
- **Pulse oximeter:** This device measures the arterial oxygen saturation of blood and the pulse rate. It operates by the principles of spectrometry, in which the amount of light that passes through a solution (blood) reveals its density. A small light source implanted in an adhesive strip or finger clip is placed in a vascular area, such as the fingertip, earlobe, or toe. This allows continuous monitoring of these parameters.

Ventilation and Perfusion

Ventilation is the exchange of carbon dioxide and oxygen between the body and the outside environment. This takes place through the respiratory system. Inadequate ventilation prevents oxygen from reaching the tissues and results in injury or death. Perfusion is the oxygen saturation in the blood. Methods of monitoring ventilation and perfusion include:

- **Observation:** The patient's thorax is observed for expansion.
- **Capnography:** Expired carbon dioxide, which is a product of ventilation, is measured. Exhaled gas is analyzed and the results displayed in waveform on a monitor.
- **Anesthesia alarm:** When an anesthesia machine is in use during general anesthesia, an alarm is triggered whenever the ventilation system is interrupted.
- **Clinical evaluation:** Trained, licensed personnel are required to monitor the patient for clinical signs of **cyanosis** (lack of oxygen in the blood). Cyanosis is a characteristic blue-gray appearance of the skin and mucous membranes. Other clinical signs are also assessed, such as the level and type of respiration, skin mottling, and breath sounds.
- **Arterial blood gas:** Blood gases may be assessed through an arterial sample. This test measures the patient's ventilation, electrolytes, and renal (acid-base) status. Ventilation is measured by evaluating the partial pressure of carbon dioxide in the blood.
- **Pulse oximetry:** As mentioned previously, the pulse oximeter is a digital sensor that detects oxygen saturation through the skin. The device is placed on a highly vascular area of the body (digit or earlobe), which makes continuous readings available.

Circulation and Fluid Balance

The ACP maintains intravascular volume and pressure using drugs and IV solutions. IV solutions are classified as *hypertonic* (greater solute concentration than plasma), *hypotonic* (lower solute concentration than plasma), or *isotonic* (equal in solute concentration to plasma). During surgery, the scrub and circulating nurse track the amount of irrigation fluid and suctioned blood to assist in computation of total fluid loss and replacement needs. Fluids are administered by a mechanical/digital pump, which delivers the exact rate of fluids programmed into the pump's computer.

Circulation is heart action that results in the delivery of blood to all tissues of the body. Circulatory assessment includes monitoring of heart function, which provides the pumping action needed to move blood through the tissues and peripheral circulation, as measured by the blood pressure and pulse rate.

Two types of methods are used to monitor circulation, direct (invasive) methods and indirect (noninvasive) methods. Direct monitoring requires the insertion of a measuring device (such as an internal pulmonary artery catheter) inside the patient's body.

- **Electrocardiography:** Electrocardiography (ECG) measures the electrical activity of the heart, which is projected into a waveform. ECG leads generally are placed on the thorax in a pattern that accurately detects and transmits the electrical impulses of the heart to the monitor (Figure 12-4).
- **Arterial blood pressure monitoring:** Blood pressure is measured manually with a mechanical sphygmomanometer and blood pressure cuff or automatically using a digital blood pressure monitoring system.

- **Transesophageal monitoring:** A transesophageal ("through the esophagus") stethoscope may be inserted to monitor the heart's rhythm, intensity, pitch, and frequency during general anesthesia. Respiratory sounds and rate also are monitored through the stethoscope, which is attached to a small earpiece.
- **Direct arterial monitoring:** Direct measurements of blood pressure may be obtained through an arterial line. The pulmonary artery catheter (also known as a *Swan Ganz line*) is used for critical care monitoring in selected patients. This allows direct assessment of pulmonary artery pressure and indirect left ventricular filling pressures. Central venous pressure is obtained by catheterization of one of the large veins, such as the subclavian vein. The catheter is advanced into the superior vena cava, where direct measurements of the right atrium and vena cava can be obtained.

Body Temperature

The normal body temperature is 97°F to 99.5°F (36° to 37.5°C). The body can tolerate environmental temperatures outside this range, but only with protection. The core temperature must be maintained within a range compatible with life. Perioperative personnel provide methods of maintaining body temperature, and the ACP monitors the temperature.

During general anesthesia, the body temperature is measured with various types of internal and external devices. Tympanic, esophageal, skin, rectal, bladder, and axillary thermometers are used. During cardiac surgery, probes can be inserted into the myocardium to monitor the temperature of the heart. A temperature sensor may also be contained with the pulmonary artery catheter used for direct measurement of arterial pressure.

Maintaining the Patient's Temperature

The patient's normal temperature is maintained with a forced air blanket or pad, warm fluids, and environmental control. The forced air blanket is a baffled air mattress that rests lightly on the patient's body. Warmed air is pumped into sections of the blanket via a flexible hose. The warm air blanket must be monitored to prevent burns. These risks are greatest when the patient is unconscious or semiconscious and unable to respond to pain. The temperature setting and the air hose-to-blanket connection should be checked before the unit is activated and thereafter at regular intervals throughout the surgical procedure.

The device should be activated only after the correct temperature has been verified with the ACP. If the connection is loose and the air hose becomes detached during surgery, the patient's skin may be exposed to a column of heated air. This might go unnoticed under the surgical drapes. Pediatric and geriatric patients and patients who are thin or debilitated are at particular risk for burns. Meticulous attention to any device that creates heat is the collaborative responsibility of everyone on the operating team.

Deliberate Hypothermia

Deliberate **hypothermia** (lowering of the patient's core body temperature) is used during **malignant hyperthermia**. This

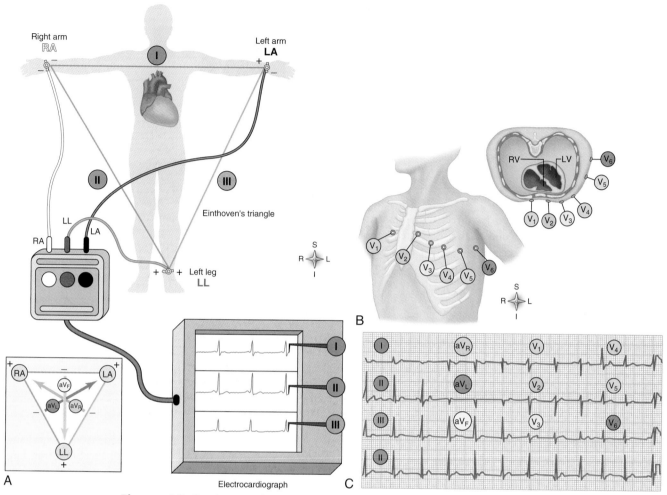

Figure 12-4 Electrocardiogram leads and output. Here, the electrodes are placed on right and left arms and the left leg to measure the electrical activity of the heart. The leads are placed on the chest wall during surgery. *(From Thibodeau GA, Patton KT:* Anatomy and physiology, *ed 3, St Louis, 2007, Mosby.)*

is a physiological reaction to specific anesthetics and neuromuscular blocking agents in which the body temperature is critically elevated (discussed later in the chapter). Hypothermia may also be initiated when normal blood flow presents a severe, uncontrollable risk. In cardiac surgery, surgical repair of large vessels, organ transplantation, and neurosurgery, **controlled hypothermia** produces a margin of safety while particular surgical procedures are performed.

Methods of Achieving Hypothermia

Hypothermia is obtained by a number of methods. Blood may be diverted to a cooling system, as during cardiopulmonary bypass. Other methods include IV administration of a cold solution and irrigation of body cavities with a cold fluid. During cardiac surgery, saline ice slush is packed around the heart to produce localized cooling. Target temperatures are no lower than 78.8° F (26° C).

Complications of induced hypothermia include cardiac arrhythmia, which occurs when normal conduction is interrupted. This can lead to heart block and cardiac arrest. Other organs of the body also may suffer damage as a result of inadequate blood supply.

Rewarming is achieved with a heating blanket, heating mattress, warm IV fluids, and warm cotton blankets. Shivering, which increases the body's requirements for oxygen, is controlled with muscle relaxants, selected analgesics, and further rewarming. The patient is rewarmed slowly to reduce the risk of circulatory collapse or sudden dilation or constriction of blood vessels.

Neuromuscular Response

During general anesthesia, neuromuscular blocking agents are administered to relax skeletal muscles. Without adequate muscle relaxation or paralysis, retraction of the body wall and other tissues is difficult, and this prevents adequate exposure of the operative site. Controlled (mechanical or manual) ventilation is required whenever a neuromuscular blocking agent is used, because the respiratory muscles are paralyzed.

A peripheral nerve stimulator is used to monitor the level of neuromuscular blocking. The stimulator delivers a series of painless electrical impulses. Muscle twitching in response to the stimuli produces a means of evaluating the degree of neuromuscular blockade.

Level of Consciousness

The patient's level of consciousness is monitored to prevent **intraoperative awareness (IOA)**. This is a rare phenomenon in which the patient retains some degree of consciousness (including sensory awareness) but lacks motor ability. The **bispectral index system (BIS)** is used to prevent patient recall of pain perceived during surgery. BIS electrodes are attached to the head to measure the level of hypnosis during anesthesia. Although intraoperative awareness is rare, the psychological consequences are serious and include post-traumatic symptoms.

Renal Function

Renal function can be assessed by direct measurement of urine output and through blood analysis. Selected surgical patients are catheterized before surgery so that fluid balance (input and output) can be measured during lengthy procedures.

METHODS OF ANESTHESIA

GENERAL ANESTHESIA

Description

General anesthesia is *reversible loss of consciousness*, which is accompanied by the *absence* of:

- Pain
- Sensory perception
- Cognition (thought, learning, language)
- Memory of experiences during the period of unconsciousness
- Some autonomic reflexes

During general anesthesia, different types of drugs are used to achieve the effects needed for surgery. For example, the anesthetic may cause loss of consciousness but not muscle relaxation. In this case, a separate muscle relaxant is administered during surgery. Other drugs are given to inhibit secretions (saliva). This combination of drugs and anesthetic agents is sometimes referred to as **balanced anesthesia**.

An inhalation anesthetic is used for prolonged surgery. IV agents are used to induce unconsciousness or to maintain deep sedation during short procedures. During inhalation anesthesia, an IV drug is used for **induction** (causing unconsciousness), and the inhalation anesthetic is used to maintain unconsciousness.

Anesthesia Machine

General anesthesia requires the use of an anesthesia machine (Figure 12-5).

The **anesthesia machine** is a complex biotechnical device used in patient monitoring, respiratory function, and administration of inhalation anesthesia. An inhalation anesthetic is administered in the form of a volatile liquid that is changed into a gas in the vaporizer. The basic mechanism is a return flow system that includes the patient's inspiratory and expiratory functions. Important components are the vaporizer, ventilator, breathing apparatus, and **gas scavenging** system.

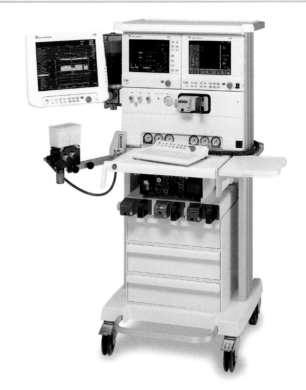

Figure 12-5 Anesthesia machine. *(Courtesy Datex-Ohmeda, Madison, Wis.)*

The anesthesia machine allows the patient to be mechanically ventilated or hand ventilated with the **breathing bag**, which is part of the ventilator and valve system. Gases enter the bag and then are delivered to the patient through a tube, which is connected to an invasive airway or face mask. Exhaled carbon dioxide is captured from the system measured, and absorbed by a soda lime reservoir.

The anesthesia face mask is used to deliver positive-pressure ventilation with anesthetic gas and oxygen. An anesthesia face mask generally is not used in place of an invasive airway device except for administration of oxygen or brief sedation or to induce anesthesia in pediatric patients (Figure 12-6).

Cleaning, disinfection, and basic troubleshooting of the anesthesia machine are the responsibilities of the anesthesia technologist. Maintenance and testing of the machine are performed by the bioengineering department. All equipment that comes in contact with the patient must be decontaminated to prevent cross-contamination. Standard Precautions are followed whenever equipment is handled and used. The hoses, soda canister, masks, and airways are sources of high bacterial contamination. The intricate valve mechanisms may also harbor large colonies of pathogenic bacteria. The use of disposable patient air hoses, masks, and airways is preferred whenever possible. Nondisposable items are decontaminated and sterilized.

Scavenging System

Escape of anesthetic gas into the surgical suite is an environmental hazard for health care workers. Scavenging systems capture escaped gases and vent them through a vacuum line.

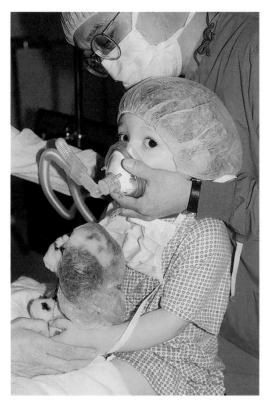

Figure 12-6 Pediatric patient with an anesthesia mask. *(From Leibert PS: Color atlas of pediatric surgery, ed 2, Philadelphia, 1996, WB Saunders.)*

The National Institute for Occupational Safety and Health (NIOSH) and the Occupational Safety and Health Administration (OSHA) regulate the allowable percentage of environmental anesthetic agent in the air. Scavenging equipment can reduce health care worker exposure up to 95%.

More information on the hazards of environmental exposure to anesthetic gas are available at http://www.cdc.gov/niosh/docs/2007-151/.

Medical Gases

Medical-grade gases include oxygen, nitrogen, air, and nitrous oxide. These are obtained through an in-line hose from wall outlets or from metal tanks (cylinders). Hoses for gas delivery to the anesthesia machine originate through in-line sources. Portable oxygen tanks are available for use during transportation of the patient recovering from anesthesia. (Chapter 14 presents a complete discussion on the safety and handling of gas tanks.)

AIRWAY MANAGEMENT

Managing the patient's airway is a primary concern during general anesthesia or an emergency in which the patient is unable to maintain respiration. During an emergency, such as cardiac or respiratory arrest, securing the patient's airway is the first priority. During surgery, the unconscious patient requires an invasive artificial airway to provide a sealed connection between the source of air, oxygen and anesthetic gases, and the patient's lung. It also supports the patient's natural

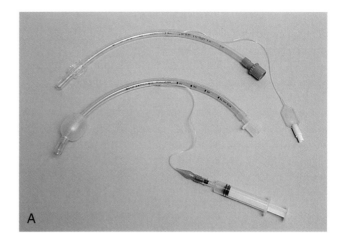

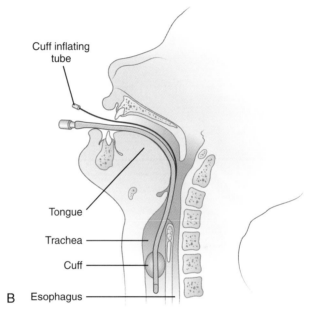

Figure 12-7 **A,** Endotracheal tubes. **B,** Endotracheal tube in position. *(**A** from Elkin MK, Perry PA: Nursing interventions and clinical skills, ed 3, St Louis, 2004, Mosby; **B** redrawn from Rothrock JC: Alexander's care of the patient in surgery, ed 12, St Louis, 2003, Mosby.)*

airway structures. The process of placing the invasive airway is called **intubation** (discussed later in the chapter). Less invasive airways are used to maintain the position of the tongue and support the soft tissues of the pharynx and larynx.

Types of Airways
Endotracheal Tube
The **endotracheal tube** (ET tube) is an invasive airway that extends from the mouth to the trachea. It is inserted orally or, less commonly, through the nose. The tube has a balloon or cuff at the tip that acts as a barrier between the upper and lower airways and prevents aspiration of fluid into the respiratory tract (Figure 12-7). The ET tube is inserted with the aid of a rigid or flexible **laryngoscope**, a lighted instrument that is inserted into the trachea during intubation (Figure 12-8).

Laryngeal Mask

The **laryngeal mask airway (LMA)** is inserted without the aid of a laryngoscope and fits snugly over the larynx. The LMA is used in patients with a difficult airway condition. However, it does not protect against aspiration (Figure 12-9).

Oropharyngeal Airway

The oropharyngeal airway (OPA) is inserted over the tongue to prevent the tongue or epiglottis from falling back against the pharynx (Figure 12-10, *A*). The OPA is commonly used when the patient is semiconscious, such as during the recovery period in general anesthesia or during an airway emergency. The OPA is used in patients who have respiratory function but need upper airway support (Figure 12-10, *B*).

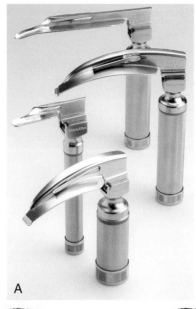

A

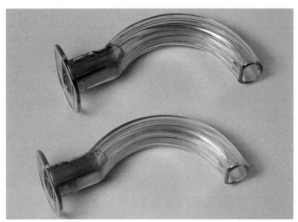

Figure 12-8 Various sizes of laryngoscopes. *(From Elkin MK, Perry PA: Nursing interventions and clinical skills, ed 4, St Louis, 2007, Mosby.)*

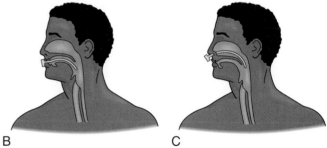

B   C

Figure 12-10 **A,** Oropharyngeal airway used in conscious patients who require support of the pharynx. **B,** Position of the oropharyngeal airway. **C,** Nasopharyngeal airway. *(**A** courtesy Welch Allyn, Skaneateles Falls, NY; **B** and **C** modified from Sorrentino SA: Mosby's textbook for nursing assistants, ed 5, St Louis, 2000, Mosby.)*

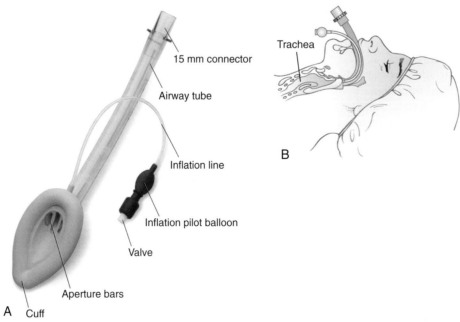

15 mm connector

Airway tube

Inflation line

Inflation pilot balloon

Valve

Aperture bars

A   Cuff

Trachea

B

Figure 12-9 **A,** Laryngeal mask. **B,** Laryngeal mask in place. Note the position over the larynx. *(**A** courtesy LMA North America; **B** redrawn from Phillips N: Berry and Kohn's operating room technique, ed 10, St Louis, 2004, Mosby.)*

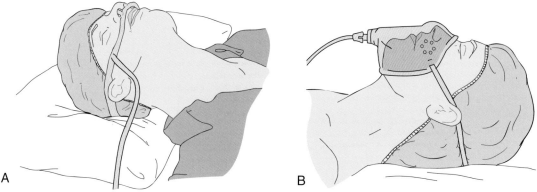

Figure 12-11 Oxygen delivery. **A,** Nasal cannula. **B,** Oxygen face mask for passive delivery of oxygen. *(Modified from Sorrentino SA: Mosby's textbook for nursing assistants, ed 5, St Louis, 2000, Mosby.)*

Nasopharyngeal Airway

The nasopharyngeal airway provides passage between the nostril and the nasopharynx. This type of airway is used in a semiconscious patient when an OPA causes gagging or when a mouth injury (e.g., fracture) is present (Figure 12-10, *C*).

Oxygen Delivery

Patients that do not need assisted ventilation receive oxygen by a nonocclusive mask or nasal cannula (Figure 12-11). These systems deliver a small amount of oxygen combined with room air. Face masks cover both the nose and mouth and can be adjusted to regulate the ratio of oxygen to air. This is passive delivery of oxygen, because the patient retains respiratory function.

Intubation

As mentioned previously, insertion of an invasive airway is called *intubation*. Intubation is a routine procedure during general anesthesia and is performed during respiratory and cardiac arrest. The patient usually is unconscious (e.g., during general anesthesia). However, conscious intubation also is performed when the patient is awake but requires airway support. Intubation with an ET tube requires a rigid or flexible laryngoscope to guide the ET tube into the trachea (Figure 12-12).

During general anesthesia, the patient is intubated immediately after *induction* (administration of a drug that causes unconsciousness). Intubation is a critical process, because the patient's respiratory status may be unstable. During general anesthesia, the circulator stands at the patient's head and assists as needed during intubation.

The ACP may ask the circulator to apply cricoid pressure to prevent aspiration during induction of the ET tube. **Cricoid pressure** is digital occlusion of the esophagus by applying external pressure over the cricoid cartilage during intubation. Pressure is directly applied on the cricoid cartilage located just inferior to the thyroid cartilage and cricoid notch (Figure 12-13). When the airway is in place, it is connected to the anesthesia machine and the inhalation drug is initiated.

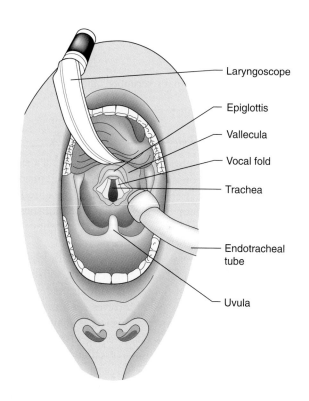

Figure 12-12 Endotracheal intubation is performed immediately after induction of general anesthesia. The airway is inserted with the aid of a laryngoscope. *(From Garden O, Bradbury A, Forsythe J, Parks R: Principles and practice of surgery, ed 5, Edinburgh, 2007, Churchill Livingstone.)*

The scrubbed surgical technologist should always remain to assist in case of cardiac arrest, aspiration, or other anesthetic emergency. The exact role of the surgical technologist during any emergency depends on the nature of the event. This is a critical period during surgery, and the scrub shares responsibility for the patient's safety. During this period, attention should be focused on the patient and ACP until an airway is secured and the patient is stabilized. The surgical

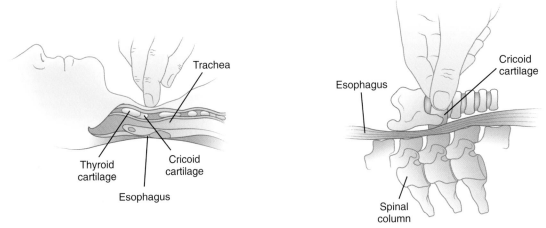

Figure 12-13 Application of cricoid pressure during intubation (Sellick maneuver). This procedure collapses the esophagus and helps ensure correct insertion of the airway into the trachea. *(Modified from Phillips N: Berry and Kohn's operating room technique, ed 10, St Louis, 2004, Mosby.)*

technologist should remain scrubbed and attentive in case assistance is needed.

PHASES OF GENERAL ANESTHESIA

The most prominent physiological effect of general anesthesia is reversible loss of consciousness, which is maintained while the anesthetic agent is administered. When the anesthetic is withdrawn, the patient quickly regains consciousness. The time and event-related phases of general anesthesia are as follows:

1. **Induction:** General anesthesia begins with loss of consciousness. An induction agent (IV drug, inhalation gas, or combination of the two) is administered.
2. **Maintenance:** This phase involves continuation of the anesthetic agent; unconsciousness is maintained with the inhalation agent and adjunct agents.
3. **Emergence:** This phase is the cessation of the anesthetic. Reversal drugs may be administered, and the patient regains consciousness.
4. **Recovery:** Postanesthesia care is provided in this phase.

Preinduction

The process of general anesthesia starts when all perioperative team members are present and preparations to start surgery have been completed. The patient is brought into the surgical suite, and noninvasive monitoring devices are put in place. If the patient does not have an IV line, the ACP inserts one when the patient arrives and ensures that the patient is comfortable and relaxed. The patient is positioned supine (lying face up), and the head is elevated slightly to facilitate respiration and immediate intubation after induction.

General anesthesia begins only after patient monitoring devices are in place and the operating team is present. The ACP assembles all needed drugs and equipment and reassures the patient while evaluating the individual's physiological status. Preoperative drugs that provide sedation and reduce anxiety may be given during this period.

Suction must be available to the ACP at all times. As long as the patient is in the operating suite, suction must remain operative. In-line suction is available from ceiling posts, cables, or wall outlets. When connecting suction cables, match the two ends of the connector, push, and turn the connector to secure it. This locking mechanism prevents the cables from separating.

Suction is delivered through a rigid or flexible suction tip. The *suction catheter* is a flexible tube that can be inserted through an airway (oral or nasal) to remove secretions below the pharyngeal cavity. The rigid suction tip has a blunt end and is used to sweep the oral and pharyngeal cavity.

Just before induction, the ACP may administer 100% oxygen to the patient through a face mask. The purpose of this is to ensure that tissues are fully oxygenated from the start of the procedure. If a temporary airway obstruction occurs, the reserve oxygen will already be in the system for rapid uptake into tissues.

Induction

During induction, the patient passes through stages from consciousness to deep surgical anesthesia. Modern anesthetics and adjunct drugs allow the patient to pass through these stages very quickly, and they are seldom distinct. The stages are:

- Stage I: The patient is conscious.
- Stage II: Delirium ensues, marked by unconsciousness and exaggerated reflexes. The airway remains intact and under the patient's control. Hearing is maintained. The pupils are dilated.
- Surgical anesthesia: The patient is relaxed, and protective reflexes (gagging, blinking, and swallowing) are lost. The patient is unable to maintain an open airway, and the respiratory response fails.

The patient is induced with an inhalation anesthetic by mask or with an IV **sedative**, which causes unconsciousness within seconds. During induction, perioperative staff members must carry out their tasks as quietly as possible. Although induction takes place very quickly, the patient is able to hear well into the induction period. Conversation should stop, and care should be taken to minimize noise. The patient can easily misinterpret sounds and verbal exchanges during induction, because the ability to interpret the environment accurately recedes. Immediately after induction, the patient is intubated.

Maintenance

Anesthesia maintenance begins when the patient's airway is secured and inhalation drugs can be administered. During maintenance, which represents the period of surgery itself, the ACP *titrates* (calculates and measures) the appropriate ratio of anesthetic agents and oxygen. These are delivered into the ventilatory system of the anesthesia machine and delivered to the patient via the airway. The level of consciousness, analgesia, and sedation are continually monitored, along with physiological parameters. All drugs and procedures are documented in the anesthesia record throughout the procedure.

Inhalation anesthetic is delivered through the airway (mask, laryngeal mask, or ET tube. The patient's ventilation is controlled by the ACP using a respirator. The ratio of oxygen to other anesthetic gases is adjusted and controlled through the anesthesia machine's ventilation system.

Neuromuscular Blockade ("Muscle Relaxation")

Adequate muscle relaxation is necessary during general anesthesia to allow manipulation of the body wall and other tissues in the operative site. Anesthetic agents vary in their effect on skeletal muscles. Most do not provide sufficient relaxation for surgery, and a separate drug must be administered. A muscle relaxant drug is called a **neuromuscular blocking agent**. This category of drugs causes paralysis by blocking neurotransmission to the muscle tissue. The level of paralysis is monitored continually throughout the procedure with a nerve stimulator. The level of relaxation is maintained at a minimum to prevent overdose. If increased relaxation is needed (e.g., during deep retraction), incremental doses can be administered.

Emergence

Termination of anesthesia and the process of regaining consciousness is called **emergence**. The ACP controls emergence by withdrawing (stopping) the anesthetic agents and reversing the effects of adjunct drugs as necessary. Narcotic reversal drugs are administered as needed to block the action of specific drugs administered during the maintenance phase of anesthesia.

When the patient regains consciousness, protective airway responses resume and the ACP may remove the artificial airway. Removal of the airway is called **extubation**. A nasal or oral airway may be inserted at this time. Emergence can occur quickly and generally proceeds smoothly. Occasionally the patient (especially children) may enter a state of temporary delirium during emergence. However, this is rare in adults.

Reversal drugs (discussed later) may be administered to hasten emergence.

Recovery

When stable, the patient is transferred to a stretcher and transported to the **postanesthesia recovery unit (PACU)**. During transportation, oxygen may be administered from a portable tank. Patients who require continuous cardiac monitoring are transported with a portable unit. On arrival in the PACU, the staff nurse receives the patient. Oxygen tubing is transferred from the portable unit to a wall outlet, and cardiac leads or other monitoring devices are connected to the PACU system. Suction is made immediately available for airway clearance. The nurse receives a report of the operative procedure, the patient's physiological status, and the anesthesia process from the ACP. The patient remains in the PACU until physiologically stable and conscious so that critical care personnel can respond to any emergency that may arise during recovery.

DISSOCIATIVE ANESTHESIA

Dissociative anesthesia is caused by the drug *Ketamine*, which blocks sensory neurotransmission and associative pathways. The patient's eyes remain open and the person appears to be awake, but he or she is unaware of the environment. The drug produces retrograde amnesia. Ketamine is administered intravenously or intramuscularly and is used for short procedures. It is used mainly in pediatric surgery. It is combined with other drugs to produce desired effects and reduce side effects such as excessive salivation and delirium during emergence. Muscle relaxants often are used in conjunction with ketamine to increase muscle tone.

The advantages of ketamine are rapid induction and metabolism. The disadvantages are related mainly to cardiac stimulation and potential psychological effects, including delirium and hallucinations, which occur in adults more often than in children. Ketamine is contraindicated in surgery of the upper respiratory system because it does not suppress laryngeal and tracheal reflexes.

CONSCIOUS SEDATION

Conscious sedation is used for short diagnostic and minor surgical procedures that do not require deep anesthesia. In this process, a combination of sedatives, hypnotics, and analgesics is administered intravenously. The patient can respond to verbal commands and breathe independently but is sedated to tolerate the procedure. Patients undergoing conscious sedation are monitored continuously throughout the procedure.

Minimal sedation is a state in which the patient can respond to verbal commands. Cognitive function and muscular coordination may be impaired. The patient's ventilatory and cardiovascular systems remain unaffected.

In *moderate sedation*, the patient's consciousness is depressed. However, the person can respond to verbal commands when stimulated. Airway support is not needed, and

Table 12-1

Characteristics of Levels of Sedation

Sedation Level	Level of Consciousness	Airway	Verbal Response	Response to Touch
No sedation	Aware of environment and self	Normal or adequate	Normal or adequate	Normal or adequate
Light sedation	Sedated but aware of environment and self	Normal or adequate	Adequate or limited Abnormal	Normal or adequate
Moderate sedation	Sleepy but easily aroused, slight awareness of environment	May require airway support	Limited or none	Adequate or limited Abnormal
Deep sedation	Unaware of environment or self	May be mildly abnormal or absent	None	Only partially responsive to pain
Surgical general anesthesia	Unconscious; does not respond to pain	Limited or absent	None	No response to touch or pain

the patient can breathe independently. The cardiovascular system usually is unaffected.

During *deep sedation*, the patient cannot be roused easily but responds to pain stimulation. Ventilatory function is intact but may be depressed. Cardiovascular functions remain intact.

Table 12-1 shows the levels of sedation.

DRUGS USED IN GENERAL ANESTHESIA AND CONSCIOUS SEDATION

Inhalation Anesthetics

In the past, highly flammable anesthetic gases such as cyclopropane and vaporized ether were commonly used during surgery. These agents were highly flammable and explosive. Conductive shoes, nonstatic flooring, and high environmental humidity were necessary to prevent surgical fires, which were relatively common compared with today. These potent agents caused serious side effects, and the risk of anesthesia was significant. Flammable anesthetic agents are no longer permitted in surgery, which creates a much safer environment for both patients and personnel.

Inhalation anesthetics are stored as liquids and administered as a vapor (gas). Only nitrous oxide is both stored and delivered in gaseous form. All other agents must be vaporized in the anesthesia machine before administration. The agent enters the lungs, where it crosses the alveoli and is made available to the nervous system, producing deep sedation and unconsciousness.

All anesthetics cause some respiratory and circulatory depression. Other side effects are considered when a particular agent is selected for a patient. Inhalation agents are commonly administered after induction with an IV drug (induction agent).

Nitrous Oxide

Nitrous oxide is a colorless, odorless gas in its natural state. It has low potency, but adjusting its concentration provides a range of anesthetic effects. It has strong analgesic properties

and is quickly dissipated from the body, usually within minutes. Nitrous oxide is not flammable, but it supports combustion.

Nitrous oxide does affect the major body systems, including the heart. In some patients it can cause severe cardiovascular depression, leading to shock. It does not affect the respiratory system or the action of neuromuscular blocking agents. It causes rapid induction, and it is used mainly with other agents. It may be used alone for short procedures. The main advantages of nitrous oxide are a decreased incidence of nausea and rapid absorption and clearance from the body. Disadvantages include low potency and lack of muscle relaxation.

Isoflurane

Isoflurane is widely used for many different types of surgery. It causes rapid, smooth induction and good muscle relaxation. It is nonflammable and has a strong odor. The systemic effects of isoflurane are superior to those of other inhalation agents. Cardiac and respiratory depression are minimal. Unlike many other agents, it does not cause bronchial spasm. Another advantage of this agent is its low metabolism, which reduces or eliminates liver and kidney toxicity. It does potentiate (increase the effects) of neuromuscular blocking agents.

Sevoflurane

Sevoflurane is very similar to isoflurane. It is nonflammable and nonirritating. It can be used safely for induction in both pediatric and adult patients. It is commonly used for anesthesia and maintenance, especially in short procedures when little postoperative pain is expected. Patients emerge rapidly from sevoflurane, making it useful for outpatient surgery. It does cause increased postoperative nausea and vomiting compared with other agents.

Desflurane

Desflurane is only partly metabolized and provides rapid emergence. This advantage makes it popular for outpatient surgery when a short recovery time is important. However, it is irritating to the upper respiratory tract and can cause gagging, coughing, laryngospasm, and **bronchospasm**. This makes it a poor induction agent.

The systemic effects of desflurane are minimal. It undergoes little metabolism by the liver and is quickly eliminated by the lungs. It may not be suitable for patients with a history of cardiac disease, because it can increase the heart rate. Desflurane must be heated during vaporization.

Halothane and Ethrane

Halothane was among the first volatile anesthetics developed in the 1960s.

In the past, halothane was widely used for most types of surgery. However, it is highly toxic to the liver and may cause hepatic failure in some individuals. Halothane causes decreased cardiac output and is known to trigger malignant hypothermia, a potentially fatal anesthetic reaction (see later discussion). Halothane is a powerful depressant that produces deep anesthesia. Ethrane is similar in chemical structure and side effects to halothane. Both have been replaced by safer, more efficient volatile anesthetics.

Sedative and Hypnotics (Induction Agents)

Sedative and hypnotic drugs are used to induce unconsciousness during general anesthesia. Drugs that cause sedation are dose related, and increasing the amount of the drug usually produces a deeper level of sedation or even unconsciousness. Under mild and moderate sedation, a person can respond to verbal commands. Respiratory and cardiovascular functions remain intact. A deeply sedated patient cannot be easily roused and ventilation may be decreased, but cardiovascular functions remain intact.

Desirable qualities for an induction agent are rapid onset, minimal or no cardiovascular depression, and rapid clearance from the body. Selected drugs in this category may also be used for maintenance of anesthesia during short procedures.

Some commonly used induction agents are propofol, etomidate, thiopental, and ketamine.

Adverse Effects of Sedatives and Hypnotics

- Respiratory depression, synergistic action with CNS depressants
- Bronchospasm
- Cardiac arrhythmia, tachycardia
- Hypotension and peripheral vasodilation
- CNS excitement (during induction and emergence)

Characteristics of Propofol

- Most commonly used induction agent
- Rapid onset (within 1 minute)
- Short duration of action (5 to 10 minutes)
- Side effects rare
- Antiemetic properties

Characteristics of Etomidate

- Onset within 1 minute
- Duration of 3 to 10 minutes
- Produces increased involuntary movement

- Can be used in trauma cases because it maintains cardiac output
- Suppresses adrenal function

Characteristics of Thiopental

- Rapid onset (1 to 2 seconds)
- Duration of 5 to 15 minutes
- Bronchospasm possible
- Poor analgesic

Characteristics of Ketamine

Ketamine is a rapidly acting sedative that produces isolation of the sensory parts of the brain, resulting in a trancelike state (dissociative anesthesia) and amnesia. Ketamine is valuable for sedation requiring profound analgesia (e.g., during debridement of burns).

Distinctive adverse affects of ketamine are:

- Seizure
- Increased secretions
- Respiratory depression
- Hypertension
- Hallucinations and delirium
- Increased intracranial pressure
- Nausea and vomiting

Benzodiazepines

Benzodiazepines have many clinical uses because of their versatility. They cause desirable **antegrade amnesia** (loss of recall of events) for up to 6 hours from the onset of drug action. This group of drugs effectively prevents and treats anxiety. The drug is given intravenously during procedures that do not require analgesia and as a preoperative medication in pediatric surgery (administered by rectal suppository). However, in combination with other CNS depressants, benzodiazepines can cause significant respiratory depression and can increase recovery time.

Some commonly used benzodiazepines are diazepam, midazolam, lorazepam, and alprazolam.

Uses of Benzodiazepines

- In combination with opioids and muscle relaxants to achieve balanced anesthesia
- For preoperative anxiety
- During endoscopy
- During cardioversion
- During cardiac catheterization

Adverse Effects

- Respiratory and cardiac depression
- Increased anesthesia recovery time
- Synergistic action with CNS depressants

Neuromuscular Blocking Agents

Neuromuscular blocking agents are used to paralyze skeletal muscles, an essential component of general anesthesia. Even during profound general anesthesia, autonomic muscle response can interfere with the manipulation of tissues. Neuromuscular blocking is a complex, controlled process that is chemically reversed at the close of surgery or whenever necessary during an emergency. The drugs cause paralysis of the respiratory muscles, and mechanical ventilation is required during their use. The effect of neuromuscular blocking drugs is adjusted during surgery according to the level of relaxation needed.

Neuromuscular blocking agents are classified as *polarizing* and *nondepolarizing*, according to their chemical action. Each group of drugs is further classified by duration of action, although this is also dose dependent.

Polarizing Agents
Polarizing agents cause muscle paralysis by stimulating involuntary muscles, which is followed by muscle fatigue. Drugs commonly used for this purpose are succinylcholine and decamethonium.

Nondepolarizing Agents
Nondepolarizing muscle blockers prevent muscle contraction by binding to the muscle's cholinergic receptor. An increase in nondepolarizing relaxant at the neuromuscular junction causes an increase in muscle paralysis. Agents commonly used for this purpose are subclassified according to their duration of action:
- Short acting (mivacurium)
- Intermediate duration (atracurium, cisatracurium, vecuronium, rocuronium)
- Long duration (tubocurarine, gallamine, metocurine, pancuronium, pipecuronium)

Reversal Drugs
Neuromuscular blocking agents are reversed when they are no longer required during surgery. Three drugs are commonly used for reversal:
- Neostigmine
- Edrophonium
- Pyridostigmine

Narcotics
Narcotics are a specific group of drugs within a class of analgesics. As mentioned previously, analgesics are drugs that reduce pain. They are classified according to source. *Opioids* are drugs derived from natural opium, such as codeine and morphine. Synthetic derivatives include hydromorphone and oxycodone. The central nervous system has many receptors for narcotic analgesics that mimic the brain's naturally occurring endorphins and easily attach to the body's receptors.

All narcotics produce analgesia by altering the patient's perception of pain. They also produce unconsciousness at high dosages. They reduce the work of the heart and may prevent elevated blood glucose and reduce postoperative pain.

During conscious sedation, a combination of narcotics and sedatives is administered for analgesia and sedation. Narcotics are delivered by the IV route as a **bolus injection** (single injection), intermittently, or as an **infusion** (given continuously in solution with IV fluids). Other routes include the epidural route and subarachnoid infusion.

Narcotic Drugs
The analgesic effect of a narcotic is always compared to morphine (in the form of morphine sulfate). Some commonly used narcotics are:
- Morphine sulfate (analgesic standard): Duration, 2 to 4 hours
- Meperidine (10% as powerful as morphine): Duration, 2 to 3 hours
- Alfentanil (10 times more powerful than morphine): Duration, 10 to 15 minutes
- Fentanyl (100 times more powerful than morphine): Duration, 30 to 45 minutes
- Sufentanil (1,000 times more powerful than morphine): Duration, 1 hour

Adverse Side Effects of Narcotics
- CNS depression
- Hypotension, shock
- Respiratory depression
- Drug interaction with alcohol, amphetamines, and antihistamines
- Profound sedation, coma
- Nausea and vomiting

Narcotic Reversal Drugs
In some cases the action of a narcotic must be reversed in surgery. Narcotics bind to the body's opiate receptors to produce their effect; this is called *antagonistic activity*. Narcotic antagonist drugs reverse the effect of the narcotic and may do this by displacing the narcotic from the receptor. Commonly used narcotic antagonists are naloxone and nalmefene.

Cryoanalgesia
Cryoanalgesia is sometimes used to provide postoperative pain relief during thoracic surgery. In this process, a small probe that has been cooled to −76° F (−60° C) is inserted into the intercostal spaces above and below the incision. This blocks sensory nerve conduction for up to 3 months. Cryoanalgesia is also used in outpatient settings for the removal of small skin lesions.

Alternative Analgesia
Alternatives to conventional methods of pain control have been attempted for many years to avoid the side effects of drugs. Hypnoanalgesia and acupuncture are examples of alternative therapies. However, these therapies are unpredictable, and the effect appears to depend on the patient's acceptance of the method.

Adjunct Agents
Anticholinergics
Anticholinergic drugs inhibit parasympathetic nerve transmission and the effects of acetylcholine. Most are derived from alkaloids of belladonna, a naturally occurring anticholinergic. Anticholinergics have many different effects that correlate with interruption of parasympathetic impulses.

In the past, potent anticholinergics such as scopolamine and atropine were given routinely to all surgical patients.

Now, however, these agents are used more selectively and can be administered intravenously for rapid results. In surgery, anticholinergics usually are used to control airway secretions and to regulate the heart rate in selected patients. In ophthalmic surgery they are used to produce mydriasis (dilation of the pupil) and cycloplegia (paralysis of the ciliary muscles). Examples of anticholinergic agents include:

- Atropine sulfate
- Scopolamine
- Glycopyrrolate

The effects of anticholinergics include the following:

- Regulation of the heart rate
- Relaxation of smooth muscles in selected ophthalmic procedures
- Drying of secretions
- Reduction of gastrointestinal, bronchial, and nasopharyngeal secretions
- Emergency treatment of cardiac conduction block and sinus bradycardia
- Prevention of bronchospasm

Histamine-2 Receptor Antagonists and Proton Pump Inhibitors

Selected surgical patients at risk for aspiration are given prophylactic drugs to change the pH or reduce the volume of gastric contents. Histamine-2 receptor (H_2-receptor) antagonists reduce gastric acidity by blocking the release of gastric acid. The drugs do not change the acidity of contents already in the stomach. When given the night before surgery, they provide some protection against chemical pneumonitis, which is inflammation of the lungs caused by inspiration of gastric contents. Examples of H_2-receptor antagonists are:

- Cimetidine
- Famotidine
- Ranitidine

Gastric proton pump inhibitors (e.g., omeprazole and lansoprazole) act on the H_2 receptor to suppress gastric acid at the cellular level.

REGIONAL ANESTHESIA

Description

Regional anesthesia provides reversible loss of sensation in a specific area of the body without affecting consciousness. Regional anesthesia is also called *conductive* or *local anesthesia*. The term *regional* is preferred because it describes the process accurately. This type of anesthetic can be used in a small, superficial area of skin and subcutaneous tissue or in an entire region of the body, such as during spinal anesthesia. Patient monitoring is always provided during regional anesthesia. The level and scope of monitoring depend on the patient's condition and whether sedation is used during the procedure.

The most common uses of regional anesthesia are:

- Limb surgery in which complete nerve block is possible
- Procedures in which consciousness is desirable or required (e.g., obstetrical procedures)

- Minor superficial procedures
- Patients for whom general anesthesia poses a significant risk

Regional anesthesia can be provided to a single nerve, a group of nerves, or to an area of the spinal cord. When sensory nerve transmission is interrupted, tissues that transmit signals along that nerve are unable to receive pain signals. There are several types of regional anesthesia:

- **Topical anesthesia:** An anesthetic is applied directly to the eye, skin, or mucous membrane. This is done before injection of a regional anesthetic into sensitive areas of the body. Topical anesthesia may also be used before insertion of a tube or catheter.
- **Local infiltration:** A small amount of drug is introduced through multiple injections into the skin and subcutaneous tissue.
- **Nerve block:** A single nerve or nerve plexus (group) is anesthetized, blocking sensory stimuli to the tissue enervated by that nerve or group.
- **Spinal, caudal**, and **epidural anesthesia:** These are specific techniques for blocking transmission to the middle and lower body.

Table 12-2 lists regional anesthetic agents.

Monitored Anesthesia Care

Monitored anesthesia care (MAC) is continuous patient monitoring provided during regional anesthesia. In addition to physiological monitoring, the ACP administers sedative and **anxiolytic** (antianxiety) drugs as needed and manages any anesthetic or physiological emergencies. Monitored care is particularly important for patients receiving regional anesthesia who have underlying systemic disease or respiratory or cardiovascular risks. Basic monitoring includes the parameters listed previously and may include others, depending on the type of drugs administered.

TYPES OF REGIONAL ANESTHESIA

Topical Anesthesia

Topical anesthesia is used on mucous membranes and on superficial eye tissues during ophthalmic surgery. Topical anesthetics (Table 12-3) are used before insertion of endotracheal and LMA devices and also before laryngoscopy and bronchoscopy to prevent reflexive gagging. During regional cystoscopic procedures, transurethral instruments may be coated with a topical anesthetic gel to ease insertion. Topical agents are readily absorbed through the mucous membranes. Although the amount of agent applied is limited, the patient is monitored for toxic reactions.

Local Infiltration

Description

Local infiltration is injection of an anesthetic into superficial tissues to produce a small area of anesthesia. The combination of an anesthetic and epinephrine sometimes is used to constrict blood vessels at the infiltration site and prevent dissipation of the anesthetic through the vascular system. Epinephrine also facilitates entry of the anesthetic into the

Table 12-2

Local Anesthetics Administered by Injection

Name	Duration	Comments
Bupivacaine hydrochloride	Long	Produces long-acting epidural anesthesia in labor with no reported effects on fetus. Maximum dose is 200 mg.
Chloroprocaine hydrochloride	Short	Little systemic toxicity because of rapid hydrolysis in plasma. No effects reported on fetus after epidural anesthesia in mother. Maximum dose is 800 mg.
Etidocaine hydrochloride	Long	Highly lipid soluble. Onset for epidural block is 5 min. Profound muscle relaxation is desirable for abdominal surgery but not for labor.
Lidocaine	Intermediate	Widely used local anesthetic; can cause drowsiness, fatigue, and amnesia. Maximum dose is 300 mg (4.5 mg/kg body weight).
Mepivacaine	Intermediate	Chemically related to lidocaine. Maximum dose is 400 mg (7 mg/kg body weight).
Prilocaine	Intermediate	Used for dental procedures. Maximum dose is 400 mg.
Procaine hydrochloride	Short	Noted for its safety because of rapid hydrolysis in plasma. Duration of epidural block is unreliable. Maximum dose is 600 mg (10 mg/kg body weight).
Propoxycaine and procaine	Short to intermediate	Used for dental procedures. Dosage is 4 mg propoxycaine and 20 mg procaine.
Ropivacaine	Long	Used for epidural, field block, and major nerve block anesthesia. Dosage is 20 to 40 mg.
Tetracaine	Long	Most widely used drug for spinal anesthesia. Onset is 5 min. Available in hyperbaric, isobaric, and hypobaric solutions. Dosage for spinal anesthesia is 2 to 15 mg.

From Clark JF, Queener SF: *Pharmacologic basis of nursing practice*, ed 6, St Louis, 1999, Mosby.

Table 12-3

Topical Anesthetics

Generic Name	Eyes	Mucous Membranes	Skin	Comments
Benzocaine	0	+	+	Widely used. Included in many nonprescription preparations to relieve itching, and mild burns. Long acting and poorly absorbed.
Butamben	0	+	+	Mucosal formulation includes benzocaine and tetracaine. Also available as a nonprescription ointment to relieve itching and burning.
Cocaine hydrochloride	+	+	0	Schedule II drug. Medically used in ear, nose, and throat procedures when vasoconstriction and shrinking of mucous membranes are desired. Ophthalmic preparations anesthetize cornea and conjunctiva.
Dibucaine hydrochloride	0	+	+	Nonprescription skin ointment or cream.
Lidocaine	0	+	+	Widely used for topical anesthesia in ear, nose, and throat procedures, upper digestive tract procedures, and genitourinary procedures. Rapid onset and intermediate duration. Nonirritating and has a low incidence of hypersensitivity.
Lidocaine hydrochloride	0	+	+	
Proparacaine hydrochloride	+	0	0	Applied topically to eye to anesthetize cornea and conjunctiva.
Tetracaine hydrochloride	+	+	+	For topical administration, onset is 5 min and duration is 45 min. Usual topical dose is 20 mg; maximum dose is 50 mg because of toxicity and slow degradation. Ophthalmic preparations are dilute solutions for instillation.

From Clark JF, Queener SF: *Pharmacologic basis of nursing practice*, ed 6, St Louis, 1999, Mosby.
+, Site suitable for application; 0, site not suitable for application.

nerve cell. Examples of procedures performed with local infiltration are excision of a skin lesion and insertion of a chest tube.

Procedure

Local infiltration takes place after the patient has been prepped and draped as part of the surgical procedure. The scrub assists the surgeon during infiltration as follows:

- Make sure supplies (including the anesthetic) are available before the procedure.
- Receive the anesthetic drug from the circulating nurse and verify the amount and strength using proper technique (see Chapter 14.
- Label the drug on the instrument table and protect it from contamination.
- Provide the following:
  - At least two 25-, 26-, or 30-gauge needles
  - Two 10- or 25-mL syringes
  - Gauze sponges
- Fill one syringe to capacity and have another ready to use as necessary. Do not fill syringes part way. This may cause confusion about the amount of anesthetic used during the procedure.
- Separate all syringes and needles used for infiltration from others on the instrument table. Do not use the equipment for any purpose except infiltration of the local anesthetic.
- Note the total amount of anesthetic used and be prepared to report this to the surgeon or circulating nurse at any time during the procedure.

Nerve Block
Description

A peripheral nerve block provides anesthesia to a specific area of the body enervated by a major nerve or nerve plexus (group). The anesthetic agent is injected into the adjacent tissue, not into the nerve itself.

Procedure

The peripheral block is performed after skin prep of the injection area with antiseptic. The nerve block may be performed as part of the surgical procedure or separately before the surgical skin prep and draping. The procedure for injection is similar to infiltration anesthesia. The scrub assists when the nerve block is carried out as part of the surgery.

Intravenous (Bier) Block

Intravenous anesthesia is sometimes called a **Bier block** (Figure 12-14). In this procedure, blood is temporarily displaced from a limb and replaced by a regional anesthetic agent. To displace the venous blood, an air-filled **pneumatic tourniquet** is placed around the proximal end of the limb. The ACP then displaces blood in the limb using a latex bandage (**Esmarch bandage**). The bandage is wrapped around the entire length of the extremity, starting at the distal end and extending to the proximal end. The tourniquet is then inflated, and the Esmarch bandage is removed. Anesthetic is injected into the major vein through a previously placed IV catheter. Double tourniquets also may be

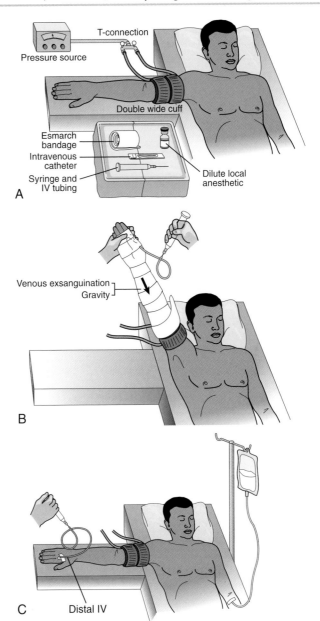

Figure 12-14 Intravenous (Bier) block. **A,** Equipment needed and position of double tourniquet. **B,** Venous exsanguination using Esmarch bandage and inflation of the tourniquet. **C,** Injection of the anesthetic into the vein. The upper tourniquet is then deflated. *(From Phillips N: Berry and Kohn's operating room technique, ed 10, St Louis, 2004, Mosby.)*

used, one proximal and one distal. The tourniquet "time" starts at the beginning of inflation and runs until the tourniquet is released. The safe tourniquet time and pressure depend on the patient's age, general condition, and size and surgical site.

Spinal Anesthesia
Description

Spinal anesthesia is injection of anesthetic into the subarachnoid space (Figure 12-15). To help facilitate correct placement of the anesthetic in the spinal canal, dextrose sometimes is added to the agent. This makes the drug heavier than the cerebrospinal fluid. In accordance with the patient's position,

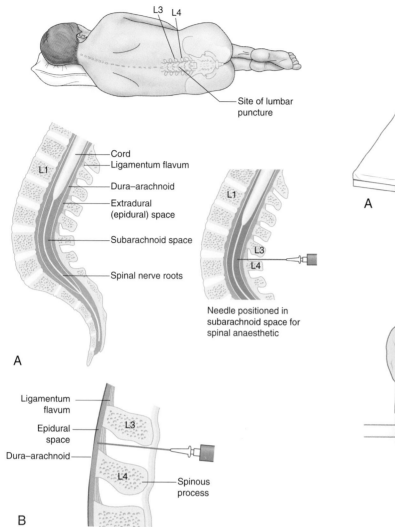

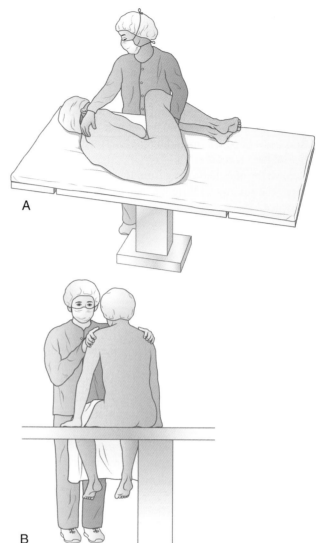

Figure 12-15 **A,** Area of injection for spinal anesthesia. The injection is made between L3 and L4 into the subarachnoid space. **B,** Epidural anesthesia. The injection is made into the epidural space. *(From Garden O, Bradbury A, Forsythe J, Parks R: Principles and practice of surgery, ed 5, Edinburgh, 2007, Churchill Livingstone.)*

Figure 12-16 Position of the patient for spinal anesthesia. **A,** The patient is side lying with the lumbar area exposed. (The patient is shown without a blanket for clarification.) **B,** Sitting position. The circulator stabilizes the patient at the shoulders.

the drug settles in the dependent areas (those affected by gravity) and is absorbed at a specific site along the spinal cord.

Conduction along the nerve roots that emerge from that location is blocked, and anesthesia is achieved. The anesthetic can be directed up, down, or laterally by tilting the operating table. Spinal anesthesia can be used for many procedures but is most often used for gynecological, obstetrical, orthopedic, and genitourinary surgery.

Patient Preparation

To facilitate exact placement of the spinal needle for injection, the patient must be positioned in a way that opens the intervertebral space. Two positions are used to achieve this—lateral (side-lying) or sitting. A knee-chest position is used with patient lying on his side and the knees drawn up. The circulator stabilizes the patient's shoulders with one

hand while providing support to the midleg with the other, as shown in Figure 12-16, *A*. The patient also may sit on the edge of the operating table and bend forward to create a rounded back. In this case, the circulator should support the patient as shown in Figure 12-16, *B*. The patient is covered with a blanket or sheet so that only the injection area is exposed. This provides warmth and protects the patient's modesty.

Procedure

When the patient has been positioned correctly, the ACP prepares the injection site with antiseptic and applies a small, sterile drape. The spinal injection site is infiltrated with a small amount of anesthetic. A spinal needle is then inserted into intervertebral and subarachnoid space, and the anesthetic injected. The patient is placed in the supine position with a slight downward tilt (Trendelenburg position) to maintain a safe level of anesthesia. The patient given spinal anesthesia receives continuous physiological monitoring throughout the procedure and is given adjunct drugs to provide mild sedation and relaxation.

Risks of Spinal Anesthesia

Risks associated with spinal anesthesia include the following:
- **Hypotension:** A severe decrease in blood pressure may occur, resulting in pooling of blood in the lower extremities.
- **Postspinal headache:** This condition is related to decreased cerebrospinal pressure resulting from a leak at the injection site in the dura mater.
- **Total spinal anesthesia:** This occurs when the hyperbaric spinal anesthetic blocks the nerves controlling the diaphragm and accessory breathing muscles.

Epidural and Caudal Block

Description

Epidural anesthesia is produced when the anesthetic agent is injected into the epidural space that surrounds the dural sac. The space contains connective tissue, an extensive vascular system, and the spinal nerve roots. Caudal and epidural anesthesia target the epidural space. However, in epidural anesthesia, the approach is through the lumbar interspace, whereas in caudal anesthesia, the caudal canal is used.

After injection, the anesthetic agent is very slowly absorbed into the cerebrospinal fluid through the dura mater. It spreads both caudally (toward the feet) and cephalad (toward the head). For a single-injection epidural, the patient's position and the molecular weight of the anesthetic have no effect on its distribution. However, with a continuous epidural, the position of the patient may affect the spread of the local anesthetic. Epidural anesthesia is often used in obstetrical, gynecological, urological, and rectal surgery. It also is used for postoperative pain control.

Procedure

The patient's skin is prepped as for spinal anesthesia. A thoracic, lumbar, or caudal puncture site is used, depending on the target site of anesthesia. The epidural needle is advanced through the skin until it enters the epidural space, and the anesthetic is injected (see Figure 12-15). Continuous or intermittent epidural anesthesia is provided through a small catheter placed in the epidural space for the duration of the surgery. This technique also is used for postoperative pain relief and for pain relief in selected patients.

In contrast to spinal anesthesia, epidural anesthesia requires a much larger amount of anesthetic agent. Accidental puncture of the dura mater can cause total spinal anesthesia. Also, because the epidural space has an extensive network of veins, overdose by accidental venous injection is a risk. If this occurs, the patient is immediately intubated and ventilated. Although the risk of hypotension exists with epidural anesthesia, the onset is slower than with spinal anesthesia and therefore easier to control and correct.

Drug Dosage

The effective dosage of anesthetic is calculated according to the individual patient's ability to absorb and metabolize the drug. The "normal" or safe dosage depends on many factors. Therapeutic ranges for all local anesthetics are considered, with knowledge of the patient's physical condition, especially the presence of cardiac disease, concurrent use of other drugs, and the patient's age, weight, and vascular status.

The rate of metabolism and response to the drug determine whether toxic levels are being reached. External monitoring is an objective method of detecting signs of toxicity. This is especially important in patients who require large amounts of anesthetic.

The surgical technologist (ST) has an intermediary role in the delivery of drugs in surgery. The ST receives the drug from licensed personnel and passes it to another person licensed to administer the drug. Because the ST does not perform nursing or medical assessment, his or her critical role is to know at all times how much drug has been delivered to the field and in what concentration.

All regional anesthetics are absorbed into the body and metabolized. This means that although regional anesthetics are relatively safe, exceeding the maximum dose may cause toxic reactions. If absorption is more rapid than metabolism, the risk of toxic reaction increases.

PHYSIOLOGICAL EMERGENCIES

The role of the surgical technologist at all times during an emergency is to protect the surgical field and provide assistance as directed. The surgical technologist may also be required to assist in cardiopulmonary resuscitation (CPR). However, CPR is meant to be a stopgap measure until biomedical intervention and medical care begin. Because these interventions are already in place in surgery, the patient is in the best location possible for a positive outcome.

REGIONAL DRUG TOXICITY AND ALLERGIC RESPONSE

Toxic reactions to local anesthetics arise most often during regional block and epidural anesthesia. This is because of the large amount of drug administered and the proximity to the vascular system. Toxic reactions related to regional anesthetics occur in two forms, central nervous system toxicity and cardiovascular toxicity.

Central Nervous System

CNS toxicity occurs in three phases. The *excitation phase* produces lightheadedness, restlessness, confusion, perioral tingling (tingling around the mouth), a metallic taste, tinnitus (ringing in the ears), and a sense of impending doom. The patient may become talkative. This phase is followed by the *convulsive phase*. Seizures can occur in this phase. The *depressive phase* is characterized by drowsiness, respiratory depression, and **apnea**.

Cardiovascular System

The first phase of cardiovascular toxicity is the *excitation phase*. The patient develops tachycardia, hypertension, and convulsions. This is followed by the *depressive phase*, which is characterized by decreased blood pressure, bradycardia, and possibly cardiac arrest.

Allergic Reaction

A true allergic reaction, which differs from reactions caused by toxicity, range from local skin irritation and itching to severe anaphylaxis, which produces life-threatening changes in the cardiovascular and respiratory systems. Maintaining verbal contact with the patient helps in the identification of symptoms. (Chapter 14 presents a complete discussion of drug hypersensitivity.)

Resuscitative equipment must be immediately available whenever a local anesthetic is administered. During any emergency, surgical technologists respond according to their training and scope of practice. Cardiopulmonary resuscitation is the minimum requirement for emergency response. Beyond this, licensed personnel are responsible for administration of resuscitative drugs, airway maintenance, and advanced life support procedures.

CARDIOPULMONARY ARREST

All health care workers must maintain current certification in CPR and be able to respond in case of a cardiac or respiratory arrest. Personnel may not be employed in a health care facility without this certification. The goal of CPR is to support and restore oxygenation, ventilation, and circulation. Restoration of intact neurological function accompanies this process. Return of spontaneous circulation is accomplished with basic life support (BLS) or advanced cardiac life support (ACLS) measures. These follow distinct algorithms that depend on the nature of the emergency. Airway, breathing, and circulation are the most basic priorities, followed by administration of cardiac drugs for emergency treatment of specific conditions.

The signs and symptoms of cardiac arrest vary according to whether the patient is fully conscious at the time or sedated. A conscious patient may feel nausea, shortness of breath, chest pain or pressure, or pain radiating from the jaw, neck, or shoulder. Sudden collapse and unresponsiveness may be the first signs of arrest. It is important to remember that resuscitative efforts must begin quickly to prevent neurological damage from lack of oxygen to the brain. Brain damage may occur as quickly as 3 minutes after circulatory collapse. Physiological monitoring during anesthesia permits immediate recognition of cardiac or respiratory failure. In these cases, medical assistance is immediately available.

Certification in CPR is the required method of ensuring complete knowledge and understanding of the procedure. All health care professionals and students are provided the opportunity for certification before beginning clinical work. To obtain information about ACLS courses and certification, students should contact the American Heart Association or consult the organization's Web site at http://www.americanheart.org/cpr.

LARYNGOSPASM

Laryngospasm is autonomic spasming of the laryngeal muscles. This usually is associated with airway secretions or stimulation of the laryngeal nerve during intubation or extubation. The condition may lead to complete airway obstruction. It is treated with positive-pressure administration of oxygen or, in severe cases, administration of succinylcholine to paralyze the muscles. Laryngospasm constitutes an emergency when an airway cannot be immediately established by positive-pressure ventilation. Patients with a difficult airway have the highest risk for a poor outcome with laryngospasm. In most cases, however, the condition can be treated with neuromuscular blocking agents and positive-pressure ventilation.

ANAPHYLAXIS

Anaphylaxis is a true allergic reaction to a material or drug that can lead to shock (see next section). In surgery, this is most commonly associated with regional anesthesia. Signs and symptoms include rash, abnormal lung sounds detected during auscultation, wheezing, and difficulty breathing. In the event of anaphylaxis, the ACP, licensed nurse, or surgeon immediately administers multiple doses of epinephrine. Other respiratory drugs and antihistamines are administered as needed. Airway assistance may be required. The on-call resuscitation team is alerted if no physician is in the room, and an airway and oxygen administration are quickly established. The preoperative examination and preanesthesia evaluation often can predict allergic response to substances or drug groups, and preventive measures are very valuable.

SHOCK

During severe shock, the supply of oxygen and nutrients to all body tissues is inadequate. This is caused by a cascade of physiological events that begins with a variety of conditions. Compensatory mechanisms in the body focus on shunting blood (and oxygen) to the most vital organs. In hypovolemic shock (caused by decreased vascular volume), the heart rate increases initially, and there is widespread vasoconstriction. Capillary flow diminishes or is shut down. The body tries to conserve fluid by reducing renal blood flow and increasing water retention in the kidneys. Urinary output is diminished or ceases. Eventually multiple organ failure occurs as a result of oxygen and nutrient starvation at the cellular level.

Types of Shock

- *Circulatory shock* is a state of inadequate blood volume for supplying the whole body. This type of shock can be caused by hemorrhage, burns (in which a dramatic shift of body fluids occurs), and severe diuresis (excretion of fluids through the renal system).
- *Cardiogenic shock* is caused by heart failure, which disables the vascular system because blood cannot be pumped adequately throughout the body.

- *Anaphylactic shock* is caused by true allergy, resulting in vasodilation and pooling of blood, which slows or halts normal circulation.
- *Neurogenic shock* is caused by failure of the autonomic nervous system to maintain vascular tone. This type of shock can be caused by specific drugs, brain injury, anesthesia, or spinal cord injury.
- *Septic shock* is caused by severe infection, which results in hypovolemia. Bacterial infection most often is the cause of septic shock, which is rapidly fatal. Disseminated intravascular coagulation is a complication of septic shock in which microcoagulation occurs in the cells. This depletes the body's platelets and other clotting factors, leading to continuous hemorrhage and death.

Treatment for shock is targeted at restoring circulatory function, electrolyte balance, and oxygenation of tissues. The immediate emergency response is related to the cause. However, in all cases circulatory balance is a priority. This may necessitate administration of fluid or blood components and drug therapy to improve the systemic blood pressure. The exact cause of the crisis is determined early in treatment so that appropriate emergency measures can be initiated.

MALIGNANT HYPERTHERMIA

Malignant hyperthermia (MH) is a rare physiological response to all volatile anesthetic agents and succinylcholine. MH causes a severe immediate or delayed hypermetabolism. The patient exhibits an extremely high core temperature, tachycardia, tachypnea, and increased muscle rigidity. Metabolic crises accompany the physical signs and include an increase in intracellular calcium ions, respiratory acidosis, metabolic acidosis, and homodynamic instability, which may lead to cardiac arrest and death.

MH is related to a familial genetic trait. Patients with family members known to have experienced MH usually report this to the ACP during the preoperative evaluation. However, no method has been devised of predicting MH when the patient has no family or personal history of the condition.

A malignant hypothermia cart is maintained in the surgical department so that all emergency equipment and drugs can be brought in immediately, because time is extremely important. The cart contains cooling equipment, including Foley catheters, plastic bags, tubing, peritoneal lavage equipment, and nasogastric tubes. Emergency drugs for MH treatment include Dantrium and agents to treat specific metabolic disorders.

If MH symptoms occur during surgery, the ACP alerts the team immediately. Treatment requires immediate cessation of anesthesia and administration of therapeutic drugs to treat the adverse metabolic symptoms. The scrub remains sterile to help protect the surgical incision. When immediate body cooling is required, the surgeon and ACP may initiate cold irrigation in open body cavities, ice packs, and a cold IV solution. The scrub receives sterile equipment, ice, and fluids to assist in lowering the body temperature. Therapy is continued until the patient is stabilized. The surgical wound may be closed when surgery must be halted. The patient is transported to the intensive care unit for further treatment and observation.

HEMORRHAGE

In the event of severe hemorrhage during surgery, blood volume is restored by giving blood substitutes, blood components, or antilogous blood (the patient's own blood previously banked or harvested at the surgical site). Allogenic (donor) blood transfusions may also be provided.

Packed red cells are mostly commonly used for transfusion, because the patient's immediate need is oxygen-carrying capacity. All blood products must be matched with the patient's blood type. A precise protocol has evolved to prevent the administration of blood of the wrong type. Whether the patient's own blood or banked blood is used, meticulous attention is given to patient identification, blood group, registration number, and date of expiration. Blood usually is brought from the blood bank shortly before surgery or, in an emergency, it is brought immediately. Blood must be stored in a location known to all personnel and protected from direct heat. Unused blood must be returned to the blood bank as soon as possible.

Intraoperative cell salvage (autotransfusion) is the immediate harvesting of blood on the surgical field and reinfusion into the patient. This may be planned in advance of a high risk surgery or implemented in an emergency. Special equipment is required for this procedure. The prototype autotransfusion system is the Cell Saver. However, other systems have been developed in recent years. Scrubs must be familiar with the cell salvage device used in their facility, because special training is required.

HEMOLYTIC REACTION

Hemolysis is the rupture of red blood cells. It is associated with ABO factor incompatibility during blood transfusion. Before any transfusion, the ABO and Rh systems are tested and cross-matched against the donor blood. However, mistakes in recording and reading blood registrations do occur, with serious consequences. Patients under anesthesia do not show the signs and symptoms seen in a fully conscious patient. ABO mismatch during transfusion outside of surgery produces the following symptoms:

- Back pain
- Chills
- Hypotension
- Dyspnea

These can lead to complete vascular collapse or renal failure. In surgery, the only symptoms likely to appear are oliguria (cessation of renal output) and generalized bleeding. Treatment requires stopping the transfusion and immediate hydration with IV fluids and forced diuresis.

DEEP VEIN THROMBOSIS

An embolus is any moving particle of the vascular system that can lodge in a small vessel. Risk factors for emboli include trauma, orthopedic fracture, burns, surgical procedures involving flexion and rotation of the hip, and use of a pneumatic tourniquet. Venous stasis, or "pooling," occurs when the patient is immobile for long periods, which can lead to clotting. A thrombus may form in proximal deep veins and subsequently break loose, preventing circulation to a vital organ such as the lung (pulmonary embolism [PE]). Symptoms may become apparent at any point in the perioperative period. Prevention of deep vein thrombosis (DVT) includes preoperative application of antiembolic stockings, use of a sequential compression device, and prophylactic medication when appropriate. Other preventive measures include slow, deliberate movement of limbs during positioning and following DVT and PE protocols according to hospital policy. These are nursing and medical interventions that are carried out by licensed personnel. Treatment for DVT includes drug therapy to prevent further embolization and treatment for the specific emergency condition, such as shock and respiratory arrest.

CHAPTER SUMMARY

- Modern anesthesia is characterized by loss of consciousness and sensory sensation.
- Neurotransmitters are responsible for the presence or absence of sensory awareness and motor control.
- Stimuli in the autonomic nervous system produce specific involuntary responses in body organs and tissues.
- The somatic nervous system is under direct voluntary control and is responsible for striated muscle response.
- The anesthesia care provider is a medical professional trained to administer anesthetic agents, perform physiological monitoring, and respond to anesthetic and surgical emergencies.
- The anesthesia machine is used to deliver inhalation anesthetic agents and for complex patient monitoring.
- Escape of anesthetic gas is an environmental hazard for health workers. Waste gases are scavenged from the system and shunted out of the operating room through a vacuum line.
- Anesthetic gas and oxygen are delivered to the patient through a semirigid airway. The patient's airway is protected at all times in the perioperative environment.
- Suction must be available and working at all times when the patient is in the operating room.
- Physiological monitoring is the continuous assessment of the patient's vital metabolic functions and is necessary whenever an anesthetic is delivered.
- Parameters of physiological monitoring include oxygenation, ventilation, circulation, body temperature, and neuromuscular response.
- Patients are fully assessed for anesthetic and physiological risks before surgery.
- The selection of an anesthetic is based on many considerations, including the patient's history and physical condition and the type of procedure. The patient's safety is the most important concern.
- Preoperative patient documentation provides a method of verifying that the correct procedure is performed on the correct patient at the correct site. Medical errors involving incorrect site and procedure occur when documentation and verification have been neglected.
- General anesthesia is reversible loss of consciousness accompanied by the absence of pain, sensory perception, cognition, memory of events during the period of anesthesia, and some autonomic reflexes.
- General anesthesia is produced and maintained using a combination of drugs.
- During general anesthesia, the patient loses many protective reflexes. The ACP must monitor and maintain all vital functions to protect the patient from injury.
- Intubation is the insertion of an artificial airway. During intubation the patient is unstable and the risk of emergency increases.
- Inhalation anesthetics are supplied as liquids and administered as a vapor. They are used to maintain general anesthesia.
- Sedatives are used to induce unconsciousness during general anesthesia.
- Benzodiazepines are used mainly to prevent and treat anxiety and produce amnesia.
- Neuromuscular blocking agents are used to paralyze skeletal muscles to allow tissue manipulation during general anesthesia.
- Narcotics provide analgesia or reduction of pain.
- Anticholinergics are commonly administered during general anesthesia to control airway secretions and regulate cardiac activity in selected patients.
- H_2-receptor antagonists and proton pump inhibitors reduce the gastric pH and volume.
- Regional anesthesia provides reversible sensation in a specific area of the body without affecting consciousness.
- Monitored anesthesia care is continuous patient monitoring provided during regional anesthesia.
- The type of regional anesthesia selected for a surgical procedure depends on the type of surgery, the length of the procedure, and the patient's condition.
- The risks of physiological emergencies related to anesthesia are lower than in the past. This is a result of safer drugs and more sophisticated physiological monitoring devices.
- The role of the scrubbed surgical technologist during physiological emergencies is to protect the surgical field and provide assistance as directed.

REVIEW QUESTIONS

1. Under what medical circumstances might regional anesthesia be used?
2. Describe the use of the Glasgow Coma Scale.
3. What educational and certification processes differentiate an anesthesiologist from an anesthetist?
4. What is the purpose of the ASA risk assessment classification?
5. Why is a musculoskeletal assessment necessary for the preoperative patient?
6. What are some considerations in selecting an appropriate method of anesthesia?
7. Define *homeostasis*.
8. What is physiological monitoring?
9. Name and define the five parameters of physiological monitoring discussed in this chapter.
10. What is the normal core temperature range for an adult?
11. What are protective reflexes? Describe four or more protective reflexes.
12. What is the function of a neurotransmitter?
13. Distinguish between the somatic and autonomic nervous systems.
14. Describe commonly used methods of regional anesthesia.
15. What are the minimum standards for monitoring during regional anesthesia?
16. To what specific tissue is a spinal anesthetic administered? An epidural anesthetic?
17. Why is it necessary to administer preoperative medications that reduce the gastric pH?
18. Describe deep vein thrombosis and pulmonary embolism. How are these conditions prevented?

BIBLIOGRAPHY

Association of periOperative Registered Nurses (AORN): *Standards, recommended practices and guidelines*, 2007 edition, Denver, 2007, AORN.

Hemmings H, Hopkins P: *Foundations of anesthesia*, ed 2, St Louis 2006, Elsevier/Saunders.

Kee J, Hayes E, McCuistion L: *Pharmacology: a nursing process approach*, ed 5, St Louis, 2006, Elsevier/Saunders.

Nagelhout J, Zaglaniczny K: *Nurse anesthesia*, ed 3, St Louis, 2005, Elsevier/Saunders.

Phillips N: *Berry and Kohn's operating room technique*, ed 11, St Louis, 2007, Mosby.

Porth C: *Pathophysiology: concepts of altered health states*, ed 6, Philadelphia, 2002, Lippincott Williams & Wilkins.

The Joint Commission: Preventing and managing the impact of anesthesia awareness. Accessed January 8, 2008, at http://www.jcipatientsafety.org/14730/.

Thibodeau G, Patton K: *Anatomy and physiology*, ed 6, St Louis, 2007, Elsevier/Saunders.

CHAPTER 13

Postoperative Recovery and Patient Discharge

CHAPTER OUTLINE

LEARNING OBJECTIVES

After studying this chapter the reader will be able to:
- Describe the layout of the PACU
- Discuss the elements of a handover from the circulating nurse to the PACU nurse
- List the elements of an assessment

- Describe the Glasgow Coma Scale
- Discuss selected types of postoperative complications
- Discuss the rationale for patient teaching
- Define the purpose of discharge planning
- Define *discharge against medical advice (AMA)*

TERMINOLOGY

Activities of daily living (ADLs): Basic activities and tasks necessary for day-to-day care, such as dressing, bathing, toileting, and meal preparation.

Arterial blood gases (ABGs): A blood test that measures the level of oxygen and carbon dioxide and the pH of the blood.

Aspiration: Inhalation of fluid or solid matter.

Auscultation: Listening to the lungs, heart, or abdomen through the stethoscope.

Bronchospasm: Partial or complete closure of the bronchial tubes.

Discharge against medical advice (AMA): Self-discharge by a patient who has not necessarily met discharge criteria.

Discharge criteria: Objective criteria used to determine whether a patient is safe for discharge from the health care facility.

Focused assessment: An assessment of the patient that focuses on specific organ systems or regions of the body.

Glasgow Coma Scale (GCS): A standardized method of measuring a patient's response to external stimuli.

Handover (hand-off): A verbal and written report from one nurse to another to provide updated patient information.

Head to toe assessment: A complete assessment of the patient, one that includes all systems.

Hypothermia: Body temperature that is below normal.

Hypoventilation: Inadequate respirations.

Hypoxia: Lack of oxygen in the tissue.

Ileus: Cessation of peristalsis in the bowel causing obstruction. Postoperative ileus is often caused by excessive handling of the bowel during surgery.

Laryngospasm: Muscular spasm of the larynx, resulting in obstruction.

Malignant hyperthermia (MH): A potentially fatal syndrome of hypermetabolism that results in an extremely high body temperature, cardiac dysrhythmia, and respiratory distress.

Perfusion: Flow of blood to tissue.

Polypharmacy: A patient care problem in which a patient is prescribed many different medications, sometimes by different health care providers; a common problem in elderly patients who have multiple health problems.

Prognosis: A prediction of the patient's medical outcome (e.g., poor prognosis, good prognosis).

INTRODUCTION

After surgery, patients are transported to the postanesthesia care unit (PACU) for recovery. Postoperative patients are at risk for immediate postoperative complications that may require an emergency medical response. The PACU is staffed by critical care nurses who are trained in postoperative recovery and emergency treatment. The unit is equipped with all necessary physiological monitoring equipment, drugs, and emergency supplies. The PACU is close to the surgical suites for rapid transfer of patients after surgery. In some facilities, the PACU also functions as an ambulatory patient recovery area.

PACU FACILITY

The floor plan of the PACU usually is one large room with separate patient stations along two or more perimeter walls. Patient beds (stretchers) are positioned in the individual care areas (or *cubicles*) on the perimeter wall in view of a central nursing station.

This arrangement allows the staff to attend to patients quickly and efficiently. Stretchers can be easily moved within the unit and around the cubicles. Because there are no walls between patients, diagnostic equipment such as portable radiograph machines, 12-lead electrocardiograph equipment, and emergency crash carts can be brought to the bedside quickly and with minimal maneuvering. The central nursing station is equipped with patient telemetry monitors, phones, and computers. Each patient cubicle has outlets for suction, oxygen, mains power, and high level lighting. Individual patient monitoring is transmitted through the department telemetry system so that staff members at the central nursing station can view each patient screen individually. Medication and supplies are dispensed from designated areas attached to the main patient area. Emergency airway equipment is kept in an easily accessible area and on crash carts.

In addition to individual patient cubicles, an isolation area provides barrier protection for selected patients, such as those with an active infection. The PACU may also have a designated area for pediatric patients.

If ambulatory patients recover in the same department as inpatients, a designated area is provided with changing rooms, a lounge, and an ambulatory discharge area. Side rooms provide space for dictation, patient and family conferences, and staff lockers.

PACU PROCEDURES

ADMISSION

Patients are admitted to the PACU immediately after surgery. When the patient arrives at the unit, an assigned PACU nurse receives the individual and assists the circulating nurse and anesthesia care provider (ACP) in setting up the patient in a cubicle. Electrocardiogram (ECG) leads, the pulse oximeter sensor, oxygen, and suction are immediately engaged. The patient's airway, circulatory status, oxygen perfusion, and temperature are then assessed.

HANDOVER (HAND-OFF)

Once all monitoring devices are in place and the patient is stable, the circulating nurse performs a **handover** (also called a **hand-off**) to the PACU nurse. The circulating nurse provides all information needed to update the PACU nurse on the patient's physiological status before and during surgery. The ACP provides specific orders for continuation of care and a smooth recovery. The circulating nurse and ACP remain with the patient until the handover is complete. The following verbal and written information is provided in the handover:

1. A brief patient history. This follows standard nursing and medical protocol and includes the patient's age, allergies, current medications, and existing pathology. This is the patient's preoperative status.

   Rationale: This information is relevant to proper assessment of current signs and symptoms and for continuity of nursing care.

2. The exact surgery that was performed, including the side and site (e.g., right colectomy with colostomy).

   Rationale: This is reported so that the PACU staff knows exactly where the surgical wounds are and the extent of the surgery for continuous postoperative care, monitoring, and assessment.

3. The total length of time anesthesia was delivered and the drugs given during that time. The amounts and routes are also reported.

   Rationale: Drugs given during the preoperative and intraoperative phase have a direct pharmacological effect on those administered postoperatively. The cumulative effect and drug interactions must be considered when additional medications are administered. The PACU nurse must know what drugs were given before the patient's arrival in the unit to anticipate physiological changes caused by the drugs.

4. Estimated blood loss and the amount and type of intravenous (IV) fluids or blood administered. If blood products were administered, the type and amount are reported.

   Rationale: The estimated blood loss is needed to determine the need for further action, such as transfusion. Total fluids given during surgery are balanced against output. This information contributes to the patient's overall medical "picture" so that evaluation is accurate. Blood loss or fluid imbalance explains specific physiological signs that trigger a nursing or medical response in the postoperative period.

5. Condition of the wound, drains, and other devices. If the surgical wound contains drains or a drainage device such as suction or closed water-seal drainage, this is reported in detail. The amount, color, and consistency of the drainage fluid are noted.

   Rationale: Wound assessment and care are of primary importance during the postoperative period. A baseline assessment provides information against which subsequent evaluations are compared. Changes in wound drainage may indicate infection or bleeding, which require an immediate medical and nursing response.

6. ASA score. Each patient is assigned a score according to the system established by the American Society of Anesthesiologists (ASA). This score reflects the patient's overall health status (see Chapter 12).
   Rationale: The ASA score is reported on postoperative records and is used in patient care planning.

7. Any surgical or medical complications that occurred during surgery.
   Rationale: This alerts the PACU staff to the patient's current condition and further complications. The information also is needed in case follow-up measures are required, such as radiographic films or blood tests.

8. Information about family members (i.e., contact numbers or location) who may be waiting in the family room.
   Rationale: The PACU staff maintains contact with the family during the postoperative period to update them on the patient's progress, condition, and discharge plans.

PATIENT ASSESSMENT

After accepting the handover, the PACU nurse performs a patient assessment. This can be either a focused assessment or a head to toe assessment. The **focused assessment**, as the name implies, focuses on specific criteria, such as respiration, circulation, pain, and level of consciousness. The **head to toe assessment** covers all or most body systems. Standard procedures are used to assess specific functions. General assessment procedures are carried out to obtain baseline information. This may lead to more complex methods of testing, such as blood tests, a 12-lead ECG, or radiographs. All findings are documented in the PACU record (Figure 13-1).

Respiratory System
* The airway is assessed by **auscultation** (listening with a stethoscope) and by observation for signs of airway obstruction.
* The respiratory rate and rhythm (patterns) are measured by observation of the thorax and accessory muscles during breathing.

Circulation
* **Perfusion** (flow of blood to tissue) is measured by pulse oximeter.
* The color of the patient's skin and mucous membranes is observed for signs of **hypoxia** (inadequate oxygen to tissues).
* The heart is monitored for rate and rhythm using ECG leads and a cardiac monitor, which produces a digital waveform.
* Heart sounds are assessed with the stethoscope and may be amplified by the cardiac monitor.
* The arterial pressure is measured directly with an arterial line or indirectly by taking the patient's blood pressure with a digital sphygmomanometer.

* **Arterial blood gases (ABGs)** (the ratio of oxygen to carbon dioxide and the blood pH) may be measured by taking a blood sample from an artery. In the modern PACU, the sample can be analyzed immediately.
* The central venous pressure may be measured with an in-line catheter or by observing the jugular veins.
* The presence or absence of a peripheral pulse is determined by palpation or by Doppler.

Core Temperature
* The patient's temperature is assessed continuously or intermittently using a digital thermometer or temperature probe.
* Hypothermia is a serious postoperative complication. The patient is continually observed for signs such as shivering.

Abdomen
* The abdomen is assessed for distention (which may indicate the presence of fluid, including blood) or air. This is done by observation, palpation, and radiographs.
* Bowel sounds are assessed by auscultation. A persistent lack of bowel sounds may indicate surgical paralytic ileus—cessation of peristalsis in the bowel leading to obstruction. Persistent paralytic ileus is a serious postoperative complication.

Fluid and Electrolyte Balance
* Fluid shifts from the vascular space to the intracellular space can occur after surgery, and the patient must be evaluated carefully.
* Assessment for dehydration includes physical signs and symptoms. Replacement fluids are administered intravenously as needed.
* Electrolyte imbalance is assessed through blood tests and specific physiological signs of imbalance, such as alteration in consciousness or cardiac dysrhythmia.

Neurological Function
Level of Consciousness
* The patient's level of consciousness is assessed using the **Glasgow Coma Scale (GSC)**. In this system, points are assigned to the response to specific stimuli (shown below). The GSC score is calculated as the total of all parameters. A score of 15 indicates the best **prognosis** (medical outcome) while a minimum score of 3 indicates a poor prognosis. The following parameters are evaluated:

Eye Opening
   (4) Spontaneously
   (3) To voice
   (2) To pain
   (1) No response

Best Verbal Response
   (5) Oriented and converses
   (4) Disorientated and converses
   (3) Inappropriate words
   (2) Incomprehensible sounds
   (1) No response

FORREST GENERAL HOSPITAL
POST ANESTHESIA CARE UNIT RECORD

POST ANESTHESIA RECOVERY SCORE		MINUTES				
		in	30	60	90	out

Activity
Able to move 4 extremities voluntarily or on command = 2
Able to move 2 extremities voluntarily or on command = 1
Able to move 0 extremities voluntarily or on command = 0

Respiration
Able to deep breathe and cough freely = 2
Dyspnea or limited breathing = 1
Apneic = 0

Circulation
BP ± 20 of Preanesthetic level = 2
BP ± 20-50 of Preanesthetic level = 1
BP ± 50 of Preanesthetic level = 0

Consciousness
Fully Awake = 2
Arousable on calling = 1
Not Responding = 0

O_2 Saturation
Able to maintain O_2 Sat > 92% on room air = 2
Needs O_2 to maintain O_2 Sat > 90% = 1
O_2 Sat < 90% even with O_2 = 0

TOTAL

Pre-op B.P. _____
Allergy _____

Airway: On Adm.
Jawthrust _____
Chin Hold _____
Endotracheal _____
Oral Airway _____
Mask Oxygen _____
Nasal Oxygen _____
Trach _____
T-Tube _____
Nasal Airway _____
Ventilator Settings _____

Addressograph

Time In _____ Time Out _____

Accompanied by _____

Type of anesthesia _____

Surgical Procedure:

PULSE - RESPIRATION - BLOOD PRESSURE

	15	30	45	15	30	45	15	30	45	15	30	45
240												
220												
200												
180												
160												
140												
120												
100												
80												
60												
40												
20												

O_2 Sat.

PAP

CODES ⊥ A-line T B.P.   V Manual or ∧ NBP   Pulse • Resp. ∘   Siderails: Yes No   Restraints:: Yes No

IV Type _____

Total IV in OR _____ cc
Blood in OR _____ units
Urinary Output in OR _____ cc
Est. Blood Loss _____ cc

RN Signature _____

RN Signature _____

Foley Cath. _____
Suprapubic _____
Ureteral _____
Levine _____

DRAINS

MEDICATIONS AND TREATMENTS

	AMT.	ROUTE	TIME
Demerol			
Morphine			
Phenergan			
Droperidol			
Zofran			
Toradol			

FORREST GENERAL HOSPITAL

DATE	TIME	DESCRIPTIVE NOTES (SIGN EACH ENTRY)

Report to Family:
Time:

	GU IRRIGANT	FOLEY OUTPUT
	TOTAL INFUSED:	TOTAL OUTPUT:

Figure 13-1 PACU record. *(From Rothrock JC: Alexander's care of the patient in surgery, ed 13, St Louis, 2007, Mosby.)*

Continued

PACU DISCHARGE SUMMARY

VITAL SIGNS ON DISCHARGE	PACU OUTCOME	COMFORT LEVEL
B/P: P: R: T:	UNEVENTFUL ☐	PAIN FREE ☐ PAIN CONTROLLED ☐
OXIMETER: PAR SCORE:	COMPLICATIONS ☐	SLEEPING BUT C/O PAIN WHEN AWAKEN ☐

REPORT TO: TIME:	SKIN CONDITION WARM COOL DRY MOIST	COLOR PINK PALE JAUNDICED DUSKY

DRESSINGS / SURGICAL SITE / PUNCTURE SITE

X-RAYS TAKEN IN PACU	LABS DRAWN IN PACU	O₂ ORDERED YES NO _____ L/MIN PER _____ O₂ TRANSPORT YES NO

TOTAL IV IN PACU	TOTAL OUTPUT IN PACU		
	URINARY	LEVINE	DRAINS
TOTAL BLOOD IN PACU			
TOTAL PO INTAKE IN PACU	IV SITE:		
	_____ cc LTC		

ORDERS FAXED TO PHARMACY YES NO	EQUIPMENT ORDERED	TRANSPORT BY: AMBASSADOR RN LPN TECHNICIAN

DIAGNOSIS (Circle number of any diagnosis made)	GOAL	Goal Achieved	
		YES	NO
1 Alteration in neurological status			
2 Alteration in comfort level			
3 Alteration in emotional status			
4 Alteration in circulation			
5 Alteration in fluid volume			
6 Alteration in mobility			
7 Alteration in respiratory function			
8 Alteration in skin integrity			
9 Alteration in temperature			
10 Alteration in elimination			
11 Alteration in gastrointestinal function			
12 Alteration in injury			
13 Alteration in bleeding			
14 Other			

RHYTHM STRIPS

Figure 13-1, cont'd.

Best Motor Response

(6) Obeys simple command
(5) Localizes to pain
(4) Flexion-withdrawal or abnormal
(3) Abnormal flexion
(2) Extension
(1) No response

Pain

- Pain is assessed using the following tools:
  Alertness: Asleep to hyperalert

Level of calmness: Calm to panicky
Movement: No movement to vigorous movement
Facial expression: Face relaxed to contortion or grimacing
Blood pressure: Baseline or below to 15% or more elevation
Heart rate: At or below baseline to 15% or more elevation
Vocalization: No vocalization to crying out

- The assessment of pain in a preverbal child is described in Table 13-1.

Table 13-1

Comfort Scale for Infants

Sign	Assessment Score*
Alertness	1 Sleeping deeply 2 Sleeping lightly 3 Drowsy 4 Fully alert 5 Hypervigilant
Calmness	1 Calm 2 Slightly anxious 3 Anxious 4 Appears panicky 5 Panicky
Crying	1 Quiet breathing no crying 2 Sobbing or gasping 3 Moaning 4 Crying 5 Screaming
Physical movement	1 No movement 2 Occasional/slight movement 3 Frequent, slight movement 4 Vigorous movement 5 Vigorous movement, including head and torso
Muscle tone	1 Muscles totally relaxed 2 Reduced muscle tone 3 Normal muscle tone 4 Increased muscle tone with flexion of fingers, toes 5 Extreme muscle rigidity with flexion of fingers, toes
Facial tension	1 Facial muscles relaxed 2 Facial muscle tone normal 3 Tension in some facial muscles 4 Tension throughout facial muscles 5 Grimacing or contortion of facial muscles
Blood pressure baseline	1 Below baseline 2 Consistently at baseline 3 Infrequent elevations 15% or more above baseline 4 Frequent elevation 15% or more above baseline 5 Sustained elevation 15% or more
Heart rate baseline	1 Below baseline 2 Consistently at baseline 3 Infrequent elevations of 15% or more above baseline 4 Frequent elevation 15% or more above baseline 5 Sustained elevation 15% or more

From the National Institutes of Health Warren Grant Magnuson Clinical Center, 2003.
*Scores are assessed as a total from 9 to 45.

Muscular Response
- Patient able to move on command
- Muscular strength (also related to neurological function)

Renal Function
- Urinary output is measured in milliliters per hour (includes intraoperative measurements). Urinary retention may be caused by neurological deficit and requires more complex assessment and treatment.
- Appearance of urine
- Selected blood tests

Wound Assessment
- Drainage amount, color, and consistency
- Incision assessment
- Swelling noted, measured for future reference

Catheters and Tubing
- Drainage amount, color
- Drains and catheters intact, open
- Intravenous lines intact

PSYCHOSOCIAL CARE

The PACU staff provides continual emotional support to the patient. Patients often need reassurance and orientation to their environment while emerging from general anesthesia or heavy sedation. Patients may be fearful of their diagnosis or the results of the surgery. Although not fully conscious, they may return emotionally to the preoperative state of anxiety. Patients need to know that, although they may not be fully functioning, they are being cared for, and they need to know who is caring for them. In some cases, the surgeon may see the patient briefly and explain the results of the surgery.

Family awaiting the results of the surgery and the patient's emergence from anesthesia also need contact with the PACU staff. The nurse may visit the family (which includes friends) in the waiting area to let them know the patient's progress and estimated time of discharge from the unit.

POSTOPERATIVE COMPLICATIONS

Postanesthesia complications occur because patients are physiologically unstable during the immediate postoperative period and may react to the procedure or drugs administered intraoperatively. They are vulnerable to pain, hemorrhage, reaction to the anesthetic agents, and rapid changes in homeostasis. The PACU staff is specially trained in critical care monitoring and response. Note that the physiological complications discussed in Chapter 12 can occur during the postoperative period.

PAIN

Although pain is expected in the postsurgical phase, not all patients respond to pain in the same way. A patient's response to pain is affected by previous experience, level of anxiety, the drugs used during surgery, and environmental factors. Patients also respond to pain according to what is acceptable in their culture. For example, in some cultures, crying out is acceptable while in others it is not. Pain management requires assessment and planning to ensure a smooth recovery. Analgesics are administered according to the patient's level of consciousness, cardiopulmonary status, and age.

RESPIRATORY

Respiratory problems are the most frequent life-threatening postoperative complication. Inadequate ventilation can be related to the effects of anesthetic drugs, muscle relaxants, or fluid-electrolyte imbalance. Inadequate intake of air and oxygen results in the accumulation of carbon dioxide in the blood. Normally, a high carbon dioxide level triggers the autonomic nervous system to stimulate breathing. However, drugs administered during the intraoperative period suppress this reflex. Pain at the operative site is another cause of **hypoventilation,** resulting in low oxygen saturation. For example, patients with abdominal or thoracic incisions do not breathe deeply because of the pain at the operative site.

Airway Obstruction

Airway obstruction most often is caused by anatomical structures or by aspiration of fluids. The tongue or soft palate can obstruct the airway in a state of deep relaxation related to anesthetic agents and adjunct drugs.

Contraction of the laryngeal muscles (**laryngospasm**) can occur whenever the larynx is irritated or stimulated by secretions, intubation, extubation, or suctioning. **Bronchospasm** is partial or complete closure of the bronchial tubes. It can be triggered by airway suctioning, aspiration of fluid, or allergy.

Aspiration or inhalation of secretions or stomach contents is associated with a weak gag reflex related to use of narcotics, sedatives, and anesthetic agents. Aspiration of gastric contents after vomiting can result in an obstructed airway and pneumonia.

Atelectasis

Atelectasis is the collapse of the lung, which can occur suddenly (as in the case of trauma to the chest wall or pulmonary obstruction). Trapped mucus or fluid in the bronchial tree can result in pulmonary obstruction postoperatively. Smokers are particularly vulnerable to atelectasis in the postoperative period. The patient is encouraged to take deep breaths and to cough frequently in the immediate postoperative period to prevent obstruction.

Pulmonary Embolism

Pulmonary embolism is blockage of a pulmonary vessel by air, a blood clot, or other substance (e.g., fragments of atherosclerotic plaque). This results in *anoxia* (decreased oxygen to the lung tissue), which can cause death of lung tissue and right heart failure. The risk of pulmonary embolism is increased in patients with a history of deep vein thrombosis (DVT). Patients are assessed for signs of DVT and pulmonary embolism in the immediate postoperative period. The patient and family are also provided with information about the signs and symptoms of DVT and pulmonary embolism so that monitoring can continue at home after discharge.

CARDIOVASCULAR

Many anesthetic agents are cardiac irritants that can sensitize the heart muscle to disturbances in rhythm, rate, and cardiac output. Hypotension and hypertension can occur as a result of fluid or electrolyte imbalance.

Hemorrhage

Hemorrhage can occur during surgery or in the postoperative period. The patient is continually monitored for signs of hemorrhage, which include pallor, hypotension, an increased heart rate, diaphoresis (sweating), cool skin, restlessness, and pain. Hemorrhage may be caused by the loss of a ligature placed during surgery, inadequate hemostasis, leakage from a vascular anastomosis, or a clotting disorder. If hemorrhage is suspected, emergency assessment measures are initiated and the patient may be returned to surgery. Chapter 12 presents a complete discussion of shock and hemorrhage.

METABOLIC COMPLICATIONS

Hypothermia

Hypothermia is a persistently low core body temperature (less than 98.6° F [37.5° C]). Elderly, pediatric, and frail patients are most vulnerable. Hypothermia can result in a longer postoperative recovery period, surgical wound infection, cardiac ischemia, and reduced ability to metabolize drugs. Most patients undergoing general anesthesia experience some level of hypothermia. However, persistent or extreme hypothermia can occur as a result of the following:

- Exposure of the body cavities to the cold ambient temperature of the operating room
- Administration of cold IV fluids
- Patient exposure before draping
- Vasodilation related to medications administered during surgery
- Decreased metabolism
- Cold irrigation solutions

Risks related to hypothermia are due mainly to physiological stress. These include:

- Shivering, which increases oxygen demand and consumption by 400% to 500%

- Excessive demand on body energy
- Decreased immune response, leading to postoperative infection
- Increased risk of adverse cardiac events, especially in patients with coronary artery disease
- Depression of the coagulation pathway
- Decreased tissue healing

Treatment for hypothermia includes use of a forced air heating mattress or placement of warm water pads under the patient. Further loss of body heat is prevented by warming IV solutions. Patients who are hypothermic during the intraoperative period may be difficult to warm postoperatively. Preoperative and intraoperative care is essential to prevent complications related to this condition.

Malignant Hyperthermia

Malignant hyperthermia (MH) is a rare condition that results in an extremely high core body temperature, cardiac dysrhythmia, tachypnea (increased respiratory rate), hypoxia, and hypercarbia. The condition is potentially fatal and occurs most commonly at the time of administration of the anesthetic. However, symptoms may appear in the postoperative period. MH can be triggered by inhalation anesthetics and succinylcholine, an anesthetic adjunct used for muscle relaxation.

MH is an extreme emergency during and after surgery, and all perioperative staff members are trained to respond appropriately according to facility protocol. Dantrolene sodium is administered as soon as the diagnosis is made by the ACP. Additional management includes total body cooling with extracorporeal ice or a hypothermia blanket, iced IV saline, and iced irrigation fluid in an open body cavity (surgical wound site). Surgery is interrupted, and the incision closed as quickly as possible. The patient is transferred immediately to the intensive care unit (ICU) for continuous care and monitoring.

NAUSEA AND VOMITING

Postoperative nausea and vomiting (PONV) are both a discomfort and a risk for the patient (see discussion of aspiration). PONV is controlled with medications in the preoperative period (as prevention) and in the postoperative period.

ALTERATIONS OF CONSCIOUSNESS

Anesthetic agents, adjunct medications, and environmental factors may cause patients to become disoriented, confused, or delirious during the immediate postoperative period. Preexisting psychiatric illness or drug abuse may contribute to these effects, which may also be due to organic causes such as electrolyte imbalance. Postoperative delirium is more common in pediatric patients and the elderly. Risk factors include the following:

- Cognitive impairment
- Sleep deprivation
- Immobility
- Sensory impairment (e.g., vision, hearing)
- Advanced age
- Electrolyte imbalance
- Dehydration
- Alcohol abuse
- Depression

ELEMENTS OF DISCHARGE PLANNING

Before an ambulatory (day case) patient is discharged to home or to an extended care facility, the PACU staff, ACP, and surgeon must determine that the patient will be safe. The patient must be able to perform **activities of daily living (ADLs)** with some degree of independence or have help in dressing, eating, mobilizing, and toileting. Discharge planning is needed to prepare the patient and caregivers for possible problems.

Discharge planning and implementation follow established roles and tasks:

1. *Discharge criteria:* These are standards that reflect the patient's physiological status and objectives for care once the patient leaves the facility.
2. *Transport or transfer plans:* Safe patient transportation is arranged, and an escort is identified.
3. *Home nursing care:* Home care objectives for the patient's recovery are established, and those who will be involved in the care are identified.
4. *Patient education:* Patients are informed and educated about their own care so that they can fully participate in their recovery. The family is instructed in specific care objectives and how to meet the patient's physical needs.
5. *Referral and follow-up:* The patient is informed of follow-up appointments. Referral numbers for emergencies or further advice are provided on a written document.
6. *Documentation:* Nursing care documentation is completed and signed off. Discharge checklists are prepared and completed.

DISCHARGE CRITERIA

Discharge criteria are physiological, psychological, and social conditions that serve as a measure of the patient's readiness for discharge. Patients are discharged from the PACU only when they meet discharge criteria. These are primarily physiological objectives, which are necessary to ensure patient safety outside the critical care unit. The health care facility establishes the discharge criteria. A number of organizations have written suggested criteria; however, the **Aldrete scale** often is used to determine whether a patient is ready for discharge to the hospital ward or unit. This is a numerical scale used to evaluate activity, respiration, circulation, consciousness, and oxygen saturation Box 13-1 shows an example of

Modified Postanesthesia Discharge Scoring System

Vital Signs	
Within 20% of the preoperative value	2
20%–40% of the preoperative value	1
40% of the preoperative value	0
Ambulation	
Steady gait/no dizziness	2
With assistance	1
No ambulation/dizziness	0
Nausea and Vomiting	
Minimal	2
Moderate	1
Severe	0
Surgical Bleeding	
Minimal	2
Moderate	1
Severe	0

From Miller R: *Miller's anesthesia*, ed 6, Philadelphia, 2005, Churchill Livingstone.

scored discharge criteria system. Modified versions of the scale have been developed for special circumstances.

Criteria for discharge include physiological criteria and the patient's psychosocial status.

Physiological Criteria

1. Vital signs are stable and reflect the patient's baseline normal.
2. Nausea and vomiting are controlled.
3. Patient is mobile with assistance or by self (the patient must be able to walk without signs of dizziness or weakness).
4. Patient is able to void (this establishes that no evidence exists of urinary retention).
5. Skin color reflects patient's baseline normal.
6. Incision site is dry, and drainage is absent or within expected limits.
7. Patient is oriented to time, place, and person.
8. Pain is controlled (patients are discharged when the level of pain is acceptable to the patient).
9. Patient is able to drink fluids.
10. Discharge orders have been written and signed by the anesthesia care provider and surgeon.

Psychosocial Status

1. Patient has transportation home (not public transport).
2. Responsible escort is available.
3. Home care is available as needed.
4. Home environment is suitable for the recovering patient.

GENERAL PLANNING

Arrangements for discharge are sometimes complex. PACU nurses not only must care for the patient during the recovery period, they also must ensure that care is in place and that safe transport has been arranged.

Patients deserve a safe discharge and transfer from the providing facility. Discharge planning must be started at the time of admission to ensure a safe and event-free return home at end of the recovery period. Home health service providers are notified, and a preoperative conference may be held with the family and discharge nurse.

When the patient is to be transferred to another care facility, a verbal and written hand-off is provided to a designated person at the receiving facility. The hand-off includes all information about the patient's physical and psychosocial status, the details of the surgery, and the care plan, including prescriptions, dressings, and drainage.

TRANSPORT

Patient transport to home or another care facility is arranged before surgery whenever possible. The patient is not discharged to public transportation, and a responsible escort must accompany the patient.

HOME NURSING CARE

In the past, patients anticipated a long recovery period both in the hospital and at home. Because of advanced surgical technology and health care economics, patients are now discharged as soon as possible after surgery. Many procedures that used to require days of hospitalization are now performed as day surgery with discharge within 1 or 2 hours of recovery. Home care during the immediate postoperative period is now more focused and has specific outcome objectives.

Discharge planning includes specific written instructions for home care and goals for the patient. This new health care philosophy has shifted the responsibility of recovery from inpatient nursing to the patient and family. In the event the patient has no assistance available, community resources, including social services and professional home nursing services, must be brought in.

PATIENT EDUCATION

Patient teaching is the responsibility of trained nursing personnel. Current surgical practice with same-day discharge and fast tracking requires that patients understand all aspects of their recovery. In theory, this allows them to be active participants in their recovery. However, the postoperative patient may not be able to understand or remember new information. Therefore patient teaching takes place before surgery and may include the family members who will assist in care.

The elements of patient teaching include both verbal and written instructions. In some facilities, video demonstration and education are available. Access to electronic information via the Internet has transformed the field of consumer medicine. However, not all patients have access to these types of resources or the ability to interpret them. And many more patients are too sick to achieve a level of self-education. For these reasons, patients' family members (when applicable) are taken through the recovery process, step by step, with thorough explanations of what to expect and what to do. This is especially important for patients who will have drains, dressing changes, and surgical appliances to maintain.

Written information is intentionally simple and easy to understand. It is written in lay language, often with illustrations for clarification. It may include information about the surgery, what it entails, and exactly what anatomical changes were made (if any). All anticipated and unanticipated events are explained. Signs of infection or other complications are written out so that patients can refer to them. Expected effects of surgery help give the patient confidence and ease anxiety when they occur.

Patients are educated fully about their prescriptions and how to take them. **Polypharmacy** is a clinical scenario in which patients are prescribed many different medications, sometimes by different primary health care providers who have no knowledge of other drugs the patient is taking. It is not unusual for a patient with a chronic disease to be taking 15 or 20 prescribed medications. Therefore it is very important that education about drugs be covered fully.

The patient's ADLs are discussed in full. These activities of daily living often determine the patient's quality of life. Even if the recovery period is rapid, patients must be able to cope with activity restrictions, special toileting needs (or problems), and meal preparation.

Patients who require dressing changes or have appliances, drains, or catheters need particular assistance and teaching to prevent infection. Patients and family may be given supplies to take home with them at the time of discharge.

Patients and family receive referral numbers for emergency care or further information. Upcoming appointments for surgical follow-up are clearly written, along with any preparation for further testing or treatment.

UNANTICIPATED PACU OUTCOME

FAILURE TO MEET DISCHARGE CRITERIA

Some patients may not meet discharge criteria after ambulatory or inpatient recovery. Further observation and care may be required, especially if the patient entered the PACU in a deteriorated condition or an adverse event occurring during recovery. Examples of such individuals are patients who are hypothermic, posthemorrhagic, or whose vital signs cannot be stabilized. Inpatients are transferred to the ICU for critical care observation and nursing. Ambulatory patients may be admitted to the ICU or surgical unit for overnight care (or longer if necessary).

DISCHARGE AGAINST MEDICAL ADVICE

Occasionally a patient may opt for self-discharge against the advice of medical and nursing personnel; this is known as **discharge against medical advice (AMA)**. Patients have a right to leave the care facility as long as they do not pose a threat to themselves or others.

Unless evidence exists of potential harm, patients must be allowed to leave. However, if possible, the facility tries to obtain a signed waiver from the patient and explain the possible outcomes of both the surgery and the consequences of early discharge. The waiver states that the consequences of early discharge have been explained, that discharge was not advised, and that the patient takes responsibility for the consequences.

DEATH IN THE PACU

Death of a patient during surgery is unusual. In the event of impending death or a rapidly deteriorating patient, surgery may be terminated and the patient taken to the PACU. Death may be pronounced (formally) in the PACU after resuscitative means have been exhausted. The patient's family is notified, and PACU staff members arrange for an immediate conference with the family and surgeon. A designated staff member stays with the family to provide emotional support. Further care is then implemented through hospital clergy and social services. Chapter 3 presented a complete discussion of death and dying.

CHAPTER SUMMARY

- Patients are transported to the postanesthesia recovery unit PACU immediately after surgery for observation and care.
- The PACU is specifically designed for rapid assessment and treatment of patients in the event of postoperative emergencies.
- A telemetry system provides continuous monitoring of patients at the bedside and at a central station in the unit.
- The PACU is staffed with nursing professionals trained in the critical care specialty.
- Upon the patient's arrival in the PACU, the anesthesia care provider and circulating nurse provide a complete handover to the assigned PACU nurse.
- Important points of the handover include the patient history, including drug allergies; a description of the surgery performed; the estimated blood loss; all drugs administered in the preoperative and intraoperative periods; the condition of the wound and drainage, the ASA score, and information about family contacts.
- A complete baseline assessment is performed at the time of admission to the PACU.
- During recovery, the patient's physiological status is monitored continually.

- Pain management is an important part of the recovery process. Pain is assessed by direct and indirect signs.
- Response to emergencies such as cardiac arrest and airway obstruction is very rapid in the PACU, because the unit is open and emergency equipment is immediately available.
- Discharge from the PACU is planned well in advance of surgery. It includes patient education, arrangement for transportation (for ambulatory patients), and communication with the family.
- Discharge criteria are established by the health care facility in consultation with health care providers and professional organizations.
- The purpose of discharge criteria is to ensure that the patient is safe once the individual has left the health care facility. Physiological and psychosocial criteria are included in the criteria.
- When a patient is transferred to another facility on discharge, a complete handover and written agreement must be made before discharge.
- Patients who do not meet discharge criteria may elect to leave the health facility (discharge against medical advice). This is their right, but they must sign a self-discharge release.

REVIEW QUESTIONS

1. Why is the PACU considered a critical care unit?
2. Why are the patient's vital signs taken immediately on arrival in the PACU?
3. What is the rationale for providing the PACU nurse with the names and amounts of all drugs administered to the patient in the preoperative and intraoperative periods?
4. Why is a patient assessment performed on arrival at the PACU, even though the patient has been under the immediate care of the surgeon and the ACP?
5. What is the Glasgow Coma Scale? What is its application in the postoperative recovery phase for a patient who had general anesthesia?
6. Hypothermia is one of the most serious complications of surgery. What procedures are necessary during the *intraoperative period* to prevent hypothermia in the *postoperative period*?
7. Which are the specific duties of the *scrubbed* surgical technologist in preventing hypothermia?
8. What is the rationale for extensive patient teaching?

BIBLIOGRAPHY

Association of periOperative Registered Nurses (AORN): Guidance statement: postoperative patient care in the ambulatory surgery setting. In *Standards, recommended practices and guidelines,* 2007 edition, Denver, 2007, AORN.

Barash P, Cullen B, Stoelting R: *Handbook of clinical anesthesia,* ed 5, Philadelphia, 2005, Lippincott Williams & Wilkins.

Good K, Verble G, Secrest J, Norwood B: Postoperative hypothermia: the chilling consequences, *AORN Journal* 83:5, 2006.

Kingon B, Newman K: Determining patient discharge criteria in an outpatient surgery setting, *AORN Journal* 83:4, 2006.

Nagelhout J, Zaglaniczny K: *Nurse anesthesia,* ed 3, St Louis, 2005, Elsevier/Saunders.

Porth C: *Pathophysiology: concepts of altered health states,* ed 6, Philadelphia, 2002, Lippincott Williams & Wilkins.

Rothrock JC: *Alexander's care of the patient in surgery,* ed 13, St Louis, 2007, Mosby.

Thibodeau G, Patton K: *Anatomy and physiology,* ed 6, St Louis, 2007, Elsevier/Saunders.

Perioperative Pharmacology

CHAPTER OUTLINE

LEARNING OBJECTIVES

After studying this chapter the reader will be able to:

- Describe the process of ensuring consumer safety for drugs
- Describe the role of the surgical technologist in handling drugs
- List drug administration routes
- Define pharmacokinetics and pharmacodynamics
- Describe immediate and delayed adverse drug reactions
- List and use the five rights of medication delivery
- Correctly identify the parts of a drug label

- Recognize different drug delivery devices
- Accurately convert values within and between measurement systems
- Perform basic arithmetic calculations accurately
- Apply the correct protocol for receiving drugs on the sterile field
- Apply the principles of safe drug handling

TERMINOLOGY

Accupuncture: An alternative health therapy in which fine needles are inserted into energy "meridians" of the body for the treatment of disease.

Adverse reaction: An unexpected reaction to a drug that is not related to dose.

Agonist: A drug that produces a response in the body by binding to the cell.

Allergy: Hypersensitivity to a substance, a response produced by the immune system.

Antagonist: A drug or chemical that blocks response in the body.

Antibiotic: A drug that inhibits the growth of or kills bacteria in living tissue.

Anticoagulant: A drug that prolongs blood clotting time.

Barium sulfate: An opaque contrast medium used in imaging studies of the gastrointestinal tract.

Bioavailability: The extent and rate at which a drug or its metabolites (products of breakdown) enter the systemic circulation and reach the site of action.

Chemical name: The name of a drug that reflects its molecular structure.

Concentration: A measure of the quantity of a substance by volume or weight.

Contraindication: A protocol, drug, or procedure that is medically inadvisable because it increases the risk of injury or harm.

Contrast medium: A radiopaque solution (i.e., not penetrated by x-rays) that is introduced into body cavities to outline their inside surfaces.

Controlled substances: Drugs that have the potential for abuse. Controlled substances are rated according to their risk potential; these ratings are called *schedules.*

Delayed drug sensitivity: Allergic reaction to a drug occurring up to 12 hours after exposure. This type of reaction is mediated by T lymphocytes.

Diuresis: Increased formation of urine by the kidneys.

Dosage: The regulated administration of prescribed amounts of a drug. Dosage is expressed as a quantity of drug per unit of time.

Dose: The quantity of a drug to be taken at one time or the stated amount of drug per unit of distribution (e.g., 0.5 mg per milliliter of solution).

Drug: A chemical substance that, when taken into the body, changes one or more of the body's functions.

Drug administration: The giving of a drug to a person by any route.

Dye: Colored substance used to stain tissue or verify the patency of a hollow or tubular structure (e.g., fallopian tube, ureter) under direct visualization.

Five rights of medication: Requirements for safe administration of drugs: right drug, right dose right route, right patient, right time.

Generation: In pharmacology, refers to a drug group that was developed from a previous prototype (e.g., first generation cephalosporin).

Generic name: The formulary name of a drug that is assigned by the U.S. Adapted Names Council.

Half-life: The time required for one half of a drug to be cleared from the body.

Immediate drug sensitivity: An allergic reaction mediated by antibodies which are released as shortly after the drug enters the circulation.

Herbal therapy: The use of medicinal herbs for the treatment of disease.

Hypersensitivity: Allergic immune response to a substance causing a range of symptoms from mild inflammation to anaphylactic shock and death.

Intraosseous: Refers to administration of a drug directly into the bone marrow.

Intrathecal: Refers to administration of a drug into the spinal canal.

Iodinated contrast medium (ICM): A radiopaque liquid injected or infused into a hollow structure to allow radiographic study of the structure.

Neurotransmitters: Chemicals that bind to target cells to produce a specific neurological effect.

Parenteral: Refers to administration of a drug by injection.

Peak effect: The period of maximum effect of a drug.

Pharmacodynamics: The biochemical and physiological effects of drugs and their mechanisms of action in the body.

Pharmacokinetics: The movement of a drug through the tissues and cells of the body, including the processes of absorption, distribution, and localization in tissues, biotransformation, and excretion by mechanical and chemical means.

Pharmacology: The study of drugs and their action in the body.

Prescription: An order for a drug written by a qualified medical staff member.

Proprietary name: The patented name given to a drug by its manufacturer.

Side effects: Anticipated effects of a drug other than those intended. Side effects may be uncomfortable for the patient or may have a positive outcome.

Stain: A substance applied directly to anatomical surfaces to differentiate normal cells from abnormal ones.

Synergistic: The interaction of agents or conditions such that the total effect is greater than the sum of the individual effects.

Therapeutic window: The difference in drug dose between the therapeutic level and toxic level.

Topical: Refers to application of a drug to the skin or mucous membranes.

Trade name: The name given to a drug by the company that produces and sells it.

Transdermal: Refers to administration of a drug through a skin patch impregnated with the drug.

U.S. Pharmacopeia (USP): An organization that establishes standards for drugs approved by the U.S. Food and Drug Administration (FDA) for their labeled use. All approved drugs have been tested for consumer safety, and written information is available about their pharmacological action, use, risks, and dosage.

INTRODUCTION

The study of drugs is called **pharmacology**. A **drug** is a substance that alters one or more functions in the body. Modern pharmacology encompasses drug composition, mechanism of action, adverse reactions, and side effects.

This chapter focuses on the surgical technologist's role in drug handling. It is not intended as an inclusive pharmacological reference. The specific categories and types of drugs and drug equipment that technologists handle are discussed in detail. Drugs used on the surgical field are emphasized, and other drugs are referenced to give the student a more widespread understanding of pharmacology.

Surgical technologists and other allied health professionals study the basics of pharmacology because they participate in the medication process. The most important points of focus in this study are drug handling, prevention of drug errors, and a basic understanding of drug categories.

Drug groups are also discussed elsewhere in this text as follows:

- Anesthetics and other central nervous system (CNS) agents: Chapter 12
- Topical hemostatic agents: Chapter 17
- Ophthalmic drugs: Chapter 26

ORIGIN OF MEDICINES

Drugs used in modern medicine are derived from a number of sources:

- Synthetic chemicals
- Animal and human proteins
- Minerals
- Elemental metals

These substances include both natural and synthetic (man-made) materials. Most medicines used in Western countries are derived from one or more synthetic molecules. These may mimic, or act like, substances found in nature, but they have been modified to alter particular physiological effects or to make them safer to use.

Throughout history, healers of all cultures have used biological (natural) substances in the treatment of medical and psychological illness. Traditional healing with plants has guided the development of modern pharmaceuticals. Today, herbal medicines have returned to modern therapy as a component of healing. Other biological substances include proteins and hormones derived from animal or human sources. These are used in many different medicinal and immunological agents and also for grafting.

Blood and blood components have a long history of use. Advanced methods of refinement and purification now allow the manufacture of fractional blood and plasma components.

Metals, salts, and other elements are also used in purified form, either alone or as components of other drugs. For example, barium is used for diagnostic procedures, and electrolytes are used to maintain fluid balance.

The term *drug* is defined in U.S. law as a substance intended for use in the diagnosis, cure, relief, treatment, or prevention of disease or intended to affect the structure of function of the body.[1] This qualification is associated with regulations that protect the public from harm caused by a medical intervention.

DRUG INFORMATION RESOURCES

Drug information, including a drug's biochemical action, the correct **dosage,** and other technical data, is available to physicians and other prescribers. Primary health care providers often use the *Physicians' Desk Reference,* which is updated yearly and contains detailed information about most drugs. Other commonly used references are the *American Hospital Formulary Service Drug Information* and the *United States Pharmacopoeia-National Formulary (USP-NF)* Nursing drug handbooks are useful for less complex information that relates directly to patient care.

The U.S. Food and Drug Administration (FDA) provides an on-line directory of all approved drug products in the United States. This can be found at http://www.fda.gov/cder/ob/default.htm or search *FDA Orange Book.*

DRUG STANDARDS AND REGULATIONS

APPROVAL AND SAFETY

In the United States, strict controls and standards are maintained for all agents used in the body. This includes not only drugs but also artificial implants, wound closure materials, and medical devices for improving or controlling body functions.

In the United States, drugs are approved for medical use after rigid testing and application to the FDA. Many years of research and testing are needed to prepare a drug for FDA approval. The FDA authorizes the sale and distribution of drugs and also is responsible for ensuring that approved drugs have met consumer safety requirements. It approves drug literature and labeling so that health care providers and the public can learn about the nature and use of a drug and the risks associated with it.

QUALITY

To protect the public from harm, all drugs must meet standards for quality, strength, packaging safety, and dosage. These standards are established by the **U.S. Pharmacopeia (USP).** All drugs that meet these standards have the initials *USP* after their generic (nonproprietary) name. Approved drugs are published in the *U.S. Pharmacopeia–National Formulary* (USP-NF), a reference that is updated every 5 years. The World Health Organization (WHO) publishes an international formulary, the *International Pharmacopoeia.* The USP also tests and registers any materials or devices that are used in the human body.

CONTROL AND CLASSIFICATION

Drugs that have the potential for *abuse* (deliberate overuse of a drug) are classified by the U.S. Drug Enforcement

Agency (DEA). The classification (called a *schedule*) is based on the risk of abuse or dependency and harmful effects:

- **Schedule I:** Drugs with no medical use that have the highest potential for abuse.
- **Schedule II:** Drugs with an accepted medical use but a high potential for abuse.
- **Schedules III** and **IV:** Drugs with less potential for abuse.
- **Schedule V:** Drugs with the least potential for abuse or dependency.

PREGNANCY CATEGORIES

Drugs are classified by pregnancy category (A, B, C, D, and X) to inform health care workers and patients of the potential risk to the fetus if a mother takes the drug. The categories are described as follows:

- A: These carry no risk to the fetus.
- B: Studies in animals show risk to the fetus; well designed studies in people do not.
- C: Inadequate studies have been done in animals and people; some studies show risk to the fetus in animals
- D: There is risk to the human fetus but the benefits may outweigh risks in certain situations
- X drugs have been proven to pose a risk that outweighs the benefit of the drug.

Most drugs are listed as category D, because it is not known whether they pose a risk and testing would be unethical under any circumstances.

DRUG HANDLING AND STATE PRACTICE ACTS

DEFINITION OF PRACTICE

The laws pertaining to prescriptions, dispensing, and administration of drugs are defined by each state's medical and nursing practice acts. The Joint Commission requires health care organizations to develop policies that agree with state laws regulating who may handle drugs and how. These policies regulate the following activities:

- Procurement, storage, and selection of drugs
- Prescription, ordering, and transcription of drug orders
- Preparation and dispensing of drugs
- Administration of drugs
- Monitoring of the patient after the administration of a drug

To prevent patient injury, all personnel who participate in these activities must be trained and specifically designated to perform them by hospital policy and individual state laws. The surgical technologist is responsible for knowing and complying with these laws and regulations. State laws do not directly cite the surgical technologists' role in the medication process, but rather specify that only licensed nurses or medical doctors may carry out specific tasks related to the administration of drugs. These medical practice acts are discussed in Chapter 4.

RESPONSIBILITY AND DELEGATION

The surgical technologist's responsibility in handling medications is defined by the medical and nursing practice acts of the particular state.

> ❖ The role of the surgical technologist in the handling of drugs is to serve as an intermediary between two professionals specifically licensed by their state to administer drugs.

The surgical technologist has defined responsibilities in the medication process:

- Accept drugs for use on the sterile field from qualified personnel only.
- Prepare and measure drugs under the supervision of a qualified nurse or physician.
- Ensure that the drug delivered to the surgeon is the one requested, in the correct strength and amount.
- Follow accepted standards of care while handling drugs to ensure safety and prevent drug errors.

IDENTIFICATION OF DRUGS

NOMENCLATURE

Drug *nomenclature* is a system of identifying drugs by name. Three methods are used in the international nomenclature system:

- Trade (or proprietary) name
- Generic name
- Chemical name

When a drug is developed, the company that produces the drug obtains a patent for it and gives it a *trade name* (brand name) under which the drug is marketed. Drug patents and their names are generally granted for 20 years. The trade name is usually easy to remember and is often associated with the effect or purpose of the drug.

The second method of drug identification is by its *generic* name, which is assigned by the United States Adopted Names council (USAN) at the time of patent. The USAN ensures that drug names do not sound or look alike, to help prevent drug errors. After the drug patent has expired, any company may produce the generic substance and provide a new trade name. By law, drugs with the same generic name must have the same chemical composition, regardless of how many companies produce it.

Generic drugs are tested and regulated by the same standards as brand name drugs. They are less expensive than brand name drugs and in general much more widely available than branded equivalents. WHO has campaigned rigorously for many years to promote the use of generic drugs and educate health consumers about their safety, effectiveness, and affordability. The third method of drug identification is by its chemical name. Chemical names are derived from the molecular formula of a drug following international convention. Some examples of drug nomenclature are listed below:

Examples of Drug Nomenclature Trade Name	Generic Name	Chemical Name
Zoloft	sertraline HCL	(1S,4S)-4-(3,4-dichlorophenyl)-IN-methyl-1,2,3,4-tetrahydro-naphthalen-1-amine
Cipro Ciproxin	ciprofloxacin	1-cyclopropyl- 6 fluoro- 7-piperazin- 1-yl-quinoline-3-carboxylic acid
Lasix	furosemide	4-chloro-2-(furan-2-ylmethylamino)- 5-sulfamoylbenzoic acid

DRUG ADMINISTRATION ROUTES

Drug administration is the actual *delivery* of the drug to the patient. There are many different methods or routes used for drug delivery. The recommended route for any drug is based on its chemical composition, the target tissue, and the condition of the patient. When a drug is prescribed, the route of administration is indicated on the label and by the prescribing health practitioner. A drug intended for one route *may not be given by another route*. The drug may be available for administration in another form, but it must be approved and labeled for that use.

The common routes of administration are as follows:
- **Parenteral drugs:** Administration is by injection (Figure 14-1).
  - Intravenous (IV): Injection directly into a blood vessel; the fastest route.
  - **Intraosseous** (IO): Injection directly into the bone marrow; used during emergencies when an IV line cannot be initiated or maintained.
  - Intramuscular (IM): Injection into a muscle.
  - Subcutaneous (SC): Injection into the adipose (fat) tissue.
  - Intradermal (ID): Injection between the dermis and epidermis.
  - **Intrathecal:** Injection into the spinal canal.
- **Oral drugs:** Administration is by mouth, abbreviated as PO (per os). Oral medications are available in tablet, capsule, or liquid form.
- **Topical drugs:** Medication is applied directly to the skin or mucous membrane, where it is rapidly absorbed into the bloodstream. A number of different methods are used to administer a topical drug.
  - Aerosol: Administration as a spray.
  - Instill: Administration by drops in the ear or eye.
  - Buccal: A tablet placed between the lip and gum.
  - Subungual: A tablet placed under the tongue.
  - **Transdermal:** Administration through the skin; the medication is applied directly to the skin for absorption or delivered through a patch.
  - Suppository: A semisolid or solid substance is introduced into the vagina or rectum, where it dissolves and is absorbed.
  - Irrigation: Washing of the skin or tissue with the medication or solution.

It is important to remember that the *route of a drug may not identify the final destination of that drug*. The chemical and

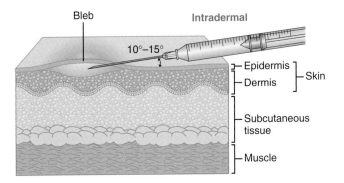
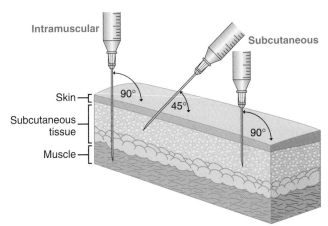

Figure 14-1 Common routes of parenteral injection. *(From Kee J, Hayes E, McCuiston L: Pharmacology, ed 5, Philadelphia, 2006, WB Saunders.)*

physical characteristics of the drug influence absorption. For example, the drug nitroglycerine is absorbed through the mucous membrane directly into the bloodstream and reaches the heart within moments. However, tablets must be broken down in the stomach and intestine before absorption. Drug contained in aerosol spray is inhaled into the respiratory system where it is quickly absorbed through the alveoli and into the bloodstream. Table 14-1 shows drug forms and routes.

DRUG ACTION

When a drug enters the body by any route, *both the body and the drug undergo change*. That is, the drug is broken down chemically (change in the drug), and the drug has a physiological effect on the patient.

Table 14-1

Drug Forms, Routes, and Packaging

Drug Form	Route	Packaging
Liquid	Parenteral administration: single-dose injection	Glass vial, ampule
	Intravenous infusion	Glass bottle or plastic pouch
	Intermittent wound irrigation	Plastic bottle
	Instillation	Dropper bottle
	Oral administration	Single-dose or multiple-dose container
	Continuous irrigation	Plastic pouch
Tablet	Oral administration	Blister pack
	Sublingual administration	Glass or metal bottle
Suppository	Rectal, vaginal insertion	Blister pack
Ointment, cream	Topical administration: skin	Pouch or tube
Ointment	Instillation administration: eye	
Water-based gel	Application to mucous membrane–lined tubular organ	
Skin patch	Transdermal administration	Dry package
Wax	Topical administration: bone	Sterile aluminum pouch
Powder	Topical administration: capillary bed	Plastic or glass jar
Absorbable collagen fiber, mesh	Topical administration: capillary bed	Glass jar
Gelatin sponge	Topical administration: capillary bed	Dry paper envelope
Gas	Inhalation via mask, endotracheal tube, laryngeal mask airway, nasal cannula	Tank or in-line supply
Aerosol droplet	Inhalation	Nebulizer or mask
Volatile liquid	Inhalation	Anesthesia machine

❖ *Changes to a drug after administration are called pharmacokinetics. The process of pharmacokinetics has several stages.*

❖ *Changes (both intended and unintended) to the body as a result of the drug are called pharmacodynamics.*

PHARMACOKINETICS

Pharmacokinetics is the action of the body on the drug itself. Once a drug is introduced into the body, as it moves through various physiological paths. This is a complex process that depends on the condition of the body as much as the drug's composition. The individual's age, genetics, physical condition, and many other factors determine how quickly the drug moves through the body, the onset (beginning) of its effects, the intensity of the effect, and how it is cleared from the tissues. Pharmacokinetics is described by mathematical formulas that take into account the rate of absorption, the volume or amount of drug in the body, and the **concentration** of the drug in the plasma.

For purposes of general study, the entire process of pharmacokinetics is divided into four processes:

- Absorption,
- Distribution,
- Biotransformation (metabolism)
- Excretion (elimination).

Absorption

Absorption is the process in which a drug enters the bloodstream following administration. The rate of absorption and the amount of drug that actually reaches the target tissue depends on many factors such as the chemical structure of the drug, method of administration, and the condition of the patient. Absorption usually involves chemical and physical breakdown of the drug. For example, oral drugs must dissolve before passing through the wall of the small intestine and liver. The substance then enters the bloodstream where it is carried to the target tissue. Drugs that are injected directly into a blood vessel reach the target tissue almost immediately, whereas one injected into the muscle or fat usually takes 15 to 30 minutes to take effect. Many drugs contain components or additives that enhance (increase the rate or amount) or delay absorption.

Distribution

After the drug enters the bloodstream, it is carried (distributed) to body tissues, where it exerts its pharmacological effect. Not all of the drug administered reaches the target tissue. The amount of drug available and the rate of availability is called the *bioavailability*. For example, some of the drug may become tightly bound to blood proteins and are released to the target tissue very slowly. Fat-soluble drugs move rapidly across the cell membranes and take effect quickly but also tend to accumulate in fatty tissue, which prolongs their effect. Water-soluble substances are much slower to act because they stay in the bloodstream longer than those that are fat soluble. In all cases, only the free unbound drug is available to tissues for pharmacological effect.

Biotransformation (Metabolism)

Biotransformation, or drug metabolism, is the chemical breakdown of a drug in the body. Most drugs are broken down into smaller, less complex chemical components by enzymes. This occurs mainly in the liver. Biotransformation prepares the drug for *excretion*, or elimination from the body. Because most biotransformation occurs in the liver, conditions that decrease liver function can alter drug metabolism, resulting in toxicity. Liver disease and advanced age are two causes of altered liver metabolism, which can affect drug metabolism.

In pharmacology and medicine, it is critical to know how long a drug is active. This is related to its rate of biotransformation, which is measured by the drug's half-life. The **half-life** is *the time it takes for one half of the drug to be cleared from the body.* Some drugs, such as antibiotics, have a short half-life and must be given repeatedly over a short period of time so that the therapeutic amount stays constant for the duration of treatment. Other drugs have a long half-life and can be given less frequently to maintain therapeutic levels.

Excretion (Elimination)

Drugs are mainly eliminated or cleared from the body through the kidneys. A small percentage is excreted through the biliary tract, breast milk, saliva, and intestine. Volatile drugs and anesthetics are excreted through the lungs during exhalation. Just as liver disease can alter drug metabolism, kidney disease can severely retard or block drug elimination and result in life-threatening toxicity.

Drugs are eliminated in their original chemical form or as the products of metabolism. In this process chemical reactions cause the drug to break down into smaller molecules or components. Metabolic components of the drug are called *metabolites.* In a healthy individual, all of the drug is excreted—either in intact form or as metabolites.

PHARMACODYNAMICS

Receptors, Antagonists, and Agonists

Pharmacodynamics is the biochemical and physiological effect of the drug on the body. Drugs exert their effect through the actions of protein receptors on the cell surface or inside the cell. Receptors have the ability to "lock on" to body chemicals, such as neurotransmitters and hormones, and thereby exert their effect. These body chemicals are involved in normal physiology and therefore are called *endogenous substances.* Drugs can take the place of the endogenous substances and either block their uptake in the cell or exert their own effect. A drug or substance that blocks endogenous substances is called an **antagonist**. A drug or substance that binds to the receptor to stimulate a specific response is called an **agonist**.

Drug action is related to the amount of drug administered. However, increasing the amount of drug beyond the therapeutic (effective) level results in toxicity. The range between the therapeutic amount and toxic dose is called the *therapeutic window.* Drugs in which the difference between the therapeutic dose and toxicity or lethal effects is small are said to have a "narrow therapeutic window." The **dose** of a drug must be carefully measured to ensure that only the amount prescribed is administered. This is very important for the surgical technologist who handles dose-dependent drugs on the surgical field.

ADVERSE REACTIONS TO DRUGS

Whenever a drug is administered, many physiological changes can take place in the body. Some of these are therapeutic (desirable) effects while others may be undesirable or potentially harmful Precautions against taking a drug under circumstances known to be harmful are stated as *contraindications.*

An **adverse reaction** is an undesirable or intolerable reaction to a drug administered at the *normal dosage.* It is important to remember that the adverse reaction occurs when the drug is given at the normal dose (normal range because other type of effects are directly related to dosage. Adverse reactions are *unexpected,* although they may be predictable in certain individuals. When a drug is tested before its release, adverse reactions are documented, and this becomes part of the drug information available to clinicians and patients. Examples of mild adverse effects include nausea and dizziness. This type of effect is usually transient and ceases when the drug is stopped. More serious adverse reactions include shortness of breath, severe itching, and swelling.

Medical and nursing personnel are trained to recognize the clinical signs and symptoms of an adverse drug event. The responsibility for assessment, evaluation, and treatment is theirs. The surgical technologist assists in emergencies as directed. Allied health personnel have two important roles in this process:

1. Keen observation of a patient's normal behavior and appearance.
2. Immediately reporting to medical and nursing personnel any signs and symptoms that seem abnormal.

❖ *Surgical technologists should make no attempt to diagnose the problem. Their time and energy should be focused on accurate reporting and responding as directed.*

When reporting a suspected drug reaction, follow these guidelines:
- What sign or signs do you observe that you believe are not normal for that patient?
- When did it start?
- What does the patient report (if applicable)?
- What comfort measures did you initiate (e.g., providing warmth, reassurance)?

Drug Allergy

True allergy to a drug is mediated by the immune system and requires previous exposure to substances in the drug or a genetic predisposition to allergy. An immune response that causes irritation, respiratory failure, or death is called *hypersensitivity.* Hypersensitivity can be mild, producing only a rash or wheezing, or it can be severe, resulting in respiratory failure and death caused by anaphylactic shock.

Allergic reactions are characterized as immediate or delayed. Delayed sensitivity can occur up to 12 hours after exposure to a drug and is mediated by T lymphocytes. Immediate reactions are mediated by antibodies. All allergic reactions are divided into the following categories:
- *Type I:* Characterized by tissue inflammation caused by the release of histamine in the body. This causes increased permeability of blood vessels and constriction of bronchioles, leading to difficulty breathing. The most extreme form of sensitivity is anaphylactic shock, which can lead to death. NOTE: The symptoms of and treatment for anaphylactic shock are described in Chapter 12.
- *Type II:* Called a *cytotoxic reaction,* the results of interaction between two antibodies and cell surface antigens. Results in the activation of powerful immune defense

mechanisms, causing injury or death. Mismatched blood transfusion reactions and hemolytic disease in newborns are type II reactions.

- *Type III:* Caused by antigen-antibody complexes, which cause tissue damage when they trigger immune response. Allergy to antibiotics is an example of a type III response. Symptoms include itching, rash, severe tissue swelling, and fever. This type of reaction usually resolves in several days.

- *Type IV:* Cell-mediated reactions (not related to antibodies) that occur 24 to 72 hours after exposure to the agent. An example of this type of delayed hypersensitivity is a positive reaction to the tuberculin skin test in which a small amount of killed *Mycobacterium tuberculosis* is injected.

MEDICATION PROCESS

The events of the medication process include the following procedures:

- **Supply and procurement:** Drugs are stored or maintained in one or more pharmacy locations in the health care facility. Medicines are obtained from these locations and distributed to other designated pharmacies. The surgical department may have one or more pharmacy locations where drugs are stored, and dispensed. Manual or electronic inventory control is maintained in all drug storage areas.

- **Prescription and selection:** Drugs are selected and obtained from the pharmacy or drug storage area by qualified personnel by means of a written or verbal prescription.

- **Measurement and preparation:** In the perioperative environment, drugs are prepared, measured, and delivered to the patient by qualified personnel. During surgery, the surgical technologist is an intermediary between two professionals qualified to administer drugs, usually the circulating nurse and the surgeon. The scrub may prepare drugs at the sterile field.

- **Administration:** Drugs are administered to the patient in the correct route, form, and amount by qualified personnel only.

- **Documentation:** Each time a drug is given, it must be documented in the patient's chart. The name of the drug, dose, route, time of administration, and person who administered the drug are recorded.

- **Evaluation:** After **drug administration,** the patient is monitored and assessed for any sign of adverse reaction or allergy.

PREVENTING DRUG ERRORS: THE FIVE RIGHTS

A drug error can occur during any stage of the medication process. An error can cause serious injury or death. Many systems have been developed to reduce drug errors. A method that has proved successful is the five rights of medication. This is a means of verifying that all parameters of drug administration are correct. The five rights are:

1. The right drug
2. The right dose
3. The right route
4. The right patient
5. The right time

A sixth right applies to medications used in the surgical field:

6. The right surgical label.

Although surgical technologists do not administer medications, they directly participate with others in selecting, receiving, dispensing, mixing, and labeling drugs. By following an exact protocol for handling drugs, the surgical technologist adapts the six rights to the practice of surgical technology.

The Right Drug

"The right drug" is the drug that has been ordered by the surgeon. This means that the correct drug must be selected from the operating room pharmacy stock before surgery. The scrub must select the right drug on the instrument table. Failure to make both selections correctly results in a medication error.

The Right Dose

"The right dose" means the right amount of drug is administered. The right dose is determined by qualified personnel based on their knowledge of the drug. The right dose is achieved on the sterile field by accurate calculation and measurement. These tasks are the responsibility of the scrub in consultation with the surgeon or circulating registered nurse.

The Right Route

"The right route" is the one intended for that drug and prescribed by the surgeon. Drugs are labeled according to approved route (e.g., "For topical use only" or "Not for use in the eyes"). A drug may not be administered by any route other than that approved; to do so may cause serious injury or death.

The Right Patient

"The right patient" means that the patient is identified as the right patient when the person enters the surgical holding area and again when the individual is brought into the surgical suite. Outside of surgery, the patient is identified immediately before a drug is administered, following a precise protocol.

The Right Time

Although "the right time" originally meant that drugs were administered according to a timed schedule, in surgery this right can mean preparing drugs at the correct time. Some drugs must be prepared immediately before use to preserve their physical properties.

The Right Label and Patient Documentation

When the scrub receives a drug from the circulator, he or she must immediately and accurately label the drug. Improper labeling (or worse, no labeling) is a violation of standard operating room procedure and is a risk to the patient. Documentation is the responsibility of the registered nurse or physician. The name of the drug, strength, dosage, administration route, and time of administration are recorded in the patient's chart.

DRUG PROCUREMENT: PRESCRIPTION AND SELECTION

The operating room uses a rotating supply of drugs from the hospital pharmacy. Drugs usually are stored in a restricted area on open shelves or in a computerized drug storage device. Most surgical departments have a dedicated pharmacy that is stocked from a central location in the facility. **Controlled substances** are always kept in a separate locked cabinet or dispenser for increased control and safety.

A **prescription** is a *written or verbal* order for dispensing and administering a drug. Only medical professionals licensed by law to prescribe drugs may give a prescription. A *drug transcription* is a handwritten or typed transfer of a drug order. Only qualified licensed personnel can give and take verbal orders for a drug. In the operating room, the surgeon usually gives a verbal order for the drugs to be used in a particular procedure. When a drug is used routinely on a particular procedure, this is noted on the surgeon's preferences, which are kept in written or computer format and constitutes an order for the drug. The prescription must include the name of the drug, dosage, and route.

Selecting the correct drug is a critical activity in the medication process. Qualified personnel select necessary drugs from the operating room stock on a case by case basis according to the surgeon's orders.

DRUG PACKAGING

Drugs are commercially dispensed to benefit the patient and health care personnel. Newer dispensing technologies have been developed to reduce medication errors and lower the risk of injury by needles and broken glass. Needleless transfer systems provide a method of mixing powder and liquid drug components without using a syringe. Drugs are transferred with a delivery device that ejects fluid from the commercial container directly into a sterile basin or bowl.

GLASS VIAL

Liquid drugs are supplied in a glass vial or an ampule (Figure 14-2). Some dry agents such as hemostatic products and biosynthetic grafting materials are also supplied in vials. The glass vial is capped with a rubber stopper and protective metal cap. The liquid drug is withdrawn from the vial with a syringe and needle. Sterile powdered and mesh hemostatics are also supplied in a glass vial to protect them from moisture and to maintain sterility. Dry materials are removed with sterile forceps.

GLASS AMPULE

A glass ampule is a hollow glass bulb with a narrow neck. Because the entire container is glass, the top must be broken off to allow withdrawal of the drug.

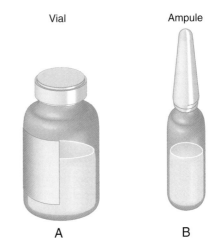

Figure 14-2 **A,** Glass vial. **B,** Glass ampule. *(From Kee JL, Marchal SM: Clinical calculations: application to general and specialty areas, ed 5, Philadelphia, 2004, WB Saunders.)*

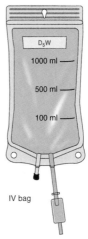

Figure 14-3 Collapsible intravenous solution bag.

COLLAPSIBLE PLASTIC BAG

Blood products and IV solutions are supplied in vacuum-sealed, collapsible plastic bags (Figure 14-3). The solution is delivered to the patient though an IV set; this is high-grade plastic tubing fitted at one end with a plastic spike for insertion into the bag. The other end fits into a standard Luer-Lock or IV catheter tip. The IV set is fitted with a clamp for releasing and stopping the flow of liquid.

RIGID PLASTIC CONTAINER

Irrigation solutions not intended for IV use are commercially dispensed in rigid plastic bottles. These are fitted with a special cap that protects the lip of the bottle from contamination during pouring. However, once a rigid container is opened, all the liquid must be dispensed.

GLASS BOTTLE OR JAR

Glass bottles are used to contain certain types of dressings, which must be kept free of moisture. Examples include gauze strips for packing the nasal cavity or vagina, and anhydrous powders used in the preparation of bone matrix.

PEEL POUCH

Agents for bone hemostasis (bone wax) and petroleum-impregnated dressings are supplied in foil peel-apart pouches. This type of packaging allows sterile distribution, from the inner surface of the square pouch, which is sealed on all four edges. The two top edges are grasped and peeled back to expose the dressings contained inside, in the same way as suture packages are delivered. This is shown in Chapter 17.

QUALITY ASSURANCE

Quality assurance is a method of providing maximum safety in the manufacturing, storage, and administration of drugs. All substances designated for use in the body are labeled to indicate their origin, designated use, and composition. This information is used to track the item from the time it leaves the manufacturer until administration or implantation in the patient. Every drug label contains the name of the drug, its chemical composition, strength, and amount. Every drug has a designated route of administration (e.g., intravenous, topical, oral). This is clearly stated on the package.

The lot number of a drug identifies the specific batch of drug prepared by the pharmaceutical laboratory. In the event of contamination or incorrect formulation of a batch, all drug samples included in the batch can be identified, recalled, and destroyed.

Drugs must not be used beyond the specified expiration date. Over time, many drugs lose their efficacy and may become toxic. The expiration date indicates when the drug must be destroyed. Administration of drugs that have passed their expiration date is a drug error.

READING A DRUG LABEL

All personnel handling drugs in the operating room must be able to correctly identify the components of a drug label, which contains the drug's name, the amount of drug, and the drug's strength, manufacturer, lot number, and expiration date (Figure 14-4).

After the drug is selected, the drug container and its contents are examined. The label is inspected to confirm that the drug and amount are correct, to verify the correct dosage, and to check the expiration date. The vial or container must be intact with no signs of cracking or chipping. The seal must be unbroken, with no sign that sterility has been breached. The drug itself must appear normal. A drug that is normally clear should have no sign of precipitation or cloudiness. The color of the drug may be an indication of changes in the chemical structure.

DRUG MEASUREMENT

All drugs and solutions are measured before administration. There is no exception to this protocol. The surgical technologist is responsible for accurate measurement throughout the entire medication process.

In surgery, drugs may be measured twice:

1. **When the scrubbed technologist receives a drug.** Drugs are distributed to the technologist before surgery begins or in the intraoperative period. Regardless of how the drug is received, the registered nurse must measure the amount accurately and the amount must be acknowledged by both individuals. Irrigation solutions are measured by the manufacturer before bottling. The amount is stated on the label, and all the solution is distributed at once (see later discussion).

2. **When the technologist delivers the drug to the surgeon.** The surgical technologist delivers the drug to the surgeon using a medical syringe, irrigation device, or container. The drug is again measured at this time. A calibrated medical syringe is always used for drugs intended for injection or infusion.

DELIVERY DEVICES

Drug delivery devices are used to measure and administer a drug to the patient. Drugs that are administered by any parenteral method must be measured by the appropriate-size syringe.

The calibrated cup is not accurate for drug administration except for household use or for oral liquids in the patient care setting. It may be used as a drug container before exact measurement and administration.

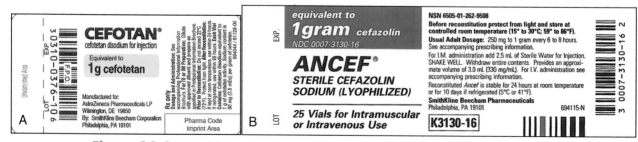

Figure 14-4   Drug labels. Note dose, strength, bar code, and use. (*From Kee J, Hayes E, McCuiston L:* Pharmacology, *ed 5, Philadelphia, 2006, WB Saunders.*)

SYRINGE

The syringe is used to measure, dispense, and administer a drug by injection and infusion. This is the most accurate method for measuring liquids. Two types of syringe tips are the locking (Luer-Lock) and catheter tips (also called plain tip or slip tip). The syringe tip accepts a hypodermic needle or a catheter. On a Luer-Lock syringe, the needle is locked in place by twisting it; the catheter tip connects to other devices without a locking mechanism (Figure 14-5).

Syringes are available in many sizes and types. All syringes except the insulin syringe are calibrated in milliliters (mL). The most common syringe sizes are 1, 3, 5, and 10 cc. The tuberculin syringe is the smallest metric syringe. The total volume of this syringe is 0.5 or 1 cc. The barrel of the syringe is inscribed with measurement hashes.

The insulin syringe is calibrated in *insulin units rather than in metric system units*. The calibrations are intended for use with insulin only. The insulin syringe can be differentiated from a normal tuberculin syringe by its orange sheath.

NEEDLES

Hypodermic needles are sized according to gauge (lumen or bore size) and length (Figure 14-6). The larger the gauge, the smaller the needle bore. Because of the risk of blood-borne diseases, the National Institute for Occupational Safety and Health (NIOSH) requires that syringes have some feature that allows the needle to be retracted or protected so that personnel are not punctured during or after use. Needleless systems are now in common use and should be available in all operating rooms.

It is acceptable to place the cap on the table and scoop it up with the point of the needle or use a needle-capping device. With this device, the cap is held in a rigid container and the needle and syringe combination is pushed down into the cap. *Needles must never be recapped using two hands.*

IRRIGATION DEVICES

Fluid irrigation is used on the surgical field to clear away blood and tissue debris. In specialized procedures, irrigation fluid may contain a drug such as heparin (an anticoagulant) or an antibiotic solution. Irrigation devices used to flush the surgical wound are designed to hold relatively large amounts of solution and direct it in a narrow stream. In some cases, a calibrated syringe is used (e.g., when irrigation fluid is directed into a vessel or duct). The most common general irrigation devices are the Asepto syringe and bulb syringe.

Smaller irrigation devices are required for procedures involving delicate tissues (e.g., the eye, ear, and vascular tissue) and during microsurgery. In these procedures, the solution is used directly from its container, which is fitted a fine irrigating tip. A conventional syringe and specialized tip may also be used for fine irrigation.

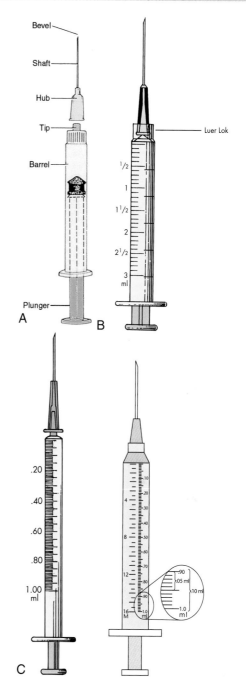

Figure 14-5 **A,** Catheter tip syringe. **B,** Luer-Lock syringes. **C,** Tuberculin syringe. *(A from Elkin M, Perry A, Potter P: Nursing interventions and clinical skills, ed 2, St Louis, 2000, Mosby; B from Potter PA, Perry AG: Fundamentals of nursing, ed 5, St Louis, 2001, Mosby; and C from Clayton B, Stock Y: Basic pharmacology of nurses, ed 12, St Louis, Mosby.)*

PARTS OF A NEEDLE

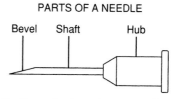

Figure 14-6 Parts of a hypodermic needle. *(From Kee JL, Marchall SM: Clinical calculations: application to general and specialty areas, ed 5, Philadelphia, 2004, WB Saunders.)*

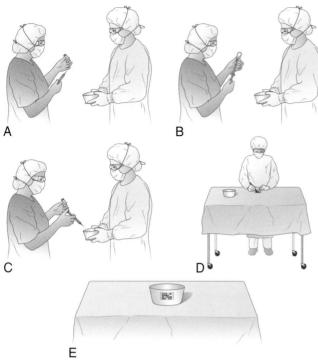

Figure 14-7 Protocol for receiving drugs on the sterile field; drug delivery to the field. **A,** The circulator shows the drug label to the scrub for verification. **B,** The circulator draws up the drug. **C,** The circulator distributes the drug into a sterile container. The circulator again shows the label to the scrub. **D** and **E,** The scrub immediately labels the drug.

DELIVERING DRUGS TO THE STERILE FIELD

The scrub commonly receives drugs or other pharmaceuticals that will be used during surgery from the circulating nurse. This may take place before surgery begins or intraoperatively. When the registered nurse (RN) dispenses a drug to the sterile field, both the RN and the surgical technologist participate (Figure 14-7).

RECOMMENDED PROTOCOL TO PREVENT DRUG ERRORS

1. The circulator holds the drug container so that the scrub can read it easily.
2. The scrub reads and *recites out loud* the name, dose, amount, strength, and expiration date of the drug.
3. The circulator verifies the drug at the same time.
4. The circulator *again shows* the drug container to the scrub, and both acknowledge the information.
5. The drug is immediately labeled.
6. When any drug is passed to the surgeon, the name and concentration or strength is again repeated out loud so that the surgeon knows what has been dispensed.

GLASS VIAL

To deliver a liquid drug from a glass vial with a rubber stopper, the RN withdraws the drug with a syringe and needle. The needle is then removed and may be replaced by a transfer system. The drug is injected slowly *into a sterile container* held by the scrub or placed at the edge of the sterile field. Only containers made of glass or nonreactive plastic are used to hold medications on the sterile field because metal containers can alter some drugs. Drugs may be poured only from containers that have a safety tip, which maintains sterility during pouring.

❖ *The scrub should not insert a needle into a vial held by the circulator. This is considered poor aseptic technique by regulatory and safety organizations and places the circulator at risk for needle injury.*

GLASS AMPULE

A glass ampule is opened by placing a sponge over the top of the ampule and snapping it off *away* from the face. A syringe fitted with a filter is used to withdraw the drug. The drug is injected into a small sterile container on the field. The broken pieces and empty vial are discarded in the sharps box. The sponge is discarded because it contains glass chips. Ampule transfer devices are also available. These reduce the risk of contamination and injury from glass particles.

DRUG RECONSTITUTION

Some drugs are dispensed in dry form and must be reconstituted to liquid form before administration. The most common drugs of this type used on the sterile field are bacitracin (an antibacterial used for irrigation) and topical thrombin (an anticoagulant).

Only sterile injectable saline is used to reconstitute drugs. The surgical technologist and registered nurse participate in drug reconstitution. The procedure for drug identification and verification of dose is performed as described previously.

1. The registered nurse (in the circulating role) prepares the drug vial and sterile injectable saline vial for aseptic distribution.
2. The injectable saline is injected into the vial containing the dry drug. The vial is gently agitated until no particles of dry agent are visible.
3. A sterile transfer device is attached to the vial.
4. The technologist receives the reconstituted drug in a container after verification of the dose and amount.

IRRIGATION FLUIDS

Sterile irrigation fluids are delivered directly into a sterile basin or bowl on the field. When irrigation fluids are poured, the flow is never interrupted. *The entire contents of the container must be delivered at one time.* The rationale for this is that the lip of the container cannot be guaranteed to be sterile once the container has been recapped. Note that specific irrigation fluids, which will be in contact with the inner surfaces of blood vessels (such as saline solution for reconstitution with heparin or iodinated contrast media), requires *injectable* saline. This is distributed by the registered nurse.

DRY MATERIALS

To deliver dry drugs (mesh, powder, or fluff) to the sterile field, the cap is opened carefully to prevent contamination of the lip of the vial. The technologist removes the contents with sterile forceps. Petroleum mesh products also are removed from peel pouches with sterile forceps. Petroleum products must not be handled with gloved hands, because the drug may cause the breakdown of glove material.

MANAGING DRUGS ON THE STERILE FIELD

LABELING

Removal of drugs from their commercial containers and transferral to the sterile field increase the risk of drug error. *To reduce drug error, each and every drug container and its delivery device must be labeled.* Labels should be made before the drugs are received so that they can be identified immediately upon delivery to the sterile field. Commercially prepared or handwritten labels are acceptable. The label must state the following information:

1. Name of the drug
2. Strength or percent of the drug
3. Expiration date and time (if this occurs within 24 hours of distribution)

Writing Legibly

All health professionals must discipline themselves to write legibly. Misinterpretation of written words and numbers is one of the causes of medication error.

Recommended Practices

- Make sure labels are printed with waterproof ink on an adhesive sticker.
- Make sure the label is legible.
- Place drugs in one spot on the instrument table and kept them there throughout the case.
- If any doubt exists about the identification of a drug, *the drug must be discarded* and a fresh drug distributed to the sterile field.
- All drugs must be identified with a permanent change of scrubbed personnel, such as during shift changes. Any drugs not labeled are discarded.

DELIVERY TO THE SURGEON

The surgical technologist delivers drugs to the surgeon in the intraoperative period. The surgeon asks for the drug by name. The technologist is responsible for identifying the correct drug from those on the sterile table, preparing the drug for administration, and passing it to the surgeon. When passing the drug, the technologist identifies the drug and its strength *out loud.*

IRRIGATION SOLUTIONS

Irrigation solutions must be kept clean and separate from sterile water used to soak instruments. Irrigation solutions are maintained at body temperature to prevent hypothermia. This is especially important for pediatric, elderly, and very thin patients. Sterile saline and water for irrigation can be kept at a controlled temperature in a solution warmer. Chilled solutions for cardiac and transplant surgery are maintained as sterile ice slush.

DRUG CALCULATIONS

Although surgical technologists do not directly administer medications to the patient, they must calculate solutions used in surgery. The circulator may distribute several types of medications to the surgical technologist, who must mix them in the proper proportions. When the surgical technologist receives any medication from the nurse, the technologist should be able to identify the drug and determine the exact amount received. This may require conversion within one system of measurement or from one system into another.

MATH REQUIREMENTS

This chapter assumes that the reader has achieved at least high school competency in mathematics. All students must be comfortable performing the following basic mathematical operations before scrubbing in surgery. This ability is a prerequisite for performing the drug calculations presented in this chapter:

1. Arithmetic of whole numbers (addition, subtraction, multiplication, division)
2. Rounding off
3. Computations involving fractions, including proper, improper, whole, and mixed fractions
4. Computations involving ratios and proportions
5. Computations involving decimals
6. Computation of percentages and conversion of percentages to decimals, fractions to percentages, and percentages to fractions

SYSTEMS OF MEASUREMENT

Two measurement systems are commonly used in pharmacology, the metric system and the apothecary system. The household system, a third method of measuring, is not used in medicine or surgery because it lacks precision. The English system (also known as *U.S. customary units*) is used in the United States, which up until now has not adopted the metric system except for scientific measurement.

METRIC SYSTEM

The metric system of weights and measures is an international system. It is commonly used in every country except the United States and is the accepted standard for scientific mea-

Box 14-1

Metric System: Mass and Volume

Units of Mass	Units of Volume
1 kiligram (kg) = 1,000 grams (g)	1 liter (L) = 1,000 mililiters (mL)
1 gram (g) = 1,000 miligrams (mg)	1 mL = 1,000 microliters
1 miligram = 1,000 micrograms	

surement. It was introduced in 1960 to standardize world trade and science. The system is based on units or powers of 10 (Box 14-1), which are applied to each type of quantity measured (volume, mass, and length).

Prefixes are used to express multiples of the metric system. Therefore, to arrive at an amount, the base unit is multiplied by the amount associated with its prefix. The prefixes are:

Kilo—1000
Hecto—100
Deca—10
Deci—0.1 (one tenth)
Centi—0.01 (one hundredth)
Mili—0.001 (one thousandth)

Examples:

1 *kilo*meter = 1,000 meters
1 *kilo*gram = 1,000 grams
1 *mili*gram = $^1/_{1,000}$ of a gram
1 *mili*liter = $^1/_{1,000}$ of a liter
5 *mili*liters = $^5/_{1,000}$ of a liter

APOTHECARY SYSTEM

The apothecary system uses Roman numerals to represent measurements and symbols to represent units of measure. The basic units of weight in the apothecary system are grains and ounces. Volume is expressed in drams and minims. Because of errors in measurement and lack of familiarity with the apothecary system, the metric system is now the common system of measurement.

INTERNATIONAL UNITS

International units (IU) are used in the measurement of selected drugs. Any measure that is expressed as units describes the number of units per milliliter after addition of a diluent. For example, if a label states that a vial contains 400,000 international units of a drug, the concentrations of the drug can be altered by adding different amounts of diluent. Remember, however, that the same number of units is contained in the vial, regardless of how much diluent is added. Only the concentration changes.

ROMAN NUMERALS

Roman numerals are based on units of 10 and use letters to represent numbers. Roman numerals are used in the apoth-

ecary system for writing prescriptions. The surgical technologist should be able to convert Roman numerals to the Arabic system (common system).

The numeral is a symbol that represents a number in the Arabic system (0 to 9) as follows:

Roman Numeral	Arabic Number
I	1
V	5
X	10
L	50
C	100
D	500
M	1,000

When numerals are printed in succession, they are added:

$$III = 3$$
$$XXX = 30$$

When a smaller value is positioned in front of a larger one, the smaller one is subtracted from the larger one:

$$IX = 9$$
$$IV = 4$$

Other rules apply for subtracting numerals:
- Subtract only powers of 10 (e.g., XLV = 45).
- Subtract only a single numeral from another single numeral (e.g., 19 = XIX, not IXX).
- Do not subtract a numeral from one that is more than 10 times greater.

MILITARY TIME

Military (or international) time is used in health care facilities to prevent errors. It is based on a 24-hour clock. When military time is written, the colon (:) and common references to time of day (AM and PM) are unnecessary.

Military time begins at 0100 "zero one hundred hours," or 1 AM, and ends at 2400 "twenty-four hundred hours," or 12 midnight. To convert to military time, remove the colon from customary time and use the total number of hours and minutes lapsed from 1200 for day time and 2400 for night time (Figure 14-8).

REVIEW OF ARITHMETIC

FRACTIONS

A fraction defines a number by specifying the division necessary to create that number. For example, the fraction ¾ is the number that results by dividing the top number (the numerator), 3, by the bottom number (the denominator), 4. When the numerator is smaller than the denominator, the result is less than 1; when the numerator is larger than the denominator, the result is greater than 1. When the numerator and denominator are the same, the result is 1.

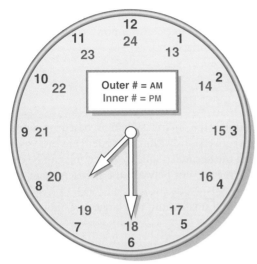

Figure 14-8 Reading military time. *(From Kee J, Hayes E, McCuiston L: Pharmacology, ed 5, Philadelphia, 2006, WB Saunders.)*

Addition and Subtraction

To add or subtract two fractions, the fractions must have the same denominator. Therefore, to complete ⅓ + ⅓, simply add the numerators; the answer is ⅔. Adding or subtracting fractions that have different denominators involves an extra step that requires an understanding of the concept of equivalent fractions. That is, if both the numerator and denominator of a fraction are multiplied (or divided) by the same number, the resulting fraction is equal to the original one. Therefore, if both the numerator and denominator of the fraction ⅓ are multiplied by 2, the resulting fraction is ²⁄₆. The fraction ²⁄₆ is exactly equal to the fraction ⅓. Therefore, adding or subtracting fractions of different denominators requires an equivalent fraction of each that has the same denominator. The denominator selected should be the lowest common denominator (LCD); that is, the lowest number that can be divided by the two denominators of the fraction that must be added or subtracted.

Examples:

Addition

$$\frac{1}{2} + \frac{1}{3} \ (LCD = 6)$$

$$(1 \times 3)/(2 \times 3) = \frac{3}{6}; (1 \times 2)/(3 \times 2) = \frac{2}{6}$$

$$\frac{3}{6} + \frac{2}{6} = \frac{5}{6}$$

$$\frac{3}{4} + \frac{1}{5} \ (LCD = 20)$$

$$(3 \times 5)/(4 \times 5) = \frac{15}{20}$$

$$(1 \times 4)/(5 \times 4) = \frac{4}{20}$$

$$\frac{15}{20} + \frac{4}{20} = \frac{19}{20}.$$

Subtraction

$$\frac{7}{8} - \frac{3}{16} \ (LCD = 16)$$

$$(7 \times 2)/(8 \times 2) = \frac{14}{16}; (3 \times 1)/(16 \times 1) = \frac{3}{16}$$

$$\frac{14}{16} - \frac{3}{16} = \frac{11}{16}$$

$$\frac{4}{7} - \frac{1}{9} \ (LCD = 63)$$

$$(4 \times 9)/(7 \times 9) = \frac{36}{63}; (1 \times 7)/(9 \times 7) = \frac{7}{63}$$

$$\frac{36}{63} - \frac{7}{63} = \frac{29}{63}$$

Multiplication and Division

To multiply, simply multiply the numerators of the two fractions and then multiply the denominators:

$$\frac{2}{3} \times \frac{5}{8} = (2 \times 5)/(3 \times 8) = \frac{10}{24}$$

Any fraction can be reduced (simplified) by dividing both the numerator and denominator by the same number:

$$\frac{10}{24} = (10 \div 2)/(24 \div 2) = \frac{5}{12}$$

The numbers 5 and 12 cannot be divided evenly by any number, therefore 5/12 is a fully reduced fraction.

To divide a fraction, first write the division as a big fraction:

$$\frac{2}{3} \div \frac{5}{6} = \left(\frac{2}{3}\right) \bigg/ \left(\frac{5}{6}\right)$$

Then multiply both numerators of the fractions that make up the big fraction:

$$\left(\frac{2}{3}\right) \bigg/ \left(\frac{5}{6}\right) = \left(\frac{2}{3} \times 6\right) \bigg/ \left(\frac{5}{6} \times 6\right) = \left(\frac{12}{3}\right) \bigg/ \left(\frac{30}{6}\right) = \frac{4}{5}$$

Another method is to invert the divisor and multiply:

$$\frac{2}{3} \div \frac{5}{6} = \frac{2}{3} \times \frac{6}{5} = \frac{12}{15} = \frac{4}{5}$$

Examples:

Multiplication

$$\frac{1}{13} \times \frac{2}{3} = (1 \times 2)/(13 \times 3) = \frac{2}{39}$$

$$\frac{3}{7} \times \frac{4}{535} = (3 \times 4)/(7 \times 5) = 12$$

Division

$$\frac{1}{3} \div \frac{5}{8} = \frac{1}{3} \times \frac{8}{5} = \frac{8}{15}$$

$$\frac{1}{4} \div \frac{1}{16} = \frac{1}{4} \times \frac{16}{1} = \frac{16}{4} = 4$$

DECIMALS

The decimal system is based on powers (multiples) of 10. Each position to the left or right of the decimal point is a higher or lower power of 10.

To convert a fraction, such as ⁴/₅, to a decimal, simply divide the numerator by the denominator (⁴/₅ = 0.8). Some fractions do not result in simple decimal numbers. For example, ⅓ is .33333 ... , and so on forever. For most purposes, the number can be simply rounded off after three figures. To round off, raise the last digit by 1 if it is 5 or higher. Thus .33333 ... is .333, but .66666 ... is .667.

PERCENTAGE

A percentage is a fraction expressed as parts of 100. To convert a fraction to a percentage, convert to a decimal and multiply by 100:

$$\frac{4}{5} = 0.8 \times 100 = 80\%$$

RATIO

A ratio is similar to a fraction. A ratio of 1 to 2 (written 1:2) means that there is 1 unit for every 2 units out of each 3 units (1 + 2) of the item described. To convert a ratio to a fraction, add the two terms to make the denominator, and use the first term as the numerator:

$$1:2 = \frac{1}{3}$$

PROPORTIONS

A proportion is an expression of equality between two fractions. For example, one can write 1:3 = ²/₆. This is the same as ¼ = ²/₈. Proportions are most commonly used for dilutions. Dilution usually is expressed as a percentage, such as a 1% solution. A common problem is determining how much of a chemical to add to a given quantity of liquid to produce a particular dilution. The unknown amount is written as *X*. For example, to make a 1% solution using 500 mL of water, how much chemical is needed? Written as a proportion, it is:

$$X/500\,mL = \frac{1}{100}$$

To solve, multiply the numerator of the first term (X) by the denominator of the second (100) and vice versa (500 × 1). In this case, 100X = 500 mL × 1. Multiplying a number by 1 gives the same number, therefore 100X = 500 mL. To solve for X, divide both sides by 100. Thus:

$$X = \frac{500}{100} = 5\,mL$$

Adding 5 mL of the chemical produces 505 mL of a .0099 solution, which can be rounded off to 1% solution.

UNIT CONVERSION

To perform any drug calculation, all values must be converted into units of the same system. Therefore surgical technologists must be competent in unit conversion. To convert values from one system to another, you must use unit conversion tables. Common conversion formulas should be memorized.

MOVING THE DECIMAL IN THE METRIC SYSTEM

As mentioned, the metric system is based on units of 10. Therefore conversions within the system are easily performed by moving the decimal point. However, this can be done only *within* the metric, not between the metric system and other systems.

To convert a smaller unit to a larger one, move the decimal point to the left.

Example: 250 mg = how many grams?
Recall that 1 g = 1,000 mg. Therefore 250 is divided by 1,000 by moving the decimal point three places to the left: 250.0 mg = 0.25 g.

To convert a larger unit to a smaller one, move the decimal point to the right.

Example: 0.980 L = how many mL?

Using the conversion factor 1 L = 1,000 mL, move the decimal point three places to the right: 0.980 L = 980 mL

To convert a larger unit to smaller units in the metric system, multiply the units that are needed by the equivalent value in the conversion chart.

Example:
You have 1 L of saline solution. You are asked to deliver 500 mL to the surgeon. How many liters is this?
- Convert the two numbers to the same units
- 1 L = 1,000 mL (from the conversion table)
- The desired unit is liters. Liters are larger than milliliters, therefore the conversion will result in a fraction of a liter. Divide the smaller amount by the larger amount:

$$X\,L = 500\,mL/1,000\,mL = 0.5\,L \text{ or } \frac{1}{2}\,L$$

Example:
Convert 120 grains (g) to drams.
- Convert the two numbers to the same units:

$$60\,g = 1\,dram$$

$$X\,drams = 120\,g/60\,g = 2\,drams$$

To convert a large unit to a smaller one in the apothecary system, multiply the unit that is needed by the equivalent value.

Example:
Convert 5 drams to grains.
- Convert both numbers to the same unit using the following conversion factor:

$$1\,dram = 60\,grains\,(g)$$

- Grains are smaller than drams. The desired units are grains. The answer in grains will be larger than the dram amount. You must multiply:

$$60 \text{ grains} \times 5 = 300 \text{ drams}$$

RATIO SYSTEM VERSUS FORMULAS

Formulas are a quick way to measure and calculate drugs. However, formulas can be forgotten or misused. Another danger with formulas is that they cannot be easily validated. If the formula is wrong, the answer is wrong. If you must rely on a formula, you may not fully understand the mathematics required.

Using ratio calculations is better than relying on formulas. Ratio calculations can be validated, and you do not need to memorize formulas. If you understand ratio calculations, you will understand exactly how you derived your answer. To perform ratio calculations, you must understand how to cross-multiply fractions.

This system of calculations uses the relationship of one value to another to solve a problem. Remember that the words *in*, *per*, *of*, and the symbols ":" and "/" denote a ratio. A ratio is a way of expressing a fraction. Study the following example:

The label on a 2-mL ampule reads 50 mg/mL. How many mg are contained in 1.5 mL?

- You are asked about concentration. Concentration is expressed in weight per amount of liquid, such as milligrams per milliliter.
- The known ratio of mg to mL is:

50 mg per 1 mL, *or*

50 mg:1 mL, *or*

50 mg/1 mL

- The unknown ratio is:

X mg per 1.5 mL, *or*

X mg:1 mL, *or*

X mg/1.5 mL

- Set up the ratio as an equation:

50 mg:1 mL = X mg:1.5 mL

- A ratio is 50 mg/1 mL as a fraction:

X mg/1.5 mL

- Cross-multiply:

50 mg/1 mL × X mg/1.5 mL

- Solve for X:

$$X(1) = 50(1.5)$$
$$\text{Answer}: X = 75 \text{ mg}$$

CALCULATION OF SOLUTION STRENGTH

Many of the drugs used in surgery are in solution. A *solution* is a specific substance (solute) dissolved in a specific volume of liquid (solvent or diluent). Expressions of equivalent concentrations are shown in Table 14-2.

A solution can be described in two ways:

- By concentration: weight per volume

Concentration = Mass (weight) of the drug/Volume of solution

- By percent solution: volume per volume, solution, or strength. This is expressed as a percentage or as a ratio. For example, a 6% solution has 6 g of drug in each 100 mL of solution. A drug that is labeled 1:1,000 means that 1 g of medication is dissolved in 1,000 mL of diluent. The strength of the solution is 1 mg/mL.

Example:

Prepare 1 L of a 6% solution.

- Known:

$$6\% = 6 \text{ g per } 100 \text{ mL}$$
$$1 \text{ L} = 1,000 \text{ mL}$$
$$6 \text{ g}:100 \text{ mL} = X \text{ g}:1,000 \text{ mL}$$

- Cross-multiply:

6 g/100 mL × X g/1,000 mL

- Solve for X:

$$100(X) = 6(1,000)$$
$$\text{Answer}: X = 60 \text{ g}$$

Table 14-2

Equivalents for Concentration Expressions

%	Ratio	g/L	g/dL	mg/mL	mg/dL	mcg/mL
10	1:10	100	10	100	10,000	100,000
1	1:100	10	1	10	1,000	10,000
0.1	1:1,000	1	0.1	1	100	1,000
0.01	1:10,000	0.1	0.01	0.1	10	100
0.001	1:100,000	0.01	0.001	0.01	1	10
0.0001	1:1,000,000	0.001	0.0001	0.001	0.1	1

Example:

There are 400,000 units of antibiotic per mL. If 1 mg equals 1,600 units, what is the dose (mL) containing 200 mg?

- Known:

$$1\,mg = 1,600\,units$$
$$200\,mg = 320,000\,units$$
$$1\,mL : 400,000\,units = X\,mL : 320,000\,units$$

- Cross-multiply:

$$6\,g/100\,mL \times X\,g/1,000\,mL$$

- Solve for X:

$$X(400,000) = 1(320,000)$$
$$Answer: X = 0.8\,mL$$

CALCULATION OF DOSAGE BY WEIGHT

Drugs administered to pediatric patients and infants are calculated based on the patient's weight or body surface. This is extremely important because even small errors in dosage can be dangerous to the infant or child. Most adult dosages are based on average adult size. The weight of an adult patient is calculated when critical drugs are being administered or when there are special medical or circumstances to consider. The proper calculation is the amount of drug per kilogram of body weight. The recommended dosage for drugs is obtained from the package insert or a reliable pharmacology reference. Calculations are written out, and the safe range is verified whenever drugs are administered to pediatric patients.

Example:

A child weighing 76 lbs. is ordered to receive 150 mg of Clindamycin every 6 hours. The recommended dose is 8-20 mg/kg/day in four divided doses. The Clindamycin is supplied in 100-mg scored tablets.

1. What is the weight in kg?

$$76\,lbs. \div 2.2\,kg/lb. = 34.5\,kg$$

2. What is the safe total daily dose?

$$Minimum: 8\,mg/kg/day \times 34.5\,kg = 276\,mg/day$$
$$Maximum: 20\,mg/kg/day \times 34.5\,kg = 690\,mg/day$$

3. Is this a safe dose?

$$150\,mg/dose \times 4\,doses/day = 600\,mg/day$$

Yes this is within the recommended safe range.

SELECTED DRUGS USED DURING SURGERY AND INTERVENTIONAL RADIOLOGY

The scrubbed technologist is required to handle and deliver several categories of drugs used on the sterile field and during interventional radiology. In practical terms, the surgical technologist should give priority to these particular drugs and agents. (Refer to Table 14-4 at the end of this chapter for a list of medications and other pharmaceuticals commonly used in surgery and their actions.)

IODINATED AND OPAQUE CONTRAST MEDIA

Indication

Iodinated contrast media are used to fill and outline hollow spaces of the body during plain radiograph and other types of interventional radiology. Examples of iodinated contrast media are:

- Diatrizoate
- Metrizoate

How Supplied

Iodinated contrast media are clear fluids supplied in a glass vial for distribution to the sterile field.

Discussion

An **iodinated contrast medium (ICM)** is a clear, injectable, *radiopaque* liquid (i.e., it is impenetrable to x-rays). An ICM is commonly used in the structural assessment and diagnosis of nearly all hollow spaces of the body. The various types differ in *osmolality* (the amount of iodine by weight in solution). In general, contrast media with high levels of iodine are associated with increased adverse effects whereas those with lower levels of iodine are safer. The modern iodinated contrast media are generally very safe as compared to prototypes used in the past. However, allergy, kidney damage, and anaphylactoid reactions can occur. Reactions can be delayed up to 7 days following administration. Toxic reaction is a risk in patients with impaired renal function. In these inpatients an alternative contrast media is used. As with all drugs used in surgery and interventional radiology, the surgical technologist must keep track of the total amount and concentration (dose) of contrast medium passed to the surgeon during a case.

The scrub prepares this drug by drawing it into a syringe fitted with intravenous tubing. A stopcock may also be attached at the syringe hub. All air must be removed from the tubing before injection as any bubbles appear as black or gray spots on x-ray and may obscure the diagnosis.

NOTE: No association has been proved between allergy to shellfish and sensitivity to an ICM.[2]

Intravascular Uses
Intravenous Uses

- Computed tomography (CT)
- Intravenous urography
- Venography (vena cavae, visceral, peripheral, epidural veins)

Arterial Uses

- Aortography
- Cardiopulmonary angiography
- CNS (cerebral, vertebral, and spinal angiography)
- CT
- Visceral and peripheral arteriography

Intrathecal Uses

- Cisternography
- Myelography

Other Uses
- Arthrography
- Breast ductography
- Cholangiography
- CT
- Cystography
- Endoscopic retrograde cholangiopancreatography
- Fluoroscopy
- Gastrointestinal studies
- Hysterosalpingography
- Nephrostography
- Sialography (salivary ducts)
- Sinus tract studies

Adverse Reactions

Adverse reactions to an ICM can range from mild to fatal. All patients are screened and assessed before surgery, but intraoperative monitoring is required whenever an ICM is used. Categories of

Mild Reaction
- Altered taste
- Anxiety
- Chills
- Cough
- Dizziness
- Flushing
- Headache
- Itching
- Nausea and vomiting
- Pallor
- Rash
- Shaking
- Sweating
- Warmth

Moderate Reaction
- Bronchospasm
- Hypertension
- Hypotension (mild)
- Mild dyspnea
- Tachycardia or bradycardia
- Wheezing

Severe Reaction
- Cardiopulmonary arrest
- Convulsions
- Heart arrhythmias
- Laryngeal edema (severe)
- Severe hypotension
- Unresponsiveness

The list of adverse reactions demonstrates that although iodinated contrast media are frequently used and common to many areas of medicine, the risk of a severe adverse reaction should be considered with every patient.

Barium sulfate is an opaque medium used in radiological studies of the gastrointestinal tract as a **contrast medium** (barium enema or barium swallow). These studies are performed in the GI clinic or interventional radiology depart-

ment and are not part of a sterile procedure. However, the surgical technologist may occasionally work in these areas of the health care facility and should be familiar with the use of barium. Barium is supplied as a liquid for oral administration or rectal infusion. Following ingestion or infusion, barium x-rays reveal well-defined areas where the substance has filled the GI tract, including small surface irregularities, outpockets of tissue, stricture, and other anomalies. Barium is not absorbed through the tissues but is excreted through the normal GI tract in its intact form.

HEMOSTATICS

Examples
- Absorbable gelatin USP (Gelfoam, Gelfilm, Surgifoam)
- Beeswax (bone wax)
- Collagen absorbable hemostat (Avitene, Instat)
- Ethylene oxide and propylene oxide (Ostene)
- Oxidized cellulose USP (Surgicel)
- Topical thrombin USP

Indication
Topical hemostatic agents are used to control bleeding on capillary surfaces where other means of hemostasis are not practical or possible (e.g., ligation or electrosurgery).

How Supplied
Topical hemostats are supplied as a liquid drug, foam, fabric, powder, or wax substance.

Discussion
A topical hemostatic agent is used to control bleeding from a small capillary complex. Larger vessels can be ligated or coagulated by electrosurgery or other physical means. However, bleeding from capillary surfaces requires other, more refined means. (A complete discussion of hemostatic agents is presented in Chapter 17 under Homeostasis.)

ANTICOAGULANTS

Examples
Heparin sodium

Indication
- Used as an irrigation solution in vascular and cardiac surgery to prevent clotting at the surgical site.
- Prior to opening blood vessels during cardiac and vascular surgery, systemic heparin is administered to the patient to prevent clotting and thrombosis during the procedure..
- Heparin is administered systemically as a preliminary treatment to deep vein thrombosis (DVT which can lead to pulmonary embolism and death.
- Heparin is used to prime cardiac bypass tubing and blood interface surfaces prior to bypass procedures and kidney dialysis to prevent clotting and cell aggregation on the inner surfaces of the bypass machine.

How Supplied
Solution

Discussion
Heparin sodium is used for irrigation during cardiovascular surgery to prevent clotting at the surgical site. Heparin is mixed with injectable 0.9% sodium chloride and used as a local irrigation fluid to flush blood vessels which are clamped. The drug solution used at the surgical site is therefore not being injected into the system circulation but only in a localized area to prevent clot formation during surgery. An **anticoagulant** does not dissolve blood clots, but only inhibits their formation. The surgical technologist receives heparin and injectable saline to formulate the appropriate strength ordered by the surgeon.

Heparin exerts a strong anticoagulation effect when given systemically or regionally. These effects allow the surgeon to perform vascular surgery with minimal risk of clot formation at the site of the surgery. If not prevented, clots not only obscure the surgical site (repair of blood vessels, or heart structures) but can detach from the vessel walls and become released into the systemic blood system. Even a small blood clot may become lodged in a critical area of the body such as the lung or brain, blocking the flow of blood to that area and result in death.

Patients who have been on routine anticoagulation therapy (warfarin) for the prevention of deep vein thrombosis may require a decrease in dosage several days before surgery to prevent the opposite effect, which is uncontrollable hemorrhage during or after surgery. NOTE: Intravenous heparin is administered before cardiac bypass. Heparin for irrigation is prepared by the surgical technologist and registered nurse. IV heparin is administered by the anesthesia care provider. (See Systemic Anticoagulants later in the chapter.)

ANTIBACTERIALS

Examples
- Bacitracin topical powder is reconstituted
- Bacitracin with polymyxin B ointment.
- Polymyxin B ophthalmic ointment and solution.
- Iodophor and bismuth tribromophenate gauze (Xeroform) available for wound dressing.

Indication
Topical antibacterial agents are used to inhibit the growth of bacterial organisms in the surgical wound.

How Supplied
- Bacitracin powder is reconstituted with normal saline for irrigation of the surgical wound.
- Gauze strips or squares are impregnated with an antibacterial agent. These are available in petroleum-based compound or in dry form.
- Available as topical ointment and ophthalmic solution.

Discussion
Antibacterial agents are used during surgery to inhibit the growth of bacteria in the wound. Systemic antibiotics may also be administered to selected patients in the perioperative period. A topical bacitracin is frequently used for wound irrigation when infection is present or the risk for infection is high. Some surgeons routinely irrigate the wound with antibiotic solution after GI, cardiac, and orthopedic surgery.

Bacitracin topical antibacterial is supplied in dry form for reconstitution with 0.9% sterile saline. The technologist receives the reconstituted solution from the circulating nurse. The solution must be discarded after 3 hours, because its potency decreases after that period.

Dressings impregnated with antibacterial or antiseptic agents (e.g., iodophor and bismuth tribromophenate [Xeroform gauze]) are supplied for use on skin and also for packing body cavities (e.g., nasal, vagina, and open wounds).

DIAGNOSTIC DYES AND SUBSTANCES

Examples
Methylene Blue
Indigo Carmen
Gentian Violet

Indication
Colored **dyes** are instilled into hollow structures to enhance direct visualization, to trace the path of a duct, and to determine *patency* (whether the structure is open or blocked). Dyes are also used in skin markers for preoperative demarcation of the wound or incision site.

How Supplied
Dyes are supplied in glass vials or as a marking pen (referred to as a skin marker or skin scribe).

Discussion
Dyes are most commonly used to assess the patency of the fallopian tubes and urethra.

TISSUE STAINS

Examples
- Ferric subsulfate solution (Monsel solution)
- Iodine, potassium iodide, and distilled water (Lugol solution)
- Acetic acid (white vinegar)

Indication
Used to stain the cervix to detect abnormal or precancerous cells.

How Supplied
Tissue stains are supplied as a liquid in a glass bottle.

Discussion
A **stain** is used as a diagnostic tool to differentiate normal cells from abnormal ones. Clinical laboratories use a variety of

staining agents. In the surgical setting, several types of stains are used to enable surgeons to see areas of diseased tissue appropriate for destruction or excision. Stains typically are applied under direct visualization with a sterile sponge or cotton-tipped applicator. The stain generally is absorbed by the abnormal cells, giving these cells a different appearance from the healthy surrounding cells.

- Lugol solution is used to perform the Schiller test to identify cervical dysplasia.
- Monsel solution is used to identify abnormal tissue cells in gynecological and urogenital procedures.
- Acetic acid is used to enhance the detection of cervical neoplasia during colposcopy.

COMMON MEDICATIONS USED IN PATIENT CARE

Drugs used in the perioperative process but not usually handled directly on the surgical field, such as fluid and electrolyte replacement, blood and blood products, and others, are given as a *prophylactic* measure (to prevent a condition) or to treat a condition related to the surgical problem.

INTRAVENOUS FLUIDS

Examples
- *Crystalloids:* Lactated Ringer solution, 0.9% sodium chloride, dextrose 5% in water
- *Colloids:* Dextran solution, hetastarch, Plasmanate
- *Blood and blood products:* Whole blood, packed red blood cells, platelets, plasma, albumin

How Supplied
- Intravenous fluids and blood products are available in collapsible plastic pouches.

Indication
Intravenous fluids are administered in the perioperative period according to the medical and physiological needs of the patients. These include the following:
- Correct electrolyte imbalance
- Restore intravascular volume
- Correct fluid shifts

Examples
- Crystalloids
   0.9% Saline
   5% Dextrose
   0.18% Saline in 0.45% Dextrose
   Other electrolyte solutions
- Colloids
   Blood
   Plasma or albumin
   Synthetics

Discussion
Approximately 2/3 of the body mass is made up of water. Water is gained normally through ingestion (eating and drinking) and lost through normal physiological processes, trauma, or disease. (vomiting, diarrhea, burns, hemorrhage) The total body water is contained in three space: the intracellular spaces (inside the cells), interstitial space (between the cells), and intravascular space (within the blood vessels).

Fluid is maintained in the proper body spaces by oncotic pressure (movement controlled by presence of large molecules such as plasma proteins) and by the process of osmosis. The total volume of body fluid must remain stable in order to sustain life and fluid shifts from one compartment (space) to another as the body maintains homeostasis. Usually, fluids move with electrolytes.

In surgery we track fluid loss mainly by measuring urine and blood loss. If fluids are needed, the choice is very specific according to the patient's physiological state at the time. Errors in fluid administration can result in fluid overload and heart failure. Administering the wrong dilution (osmolarity) of an electrolyte solution can cause serious injury or death related to the chemical reactions caused (or prevented) by the presence of the electrolytes.

Fluids are administered routinely in surgery and medicine. Many different types of solutions are used, There are two general categories of intravenous fluids—Crystalloids and Colloids.

Crystalloids are solutions which contain a small amount of solutes (dissolved substances). These solutions are mainly administered to correct phyiological imbalance related to electrolytes, blood pH, and to restore fluids lost through disease (dehydration). . Commonly used crystalloids are 0.9% saline solution (sometimes called "normal saline" and dextrose solution. Another crystalloid used frequently is Lactated Ringers whose chemical composition is close to that of human plasma. Other crystalloids contain specific electrolytes such as potassium and calcium, which are prescribed according to the patient's needs. For example, electrolyte imbalance or deficit may be corrected through the administration of specific crystalloid solutions.

Colloids are crystalloid based and contain water and electrolytes. However, they also have additional components which cause the fluid to move in a specific way. A colloid is a particle or substance which is dispersed throughout the fluid but not dissolved in it. In medicine, colloids are administered to prevent fluids from escaping the closed vascular system across the cell membrane. So, patients who need intravascular fluid replacement for may be administered a colloid. This solution increases the intravascular (oncotic) pressure but the colloid particles do not allow the fluid to escape into the other body compartments.

Common colloids are blood, plasma, and synthetic substances which have large "macromolecules," to prevent the escape of the fluid outside the vascular system. A colloid may be given, for example, as a life saving means when blood is not yet available In this case we would not administer saline because it would quickly become dispersed among the other body compartments and not exert oncotic pressure in the vascular system. During massive blood or plasma loss(as occurs during severe burns) the oncotic pressure of the vascular system must be raised to enable the heart to move the blood through the body effectively. Colloids are vascular volume expanders. *Dextran* solutions have properties similar to those of human albumin. *Hetastarch* is a hypertonic synthetic starch. These colloidal fluids increase osmotic pressure, which controls the movement of water into and out of the intravascular space.

BLOOD AND BLOOD PRODUCTS

How Supplied

Blood and blood products are mainly supplied in collapsible plastic pouches.

Indication

- Blood replacement if a significant amount of blood has been lost due to trauma or disease. It is used only when the patient's blood loss exceeds 30% of total blood volume (approximately1,500 mL in an adult).
- Specific blood products are needed according to the patient's condition. For example, some patients need only platelets, while others may require one of the blood-clotting factors because of disease conditions in which the body is unable to produce them.

Examples

- Whole blood—contains serum and blood cells plus anticoagulant and preservative. Whole blood is not commonly given because it can be broken down into components that can be administered separately and may waste products which are not needed.
- Red blood cells—A unit of red blood cells contains 150 to 210 ml of red cells, plus a small amount of plasma and preservative. Packed red blood cells (PRBCs) are administered to increase the oxygen-carrying capacity of the blood. A combination of packed red blood cells and plasma expanders is effective in increasing the total intravascular volume and oxygen-carrying capacity. All cell transfusions must be ABO—Rh compatible with the recipient. Packed cells are handled and monitored in the same way–gm/dL.
- Washed red blood cells—are normal RBCs that have been washed to remove the plasma and are administered to patients who demonstrate repeated hypersensitivity to blood or components.
- Leukoreduced red blood cells—contain leukocytes in reduced volume within red blood cells. Leukoreduced RBCs are used in patients with a history of non-hemolytic febrile transfusion reactions.
- Platelets—are essential for blood coagulation and contain coagulation factors, red blood cells, and white blood cells. Platelets are administered to patients with bleeding disorders such as thrombocytopenia, platelet dysfunction, or other conditions.
- Granulocytes (neutrophils)—are obtained from an ABO-Rh compatible donor and used in the treatment of severe neutropenia.
- Fresh frozen plasma (FFP)—is the plasma that has been removed from whole blood and contains normal amounts of coagulation factors. This blood product is used for patients who have coagulation deficiencies, active bleeding, and require invasive procedures.
- Cryoprecipitate—is a concentration of several hemostatic proteins that have been prepared from whole blood. The hemostatic proteins contained in cryoprecipitate are Factor VIII, von Willebrand factor, factor XIII, and fibrinogen. Cryoprecipitate is used for patients with significantly decreased fibrinogen who are actively bleeding or require invasive procedures. Cryoprecipitate is also used in the preparation of fibrin glue, orthopedic procedures, ENT, and neurosurgical procedures.
- Factor concentrates—contain Factor VIII, IS, and antithrombin III. This product is used in patients with hemophilia who require invasive procedures.

Discussion

When blood and blood products are used, an exact protocol must be followed Cross-checking of products that are ABO-Rh specific is performed by two people before administration, which must be performed by medical or nursing staff. Blood products must be stored at temperatures between 33.8° and 42.8°F (1° and 6°C). External temperature tape may be used to monitor the temperature of individual units. Units must be used within 30 minutes in a noncontrolled environment. Unused blood is returned to the blood bank.

SYSTEMIC ANTIMICROBIALS

Examples

- Antibacterials
  - Penicillin and cephalosporin
  - Tetracycline and macrolides
  - Aminoglycosides
  - Fluoroquinolones
  - Sulfonamides
- Antifungals

Indication

Antimicrobials are used for the treatment or prevention of microbial infections.

Discussion

Antimicrobial drugs are administered to treat or prevent infection. It should be noted that *antibiotics* and *antimicrobials* are not synonymous. The term *antibiotics* refers to drugs that target bacteria specifically, whereas the term *antimicrobials* refers to drugs that target any type of microbe. Antimicrobials are studied according to their chemical group or the microbes they target. This discussion focuses on the microbial groups.

ANTIBACTERIALS

The mechanisms of antibacterial action are:
- Inhibition of synthesis of the cell wall
- Alteration in the permeability of the cell membrane
- Prevention of the synthesis of cellular proteins

- Inhibition of the cell's genetic material (i.e., deoxyribonucleic acid [DNA] and ribonucleic acid [RNA]), which is needed for replication
- Interference with cell metabolism

Penicillins

Penicillin was developed during the early 1940s. It was the first true antibiotic, and many different categories of penicillin have emerged, all arising from the prototype. Penicillins are divided into two types: broad spectrum (effective on gram-positive and some gram-negative bacteria) and narrow spectrum (effective only on gram-positive bacteria). Other classes of penicillin are distinguished by their ability to target specific bacterial defense mechanisms or groups of bacteria.

Examples

Procaine penicillin
Benzathine penicillin
Penicillin V potassium
Ampicillin
Cloxacillin
Methicillin
Carbenicillin
Piperacillin

Cephalosporins

Cephalosporins were first developed in the 1960s. Each subsequent group has been broader in spectrum than the previous group. These groups are called *generations* of cephalosporins, because they emerged from the previous parent prototype. First-, second-, third-, and fourth-generation cephalosporins have been developed (Table 14-3).

Macrolides

Macrolides are bacteriostatic at low levels and bactericidal in high doses. These are broad-spectrum drugs, but they are most active against gram-positive bacteria. They most commonly are used to treat respiratory tract infections and sexually transmitted diseases.

Examples

Azithromycin
Clarithromycin
Erythromycin

Lincosamides, Vancomycin, and Ketolides

Lincosamides, vancomycin, and ketolides have a similar action. They are bacteriostatic and bactericidal, and they inhibit protein synthesis in bacteria. Vancomycin was used extensively in the 1950s, but its use has decreased in recent years.

Examples

Clindamycin
Vancomycin

Tetracyclines

Tetracyclines are broad-spectrum antimicrobials that inhibit bacterial protein synthesis. They are supplied almost exclusively for oral administration against specific microbes such as rickettsiae and mycobacteria.

Examples

Doxycycline
Minocycline
Methacycline

Aminoglycosides

Aminoglycosides are effective against gram-negative bacteria, in which they inhibit protein synthesis. This group of antibiotics is used selectively and carefully because of adverse reactions.

Examples

Gentamicin
Paromomycin
Amikacin

Fluoroquinolones

Fluoroquinolones are broad-spectrum antibacterials that inhibit DNA synthesis. They are used in a variety of infections, including respiratory, arthritic, urinary tract, and GI conditions.

Examples

Ciprofloxacin
Levofloxacin
Sparfloxacin

Sulfonamides

Sulfonamides were first introduced in the 1930s. They are bacteriostatic only. Because of their limited use and the emergence of increasingly drug-resistant bacterial strains, they have been replaced by drugs that are more effective. Sulfonamides are most commonly used to treat acute urinary tract infections.

Examples

Sulfamethoxazole
Trimethoprim
Co-trimoxazole

Table 14-3

Cephalosporins

First Generation	Second Generation	Third Generation	Fourth Generation
Cefazolin	Cefaclor	Cefixime	Cefepime
Cephalexin	Cefuroxime	Ceftriaxone	

ANTIFUNGALS

Antifungal drugs are used for superficial and systemic fungal disease. Skin infections are treated mainly with over-the-counter (OTC) topical medications, although resistant strains may require oral administration. Systemic fungal infection is difficult to treat and can be fatal. Intravenous administration is required for many antifungal medications.

Examples
Amphotericin
Miconazole
Flucytosine

SYSTEMIC ANTICOAGULANTS

Examples
Heparin sodium (IV and SC administration)
Warfarin (oral administration)

Discussion
Intravenous heparin is administered prophylactically to prevent thrombosis (blood clotting). The normal blood-clotting mechanism is triggered by injury to the endothelial wall of a blood vessel. This causes two biochemical responses, known as the *extrinsic pathway* and the *intrinsic pathway*. In these chemical reactions, prothrombin is converted to thrombin, and fibrinogen is converted to fibrin, a sticky substance that promotes platelet clumping and clot formation. Heparin inactivates thrombin and inhibits its conversion to fibrinogen, thus preventing clot formation.

Heparin is administered to patients before cardiac bypass and other selected procedures because the blood is shunted outside the body through a series of cannulas. At the close of the procedure, the effects of heparin are reversed with the antiplatelet drug *protamine sulfate*.

Anticoagulant therapy is prescribed for individuals with a history or known risk of deep vein thrombosis (DVT). During oral anticoagulant therapy, two tests are used to assess clotting and platelet formation: the prothrombin time (PT) and the international normalized ratio (INR). Adjustments are made in the dose of the anticoagulant as needed. Patients who are to undergo surgery must stop taking anticoagulants before the procedure to prevent excess bleeding intraoperatively and postoperatively.

DIURETICS

Examples
Hydrochlorothiazide
Bumetanide
Furosemide
Mannitol
Acetazolamide

Discussion
Diuretics stimulate the production of urine by the kidneys. This creates a shift of body fluids. They are most commonly used in the treatment of hypertension and pulmonary edema. However, they are also used for emergency treatment of intraocular pressure and increased cerebral pressure (ICP). Diuretics reduce the total vascular volume by depressing reabsorption of sodium in the kidneys and increasing water excretion from the nephron. This results in increased **diuresis** (increased urinary excretion).

Specific classes of diuretics function differently. Many cause excess excretion of potassium, an electrolyte necessary for cardiac and cell function. Potassium-sparing diuretics are preferred for this reason. Loop diuretics are extremely potent and cause rapid diuresis and loss of electrolytes. The osmotic diuretics also are very potent and are used to reduce intraocular pressure and cerebral edema. This class of diuretics is given during neurosurgical procedures. Carbonic anhydrase inhibitors are used specifically for reducing intraocular pressure in patients with open angle glaucoma. They inhibit the enzyme carbonic anhydrase, which partly controls the acid-base balance in the blood. Thiazide diuretics are weaker and do not cause immediate diuresis. They are used in the treatment of hypertension because they cause arteriole dilation and reduce cardiac output.

GASTRIC MEDICATIONS

Examples
Histamine antagonist
Proton pump inhibitor
Serotonin antagonist
Dopamine antagonist
Anticholinergic
Antihistamine

Discussion
Gastric medications have specific uses in surgery. During general anesthesia, the risk exists that the patient may aspirate stomach contents after regurgitating or vomiting. Complication of aspiration can be extremely serious and include airway obstruction, chemical destruction of lung tissue, and increased risk of pneumonia as a result of tissue damage. Preoperative administration of gastric medications reduces the pH of gastric secretions and lowers the risks of chemical destruction and pneumonia. Proton pump inhibitors suppress gastric secretions in the parietal cells. Histamine antagonists (H$_2$ antagonists) block the secretion of stomach acid.

Postoperative nausea and vomiting (PONV) is managed with several groups of medications. The exact drug group depends on the root cause of the nausea and other drugs given in the perioperative period. Medications used for the management of PNOV include serotonin antagonists, dopamine antagonists, anticholinergics, and antihistamines.

DRUGS USED DURING LABOR

Examples
Oxytocin
Dinoprostone
Methylergonovine maleate
Misoprostol

Discussion
Drugs that enhance uterine contractions are called *uterotropics*. The most common uterotropic is *oxytocin*, which is

produced naturally by the hypothalamus. Synthetic oxytocin (Pitocin) is used to induce (initiate) and intensify labor. Prostaglandin (dinoprostone, carbroprostomethamine) is used to soften and efface the cervix; this naturally occurring substance is used in combination with oxytocin.

Anesthetics and pain medications were discussed in Chapter 12. After delivery, misoprostol (Cytotec) or methylergonovine maleate (Methergine) may be administered to reduce blood loss.

AUTONOMIC NERVOUS SYSTEM AGENTS

Examples

Adrenergic Drugs
- Epinephrine
- Albuterol
- Isoproterenol

Antiadrenergic Drugs
- Atenolol
- Metoprolol tartrate
- Propranolol HCl

Cholinergic Drugs
- Bethanechol
- Carbachol
- Pilocarpine

Anticholinergic Drugs
- Atropine sulfate
- Glycopyrrolate

Discussion

CNS agents (which were discussed in Chapter 12) affect the brain and spinal cord. The *peripheral nervous system* receives stimuli via the central nervous system and is divided into two important subcategories, the autonomic nervous system and the somatic nervous system. The autonomic system is not under voluntary control.

Autonomic System

The autonomic system is further divided into the sympathetic and parasympathetic systems. Many essential physiological functions are controlled by the sympathetic system, including thermoregulation, heart rate, peristalsis, and vascular constriction or dilation.

The sympathetic system controls the "fight or flight" responses of the body. Responses in this system include bronchiole dilation, increase cardiac output, dilation of blood vessels, and increased availability of blood glucose.

The parasympathetic system is more active when the body is at rest. The heart rate is slower, and cardiac output is decreased. Digestion is increased to store glycogen for energy.

Specific chemicals in the body, called **neurotransmitters,** are responsible for the sympathetic and parasympathetic responses (Figure 14-9). Neurotransmitters lock on or bind to the neuron to produce the response:

- *Adrenergics* stimulate the responses of the sympathetic system. The natural chemical norepinephrine creates the response.
- *Antiadrenergics* block the effects of norepinephrine.
- *Cholinergics* stimulate the parasympathetic response. The neurotransmitter is acetylcholine.
- *Anticholinergics* block the effects of acetylcholine.

Drugs that block a neurotransmitter also block its effect. The *binding site* or *receptor* of the nerve also determines the responses. For example, alpha-adrenergic receptors increase cardiac contraction, and beta sites increase blood pressure and dilation of the bronchioles. Drugs that act like (mimic) neurotransmitters can create the same effect as the neurotransmitter itself.

Drugs are administered to selectively increase or block these responses to produce the desired effect. For example, a patient's blood pressure can be lowered by administering either a drug that blocks vasoconstriction or one that increases the effect of vasodilation. These drugs are called *antihypertensives.*

CARDIAC DRUGS

Examples

Glycoside
Antianginal
Antiarrhythmic

Discussion

Cardiac drugs are most commonly used to treat dysfunctions of the strength of pumping action, heart rate, and rhythm. The cardiac *glycosides* have inotropic and chronotropic effects on the heart.

- *Inotropic drugs:* Affect the stroke volume (amount of blood pushed through the heart with each cardiac cycle), which is related to the strength of the muscle.
- *Chronotropic drugs:* Affect the heart rate.

Glycosides also affect the heart rhythm, resolving unproductive or disorganized muscle contractions.

Angina is sudden chest pain caused by insufficient blood flow through the coronary arteries that supply the heart. Prolonged, severe angina can lead to ischemia of heart tissue and cardiac arrest. Antianginal drugs cause vasodilation and relaxation of the vessels. The most common antianginal drug is nitroglycerine. Other common drugs are beta blockers, which interrupt sympathetic neurotransmission. Calcium channel blockers reduce the oxygen demand of the heart.

ENDOCRINE DRUGS

Examples

Pituitary
Growth hormone (sermorelin acetate, somatropin)
Thyroid-stimulating hormone (corticotropin, cosyntropin)

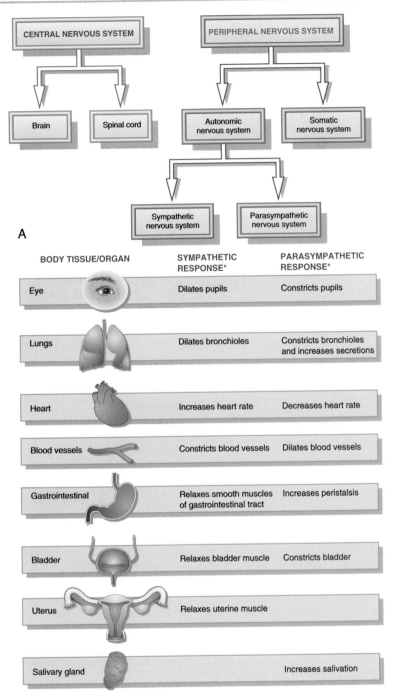

Figure 14-9   A, Divisions of the peripheral nervous system. **B,** Sympathetic and parasympathetic responses. *(From Kee J, Hayes E, McCuiston L: Pharmacology, ed 5, Philadelphia, 2006, WB Saunders.)*

Posterior Pituitary
Desmopressin acetate
Vasopressin

Thyroid
Levothyroxine sodium

Parathyroid
Calcifediol
Calcitriol

Adrenals (Glucocorticoids)
Hydrocortisone
Methylprednisolone
Betamethasone
Dexamethasone

Discussion
Endocrine drugs replace or inhibit the effects of hormones produced by the adrenal glands, parathyroid, thyroid, and pituitary. The prototype drugs in this category are:

- *Prednisone:* Adrenal hormone glucocorticoid; used to reduce the inflammatory response and as an immunosuppressant.
- *Calcitriol:* Parathyroid; promotes calcium absorption. Parathyroid regulates calcium levels for cellular metabolism.
- *Levothyroxine sodium:* Thyroid hormone; used to treat hypothyroidism.
- *Corticotropin:* Pituitary adrenocorticotropic hormone; simulates the adrenal cortex to secrete cortisol.

REPRODUCTIVE SYSTEM DRUGS

Examples
Estrogen
Progestin
Testosterone

Discussion
Reproductive system hormones are secreted by the gonads (i.e., the ovaries and testicles). The female reproductive system is under the control of many different hormones triggered by the hypothalamus, anterior pituitary, CNS, and other tissues. The steroid sex hormones produced by the ovaries are estrogen, progesterone, and androgens. These directly influence reproductive ability and indirectly influence other physiological processes. For this reason, hormones, including those produced by organs other than the ovaries, are prescribed in the treatment of hormone dysfunction or for symptoms of their absence, such as during menopause. Estrogen and progestin are prescribed as replacements and for birth control.

The male androgens are responsible for sexual function, bone and muscle development, and secondary sexual characteristics. Testosterone is the male androgen. It is used in the treatment of testosterone deficiency caused by testicular dysfunction. Deficiency may be related to diseases of the hypothalamus or pituitary gland. Androgens also are used in women in the treatment of endometriosis and carcinoma of the breast.

ANTINEOPLASTIC DRUGS

Anticancer drugs are called *antineoplastic agents.* Multiple drugs are used in chemotherapy to treat a primary tumor or metastatic disease. Cancer cells are not specifically targeted during chemotherapy. All cells are affected by the drug. However, normal cells undergo repair, which cancer cells are unable to do.

Many different types of chemotherapy are used. The significance of all types for a discussion of surgical pharmacology is the added physiological stress on the body and the immune suppression caused by anticancer drugs. The adverse effects of cancer therapy are destruction of healthy cells and disabling of the body's intrinsic immune system. Consequently, patients undergoing treatment are at risk of infection, pneumonia, and other complications related to the body's inability to defend itself.

ALTERNATIVE HEALING THERAPIES

Alternative healing therapies are now an accepted component of Western medicine. Many patients request nondrug or herbal treatment in place of or in addition to conventional medicine. Alternative therapies include:
- Herbal medicine
- Acupuncture
- Aroma therapy

Although these are not practiced within the perioperative setting, they represent a part of many patients' medical regimen. Many naturopathic practices originate in non-Western cultures and are not considered alternative healing methods. Several alternative or complementary therapies have gained popularity in Western culture. These include practices that provide deep relaxation, such as music therapy, yoga, aromatherapy, and massage, which are important complements to traditional therapy.

Herbal therapy is an ancient method of healing and well-being based on plant substances. Herbal substances can be both beneficial and harmful. These substances are not regulated in the United States, although they are prescribed by individuals who practice natural healing. They are classified as dietary supplements, and suggested dosages are available for commonly used remedies.

Acupuncture is a practice of traditional Chinese medicine. To produce analgesia or achieve healing. The needles are inserted into acupuncture points that are distant from the source of disease but lie along body *meridians* or pathways. Many people perceive benefit from acupuncture; however, it is not an evidenced-based practice.

SAMPLE PROBLEMS

1. To produce 30 cc of 50% Hypaque solution, how much 100% Hypaque and how much sterile saline solution are required?
2. How much alcohol is required to prepare a 1-L solution of alcohol in water in a ratio of 1:70?
3. To prepare a single solution in which the ratio of bacitracin to neomycin is 1:3 and the ratio of the bacitracin/neomycin mixture to sterile solution is 1:1, how much bacitracin, neomycin, and sterile saline solution do you need to make a total of 100 cc of solution?
4. To produce 30 cc of 0.5% Xylocaine, how much sterile saline solution and how much 1% Xylocaine are required?
5. To produce a 100-cc solution of Hypaque in a ratio of 1:3, how much 50% Hypaque solution and how much sterile solution should you use?

Table 14-4

Common Surgical Medications

Generic (Brand) Names	Uses	Action
Anticoagulant		
Heparin	Prolong the clotting time of blood; to prevent and treat deep vein thrombosis (DVT) and pulmonary embolism; as an irrigant in cardiovascular surgery to prevent the formation of clots in the wound.	Inhibits thrombosis by inactivating factor X and inhibiting conversion of prothrombin to thrombin.
Hemostatics, Coagulants, Reversal Drugs		
Avitene (microfibrillar collagen hemostat)	Direct topical application to areas of active bleeding to control the bleeding.	When Avitene comes in contact with a bleeding surface, it attracts platelets, which adhere to the fibrils. The platelets then aggregate, beginning the clotting cascade. Available as a loose fibrous form or a compact, nonwoven web form.
Gelfoam (absorbable gelatin sponge)	Same as Avitene.	A pliable gelatin sponge that absorbs fluid, expands, and exerts pressure on adjacent structures.
Surgicel (oxidized regenerated cellulose)	Same as Avitene.	An absorbable, white, knitted fabric; when saturated with blood, it swells into a dark, gelatinous mass, which aids the formation of clots.
Protamine	Neutralize the effects of heparin (1 mg of protamine neutralizes 100 units of heparin).	Protamine by itself is an anticoagulant and increases clotting time. When mixed with heparin, the drugs are attracted to each other and form a stable salt that neutralizes the effects of heparin.
Thrombin	As a topical hemostatic agent, usually used in combination with an absorbable gelatin sponge.	Induces clotting on bleeding surfaces where conventional methods of hemostasis are contraindicated, such as friable and delicate tissue.
Oxytocics		
Oxytocin (Pitocin)	Induce and maintain labor and prevent or control hemorrhage postpartum.	Stimulates contractions of uterine smooth muscle.
Methylergonovine (Methergine)	Prevent postpartum bleeding.	Same as oxytocin.
Corticosteroids		
Betamethasone sodium phosphate (Celestone)	As a treatment of many inflammatory diseases and conditions.	Mostly used for antiinflammatory properties, both systemic and local.
Betamethasone sodium phosphate (Celestone phosphate)	Same as betamethasone sodium phosphate.	Same as betamethasone sodium phosphate.
Dexamethasone (Decadron, Dexamethasone, Hexadrol)	Same as betamethasone sodium phosphate.	Same as betamethasone sodium phosphate.
Hydrocortisone sodium succinate (Solu-Cortef)	Same as betamethasone sodium phosphate.	Same as betamethasone sodium phosphate.
Methylprednisolone acetate (Depo-Medrol)	Same as betamethasone sodium phosphate.	Long-acting corticosteroid.
Methylprednisolone sodium succinate (Solu-Medrol)	Same as betamethasone sodium phosphate.	Same as betamethasone sodium phosphate.
Triamcinolone acetonide (Kenalog)	Same as betamethasone sodium phosphate.	Same as betamethasone sodium phosphate.
Triamcinolone diacetate (Aristocort)	Same as betamethasone sodium phosphate.	Same as betamethasone sodium phosphate.

Table 14-4

Common Surgical Medications—cont'd

Generic (Brand) Names	Uses	Action
Antibiotics, Antimicrobials, and Antiinfectives		
Cefazolin (Kefzol, Ancef)	Prevent postoperative wound infections caused by gram-negative organisms (e.g., *Staphylococcus epidermidis*); treat respiratory, genitourinary, skin/soft tissue, and blood infections caused by gram-positive and certain gram-negative organisms.	Inhibits bacterial cell wall synthesis (bactericidal).
Clindamycin (Cleocin)	Treat infections caused by susceptible aerobic and anaerobic gram-positive organisms.	Inhibits bacterial protein synthesis (bacteriostatic).
Gentamicin (Garamycin)	Treat respiratory, genitourinary, gastrointestinal, ophthalmic, and blood infections caused by gram-negative organisms.	Inhibits bacterial protein synthesis (bactericidal).
Vancomycin	Treat respiratory, genitourinary, bone, skin/soft tissue, and blood infections caused by gram-positive organisms.	Inhibits bacterial cell wall synthesis (bactericidal).
Levofloxacin (Levaquin)	Treat respiratory, genitourinary, ophthalmic, skin/soft tissue, and blood infections caused by certain gram-positive organisms (e.g. pneumococci), gram-negative organisms, and atypical organisms (e.g. *Mycoplasma*).	Inhibits bacterial DNA replication and transcription (bactericidal).
Metronidazole (Flagyl)	Treat infections caused by anaerobic organisms.	Inhibits bacterial protein synthesis (bactericidal).
Irrigation Solutions		
Bacitracin	As an irrigation solution to prevent gram-positive infections at the site of the surgical procedure.	Inhibits bacterial cell wall synthesis (bactericidal).
Neomycin	As an irrigation solution to prevent gram-negative infections at the site of the surgical procedure.	Inhibits bacterial protein synthesis (bactericidal).
Polymyxin B	As an irrigation solution to prevent gram-negative infections at the site of the surgical procedure (urological).	Binds to phospholipids, alters permeability, and damages bacterial cytoplasm membrane, permitting leakage of its components.
Diagnostic Imaging Agents		
Renografin	For cholangiography and hysterosalpingography.	When injected, shows as white on radiographs.
Cystografin (Cysto-Conray)	For radiographs of the urinary tract.	Same as Renografin.
Hypaque	For radiographs of the biliary tract, kidney, and other internal structures.	Same as Renografin.
Hyskon	In hysteroscopy, as an aid in distending the uterine cavity and irrigating and visualizing surfaces.	An electrolyte-free, nonconductive solution.
Dyes		
Methylene blue	Mark a specific surface or area; color solutions; and test the patency of specific organs.	Turns skin blue when used topically and turns urine a greenish color when used systemically.
Indigo carmine	Same as methylene blue.	Same as methylene blue.

Continued

Table 14-4
Common Surgical Medications—cont'd

Generic (Brand) Names	Uses	Action
Diuretic		
Mannitol	Promote diuresis and treatment of oliguric phase of acute renal failure after cardiovascular surgery; reduce elevated intraocular and intracranial pressure.	Inhibits water/electrolyte reabsorption in the kidneys and increases urinary output.
Analgesics		
Fentanyl (Sublimaze)	As a preoperative medication; as an adjunct therapy during local, regional, and general anesthesia.	Narcotic analgesic that increases the pain threshold and alters pain perception. Rapid onset and short duration.
Alfenta (Sufenta)	Same as fentanyl.	Narcotic agonist analgesic with a rapid onset and short duration.
Morphine sulfate	Same as fentanyl.	Same as fentanyl, but slightly longer onset (5–15 min) and longer duration (4–5 hr).
Meperidine (Demerol)	Same as fentanyl.	Same as fentanyl, but slightly longer onset (5–15 min) and longer duration (3 hr).
Hydromorphone (Dilaudid)	Relieve moderate to severe pain (alternative to morphine).	Mechanism of action is similar to fentanyl, but analgesic effect is eight to 10 times more potent than morphine. Onset 10–15 min, duration 4–5 hr.
Benzodiazepines		
Diazepam (Valium)	Provide sedation or muscle relaxation, and/or alleviate anxiety before surgery; treat seizures.	Central nervous system (CNS) depressant; long-acting benzodiazepine with sedative, hypnotic, and anticonvulsant properties.
Midazolam (Versed)	Provide sedation or muscle relaxation, and/or alleviate anxiety before surgery; impair memory of perioperative events.	CNS depressant; intermediate-acting benzodiazepine with sedative, hypnotic, and anticonvulsant properties; also has anterograde amnestic effects.
Lorazepam (Ativan)	Same as diazepam.	Same as midazolam, except with no anterograde amnestic effects.
Emergency Drugs		
Epinephrine (Adrenalin)	Treat cardiac arrest/asystole; treat severe bradycardia or hypotension.	Causes vasoconstriction; increases blood pressure, heart rate, and cardiac output.
Norepinephrine (Levophed)	Treat severe hypotension associated with cardiogenic or septic shock.	Causes vasoconstriction; increases blood pressure.
Dopamine	Treat severe hypotension associated with cardiogenic or septic shock; increase urinary output (lower doses should be used).	Low dose increases urinary output; intermediate dose increases cardiac output and blood pressure; high dose reduces vasoconstriction and increases blood pressure and heart rate.
Nitroprusside (Nipride)	Treat hypertensive emergencies.	Arterial and venous vasodilator; reduces blood pressure very quickly; reflex increases heart rate and cardiac output.
Amiodarone	Treat life-threatening ventricular arrhythmias (Vfib/Vtach); in cardiac arrest with persistent Vfib; for treatment of atrial arrhythmias (atrial fibrillation).	Prolongs conduction and refractory period in ventricles (increases electrical stimulation threshold); also decreases AV/SA node conduction and therefore is beneficial in patients with atrial fibrillation.
Lidocaine	Treat ventricular arrhythmias (Vfib/Vtach); in cardiac arrest with persistent Vfib.	Increases electrical stimulation threshold; prolongs conduction and refractory period in ventricles during diastole.
Atropine	Treat sinus bradycardia.	Competitive antagonist of acetylcholine in smooth and cardiac muscle; increases heart rate.

Table 14-4

Common Surgical Medications—cont'd

Generic (Brand) Names	Uses	Action
Sodium bicarbonate	Treat metabolic acidosis.	Neutralizes hydrogen ion concentration and raises blood and urinary pH.
Magnesium sulfate	Treat ventricular arrhythmia, torsades de pointes.	Prolongs conduction through ventricles and slows SA node conduction.
Digoxin (Lanoxin)	Slow the rate of tachyarrhythmias such as Afib/A flutter or supraventricular tachycardia; relieve signs and symptoms of congestive heart failure (CHF).	Suppresses AV node conduction to increase refractory period and decrease conduction velocity; inhibits Na+/K+ ATPase pump, which increases intracellular Ca++ to increase myocardial contractility.
Blood and Blood Substitutes		
Hetastarch (Hespan)	Blood volume expander used in treatment of shock or impending shock (e.g., as a result of hemorrhage) when blood or blood products are not available. Not a substitute for blood or plasma because it does not have oxygen-carrying capability.	Produces plasma volume expansion by virtue of its highly colloidal starch structure.
Albumin	Expand plasma volume and maintain cardiac output in shock or impending shock.	Produces plasma volume expansion by virtue of its structure; increases intravascular oncotic pressure and causes mobilization of fluids into intravascular space.
Fresh frozen plasma, washed packed cells, whole blood, cryoprecipitate, and factor VIII	Blood and blood components to restore cell volume.	Maintain blood volume; improve coagulation.
Solutions		
Sodium chloride 0.9% (normal saline solution)	Restore blood volume in hemorrhage and blood pressure in shock; compensate for fluid loss from burns, dehydration, and many similar conditions; as a means of giving needed intravenous medications.	Electrolyte solutions are given to maintain balance; the type used depends on the needs of the patient.
Lactated Ringer's solution	Same as sodium chloride 0.9%.	Same as sodium chloride 0.9%.
Dextrose solution	Same as sodium chloride 0.9% but with added nutrients/calories.	Prepared in isotonic sodium chloride, lactated Ringer's solution, and distilled water for use as patient's condition indicates.

CHAPTER SUMMARY

- Surgical technologists handle drugs on the sterile field and are therefore required to have a basic knowledge of pharmacology.
- Surgical technologists do not administer prescription drugs to the patient, but they prepare them for the surgeon to administer.
- Protocols for safe handling of drugs in the perioperative environment are established by the Joint Commission and AORN. These guidelines are the accepted standard for surgical practice.
- All drugs are approved for administration by a specific route, such as the oral, parenteral, or topical route.

- *Pharmacokinetics* is the process by which a drug is modified as it is broken down, absorbed, and excreted by the body.
- *Pharmacodynamics* is the biochemical and physiological effect of a drug on the body.
- Adverse reactions to drugs include side effects and true allergy.
- The medication process includes supply and procurement of the drug in the health care facility, prescription and selection, administration, and documentation.
- Drug errors are responsible for thousands of deaths each year in health care facilities. Surgical technologists

participate in drug handling and therefore are responsible in drug errors.

- One method of preventing drug errors is to follow the "five rights" of medication: the right drug, dose, route, patient, time; a sixth right, with surgical procedures, is proper identification of the drug on the sterile field.
- The registered nurse is responsible for proper procurement and selection of the drugs used in surgery.
- Drugs are packaged in a way that facilitates their safe administration to the patient. The surgical technologist must be familiar with drug packaging and measurement to participate in drug handling.

- Drugs are delivered to the sterile field according to a prescribed method. The registered nurse and surgical technologist coordinate this process.
- A common cause of patient injury is mislabeling of drugs on the sterile field. Drugs must be labeled by name, strength, and expiration date within 24 hours of distribution.
- Surgical technologists are required to have basic math skills. Miscalculation of drug dosage is one of the primary causes of drug error and patient injury.

REVIEW QUESTIONS

1. What particular drug policies are regulated by the Joint Commission?
2. What is the "intermediary role" of the surgical technologist in the handling and distribution of drugs?
3. What is a generic drug? How does it differ from a nongeneric drug?
4. If the surgical technologist suspects that a patient is having an adverse reaction to a drug, what information is most important to give the surgeon or nursing personnel in the room?
5. What is an allergy?
6. Outline the headings of the medication process and describe them briefly.
7. How does the surgical technologist ensure that a drug is given by the right route?
8. What units are marked on an insulin syringe?
9. What is the rationale for pouring all of a liquid from its sterile container when it is distributed to the scrub?
10. What is the difference between a contrast medium and a dye?
11. What ways might you collaborate with the circulating nurse to keep track of the amount of irrigation solution used during a surgical procedure?

REFERENCE

1. http://www.merck.com/mmhe/sec02/ch010/ch010a.html. Accessed April 11, 2009.
2. American Academy of Allergy, Asthma, and Immunology: The risk of severe allergic reactions from the use of potassium iodine for radiation emergencies. Retrieved June 12, 2008, at http://www.aaaai.org/media/resources/academy_statements/position_statements/potassium_iodide.asp.

BIBLIOGRAPHY

American College of Radiology: Manual on contrast media, version 6. Retrieved June 1, 2008, at http://www.acr.org.
Association of periOperative Registered Nurses (AORN): Guidance statements: safe medication practices in perioperative practice settings. In Standards, recommended practices and guidelines, Denver, 2007, AORN.
Hendrickson T: Verbal medication orders in the OR, J AORN 86:4, 2007.
Kee J, Hayes E, McCuistion L: Pharmacology: a nursing process approach, ed 5, St Louis, 2006, Mosby.
Porth C: Pathophysiology: concepts of altered health states, ed 6, Philadelphia, 2007, Lippincott, Williams & Wilkins.
Wanzer L: Perioperative initiatives for medication safety, J AORN 82:4, 2005.

CHAPTER **15**

Environmental Hazards

CHAPTER OUTLINE

LEARNING OBJECTIVES

After studying this chapter the reader will be able to:
- Describe toxic substances in smoke plumes
- Identify safe use of the smoke evacuator
- Recognize international hazard communication signs
- Describe the difference between latex allergy and allergic dermatitis
- Describe the symptoms of true latex allergy
- Identify necessary precautions to prevent latex reaction in allergic patients
- Discuss fuels and sources of ignition commonly found in the operating room
- Identify methods associated with preventing fires in the operating room
- Describe how to respond appropriately to a patient fire
- Describe how to respond appropriately to a structural fire

- Identify the practice of Standard Precautions
- Identify the practice for transmission-based precautions
- Describe proper body mechanics for lifting, pulling, and pushing objects
- Discuss various techniques to prevent sharps injuries
- Describe measures to safely store, transport, and use compressed gas cylinders
- Identify methods of properly handling and disposing of hazardous waste in the operating room
- Identify precautions to prevent exposure to ionizing radiation
- Identify precautions to prevent patient burns caused by electrical equipment
- Describe methods to avoid chemical injury
- Analyze a chemical label

TERMINOLOGY

Airborne transmission precautions: Precautions that prevent airborne transferral of disease organisms in the environment.

Blood-borne pathogens: Harmful microorganisms that may be present in and transmitted through human blood and body fluids (e.g., the hepatitis B virus [HBV] and the human immunodeficiency virus [HIV]).

Current: The rate of electrical flow through a conductive material.

Electrocution: Severe burns, cardiac disturbances, or death as a result of electrical current discharged into the body.

Electrosurgical unit (ESU): Medical device commonly used in surgery to coagulate blood vessels and cut tissue.

Eschar: Burned tissue fragments which can accumulate on the electrosurgical tip during surgery; eschar can cause sparking and become a source of ignition.

Flammable (inflammable): Cable of burning.

Genetic mutation: A permanent change in the DNA makeup of a gene.

Grounding: A path for electrical current to flow unimpeded through a material and dispersed back to the source or dispersed into the ground.

Hypersensitivity: A cell-mediated immune response to a substance in the body.

Impedance/resistance: The ability of a substance to stop or alter the flow of electrons through a conductive material.

Latex: A naturally occurring sap obtained from rubber trees that is used in the manufacture of medical devices and other commercial goods.

Needleless system: A system of parenteral access that does not use needles for the collection or withdrawal of body fluids through venous puncture.

297

Neutral zone (no-hands) technique: A method of transferring sharp instruments on the surgical field without hand-to-hand contact. A neutral zone is identified, and sharps are exchanged in this zone.

Occupational exposure: Exposure to hazards in the workplace; for example, exposure to hazardous chemicals or contact with potentially infected blood and body fluids.

Oxidizer: An agent or substance capable of supporting fire.

Oxygen-enriched atmosphere (OEA): An environment that contains a high percentage of oxygen and presents a high risk for fire.

Personal protective equipment (PPE): Clothing or equipment that protects the wearer from direct contact with hazardous chemicals or potentially infectious body fluids.

Postexposure prophylaxis (PEP): Recommended procedures to help prevent the development of blood-borne diseases after an exposure incident such as a needle stick injury.

Risk: The statistical probability of a given event based on the number of such events that have already occurred in a certain population.

Sharps: Any objects that can penetrate the skin and have the potential to cause injury and infection. Sharps include but are not limited to needles, scalpels, broken glass, broken capillary tubes, and exposed ends of dental wires.

Smoke plume: Smoke created during the use of an electrosurgical unit (ESU) or laser. This smoke contains toxic chemicals, vapors, blood fragments, and viruses.

Standard Precautions: Guidelines recommended by the Centers for Disease Control and Prevention (CDC) to reduce the risk of transmission of blood-borne and other pathogens.

Transmission-based precautions: Standards and precautions to prevent the spread of infectious disease by patients known to be infected.

Underwriters Laboratories: A nonprofit agency that tests and certifies electrical equipment in the United States.

Volatile: A substance with a low boiling point which therefore converts easily to a vapor such as alcohol.

INTRODUCTION

The potential for accident and injury in the operating room (OR) is one of the highest in the health care setting. High voltage equipment, chemicals, exposure to blood and body fluids, and stress injury are some of the risks that perioperative personnel encounter daily.

Management of environmental risks requires a knowledge of the risk, a plan of action, and continuous monitoring. A successful injury reduction plan must consider both the human factor and the technological aspects. Education, awareness, and compliance with recommendations and safety protocols are equally important. This chapter discusses hazards in the OR environment and provides a basis for knowledge and understanding of the hazards for patients and personnel. Many topics in this chapter are discussed in greater detail elsewhere in the text, such as risks related to electrosurgery, anesthetic agents, and disease transmission.

RISK AND SAFETY

A discussion on safety must include the concept of risk. Risk is the statistical probability of a harmful event; it is defined as the number of harmful events that occur in a given population over a stated period. In other words, risk represents the number of times an event actually occurs under specified conditions in a specific environment. For example, the risk of contracting HIV as a result of working in the health care environment is based on the number of people who have contracted HIV through occupational exposure in the past (based on yearly statistics). Risk and probability are not difficult to measure when reporting is carried out each time there is an accident injury in the workplace is documented as a sentinel event by those involved. Other organizations may also be notified, depending on the type of accident or injury. Statistics that are collected and analyzed so that risk can be measured and policies put in place to prevent future accidents. People often ignore risk factors because they believe they somehow will escape harm. They know that risk exists, but not for themselves. Taking risks means trying to beat the odds, but it does not change the probability that a given event will occur.

In the health care setting, taking a risk for oneself often means risking the safety of the patient and other staff members.

Most of the discussions in this chapter focus on the technical aspects of accident and injury. However, human factors also contribute to risk. Some of the human causes of injury include:

- Frequent lifting and long hours of standing, resulting in fatigue
- A work culture focused on completion of tasks rather than the methods used to complete the tasks safely
- Rushing through tasks to get the work done
- Lack of knowledge about the risks involved
- Emotional strain and stress, which may influence work habits

A culture of safety is critical to injury reduction in the workplace. This means that staff members must have *knowledge* of the risk, *accept* the responsibility for harm reduction, and *act* on prevention measures.

The risks discussed in this chapter focus on three types of potential injury, posed by:

- *Technical risk factors:* Hazards related to medical devices and energy sources.
- *Chemical risk factors:* Hazards related primarily to liquid, gas, and solid chemicals in the perioperative environment.
- *Biological risk factors:* Hazards related to the transmission of infectious disease.

SAFETY STANDARDS AND RECOMMENDATIONS

Environmental safety standards are designed to protect patients and staff members. Safety standards are evidence based. They are developed with consideration for human factors and technical error.

A number of private, professional, and government organizations create standards and recommendations aimed at reducing injury in the health care setting:

- The Association of periOperative Registered Nurses (AORN): http://www.aorn.org
- The Association for Professionals in Infection Control and Epidemiology (APIC): http://www.apic.org
- The Centers for Disease Control and Prevention (CDC): An agency of the federal government and the central authority on infectious diseases. http://www.cdc.gov
- ECRI Institute: A nonprofit research organization designated as an evidence-based practice center by the U.S. Agency for Healthcare Research and Quality and a collaborating agency of the World Health Organization. http://www.ecri.org
- The U.S. Environmental Protection Agency (EPA): http://www.epa.gov
- The U.S. Food and Drug Administration (FDA): http://www.fda.gov
- The Joint Commission: http://www.jointcommission.org
- The Occupational Safety and Health Administration (OSHA): http://www.osha.gov

These organizations can be contacted for further information on occupational risks in surgery. Standards are periodically updated and renewed. The surgical technologist should remain current, because hazards and risks change as new technologies develop.

RISKS RELATED TO MEDICAL DEVICES AND ENERGY SOURCES

FIRE

Fire in the operating room historically has been a great risk. In the past, many fires were associated with flammable anesthetics and unregulated combustible materials. Although these are no longer used, fire is still a real risk.

Fire Triangle

Fire requires three components:

- **Oxygen** (available in the air or as a pure gas)
- **Fuel** (a combustible material)
- **Source of ignition** (usually in the form of heat)

These components are commonly present in the operating room (Figure 15-1).

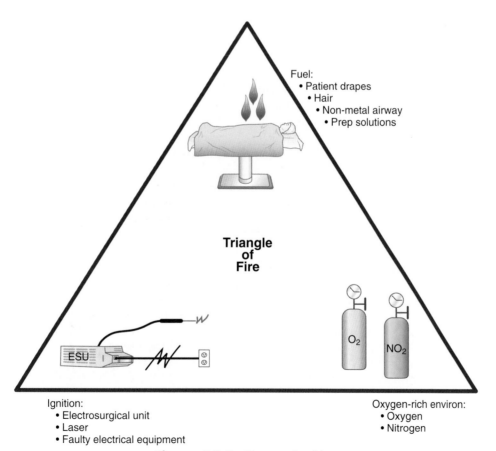

Figure 15-1 The triangle of fire.

Oxygen

Normal air contains about 21% oxygen. An environment that contains a greater concentration of oxygen is called an **oxygen-enriched atmosphere (OEA)**. The operating room is an OEA because oxygen is used in conjunction with general anesthetics and in patient care. Consequently, the risk of fire is high. Oxygen is heavier than air and settles under drapes and in confined areas, such as body cavities, where it remains trapped. When nitrous oxide decomposes in the presence of heat, oxygen molecules are produced.

As the concentration of oxygen increases in the environment, so does the speed of ignition, duration, and temperature of a fire. Items that normally would not burn in atmospheric air are highly flammable in the presence of oxygen. Oxygen and nitrous oxide are called *oxidizers*, because they are capable of supporting fire.

Fuel

Any material capable of burning is potential fuel for a fire. Materials and substances that burn are called *flammable*. Note that the words *flammable* and *inflammable* have the same meaning; both indicate combustibility. Sources of fuel commonly found at the surgical site are listed in Table 15-1. Although many items used in the surgical setting are considered "flame resistant" or "flame retardant," they may readily catch fire when ignition occurs in an OEA.

Flammable Chemicals

Skin prep solutions, especially alcohol, are a common source of fuel in surgical fires. An alcohol concentration greater than 20% is flammable and highly *volatile* (i.e., vaporizes at a low temperature). Most skin prep solutions contain 70% alcohol.

Vapor from volatile prep solutions such as alcohol can be trapped under drapes. When the vapor is ignited, the fire is hidden from view. Second- or third-degree burns can occur within moments of ignition. Most fires arising from alcohol prep solutions occur in combination with an electrosurgical spark (ignition). Although alcohol is highly volatile, it is widely used because it is inexpensive, readily available, and effective.

Chemicals such as cyanoacrylates (fibrin glue), used as tissue glue and for taking tissue grafts, and methylmethacrylate (bone cement) are volatile and flammable. Petroleum products, such as ointments, also can ignite.

Medical Devices

Rubber, plastic, Silastic, and vinyl materials are flammable. Medical devices made of these materials are common in surgery. Disposable anesthesia equipment, such as endotracheal tubes, airways, masks, cannulas, and corrugated tubing are hazardous sources of fuel.

Endotracheal tubes, except those made especially for laser surgery, frequently are the cause of patient fires during laser surgery of the head, neck, and face. An endotracheal fire can begin as an explosion, causing extensive burns within moments. The fire moves quickly along the oxygen path and spreads to the lungs, face, hair, and drapes.

Drapes and Gowns

Surgical drapes and gowns are flame resistant. However, in an OEA they can ignite easily. The operating table mattress and positioning devices made of foam and liquid gels also are potential fuel. As these items burn, they release toxic gases which are an additional source of injury.

Intestinal Gases

The intestine normally produces hydrogen, oxygen, nitrogen, carbon dioxide, and methane. Some gases are produced by normal bacteria in the gastrointestinal (GI) tract, and others are ingested with food. Forty percent of these gases are contained in the large bowel. Hydrogen and methane are present in sufficient quantities and concentration to be an important risk. Methane is explosive at concentrations of 5% to 15%.

Sources of Ignition

Any heat-producing device has the potential to cause a fire. The more intense the heat, the more rapidly oxidation and ignition are likely to occur. Many potential sources of ignition can be found in the operating room.

Table 15-1

Fuel Sources at the Surgical Site

Fuel Source	Fire Prevention
Oxygen-rich environment (OEA)	Tent drapes away from the patient's head during surgery.
Dry sponges and drapes	Place the tip of the electrosurgical unit (ESU) in a holder.
	Use wet towels, wet sponges, or nonflammable drapes at the operative site.
Endotracheal tube and other flammable anesthesia equipment	Use only laser-approved airways and endotracheal tubes.
	Use a reflective shield between the patient's head and the surgical field.
Volatile prep solutions	Drape the patient only after all prepping solutions are dry.
	Tent drapes to allow the escape of vapors when an alcohol-based prep is used.
	Always check for solutions pooling under the patient before draping.
Lanugo (fine body hair on the patient)	Use a water-based gel on lanugo near laser or ESU sites.
Petroleum-based products	Do not use around laser or ESU sites.
Suction catheter and other peripheral venous catheter (PVC) devices	Do not use around ESU or laser sites.
Smoke plume evacuator tip	Use noncombustible evacuator tip.
	Use moist sponges around laser area.
Gastrointestinal gas	Use suction to remove gases at operative site.

Laser

Approximately 13% of surgical fires involve lasers.[1] Laser surgery of the trachea and adjacent structures is performed in an OEA close to flammable material. During laser surgery of the neck and throat, a nonflammable endotracheal tube and aluminum-coated drapes are used. In spite of these precautions, laser energy remains a potent source of ignition in an OEA during surgery.

Electrosurgical Unit

The electrosurgical unit (ESU) uses electrical energy to coagulate and cut tissue. The active electrode can reach 1,292°F (700°C), hot enough to ignite surgical drapes and other supplies. The tip of the active electrode can become coated with eschar (oxidized tissue residue), which holds heat in much the same way as charcoal. Eschar can cause sparking and ignition. Small bits of eschar can be released into the wound as burning embers (e.g., into the throat during neck surgery).

Sparking can occur when the active electrode comes in contact with metal. Sparks can ignite volatile gases, liquids, drapes, and sponges, especially in the presence of oxygen. (Chapter 19 presents a complete discussion of the hazards associated with the ESU.)

High-Speed Instruments

Other, less obvious devices can ignite combustible materials in surgery. These include power instruments, burrs, drill bits, saws, and the harmonic scalpel, which uses high-frequency sound waves to cut and coagulate tissue. When high-speed drills are used, the active tip is irrigated to prevent the buildup of heat created by friction between the metal tip and the bone. Hot drill bits, saw blades, and other metal tips should never be placed in contact with drapes or other combustible materials.

High-Intensity Light

Light sources used in surgery are intense and bright. Although modern surgical light is cooler than in the past, these light sources are still a risk. Fiberoptic light, used in endoscopic instruments, is particularly intense. The light source is delivered through a fiberoptic cable. When the cable is detached from the endoscope, light emitted from the cable can easily ignite drapes, cloth, or other materials. (The safe use of fiberoptic light is fully described in Chapter 19.)

Electrical Malfunction

An electrical short or other malfunction can cause sparking (electrical arcing), which can ignite combustible materials on the surgical field. If an electrical device malfunctions during surgery, it must be removed from service immediately and labeled for repair by the bioengineering department or manufacturer. Perioperative staff must never attempt to repair malfunctioning electrical equipment.

Fire in the Operating Room

Patient Fire

Patient fire is a rare but devastating event. Fires can occur inside the body or on the skin surface. Approximately 21% of patient fires occur in the airway, 44% on the face, 8% inside the patient, and 26% on the skin.[2] It takes only moments for a flash fire to engulf the patient. To stop the progression of the fire, *the triangle of fire must be broken*. This means that one or more components (fuel, oxygen, or ignition) must be removed from the fire.

During a patient fire, time is critical. Three steps are immediately taken to protect the patient and stop the fire:

1. Shut off the flow of all gases to the patient's airway.
2. Remove any burning objects from the surgical site.
3. Assess the patient for injury and respond appropriately.

The anesthesia care provider (ACP) reduces the flow of oxygen in the event of fire around the airway. At the same time, burning objects are removed from the field as safely as possible. The surgical technologist must stand by for direction from the surgeon and other staff members in the room. Patient fires usually can be contained when one of the elements of the fire has been removed. The next phase of the emergency focuses on the patient's injuries.

Structural Fire

If the fire extends beyond the immediate patient area, the surgical team must activate the hospital fire plan. This plan is based on four immediate actions, which are easily remembered by the acronym **RACE:**

Rescue patients in the immediate area of the fire.

Alert other people to the fire so that they can assist in patient removal and response. Activate the fire alert system.

Contain the fire. Shut all doors to slow the spread of smoke and flame. Always shut off the zone valves controlling in-line gases to the room.

Evacuate personnel in the areas around the fire.

If the fire is limited to a small area, appropriate extinguishing agents may be used to put it out. Personnel should never let a fire get between them and the exit.

Fire Drills and Extinguishers

- Fire drills are held regularly in all health facilities, and new staff members are trained during orientation. Staff training includes emergency response, the location of fire extinguishers and fire escape routes, and how to activate the fire alert system. Most fire extinguishers used in the OR are water-based, carbon dioxide, or dry powder. Carbon dioxide is the preferred type for OR fires.

To activate the fire extinguisher, pull the ring from the handle, aim the nozzle at the base of the fire, squeeze the handle, and sweep the fire with the tank contents. These steps can be remembered by the acronym **PASS:**

Pull

Aim

Squeeze

Sweep

Fire Prevention

- Fire prevention is the responsibility of everyone working in the operating room. Risk reduction strategies have been developed by the Joint Commission, AORN, and other professional organizations concerned with the protection of patients and staff members. AORN has established guidelines for yearly fire prevention activities (AORN Guidance Statement, 2006. "AORN Guidance statement: Fire prevention in the Operating Room: in Standards, Recommended Practices, and Guidelines. Denver: AORN)

- Participation in fire drills
- Demonstration of the use of firefighting equipment
- Methods for rescue operation
- Gas shutoff procedures
- Location of ventilation and electrical systems
- Review of code "red" (fire alert) policies
- Fire department procedures
- Developing a safety culture

Risk Management

AORN has established fire risk management strategies for perioperative personnel that are intended to minimize or remove the risks (Table 15-2). These risk management strategies should be carefully studied by all students and reviewed yearly by experienced personnel.

COMPRESSED GAS CYLINDERS

Gases such as oxygen, nitrous oxide, argon, and nitrogen are compressed into metal cylinders for medical use:

- *Oxygen* is contained in portable tanks and is used when in-line systems are not available or when patients are transported.
- *Compressed* nitrogen is used as a power source for instruments such as drills, saws, and other high-speed tools.

- *Argon* is used during laser surgery.
- *Nitrous oxide* is an anesthetic gas.
- *Carbon dioxide* is used for insufflation during laparoscopy or pelviscopy.

Tank Components and Specifications

A compressed gas tank is made of heavy steel that is able to withstand the pressure of the gas and to resist puncture or breakage. The wall of a large tank is approximately ¼-inch (0.63 cm) thick, and the gas is pressurized to 2,200 pounds per square inch (psi). A regulator is fitted into the cylinder by a threaded connection. The regulator contains two gauges; one displays the flow of gas from the regulator to the equipment being used, and the other shows the amount of gas in the tank (in psi). The regulator is activated by a valve handle. A valve stem or hand wheel is fitted into the top of the tank. Gas flows through the regulator when the tank valve is opened.

Hazards

Two types of hazards are associated with compressed gas cylinders: physical hazards, which are related to the high pressure in the cylinder, and chemical hazards, which are related to the flammability or oxidative qualities, toxicity, or other properties of the contents of the tank.

Any compressed gas cylinder can explode or rupture, because the tank is under extremely high pressure. If the gas is also flammable or supports combustion (e.g., oxygen and nitrous oxide), the risk increases significantly. Tanks must be handled with caution. A leak in a tank or separation of the valve from the tank can propel the tank with the force of a missile, sending it through walls and into objects and people. All surgical personnel must be familiar with the proper handling of gas cylinders (Figure 15-2).

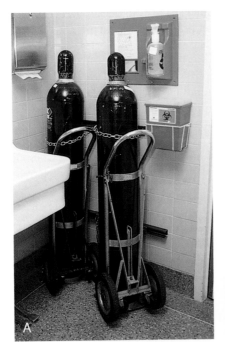 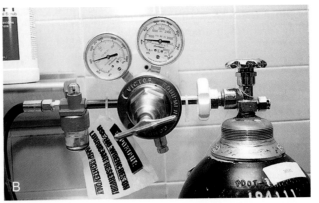

Figure 15-2 Handling of compressed gas cylinders. *(From Ignatavicius DD, Workman L: Medical-surgical nursing: critical thinking for collaborative care, ed 4, Philadelphia, 2002, WB Saunders.)*

<u>Table 15-2A</u>

Fire Management Strategies: Ignition

FIRE RISK—IGNITION

Risk	Management
Electrosurgical unit (ESU)	• Use the lowest possible power setting. • Place the patient return electrode on a large muscle mass close to the surgical site. • Large reusable return electrodes should be used according to the manufacturer's instructions. • Always use a safety holster. • Do not coil active electrode cords. • Inspect the active electrode to ensure its integrity. • Do not use the ESU in the presence of flammable solutions. • Ensure that electrical cords and plugs are not frayed or broken. • Do not place fluids on top of the ESU. • Do not use the ESU near oxygen or nitrous oxide. • Ensure that the ESU active electrode tip fits securely into the active electrode handpiece. • Ensure that any connections and adaptors used are intended to connect to the ESU and fit securely. • Do not bypass ESU safety features. • Ensure that the alarm tone is always audible. • Remove any contaminated or unused active accessories for the sterile field. • Keep the active electrode tip clean. • Use wet sponges or towels to help retard fire potential. • Never alter a medical device. • Do not use rubber catheters or protective covers as insulators on the active electrode tip. • Use *Cut* or *Blend* instead of *Coagulation* when possible. • Do not open the circuit to activate the ESU. • Make sure the active electrode is not activated near another metal object that could conduct heat or cause arcing. • After prepping, allow the prep solution to dry and the fumes to dissipate. Wet prep and fumes trapped beneath drapes can ignite. • Provide multidisciplinary in-service programs on the safe use of ESUs based on the manufacturer's instructions
Argon beam coagulator	• Argon beam coagulators combine the ESU spark with argon gas to concentrate and focus the ESU spark. Argon gas is inert and nonflammable, but because it is used with an ESU, the same precautions as with an ESU should be taken. • Always use a safety holster. • Make sure the active electrode is not activated near another metal object that could conduct heat or cause arcing.
Laser	• Use a laser-specific endotracheal tube (i.e., a tube that has laser-resistant coating or contains no material that will ignite) if head, neck, lung, or airway surgery is anticipated. • Wet sponges around the tube cuffs may provide extra protection to help retard fire potential. Moist towels around the surgical site also may retard fires. • Keep towels moist and away from the edge of the surgical site to retard fires. • Do not use liquids of ointments that may be combustible. • Inflate cuffed tube bladders with tinted saline so that inadvertent rupture may be detected during chest or upper airway surgery. • Do not use uncuffed, standard endotracheal tubes in the presence of a laser or the ESU. • If an endotracheal tube fire occurs, oxygen administration should be stopped and all burning or melted tubes should be removed from the patient immediately. • Prevent pooling of skin prep solutions. • Have water and the correct type of fire extinguisher available in case of a laser fire. • Ensure that the alarm tone is always audible.
Fiberoptic light sources and cables	• Ensure that the light source is in good working order. • Place the light source in standby or turn it off when the cable is not connected. • Place the light source away from items that are flammable. • Do not place a light cable that is connected to a light source on drapes, sponges, or anything else that is flammable. • Do not allow cables that are connected to hang over the side of the sterile field if the light source is on. • Make sure light cables are in good working order and do not have broken light fibers.

Continued

Table 15-2A

Fire Management Strategies: Ignition—cont'd

FIRE RISK—IGNITION

Risk	Management
Power tools, drills, and burrs	• Instruments and equipment that move rapidly during use generate heat. Always make sure they are in good working order. • A slow drip of saline on a moving drill or burr helps reduce heat buildup. • Do not place drills, burrs, or saws on the patient when they are not in use. • Remove instruments and equipment from the sterile field when not in use.
Defibrillator paddles	• Select paddles that are the correct size for the patient (e.g., pediatric paddles on a child). • Ensure that the gel recommended by the paddle manufacturer is used. • Adhere to appropriate site selection for paddle placement. • Contact between the paddles and the patient should be optimal, and no gaps should be present before the defibrillator is activated.
Electrical equipment	• Ensure that all equipment is inspected periodically by biomedical personnel for proper function. • Check the biomedical inspection stickers on the equipment; they should be current. • Do not use equipment with frayed or damaged cords or plugs. • Remove any equipment that emits smoke during use.

Modified from the Association of periOperative Registered Nurses (AORN): Fire prevention in the operating room. In *Standards, recommendations, practices and guidelines,* 2007 edition, Denver, 2007, AORN.

Handling of Gas Cylinders

Many modern operating rooms have in-line gas outlets that dispense oxygen, nitrogen, and air. Even so, gas cylinders, especially oxygen and nitrogen, are common in the hospital environment. The surgical technologist should be familiar with the following procedures for opening, adjusting, and connecting the cylinder to a power hose.

1. The gas cylinder has two valves. One opens the cylinder and allows gas to flow to the regulator. This valve is located on top of the cylinder.
2. The second valve is located on the regulator. This valve controls the flow from the regulator to the power instrument. It must be adjusted according to the requirements of the instrument.
3. The right-hand gauge displays the pressure in the cylinder. The left-hand gauge displays the pressure in the power hose connected to the instrument.
4. If the regulator is already attached to the cylinder, slowly turn the tank valve to its full open position. With the valve in this position, the tank pressure is displayed on the right-hand pressure gauge.
5. Do not use the tank if the pressure is less than 500 psi. This means there is insufficient gas remaining in the tank. A small amount of residual gas (and pressure) in the tank prevents debris (e.g., rust and dust) from entering the hose. Particles entering the hose can damage the equipment or cause injury.
6. Attach the power hose securely to the regulator outlet. Most connectors can be attached by pushing and turning firmly.
7. Turn the regulator wheel handle to set the pressure at the correct level. The required pressure level depends on the instrument manufacturer's specifications. Some instruments must be running to set the correct pressure. Make sure the correct pressure is maintained throughout use.
8. After use, turn off the tank pressure valve. Then bleed the gas remaining in the air hose by activating the instrument.
9. Close the regulator valve by rotating the regulator dial. The pressure should now read zero.
10. Do not return a tank to storage if the pressure is below 500 psi. The tank must be replaced.
11. *Regulators are gas specific and are not interchangeable.* Do not attempt to modify a regulator gauge to fit the gas you are using.

Storage and Transport

All personnel should be familiar with safety precautions used for the storage and transport of gas cylinders (Box 15-1).

ELECTRICITY

Risk

Electrical malfunctions are a leading cause of hospital fires in the United States. Accredited hospitals are required to install explosion-proof outlets and to comply with building and environmental codes enacted to prevent electrical fire. However, electrical equipment also must be maintained. The probability of malfunction increases as devices become technologically more sophisticated and have greater requirements for repair and maintenance.

Characteristics of Electrical Energy

The characteristics of electricity (the flow of electrons) are current, voltage, impedance (resistance), and grounding.

Table 15-2B

Management Strategies: Fuel and Oxidizers

FIRE RISK—FUEL

Fuel Sources	Management Strategies
Bed linens Caps, hats Drapes Dressings Gowns Lap pads Shoe covers Sponges Tapes Towels Prep solutions	• Assess the flammability of all materials used in, on, or around the patient. Linens and drapes are made of synthetic or natural fibers. They may burn or melt, depending on the fiber content. • Do not allow drapes or linens to come in contact with activated ignition sources (e.g., laser, electrosurgical unit [ESU], light sources). • Do not trap volatile chemicals or chemical fumes beneath drapes. • Moisten drapes, towels, and sponges that will be near ignition sources. • Ensure that oxygen does not accumulate beneath drapes. • If drapes or linens ignite, smother small fires with a wet sponge or towel. Remove burning material from the patient. • Extinguish any burning material with the appropriate fire extinguisher or with water, if appropriate. • Use flammable prep solutions with extreme caution. • Do not allow prep solutions to pool on, around, or beneath the patient. • After prepping, allow the prep solution to dry and the fumes to dissipate. Wet prep and fumes trapped beneath drapes can ignite. • Do not activate ignition sources in the presence of flammable prep solutions. • Do not allow drapes that will remain in contact with the patient to absorb flammable prep solutions.
Skin degreasers	• Skin degreasers may be used before skin prep to degrease or clean the skin or as part of the dressing. These products may contain chemicals that are flammable. Allow all fumes to dissipate before beginning surgery. The laser or ESU should not be used after the dressing is in place.
Body tissue and patient hair	• The patient's own body can be a fuel source. Coat any body hair that is near an ignition source with a water-based jelly to retard ignition. • Ensure that surgical smoke from burning patient tissue is properly evacuated. Surgical smoke can support combustion if allowed to accumulate in a small or enclosed space (e.g., the back of the throat).
Intestinal gases	• The patient's intestinal gases are flammable. The ESU or laser should be used with caution whenever intestinal gases are present. Do not open the bowel with the laser or ESU when gas appears to be present. • Use suction during rectal surgery to remove any intestinal gases that may be present.

FIRE RISK—OXIDIZERS

Oxidizers	Management Strategies
Oxygen	• Oxygen should be used with caution in the presence of ignition sources. Oxygen is an oxidizer and is capable of supporting combustion. • Ensure that anesthesia circuits are free of leaks. • Pack wet sponges around the back of the throat to help retard oxygen leaks. • Inflate cuffed tube bladders with tinted saline so that inadvertent ruptures can be detected. • Use suction to help evacuate any accumulation of oxygen in body cavities such as the mouth or chest cavity. • Do not use the laser or ESU near sites where oxygen is flowing. • Use a pulse oximeter to determine the patient's oxygenation level and the need for oxygen. • Allow oxygen fumes to dissipate before using the laser or ESU. • Oxygen should not be directed at the surgical site. • Ensure that drapes are configured to help prevent oxygen accumulation when mask or nasal oxygen is used. • With a large fire, turn off the gases; with an airway or tracheal fire, disconnect the breathing circuit and remove the endotracheal tube. • Stop supplemental oxygen for 1 min before using electrocautery or laser for head, neck, or upper chest procedures.
Nitrous oxide	• The strategies to manage oxygen also should be used to manage risks associated with nitrous oxide.

From the Association of periOperative Registered Nurses (AORN): Fire prevention in the operating room. In *Standards, recommendations, practices and guidelines,* 2007 edition, Denver, 2007, AORN.

Box 15-1
Guidelines for Storage and Transport of Gas Cylinders

1. Label storage areas with the names of the gases stored there.
2. Never use a gas cylinder that is not labeled properly.
3. A gas cylinder must be secured at a point approximately two thirds of its height at all times. Each cylinder should be secured individually with a chain, wire cable, or cylinder strap.
4. Store cylinders so that the valve is accessible at all times.
5. Never store oxygen cylinders in the same area as flammable gases.
6. Cylinders must never be stored in public hallways or other unprotected areas.
7. Never use grease or oily materials on oxygen cylinders or store them near these cylinders.
8. Always secure a gas cylinder before transporting it. Use a caged rack, chain, or other secure device designed to prevent the cylinder from falling or tipping over.
9. Do not store cylinders of different gases together or allow one to strike another.
10. Never store gas tanks near heat or where they might come in contact with sources of electricity.
11. Never roll, drag, or slide a gas cylinder. Always use a handcart to transport a tank.
12. Do not tamper with tank safety devices.
13. Always read the identification label of any gas cylinder. Do not rely on the color for identification.
14. Do not attempt to repair a cylinder or valve yourself. The tank must be returned to the bioengineering department or regulator supplier for repair.
15. Never use pliers to open a cylinder valve. Cylinders are equipped with a wheel or stem valve to initiate the flow. Operation of stem valves requires a key, which must remain with the cylinder at all times.
16. Make sure all compressed gas storage areas have adequate ventilation.

- Current is the rate of electrical (electron) flow. Direct current (DC) is low voltage and originates from a battery. Alternating current (AC) is transmitted by a 220- or 110-V line, such as that normally found in wall outlets. The available power is much higher with AC than with DC.
- Voltage is the driving force behind the moving electrons.
- Impedance (resistance) describes the ability of a substance to stop the flow of electrons (electricity). Electricity follows the path of least resistance. Nonresistant materials include metal, water, and the human body. When electricity enters the body and is not directed back to the source, severe burns and cardiac arrest can result. This is commonly referred to as *electrocution*.
- Grounding is the discharge of electrical current from the source to ground, where it is dispersed and rendered harmless. As long as electrical current can travel unhindered through the body and is directed back to its source, electrocution does not occur. An improperly grounded electrical device can send electricity through the patient but does not control its dispersal to the ground. Normal grounding is established by the use of a three-prong plug. Two of the prongs send the current through the device. The ground wire, or third prong, connects the device to the ground. If no ground wire is used, current can leak into other conductors and will follow a nonresistant path.

Preventing Electrical Malfunction

- Equipment with frayed cords or devices with exposed wires must never be used.
- Cords must not be spliced or threaded through solid obstacles.
- All switches must be protected from moisture.
- Only devices intended for use around fluids should be used.
- All equipment must be properly grounded.
- Any instrument or device must be switched to the Off position before the power plug is removed.
- All equipment used in the operating room must be inspected and must be approved by Underwriters Laboratories (UL). This agency develops and maintains standards of safety for consumer electrical products. Electrical items that do not have a UL approval rating must not be used.

❖ *The most common source of electrical injury to the surgical patient is the electrosurgical unit (ESU).*

Chapter 19 presents a complete discussion of the risks and proper use of electrosurgical equipment.

IONIZING RADIATION

Risk
Radiograph machines, fluoroscopes, and unshielded radioactive implants produce ionizing radiation in amounts high enough to damage tissue. Exposure occurs when workers are not protected during procedures that use radiography or fluoroscopy. Hazard warnings should be posted whenever radiographic or fluoroscopic studies are in progress (Figure 15-3).

The extent of tissue damage depends on the duration of exposure, the distance from the source of radiation, and the tissue exposed. Repeated exposures have cumulative effects. Among the risks of overexposure to radiation are **genetic mutation**, cancer, cataract, burns, and spontaneous abortion. Certain areas of the body are more vulnerable than others. These are the areas in which cell reproduction is the most rapid, including the ovaries, testes, lymphatic tissue, thyroid, and bone marrow.

Injury Prevention
Radiography and fluoroscopy frequently are used in diagnostic areas and in the operating room. Lead shields are the most effective method of blocking radiation. The distance from the radiation source, the duration of exposure, and the quality of the shielding are the most important parameters determining risk and protection.

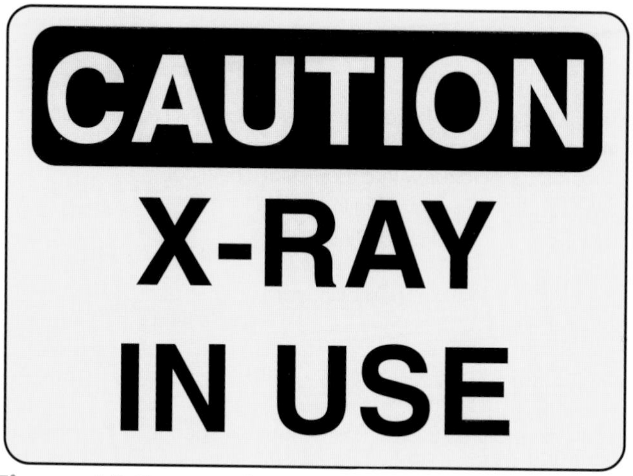

Figure 15-3 Hazard warnings that radiographic equipment is in use.

Safety Precautions During Use of Ionizing Radiation

- Although lead aprons are uncomfortable and heavy, team members should wear them under their sterile gowns during any procedure that requires radiation. Many lead aprons shield only the front of the body, therefore workers should face the radiation source during exposure.
- A lead apron must be worn during fluoroscopy to prevent exposure to scatter radiation.
- Lead aprons must be stored flat or hung in a manner that prevents bending of the material.
- Remember that a lead apron protects only the areas of the body that are covered by the apron. The eyes and hands are not protected.
- Lead glasses should be worn during exposure to a fluoroscope.
- Neck shields are available to protect the thyroid, which is sensitive to radiation, during fluoroscopy.
- Nonsterile workers should step outside the range of exposure, either behind a lead screen or outside the room. Those who must remain in the room during exposure must maintain a distance of at least 6 feet (1.8 m) from the patient. The safest place to stand is at a right angle to the beam on the side of the radiograph machine or origin of the radiation beam.
- In the radiology department, the walls are lined with lead to protect workers when diagnostic studies are performed. In this circumstance, personnel may be able to step behind the lead wall while the equipment is in operation.
- Whenever possible, a mechanical holding device should be used to support radiograph cassettes to prevent exposure of the hands.
- Lead-impregnated gloves must be worn any time the hands are directly exposed to the radiation beam, such as during fluoroscopy or when radioactive implants or dyes are handled.

- Dosimeters are available to measure the cumulative radiation dose for those who are often exposed to radiation.
- Perioperative staff members should rotate through cases involving ionizing radiation. This prevents overexposure of the same staff members.

MAGNETIC RESONANCE IMAGING

Risk

Perioperative staff members may assist during magnetic resonance imaging (MRI) procedures. MRI provides a three-dimensional view of the patient's anatomy using radiofrequency. Whenever MRI is used, the primary risk is the presence of metal, which can be drawn from its source and into the path of the powerful magnetic field. For this reason, absolutely no metal objects are permitted in the environment during this process. Also, a substantial risk of injury exists from certain types of metal implants in the patient or staff members and personal items, such as scissors or jewelry. Only plastic and titanium objects are safe to use during MRI procedures.

CHEMICAL RISKS

TOXIC CHEMICALS

Risk

Operating room workers are exposed to many different types of chemicals. Many of these are hazardous and can produce serious long-term effects, such as respiratory or skin problems, genetic changes, and fetal injury. It is important to remember that, although exposure to a particular chemical may be brief, constant exposure to chemicals in a variety of work situations has a cumulative effect. For example, in a given day a surgical technologist might be exposed to glutaraldehyde disinfectant, vapor from methylmethacrylate cement, formaldehyde used as a specimen preserver, a phenolic agent used during environmental cleaning, and peracetic acid used as a sterilizing agent. Although the effects of any single exposure may be limited, the cumulative and synergistic effects can be much greater.

Standards and guidelines for handling chemicals are designed to reduce the risk of occupational exposure and associated injuries. All hazardous chemicals approved for use in the United States are issued a Material Safety Data Sheet (MSDS). The MSDS describes the chemical, precautions for handling the chemical, hazards associated with the chemical, and firefighting techniques and first aid for exposure. Each department in the health facility is required to maintain an MSDS for chemicals used in that department, and employees must have access to these.

Exposure

Toxic chemicals can enter the body through the respiratory tract, by direct skin contact, by splash contact, or by ingestion. **Personal protective equipment** (PPE) protects personnel against high concentrations of chemicals. Exposure to an airborne chemical (vapor) is measured by concentration, in parts

Box 15-2
Reading a Chemical Label

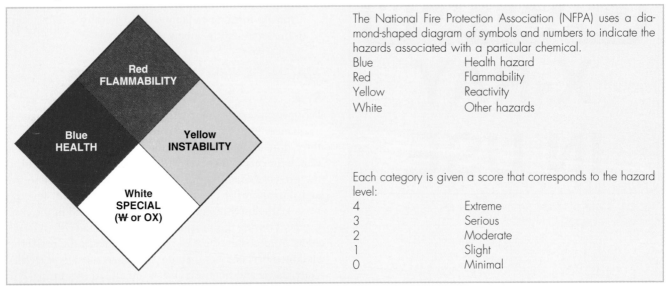

The National Fire Protection Association (NFPA) uses a diamond-shaped diagram of symbols and numbers to indicate the hazards associated with a particular chemical.

Blue   Health hazard
Red   Flammability
Yellow   Reactivity
White   Other hazards

Each category is given a score that corresponds to the hazard level:

4   Extreme
3   Serious
2   Moderate
1   Slight
0   Minimal

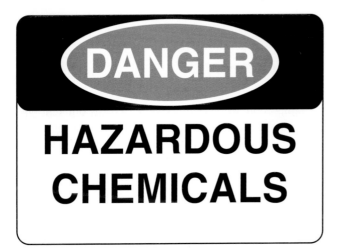

Figure 15-4 Hazard warning for chemicals.

per million (ppm) or milligrams of substance per cubic meter of air (mg/m^3). Every chemical used in the health care setting has a safe limit of exposure, which is determined by government agencies.

Prevention

Chemicals used in the health care setting must carry a label containing information about the chemical, including its intended safe use, toxicity, and postexposure measures. All personnel must be familiar with chemical labels and know how to interpret them (Box 15-2). When working with any chemical, you must know and use the appropriate concentration and the proper procedure (e.g., glutaraldehyde must be used under a hood to prevent respiratory irritation). Hazard warning labels are posted on the container and in storage areas (Figure 15-4). Chemicals transferred from larger containers to smaller ones must be labeled with the exact information found on the original container. Table 15-3 lists the chemicals commonly found in the operating room environment.

SMOKE PLUME

A **smoke plume** is created during laser surgery and electrosurgery. It contains harmful toxins that must be removed from the immediate surgical environment. Smoke plumes are known to contain benzene, hydrogen cyanide, formaldehyde, blood fragments, and viruses. These materials pose a risk for perioperative personnel who breathe the plume. NIOSH recommends an efficient evacuation and filtering system. This includes a suction tip and tubing at the site of smoke plume generation and filters designed to absorbed the minute toxic particles and vapors. This equipment must be used according to manufacturer's instructions. Filters are considered toxic waste and are handled according to institutional and government policy. (The details of smoke plume control and risks are discussed in Chapter 19.)

BIOLOGICAL RISKS

DISEASE TRANSMISSION IN THE PERIOPERATIVE ENVIRONMENT

Sources of infection and the ways diseases are spread from one person to another are discussed in Chapter 7 In this section, transmission precautions and recommendations are linked with tasks and duties in the perioperative environment.

❖ *The primary focus of disease control in the health care environment is on preventing contact with blood and body fluids.*

Standard Precautions

Contact with blood and body fluid has always been avoided (in recent history) in the surgical environment. However, at the start of the crisis over the human immunodeficiency virus (HIV) and acquired immunodeficiency syndrome (AIDS), the CDC and other agencies involved in public health safety became concerned about the possibility that health care workers might

Table 15-3

Hazardous Chemicals Commonly Used in the Operating Room Environment

Substance	Use	Precaution
Anesthetic gases	General anesthesia	Must be scavenged by anesthesia machine. Be wary of possible fetal injury.
Ethylene oxide	Sterilization	Objects must be aerated in chamber. Personnel should wear dosimeters to measure exposure. Do not handle objects until aeration is complete.
Peracetic acid	Sterilization	Use goggles, face shield, and gloves when operating sterilizer.
Glutaraldehyde	Disinfection	Use only under hood. Wear gloves, mask, and goggles.
Phenolic compounds	Decontamination (environmental)	Use proper dilution. Wear gloves and goggles.
Sodium hypochlorite (1 ppm)	Decontamination (environmental)	Use proper dilution. Wear gloves and goggles.
Formaldehyde	Tissue preservative	Wear masks, gloves, and goggles.
Methylmethacrylate	Bone cement	Do not wear soft contact lenses around this substance; it causes corneal burns and melts contact lenses. Wear mask, gloves, and goggles.
Fibrin glue	Tissue glue	Wear goggles, gloves, and mask.

contract or transmit blood-borne disease in the course of their work. The result of this response was a set of recommendations called *Universal Precautions*. Initially these guidelines applied only to body fluids capable of transmitting blood-borne viruses. Later the concept was expanded to include any body substance capable of harboring pathogenic microorganisms.

The current guidelines for preventing disease transmission are called *Standard Precautions*. **Standard Precautions** are behaviors and methods of working in the health care setting that reduce exposure to blood and body fluids. All patients are considered *potential* sources of disease transmission, therefore Standard Precautions are used at all times and with all patients.

Guidelines

Box 15-3 presents AORN's guidelines for preventing transmissible infections in the perioperative environment.

Specific Practices of Standard Precautions

Hand Washing

Hand washing is the most important method of preventing disease transmission in the health care setting.

- Wash your hands after touching blood, body fluids, secretions, excretions, and contaminated items, regardless of whether gloves are worn. Wash your hands immediately after removing your gloves between patient contacts. You may need to wash your hands between tasks and procedures on the same patient to prevent cross-contamination of different body sites.
- Use a plain soap (not an antimicrobial soap) for routine hand washing.
- Wear gloves (clean, nonsterile gloves are adequate) when touching blood, body fluids, secretions, excretions, and contaminated items. Put on clean gloves just before

touching mucous membranes and nonintact skin. Change gloves between tasks and procedures on the same patient after contact with material that may contain a high concentration of microorganisms. Remove your gloves immediately after use, before touching uncontaminated surfaces, and before going to another patient.

Face, Eye, and Body Protection

- Wear a mask and eye protection or a face shield to protect against splash contamination. Prescription eyeglasses are not considered adequate, because they do not shield the sides of the eyes.
- A clean, nonsterile cover jacket should be worn to protect the skin and prevent soiling of clothing during procedures and patient care activities likely to generate splashes or sprays of blood, body fluids, secretions, or excretions.
- Remove a soiled gown as promptly as possible and wash your hands to prevent the transfer of microorganisms to other patients or environments.

Patient Care Equipment and Linen

Patient care equipment and linens must be handled in a way that prevents contact with skin and clothing. Handle soiled linens with gloved hands only. Hold soiled linen away from your body and place it in a biohazard laundry bag for disposal. Always wear gloves when handling patient care items.

SHARPS INJURY

The most common means of transmission of **blood-borne pathogens** to health care workers is sharps injuries. **Sharps** are such a threat to health care personnel that OSHA has issued the Blood-Borne Pathogen Rule, a special set of regulations for handling and disposing of sharps. More information

Box 15-3

Recommended Practices for Preventing Transmissible Infections in the Perioperative Setting

1. Health care workers should use Standards Precautions when caring for all patients in the perioperative setting.
2. Hand hygiene should be performed before and after each patient contact.
3. Protective barriers must be used to reduce the risk of skin and mucous membrane exposure to potentially infectious material.
4. Health care practitioners should double-glove during invasive procedures.
5. Contact precautions should be used in providing care for patients who are known or suspected to be infected or colonized with microorganisms that are transmitted by direct or indirect contact with patients or items and surfaces in patients' environments.
6. Droplet precautions should be used when caring for patients who are known or suspected to be infected with microorganisms that can be transmitted by infectious large-particle droplets that generally travel short distances (i.e., 3 feet [0.9 m] or less); diseases caused by such microorganisms include diphtheria, pertussis, influenza, mumps, and pneumonic plague.
7. Airborne precautions should be used when caring for patients who are known or suspected to be infected with microorganisms that can be transmitted by the airborne route; diseases caused by such microorganisms include rubella, varicella, tuberculosis, and smallpox.
8. Health care workers should be immunized against epidemiologically important agents according to the regulations of the Centers for Disease Control and Prevention (CDC).
9. Work practices must be designed to minimize the risk of exposure to pathogens.
10. Personnel must take precautions to prevent injuries caused by needles, scalpels, and other sharp instruments.
11. The activities of personnel with infections, exudative lesions, nonintact skin, and/or blood-borne diseases should be restricted when these activities pose a risk of transmission of infection to patients and other health care workers.
12. Policies and procedures that address responses to threats of intentionally released pathogens should be written, reviewed periodically, and readily available within the practice setting.
13. Policies and procedures that address responses to epidemic or pandemic pathogens should be written, reviewed periodically, and readily available within the practice setting.
14. Personnel should demonstrate competence in the prevention of transmissible infections.*

Modified from the Association of periOperative Registered Nurses (AORN): Transmission of transmissible infections. In *Standards, recommended practices and guidelines*, 2007 edition, Denver, 2007, AORN.

on the OSHA standards is available at http://www.osha.gov/SLTC/bloodebornepathogens/standards.html.

Sources of Injury

- Hypodermic needles
- Suture needles
- Scalpel blades
- Needle-point electrosurgical tips
- Trocars, such as those used to perform endoscopic surgery or to place wound drains
- Sharp instruments, such as skin hooks, rakes, and scissors
- Metal guide wires and stylets
- Orthopedic drill bits, screws, pins, wires, and cutting tips, such as saw blades and burrs

Certain tasks are associated with a high risk of sharps injury:

- Passing and receiving a scalpel
- Preparing and passing sutures
- Collision of two individuals' hands when they reach for the same sharp instrument
- Mounting or removing a scalpel blade from the handle
- Manually retracting tissue
- Suturing

The risk of sharps injury can be reduced if team members follow recommended guidelines and standards. This usually means changing the way a task is carried out. All health care workers are responsible for their own safety and the safety of others on the team. Therefore compliance with guidelines is an ethical issues as well as a safety issue.

Risk Reduction

- Whenever possible, retractable or self-sheathing needles and scalpels should be used.
- Blunt suture needles are now recommended over sharp needles.
- If hollow-bore hypodermic needles are used, they must never be recapped by hand. The cap is replaced by grasping it with an instrument. Removable needles must be handled only with an instrument, never by hand. Self-sheathing needles have nonremovable parts.
- Scalpel blades must be mounted and removed with an instrument.
- Used disposable syringes and needles, scalpel blades, and other sharp items should be placed in appropriate puncture-resistant containers located as close as practical to the area where the items were used. The container must be removed and replaced at frequent intervals to prevent overflow, another common source of sharps injury.
- During surgery, sharps are contained on a magnetic board or in a special holder that can be contained and disposed of properly.
- All health care employees should be immunized against the hepatitis B virus (HBV).

Neutral Zone (No-Hands) Technique

The **neutral zone (no-hands) technique** was developed because the evidence showed that most sharps injuries in surgery occurred when instruments were passed and received on the field. OSHA, the CDC, AORN, and the Association of

Surgical Technologists (AST) now strongly recommend that the neutral zone technique be adopted in surgical settings whenever possible. The technique uses a hands-free space (designated receptacle) on the sterile field where sharps can be placed and retrieved so that the surgical technologist and surgeon do not hand instruments to each other directly. (This technique is described in Chapter 16.)

HUMAN FACTOR

Although the nature of blood-borne disease, its transmission, and prevention methods are known, the human factor must be included in the planning and implementation of any risk reduction program. The following are some reasons people have difficulty with risk reduction:

- Working too quickly
- Distraction from the task at hand
- Failure to comply with precautions and standards ("It can't happen to me")
- Extreme fatigue
- Lack of support in designing and maintaining a prevention program
- Difficulty abandoning old and valued methods of working
- Difficulty adapting to newer, safer medical devices

POSTEXPOSURE PROPHYLAXIS

Postexposure prophylaxis (PEP) is a risk reduction strategy that is used after exposure to blood or other body fluids. It involves the administration of drugs and testing. PEP is voluntary; no health care worker should be coerced into receiving it. However, the decision must be made quickly, because the preventive drugs are most effective when given within 24 hours after exposure.

Components of Postexposure Prophylaxis

Individuals exposed to HBV should be tested for HBV surface antigen, and an immunization series should be initiated. Health care workers who have not been previously vaccinated should be given hepatitis B immune globulin (HBIG) if the incident involved mucous membrane exposure or penetrating exposure to a patient's blood or other body fluids.

PEP for HIV consists of a regimen of antiviral drugs followed by regular testing. PEP must be initiated soon after exposure and has a limited effect, and additional health risks are associated with the medications used. Because PEP must be initiated within a brief period after exposure, it is vital that health care workers be evaluated rapidly and that the patient is screened for HIV before leaving the health care setting.

Antibodies generally take 25 days to 3 months to appear on standard HIV tests. The attending physician assesses the patient's HIV exposure risks. PEP includes the use of two or three antiretroviral agents to prevent the virus from attacking the immune system. These drugs are administered orally, and the regimen usually lasts for 1 month. These antiretroviral agents have a number of side effects that must be considered before PEP is initiated.

TRANSMISSION-BASED PRECAUTIONS

Transmission-based precautions are implemented when a patient *is known or suspected to have a highly infectious disease and Standard Precautions are insufficient to prevent transmission to others.* These guidelines are used in addition to Standard Precautions.

Airborne Transmission

Airborne transmission precautions reduce the risk of transmission of airborne agents by droplet nuclei up to 5 µm in size (see Chapter 7). Because of their small size, such droplets remain suspended in the air and disperse widely in the environment.

A patient with a disease that can be spread by airborne transmission must wear a surgical mask during transport. Health care personnel must wear respiratory protection when within 3 feet (0.9 m) of such a patient. Masks must pass NIOSH-approved high-efficiency particulate air (HEPA) standards to be completely effective.

Airborne transmission precautions must be taken for the following diseases:

- Measles
- Varicella (including disseminated herpes zoster)
- Tuberculosis

NOTE: More detailed information on tuberculosis can be obtained from the CDC publication, *Guidelines for Preventing the Transmission of Tuberculosis in Health Care Facilities.*[3]

Droplet Precautions

Droplet precautions are implemented to reduce the risk of infectious disease transmission by large, moist, aerosol droplets. These are spread from the mouth, nose, oropharynx, and trachea to a susceptible host. The traveling distance of droplets is 3 feet (0.9 m) or less, and they do not remain suspended in the air. Patients with any of the diseases that can be transmitted in this way must be separated from other patients by at least 3 feet (0.9 m), and health care workers must wear a mask when within 3 feet (0.9 m) of the patient.

A partial list of the infections for which droplet precautions should be implemented includes:

- Invasive infection with *Haemophilus influenzae* type B
- Invasive infection with *Neisseria meningitidis*
- Streptococcal pharyngitis
- Rubella

Contact Precautions

Contact precautions are used with patients known or suspected to harbor an infection transmitted by direct contact. In addition to Standard Precautions, the following steps are required:

- Gloves must be worn and hands must be washed before and after contact with the patient.
- Health care personnel must wear protective gowns.
- All items that come in contact with the patient must be disinfected or sterilized.

Contagious conditions for which implementation of contact precautions is required include:

- Infection with the herpes simplex virus
- Impetigo
- Noncontained abscesses, cellulitis, or decubitus ulcers
- Disseminated herpes zoster
- Infection with *Clostridium difficile*
- Infection with any multidrug-resistant bacterium

HAZARDOUS WASTE

Definition

The EPA defines medical waste as any solid waste generated in the diagnosis, treatment, or immunization of humans or animals, in research that involves people or animals, or in the production or testing of biologicals. This includes, for example:

- Soiled or blood-soaked bandages
- Culture dishes and other glassware
- Discarded surgical gloves after surgery
- Discarded surgical instruments and scalpels
- Needles used to give shots or draw blood
- Cultures, stocks, and swabs used to inoculate cultures
- Removed body organs (e.g., tonsils, appendices, limbs)

Besides the EPA, the federal agencies associated with the regulation of various aspects of medical waste include the FDA, OSHA, and the Nuclear Regulatory Commission (NRC). Medical waste disposal also is regulated at the state level, and each state has laws that apply specifically to medical waste.

Waste Handling

Infectious waste is separated from all other waste and placed in red biohazard disposal bags. (The common term for medical waste is "red bag" waste.) The biohazard symbol (Figure 15-5) may or may not appear on the bag. The bag color and biohazard symbol are a form of hazard communication to anyone who later handles the waste material. Any person handling infectious waste, from the point of generation until its destruction, must wear PPE (see Chapter 8). Gloves must be worn at all times. Face shields and protective gowns protect the handler from splash hazards.

Guidelines for the handling and disposal of waste in the operating room environment include the following:

- Always wear gloves when handling any object contaminated with blood or body fluids.
- Red waste bags for infectious material must be available during case cleanup.
- Do not place noninfectious waste in red bags. The cost of processing is 10 times higher for infectious waste than for noninfectious waste.
- Place all sharps in an impenetrable sharps container.

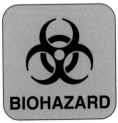

Figure 15-5 Biohazard warning label.

- Do not overload sharps containers. Container overflow is one of the major causes of blood-borne disease transmission among health care workers.
- If it is necessary to examine items in a refuse bag, separate the items carefully by spreading them on an impermeable sheet or drape. Never handle waste material unless you can see what is contained in the refuse bag. Sharps may be present among trash and cause serious injury.
- Handle suction canisters and other blood containers with extreme caution. The practice of opening suction canisters used during surgery and pouring the contents into an open hopper puts workers at extremely high risk for disease transmission. Blood and fluid solidifiers are available. After fluids are solidified, they can be placed in tear-resistant plastic bags.
- Bags must not be loaded beyond their tensile strength. Double bagging may be necessary.
- Separate soiled reusable linen from disposable paper products and unsoiled items at the point of use.
- Keep all contaminated (soiled) or potentially contaminated waste separate from uncontaminated goods.
- Do not compact waste contained in plastic bags. Pack loosely and secure the open end.
- When transporting medical waste, do not use trash chutes or dumbwaiters. Use a transport cart.

A designated area of the operating room is reserved for the disposal of infectious waste. This must be completely separated from restricted and semirestricted areas of the department. Biohazard signs should be posted in areas of waste disposal.

LATEX ALLERGY

Sensitivity and true allergy to latex rubber are risks to both patients and personnel. True allergy is differentiated from other types of immune response. True allergic response, which is mediated by the immune system, was described in Chapter 14. Table 15-4 lists three types of skin reactions.

Allergy and Sensitivity

Latex is a naturally occurring sap obtained from rubber trees. It is used commercially in the manufacture of many products, including medical devices. True allergy is an abnormal immune response to a substance. Previous exposure and sensitization are required for the body to initiate the formation of antibodies against the allergen.

Latex allergy is a local or systemic reaction mediated by the body's immune system. The reaction causes the release of histamines, which occur normally in the body. This causes edema (swelling) and redness. When histamines are released in massive amounts, the reaction can be life-threatening. The extent of the reaction depends on the exact location and nature of the contact. Allergies are a response to proteins within a substance.

Hypersensitivity is a cell-mediated response. It is a type of delayed reaction that causes dermatitis on contact with the object. In the case of latex gloves and medical devices, this reaction generally is related to chemicals in the latex product rather than the latex itself.

Table 15-4

Allergic and Nonallergic Skin Reactions

Type of Reaction	Symptoms/Signs	Cause	Prevention/Management
Contact dermatitis (nonallergic)	Scaling, drying, cracks in skin. Bumps and sores, especially on the dorsal side of the hand, caused by gloves.	Skin irritation caused by gloves, powder, soaps, and detergents. Incomplete rinsing after hand washing and surgical scrub. Incomplete hand drying.	Use alternative products. Rinse hands thoroughly after exposure to detergents and antiseptics. Dry hands completely before donning gloves.
Allergic contact dermatitis (delayed hypersensitivity or allergic contact sensitivity)	Blistering, itching, crusts, similar to a poison ivy reaction. Cracks that occur on hands or arms after skin exposure, caused by gloves.	Chemicals used in latex processing, including accelerators (thiurams, carbamates, and benzothiazoles).	Correctly identify cause. Use gloves that do not contain these chemicals.
Natural rubber latex (NRL) allergy (IgE/histamine mediated) (Type I immediate hypersensitivity)	Hives in the area of contact with NRL. Generalized redness nasal irritation, wheezing, swelling of the mouth, and shortness of breath. Can progress to anaphylactic shock.	Direct contact with or breathing of natural latex proteins, including those contained in glove powder or found in the environment.	Eliminate or drastically reduce exposure to NRL protein. Use nonlatex, powder-free gloves.

Nonallergic dermatitis (skin inflammation) is caused by many irritants found in the operating room environment. Chemicals, antiseptic residue from surgical scrub or hand washing, and glove powder are known to cause irritation in some sensitive individuals.

All health facilities have a latex-safe cart available for patients known to be allergic to latex. The cart contains supplies needed for management of the patient with latex sensitivity. Latex cannot be eliminated from the medical environment completely, but risk reduction is an important factor in preventing injury.

Exposure and Symptoms

Patients and perioperative personnel can be exposed to latex through the skin, circulatory system, respiratory system, and mucous membranes. Gloves and glove powder containing latex molecules are a major concern, but many other medical devices contain latex as well.

Latex can cause skin reactions, including sores, skin cracks, lumps, and itching. Latex can come in contact with the circulatory system through intravenous catheters, tubing, and other intravascular devices. If the latex reaches the bloodstream, large amounts of chemical mediators are released. These can cause severe bronchial obstruction, pulmonary edema, and death.

Individuals at Risk

- People who have had repeated surgeries or frequent contact with medical devices, especially in early childhood.
- Individuals who have a positive reaction to a serum latex antibody test.
- Anyone with a history of asthma or allergies to particular foods.
- Individuals with a history of undiagnosed allergic symptoms after contact with medical devices.

Box 15-4

Common Sources of Latex

Blood pressure cuffs
Blood pressure tubing
Bulb syringe
Catheters, internal and external
Esmarch bandages (used with pneumatic tourniquet)
Gloves, sterile and nonsterile
Intravenous catheters
Medical tape
Needles
Oxygen delivery systems
Pneumatic tourniquet
Rebreathing bag for anesthesia machine
Respiratory tubing and all connectors
Stethoscope
Syringes
Tubing
Urinary drainage systems
Wound drains

Sources of Latex in the Operating Room

The operating room environment has many potential sources of latex. The most common concern among surgical personnel is latex gloves. Most surgical and examination gloves contain latex because of its strength and resilience. However, nonlatex gloves are available. Box 15-4 lists common sources of latex.

Prevention and Risk Reduction

Prevention of latex injury requires identification of those at risk and avoiding contact with devices that contain latex. A supply area containing latex-free devices should be maintained for patients known to be allergic to latex. If the patient is known to be latex sensitive, a warning sticker is placed on the person's chart. The information also is included in the patient information.

Workers who believe they are sensitive or allergic to latex should be tested. The use of low-allergen latex and powder-free gloves is recommended by NIOSH and other organizations concerned with the health risks of latex in the health care setting.

MUSCULOSKELETAL RISKS

CAUSES OF MUSCULOSKELETAL INJURY

Musculoskeletal injury is a risk to all personnel working in the operating room. The lumbosacral area, wrist, shoulder, and neck are particularly vulnerable. The causes of musculoskeletal injury are classified according to the types of movement and the workload involved.

Exertion is the amount of physical effort needed to perform a task, such as moving an object. The amount of exertion required for a task varies with the duration and nature of the task; it also can be modified by changing one's posture or grip.

Posture is a critical component of musculoskeletal stress. Twisting or turning the body disrupts normal balance. Other high-risk positions include bending, kneeling, reaching overhead, and holding a fixed position for a long time.

Repetitive motion places stress on tendons and muscles. Factors that affect the risk are the speed of the movement, the required exertion, and the number of muscles needed to complete the action.

Contact stress is excessive direct pressure against a sharp edge or hard surface. Increasing the pressure increases the risk of damage to nerves, tendons, and blood vessels.

INJURY PREVENTION IN THE ENVIRONMENT

In the operating room, musculoskeletal injuries most often occur as a result of the following:

- Lifting, positioning, transporting, and transferring the patient (see Chapter 10)
- Retrieving and shelving heavy instrument trays overhead or near the floor
- Moving heavy equipment (e.g., the operating table, operating microscope, or video tower)
- Catching items that are falling
- Tripping over tubing or electrical cords
- Balancing a heavy instrument tray in the hand while distributing it onto the sterile field
- Attaching cords to wall sockets or overhead in-line connectors
- Climbing over operating room clutter or trying to retrieve a heavy item from a cluttered environment

Prevention of musculoskeletal injuries involves creating a safe work environment and using good body mechanics.

Clutter

When the surgical suite is crowded with equipment, workers are inclined to shift their weight off balance to move around. Tubing and power cords are added risks. Reducing clutter usually requires better planning. Extra space may not be available for the equipment needed, but clutter can be consolidated. Bring in only what is needed for immediate use. Avoid draping cords over furniture and equipment. Consolidate extra supplies on a designated cart, which can be placed away from traffic areas. Create alternate storage systems.

Supporting the Body

Fatigue and stress affect muscle control, which can lead to injury. Standing and walking for long periods puts extra stress on muscles, tendons, and joints.

Perioperative personnel can reduce muscle fatigue while standing by placing the feet shoulder width apart. If a lift (raised platform) is used, it should accommodate a wide stance. Two lifts may be needed so that the scrubbed technologist is required to step up and down while working between the instrument table and the patient.

Shifting the weight back and forth on a level surface can reduce muscle strain. Standing on one foot for long periods, however, increases stress and puts the body off balance. Elevating the feet during breaks helps increase circulation to the legs.

Support stockings and leggings significantly reduce muscle ache. These can be purchased in medical supply stores. Supportive shoes distribute pressure on the foot to prevent heel spurs and arch problems.

Storage Systems

Heavy items such as large instrument trays must be stored at elbow height, never above the head or at floor level. If they must be stored at floor level, attention to good body mechanics in retrieving these items helps prevent lower back injury. The appropriate way to shelve equipment is to place the heaviest items even with the elbows and smaller items on shelves above and below this height.

Safe Body Mechanics

Developing good body mechanics is a conscious activity. Students and new employees should learn these methods before entering the clinical area for work. If you are injured on the job, obtain medical care as soon as possible.

Lifting

When lifting an object, keep it close to your body. This reduces the force of exertion. Figure 15-6 demonstrates force exerted on the back in various lifting positions. Figure 15-7 illustrates safe and unsafe lifting techniques.

- Always bend at the knees when raising or lowering a heavy object. This takes pressure off the lower back and uses the body's heaviest muscles to do the work. Remember to keep your back straight and legs wide apart with both feet flat on the floor for balance.
- Never lock the knees and bend over to pick up an object (Figure 15-8). This puts stress on the lower back and does not permit use of the thigh muscles to help lift the body.

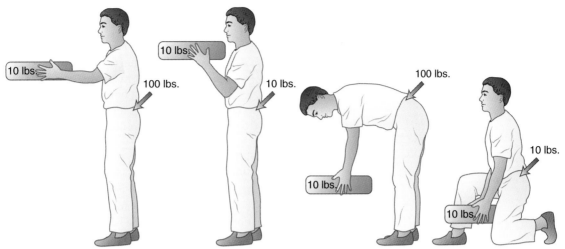

Figure 15-6 Weight on the back in various lifting positions. *(Redrawn from Saunders DH, Saunders R: Evaluation, treatment, and prevention of musculoskeletal disorders, vol 1, ed 3, Chaska, Minn, 1995, Saunders Group.)*

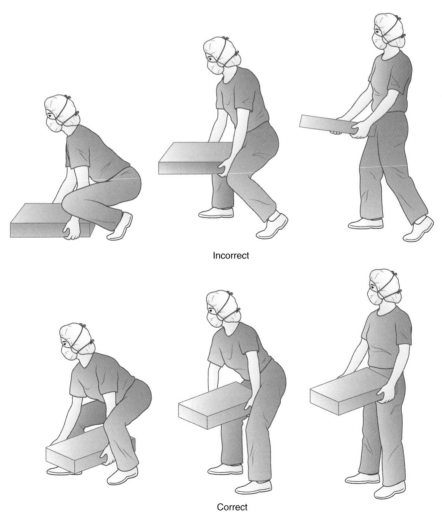

Incorrect

Correct

Figure 15-7 Body mechanics: Correct and incorrect lifting techniques. *(Redrawn from Saunders DH, Saunders R: Evaluation, treatment, and prevention of musculoskeletal disorders, vol 1, ed 3, Chaska, Minn, 1995, Saunders Group.)*

Pushing and Pulling

When pushing a cart ahead of you from a standstill, place one foot behind the other. The back foot should be braced comfortably (Figure 15-9). Use the back foot to push off while transferring your weight to the front foot. Pushing is the preferred method of transporting objects rather than pulling. Make sure you can see any obstacles in your path.

- When pulling a cart toward you, use the same stance as in pushing. Use your front leg to exert backward pull while the back foot maintains balance and support.
- When performing a horizontal transfer (straight across from one surface to another), use abdominal and arm muscles actively. Do not simply lean back and pull.

Bending

- When you must bend or reach upward to connect an electrical outlet or in-line gas connection, never twist your body or balance on one foot (Figure 15-10). This combination not only places the body off balance, it also increases the risk of back injury, because the standing leg is locked in position.

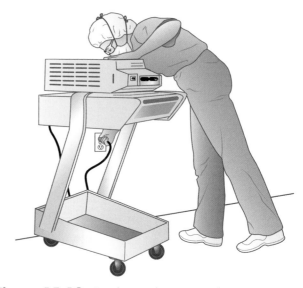

Figure 15-10 Bending and twisting at the same time creates the risk of back injury. Avoid putting weight on one foot, which decreases balance.

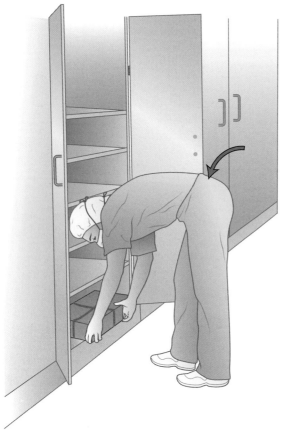

Figure 15-8 Unsafe body mechanics: Locking the knees creates the potential for back injury.

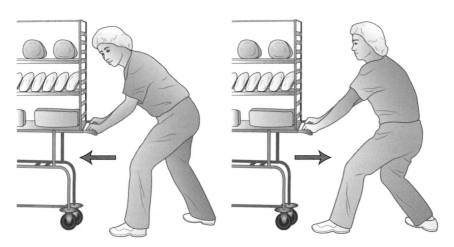

Figure 15-9 Safe methods of pushing and pulling a cart. Note the position of the brace foot.

To lift or transfer a patient, use your abdominal muscles to hold the weight of your upper body. When the abdominal muscles are not engaged in exertion, the back muscles, especially those in the sacral and lumbar region, must support the entire trunk; this is a common cause of back injury. Tighten your abdominal muscles as you lift and notice that your back feels much more supported.

CHAPTER SUMMARY

- The potential for accident and injury in the operating room is one of the highest in the health care setting.
- Management of environmental risks requires a knowledge of the risks, a plan of action, and monitoring.
- Risk is the statistical probability of a harmful event and is defined as the number of harmful events that occur in a given population over a stated period.
- A work culture of safety is critical to injury reduction.
- Fire requires three components: oxygen, fuel, and a source of ignition.
- The operating room is an oxygen-enriched environment that supports combustion and fire.
- As the concentration of oxygen increases in the environment, so do the speed of ignition, duration, and temperature of a fire.
- Medical devices made of flammable materials are common in surgery.
- Any heat-producing device has the potential to cause a fire.
- Sparking can occur when an active electrode comes in contact with metal. Sparks can ignite volatile gases, liquids, drapes, and sponges, especially in the presence of oxygen.
- During a fire, the most important priority is protecting the patient.
- Immediate action during a fire is described by the acronym RACE: **r**escue patients in the immediate area of the fire; **a**lert other people to the fire so that they can assist in patient removal and response; **c**ontain the fire; **e**vacuate personnel in the areas around the fire.
- Compressed gases in steel cylinders are associated with serious accidents and fatalities related to explosion or rupture of the tank.
- A ruptured gas cylinder can become a projectile capable of penetrating walls. Safe handling techniques can prevent rupture.
- The most common source of electrical injury to the surgical patient is the electrosurgical unit (ESU). (Chapter 19 presents a complete discussion of the risks and proper use of electrosurgical equipment.)
- Ionizing radiation used in the operating room and interventional radiology departments can cause tissue damage. The most important method of reducing risk is to prevent exposure by using lead shields, aprons, and other protective devices.
- Magnetic resonance imaging uses radiofrequencies to provide a three-dimensional view of the patient's anatomy. Metal can be drawn into the magnetic field, causing severe injury or death.

- Dangerous chemicals are used in the perioperative environment for disinfection, sterilization, specimen preservation, and preparation of surgical implants.
- All staff members must have access to information about specific chemicals in their work environment. Precautions, hazards, and safety information are contained in the Material Safety Data Sheet (MSDS).
- A smoke plume is created whenever tissue is burned, such as during electrosurgery and laser surgery. Smoke plumes are known to contain toxins and therefore must be removed from the immediate surgical environment.
- Transmission of blood-borne disease organisms is a primary risk to personnel working in the surgical environment.
- The risk of disease transmission is significantly reduced when personnel follow Standard Precautions.
- All patients are considered potential sources of disease transmission. For this reason, Standard Precautions are used at all times and with all patients.
- The most common source of transmission of blood-borne pathogens to health care workers is sharps injuries. To reduce the risk of blood-borne disease transmission by sharps injuries, OSHA has established a set of rules pertaining to their handling and disposal, the *Blood-Borne Pathogen Rule*.
- A neutral zone technique prevents injury from sharps on the surgical field. With this method, no sharps are passed from one person to another by hand. Instead, a no-hands zone is established in which the surgeons and scrub pass and retrieve sharp items.
- Postexposure prophylaxis (PEP) is used after injury with a contaminated instrument. PEP includes a regimen of antiviral drugs and testing for hepatitis B.
- Transmission-based precautions are implemented when a patient is known to have or suspected of having a highly infectious disease and Standard Precautions are insufficient to prevent transmission to others.
- Hazardous waste is specifically defined by the Environmental Protection Agency (EPA). Disposal of medical waste is highly regulated by state laws. Medical personnel must handle medical waste according to facility policies, which are based on state regulation.
- Latex allergy is an immune response to latex rubber and can result in serious injury or death. Previous exposure and sensitization are needed for the body to initiate formation of antibodies to the allergen.
- Many medical and surgical devices contain latex. Prevention of latex injury requires identification of those at risk and avoidance of contact with devices containing latex

- Musculoskeletal injury is a risk to all personnel working in the operating room. The lumbosacral area, wrist, shoulder, and neck are particularly vulnerable.
- The primary causes of musculoskeletal injury are stress, lack of balance, overexertion, and repetitive motion.

- Proper body mechanics prevents musculoskeletal injury. However, staff members often neglect good mechanics because of personnel shortages, rushing, or fatigue.

REVIEW QUESTIONS

1. What is the definition of risk? What is meant by risk management?
2. Why are perioperative personnel likely to ignore safety precautions?
3. Describe the elements of the fire triangle.
4. What characteristics of oxygen make it particularly dangerous in the perioperative environment?
5. What is an endotracheal fire?
6. Define the RACE procedure during a fire.
7. What are the elements of the PASS procedure for use of fire extinguishers?
8. What is the rationale behind Standard Precautions?
9. Why were Standard Precautions developed?
10. Describe postexposure prophylaxis.
11. Define hazardous waste.
12. What is the minimum safe distance from a source of ionizing radiation during radiographs?
13. What is a Material Safety Data Sheet?
14. What is the safest way to lift a heavy object from floor level?
15. How can you protect against musculoskeletal stress when standing for long periods?

CASE STUDIES

1. You are scrubbed on a tonsillectomy. The patient is fully covered by drapes, and the case has started. The surgeon is using electrosurgery to coagulate a bleeding vessel in the throat. Suddenly there is an arc of fire emanating from the patient's throat, igniting the head drape. What are your initial responses as a surgical technologist?
2. In the above case, there is a *mouth gag* (a type of retractor that attaches to the Mayo stand and holds the patient's mouth open) firmly in place. Does this change your response?
3. You have been asked to retrieve a nitrous oxide tank from the store room and bring it to the surgical suite. You load the tank on a transportation cart. While in transit through the hallway, the tank falls to the floor and you suddenly hear a loud hissing sound from the top of the tank. What is your response?
4. You have finished a busy day at work and are passing through one of the hospital wards to see a friend. As you walk past a utility room, you see that a small fire has started near the linen cart. What do you do?
5. After a case in outpatient surgery, you are hurrying to clean up so that you can scrub on the next case. You suddenly cut your hand on a sharp retractor that has been soaking in an instrument basin. You decide not to tell anyone because you are sure there won't be any consequences, and you don't have time to fill out an incident report or go the ER. Two weeks later you regret your decision, and are worried about the incident. You may face disciplinary action for not reporting the injury, but you are extremely worried. What do you think you would do?

REFERENCES

1. ECRI Institute: A clinician's guide to surgical fires: how they occur, how to prevent them, how to put them out. Retrieved June 10, 2008, at http://www.guideline.gov/summary/summary.aspx?ss=15&doc_id=3688&nbr=2914.
2. ECRI 2006.
3. Shuster L, Chinn RYW: Guidelines for preventing the transmission of tuberculosis in health care facilities, *Morbidity and Mortality Weekly Report*. The Centers for Disease Control and Preventions June 6, 2003.

BIBLIOGRAPHY

Association of periOperative Registered Nurses (AORN): Fire safety in perioperative settings, *AORN Journal* 86, Supplement 1, Pages S141-S145 December 2007.

Association of periOperative Registered Nurses (AORN): *Standards recommendations, practices and guidelines,* 2007 edition, Denver, 2007, AORN.

Bruley ME: Surgical fires: perioperative communication is essential to prevent this rare but devastating complication. Retrieved January 4, 2006, at http://qhc.bmjjournals.com/cgi/content/full/13/6/467.

Centers for Disease Control and Prevention (CDC): Bloodborne pathogens in healthcare settings: bloodborne pathogens and needlestick prevention. Retrieved January 15, 2008, at http://www.dcd.gov/ncidod/dhaq/bp.html.

ECRI: A clinician's guide to surgical fires: How they occur, how to prevent them, how to put them out. *Health Devices.* 2003;32(1):5-24.

Graling P: Fighting fire with fire safety, *AORN Journal* 84(4), 2006.

Groah L: Is there a relationship between workplace and patient safety? *AORN Journal* 84(4), 2006.

Joint Commission on Accreditation of Healthcare Organizations. Special report: 2005 Joint Commission National Patient Safety Goals. *Joint Commission Prespectives on Patient Safety.* September 2004. Available online at http://www.jcrinc.com/

Lyczko E: Anesthesia and medical gas systems safety, *AORN Journal* 84(5), 2006.

McCarthy P, Gaucher K: Fire in the OR—developing a fire safety plan, *AORN Journal* 79(3), 2004.

Occupational Safety and Health Administration (OSHA): *Revision to OSHA' s bloodborne pathogens standard: technical background and summary*, April 2001.

Occupational Safety and Health Administration(OSHA): Hazard recognition. Retrieved January 15, 2008, at http://www.osha.gov/SLTC/bloodbornepathogens/recognition.html.

Salmon L: Fire in the OR: Prevention and preparedness. *AORN Journal* (80) 42-54, July 2004.

Smith C. Surgical fires: learn not to burn. *AORN Journal* (80):24-46, July 2004.

CHAPTER 16

Case Planning and Intraoperative Routines

CHAPTER OUTLINE

LEARNING OBJECTIVES

After studying this chapter the reader will be able to:

- Explain the rationale for a sterile setup
- Describe the correct process for performing sponge, needle, instrument, and sharps counts
- Define *timeout*
- Demonstrate the neutral zone (no-hands) technique

- Describe how sponges are managed during surgery
- Demonstrate how to pass instruments
- Describe the methods used to protect the wound during surgery
- Discuss the consequences of losing or mislabeling a specimen
- Identify methods of caring for specimens correctly

TERMINOLOGY

Assignment board: A large, erasable board that lists scheduled surgical cases and assigned personnel. The board is kept in a central location in the restricted area of the surgical department.

Biopsy: Removal of a sample of tissue for pathological analysis.

Bleeder: A bleeding vessel.

Blunt dissection: The technique of separating tissue layers by teasing them apart with a rough sponge dissector.

Case cart: A closed stainless steel transport cart equipped with wheels. The case cart is used to transport instruments and supplies needed for surgery into the operating room and take them to the decontamination area after surgery.

Case planning: The process of organizing the tasks and equipment required for a surgical procedure. Case planning requires the ability to prioritize, organizational skills, and a knowledge of the procedure.

Case setup: A time-related set of procedures in which sterile supplies are distributed and arranged on the sterile table.

Cottonoid sponge: A flat neurosurgical sponge available in numerous small sizes and constructed of compressed synthetic and natural fibers. Sometimes called a *patty.*

Count: A systematic method of accounting for all sponges, needles, instruments, and other items that can be retained in the patient. Counts are performed in all cases in which a possibility of leaving an item in the surgical wound exists.

Culture: A process in which a sample of exudate, pus, or fluid is grown in culture media and analyzed for the presence of infectious microorganisms. If microorganisms colonize the sample, they are examined for type and sensitivity to specific antibiotics. This procedure is called a *culture and sensitivity* (C & S).

Event–related: An activity or process linked with an event. For example a sponge, needle, and instrument count is always taken before the closure of a body cavity during surgery, to ensure that no items are left inside. This is an even-related process.

Free–tie suture: A length of suture material used to tie around a bleeding blood vessel in surgery.

Frozen section: A microscopical slice of frozen anatomical tissue that is evaluated for the presence of abnormal cells. Frozen section analysis is performed during surgery to diagnose malignancy.

Graft: An implant used to replace or augment existing tissue. A graft may be obtained from the patient, another person, animal source, synthetic, or biosynthetic materials.

Implant: A synthetic or metal replacement for an anatomical structure, such as a joint or cranial bone.

Laparotomy sponge: A large padded sponge used in major surgery for absorption and during retraction; also called a *lap tape* or *tape*.

Paralytic ileus: Loss of peristalsis to the bowel as a result of excess handling during surgery.

Radiopaque: Any object that is not penetrable by x-rays. Surgical sponges and radiopaque (detectable on x-ray).

Raytec: A surgical sponge folded to 4 inches by 4 inches. The Raytec, also called a "four by four" derives its name from one of the companies which manufacture surgical sponges.

Sharps: Any objects that can penetrate the skin and have the potential to cause injury and infection; these include but are not limited to needles, scalpels, broken glass, broken capillary tubes, and exposed ends of dental wires.

Sponge dissector: A small compact sponge used to dissect soft tissue planes. The sponge dissector is always mounted on a clamp for use in the surgical wound.

Sponge stick: A Raytec sponge folded and mounted on a sponge forcep for use deep in the body. Raytec sponges are not permitted in or around the surgical wound when a body cavity is open or a sponge could be lost in the wound, unless mounted on an instrument.

Sterile setup: The process of organizing and arranging sterile supplies and equipment before surgery. The setup is performed by the scrubbed surgical technologist.

Surgeon's preference card: A database or card system containing the methods and materials used by each surgeon for specific surgeries. The preference card contains their choice of suture, special equipment and settings, and other information used to prepare the patient and supplies before surgery.

Time–related: An event or activity linked with a specific time or process (e.g., timeout for verification of the patient's identity, correct operative site and side is time-related, occurring just before surgery starts.

Timeout: A procedure for verifying the patient's identity, correct surgical procedure, site, and side. Timeout takes place after the patient has been positioned, prepped, and draped but before the first incision. The procedure is promoted by the AST and described in detail by the AORN and the WHO.

Tonsil sponge: A rounded sponge approximately walnut size, with string attached; used for absorption during tonsillectomy.

INTRODUCTION

The purpose of this chapter is to orient the surgical technologist to the flow of a surgical procedure from the time of preparation to the close of surgery. Many activities require coordination between the scrub, the circulator, and other team members. Table 16-1 presents descriptions of the activities of the scrubbed surgical technologist, circulator and surgeon.

Box 16-1 lists the sequence of events in surgery.

CASE PLANNING

Good case planning is a learned skill that develops with experience. Attention to detail and efficient use of time, energy, and space improve the technologist's ability to perform the tasks required.

Case planning combines knowledge of a surgical procedure and surgical techniques. As students become familiar with procedures, they should start to think strategically about each case. This means analyzing the situation and looking at available resources. The following is an example of how to analyze surgical cases.

Surgical procedures can be classified into five categories. A knowledge of these categories can aid case planning, because different surgical procedures within a specific category require common skills and techniques. The five categories are:

1. Diagnosis
2. Reconstruction
3. Repair
4. Removal
5. Replacement or implantation

DIAGNOSTIC PROCEDURE

The results of a diagnostic procedure provide information about the nature of a medical problem and the options available for treatment. Diagnostic procedures may be performed as a part of surgery or as a separate procedure.

Questions for Planning

- What is the target structure or tissue? What technique will be used to perform the diagnosis (e.g., radiography, biopsy, dye study)?
- What special equipment is needed for the planned technique (e.g., endoscope and accessories, contrast medium, syringes)?
- How will the information be documented (e.g., radiograph, pathologist's report, video record, fluoroscopic image)?
- Is the procedure scheduled to take place in a procedure room or in the operating room (OR)? Has the radiology staff been notified that they will be needed (if the procedure is to take place in the OR)?
- Will the surgeon need other diagnostic films or reports during surgery and are those available in the room?
- What kind of anesthesia will be required?

RECONSTRUCTIVE SURGERY

In surgical reconstruction, tissue is remodeled or replaced for functional or aesthetic reasons. The procedure may be performed in a single operation or may require multiple surgeries. This type of procedure requires specialty instruments. For example, a cranioplasty requires neurological and orthopedic

Table 16-1

Tasks and Duties of the Scrubbed Technologist Circulator, and Surgeon

Scrubbed Technologist	Circulator *Licensed RN responsibility	Surgeon
Before Surgery Receives case cart for surgery or selects individual items needed from instrument and supply rooms. Assembles all items needed for surgery according to surgeon's case information. Orients furniture in the room in accordance with surgery. Opens sterile equipment and instruments using aseptic technique. Protects the sterile equipment from contamination. Performs surgical hand scrub. After scrub, surgical technologist is a "sterile" team member.	Positions the OR table and prepares foam pads and accessories according to the surgery. Assembles needed equipment. Connects suction canisters to ceiling or wall mounts. Tests suction and in-line gas. Keeps the OR doors closed. Obtains radiographs or other diagnostic reports needed during surgery. Opens sterile supplies. *Selects medications and drugs for use during surgery. *Reviews operative checklist. *Witnesses signing of operative or anesthesia permit. *Checks all permits. Notes operative side and surgeon's mark or signature on operative side. Assesses patient's psychosocial condition. *Measures vital signs and performs assessment. *Answers patient's questions about surgery and postoperative care. Transfers patient to OR. Transfers patient to OR bed using safe technique. Applies safety strap over patient. Provides warm blankets for patient.	Greets patient in holding area. Orients patient and family. Answers patient's questions. Ensures that permits are signed and witnessed. Identifies operative side and site. If patient is to be placed in prone position, assists in transfer after anesthesia induction. Patient undergoes induction in supine position and is then turned to prone. Along with surgical assistants, performs surgical hand scrub or may scrub after positioning patient following induction.
Before the First Incision Is Made Gowns and gloves self using aseptic technique. Drapes Mayo stand. Places sterile instrument trays in position on back table. Separates sharps (e.g., scalpel blades, needles) from other equipment to avoid injury during setup. Sorts drapes and surgical gowns in order of use. According to the specific surgery, prepares instruments, sutures, devices, solutions, and medications. Protects the surgical setup from contamination. Performs the initial instrument, sponge, and needle count. Receives medications from circulator using proper technique. When setup is complete, waits *within the sterile field.* Hands each surgeon/assistant a sterile towel to dry hands. Gowns and gloves each sterile team member. Hands individual draping materials to surgeon and assistants. Participates in draping, maintaining sterility. Moves Mayo stand into position. Secures suction tubing and power and light cords to top drape. Hands or drops ends off OR table for attachment to power sources. Hands light handle covers to surgeon.	Secures scrubbed surgical technologist's gown. Secures surgeons' gowns. *Performs the instrument, sponge, and needle count with the scrubbed surgical technologist. *Distributes medications to scrubbed surgical technologist. Prepares nonsterile equipment. *Assists anesthesiologist during anesthesia induction and intubation. *Assists in the correct positioning of the patient for surgery. *Carefully applies grounding pads to the patient for use of electrocautery. *May perform skin preparation. *Completes hook up of suction, power, electrocautery, and light cords to be used. Advocates for patient safety during the procedure.	May perform skin preparation. With assistants, enters OR suite from scrub area. Along with assistants, is gowned and gloved by surgical technologist. With assistants and surgical technologist, drapes patient.

Continued

Table 16-1

Tasks and Duties of the Scrubbed Technologist Circulator and Surgeon—cont'd

Scrubbed Technologist	Circulator *Licensed RN responsibility	Surgeon
From Incision to End of Surgery Places two sponges on incision site. Passes marking pen or scalpel to surgeon. Gives retractors to assistant after skin incision. Participates in all instrument, sponge, and needle counts with circulator. Passes sterile equipment to surgeons and assistants using correct orientation and technique. Listens for direction and anticipates each step of the surgery. Maintains a sterile field, notifying others when aseptic technique is broken. Deposits soiled sponges in designated receptacle. Maintains a safe surgical field by exercising all precautions when electrosurgical devices, lasers, and sharps are in use. Requests additional equipment as needed. Secures intraoperative tissue and fluid specimens provided by the surgeon. Obtains grafts and implants as required by the surgery. Prepares dressings and begins to separate soiled from clean instruments. Participates in final instrument, sponge, and needle count. Notifies surgeon if count is incorrect. If count is incorrect, searches for missing item. Applies sterile dressings as directed by surgeon. Maintains sterility until patient leaves the room. Keeps basic instruments on Mayo stand in case of emergency. Prepares instruments on back table for decontamination.	*Records time of incision on patient record. *Distributes sterile solutions and medications to scrubbed person. Provides additional equipment as needed by the surgical technologist and surgeons. Operates nonsterile equipment. Adjusts lighting. Flash sterilizes instruments as needed. Answers surgeon's pages and relays messages. Anticipates flow of surgery and equipment needs of surgeon and surgical technologist. *Monitors urinary output. Responds to medical emergencies. Directs instrument, sponge, and needle counts at appropriate times. *Labels specimens obtained from the scrubbed person for the pathology department. Wearing gloves, separates sponges and places them in counting area or isolates them in groups of 5 or 10. Maintains safe environment. Keeps doors closed; maintains quiet. Replaces equipment that is unsafe or malfunctions. Assesses the patient's physical status and assists ACP as needed. Near completion of surgery, calls for next patient. Checks on equipment for next procedure. Participates in count. Notifies surgeon if count is incorrect. At completion of surgery, assists in removing drapes and disconnecting hoses and tubing. Suction remains connected until patient leaves the room. Applies tape to dressings and connects nonsterile ends of drainage devices. Removes dispersive electrode pad and assesses site. *Completes intraoperative record. Transfers patient to stretcher. Calls for orderlies to prepare for room turnover. *Accompanies patient and ACP to postoperative recovery unit and gives report to PACU nurse.	Marks incision area or begins skin incision. Performs surgery according to plan and intraoperative events. Directs the surgical team during emergency. If count is incorrect and missing item is not found, takes responsibility for further action (e.g., radiography, reopening of wound) Removes gown and gloves, signs patient care documents, and gives any instructions to RN and ACP. Assists in transferring patient to stretcher.
After the Patient Leaves the Operating Room Separates single-use from reusable items. All soiled disposables are placed in biohazard bags. Linens are also placed in biohazard bags. Aspirates all solutions in closed suction containers. Removes containers from room. Places sharps in secure closed sharps container. Places all contaminated materials in biohazard bags. Removes soiled gown and gloves and places them in biohazard waste bag. Removes mask by handling only strings. Removes face shield without touching bare skin. Puts on nonsterile gloves to transport covered equipment to decontamination area. Follows hospital policy for equipment decontamination. Is responsible for correct destination of instruments and supplies. Assists with proper cleaning of OR suite.	Checks on equipment for next case. May begin to open the next case after the OR suite is cleaned. Receives next patient in the holding area.	Notifies the family of the patient's condition. Dictates the operative report.

ACP, Anesthesia care provider; *OR*, operating room; *PACU*, postanesthesia care unit; *RN*, registered nurse.

Box 16-1

Sequence of Events in Surgery

Routine surgical events follow a sequence that is common to most procedures. Routines are time or event related (or both); that is, a task is performed at a particular time or in a particular sequence or is associated with an event.

Preoperative Sequence

Equipment and supplies for the surgical case are brought into the surgical suite.
1. The scrub and circulator open the case.
2. The patient arrives from the holding area and is transferred to the operating bed.
3. The anesthesia care provider (ACP) and circulating nurse prepare the patient for anesthesia.
4. The patient is positioned for surgery.
5. The scrub performs hand antisepsis or scrub.

Intraoperative Sequence

1. The scrub gowns and gloves and immediately sets up sterile supplies.
2. The first sponge, sharps, and instrument count is performed.
3. General anesthesia is initiated (if applicable).
4. The circulator continues to distribute sterile supplies as needed.
5. The patient is draped.
6. Sterile tables are moved into position.
7. Suction, the electrosurgical unit (ESU), and sponges are secured on the surgical site.
8. A timeout is allowed to verify the correct side and site of the surgery.
9. Surgery is begun and the time noted.
10. The scrubbed technologist anticipates the need for instruments, equipment, and supplies for the surgeons.
11. Counts are performed per protocol.
12. Specimens may be collected at any time.
13. The wound is closed.
14. When the procedure is complete, anesthesia is withdrawn and the time noted.
15. Dressings are applied.
16. Drapes are removed and the dressings secured.
17. The patient is stabilized for transport.

Postoperative Sequence

1. The patient is transferred to the postanesthesia care unit (PACU).
2. Surgical instruments and supplies are sorted and prepared for decontamination.
3. All disposable items are disposed of in designated containers.
4. Documentation is completed and signed off (circulating nurse and scrubbed technologist).
5. Soiled instruments and reusable supplies are transported to the decontamination area.
6. Specimens are documented and transported to a designated area for pick up.
7. The surgical suite is cleaned and decontaminated for the next case.
8. Equipment and furniture are returned to their normal locations.

---

instruments, implants, and possibly tissue cement. A procedure to reconstruct the nose requires plastic surgery and nasal instruments.

Questions for Planning

- What specialty instruments are needed for the surgery?
- What patient position will be used?
- Will grafts be taken? If so, what tissue will be selected?
- Does the procedure require more than one operative site?
- What is the age of the patient? Congenital defects often are corrected during infancy or childhood, and these procedures require pediatric-size instruments.
- Does the reconstruction require external support, such as special dressings, a rigid cast, or traction?
- If implants are to be used, are they available?

REPAIR

The goal of repair is to restore function to a structure, organ, or system Repair can involve any type of tissue. The type of repair and the tissue involved determine what instruments or special equipment is needed.

Questions for Planning

- What will be repaired?
- What special instruments are needed?

- What materials will be used to make the repair (e.g., sutures, plates, synthetic mesh)?
- How will the repair be held in place (e.g., sutures, screws, fibrin glue)?
- Does the patient have recent injuries and movement limitations?
- Will radiographs be required? Many orthopedic cases require radiographic or fluoroscopic imaging.
- Is the repair area particularly vascular (will additional hemostasis be required)?

REMOVAL

Removal may involve tissue, an organ, or a foreign body (e.g., a bullet or debris embedded during trauma).

Questions for Planning

- What will be removed, and what tissue is involved?
- What surgical approach will be used (e.g., abdominal, thoracic)?
- Will a specimen be taken for frozen section analysis (immediate tissue analysis to determine malignancy)?
- Is the wound contaminated? (Many trauma cases require extraction of metal, glass, or wood. In these cases the wound is contaminated, and antibiotic irrigation solutions are used.)

REPLACEMENT OR IMPLANTATION

Tissue replacement involves implantation of an organ or other anatomical structure that has lost function through disease or trauma. An **implant** usually is a metal or synthetic prosthesis or medical device. A *graft* is a an implant derived from the patient or from another person or an animal, or biosynthetic material.

Questions for Planning

- What will be replaced or implanted (e.g., skin, heart valve, joint, pacemaker)?
- What organ system or tissue is involved (e.g., bone, ligament, blood vessel, heart muscle)?
- What is the nature of the implant? Will it require trial sizers?
- If nonfunctioning tissue is to be removed, how will this be done (e.g., dissection, bone cutting, laser)?
- How will the implant be held in place (e.g., sutures, orthopedic devices)?

CASE PREPARATION

ASSIGNMENTS

Surgical cases are assigned to individual staff members before the procedure, at the beginning of the day, or on a rolling basis. A printout of the schedule usually is available to all staff members and is posted in central locations. An **assignment board**, located near the entrance to the restricted area, lists cases and assigned personnel. After receiving the schedule, the surgical technologist plans his or her time and tasks so that instruments and supplies are ready close to the time of surgery.

GATHERING SUPPLIES AND INSTRUMENTS

The method used to gather supplies for a case depends on the system established by the health facility. The case cart method is most commonly used. Wrapped sterile supplies are prepared by the central supply (central processing) department and placed on a stainless steel case cart (see Chapter 8), which is transferred to the surgical department when ready or when called for. Case carts are kept in the substerile area to protect them from contamination.

After the case cart is received in the operating room, the surgical technologist is responsible for completing it by using the surgeon's preference card (see the next section). Selected case carts are kept ready for emergency cases, such as trauma or a cesarean section (C-section). Basic items, such as instrument sets and linen packs, are assembled. Special items can be quickly added shortly before surgery.

SURGEON'S PREFERENCE CARD

Specific instrument sets, equipment, and supplies needed for a procedure are listed on the surgeon's preference card. Before computerized documentation, a card system was maintained for surgeons' preferences. Many facilities still use a card

system, whereas others maintain a computerized database containing each surgeon's particular routines for a specific surgery. The data on file include the following:

- Instrument sets and special instruments required for the case
- Special equipment
- Suture preferences
- Glove and gown size
- Skin prep and draping routine
- Intraoperative drugs, including dose and strength
- Surgeon's individual techniques
- Dressings

OPENING A CASE

PREPARING NONSTERILE EQUIPMENT

The scrub and circulator arrange the furniture in the room in a logical manner to build the sterile field. Nonsterile equipment (e.g., the operating microscope or digital imaging cart) is brought in at this time. After all wrapped supplies have been assembled, they are transported on the case cart to the assigned room.

Preparing the Room

1. Arrange the room furniture so that the head of the OR table is in a proper position to accommodate the surgery (Figure 16-1). The table may require rotation to accommodate large equipment such as a radiograph machine or C-arm fluoroscope. Make sure the OR table is positioned directly under the overhead surgical lights.
2. Arrange the room in a manner that prevents contamination of sterile surfaces by traffic and nonsterile equipment and to prevent clutter.
3. Place furniture so that draped (sterile) tables are no closer than 18 inches (45 cm) to a nonsterile surface.
4. Place clean linen on the OR table and ensure that arm boards and other attachments are available in the room. Secure one end of the patient safety strap to the table.
5. Connect suction tubing to canisters, making sure that the connections are tight. Pretest the suction lines for adequate pressure.
6. Gather diagnostic studies (e.g., radiographs, magnetic resonance imaging [MRI] scans) or other data the surgeon will need during the case.
7. If an anesthesia technician is unavailable, the circulator assembles monitoring equipment and other accessories, such as cardiac leads, airway equipment, compression devices, and warming or cooling blankets.
8. If power equipment is to be used during surgery, the in-line or tank gas sources must be tested and the gauges set according to the manufacturer's recommendations.

OPENING STERILE SUPPLIES

Sterile supplies are opened in sequence from large to small. The basic pack containing towels, drapes, and gowns is centered on the back table and opened using aseptic technique.

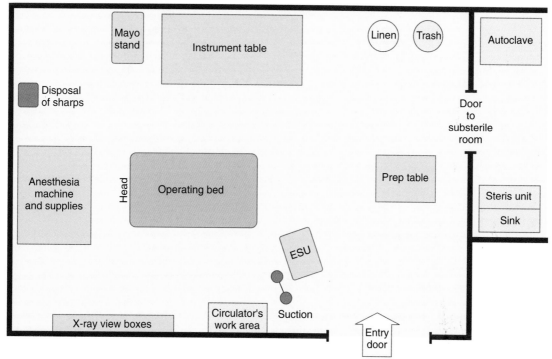

Figure 16-1 Room setup for surgery. *(Modified from Phillips N:* Berry and Kohn's operating room technique, *ed 10, St Louis, 2004, Mosby.)*

As the wrapper is unfolded, the inner sterile surface is exposed. This provides a sterile surface for other items to be distributed. Small items are opened by removing the outer wrapper. The item is then gently but purposefully tossed onto the sterile table. Wrapped basins are opened in the ring stand. Anticipate the need for smaller tables for supplementary instrument trays, drills, and orthopedic components as needed.

Recommendations for Opening a Case

1. Always maintain a safe distance from sterile surfaces to avoid contaminating them, but stand close enough to project the item you are opening accurately.
2. When opening packages sealed with tape, break the tape rather than tearing it. This prevents the outer wrapper from ripping and causing contamination.
3. Packages wrapped in sealed pouches may contain an inner wrapper. Open the outer pouch and distribute the item with its inner wrapper intact.
4. Never unwrap a heavy item while holding it in midair. Instead, place the item on a small table and open the wrapper using aseptic technique.
5. When opening instruments in closed sterilization trays, break the seal and lift the top straight up and away from the tray. Remember that the edges of the tray are not sterile. Do not open any sterile goods into this tray. If the smaller item is contaminated during opening, the whole tray is considered contaminated.
6. When opening sterile goods, place clean wrappers in clean trash receptacles. Do not use kick buckets or biohazard bags for clean waste.
7. Extra sutures, special equipment, and implants should be held unopened until the surgeon asks for them. This prevents waste.

8. Sharps are opened during the setup. The circulator opens the outer package, and the scrubbed technologist removes them and places them in a sharps holder.
9. Open the scrub person's gown and gloves onto a small table or Mayo stand, not on the back table.

STERILE SETUP

After the case has been opened, the surgical technologist or scrub nurse performs the surgical scrub (or hand antisepsis). The person then re-enters the surgical suite *without contaminating the hands or arms* and proceeds to gown and glove.

Immediately after gowning and gloving, the technologist must organize the sterile items on the back table and Mayo stand. This is called the *sterile setup* or *setting up a case.* Students and even experienced surgical technologists in a new specialty can feel overwhelmed by the amount of equipment that must be organized and ready by the time the surgeons arrive to start the case. Using a methodical approach to all setups improves efficiency.

As you first approach the pile of sterile equipment, do not move anything until you have a plan. The following are general guidelines that are efficient and time saving.

Recommendations for Sterile Setup

- **Increase the size of the sterile working area.** Before organizing and preparing supplies, increase the size of the sterile area. Drape the Mayo stand first (Figure 16-2). If you need additional work space, the circulator will provide smaller tables that can be draped. For example, power equipment or other specialty items can be placed on a separate table. If multiple tables are used, they should be placed close to the back table so that a

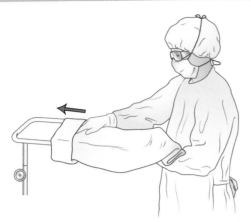

Figure 16-2 *Draping the Mayo stand. (Redrawn from Phillips N: Berry and Kohn's operating room technique, ed 10, St Louis, 2004, Mosby.)*

continuous sterile field is created. This saves steps and motion.

- **Avoid shifting items around from one place to another. Try to handle an item only once.** Shifting items from one location to another without purpose increases the chance of contamination and is not productive. Retrieve the item you need and place it in its final location.

- **Prepare items that are needed at the beginning of the procedure first.**

- **Try to avoid doing several things at once. Think and act strategically.** Perform one task and then proceed to the next. Set your mind to the priority of items as they will be needed in the case.

TIME- AND EVENT–RELATED SUPPLIES

Before you begin to set up any equipment, ask yourself, "What items are needed at the beginning of the case?" Most procedures follow this sequence:

1. Towels are distributed to team members, and they are gowned and gloved.
2. The patient is prepped.
3. The patient is draped.
4. Suction tubing and the electrosurgical pencil are set up.
5. Sterile light handles are attached.
6. Two sponges are placed on the field.
7. The incision is made.

Knowing this sequence, retrieve and prepare the following items in this order:

1. **Towels, gowns, gloves, drapes.** Arrange towels, gowns, and gloves in order of use. Pull the drapes out from the pile and stack them in order of use from the top down. If you plan to place the drapes, gowns, and gloves on the back table, you may have to shift things over to make room. If you do, just move them slightly, but do not start arranging other things.

2. **Light handles, suction tubing, and electrosurgical pencil and holder.** You might place these in a dry instrument basin. They will be placed on the field as soon as the patient is draped.

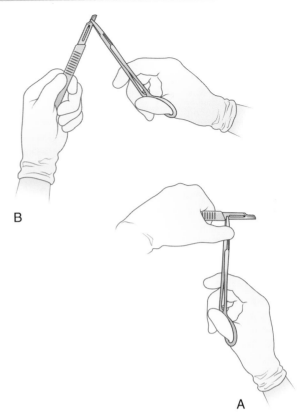

Figure 16-3 **A,** *Mounting the knife blade on the handle. Brace the thumb against the clamp to stabilize it.* **B,** *Removing the knife blade. Always point the blade away from the body.*

3. Knife and basic instruments. These consist of clamps, scissors, shallow retractors, and nonpenetrating towel clamps. Locate knife handles, dissecting scissors, forceps, and retractors. Mount knife blades (Figure 16-3). Place these, along with a few necessary instruments, on the Mayo stand. Place all other sharps together on a magnetic board or in a sharps holder (Figure 16-4).

4. Sponges and sutures. Put all sponges in one location, organized by type, so that you are ready to count when the circulator is free to do so. Place suture packets and other small items together in one or more small basins.

5. You now have all the "priority" equipment you need to start a case. All other equipment can be set up as "secondary preparation." This concept is very important during an emergency, when there may not be time to organize any equipment

SUTURE PREPARATION

The selection of suture material is almost always *prescriptive* (i.e., written on the surgeon's case plan ahead of time). Although many different types of suture materials and needles are available, actual preparation is not difficult. After working in a particular specialty, you will become familiar with the types of sutures used during those procedures. Few people memorize every single suture-needle combination.

- Suture ties (strands) may be needed shortly after the surgery begins. Many scrubs place free ties on the Mayo stand between two towels, under the instruments. This system allows ready access to the ties but also requires instruments to be moved as new suture ties are added.

- Suture reels can remain on the Mayo stand, and individual ties can be removed as needed. An alternative method is to make a "suture book" with towels. Suture ties can be put between sections of a fan-folded towel and placed on the Mayo stand. Each fold can accommodate a different size or type of suture.
- Swaged (atraumatic) needles can be placed in a small basin on the back table until needed.

INSTRUMENTS

You may have up to 10 trays on a complex case. This is why it is important to think about what you need, locate it among

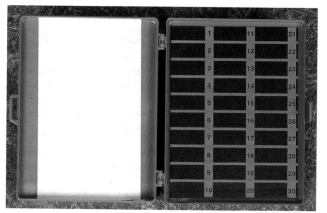

Figure 16-4 Magnetic sharps container with closing lid. *(Courtesy DeRoyal Industries, Powell, Tenn.)*

all the supplies, and then put it in a specific place. If instrument trays must be stacked, place heavier ones on the bottom. Instruments can be arranged on the back table in many ways. Regardless of the method you use, make sure you know each instrument's specific or general location.

MAYO STAND

The Mayo stand is used for instruments and supplies that are needed frequently during surgery. Supplies are exchanged from the back table to the Mayo stand as the case progresses. Many ways and methods can be used to set up the Mayo stand. *The method that works for the individual is the best one.* However, some health facilities use a standardized setup so that personnel taking over at shift changes or breaks know the location of all supplies and instruments. The Mayo stand should be kept neat and orderly. Figure 16-5 shows a classic Mayo setup.

SOLUTIONS AND DRUGS

Irrigation and soaking solutions usually are distributed after the case is underway or just before the case begins. These are distributed into basins in a ring stand, a solution warmer, or a slush basin (Figure 16-6). Medications are distributed into labeled containers on the back table. (The procedure for receiving medications is detailed in Chapter 14)

COMPLETING THE SETUP

Once the Mayo stand and back table have been set up for the start of the case, the remaining supplies can be arranged and

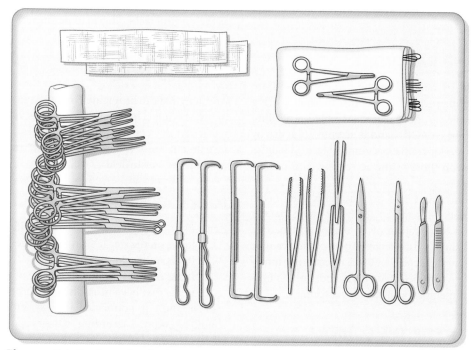

Figure 16-5 Example of a Mayo tray setup. *(Redrawn from Phillips N: Berry and Kohn's operating room technique, ed 10, St Louis, 2004, Mosby.)*

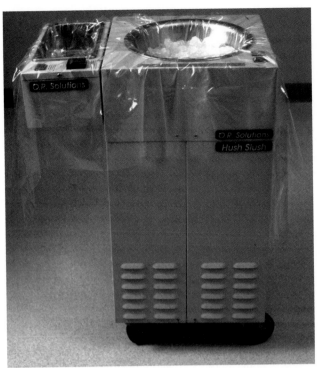

Figure 16-6 Slush basin draped with clear sterile plastic. *(Courtesy DeRoyal Industries, Powell, Tenn.)*

prepared. The sponge, sharps, and instrument count is performed during the setup.

After the setup is complete, instruments and supplies should not be handled, because this increases the risk of contamination. Unless the case is delayed, the technologist should *remain in the room.*

SPONGE, SHARPS, AND INSTRUMENT COUNT

DEFINITION AND RATIONALE

All items that could be retained in the surgical wound are counted in an exact manner before the first incision, during surgery, and before the wound is closed. Accepted procedure for the **count** is published AORN and is accepted practice by surgeons and other perioperative personnel. Health facilities create policies based on those of the accrediting and professional organizations.

The purpose of the count is to prevent items from being retained in the patient. A retained item can cause patient injury from infection, perforation of an organ, obstruction, and scarring. Repeat surgery for a retained item causes trauma, a longer recovery time, and expense. Severe infection or injury may result in death. A retained item is grounds for a negligence charge against members of the surgical team.

RESPONSIBILITY FOR THE COUNT

All team members are responsible for ensuring that no item is left in a patient. The active responsibility lies with the scrub and circulating nurse. It is their responsibility to perform counts and to notify the surgeon when the count is incorrect. Action taken to resolve the count is then the team's responsibility. During surgery the scrub person should know at all times how many sponges, instruments, and other items are inside the patient. The scrub must know the location of counted items on the back table and Mayo stand and is responsible for the handling of items. The scrubbed surgical technologist should be ready for a count at any time during surgery.

WHEN TO PERFORM THE COUNT

A count is performed at the following times:
1. Before surgery begins to establish a baseline count
2. Before closure of a hollow organ
3. Before closure of a body cavity
4. Before skin closure
5. Whenever suspicion of a retained item arises
6. Whenever a permanent change in personnel occurs (e.g., during a shift change or when relief personnel come into a case)

WHO PERFORMS THE COUNT

The count is performed by two people. The professional standard for counts, as published by AORN (Association of periOperative Registered Nurses (AORN): Recommended practices for counts: sponges, sharps, and instruments. In *Standards, recommended practices and guidelines,* 2007 edition, Denver, 2007, AORN(Association of periOperative Registered Nurses (AORN): Recommended practices for counts: sponges, sharps, and instruments. In *Standards, recommended practices and guidelines,* 2007 edition, Denver, 2007, AORN, requires a licensed registered nurse and another health care worker, such as the surgical technologist, to perform the count. One person must be in the scrub role.

COUNTED ITEMS

Any item that can be retained in the surgical wound is included in the count. This includes sponges, sharps, instruments, retraction devices (e.g., umbilical tapes, elastic vessel loops), instrument bolsters, suture reels, and any other small items used on the sterile field.

PROCEDURE FOR THE COUNT

Items usually are counted in the a specific order:
1. Items on the sterile field (i.e., those on or in the patient)
2. Items on the Mayo stand
3. Items on the instrument table
4. Items that have been discarded from the field

The count is performed in a systematic manner. Items should be counted according to their type. For example, count all laparotomy sponges, and then count all Raytec sponges; continue to count all other types of sponges on the field according to their classifications.

Count suture needles, blades, and instruments (and their loose parts) as separate groups. The items being counted should be grouped together and readily accessible for the initial count.

The count is performed systematically and audibly, with the circulator and the scrub person participating equally. The recommended practice for the count is shown in Box 16-2.

DOCUMENTATION

The circulator and scrub are required to sign the count on the patient's operative record. This is a legal document that attests to the outcome of the count. Anyone who performs a count, including relief personnel, must sign their count.

LOST AND RETAINED ITEMS

Loss of sponges, needles, instruments, or other surgical equipment extends anesthesia time, increases the risk to the patient, raises costs, and increases stress on the surgical team.

How Items Are Lost

Sponges can be lost when the following occur:

- A sponge is used inappropriately (i.e., outside of the usual protocol). For example, a Raytec (4 × 4) sponge is not mounted on a clamp for use in a large body cavity).
- The team has not kept track of sponges as they are used.
- The surgical field is cluttered or disorganized.
- The sponge count is performed improperly or not at all.

The scrub must be accountable for sponges *as they are used.* This requires keen attention to the operative site and concentration on what items are in use. Sponges (and instruments) can easily become "lost" in the body cavity of a large patient. Sponges often are found in the folds of drapes, under basins, among preparation sponges, or on the floor under the table. Small needles are lost when they snag on drapes or other linen and spring off the field. Small items, such as instrument parts, can easily drop into the wound.

How to Search for a Lost Item

If the count is incorrect, the surgeon is notified and the count is repeated. If the count is still incorrect, a search is initiated. All trash and waste receptacles are emptied on an impervious drape, and each piece is searched. As each bag is searched, the contents are rebagged systematically. Equipment on the back table must be shifted to allow a search under instrument trays and basins. The floor around the operating table is thoroughly examined, and team members are asked to step away from the field. Sponges often are found between the team member and the table or patient. A rolling magnet is used to search all floor spaces. Team members must show the bottoms of their shoes for inspection, because this is another place where lost needles often are found. Very small needles are not visualized by radiographs or the naked eye.

If a sponge or needle is not found, a radiograph usually is ordered. If the item is lost during closure, the procedure may be halted until the radiograph is read. However, not all retained items are easily seen on a radiograph. If a lost item is

---

Box 16-2

Recommended Practices for Sponge, Sharps, and Instrument Counts

- Each sponge is separated fully from the others in a stack or group and counted audibly.
- Sponges are commercially prepared in packs of 10. However, never assume that a pack contains the designated number of sponges.
- If a package contains an incorrect number of sponges, it should be removed from the field, bagged, and isolated from the rest of the sponges in the operating room.
- All sponges used in a surgical procedure must be radiopaque (detectable by radiographs).
- Never cut a surgical sponge for any reason. Do not use surgical sponges as dressings.
- All counted sponges must remain in the room during the entire procedure. Do not remove any linen or waste from the room until after the last count of the procedure.

Sharps and Small Items

- All sharps should be mounted on an instrument or medical device or contained on a magnetic board or other sharps holder. Sharps should never be loose on the field.
- Sharps counts are performed at the same time and in the same manner as sponge counts: audibly and visually.
- If a sharp breaks during surgery, all parts must be retained and isolated from the surgical field.

- A counted sharp must never be removed from the room until the after the final count.
- Any item that may become lost among equipment or supplies should be kept in a small bowl or container.
- Sharps must be disposed of in a designated sharps container at the close of surgery.

Instruments

- Instruments are counted in a systematic manner; that is, always count instruments in the same order for each count and each case.
- Some hospitals attach a list of instruments and the number of each type to the outer wrapper of the instrument tray. This list is not intended to replace a physical count in surgery.
- During the count, the instruments must be separated. The name of each instrument is stated out loud, and the instrument is counted audibly. Both the circulator and the scrub must see each instrument during the count.
- Additional instruments distributed to the field during surgery must be added to the count.
- No instrument should be removed from the room until the final count is complete.
- If an instrument breaks during a case, all parts must be retained and isolated from the surgical field.

From the Association of periOperative Registered Nurses (AORN): Recommended practices for sponge, sharps, and instrument counts. In *Standards, recommended practices and guidelines,* 2007 edition, Denver, 2007, AORN.

neither found in the room nor revealed on a radiograph, it may still be retained in the wound. In such a case, all layers of the surgical wound may be reopened and searched. If the item still is not recovered, the radiograph may be repeated. An incident report is filed *whether or not* the item is recovered and the count rectified.

Reporting Lost Items

A lost item is reported as a sentinel event (see Chapter 4). This requires documentation on an incident report. In the event of an adverse event related to a retained item, hospital administration and legal services become involved in investigation.

STARTING THE CASE

The patient usually is brought into the surgical suite during the latter part of the setup. The anesthesia care provider and circulator then focus on preparing the patient for anesthesia. (The role of the circulator during these activities is detailed in chapters 10 and 12.) Anesthesia begins only after the surgeon has arrived and is ready to scrub. The surgeon and assistant (or assistants) perform hand antisepsis and enter the surgical suite to be gowned and gloved by the scrubbed technologist.

The circulator performs the patient skin prep at this time. (If the surgeon performs the skin prep, he or she requires regloving.) Draping of the patient follows immediately afterward.

As soon as the drapes are secured, the instrument tables are brought into position (Figure 16-7). The patient now is the center of the surgical field, and all equipment is placed close by.

Suction tubing, the electrosurgical unit (ESU) pencil and holster, light cords, and hoses are secured to the top drape, allowing sufficient slack between the instruments and the edge

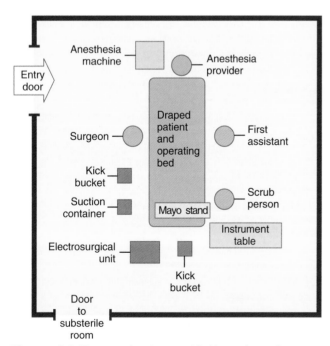

Figure 16-7 Completed surgical field. *(Redrawn from Phillips N: Berry and Kohn's operating room technique, ed 10, St Louis, 2004, Mosby.)*

of the sterile field. After tubing and cords are in place, the ends cannot be brought back up to the field. The technologist places one or two sponges on the field, along with the scalpel or marking pen as needed.

TIMEOUT

Wrong site surgery and wrong surgery occur frequently in the United States. Statistics from the Joint Commission indicate that wrong site surgery accounts for 13.1% of all sentinel events and represents the single largest group of sentinel events reported.[1] The highest incidence of wrong site or wrong surgery occurred in 2007.

In human terms, this represents needless trauma and suffering for many patients. In 2004 the Joint Commission released a universal protocol for preventing wrong site surgery. The protocol establishes a **timeout** period for every surgical procedure to allow verification of information, which helps prevent wrong site surgery and other related events.

Timeout is observed by surgeons, nurses, and surgical technologists, all of whom are responsible for injury prevention and patient safety. Timeout is a team event, with everyone participating. It takes place immediately before the start of surgery and includes the following mandatory steps:

1. Verification that the correct patient is present
2. Verification of the correct side and site
3. Agreement on the procedure to be done
4. Verification of the correct patient position
5. Verification of the availability of correct implants and any special equipment or requirements[2]

Timeout is preceded by the preoperative verification process and by marking of the operative site. Final verification of the site mark is done during timeout. (To view the entire protocol for timeout, see the Joint Commission Web site at http://www.jointcommission.org/SentinelEvents/SentinelEventAlert/)

MANAGING THE SURGICAL FIELD

MAINTAINING AN ORDERLY SETUP

One of the responsibilities of the scrubbed surgical technologist is to maintain a clean and orderly instrument table and sterile field. Paper wrappers and protective caps must be cleared from the setup. Cut suture ends are cleared from the field and placed in a trash receptacle. Small bits of tissue should be removed from the drapes. If the drapes become soaked around the incision, a small impervious drape can be placed over the site.

Instruments should be kept off the patient when not in use. As instruments are passed back from the field, they should be wiped clean to prevent blood and body fluids from drying on the surface. Suction tips are cleared by running small amounts of water through them. An extra suction tip should be available for use while one is being cleared. A metal stylet is used to remove solidified clots that cannot be removed with water. A sterile basin of water is placed near the back table for soaking soiled instruments during surgery.

Try not to overmanage the sterile field. Too much movement and rearranging of instruments can create distraction and increases the risk of contamination.

Remove instruments that are not in use and replace sponges when they become soiled. However, do this with as little movement as possible. When replacing a sponge, pick up the soiled sponge and lay the clean one on the field at the same time. Do not pull sponges out from under instruments or the surgeon's hand; this disrupts concentration and displaces instruments on the field. If instruments begin to pile up out of reach, wait for a pause in the surgery before asking the surgeon or assistant to place them within reach. Do not reach around behind the surgeon to retrieve the instruments.

Surgery requires extreme concentration. If the surgeon asks for an instrument that is already on the field, pick it up and pass it. Do not simply state where it is, unless it is out of your reach.

LIGHTING

Inadequate lighting increases the risk of error. The surgical technologist adjusts lights as needed. Overhead lights produce a small, shadowless beam that spreads peripherally to focus on a large or small area as needed. If the surgeon is working high in the abdominal cavity or low in the pelvis, the light must be lowered vertically and directed horizontally to angle the beam correctly.

SPONGES

Surgical sponges are available in a variety of sizes, shapes, and materials (Figure 16-8). Because of their compatibility with human tissue and their pliability when wet, sponges can become lodged in the surgical wound and become difficult to differentiate from tissue. Therefore every surgical

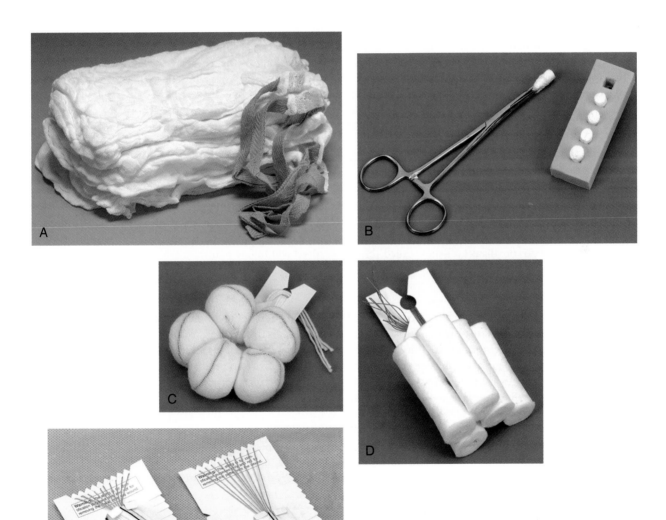

Figure 16-8 Surgical sponges. **A,** Laparotomy sponge. **B,** Small dissector. **C,** Tonsil sponge. **D,** Cotton roll. **E,** Neurosurgical patty. *(Courtesy DeRoyal Industries, Powell, Tenn.)*

sponge is sewn or impregnated with a radiopaque strip that helps identify by x-ray its location in the wound in case it is retained or lost.

4 × 4 (Raytec) Sponge

The 4 × 4 sponge (also called a "four by four" or *Raytec*) is a large square of loosely woven gauze folded into a 4-inch-square pad. When used in a deep incision, the Raytec sponge is always mounted on a sponge forceps, commonly called a *sponge stick.* To mount a 4 × 4 sponge, fold it in equal thirds in one direction and in half in the other direction. Mount the sponge with the folded edge exposed at the tip of the sponge forceps.

❖ *Only mounted 4 × 4 sponges are to be placed on the field when a body cavity is open.*

Laparotomy Sponge

The laparotomy sponge, also called a *lap* or *tape,* is used in major surgery, including procedures in which the abdominal or thoracic cavity is opened, during major orthopedic surgery, and in procedures in which large blood vessels are encountered. Laparotomy sponges are used to absorb blood and fluids and for padding beneath the blades of large retractors. This helps prevent injury from direct contact of the retractor blade.

Lap sponges usually are moistened before use. A basin of warm saline is used for this purpose. The sponge is immersed in saline and then wrung dry.

Sponge Dissector

A sponge dissector (also called a *peanut,* a *pusher,* and various other names) is a small, round or oval sponge covered with gauze. The sponge dissector is always mounted on a clamp and is used to separate or dissect tissue—called blunt dissection.

Round Sponge

A *tonsil sponge,* is covered with gauze and has a string attached for retrieval. This sponge is commonly used in throat surgery and often is used to control bleeding in the tonsillar fossae after tonsillectomy. The string is draped outside the patient's mouth. Use of round sponges without strings is extremely dangerous in throat surgery. Such sponges can easily drop into the trachea and cause complete airway blockage. Asphyxia and death can occur very quickly, especially in pediatric patients. When the round sponge is returned after use, always make sure the string is attached.

Surgical Cotton Balls

The surgical cotton ball is specially manufactured to resist shredding and is commonly used in neurosurgical procedures, especially around fragile brain and spinal cord tissue. Cotton balls may be dipped in normal saline or topical thrombin to aid hemostasis.

Flat Neurosurgical Sponges

The flat sponge, also called a *cottonoid* or *patty,* is a compressed square of synthetic or cotton material with a string attached. Flat sponges are available in many different sizes for use during neurosurgical, ear, and vascular procedures. They usually are offered to the surgeon moistened with saline or topical thrombin rather than dry. The flat sponge is used to maintain hemostasis or as a filter over delicate tissue requiring suction. When flat sponges are exchanged on the field, make sure every sponge is returned intact with the string attached.

MANAGING SPONGES FOR A COUNT

Used laparotomy and Raytec sponges are dropped into the kick bucket. The circulator retrieves the sponges with gloved hands or an instrument and isolates them in a sponge holder or impervious container. Used dissection sponges are retained in their holders on the sterile field. Neurosurgical sponges are placed on a small container or towel on the back table or on a separate prep table near the back table.

Regardless of the type of sponge to be counted, the circulator places used sponges where the scrub can see them so that both can participate in the counts. As additional sponges are needed during surgery, they are counted as soon as the scrub receives them. The circulator adds these to the count on the operative record. When blood loss must be estimated, the circulator may be required to weigh each sponge. The amount of irrigation fluid used is factored into this calculation.

HANDLING AND PASSING INSTRUMENTS

Handling and passing instruments are important tasks of the scrubbed technologist. As with all manual skills, time is needed to develop speed and coordination. As you gain coordination, speed will follow naturally. Do not attempt to increase speed until coordination is secure. Rushing results in dropped instruments, mistakes on the field, and injury. Work at a pace that feels safe and comfortable.

All instruments are passed in their closed (locked) position unless the surgeon requests otherwise. Instruments must be oriented spatially so that the person using the instrument does not have to reposition it or look away from the operative site to receive it. General surgical and medium-weight to heavy instruments are passed firmly. When delicate instruments are passed, they are placed lightly in the surgeon's hand. When a specific instrument is required, the surgeon positions his or her hand as if using the instrument. Some surgeons use specific hand motions to indicate whether forceps, scissors, or suture is needed (Figures 16-9 through 16-14).

Long Instruments

When the surgical wound is deep, replace short instruments on the Mayo stand with longer clamps, dissecting scissors, forceps, needle holders, and sponge clamps. Some instruments are passed with the tips facing downward (e.g., ligation clips and mounted sponge clamps). If you see the surgeon repositioning an instrument each time you pass it, adjust your passing technique to match.

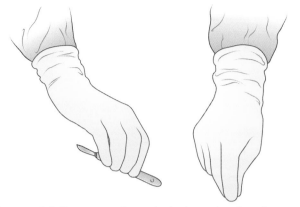

Figure 16-9 Passing the scalpel. The no-hands technique is used whenever possible.

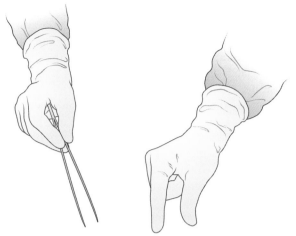

Figure 16-10 Hand signal: forceps.

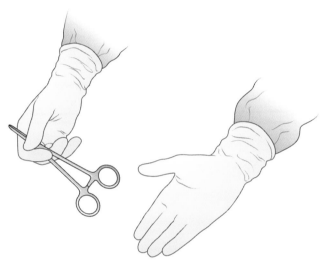

Figure 16-11 Hand signal: clamp.

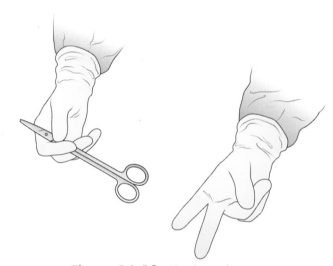

Figure 16-12 Hand signal: scissors.

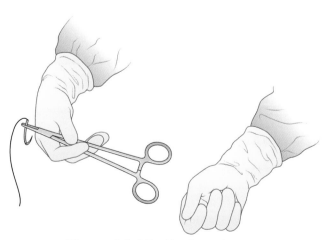

Figure 16-13 Hand signal: suture.

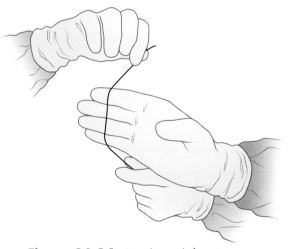

Figure 16-14 Hand signal: free tie suture.

Microsurgical Instruments

When receiving microsurgical instruments, the surgeon does not remove his or her eyes from the microscope. The scrub must place the instrument in the surgeon's hand in exactly the correct position without touching the microscope.

Do not jar the microscope or the surgeon's hand when passing microsurgical instruments; the patient may be injured by an instrument in the surgeon's opposite hand or by sudden movement of the microscope. Jarring the microscope also moves the field of vision. Even a small unexpected movement of the lens can be disturbing for the surgeon and may require repositioning of the microscope.

Because instruments must be oriented according to use, the surgeon rotates the receiving hand into various positions. The technologist must adjust the instrument to complement the hand position. To determine the correct orientation, imagine yourself in the surgeon's place looking through the microscope. For example, if the instrument tip is needed at the 12 o'clock position, the surgeon must reach around the front of the microscope to receive it. If the instrument tip is needed at the 3 o'clock position, it is passed to the side of the focal point. The surgeon indicates the correct position of the instrument by the position of his or her hand.

Do not handle the tips when passing microsurgical instruments. Grasp the middle of the instrument (Figure 16-15, *A*). Bayonet forceps usually are oriented with the middle break of the instrument curved upward (Figure 16-15, *B*).

Sharps

Sharps are any items or instruments that can potentially puncture or cut through tissue. Examples are scalpels, hypodermic needles, cut wire, and suture needles. Glass shards from medicine ampules are also considered as sharps. These are counted separately as part of the sponge, needle, and instrument count. All sharp instruments or small sharps should be passed on the sterile field using the neutral zone (no-hands) technique. If hospital policy or an individual surgeon has not implemented this technique, the scrub must pass sharps in the traditional manner.

In the neutral zone technique, a designated area is established on the surgical field near the surgical wound. The site must be easily accessible to both the scrub and the surgeon. Whenever sharp instruments are exchanged, they are placed in this zone rather than directly into the hands of the team members. The neutral zone can be a magnetic pad with a recessed reservoir or a shallow basin used to receive the instruments. This eliminates hand-to-hand contact (Figure 16-16).

Establishing the practice of neutral zone instrument exchange requires collaboration among all team members. For the technique to be effective, everyone must agree that it is worthwhile, because use of the technique requires changing time-honored practices. The procedure for establishing and using a neutral zone is described in Box 16-3.

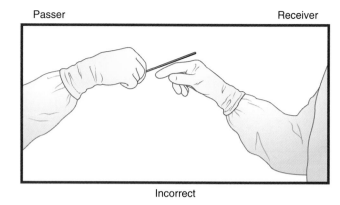

Passer   Receiver

Incorrect

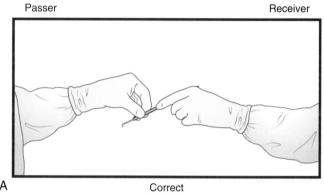

Passer   Receiver

Correct

A

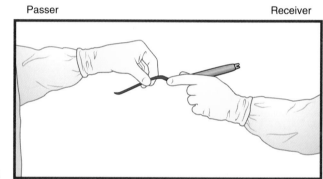

Passer   Receiver

B

Figure 16-15   A, Passing microinstruments. **B,** Bayonet forceps.

Scalpel

If operating room policy has not specified a neutral zone (no-hands) technique, the scrub passes the scalpel (commonly called "the knife") by grasping the handle in the middle with the cutting side of the blade down. Your hand should always be above the handle. The scalpel should not be released until the surgeon has complete control of the handle. The scalpel is returned by placing it on a folded towel or in a small basin. Never leave the knife on the surgical field.

If sharps are passed in the traditional manner, without regard to a neutral zone, extreme caution should be exercised. The surgical scalpel blade is a precision instrument, designed to cut smoothly and easily through tissue. A truly sharp scalpel should glide through tissue with minimal pressure.

The blade of the surgical scalpel loses its "buttery" feel after several passes through tissue, especially through skin and fibrous tissue, such as cartilage and periosteum. Surgeons who

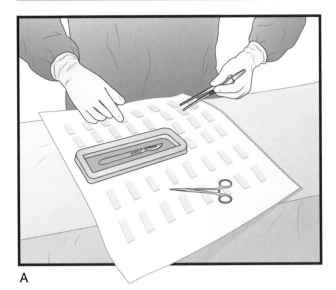

A

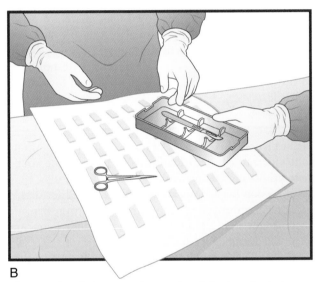

B

Figure 16-16   Neutral zone (hands-free) method of passing sharps. A magnetic pad and square pan for scalpels are placed on the field.

removes it from the wound. Again, always make sure to pass sharp retractors with your hand above the instrument.

Suture Needles

Many needlestick injuries occur during suturing. To prevent injury, pass the needle holder to the surgeon on an exchange basis; that is, when the surgeon returns the needle holder and needle, pass another. Do not use more than two needle sutures on the field at one time unless two surgeons are suturing. If double-armed sutures are used (i.e., sutures with a needle at each end), clamp one needle in the needle holder and the other with a fine forceps to prevent snagging. (Chapter 17 presents a complete discussion of suture handling techniques.)

TISSUE MANAGEMENT

Surgery is by nature traumatizing to tissue. The manner in which the surgical team and postsurgical caregivers manage this traumatized tissue contributes to the success or failure of the surgery. Never forget that tissues are alive, functioning, and very much subject to unintentional physiological and physical injury. Wound management is the process the entire surgical team uses to care for tissues during surgery. A favorable outcome in wound management reflects strict surgical technique.

The tissues within and around the surgical wound are at risk for injury during surgery. The surgical technologist contributes directly to tissue care by:
- Providing correct instrumentation
- Observing tissues for drying and offering irrigation as needed
- Assessing the potential for patient injury from devices and instruments

favor the scalpel over other cutting instruments may need many fresh blades during surgery. The surgical technologist should know this in advance from working with a particular surgeon or from the surgeon's preference card.

Whenever you pass a scalpel with a new blade to the surgeon, you must announce, "New blade." This alerts the surgeon to exactly how much pressure is required to make a cut. There is almost no circumstance in which a dull blade is advantageous. Anticipate when a blade is getting dull and replace it. If you see the surgeon "sawing" through tissue with a scalpel blade, the blade probably is dull (or will be after being used in this manner).

Sharp Retractors

Skin hooks and rakes can easily puncture a glove or sleeve. When passing a sharp retractor, always keep the tips facing downward. Do not grasp the retractor near the sharp end. Remove the retractor from the field as soon as the surgeon

- Preventing incidents that interrupt the flow of the procedure
- Preparing sutures, medications, and irrigation solutions correctly
- Offering wound management assistance and materials at the appropriate time
- Participating directly in a procedure (e.g., tissue retraction) as permitted by hospital policy and state practice codes

PREVENTING TISSUE INJURY

Controllable factors that contribute to tissue injury include the following:

- Excessive bruising from too much handling or rough handling
- Tissue dehydration from heat and exposure to the environment
- Hemorrhage
- Pooling of serous fluid as a result of inflammation and edema
- Unintentional blunt, sharp, or burn injury

Rough or Excessive Handling of Tissues

Rough handling of deep tissues (e.g., bowel, blood vessels) and other delicate structures can cause extensive bruising, tissue swelling, and ischemia. This results in an increased inflammatory response and delayed healing. Gentle handling of tissues and prevention of drying, heating, hemorrhage, and trauma reduce inflammation and lead to faster recovery.

During surgery, tissue must be handled as little as possible. Any physiological stress on the body, including surgery, causes an increased release of catecholamines (e.g., epinephrine). This produces local swelling and fluid accumulation. This stagnant fluid can become a reservoir for microorganisms in the postoperative period. Excessive or rough handling of bowel tissue can cause a sympathetic nerve response called *paralytic ileus,* in which peristalsis ceases, possibly leading to intestinal obstruction.

Irrigation

Tissues must not be allowed to dry out during surgery. Extremely dry tissues cannot withstand handling and may slough during the healing phase. Wound edges, bowel tissue, muscle, and subcutaneous tissue are particularly sensitive to dehydration and bruising. Intermittent irrigation is necessary to protect delicate tissues, or tissues may be covered with a sponge moistened in normal saline.

The technologist offers irrigation fluid when the surgeon asks for it and whenever tissues appear to be dehydrated. Signs of dehydration in internal tissues are dullness, loss of surface elasticity, and tissue fraying. Warm normal saline is used for irrigation. Antibiotic irrigation is used to prevent infection in selected cases.

Solution is distributed to the surgeon with an Asepto or a bulb syringe (Figure 16-17). Two syringes may be required; while one is in use, the other is being filled. Irrigation solution

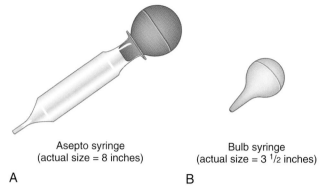

Asepto syringe
(actual size = 8 inches)

Bulb syringe
(actual size = 3 ¹/₂ inches)

A   **B**

Figure 16-17 Wound irrigation. **A,** Asepto syringe. **B,** Bulb syringe for smaller wounds.

is removed from the wound with the suction tip. A perforated suction guard, such as a Poole suction guard, must be used whenever delicate tissues are exposed. This guard is a perforated sleeve that distributes the total suction pressure over many openings and prevents tissue trauma. The surgical technologist must keep track of the amount of irrigation fluid used in the wound so that the estimated blood loss can be calculated.

Retraction

As tissue planes are is dissected or opened, the surgical wound becomes increasingly deep. Retractors are placed at the wound edge to expose underlying tissue.

As the wound gets deeper, anticipate the need for deeper retraction. Sharp-tipped retractors are used only on skin and subcutaneous tissue, almost never in deep tissues. Retractors may be self-retaining or handheld. Examples of large self-retaining retractor are the Balfour retractor (for abdominal surgery) and the Finochietto retractor (thoracic surgery). Smaller self-retaining retractors (e.g., the Weitlaner retractor) are used in the groin.

Occasionally the scrub is asked to retract during surgery. Retraction almost always involves delicate tissues such as internal organs, tendons, muscle, and skin. Nerve damage resulting from excess pressure or inattention to the retractor blade or tip can result in loss of mobility and sensation for the patient. Excess pressure on tissue can cause bruising, local ischemia (loss of blood supply), and necrosis.

Retraction does not require excessive pressure. The blade of the retractor is used as a backstop to prevent tissue from obstructing the open incision. In the proper method of retraction, the surgeon places the retractor, and the surgical technologist then holds it in place without toeing the blade inward unless instructed by the surgeon (Figure 16-18). The blade should be maintained in a constant right-angle position to prevent tissue damage.

Never look away from the wound if you are retracting. You must remain alert to prevent tissue injury. Retraction requires a balance between gentle tissue displacement and minimization of fatigue so that the tissue does not slip back and obscure the surgeon's view.

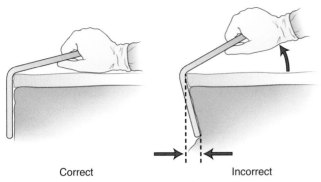

Correct   Incorrect

Figure 16-18 Correct method of retraction to prevent tissue bruising.

MANAGEMENT OF SURGICAL SPECIMENS

RESPONSIBILITY FOR SPECIMENS

During surgery, tissue, fluid, or objects often are removed for pathological analysis. Any item removed from a patient must be registered and submitted for analysis. Critical medical decisions are based on specimen analysis. Every person who handles a specimen is responsible for its protection, preservation, and accurate identification.

Damage to or loss of specimens is a serious concern in patient safety. Mishaps related to specimen loss include incorrect identification, loss of a specimen in the laundry (a result of placing the specimen in a towel), specimens thrown away in the trash, and failure to correctly identify anatomical margins or the tissue of origin. The consequences of such negligence can be devastating. The result may be an incorrect diagnosis, repeat or needless surgery, or delayed treatment for malignancy.

The scrub is directly responsible for receiving and handling specimens on the surgical field. It is the scrub's duty to correctly identify, with the surgeon, the tissue of origin, the orientation of margins for malignancy, and the correct side (right or left). This information is communicated to the circulating nurse at the time of removal.

In addition to medical accountability for specimens, a legal responsibility exists. The serious consequences of loss of or damage to specimens can rapidly result in litigation. Each person handling the specimen is part of the chain of custody and liable for errors.

Recommendations

1. The surgeon may place a suture in the specimen to indicate the anatomical margins of the tissue. Never remove any suture material from a specimen.
2. When multiple specimens are anticipated, the scrubbed surgical technologist must be prepared to identify each specimen separately. The scrubbed surgical technologist is responsible for correctly identifying each specimen. Follow a protocol of "write down, read back" to prevent errors.
3. Never remove a specimen from the sterile field without the surgeon's specific permission to do so.

4. *Do not use sponges* to wrap a specimen. Instead, use a moist Teflon pad to protect a bone or tissue specimen. Place the specimen in a conspicuous protected area until it can be passed to the circulator.
5. Maintain the specimen in a condition conducive to pathological examination per the facility's protocol. The surgical technologist is expected to know these protocols.
6. Never discard any tissue.
7. Do not use bone clamps, hemostats, or other crushing instruments on specimens, because this can destroy cells.

RECEIVING SPECIMENS FROM THE STERILE FIELD

Specimens obtained during surgery are identified by the surgeon and then passed off to the scrubbed technologist or nurse. The circulator receives the specimen in a designated container. Containers should be prepared ahead of time.

- Specimens are received and immediately placed in the appropriate container.
- Communication and documentation of the precise tissue origin (and side, if applicable) are completed immediately.
- The specimen is contained in a specific medium according to institutional protocol. The circulator is expected to know these protocols for protection of the specimen.
- When a specimen is handed off the field, the surgeon identifies the origin, side, and site. The scrub or nurse repeats the information back to the surgeon to ensure that it is correct.

Identification of Specimens

Identification of specimens is a critical aspect of surgery. Each specimen must be identified with the following information:

1. Identification of the patient with two distinct identifiers (the patient's name and one other, such as the individual's hospital number)
2. Type of tissue
3. Origin (site) of the specimen (e.g., right breast, left leg, left tonsil)
4. Clinical diagnosis and other clinical information
5. Any special markings and their significance (e.g., suture at 1 o'clock)
6. Other registration information, date and time of removal, surgeon's name

Specimen Types

Tissue Biopsy

Biopsy is the removal of tissue or cells for analysis by a pathologist. Microscopic analysis results in a definitive diagnosis, such as malignancy, or is used to determine the nature of an abnormality. The surgeon performs a biopsy during endoscopic or guided imagery surgery or as part of an open procedure. Tissue usually is contained and submitted in saline or a fixative solution unless the surgeon specifies another method.

Several types of tissue biopsy can be done:

- *Excisional (incisional) biopsy* is used when a large, deep section of tissue is required for analysis.
- *Fine-needle aspiration (FNA)* uses a long, fine needle to aspirate (suction) small pieces of tissue from a tumor.
- *Needle biopsy* is similar to FNA, but a large-bore, hollow trocar or needle is used to collect tissue. The needle is inserted into an organ, such as the liver, and tissue is removed for analysis.
- *Brush biopsy* is performed during flexible endoscopic procedures. A fine brush is used to collect cells on the surface of mucous membrane tissue.

Fluids

Body fluids, such as urine and blood, are usually obtained in the outpatient setting. Fluids occasionally are collected during surgery. For example, cord blood obtained during a cesarean section is submitted for analysis. Free fluid in a body cavity may also be sent for microscopic analysis. During surgery, fluid can be collected through a syringe and then transferred to a sterile tube or collection vial.

Stones

Stones are removed from the urinary tract, salivary ducts, and gallbladder. Stones are submitted in a dry container.

Foreign Body

A *foreign body* is a nontissue item obtained from the patient's body. Some specimens, such as bullets and knife blades, are critical as forensic evidence and may be used for legal purposes. A retained item from a previous surgery has obvious legal importance. Other items, such as implants and fragments of metal, glass, wood, or any other foreign material, also are retained as specimens. All foreign bodies are submitted dry unless the surgeon requests another method.

Items that may be part of forensic evidence may be handed over to the police for analysis. All items must be registered according to hospital policy pertaining to forensic evidence. No specimen can be released without specific documentation issued by the hospital.

Amputated Limb

After an amputation, the surgeon passes the limb to the scrub to pass off the field. In all cases the patient must be protected from witnessing this procedure. The limb can be wrapped in a paper drape and placed in a protected location on the back table until the circulator is prepared to receive it from the scrub. It is then wrapped in plastic or according to hospital policy. Final disposition of the limb depends on the patient's wishes. The limb may be sent on to the mortuary and retained until the patient's death. Initially the limb must be registered and sent for analysis like other specimens. Special disposition is noted in the patient's record and documents accompanying the specimen.

Frozen Section

In surgical cases that require analysis of tissue for cancer, immediate examination of the tissue may be needed. Surgery may be extended according to the results of the analysis. This immediate analysis is accomplished by freezing the tissue and then making fine sectional slices that can be examined microscopically. The process is called **frozen section**.

Frozen section analysis is usually schedule ahead of the surgery to ensure that the pathologist is available for consultation. Often the orientation of the specimen in relation to the wound margins must be identified. This is done with fine sutures placed in strategic locations around the specimen. A suture should never be cut or removed from a specimen.

The specimen is passed to the scrub, who immediately hands it off the field to the circulating nurse. Frozen section specimens are kept moist but not wet. After the pathologist is consulted, additional specimens may be required to ensure that no abnormal cells exist at the wound margins.

Cultures

Tissue or fluid suspected of being infected is cultured. In this process, a small sample is collected from the wound and sent for **culture** and sensitivity (described in chapters 8 and 20). Suspected infection is treated immediately until the confirmed diagnosis is returned.

Sampling is performed with a culture tube, dry container, or liquid medium. A culture tube contains one or two cotton-tipped swabs, which are swiped across the suspect tissue and replaced in the tube. Some culture tubes contain a preservative at the bottom, which is released when the tube is squeezed.

Two types of bacterial cultures are commonly taken during surgery: aerobic and anaerobic bacterial specimens are cultured. These are discussed in Chapter 8. Each requires a designated type of transfer tube. Take care not to contaminate the outside of the tube.

Cultures should be removed from the sterile field immediately after collection and sent for analysis. Special con-tainers for anaerobic specimens are available from the laboratory, and these should be used for the appropriate type specimen.

Table 16-2 lists common specimen locations and types of tissue obtained.

WOUND CLOSURE

When the surgical procedure is complete, the wound is irrigated and closed. The surgical technologist begins preparing sutures for closure before they are needed. This usually occurs toward the end of surgery, before irrigation.

Before closure, all excess instruments are removed from the operative site. A clean surgical towel can be placed at the wound edge to prevent any tissue debris on the drapes from re-entering the wound. Closure materials are placed on the Mayo stand, along with suture scissors and clean sponges.

Table 16-2

Important Specimens from Various Sites and Types of Infections

Site/Type of Infection	TYPE OF SPECIMEN			
	Fluid	Tissue	Swab	Other
Urinary Tract				
Bladder	Urine			
Kidney	Urine	Renal biopsy		
Intestine			Rectal swab	Feces
Mouth	Washings			
Liver		Liver biopsy		
Biliary tract	Bile			
Abdomen	Pus			
	Peritoneal aspirate			
	Ascitic fluid			
Respiratory Tract				
Nose			Nasal swab	
Ear			Ear swab	
Eye			Eye swab	
Nasopharynx, throat	Washings			
Lung	Sputum			
	Alveolar lavage			
Pleural space	Pleural fluid	Lung biopsy		
Central Nervous System				
Meninges encephalitis (herpes)	Cerebrospinal fluid (CSF)	Brain biopsy		
Brain abscess	Pus; CSF			
Genital Tract				
Urethra			Urethral swab	Direct microscopy and culture in clinic
Vagina			Vaginal swab	
Cervix			Cervical swab	
Endometrium		Endometrial biopsy		
Skin and Soft Tissue				
Skin	Vesicle fluid	Skin biopsy	Skin swab	
Wound	Pus	Scrapings	Wound swab	
Bone and Joint				
Osteomyelitis	Pus	Bone		
Joint	Aspirate			
Septicemia	Blood			
Endocarditis	Blood	Heart valve		

From Mims C et al: *Medical microbiology*, ed 2, London, 1998, Mosby.

Drains and drain tubing are also prepared at this time. The wound then is closed according to the surgeon's protocol. Dressings are not brought to the Mayo stand until the superficial wound layers have been closed and the final sponge counts have been completed.

When closure is complete, the wound site is cleansed with moist sponges, and the dressings are applied. These are held in place manually while drapes are removed. Dressings are secured and other wound materials are applied, depending on the procedure performed. The patient is covered with warm blankets and stabilized for transfer to the postanesthesia care unit (PACU).

All surgical instruments and supplies are sorted and assembled for transfer to the decontamination area.

CHAPTER SUMMARY

- Case planning is preparing for a surgical case. Planning requires a knowledge of the procedure, the equipment needed, the surgeon's preferences, and specific patient needs.
- The surgeon's preference card is a computer-generated document or card that describes the specific instruments, sutures, drugs, and special techniques used by a particular surgeon. It is used during case preparation to ensure that all needed supplies are on hand at the time of surgery.
- Sterile supplies selected or picked for a surgical case are transported on a cart to the assigned room.
- A case is "opened" after nonsterile operating room equipment has been arranged in a logical manner.
- Sterile supplies and instruments are opened in a way that protects them from contamination.
- The sterile set up is performed by the scrubbed technologist or nurse. Equipment, instruments, and supplies are organized and prepared for surgery during the setup.
- All items that might be retained in the surgical wound are counted using the accepted protocol.
- All team members are responsible for an accurate count. However, the count is performed by the scrub and circulator, and it is their duty to perform the count in the prescribed manner.
- The scrub must keep track of all counted items throughout a surgical procedure. The scrub must know what kind of and how many items are inside the patient at any point during the procedure.
- Counted items can become "lost" when established protocols for their handling and use are not followed. This may be due to adverse events during surgery or negligence.
- If a counted item remains unaccounted for, the incident is reported to the surgeon. An incident report is filed with the health care institution regardless of whether the item is found.
- Many thousands of patients are injured each year in incidents involving the wrong side, wrong surgery, or wrong patient. To reduce the number of injured patients, a timeout is performed before the procedure begins. This protocol involves everyone on the surgical team.
- During the timeout, the identity of the patient and the side, site, and intended procedure are verified with legal documentation that accompanies each patient to the operating room. If any discrepancy is noted, surgery is halted.
- The scrub is responsible for maintaining a safe, organized surgical field.
- Surgical sponges are used in all procedures involving an incision. They are used mainly for hemostasis and tissue dissection. All sponges are impregnated with a radiopaque strip so that they can be seen on radiographs.
- Small dissecting sponges are used only when mounted on a clamp to prevent loss of the sponge in the surgical wound.
- The scrub is responsible for handing the correct instrument at the right time during surgery. Instruments are kept clean of tissue debris and blood and protected from damage.
- Instruments are passed using accepted methods that allow the surgeon to remain focused on the surgical wound while receiving an instrument.
- Sharp items are passed to the surgical field using a hands-free zone. This is a basin or magnetic pad close to the surgical wound on which sharp instruments are placed.
- Any tissue or item removed from the patient's body during surgery is a specimen. Specimens are maintained in a specific way on the surgical field to prevent loss of or damage to them.
- Surgical specimens are often used to determine the boundary of malignancy in the body. Markers are used to orient the specimen with regard to its anatomical position in the body.
- Care of specimens on the sterile field is the responsibility of the scrub. Errors in handling or identification can have devastating repercussions.
- Thorough documentation accompanies all specimens for pathological analysis. To prevent errors, specimen containers are labeled before receiving the tissue.

REVIEW QUESTIONS

1. What do you think is the most difficult part of setting up a surgical case? How do you intend to improve this process for yourself?
2. What is the rationale for opening large, heavy items first when preparing for a surgical case?
3. During the surgical case setup, there often seems to be insufficient space to place items on the sterile table. What strategies will you use to solve this problem?
4. What is the rationale for handling sterile items as little as possible during the setup?
5. What is the rationale for surgical counts?
6. Who can perform a count?
7. When are counts performed?
8. Who is legally responsible for the surgical count?
9. What is the rationale for a hands-free technique when handling sharps?
10. What are the specific responsibilities of the scrubbed surgical technologist in handling tissue specimens?
11. Discuss the consequences of (a) losing a specimen; (b) misidentifying a specimen.

REFERENCE

1. Joint Commission: Sentinel event statistics: March 31, 2008. Retrieved June 10, 2008, at http://www.jointcommission.org/SentinelEvents/Statistics/.
2. Joint Commission: Universal protocol for preventing wrong site, wrong procedure, wrong person surgery. Retrieved June 16, 2008, at http://www.jointcommission.org/PatientSafety/UniversalProtocol/.

BIBLIOGRAPHY

Association of periOperative Registered Nurses (AORN): Guidance statements for sharps injury prevention in the perioperative setting. In *Standards, recommended practices and guidelines,* 2007 edition, Denver, 2007, AORN.

Association of periOperative Registered Nurses (AORN): Recommended practices for specimen care and handling. In *Standards, recommended practices and guidelines,* 2007 edition, Denver, 2007, AORN.

Association of periOperative Registered Nurses (AORN): Recommended practices for counts: sponges, sharps, and instruments. In *Standards, recommended practices and guidelines,* 2007 edition, Denver, 2007, AORN.

Phillips N: *Berry and Kohn's operating room technique,* St Louis, 2007, Mosby.

Watson D: Improving specimen practices to reduce errors, *AORN Journal* 82:6, 2005.

CHAPTER 17

The Surgical Wound

CHAPTER OUTLINE

LEARNING OBJECTIVES

After studying this chapter the reader will be able to:
- Describe surgical methods of hemostasis
- Discuss the structure and properties of suture
- Describe the sizing system used for sutures
- Identify surgical needles by their shape and type of point
- Identify safety precautions to prevent needlestick injuries during suture use

- Discuss types of dressings and the circumstances in which they are used
- Describe common wound drains and the circumstances in which they are used
- Explain the process of healing
- Discuss postoperative wound complications

TERMINOLOGY

Absorbable suture: Suture material that is broken down and digested by the tissues. It is then absorbed by the body.

Adhesion: Scar formation, particularly of the abdominal viscera.

Anastomosis: The surgical creation of an opening between two blood vessels, hollow organs, or ducts.

Approximate: To bring tissue together by sutures or other means.

Autotransfusion (blood salvaging): A method of retrieving blood lost at the operative site, reprocessing it and infusing it back to the patient. There are many different types of devices available. The most well known commercial device is called a *Cell Saver.*

Bioactivity: In describing suture use, the way the body reacts to the presence of the suture material.

Blunt needle: A curved, tapered needle with a blunt point that is used for highly vascular organs, such as the liver.

Bolsters: Tubing through which retention sutures are threaded to prevent them from cutting into the patient's skin.

Bone wax: A pliable, waxy dough made from synthetic material used to control capillary bleeding on the surface of bone.

Brown and Sharp (B & S) sizing system: A sizing standard used to measure the diameter of wire or stainless steel.

Capillary action: The ability of suture material to absorb fluid.

Chromic salt: A chemical used to treat surgical gut to make it resistant to absorption by tissue.

Collagen: The protein matrix of connective tissue.

Continuous suture: A technique of suturing in which one long strand of suture is used to sew tissue edges together, with no interruption or separate knots.

Contracture: Tissue that heals without scar formation, causing limited mobility.

Control-release: A suture-needle combination designed to release the suture easily.

Cutting needle: A suture needle with a cutting edge along one side of the shaft. The conventional cutting needle has a cutting edge on the outside curve.

Debridement: Chemical or mechanical removal of necrotic tissue after infection or trauma.

Dehiscence: Separation of the layers of a surgical wound.

Detachable needle: A specialty suture-needle combination in which the suture can be quickly disengaged from the needle by pulling it straight back and away from the swage.

Double-armed suture: Suture-needle combination that contains a needle at each end of the suture; it is used to join circular or tubular structures.

Esmarch bandage: A 2 to 4 inch wide rubber bandage wrapped around a limb to sequentially push blood away (exsanguinate) from the limb (toward the heart) just before the tourniquet is tightened. The tourniquet keeps blood from flowing back into the limb and provides a bloodless field during surgery. The tourniquet is released after surgery is completed.

Evisceration: The protrusion of abdominal viscera through a wound or surgical incision.

Fistula: A complication of wound infection in which one or more hollow, skin-lined tracts form at the wound site and continue to drain pus and fluid. This prevents the wound from healing.

Hematoma: A blood-filled space in tissue, the result of a bleeding vessel.

Hemostatic (vessel) clip: A fine V-shaped clip made of stainless steel, titanium, biosynthetic material or suture material, used to occlude a bleeding vessel.

Inert: Causing little or no reaction in tissue or with other materials.

Interrupted sutures: A technique of bringing tissue together by placing individual sutures close together.

Keloid: Excessive scar formation, which can result in a cosmetic or functional defect.

Ligate: A loop or tie placed around a blood vessel or duct.

Memory: In suture material, the tendency of suture to recoil to its original shape during packaging.

Monofilament suture: Extruded suture of a single fiber.

Multifilament suture: Braided or twisted suture.

Nonabsorbable sutures: Suture materials that resist breakdown in the body.

Occlusive dressing: Wound dressing which prevents air, moisture, and contaminants from entering the tissues.

Plain catgut: A suture made from animal protein which is quickly absorbable in tissue.

Pliability: The flexibility of a suture material.

Primary intention (wound healing): The healing process after a clean surgical repair.

Purse-string: A suturing technique in which a continuous strand is passed in and out of the circumference of a lumen and then is pulled tight, like a drawstring.

Resection: A surgical technique in which a portion of tissue or an organ is removed and rejoined in another configuration.

Retention sutures: Heavy, nonabsorbable sutures that are placed behind the skin sutures and through all tissue layers to give added strength to the closure. Also called a *secondary suture line*.

Reverse cutting needle: A curved surgical needle with three honed edges, one on the outside curve of the needle.

Running suture: A method of suturing that uses one continuous suture strand for tissue approximation.

Scar: The formation of permanent connective tissue at the site of tissue trauma.

Secondary intention (wound healing): Natural healing of a wound without sutures or other means of approximating tissue.

Serosanguinous fluid: Exudate or discharge containing serum and blood.

Spatula needle: A side cutting suture needle with flat top and bottom, used in ophthalmic surgery.

Stent dressing: A specialty dressing used on skin grafts to maintain contact between the graft and wound base.

Stitch: Term commonly used by surgeons when requesting a suture.

Subcuticular (buried) suture: A technique of suturing tissue edges in which the needle enters the dermis from the edges from side to side of the wound. No sutures are visible from the skin surface and there is little or no scarring.

Swage: The area of an atraumatic suture where the suture strand is fused to the needle. Also called an atraumatic suture.

Taper cut needle: A suture needle with a reverse cutting edge at the tip and a round body. Taper cut needles are used for suturing dense fibrous connective tissue, such as the fascia, tendon, and periosteum.

Tapered needle: A suture needle that has a round body that tapers to a sharp point. It punctures tissue, making an opening for the body of the needle to follow.

Tensile strength: The amount of force or stress a suture can withstand without breaking.

Third intention (wound healing): Delayed primary wound closure. Routine wound closure after a period of healing.

Throw: A loop that forms a knot.

Tie on a passer: A strand of suture material attached to the tip of an instrument.

Tissue bank: A repository located in the community and/or in the health facility where donor tissue is registered, processed, and stored.

Tissue drag: A characteristic of some suture material that results in friction between the suture and the tissue.

Topical hemostatic agent: A substance applied to bleeding arising from the surface of tissue to enhance rapid coagulation (e.g., topical gelatin sponge applied on area of capillary bleeding on the spleen).

Tourniquet time: The amount of time a tourniquet may be safely left in place (tightened) during surgery. The time depends on the patient's condition, location, and type of tourniquet.

Water-sealed drainage system: A wound drainage system used to pull fluid or air from the thoracic cavity after thoracic surgery or trauma to the thorax.

INTRODUCTION

Management of the surgical wound is a team responsibility that involves many different skills. From the time the incision is made until healing is complete, many steps are required to produce in a successful surgical outcome. These include hemostasis, suturing and other forms of tissue approximation, use of implants, wound drainage, and dressings. This chapter covers these topics as they apply to the intraoperative period. The process of wound healing and complications are included for a holistic understanding of wound management.

Successful wound management is based on a few essential principles:

1. Handling the tissues gently
2. Controlling bleeding as efficiently as possible
3. Using the correct instruments and sutures for the tissue

4. Careful but efficient use of time to minimize tissue exposure
5. Meticulous aseptic technique to prevent infection

HEMOSTASIS

One of the most important goals during surgery is to maintain hemostasis. In technical terms, *hemostasis* means controlling bleeding with sutures, surgical instruments, thermal energy (e.g., electrosurgery), and drugs. In physiological terms, it means conserving the body's total blood volume, which is necessary for life. Bleeding is controlled in the surgical wound to control infection and promote healing. Blood can be a barrier to healing, because it forms a physical barrier between tissue edges. Uncontrolled oozing or insecure hemostasis can lead to a hematoma. This is a collection of blood that may become a source of infection. In addition, a large hematoma can impinge on regional nerves and vessels.

PROCESS OF COAGULATION

The body's natural coagulation process takes place through a series, or "cascade," of events, each triggered by the one preceding it. The mechanism begins when a blood vessel is injured. The subsequent events are:

1. *Vasospasm occurs.* The blood vessel retracts and constricts. This reduces blood flow through the vessel.
2. *A platelet plug forms.* Platelets aggregate in the area and form a plug. The presence of platelets initiates the release of coagulation factors in the plasma.
3. *Coagulation begins.* A meshwork of fibrin strands forms around the blood cells, creating a clot. This process is initiated by coagulation *factors* (organic substances present in the blood) (Box 17-1). Coagulation is activated by two pathways, the e*xtrinsic pathway* and the *intrinsic pathway.* The intrinsic pathway is activated by factors present in the blood. The extrinsic pathway occurs in the tissues.

Box 17-1
Coagulation Factors

Factor	Nomenclature
I	Fibrinogen
II	Prothrombin
III	Thromboplastin, thrombokinase
Factor IV*	—
V	Proaccelerin, labile factor
Factor VI*	—
VII	Serum prothrombin conversion accelerator (SPCA)
VIII	Antihemophilic globulin (AGH)
IX	Plasma thromboplastin component
X	Christmas factor
XI	Stuart factor
XII	Hageman factor
XIII	Fibrin-stabilizing factor

*Factors IV and VI are now obsolete.

Coagulation involves many chemicals that interact in an elaborate feedback mechanism. If any of the factors are missing, through genetic anomaly or disease, hemostasis is altered. Naturally, in severe trauma hemorrhage may overwhelm the body's natural mechanisms for controlling bleeding. Therefore surgical hemostasis is needed.

HEMOSTATIC DRUGS AND AGENTS

Topical Thrombin USP

Topical thrombin USP (United States Pharmacopoeia) is commercially prepared as a dry powder or solution derived from bovine or human sources (recombinant human thrombin). When applied to oozing tissue, it combines with fibrinogen to promote coagulation.

Topical powder is applied directly to an oozing surface or mixed with injectable isotonic saline for use as a spray or for soaking hemostatic sponges. Dry hemostatic materials, such as *Gelfoam* (absorbable gelatin sponge USP), or flat sponges, such as those used in neurosurgery, can be saturated in thrombin solution and applied to bleeding tissue.

❖ *Thrombin is never injected into blood vessels.*

Absorbable Gelatin USP

Absorbable gelatin USP is a dry sponge material derived from porcine tissue. It is used to promote coagulation in bleeding capillaries. When applied to tissue, it absorbs blood quickly and forms an artificial clot. The clot is the result of mechanical rather than chemical action of the material. Absorbable gelatin is most commonly supplied under the proprietary names *Gelfoam, Gelfilm, and Surgifoam.* These are available in squares, which are cut to size as needed.

❖ *Absorbable hemostatic agents are not left in place over neural or bony tissue, because serious injury can result.*

Preparation of Gelatin Hemostat

The scrubbed surgical technologist receives gelatin sponge as a sterile drug in small, square sheets. These are cut into smaller pieces, according to the surgical application, as requested by the surgeon. The pieces are soaked in normal saline or topical thrombin or are used in dry form.

After gelatin sponge pieces are soaked in saline, they should be removed and compressed to remove the air. They then are returned to the solution and kept there until use. If the sponge does not expand, it should be taken out of the solution and compressed again. The technologist can offer the sponge pieces in a small basin.

❖ *Unused or discarded pieces of Gelfoam must be kept away from the surgical wound so that they do not enter the surgical wound.*

Oxidized Cellulose USP

Oxidized cellulose USP is available in mesh and powder form. Oxidized cellulose is always applied dry. On contact with blood, it rapidly forms a gelatin clot, which is absorbed by the body during the healing process. Oxidized cellulose is manufactured as *Surgicel*.

Preparation of Oxidized Cellulose

Surgicel must be kept dry before use on tissue. If allowed to become wet, it is difficult to handle and loses its shape. It is available in small strips or squares, which may need to be cut with suture scissors. The pieces can then be offered to the surgeon in a small basin or container. Any discarded material should be cleared from the surgical site so that it does not enter (or re-enter) the wound.

Collagen Absorbable Hemostat

Collagen absorbable hemostat is manufactured from bovine collagen and supplied in dry form as powder, sheets, and sponges. *Avitene* is approved for use in all surgery and is also supplied in preloaded applicators for endoscopic use. In powder form, it is applied directly to capillary surfaces. The sheets may be wrapped around sites of **anastomosis** in vascular surgery to help form a coagulated seal. *Instat* absorbable collagen is available in powder, sheets, and pads. This product is not approved for all surgical tissue. Preparation and use of collagen absorbable hemostat is the same as for oxidized cellulose.

Bone Hemostasis

Hemostasis in bone is achieved by occlusion using a waxy substance commonly called *bone wax*. This material traditionally has been made from a combination of beeswax and other additives. A new material derived from ethylene oxide and propylene oxide (*Ostene*) is now available as an alternative to beeswax preparations. All bone hemostasis materials must be warmed slightly before use. This is done by kneading them between the gloved fingers. They then can be offered to the surgeon in small pieces in a small basin or container.

AUTOTRANSFUSION

Autotransfusion is the salvaging to blood at the operative site and reinfusion into the patient. Special equipment, such as the *Cell Saver* device, is required for this. Blood is collected through a special suction tip and routed through tubing directly attached to the device, which rinses, anticoagulates, and separates the blood cells from unwanted components. Autotransfusion is acceptable to patients who, for religious, cultural, or other reasons, decline transfusion of blood from another person. Patients may elect to have their own blood drawn and banked for use at a later date when surgery is schedule. However, there is some difference of opinion about whether this weakens the patient ahead of major surgery and may not be beneficial.

THERMAL AND HIGH-FREQUENCY COAGULATION

Coagulation is performed surgically using a number of technologies, including the electrosurgical unit (ESU), laser, high-frequency electricity, and ultrasound. These are discussed in detail in Chapter 19.

PNEUMATIC TOURNIQUET

The pneumatic tourniquet (Figure 17-1) is used in limb surgery to create a bloodless surgical site. The tourniquet cuff is a nonlatex air bladder encased in a nylon cuff much like a blood pressure cuff. Tourniquet cuffs are manufactured in a variety of sizes and widths. Before the tourniquet is placed on the limb, the area where the tourniquet is to be wrapped is padded with soft bandaging material (Webril), which conforms to the shape of the leg or arm as it is wrapped. The tourniquet is then applied over the Webril (but not yet inflated).

To produce a bloodless surgical site, a flexible latex bandage (Esmarch bandage) is wrapped sequentially around the limb from distal to proximal up to level of the tourniquet (Figure 17-2). This exsanguinates the limb, pushing the blood proximally away from the surgical site. The pneumatic tourniquet is inflated with the Esmarch bandage in place. This prevents blood from flowing back into the vessels. Once the tourniquet

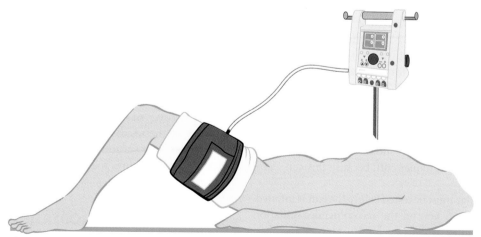

Figure 17-1   A pneumatic tourniquet. The tourniquet is applied to the limb, and the correct pressure is set on the digital control unit.

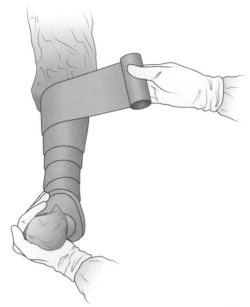

Figure 17-2 An Esmarch bandage is wrapped from distal to proximal to exsanguinate the limb before the pneumatic tourniquet is inflated.

reaches the designated pressure, the Esmarch bandage is removed.

Misuse of a pneumatic tourniquet is associated with tissue necrosis and vascular and nerve damage. These tourniquets are applied and managed only by trained personnel, who observe the following safety precautions to prevent injury to the patient.

- When the pneumatic tourniquet is inflated, the period from cuff inflation to deflation is called tourniquet time and is measured precisely. Both inflation and deflation times are documented in the patient's intraoperative chart.
- The tourniquet may remain inflated for up to 1 hour on an upper extremity and 1½ to 2 hours on a lower extremity. After that period, the patient is at risk for nerve and vascular damage and tissue necrosis related to ischemia.
- The surgeon or registered nurse circulator applies the tourniquet.
- For an adult patient, the tourniquet pressure must not exceed 50 to 75 mm Hg above the patient's systolic blood pressure for an upper extremity or 100 to 150 mm Hg above the systolic pressure for a lower extremity. For a pediatric patient, the upper limit is 100 mm Hg above the patient's systolic pressure.
- Strict policies regarding the use of tourniquets are enforced in all facilities.
- Prep solutions and moisture should be prevented from seeping under the tourniquet cuff, because this can cause burns.
- The pressure gauge must be tested before the cuff is inflated.
- If surgery continues beyond the recommended inflation time, the tourniquet is deflated for 10 minutes and then reinflated. As soon as it is deflated, the field will fill with blood, and hemostasis must be maintained.

- The surgical technologist should always roll the Esmarch bandage after it is removed, because it may be needed again during the surgical procedure.
- The circulator assesses the site for the tourniquet before it is applied. The site is assessed a second time and charted when the tourniquet is removed.

SUTURES

Suture materials are used to **approximate** tissues (i.e., hold tissue together by suture) while healing takes place and to ligate (tie) blood vessels or tubal structures. In surgery, *suture* can refer to a length of suturing thread or a suture thread and needle combination. Packages of suture material are simply called "sutures." Suture material is made from synthesized chemicals, animal protein, metal, and natural fibers. The material itself is one of the factors that determine how and where the suture is used in the body.

STUDYING AND LEARNING SUTURE USE

Suture and needles are available in a wide variety of sizes and materials (Table 17-1). The techniques and knowledge for handling these instruments are acquired over time with repetition and study. Suture manufacturers recognize that the scrub and circulator need to identify a suture type quickly. Packages are color coded by suture type, and needles often are pictured on the label to aid rapid selection and delivery to the sterile field. Difficulties may arise because of the many different types of sutures and needles, and identical suture materials made by different companies have different names. The same suture material from one company may be dyed a different color by another. These problems are overcome by working with the same surgeons and becoming familiar with their preferences.

REGULATION OF SUTURES

Drugs and materials used in the United States must be approved by the federal Food and Drug Administration (FDA) and the United States Pharmacopeia. The USP began as an organization of physicians that set minimum standards for medical products and substances. These standards were adopted by the federal government and now are included in the regulations of the FDA. All substances, including suture products, that bear the USP label must meet minimum standards. Included in the standards for suture materials are regulations for size, tensile strength, and sterility. Additional standards cover packaging, dyes used in the suture, and the integrity of the needles. The European Pharmacopoeia (EP) sets standards for sutures used in European Union (EU) countries, including sutures manufactured and distributed by U.S. companies.

STRUCTURE AND PROPERTIES OF SUTURE

It is important to become familiar with the characteristics of different kinds of sutures. These qualities, which contribute

Table 17-1

Suture Brands and Types

Name	Color	Size	Material	Structure	Absorption	Uses
Biosyn *Syneture*	Violet Beige	7-0 to 2	Polyester	Monofilament	Absorbable	General soft tissue Ophthalmic
Bondek *Deknatel*	Green Violet Beige	8-0 to 2	Polyglycolic acid	Braided Coated	Absorbable	General soft tissue Ophthalmic
Caprosyn *Syneture*	Violet Beige	6-0 to 1	Polyglytone polyester	Monofilament	Absorbable	General soft tissue
Cottony II *Deknatel*	Green White	9 to 8-0 1- to 3-mm tape	Polyester (uncoated)	Braided Twisted Tape	Nonabsorbable	General soft tissue Cardiovascular
Deklene *Deknatel*	Blue Clear	10-0 to 2	Polypropylene	Monofilament	Nonabsorbable	General soft tissue Cardiovascular
Dexon II *Syneture*	Beige Green	6-0 to 2	Polyglycolic acid	Braided Coated	Absorbable	General soft tissue Ligation Ophthalmic
Ethilon *Ethicon*	Black	10-0 thru	Nylon	Monofilament	Gradual loss	General soft tissue Cardiovascular Ophthalmic Neurosurgical
Force Fiber *Deknatel*	White	2-0 to 2	Polyethylene	Monofilament	Nonabsorbable	General soft tissue Orthopedic
Gut, chromic	Brown Blue	7-0 to 3	Bovine/ovine collagen	Monofilament Noncoated	Rapidly absorbable	General soft tissue Ligation Ophthalmic
Gut, plain	Yellow Blue	7-0 to 3	Bovine/ovine collagen	Monofilament Noncoated	Absorbable	General soft tissue Ligation Ophthalmic
Maxon *Syneture*	Green	7-0 to 1	Copolymer polyglyconate	Monofilament	Absorbable	General soft tissue Cardiovascular
Mersilene	Green White	6-0 to 5	Polyester	Braided	Nonabsorbable	General soft tissue Cardiovascular Ophthalmic Neurological
Monocryl *Ethicon*	Violet Natural	6-0 to 2	Poliglecaprone 25	Monofilament	Absorbable	General soft tissue Ligation Skin Gynecology
Novafil	Green	10-0 to 2	Polybuster	Monofilament	Nonabsorbable	General soft tissue Cardiovascular Ophthalmic
Nurolon *Ethicon*	Black Clear	6-0 to 1	Nylon	Braided	Gradual loss	General soft tissue Cardiovascular Ophthalmic Neurological
PDS II *Syneture*	Violet Blue Clear	9-0 to 2	Polydioxanone	Monofilament.	Absorbable	General soft tissue Cardiovascular Ophthalmic
Perma Hand *Ethicon*	Black	9-0 to 5	Derived from natural silk	Braided Wax coated	Gradual loss	General soft tissue Cardiovascular Ophthalmic Neurological

Continued

Table 17-1

Suture Brands and Types—cont'd

Name	Color	Size	Material	Structure	Absorption	Uses
Polydek *Deknatel*	Green White	9-0 to 7-0	Polyester	PTFE coated	Nonabsorbable	General soft tissue Cardiovascular
Polysorb *Syneture*	Violet	8-0 to 2	Lactomer glycolide/lactide	Braided	Absorbable	General soft tissue Ligation Ophthalmic
Prolene *Ethicon*	Blue Clear	7-0 to 2	Polypropylene	Monofilament	Nonabsorbable	General soft tissue Cardiovascular Ophthalmic Neurological
Pronova *Ethicon*	Blue	10-0 to 2	Hexafluoropropylene-VDF	Monofilament	Nonabsorbable	Soft tissue Cardiovascular Ophthalmic Neurological
Sofsilk *Syneture*	Black White	9-0 to 5	Natural silk	Braided Coated with wax or silicone	Nonabsorbable	General soft tissue Cardiovascular Ophthalmic Neurological
Steel	Natural silver	5-0 to 7 B & S 18 to 35	Steel alloy	Monofilament Braided	Nonabsorbable	Orthopedics: bone and soft tissue
Surgidac *Syneture*	Green	6-0 to 0	Polyethylene	Braided Monofilament Coated or uncoated	Nonabsorbable	General soft tissue Cardiovascular Opthalmic Neurosurgical
Surgipro *Syneture*	Blue Clear	10-2 to 2	Polypropylene and polyethelene	Monofilament	Gradual encapsulation	General soft tissue Cardiovascular Opthalmic
Tevdek *Deknatel*	Green White	10-0 to 9	Polyester	Braided PTFE Impregnated	Nonabsorbable	General soft tissue Cardiovascular
Ti-Cron *Syneture*	Blue White	8-0 to 5	Polyester	Braided Uncoated or coated with silicone	Nonabsorbable	General soft tissue Cardiovascular Opthalmic Neurosurgical
Vicryl *Ethicon*	Violet Natural	8-0 to 3	Polyglactin 910	Braided Monofilament	Absorbable	General soft tissue Ophthalmic Ligation

PTFE, Polytetrafluorethylene (Teflon); *B & S*, Brown and Sharp gauge.

to the surgeon's choice of suture for a particular tissue and application, include:

- *Physical characteristics:* The structure of the suture and its dimensions, strength, and size.
- *Handling qualities:* Pliability, elasticity, and memory (recoil).
- *Absorption quality:* The effect of the tissue on the suture, its resistance to digestion (degradation of the material by the lysosomal action of cellular enzymes), and absorption.
- *Bioactivity:* The effect of the suture on the tissue.

- *Composition:* The chemical makeup and origin of the material used to manufacture the suture.

Physical Characteristics

Structure

Sutures are broadly divided into two main structural categories:

- **Monofilament suture:** A single continuous fiber made of a polymer chemical (chains of the same molecule strung together) that is extruded and stretched.

- **Multifilament suture:** Many filaments that together form one strand of suture. Multifilament suture in turn is divided into two types:
  - *Twisted:* Multiple fibers twisted in the same direction.
  - *Braided:* Multiple fibers that are intertwined (braided).

Braided and twisted sutures usually are coated with Teflon or a similar chemical to reduce friction as the suture is drawn through the tissue (called **tissue drag**). Figure 17-3 shows two basic suture structures.

Capillary Action

Sutures made of multifilament strands absorb moisture and hold body fluids (called *wicking* or **capillary action**). If bacteria are present, suture materials with high capillarity are able to retain and spread infection by means of the suture fibers. Suture with low capillarity is preferred in surgery when the risk of infection is high.

Some multifilament suture is coated to reduce tissue drag and wicking. In the past, absorbable suture was coated with a nonabsorbable material such as beeswax, paraffin, or silicone. Coatings similar in composition to the suture are biocompatible and cause less tissue reaction in the patient.

Size

The size of the suture is based on its diameter. The USP numbering system indicates the suture's outside diameter and ensures that a stated size is the same regardless of the material.

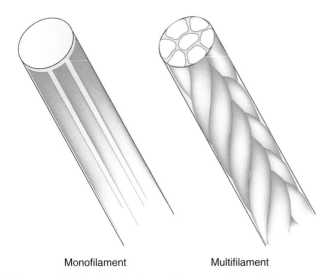

Figure 17-3 Extruded monofilament and braided multifilament sutures. *(Redrawn from Rothrock JC: Alexander's care of the patient in surgery, ed 12, St Louis, 2003, Mosby.)*

For example, size 2-0 silk suture has the same diameter as size 2-0 nylon suture.

Suture ranges in size from 12-0 (thinnest) to 5 (thickest). The greater the diameter, the larger the designated size. For example, size 2 is thicker than size 0. Sutures smaller than 0 are designated by additional zeros. For example, size 2-0 is an average size for abdominal wall tissue. Size 11-0 is used in microsurgery. This suture is light enough to remain suspended in the air. Sutures of this size are very delicate and expensive and must be handled with care.

Stainless steel suture historically has used the **Brown and Sharp (B & S) sizing system** rather than USP sizes. These numbers begin with size 38/40 gauge (the thinnest) and go up to 18 gauge (the thickest). Stainless steel now is sized according to USP standards. However, some surgeons may request the B & S number, which is printed on steel wire packages. Table 17-2 shows B & S sizes and their corresponding USP size.

Strength

The **tensile strength** of suture refers to the amount of force needed to break the suture. Tensile strength is measured by comparing different sutures of the same size. Tensile strength is influenced by many factors, such as:

- The *type of knot* used to tie the suture. Suture material becomes 10% to 40% weaker when knotted.
- The *biological environment* of the suture. Suture materials vary in strength when exposed to body fluids. Some resist digestion, whereas others are quickly degraded and absorbed. The presence of infection affects the strength of most suture materials.
- *Uniformity* (a quality control factor). Sutures must be uniform in diameter to maintain tensile strength.

Handling Qualities

The handling qualities of a suture determine its ease of use and may affect the technical quality of the wound closure. For these reasons, surgeons are careful to balance the handling qualities of a suture with its other characteristics.

Memory

Memory describes the suture's tendency to retain its shape or configuration after it is removed from the package. Most suture is packaged in coils (stainless steel is packaged straight to prevent kinking). High memory suture is springy and tends to tangle during preparation and use. This also correlates with the ability of a suture to stay knotted. Material that is stiff or retains memory tends to loosen easily. This is both annoying and time-consuming for the surgeon. Extruded monofilament

Table 17-2

Stainless Steel Suture Sizes

B & S gauge	#40	#35	#32	#30	#28	#26	#25	#24	#23	#22	#20
USP size	6-0	5-0	4-0	3-0	2-0	0	1	2	3	4	5

B & S, Brown and Sharp; USP, United States Pharmacopeia.

sutures have greater coil memory than braided or twisted fiber suture.

Pliability

A pliable suture is one that is soft and nonresistant. The knots lie flat and remain secure (called *tie-down*). **Pliability** increases the security of the knot. Pliable suture is easy to control and manipulate. Silk suture had traditionally been considered the gold standard of all suture materials for its pliability, tight knits, and ease of use. More inert suture materials have taken its place through the years, but the other qualities remain the highest standard for handling qualities.

Elasticity

Elasticity refers to the material's ability to stretch and then return to its former configuration. Elasticity can be advantageous as long as the suture retains its strength when stretched.

Absorption Qualities

Suture materials are partly categorized according to their absorption characteristics and the origin of the material. Absorption is different from bioactivity, which describes how the body reacts to the suture. *Absorption* describes how the suture reacts in the presence of body tissue. Both **absorbable suture** and **nonabsorbable suture** are available in natural (biological) and synthetic (manmade) form.

The ideal suture would be one that retains its strength throughout the healing period and then dissolves (is absorbed) when healing is complete. However, the ideal suture does not exist.

Absorbable, protein-based suture is attacked by enzyme-releasing lysosomes that digest the suture. Absorbable synthetic sutures are degraded by *hydrolysis,* a chemical reaction that occurs in the presence of water. Nonabsorbable sutures become encapsulated in connective tissue, and some (e.g., nylon and silk) eventually are absorbed. All sutures, except stainless steel, can degrade if infection is present.

Bioactivity

Bioactivity is the body's response to suture. The immune system reacts to suture as it would to any foreign material. The bioactivity depends on the chemical structure of the suture material and the condition of the patient. Sutures that cause little or no bioactivity are said to be highly inert, causing little or no inflammation. Stainless steel suture is the most inert of all materials; natural fiber and protein-based sutures cause the most tissue reaction.

Note that bioactivity is different from a tendency to cause infection, which is related to the structure of the suture rather than its chemical makeup.

NATURAL ABSORBABLE SUTURE

Surgical Gut

Surgical gut, also called *catgut,* is a protein collagen derived from the submucosal layer of beef or sheep intestine. The suture is monofilament and available in sizes 7-0 to 3. It is used on tissues that heal rapidly.

Plain surgical gut is digested quickly and absorbed by tissues, but this rapid reaction can also cause inflammation. The suture retains tensile strength in the body for 7 to 10 days. It is used primarily in mucous membrane or in tissue where stones can form, such as the biliary or urinary systems. Plain gut is straw colored in its natural bleached state. Chromic gut is treated with **chromic salt** to resist digestion and absorption. Chromic gut usually is absorbed in 7 to 21 days. Both types of gut are absorbed rapidly if infection is present, and they are not used in contaminated wounds.

Gut requires special handling to preserve its strength and pliability. The sutures are packaged in an alcohol solution, which can be a source of ignition on the surgical field. Gut dries out quickly and should be dipped in saline just before use. This prevents the suture from breaking. However, gut should not be soaked, because it absorbs water readily and becomes swollen and weak.

Dipping the strands in saline also softens them so that the coils can be removed. This is done by grasping the ends of the strand and pulling gently. It is important to pull on the strands gently, especially when they are wet, because they can overstretch and become weak. Gut should be handled as little as possible, because contact with gloves causes the strands to fray.

SYNTHETIC ABSORBABLE POLYMERS

BONDEK
BIOSYN
CAPROSYN
DEXON II
DEXON S
MAXON
MONOCRYL
PDS II
POLYGLYCOLIC ACID
POLYDIOXANONE
POLYGLACTIN 910
POLYSORB
VYCRYL

Absorbable synthetic sutures are made of polymer or copolymer chemicals. They are available in monofilament and braided form. They provide wound support for 3 weeks to 6 months, depending on the material. They are easily absorbed by the body after breakdown. These materials are pliable and easy to handle, even in the braided form. Most are coated for ease of handling and to reduce friction.

Polymer sutures are dyed to make them easier to see on the surgical field. However, they are also available in their natural color for superficial use. Absorbable synthetic sutures are used in most types of tissue and cause little tissue reaction compared to surgical gut. Polymers are handled in their dry state and have a high tensile strength.

ABSORBABLE BIOPOLYMER SUTURE

TEPHAFLEX

Absorbable biopolymer suture is manufactured through patented recombinant DNA technology (Tepha, Lexington, Massachusetts). The applications of biopolymer are similar to those for synthetic polymers, but biopolymer has 50% greater tensile strength and is biocompatible with body tissue. (For more information on this new technology, see the manufacturer's Web site at http://www.tepha.com.)

NONABSORBABLE SUTURE

Silk

PERMA-HAND
SOFSILK

Silk suture is derived from fibers produced by the silkworm. It has a long history of use. The most famous advance in suturing involved the use of very fine sutures placed in close approximation. This technique was developed by the physician William Halsted in the late 1800s. Halsted's method established the standard for excellence in surgical technique, and the principles still apply.

Silk is soft and pliable and has excellent tensile strength. It is available in braided or twisted form. Silk strands are coated to prevent wicking. Silk handles exceptionally well, and the knots remain secure and flat. Silk suture is used in most deep tissues, especially in intestinal, vascular, ophthalmic, and neurosurgical procedures. Dermal silk is used to close the skin in areas where the incision is subjected to excessive strain. Virgin silk is used mainly for ophthalmological procedures because of its pliability and performance in eye tissue. Silk is available in black or white in sizes 9-0 to 5. Silk begins to break down after about a year and usually is absent from tissue after 2 years.

Cotton

Cotton sutures are no longer marketed in the United States but are still available in other countries. Traditionally used in intestinal closure, cotton has been replaced by stronger, more inert materials.

Nylon

DERMALON
ETHILON
MONOSOF
NUROLON

Nylon was the first synthetic suture material available (1940) and is still widely used. It is available in braided or monofilament strands. The most outstanding feature of nylon is that is causes little or no tissue reaction and passes very easily through delicate tissues of the eye or blood vessels. Also, nylon has a very high tensile strength. However, in larger sizes it is stiff and may cut through tissue. Nylon suture loses its tensile strength over time. It is used when long-term strength is not required. Nylon suture is available in sizes 11-0 to 2. It is available in black, blue, green, and clear colors in braided or monofilament, coated or uncoated.

Polyester

COTTONY II
ETHIBOND
MERSILENE
NOVAFIL (polybuster)
POLYDEK
POLYSORB
SURGIDAC
TI-CRON
TEVDEK

Polyester fiber suture is extremely strong, easy to handle, and relatively inert in tissue. It is braided and is available coated or uncoated. The coated form is widely used for cardiovascular surgery, especially when grafts are used, because of its strength-to-size ratio. Polyester suture is green, blue, or white and is available is sizes 11-0 to 2.

Polypropylene

DEKLENE II
PROLENE
PRONOVA (hexafluoropropylene)
SURGIPRO

Polypropylene is an extremely inert monofilament suture. Its smooth surface makes it popular for plastic, ophthalmic, and vascular surgery. Because of its high tensile strength, it is used for retention sutures, particularly in abdominal wall closure. It is available in a wide variety of sizes and can be used when infection is present and can be left in place for extended periods. It is clear or blue in color and is available in sizes 10-0 to 2.

Stainless Steel

Stainless steel is the strongest of all suture materials. It is widely used in the approximation of bone and other connective tissue. Surgical stainless steel suture has no significant inflammatory properties. It is available in monofilament and twisted form.

Stainless steel suture requires special handling. It kinks easily, and the ends are needle sharp. The suture ends can puncture gloves, drapes, and other soft materials. Stainless steel suture is dispensed from the package as long, precut strands. The strands have considerable spring, and the ends must be handled carefully to control them. They must be kept straight and delivered without kinks or bends, which can tear through tissue as the strand is drawn through.

To prepare steel suture lengths, carefully remove a single strand from the package just before use. Place a hemostat on one end to maintain control. If the strand is to be threaded through a needle, thread the strand 1 or 2 inches (2½ to 5 cm) from the end and put a twist at the eye to secure the strand in place. Use a needle holder or wire holder to make the twist. Never use suture scissors to cut stainless steel wire. Always use wire scissors designated for this purpose.

Bits of stainless steel wire must be removed from the field and collected in a container during surgery. These are sharp items that can cause injury and must be treated as sharps on the surgical field.

SURGICAL NEEDLES

Surgical needles are made from high quality steel alloy. The combination of metals used in the manufacturing process renders the needles strong and inert. Needles are available in several types, according to their *eye* (the area where suture is threaded or attached), shape or curvature, and point style.

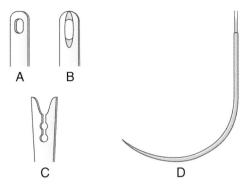

Figure 17-4 Suture eyes. **A** and **B,** Closed eye. **C,** French eye. **D,** Atraumatic eye. (Redrawn from Phillips N: Berry and Kohn's operating room technique, *ed 10, St Louis, 2004, Mosby.*)

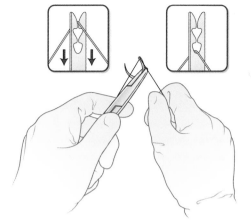

Figure 17-5 Technique for mounting suture on a French eye needle. (Redrawn from Phillips N: Berry and Kohn's operating room technique, *ed 10, St Louis, 2004, Mosby.*)

Surgical needles have three distinct parts: the point, the body, and the eye.

Needle Eye

The eye of the needle provides the attachment for the suture. Three types of needle eyes are available: the closed eye, the French eye (also called a *split* or *spring eye*), and the atraumatic (swaged) suture (Figure 17-4). The conventional closed eye needle resembles a sewing needle, and the eye hole is round, rectangular, or square. French eye needles have two eyes that are connected by a slit from the top through the eyes, with ridges that hold the sutures in place.

Few surgeons use eyed needles. However, the surgical technologist must be familiar with their use. Eyed needles are identified by their shape and by the type of eye. Threading and passing eyed needles in rapid succession are skills that require practice. When the needle is threaded, the suture must be passed from the inside of the needle curve to the outside. The short end should extend approximately 4 inches (10 cm) from the eye. Both ends must be prevented from adhering to the shank of the needle holder. When the surgeon receives the suture, both the short and long ends must be free.

Swaged (Atraumatic) Suture

Most commercial needles are now manufactured with the suture preattached. This is called a swaged, or atraumatic suture. The suture is inserted into the eye end of the needle, and the area is crimped and sealed. This produces a nearly seamless connection between the needle and the suture and also allows faster suturing with minimal tissue trauma.

The French eye (or spring eye) needle usually was used before swaged sutures became available, and some surgeons still prefer them. When the spring eye needle is threaded, the end of the suture is pressed down over the top of the spring, which causes it to snap into the eye (Figure 17-5). The suture should not be pulled through the eye after it is in place, because this strips the suture and may break it.

A detachable suture (Figure 17-6) is one in which the suture can be detached from the needle by pulling it straight

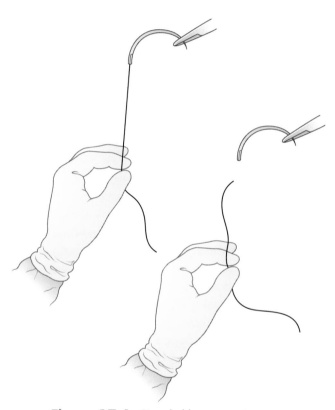

Figure 17-6 Detachable atraumatic suture.

Figure 17-7 Double-armed suture used for anastomosis or suturing of circular incisions (e.g., the eye) or in gastrointestinal and vascular surgery.

back from the **swage**. These are referred to by their proprietary names, such as *De-tach* and **Control-release**.

A **double-armed suture** is one with a needle swaged to each end. This type of suture is used for circular tissue, such as in ophthalmic surgery, or for hollow structures, such as blood vessels or the intestine (Figure 17-7).

Needle Shape

Needles are available in a number of different shapes to conform to their use. The curvature **of** a needle relates to the body and radius of the needle. The curve is measured as a circumferential fraction in a complete circle. Curvature designations are ¼, ⅜, ½, and ⅝. For example, a ½-curve needle is exactly one half the circumference a circle.

In general, deep tissue in a confined space requires a more extreme curve. The curved needle allows the surgeon to dip beneath the surface of the tissue and retrieve the point as it emerges. The shape and characteristics of a needle are shown in Figure 17-8.

Needle Size

Needle size is measured by the diameter of the shaft and the dimension from tip to eye. Historically, suture needles were identified by the curvature and name. These names are seldom used, and many have been replaced by common manufacturer codes or shape.

Needle Point

Many different types of needle points are available (Figure 17-9). However, they all are variations of the three basic types:

- Blunt
- Tapered
- Cutting

The **blunt needle** is a round shaft with a blunt tip. It pushes tissue aside as it moves through it. It does not puncture the tissue, but rather slides between tissue fibers. It is the least traumatic and safest needle point. The blunt needle traditionally has been used only for suturing and for blunt dissection of friable tissues and of organs that are soft and spongy, such as the liver, spleen, and kidneys. The blunt needle now is advocated for general suture use because it significantly reduces the risk of needlestick injury and transmission of blood-borne diseases.

The tapered needle has a round body that tapers to a sharp point. It punctures tissue, making an opening for the body of the needle to follow. Its primary use is for suturing soft tissue, such as muscle, subcutaneous fat, peritoneum, dura, and gastrointestinal, genitourinary, biliary, and vascular tissue.

The cutting needle has a cutting edge along its shaft. A needle with the cutting edge on the inside of the curve is called a *conventional cutting needle*. A needle with the cutting edge on the outside or lower edge of the curve is called a **reverse cutting needle**.

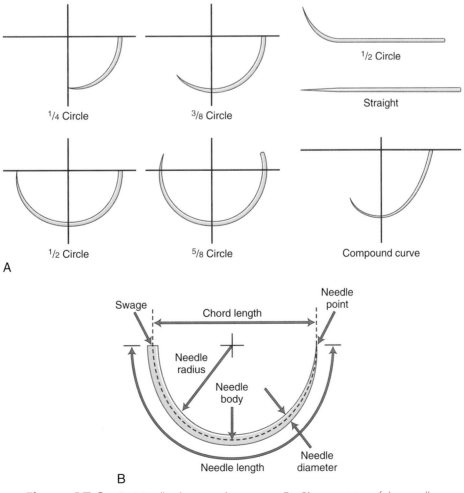

Figure 17-8 A, Needle shape and curvature. **B,** Characteristics of the needle.

POINT/BODY SHAPE	APPLICATION
Conventional cutting 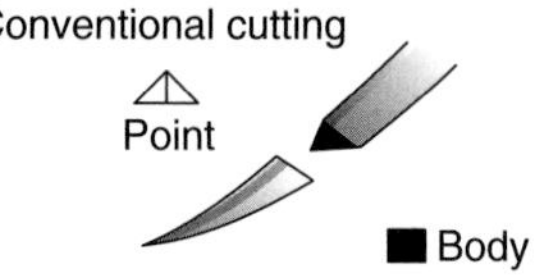 △ Point ■ Body	Skin, sternum
Reverse cutting 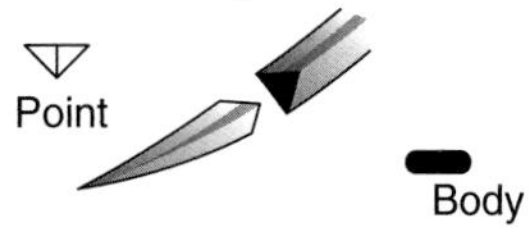 ▽ Point ▬ Body	Fascia, ligament, nasal cavity, oral mucosa, pharynx, skin, tendon sheath
Precision point cutting 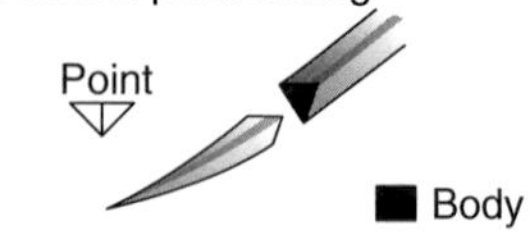 Point ▽ ■ Body	Skin (plastic or cosmetic)
PC PRIME needle 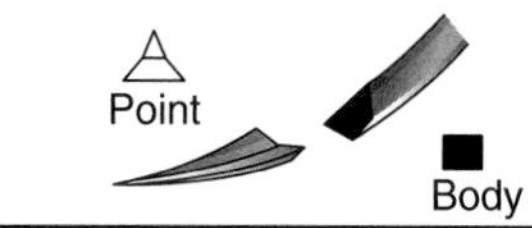 △ Point ■ Body	Skin (plastic or cosmetic)
MICRO-POINT reverse cutting needle 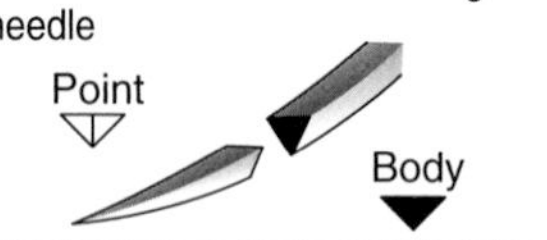 Point ▽ ▼ Body	Eye
Side-cutting spatula 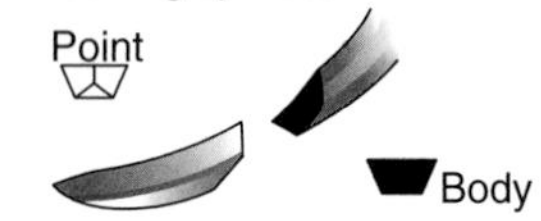 Point ▽ ▼ Body	Eye (primary application), microsurgery, ophthalmic (reconstructive)
CS ULTIMA ophthalmic needle 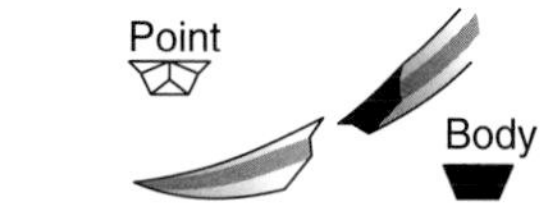 Point ▽ ▼ Body	Eye (primary application)
Taper 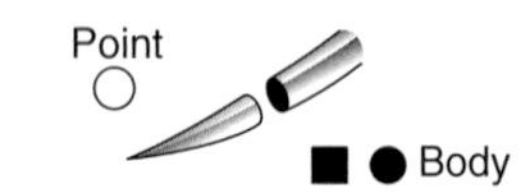 Point ○ ■ ● Body	Aponeurosis, biliary tract, dura, fascia, gastrointestinal tract, laparoscopy, muscle, myocardium, nerve, peritoneum, pleura, subcutaneous fat, urogenital tract, vessels, valve
TAPERCUT surgical needle 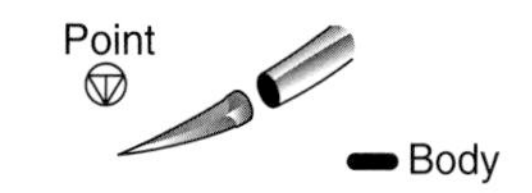 Point ▽ ▬ Body	Bronchus, calcified tissue, fascia, laparoscopy, ligament, nasal cavity, oral cavity, ovary, peri-chondrium, periosteum, pharynx, sternum, tendon, trachea, uterus, valve, vessels (sclerotic)
Blunt 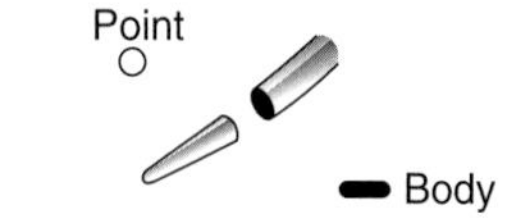 Point ○ ▬ Body	Blunt dissection (friable tissue), cervix (ligating incompetent cervix), fascia, intestine, kidney, liver, spleen

Figure 17-9 Needle points and shapes. *(From Wound closure manual, Somerville, NJ, 1999, Ethicon Inc.)*

Cutting needles are used on fibrous connective tissue, such as the skin, joint capsule, and tendon. As described above, the conventional cutting needle has a triangular-shaped shaft. Its cutting edge is on the inside curve of the needle; as the needle is drawn through tissue, the curve tends to slice tissue in an upward direction. The reverse cutting needle solves this problem by locating the cutting edge on the outside of the curve, away from the direction of tension during suturing. It is stronger than the conventional cutting needle and produces minimal scarring.

The taper cut needle has a reverse cutting edge at the tip and a round body. The point of the needle is tapered. Taper cut needles are used for suturing dense fibrous connective tissue, such as the fascia, tendon, and periosteum.

Spatula needles are side-cutting needles with a flat surface on the top and the bottom. These are used in ophthalmic surgery to separate corneal and scleral tissue.

SUTURE STORAGE, PACKAGING, AND DISPENSING

Storage
Sutures are stored in individual boxes containing multiple suture packs (Figure 17-10). Suture racks may be kept in substerile areas and in closed cabinets in the operating room. Suture carts should not be brought into the operating room, where they can become contaminated with blood and body fluids. At the start of surgery, only the minimum number needed are opened. The surgical technologist should anticipate the need for additional suture packs as the case progresses and request them in time.

Packaging
Suture manufacturers have developed innovative methods of packaging that are important to surgeons, surgical technologists, and nurses.

The following are important features of a packaging system:
- *Product protection:* The package must maintain sterility and protect sutures and needles from damage during storage and dispensing.
- *Efficient dispensing:* The design of the packaging system must ensure that the suture can be withdrawn rapidly and smoothly without tangling or knotting.
- *Selection:* Package labeling should be easy to associate with a specific suture. Rapid selection is desirable.
- *Minimal packaging:* A packaging system that produces minimal waste is desirable. Excessive wrapping and packaging are time-consuming to dispose of and create clutter on the surgical field.
- *Environmentally responsible:* Packaging should reflect an effort to promote biodegradable materials.

Reading a Suture Label
Sutures packages contain information that the surgical technologist needs to know when selecting suture. In Figure 17-11, note the name, size, and color of the suture, type and size of the needle (when applicable), lot number, and expiration date.

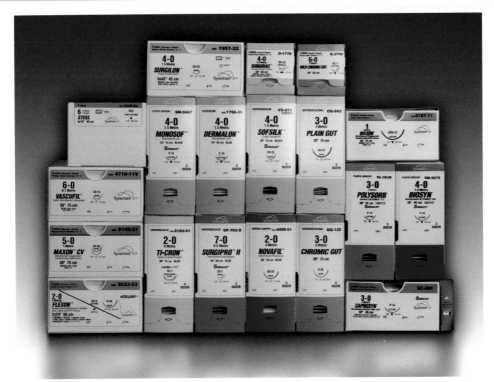

Figure 17-10 Assorted sutures. (Copyright © 2008 Covidien. All rights reserved. Reprinted with permission of Covidien.)

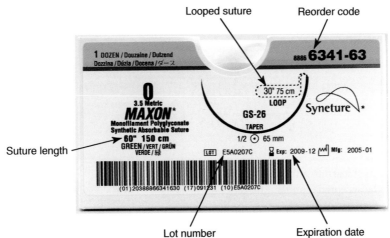

Figure 17-11 Single suture package details. (Copyright © 2008 Covidien. All rights reserved. Reprinted with permission of Covidien.)

Dispensing

Suture wrapping and dispensing methods vary among suture manufacturers. However, the products themselves are standard.

- *Suture-needle combination:* One suture-needle combination is provided per pack (Figure 17-12).
- *Multiple suture strands:* One suture package contains multiple precut strands of suture (Figure 17-13).
- *Suture reel:* A spool of suture material is wound into a round reel.
- *Multiple suture-needle combinations:* One package contains many suture-needle combinations in detachable format (Figure 17-14).

- *Double-armed suture:* One pack contains a single suture strand with a needle attached at each end.

SUTURING TECHNIQUES

The primary use of sutures is to repair or construct tissue. The process of suturing that means to hold two tissue edges together is called approximation. Suture is also used to tie, or **ligate**, bleeding vessels. Sutures are tied using special techniques to ensure that the knots are secure. Each loop of the knot is referred to as a throw. When requesting a suture-needle during a procedure, the surgeon may refer to it as a stitch.

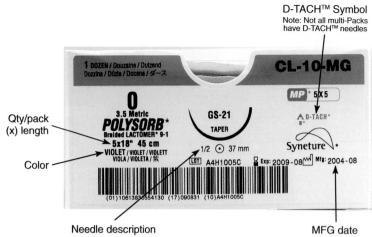

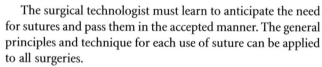

Figure 17-12 Multiple suture pack. *(Copyright © 2008 Covidien. All rights reserved. Reprinted with permission of Covidien.)*

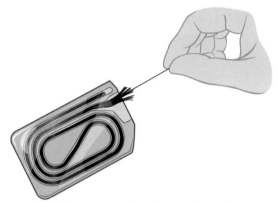

Figure 17-13 Race track packaging for single suture strands.

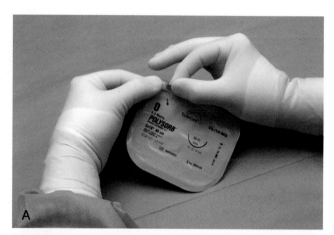

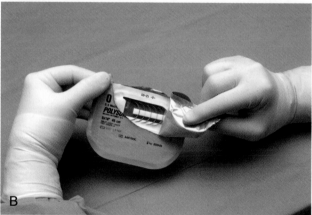

Figure 17-14 Multiple detachable needles in a single pack. *(Copyright © 2008 Covidien. All rights reserved. Reprinted with permission of Covidien.)*

The surgical technologist must learn to anticipate the need for sutures and pass them in the accepted manner. The general principles and technique for each use of suture can be applied to all surgeries.

A suture, or "sewing," technique is the method and pattern formed as tissues are approximated. Two general types of suturing technique are used: continuous and interrupted.

Continuous Suture Techniques

A continuous suture, or **running suture**, is a single long suture length that is anchored at one end of the tissues. The needle is alternated from one side of the tissue edge to the other (Figure 17-15). The advantages of this suture technique are that it is rapid and uses relatively little suture material. A disadvantage is that if one point along the suture breaks during healing, the wound may open up. This technique does not allow the surgeon to make adjustments in aligning the wound edges, which tend to pucker when a running suture is used. Compared with running sutures, interrupted sutures are easy to place, have greater tensile strength, and have less potential for causing wound edema and impaired cutaneous circulation.

Subcuticular Suture

The subcuticular or buried suture is used for cosmetic closure and in pediatric patients. The needle is placed within the dermis from side to side (Figure 17-16). This technique brings the skin edges together in close approximation and no suture material is visible from the outside. The technique produces a very fine scar or no scar, but it is time-consuming and meticulous.

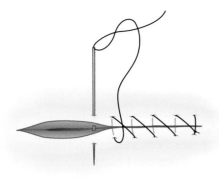

Figure 17-15 Continuous (running) suture.

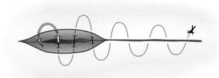

Figure 17-16 Subcuticular suture.

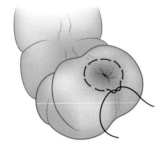

Figure 17-17 Purse-string suture.

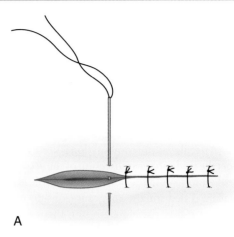

A

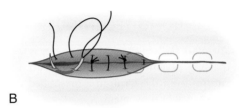

B

Figure 17-18 **A,** Interrupted suture (superficial). **B,** Deep interrupted suture.

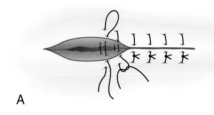

A

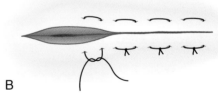

B

Figure 17-19 **A,** Vertical mattress suture. **B,** Horizontal mattress suture.

Purse-String Suture

The **purse-string** is a special continuous suture technique for closing the end of a tubular structure (lumen), such as the appendix, its most common application. In this technique, one end of the suture is anchored and stitches are placed around the periphery of the open "tube." The suture then is drawn tight around the neck of the lumen (Figure 17-17).

Locking Suture

The locking stitch provides added strength to a running suture line. As the needle is passed through each side of the wound edges, it is passed underneath one loop. This equalizes the tension between each loop of the suture and provides increased hemostasis on the wound edges.

Interrupted Suture Techniques

Interrupted sutures are individually placed, knotted, and cut (Figure 17-18). The finished suture line is very strong, because the tension of the wound edges is distributed over many anchor points. This technique is detailed and time-consuming. Many interrupted stitches produce a secure suture

line with minimal scarring. Interrupted sutures placed far apart are used in areas of less wound tension. The vertical mattress suture (Figure 17-19, *A*) and the horizontal mattress suture (Figure 17-19, *B*) increase wound strength.

Retention Sutures

Retention sutures are a type of interrupted technique used to provide additional support to wound edges in abdominal surgery. In this technique, heavy sutures are placed though all the tissue layers of the body wall several centimeters from the primary suture line. The sutures are placed perpendicular to the incision. As each suture is drawn tight, it pulls the edges of the incision into approximation without cutting into the tissue. Plastic or rubber **bolsters**, or small lengths of tubing, are threaded through the suture to prevent it from cutting into to the patient's skin (Figure 17-20).

Suture Ligature

A suture ligature is used to ligate a large bleeding vessel. The purpose of the technique is to prevent the ligature from sliding off the vessel. A needle-suture combination is used. The surgeon passes the needle through the midsection of the vessel and adds an additional wrap around the outside. The needle is removed, and the ligature is tied snugly. Many surgeons do not cut the suture ends, but rather place a clamp on them (tagging the suture) until they are certain that no bleeding will occur. A suture ligature may be referred to as a *stick tie* (Figure 17-21).

SUTURE HANDLING TECHNIQUES

One of the primary skills in surgical technology is the preparation and passing of sutures. Surgeons are accustomed to receiving sutures from the scrub in a prescribed manner for safety and efficiency of movement.

Safety

1. Suture needles are hazardous on the sterile field. They increase the risk of blood-borne contamination related to accidental puncture of a team member.
2. Good technique in handling sutures prevents their loss in the surgical wound. Lost items are a safety hazard and increase operative time and team stress.

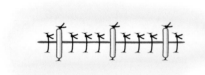

Figure 17-20 Retention sutures.

3. Inappropriate tissue-needle combinations can cause unnecessary trauma to tissue.
4. Proper preparation of sutures increases their potential to facilitate uncomplicated healing.

Efficiency of Movement

1. An efficient process for passing sutures reduces operative time.
2. Sutures are very expensive. Conservative use lowers the total cost to patients and facilities.
3. Poor technique in preparing sutures can result in waste, because sutures break, disengage from the needle, and are lost on the sterile field.

Suturing Instruments

Curved suture needles are mounted on a needle holder (also called a *needle driver*) for use. Select a needle holder that is the correct length for the depth of the wound and the correct weight (heavy or delicate). The jaws of the needle holder must be selected according to the delicacy of the needle. Needle holders used in general surgery have diamond or carbon steel inserts over the portion that holds the needle. This prevents the needle from slipping or rotating. The type and size of the needle holder is adjusted to the size of the needle.

The surgeon nearly always uses tissue forceps to stabilize the tissue while suturing. The scrub selects the forceps by length, weight, and type of jaws according to the tissue to be sutured. The general categories of jaws are smooth and toothed (Figure 17-22). The most delicate needle holders are those used in microsurgery and ear and ophthalmic surgery (Figure 17-23).

- *Smooth forceps* are used on mucous membrane organ tissue (e.g., the spleen and kidneys) and on any tissue that bleeds easily.
- *Toothed forceps* are used on connective tissue, including the skin.
- *Vascular forceps* are specially designed with a scored insert at the working tip; this prevents puncturing of the blood vessel but provides sufficient friction to hold.

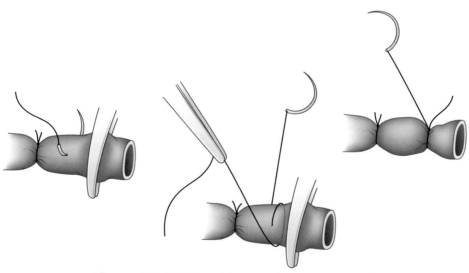

Figure 17-21 Use of the suture ligature on a vessel.

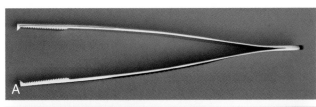

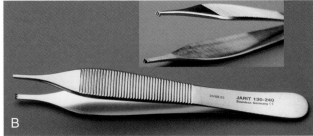

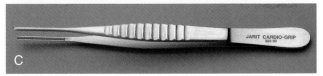

Figure 17-22 Tissue forceps. **A,** Toothed forceps for general use. **B,** Adson forceps for skin. **C,** DeBakey forceps for vascular tissue. *(Courtesy Jarit Instruments, Hawthorne, N.Y.)*

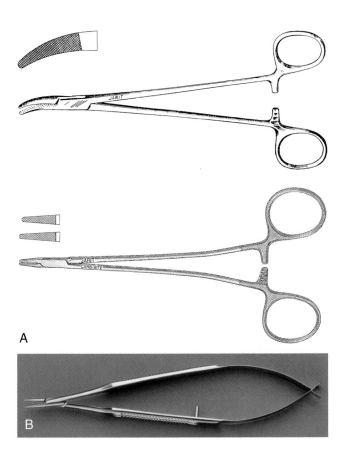

Figure 17-23 Needle holders. **A,** Standard needle holders. **B,** Needle holder for delicate tissue. *(Courtesy Jarit Instruments, Hawthorne, N.Y.)*

Technique for Passing Sutures

Mount the needle about 0.5 mm from the end of the swaged section. Do not clamp the swage, because this weakens it and places the needle holder too far back for correct balance. Drape the suture end over the back of your hand before you pass it. This prevents it from becoming caught in the surgeon's hand as he or she receives the suture. The "armed" needle holder must be passed so that the surgeon does not have to reposition it in the hand or look up from the surgical site. It must be oriented correctly.

The position of the needle holder in relation to the suture needle depends on whether the surgeon is right-handed or left-handed. The long end of the suture should not come in contact with the surgeon's palm. It may be draped over the scrub's hand or allowed to hang downward (Figure 17-24).

The position of the needle holder in relation to the suture needle depends on:

- Whether the surgeon is right-handed or left-handed
- Whether the surgeon stands opposite the scrub or next to the scrub
- Whether the suture is back-handed

Regardless of where the surgeon stands in relation to the scrub, the needle must always be positioned so that it does not have to be repositioned for use. A left-handed surgeon sutures by driving the needle into the tissue in a counterclockwise direction. A right-handed surgeon drives the needle clockwise. *An exception to this is the back-handed suture, in which the direction is reversed.*

One method of learning the correct orientation of the mounted needle holder is to practice the movements as if you were the one suturing. Work with a colleague and position yourself as the surgeon would be. The logic of presenting the suture in correct spatial orientation will be immediately apparent.

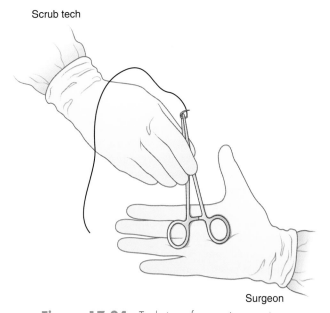

Figure 17-24 Technique for passing a suture.

Multiple Sutures

Since the adoption of swaged needles in surgery, the technique of rapid-sequence threading has been replaced by multiple needle-suture packs. The manner in which the needle is packaged often determines how quickly and safely sutures can be passed to the surgeon. More paper and many more needles are generated than in the past, increasing the risk of a lost or retained needle.

To prevent needle injury and keep pace with the surgeon, follow these guidelines:

1. Keep suture packs organized. Know where each type of suture is. As soon as a free needle is returned, immediately place it on the magnetic board or sharps holder.
2. Sutures are passed on an exchange basis. Have a loaded needle prepared at all times.
3. Load the needle holder before removing the entire needle-suture from its package.
4. Do not use the sponge bucket for suture wrappers. A needle may be lost among the sponges, and it is extra work for the circulator to pick out the wrappers.
5. If you find you are not keeping pace with the surgeon, try to focus on the job at hand and avoid becoming frustrated while working.

Suture Ties

Suture strands are available in precut or full-length strands ranging from 12 to 60 inches (30 cm to 1.5 m). The scrub must cut full-length sutures according to the surgeon's requirements. The following technique is used to cut full-length suture into thirds:

1. Remove the coiled suture from its package. Place the coil over one hand and pull the free end slowly to uncoil the strand.
2. Grasp each end of the strand and pull the center into thirds (Figure 17-25).

Continuous reels or rolls of suture are also used for repeated blood vessel ligation. The surgeon holds the reel and uses the amount needed. The reels contain 54 inches (135 cm) of suture material. When suture reels are used, the entire reel is passed (placed in the surgeon's palm). The surgeon usually replaces the reel in the Mayo tray after use, or the technologist can retrieve it from the surgical field after use.

A suture may be passed around a vessel or duct with a clamp. This type of tie is passed by securing one end of the suture to the end of the clamp. The clamp is passed in the normal manner, but the suture length should be draped over the scrub's hand in the same way a mounted needle is passed. If this type of tie is needed during a procedure, the surgeon may ask for a **tie on a passer** or simply a tie. The scrub is expected to assess whether a passer is required. Commonly a right-angle or long, curved clamp is used to pass a tie. When mounting a tie, insert the tip of the suture into the nose of the clamp (Figure 17-26).

Double-armed sutures are used on circular or tubular suture lines. When a double-armed suture is passed, only one needle is mounted on the needle holder. The surgical technologist must take care that the unsecured needle does not snag on drapes or other items on the surgical field.

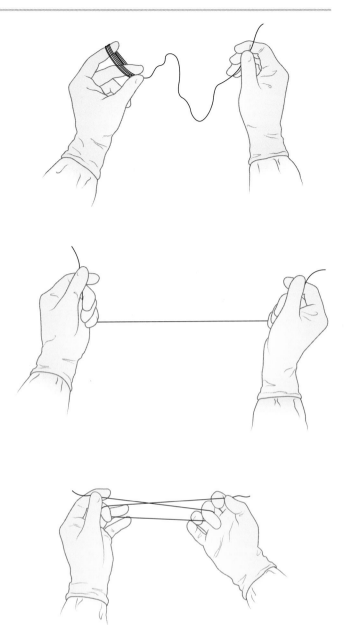

Figure 17-25 Dividing long suture into thirds. *(Redrawn from Phillips N: Berry and Kohn's operating room technique, ed 10, St Louis, 2004, Mosby.)*

Cutting Sutures

Occasionally the surgeon asks the surgical technologist to cut suture ends when tying a knot. When sutures are cut, the ends must be short to reduce the amount of foreign material in the wound, but long enough that the knot does not untie. When the suture is cut too short, the knot may actually be cut. If this happens, the surgeon replaces the suture with another.

The proper technique for cutting sutures is as follows:

1. Use only sharp suture scissors; never use tissue scissors on suture material.
2. To cut the suture, open the scissors slightly. Use the tip of the scissors to cut.
3. Hold the scissors as shown in Figure 17-27.
4. Place your index finger over the top of the scissors to steady the blades. Turn the scissors at a 45-degree angle.

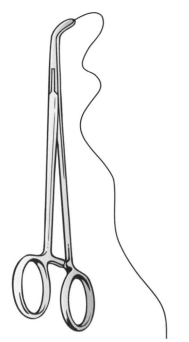

Figure 17-26   Suture tie on a passer. *(Redrawn from Phillips N: Berry and Kohn's operating room technique, ed 10, St Louis, 2004, Mosby.)*

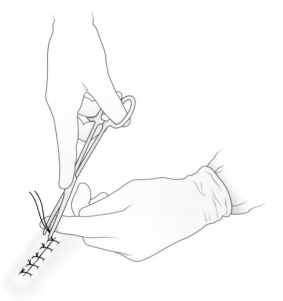

Figure 17-27   Cutting sutures. Note the use of the ring finger through the ring handle. This provides the best control on.

This creates a small "whisker." Cut the suture ends while keeping the scissors at an angle.

5. When cutting sutures and performing other tasks at the same time, it is convenient to "palm" the scissors in one hand (Figure 17-28).

6. Remove any cut suture ends from the wound area to prevent them from falling into the wound.

Suture Removal

When the surgeon needs to remove old (deep) sutures from a previous surgery, the knots usually are embedded in scar

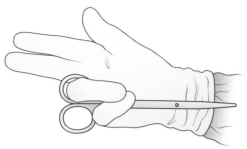

Figure 17-28   Palming the suture scissors.

tissue and may be difficult to grasp and cut. A straight, fine-tipped hemostat works best for pulling out old suture. The scrub should provide a towel into which the extracted suture pieces can be deposited so that they do not drop back into the wound.

SURGICAL STAPLING AND LIGATING DEVICES

Stapling

Surgical stapling instruments (Figure 17-29) are used to perform multiple suture and resection maneuvers. Staplers are available as single-use medical devices or as stainless steel instruments. Both types use manufactured cartridges or staples made of steel or nylon. The cutting assembly includes an anvil, which clamps the tissue against the staple cartridge. The cartridge contains staples that fire individually or together in single, double, triple, or quadruple lines. Surgical staples have many advantages:

* Tissue handling is greatly minimized, reducing trauma from manipulation and exposure.
* The suture lines are strong and dependable.
* The staples are nonreactive in tissue.
* The staples are noncrushing, preventing tissue necrosis from compromised blood and nutrient supply to the tissue edges.

The surgical technologist must become familiar with the proper handling of staplers and the loading of staple cartridges. Much aggravation can be prevented during surgery if the instruments are studied carefully before they are needed.

Several manufacturers make surgical stapling instruments. Each type of stapler is intended for a specific surgical technique and use. When passing a surgical stapling device, make sure any safety catch is activated to prevent accidental firing of staples. Any loose staples must be removed from the surgical site to prevent their loss in the wound. Remember that staples are sharp and must be handled with care. The most common types of surgical staplers are:

1. *Skin stapler:* Places a single line of staples across the incision border and is used for closing a skin incision.

2. *Ligation-dividing stapler* (LDS): Places a double row containing two staples in each row and severs the tissue between rows when fired.

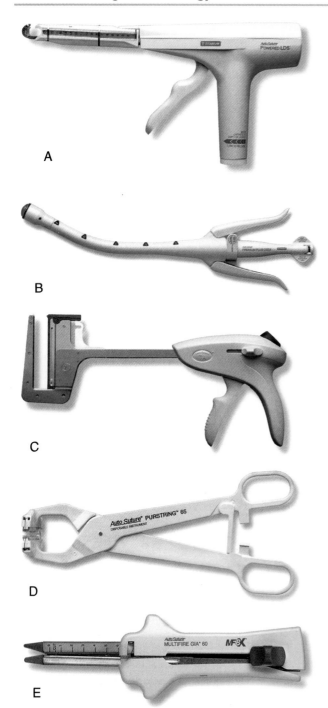

Figure 17-29 Surgical stapling instruments. **A,** Ligating and dividing (LDS). **B,** Circular or end to end (EEA). **C,** Thoracoabdominal (TA). **D,** Purse-string. **E,** Gastrointestinal anatomosis (GIA). *(Courtesy United States Surgical Corp., Norwalk, Conn.)*

3. *Circular* or *end-to-end (EEA) stapler:* Used for end-to-end intestinal resection (cutting and rejoining). It joins two arms of intestine with a double row of staples.
4. *Thoracoabdominal (TA) stapler:* Has a right-angle firing section that fits around deep structures for resection and anastomosis. It is commonly used in lung or abdominal surgery.

5. *Purse-string stapler:* Performs the same function as a purse-string suture and places circumferential nylon sutures and staples.

Hemostatic Clips

Hemostatic or vessel clips are small, V-shaped staples that close down and occlude a vessel or duct. Small, medium, and large clips are available in small cartridges that are color coded by size. Disposable and reusable systems are available. The size of the applier must be matched to the size of the clip. To load the vessel clip, grasp the proper-size clip applier at the hinge. Press the open jaws of the applier straight down over the clip; this locks the clip into the jaws (Figure 17-30). Pass the clip applier with the tip down, taking care not to squeeze the handles, which would release the clip prematurely. Clips are also available in biosynthetic materials.

SYNTHETIC TISSUE ADHESIVES

Fibrin Glue

Synthetic tissue adhesive is used to join wound edges without using sutures. It encourages the body's natural coagulation and healing process and provides adhesion during the healing process. Two cyanoacrylate products are available in dispenser form: Indermil (Covidien, Mansfield, Massachusetts) and Dermabond (Ethico, Somerville, New Jersey).

TISSUE IMPLANTS

Tissue implants are used to replace or augment the patient's own tissue. Tissue loss can be caused by a number of conditions and incidents, including trauma or injury, congenital deformity, surgical excision and resection, and any number of degenerative diseases. This loss of tissue can create a significant defect in the anatomy. Many of these tissues may be replaced or substituted with biological dressing, implanted materials, or synthetic prosthetic materials. Tissue grafts usually are obtained from a registered tissue bank (central location in the health facility or community) unless the tissue is from the patient's body. In this case, it may be used immediately or stored in the health care facility.

IMPORTANT TERMS

It is important for the surgical technologist to use the correct terms for tissue implants and grafts.

Allograft: A tissue graft derived from human tissue. Allografts are tested for infectious disease and infection before distribution from the tissue bank.

Autologous autograft: Tissue obtained from the patient's body and implanted in another site, such as a bone graft taken from the hip for implantation in the spine.

Bovine graft: Tissue graft of beef origin.

Epithelialization: The migration of epithelial cells into the wound during healing.

Implant: Any type of tissue replacement or device placed in the body.

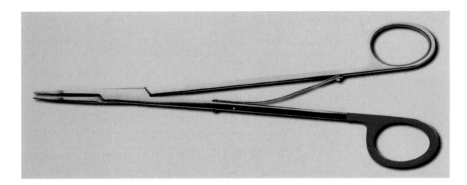

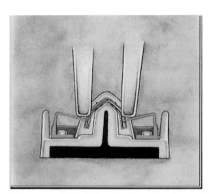

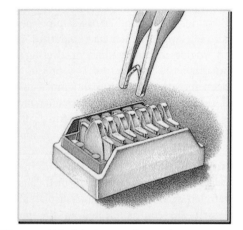

Figure 17-30 Loading the hemoclip (Weck clip). *(Courtesy Weck Industries, Research Triangle Park, N.C.).*

Porcine graft: Graft taken from pig tissue.

Wound cover: Tissue used to cover large defects in skin, usually a result of burns, trauma, or infection. Wound cover materials may be temporary until healing occurs.

Xenograft: A graft taken from a different species than that of the donor.

GRAFTS

Skin Grafts

Skin grafts are used to replace skin that has been destroyed by disease or injury. The skin is a critical barrier against infection and fluid loss. A skin substitute is needed to protect deep tissues from injury and contamination. Traditionally, skin grafts were taken only from the patient's own body, because these were the most successful. Now, other biological materials are available that can provide excellent protection again infection while reducing scarring and preventing fluid loss. Some grafting materials also aid the formation of granulation tissue in wounds. (The surgical techniques used in skin grafting are discussed fully in Chapter 29).

Porcine Dermis

Pig skin is used to temporarily cover a full-thickness injury. The graft does not develop vascularization. After 1 to 2 weeks, the graft sloughs. Porcine grafts are available in sheets and rolls and may be frozen, fresh, or dried. Some grafts are soaked in iodophor, and these should not be used on patients allergic to Betadine.

Amniotic Membrane

Amniotic membrane from human placentas can be used as a biological dressing for burns, skin ulcers, and infected wounds. This type of graft may also be used to cover spina bifida defects and in corneal surgery. The placenta has two layers or membranes: the *amnion,* which is used primarily in partial-thickness wounds, and the *chorion,* which is used primarily in full-thickness wounds. The amnion may be used fresh, frozen, or dried. Both membranes may be obtained from a tissue bank.

Engineered Skin Substitutes

Engineered skin substitutes (artificial skin) were created because of the lack of available human skin to cover large defects and wounds. All artificial skin has an outer layer that creates a barrier to infection, and many products include a dermal element that guides the cell during epithelialization. In addition to providing a barrier to infection, artificial skin reduces the severe pain associated with frequent dressing changes. It also decreases the risk of scar **contracture**.

Biobrane is a biosynthetic dressing made of a silicone film in which a nylon fabric is partially embedded. The matrix encourages blood clotting between the fibers, resulting in good contact until new skin growth takes place. Biobrane is used in clean burn wounds that do not require surgical excision (partial-thickness burns) and as a protective covering over a meshed autograft. It is not used in chronic wounds because it lacks antimicrobial properties.

TransCyte is a temporary skin substitute derived from human fibroblasts (cells that secrete collagen matrix material). It is frozen so that no cellular metabolic activity remains; however, essential structural proteins are intact. TransCyte typically is used as a temporary skin dressing before autografting over clean partial-thickness burns or for surgically excised, full-thickness and deep partial-thickness burns.

Integra Bilayer Matrix Wound Dressing is an immediate wound cover for partial- and full-thickness soft tissue injuries and chronic wounds. It is composed of a semipermeable polysiloxane (silicone) layer that acts like epidermis. It controls fluid loss and provides a flexible, adherent covering that resists shearing and tearing. The structure is a porous matrix of bovine collagen and glycosaminoglycan (similar to the structure of a cell wall). This creates a bed for cellular and capillary growth. It is replaced by a split-thickness skin graft.

Integra Dermal Regeneration Template is an alternative to allografting. It is the only approved skin substitute that regenerates the dermis. The template is positioned on the skin, and a 0.05-inch epidermal autograft is performed. The template must be protected against shearing and displacement. Both Integra products are contraindicated in the presence of infection.

Cultured epithelial autograft (*Epicel*) (Genzyme, Cambridge, Massachusetts) is an epidermal replacement generated from a biopsy of skin taken from the patient. Keratinocytes are duplicated in 2 to 3 weeks.

Foreskin grafts are obtained from neonates and used as a temporary skin barrier in the treatment of noninfected skin ulcers. *Apligraf* has two layers, a human-derived epidermis and bovine collagen dermis. The epidermis provides a barrier while the dermal layer heals. Apligraf is gradually replaced by host cells, which eliminates the need for additional split-thickness skin grafting.

Bone Graft

Bone grafts are used for structural support and to stimulate new bone growth in a defect caused by trauma or a congenital anomaly. Two types of bone are used for grafting, cancellous bone and cortical bone. Cancellous bone is porous, and tissue fluid can reach deep into it, allowing most of the bone cells to live. Cortical bone is very rigid and strong. It typically is used to repair skeletal defects because of its strength. Cortical bone is fixed into position with metal sutures or plates and screws. Many types of bone grafts can be done:

- *Autologous grafts:* Grafts made from the patient's body.
- *Allogenic grafts:* Grafts made from nonliving cadaver bone.
- *Composite grafts:* Grafts made of a combination of cadaver bone, morcelized allograft bone, and marrow.
- *Demineralized bone matrix (DBM):* A processed material made from collagen, protein, and growth factors. It is used as granules, chips, putty, or a gel.
- *Ceramic materials:* These provide structural support only.
- *Graft composites:* Grafts that contain combinations of DBM and marrow, ceramic-collagen, and ceramic-autograft-collagen combinations.

Umbilical Cord

Human umbilical cord is used in vascular surgery to replace an artery when saphenous autografting is not feasible.

SYNTHETIC IMPLANTS

Most tissue implants are derived from synthetic or biopolymer materials. Examples include artificial heart valves, pacemakers, and artificial joints. Implants are regulated by the FDA and are approved as medical devices after rigorous testing. Implants must meet certain criteria for a successful surgical outcome. They must be:

- Compatible with body tissue.
- Available as a sterile product or able to withstand a sterilization process.
- Proven safe and nonpathogenic.
- Able to provide adequate tissue coverage and vascularization around the implant.
- Able to provide adequate stability for the intended use.

The process for sterilizing implants is discussed in Chapter 8.

Metal

Stainless steel, vitalium, titanium, and other alloys have been used in the manufacture of orthopedic implants for many years. The materials are strong, resilient, and inert. Polyetheretherketone (PEEK) polymer reinforces the implant and prevents leakage and wear.

Methylethacrylate

Synthetic bone cement frequently is used to secure prosthetic implants into bone and for remodeling during cranioplasty. Bone cement is mixed on the sterile field using two components, methylmethacrylate powder and a volatile liquid. Because the fumes created by the chemical mixture are toxic, the cement must be mixed in a special closed container. The manufacturer's recommendations for proper mixing and safety precautions should be followed.

Resorbable Implants

Synthetic polymer implants composed of polyglactic acid (PLA) polymer currently are used in orthopedic and maxillofacial surgery. The newer generation of biopolymers manufactured from recombinant deoxyribonucleic acid (DNA) technology also has been approved for surgical use, including implants.

Polyethylene

Porous polyethylene implants are often used in facial reconstruction. The porous nature of the implant allows for both soft tissue and vascular ingrowth. As collagen grows into the implant, the framework of the implant becomes stronger.

Silicone

Silicone and Silastic are two very common implant materials. They are relatively inert and durable. Implants are available in many forms, including gel, sponge, film, tubing, liquid, and sheets. These implants should not be handled with bare hands, and care should be taken to ensure that they do not pick up lint or dust, because any foreign material can cause an inflammatory reaction around the implant.

Woven Synthetics

Vascular grafts are made from a number of woven synthetic materials. These include Dacron, polytetrafluoroethylene (PTFE), and polyester.

WOUND DRAINAGE AND DRESSINGS

WOUND DRAINAGE

Purpose

The presence of fluid in a surgical wound can delay healing and cause infection. Fluid sometimes accumulates as part of the inflammatory process or as a result of oozing from small capillaries. The accumulation of serosanguinous fluid (blood and serum) becomes a medium for microbial growth. To prevent this, a wound drain is inserted in selected cases before closure.

Surgery of the thoracic cavity removes negative pressure, which must be restored and maintained until the wound is closed and secure. This is done with closed chest drainage.

Surgery of the bile system or genitourinary tract may require drainage from a duct or tube. In this case, a tubular drain is threaded into the structure for a short period.

All but very simple drainage systems require a reservoir to collect the fluid. This prevents the spread of infection and allows measurement and analysis to determine the progress of healing. Drains are placed in the wound before complete closure. The surgical technologist should be familiar with common drainage systems.

Passive Drains

A passive drain creates a passage from the tissue inside the wound to the outside of the body. These usually are placed when drainage is minimal. The *Penrose* drain is a simple tubular length of nonlatex material similar to surgical glove material. Before closing, the surgeon places the drain loosely in the wound and secures it with sutures. A gauze dressing is placed over the drain to collect fluid from the wound.

A gravity drain is used in wounds or hollow structures that produce significant amounts of fluid but do not require suction for removal. Examples of gravity drainage are the *T-tube, Pezzer*, Malecot, and Foley catheters. The T-tube is used specifically for bile duct drainage and is connected to a bile bag by a length of clear tubing. The *Foley catheter*, and *Malecot* drains provide continuous drainage after genitourinary surgery. Various other types of ureteral drainage tubes may also be used after surgery of the kidney or ureter; these are discussed Chapter 25.

Suction Drains

A suction drain pulls serum and blood from the wound by a negative pressure device. A tube is placed in the center of the wound and connected to a one-way valve in the drain reservoir. Air is evacuated from the container by squeezing it to activate the negative pressure and the wound tubing attached. Two common suction drains are the Hemovac (Figure 17-31), and the Jackson-Pratt drain (Figure 17-32).

Water-Sealed Drainage System

A water-sealed drainage system is used to pull fluid or air from the thoracic cavity after thoracic surgery or trauma to the thorax. The thoracic cavity is under negative pressure. The difference between atmospheric pressure and thoracic pressure allows the lungs to expand normally. Loss of negative pressure causes the lung to collapse. After surgery or a penetrating injury to the chest wall, negative pressure must be restored. The underwater drainage system performs this task.

The drainage system has three separate water chambers sealed in a plastic unit. One or more chest drainage tubes are placed in the thorax and connected to the drainage system. When suction is applied to one of the chambers, air or fluid is pulled into the collection system. Each of the remaining chambers contains a small amount of water, which prevents the loss of negative pressure in the thoracic cavity (Figure 17-33).

When any drainage system is in use, the collection unit must remain below the level of the insertion tube. This prevents fluids from re-entering the drainage space. Chest drainage systems must never be allowed to back up into the thorax, because this can cause immediate collapse of a lung. When a patient with an underwater chest drainage system is transferred, the system must be kept upright. If the collection system falls over, it should be righted and checked for cracks. Make sure all tubes and connections are tight. If any doubt exists about the integrity of the system, seek help immediately.

DRESSINGS

Functions

Sterile wound dressings are placed over the incision site at the close of surgery. Many types of wound dressings are available, each with a specific purpose. For example, dressings:

- Prevent environmental contamination of the incision
- Collect exudate from the wound
- Provide mechanical support of the operative site
- Prevent the accumulation of necrotic tissue
- Provide continuous contact with an antiseptic or antibacterial agent

Elaborate dressings have multiple components. In most cases, the initial layer comes in direct contact with the wound. Additional dressings are added to protect and support the operative site.

Dressing Materials

Materials in direct contact with the surgical wound usually have a nonstick surface. Telfa and various petroleum-based

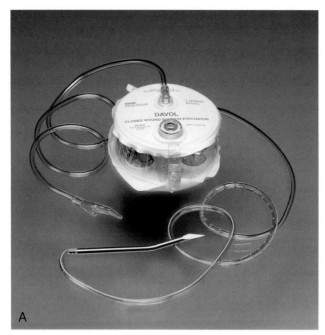

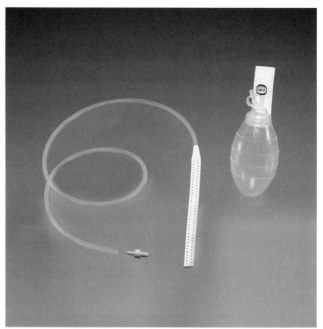

Figure 17-32 Jackson-Pratt suction-reservoir drain. The perforated tubing is placed inside the surgical wound, and the distal end is connected to the hand suction device. *(From Rothrock JC: Alexander's care of the patient in surgery, ed 13, St Louis, 2007, Mosby.)*

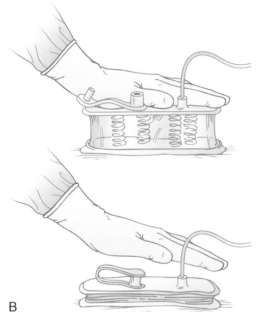

Figure 17-31 **A,** Hemovac suction drain. The proximal end of the drain tubing is placed in the open surgical wound. The distal end is attached to the metal trocar. This is used to make a tunnel for the tubing. **B,** The tubing is connected to the reservoir. After wound closure, the reservoir is compressed, creating suction within the wound and drawing fluid out. *(A from Rothrock JC: Alexander's care of the patient in surgery, ed 13, St Louis, 2007, Mosby; B redrawn from Phillips N: Berry and Kohn's operating room technique, ed 10, St Louis, 2004, Mosby.)*

products are impregnated into gauze to prevent the edges from splitting when the dressing is removed.

Flat dressings generally are made with loose gauze fabric. Absorbent gauze "fluffs" can be used to cushion the wound site and provide extra protection. Absorbent dressings are layered over the primary dressing and designed to isolate wound exudate. The *ABD* (abdominal) pad is a large absorbent dressing used to cover draining wounds (Figure 17-34, *A*).

Rolled dressing materials are used for wrapping a limb. They may be plain gauze or an elasticized material (Figure 17-34, *B*). Kling gauze is very pliable and soft and can be molded over a limb to provide uniform coverage. Elastic roller bandage is used when compression is needed. *Elastoplast* roller bandage is a highly adherent dressing that provides compression and mild support to the wound. *Tube stockinet* is a thin, socklike sleeve that fits over the limb to protect a gauze bandage or provide protection under a plaster cast.

Gauze packing is used in a cavity, such as the nose or an open wound. It is available in a long, thin strip and packaged in a bottle or similar container. This type of dressing usually is removed early in the recovery period, because it can rapidly become a source of infection.

Ointments and other medicines are not usually applied over a surgical wound. However, the dressing itself may be impregnated with an antibacterial agent, such as iodophor or povidone (*Xeroform, Nu Gauze*) (Figure 17-34, *C*). These are used only when infection is a risk. Narrow gauze strips used are used for this purpose (Figure 17-34, *D*).

Adhesive tape is needed for most dressings. Tape is used to secure a flat dressing. Paper "silk" tape is lightweight and has minimal adhesive properties. Plastic tape is pliable and has more adhesive strength. Cloth tape is seldom used for surgical wounds.

Steri-Strips are used to approximate small incisions and protect the wound. These are used in minor surgery and for minor wounds (Figure 17-35). A small amount of biological adhesive, such as benzoin liquid or spray, may be applied to the skin for extra adhesion before the strips are applied. In

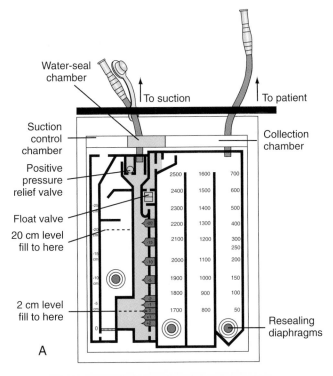

Water-seal chamber

To suction | To patient

Suction control chamber

Collection chamber

Positive pressure relief valve

Float valve

20 cm level fill to here

2 cm level fill to here

Resealing diaphragms

A

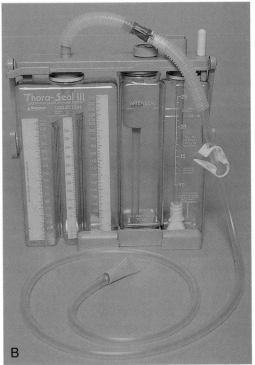

B

Figure 17-33 Underwater sealed chest drainage. **A,** Pleur-evac disposable chest suction system. **B,** *(A from Lew SM, Heitkemper MM, Kirksen SE: Medical-surgical nursing: assessment and management of clinical problems, ed 6, St Louis, 2004, Mosby; B from Elkin MK, Perry AG, Potter PA: Nursing interventions and clinical skills, ed 3, St Louis, 2004, Mosby.)*

some minor wounds, Steri-Strips serve as a dressing because they protect the incision line.

A simple occlusive film dressing (*OpSite*) is one that prevents most environmental exposure. The film is semipermeable to air but prevents direct contact with the incision site.

Film dressing is contraindicated for use in deep cavity wounds and is and is and is normally used on superficial wounds, burns, and abrasions.

SIMPLE AND COMPOSITE DRESSINGS

Flat Dressing

The most common and simplest type of surgical wound dressing is a thin, nonstick pad covered by one or two layers of flat gauze secured with tape. Additional layers of gauze or ABD pad are used if the surgeon anticipates drainage. If a mechanical drain has been inserted into the wound, layers of absorbent gauze are placed around the drain. An ABD pad may be placed over this and secured with tape.

Pressure Dressing

A pressure dressing most often is used over a skin graft. The graft must remain in close contact with the underlying tissue to retain its vitality and become integrated into the new site. Slight pressure on the graft site prevents serous fluid from lifting the skin graft away from the recipient site. A stent dressing is a type of pressure dressing in which gauze or other material is molded into a thick pad that fits the graft area. Sutures are placed around the graft site. The long suture ends are then tied over the pad to secure it in place (Figure 17-36).

Support Dressing

Supportive dressings are used to prevent or limit movement of the surgical wound during healing. Orthopedic procedures often require the use of supportive dressings and appliances. Thick cotton covered with stretch gauze is used for soft support. Hard casting materials are used when complete immobility is required. (Casting and other orthopedic techniques are discussed in Chapter 30)

WOUND HEALING AND COMPLICATIONS

CLASSIFICATION OF WOUNDS

The wound healing process (Figure 17-37) is classified according to whether it is clean or contaminated, sutured or left open. Surgical wounds are classified by the potential risk for infection (Box 17-2).

A surgical wound that is sutured together heals by **primary intention**. This means that the cut tissue edges are in direct contact.

A wound that is not sutured must heal by **secondary intention**. This type of wound heals from the base. The healing process involves filling the tissue gap with granulation tissue. It is much slower, and the resulting scar can be quite large compared with primary intention closure. Sometimes a skin graft is necessary because the wound is too large to heal without risk of contamination and infection. Wounds that are infected or grossly contaminated (e.g., those caused by a traumatic injury) also require secondary intention healing.

Third intention healing, or delayed closure, is a process in which an infected or a contaminated wound is treated and the

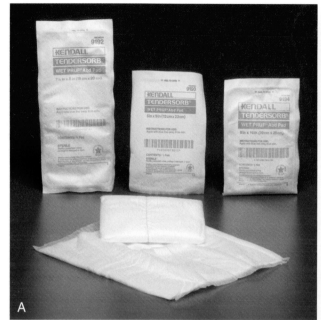

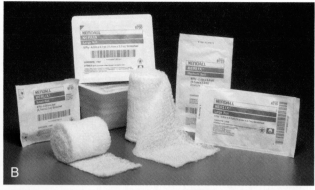

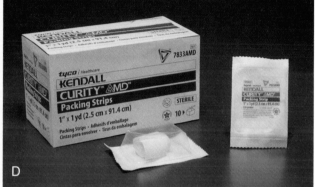

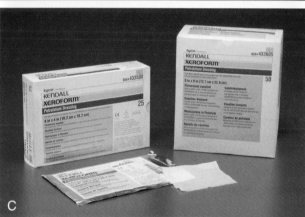

Figure 17-34 A, ABD pad used for draining wounds. **B,** Rolled dressing material. **C,** Dressings with antibacterial agents. **D,** Gauze strips. *(Copyright © 2008 Covidien. All rights reserved. Reprinted with permission of Covidien.)*

wound space is packed to prevent serum accumulation and to protect it against environmental exposure. When sufficient granulation tissue has filled in the wound, it is sutured.

PROCESS OF WOUND HEALING

Two types of tissue repair occur naturally. Parenchymal tissue heals by replication of special cells. Parenchymal cells are found in epithelial tissue, such as the mucous membranes, fallopian tubes, vagina, gastrointestinal tract, and urinary tract. Bone marrow cells are also parenchymal cells. Other cells, such as those found in the liver, also multiply, but division stops once growth and development are complete. These tissues are referred to as *stable cells*.

The permanent cells of the body do not regenerate or divide when they are injured. Permanent cells make up muscles (including heart muscle) and nerves. Tissues that cannot regenerate or repair themselves are replaced by connective tissue after injury. This connective tissue is com-

monly called *scar tissue*. Scar tissue has few of the characteristics of the original tissue. It has none of the special functions of the permanent cells, such as nerve transmission or secretion. It simply fills the gap left by the injury. The process of tissue repair involves the growth and modeling of scar tissue.

PHASES OF HEALING

The healing process, which involves the growth of new cells and replacement with connective tissue, is divided into three primary phases: the inflammatory phase, the proliferative phase, and remodeling. Under normal healing conditions, these phases progress naturally from the moment of injury until the wound is healed.

Inflammatory Phase

The inflammatory phase of healing begins as soon as tissue is injured. The natural process of hemostasis described previ-

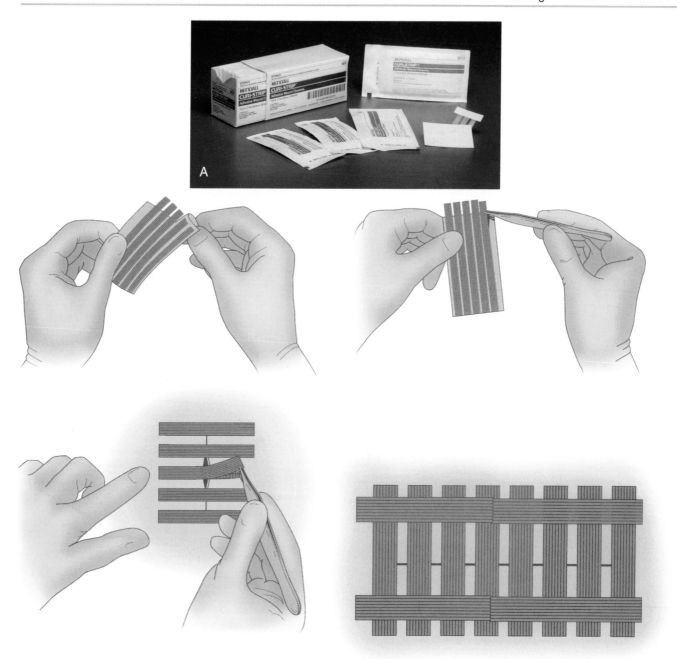

Figure 17-35 **A,** Skin closure strips packaged. **B,** Skin closure strips in use. (**A** Copyright © 2008 Covidien. All rights reserved. Reprinted with permission of Covidien. Covidien, Mansfield, Mass; **B** from Rothrock JC: Alexander's care of the patient in surgery, ed 13, 2007, Mosby.)

ously begins the healing process. Inflammation, platelet aggregation, and the formation of a scab are followed by the cellular phase.

During inflammation, phagocytes migrate to the wound site and digest excess fibrin, bacteria, and cell fragments, a process that usually takes 3 to 4 days. The phagocytes are replaced by macrophages, which remain in the wound for a much longer period. Macrophages attract fibroblasts and release growth factors, which initiate the proliferation of epithelial cells and the growth of new blood vessels. During this period, tissue debris is continually removed by the macrophages.

Proliferative Phase

The proliferative phase begins about day 4 or 5 and continues for approximately 2 weeks.

During this phase, fibroblasts synthesize **collagen** and other cell matrices. These form the ground substance of the new tissue, providing support and strength. This new tissue is called *granulation tissue*. Epithelial cells begin to form at the edges of the wound and migrate to the middle, forming a new wound surface. When sufficient epithelial cells have filled in the wound, the scab sloughs away, leaving the new layer. Wound strength increases steadily, and sutures are removed at the end of this phase.

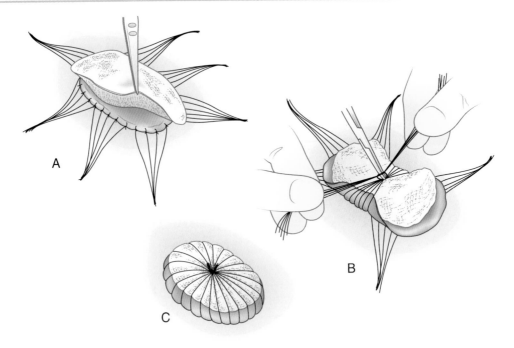

Figure 17-36 Stent dressing used to cover a skin graft.

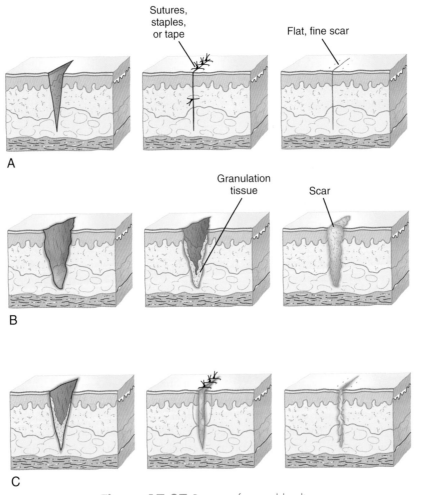

Figure 17-37 Process of wound healing.

Box 17-2
Wound Classification

Clean Wound (1% to 5% Risk of Postoperative Infection)

Example
Total hip replacement, vitrectomy, nerve resection

Characteristics
Uninfected
Clean
No inflammation
Closed primarily (all tissue layers sutured closed)
Respiratory, gastrointestinal, genital, and uninfected urinary tracts were not entered.
May contain closed drainage system.

Clean-Contaminated Wound (3% to 7% Risk of Postoperative Infection)

Example
Cystoscopy, gastric bypass, and removal of oral lesions

Characteristics
Respiratory, gastrointestinal, genital, and urinary tracts were entered without unusual contamination.
No evidence of infection or major break in aseptic technique.
Includes surgery of the biliary tract, appendix, vagina, and oropharynx.

Contaminated Wound (10% to 17% Risk of Postoperative Infection)

Example
Removal of perforated appendix, removal of metal fragments related to an explosion

Characteristics
Open, fresh, accidental wound.
Major break in aseptic technique occurred during the surgical procedure.
Gross spillage from the gastrointestinal tract occurred.
Presence of acute, nonpurulent inflammation.

Dirty or Infected Wound (>27% Risk of Postoperative Infection)

Example
Incision and drainage of an abscess

Characteristics
Old traumatic wounds with devitalized tissue
Existing clinical infection
Perforated viscera

Remodeling

The last stage of wound repair begins after about 3 weeks. During the remodeling phase, which lasts 22 days to 1 year, the collagen is continually replaced and absorbed in stress areas. As the wound heals, it contracts slightly. However, large wounds (e.g., those caused by a burn injury on the back, buttocks, or posterior neck) contract as they heal. Contracted tissue prevents mobility and causes cosmetic defects. The contracture can be released surgically or prevented with physical therapy and the use of specialized dressings during healing. When the proliferation of collagen is excessive, the **scar** is called a **keloid**. Keloids most commonly develop in individuals of African descent.

CONDITIONS THAT AFFECT WOUND HEALING

Complications can occur anytime in the wound healing process but usually are evident in the first week after surgery. Wound complications can occur at the surface incision or in deep tissue, resulting in delayed healing or breakdown of the wound.

Immune System

The body's ability to heal depends on the immune response. Radiotherapy and other types of cancer therapy lower immune resistance, retard healing, and increase the risk of postoperative infection.

Chronic Disease

Diabetes, endocrine disease, and vascular disease are examples of chronic diseases that affect the healing process. A patient with a chronic disease is physiologically stressed before surgery. Tissues may be weakened, and cellular metabolism may be compromised.

Nutritional Status

During healing, the body uses extra nutrients in the form of protein for repair and carbohydrates for cellular energy. These must be continuously available throughout the healing process. A debilitated or nutritionally depleted patient may not have the reserves for this extra metabolic activity. Extensive burns and trauma require particularly high levels of nutrients for healing.

Obesity

An obese patient is at high risk for surgical complications. Added tension on the surgical site can result in incisional failure. Adipose tissue has a poor blood supply, which decreases vascularity to the wound site and prevents the cellular oxygenation and nutrition necessary for healing. The poor ventilation and respiratory deficiency common to obese patients also contribute to wound complications.

Age

The mechanisms of healing tend to become impaired as a person ages. The blood supply to tissues is reduced, which decreases oxygenation of the cells. Metabolism generally is slowed, and this affects the body's ability to regenerate tissue and build the collagen necessary for healing. Increased physiological stress can predispose an elderly patient to infection or other complications.

Surgical Technique

The surgical technique affects the health status of wound tissues. Rough handling or failure to irrigate tissues adequately during surgery can result in tissue breakdown in the postop-

Table 17-3

Dressings and Specialty Wound Care Products

Name	Other Names	Type	Description	Uses
Surgical Dressings				
Sterile gauze square	Gauze sponge Flat dressing Gauze dressing "Flat" "Topper"	Flat surgical dressing	Lightweight gauze folded into squares; sterile	For an uncomplicated surgical incision with no drainage. Used in combination with nonadherent layer and surgical tape.
Telfa pad	Telfa	Nonadherent flat fabric pad	Square of compact, felted material with an outer covering of Telfa; used for its nonstick properties.	Clean surgical wound. Also used in surgery for care of specimens.
Clear Telfa	Clear Telfa	Nonadherent flat wound covering	Single-layer clear Telfa	Used to cover delicate incisions when a nonadherent surface is required (e.g., burns, skin grafts).
Gauze fluff	Fluffs "Bulky dressing" Kerlix fluff	Diamond weave, flat wound dressing folded many times	Diamond weave, crimped, soft gauze square of synthetic material folded into squares; can be unfolded and "fluffed" to increase loft	Used to provide soft padding and drainage in simple draining wounds or in delicate surgical repair (e.g., hand surgery).
Transparent film dressing	Film; also various brand names	Film dressing	Single-layer clear adhesive square	Used primarily for intravenous (IV) sites; also used for donor skin graft sites, ulcers.
Cotton sponge	Dermacea Cotton prep sponge	100% Cotton flat sponge	Flat gauze sponge with wide "crimped" diamond weave; 100% cotton for lint-free use	For lint-free prepping and wound packing.
ABD pad	Combine dressing "Bulky dressing" ABD	Nonwoven, padded dressing	Oversize square pad; nonwoven material is contained in a lightweight, smooth outer covering that may be water repellent	Used for draining wounds when absorption is required.
Vaseline gauze	Petrolatum gauze	Impregnated nonadherent gauze	Gauze strip impregnated with Vaseline or similar petrolatum substance	Used to cover delicate incisions where tearing of tissue would disrupt repair (e.g., hand, face, minor burns, skin graft, circumcision).
Xeroform gauze	Xeroform dressing	Impregnated nonadherent gauze	Gauze strip or square impregnated with 3% bismuth tribromophenate	Used as for other nonadherent dressings; has bacteriostatic properties*; promotes moisture.
Webril	Webril Rolled cast padding	Rolled bandage; nonsterile	Soft, felted, 100% cotton	Used under pneumatic tourniquet and casts for padding and protection.
Roll gauze	Rolled gauze Roller gauze Bandage Rolled bandage	Sterile rolled gauze bandage	Gauze bandage roll, small to medium-size weave made of synthetic or 100% cotton; molds easily to shape	Used to overwrap surgical wound on a limb. Also used in conjunction with flat dressings and other padded dressings.
Kerlix rolled gauze	Kerlix Kerlix roll Kerlix roller gauze	Sterile, rolled gauze bandage	Crimped, rolled gauze bandage with a wide diamond weave	As for *roll gauze*. Diamond weave permits ease of conforming around limb.

Table 17-3

Dressings and Specialty Wound Care Products—cont'd

Name	Other Names	Type	Description	Uses
Gauze packing	Adaptic Packing strips Gauze packing	Gauze packing material	Narrow, fine weave gauze in a continuous strip; may be impregnated with a bacteriostatic agent* or petrolatum	Used for packing sinus structures, fistula tracts, or wounds healing by third intention. Single long strip allows incremental placement in the wound.
Compression bandage	Stretch bandage Ace wrap Elastic bandage	Nonsterile, rolled compression bandage	Elasticized roller bandage can be supplied as lightweight stretch gauze or heavier stretch cloth; secured with clips or tape or may be self-adhering	Used as a pressure dressing for limbs. Used over a gauze dressing or other type of dressing in direct contact with surgical wound.

Specialty Wound Care

Name	Other Names	Type	Description	Uses
Hydrocolloid	Hydrocolloid; also known by brand names	Hydrocolloid occlusive gel dressing	Contains gel-forming agents in a foam or film; self-adhesive and occlusive; adheres to wet or dry wound	Used in clean, granulating wounds with little drainage. Promotes healing by providing moisture and barrier to bacterial invasion. Also, absorbs moisture. May be used in conjunction with sterile maggot therapy.
Intersorb Mesh	Intersorb	Wide mesh burn dressing	Layered, wide mesh gauze made of 100% cotton for lint-free surface	Used as a specialty dressing for burns.
Hydrogel gauze	Hydrogen dressing	Hydrogel-impregnated dressing	Gauze square or strips impregnated with Hydrogel	Hydrogel provides moisture in the wound and supports natural lysis and absorption of necrotic tissue. Can be conformed to fit the wound.
Moist gauze	Sodium chloride dressing Wet-to-dry dressing Wet dressing	Wet-to-dry dressing	Saline-moistened, loosely woven gauze squares	Used to pack the wound and mechanically debride tissue. When gauze packing has dried, it is removed, pulling away necrotic or devitalized tissue.
Foam dressing	Foam	Padded, nonadherent dressing	Soft foam material covered with smooth, nonadherent coating	Used to cushion and protect chronic wounds and absorb exudate. Commonly used in pressure sores.
Alginates	Alginate dressing	Protective gel dressing	Gel dressing made from seaweed that is highly absorbent and biodegradable; rinses easily with saline solution	Used in deep wounds, fistulas, venous and diabetic ulcers, burns and pressure ulcers. Provides moisture and enhances epithelialization.

*Antibiotic ointments (e.g., "triple antibiotic") are no longer recommended for use on surgical wounds. Bacteriostatic agents are preferred, and these are indicated only in selected cases.

erative period. Retractors that bruise and macerate tissue can cause healing complications at the wound's edges. These can lead to *tissue edema* (fluid accumulation in interstitial spaces) and inflammation of the peritoneal layer. Inflammation causes the release of serosanguinous fluid, which becomes a medium for infection. Tissue layers must be approximated in anatomical position to prevent *dead space*, where serum can accumulate. Excessive stress on suture points can tear and bruise tissue and is very uncomfortable for the patient. All these factors contribute to postsurgical complications.

WOUND COMPLICATIONS

Surgical Site Infection

Postoperative (surgical site) infection can occur anytime in the healing process but is more likely in the first week. The first signs of infection are excess inflammation and serous discharge from the wound. At this stage, medical and nursing personnel take immediate action to halt the process of infection.

A variety of debriding agents and dressings, in addition to meticulous care of the wound, contributes to treating a surgical site infection. However, if the infection threatens to become systemic, the patient is prescribed antibiotics and may require aggressive wound care. This includes continuous wound irrigation, **debridement**, and holistic care to improve the patient's nutritional status. Wound drainage is an important factor in the healing of an infected wound. Closed suction drainage may be required to flush the wound of bacteria, pus, and tissue debris. Infections that penetrate the body wall (abdominal wall, thoracic cavity) can become life-threatening as vital organs are involved. At this level, the patient may require critical care and must face a very long and difficult recovery period.

Seroma and Hematoma

A *seroma* is a collection of fluid that develops in the wound during healing. The seroma acts as a physical barrier between the wound's edges and prevents healing. A *hematoma* is a collection of blood that forms in a surgical wound because of incomplete hemostasis during surgery. In addition to the dangers arising from an unsecured blood vessel, a hematoma increases the risk of wound infection. With both seromas and hematomas, re-entry of the wound may be required to resolve the problem.

Dehiscence

Tissue breakdown at the wound margins is called **dehiscence**. Inflammation is evident, and some serous fluid or pus may be present. Dehiscence can occur at the skin margins or may extend to deeper tissue layers. Complex infected wounds can take weeks or months to heal. A complication of infection is fistula formation. A *fistula* is a tract that leads from the point of infection to a point of eruption outside the body. One or more fistulas may form.

If infection is present, the dressing routine may be altered. A moist dressing sometimes is applied and allowed to dry between dressing changes. The dry dressing pulls away dead tissue and exudate. Many types of dressings are used in the treatment of wounds (Table 17-3).

Wound breakdown can lead to abdominal wall defects that require surgery. Scars formed after wound breakdown have little strength compared to healthy tissue, and the anatomical planes are disrupted. This can lead to a hernia or rupture in the body wall under the intact skin.

Evisceration

Evisceration is dehiscence with protrusion of the abdominal contents outside the wound. Evisceration requires immediate action to replace and hydrate the extruded tissues and prevent necrosis. Abdominal evisceration can involve a portion of the bowel or omentum. If the dehiscence is small, the viscera may slide through the defect or become trapped by it, resulting in necrosis.

Adhesions

An **adhesion** is a band of scar tissue between the abdominal or pelvic organs and the peritoneum. Adhesions usually are associated with infection or multiple abdominal surgeries. Adhesions can cause pain and discomfort. They also increase the risk of injury to organs during surgery.

CHAPTER SUMMARY

- Hemostasis is a primary goal during surgery. In technical terms, *hemostasis* means controlling bleeding with sutures, surgical instruments, thermal energy (e.g., electrosurgery), and drugs. In physiological terms, it means conserving the body's total blood volume, which is necessary for life.
- The physiological process of coagulation involves many chemical factors in an elaborate feedback mechanism. If any of the factors are missing, through genetic anomaly or disease, hemostasis is altered.
- Topical hemostatic agents are commonly used in the surgical wound to stop capillary bleeding.

- Blood vessels are coagulated using thermal and high-frequency coagulation and suture ligatures.
- The pneumatic tourniquet is used to create a bloodless field in limb surgery. The procedures and safety protocols for use of a tourniquet prevent vascular, nerve, and tissue damage.
- Suture materials are used to approximate tissues (hold tissue together by suture) while healing takes place and to ligate (tie) blood vessels or tubal structures.
- Sutures are regulated by the same standards as drugs because they are used in the body.

- The structure and properties of a particular suture type determine how and where it is used in the surgical wound.
- The handling qualities of a suture determine its ease of use and may affect the technical quality of the wound closure.
- *Bioactivity* is the body's response to suture. The bioactivity depends on the chemical structure of the suture material and the condition of the patient.
- *Absorption* describes how the suture reacts in the presence of body tissue.
- Absorbable suture is digested by cellular enzymes and absorbed within days or months. Nonabsorbable suture resists breakdown and may remain intact for years.
- Absorbable sutures are made of synthetic, natural, and biosynthetic materials.
- Nonabsorbable sutures are made of synthetic and natural materials.
- Surgical needles are made of high quality steel alloy and are available in many shapes and sizes.
- Suture needles have three distinct parts: the eye, the body, and the point.
- Atraumatic, or swaged, needles are continuous with the suture material. The suture material is incorporated into the shaft of the needle.
- A detachable needle is one in which the suture comes away from the needle when it is pulled straight back from the swage.
- A double-armed needle is used for suturing circular or tubular structures, such as in vascular or intestinal surgery.
- Needle curvature relates to the body and radius of the needle. The curve is measured as a circumferential fraction in a complete circle.
- Needle size is measured by the diameter of the shaft and the dimension from tip to eye.
- The needle point and body are designed for minimal trauma in specific types of tissue.
- Suture packaging is designed for ease of selection and rapid delivery.

- Suture handling is one of the primary skills of surgical technology. It involves preparing, passing, and anticipating the correct type of suture-needle combination during surgery.
- Safety concerns associated with sutures are the risk of needlestick injury and loss of a needle in the surgical wound.
- Stapling devices are commonly used in open and endoscopic surgery. Surgical staples can eliminate the need for multiple sutures in some types of surgery.
- Tissue implants are used to replace or augment the patient's own tissue
- Skin grafts are used to replace skin that has been destroyed by disease or injury. Materials used for grafting include natural skin from the patient's own body or from a cadaver (banked skin) or an animal, as well as biosynthetic and synthetic materials.
- Most tissue implants are derived from synthetic or biopolymer materials. These include resorbable implants, metal, polyethylene, silicone, and other synthetic polymers.
- Wound drains are used to prevent the accumulation of body fluids and blood in the surgical wound during the healing process.
- A closed water-sealed drainage device is used when the thoracic cavity has been entered. The drainage system is used to maintain negative pressure and allow the lungs to expand.
- Dressings are used primarily to protect the surgical wound, collect exudate, or provide mechanical support.
- The wound healing process comprises distinct phases, which are first triggered by the immune system. These include the inflammatory, proliferative, and remodeling phases.
- Wound healing can be complicated by many factors, including disease, poor nutrition, fluid and electrolyte imbalance, obesity, and age.
- Complications in wound healing can be prevented by strict aseptic technique, good surgical technique on the part of the surgeon, proper postoperative care, and maintaining the patient's overall well-being.

REVIEW QUESTIONS

1. Explain how suture is sized.
2. Name four types of surgical needles.
3. How are sutures regulated in the United States?
4. What is the function of a double-armed suture?
5. What is the purpose of a suture ligature?
6. Define allograft; autograft; Xenograft; autologous; and allogenic.
7. List the functions of a dressing.
8. What is the purpose of a surgical drain?
9. Explain negative pressure in the thoracic cavity and how water-sealed drainage is used to restore this after surgery.
10. What is dehiscence? How is it different from evisceration?

CASE STUDIES

Case 1

The surgeon asks you for size 2-0 silk suture. After you have given the surgeon the suture, you realize that you have mistakenly passed a 3-0 suture. The surgeon has already inserted the suture and is about to tie it. What will you do?

Case 2

You placed a package of surgical gut in a basin to rinse it and make it more pliable. You forgot that the suture was in the basin, and now it is very limp and water-logged. Is it safe to use?

Case 3

While you are passing a double-armed suture, the free needle snags on the drapes and breaks. What is the next step?

Case 4

You have been working on a vascular case for 3 hours. You are completely out of silk ties. When should you have requested more ties? After you receive the ties from the circulator, you cannot take the time to place them under the Mayo stand towel. Now you have three packages of ties in three different sizes. The ties are mixed up on top of the Mayo stand in no particular order. What problems can this cause, and how should you have prevented this problem?

Case 5

At the close of the case, the surgeon's assistant leaves to attend to another patient. The surgeon asks you to cut sutures for him. When you cut the first suture, you slice through the knot and the suture comes out. What is the next step?

BIBLIOGRAPHY

Association of periOperative Registered Nurses (AORN): *Standards, recommended practices and guidelines,* 2007 edition, Denver, 2007, AORN.

Autosuture, Inc: Surgical staplers. Retrieved June 15, 2008, at http://www.autosuture.com.

Ethicon, Inc: Wound closure manual. Retrieved May 10, 2008, at www.jnjgateway.com/public/NLDUT/Wound_Closure_Manual1.pdf.

Palao R, Gomez P, Huguet P: Burned breast reconstructive surgery with Integra dermal regeneration template, *British Journal of Plastic Surgery* 56:252, 2003.

Porth C: *Pathophysiology concepts of altered health states,* ed 6, Philadelphia, 2002, Lippincott Williams & Wilkins.

Thibodeau G, Patton K: *Anatomy and physiology,* ed 6, St Louis, 2007, Elsevier/Saunders.

Wood FM, Kolybaba ML, Allen P: The use of cultured epithelial autograft in the treatment of major burn injuries: a critical review of the literature, *Burns* 32:395, 2006.

CHAPTER 18

Biomechanics and Computer Technology

CHAPTER OUTLINE

LEARNING OBJECTIVES

After studying this chapter the reader will be able to:

- Describe the nature of the atom
- Describe the elements of motion
- Discuss different types of electromagnetic energy
- List the properties of waves
- Discuss alternating and direct current
- Describe how energy is derived from free electrons moving along a conductive path

- Describe conduction, convection, and radiation as they relate to patient safety
- Describe the relationship between a lens and light rays
- Perform basic computer tasks
- Discuss the importance of data security

TERMINOLOGY

Matter

Atom: A discrete unit made of matter consisting of charged particles.

Atomic number: The number of protons in an atom of a specific element.

Atomic weight: The combined weight of an atom's protons and neutrons.

Boiling point: The temperature of a substance when its state changes from a liquid to a gas.

Electron: A negatively charged particle that orbits the nucleus of an atom.

Element: A pure substance composed of atoms, each with the same number of protons (e.g., iron, copper, and uranium).

Isotope: An atom of a specific element with the correct number of electrons and protons but a different number of neutrons.

Liquid: One of the three states or properties of a substance; a liquid results when the temperature of the substance reaches the melting point.

Melting point: The temperature at which a substance changes from solid to liquid state.

Molecule: A specific substance made up of elements that are bonded together.

Neutron: A subatomic particle located in the nucleus of the atom. It has no electrical charge.

Nucleus: The center of an atom.

Periodic table: A standardized chart of all known elements.

Plasma: A gaseous state in which the atom's nucleus becomes separated from the electrons.

Proton: A subatomic particle that is part of the nucleus of an atom. It has a positive charge.

Solid: A state of matter in which the molecules are bonded very tightly. Characteristics of solids are hardness and the ability to break apart into other solid pieces.

States of matter: The physical forms of matter. The four states of matter are gas, liquid, solid, and plasma.

Subatomic particles: The physical components of an atom. The most common are the neutron, proton, and electron.

Motion

Amplitude: In electromagnetic wave energy, the height of a wave.

Chemical energy: The energy contained in the bonds of atomic particles and between molecules. When these bonds are broken, energy is released.

Circumference: The circular path of an object.

Crest: The greatest point of disturbance in a medium such as water or air.

Electromagnetic field: A three-dimensional pattern of force created by the attraction and repelling of charged particles around a magnet.

Electromagnetic waves: The natural phenomenon of wave energy, such as electricity, light, and radio broadcasts. The type of energy is determined by the frequency of the waves.

Gravitational energy: The natural attractive force of masses in the universe.

Kinetic energy: Energy derived from electromagnetic waves (e.g., electricity and light).

Momentum: The mathematical relationship between the weight and velocity of a mass.

Newton's laws of motion: A set of hypotheses concerning the behavior of objects in motion, proposed by Sir Isaac Newton in the 1600s. Some of these laws are used in modern physics.

Projectile motion: The path of an object in motion in which gravity acts to pull the object downward.

Energy

Energy: Power or force generated by various types of natural occurrences.

Force: In physics, the pushing or pulling of objects (e.g., gravity and magnetism).

Frequency: In physics, the number of waves that pass a point in one second. The unit of measurement for frequency is the hertz (Hz).

Magnetic field: A three-dimensional force pattern created by the positive and negative charges of a polar magnet.

Mechanics: In physics, the study of objects and motion; that is, how they behave and the natural laws that govern their behavior.

Nuclear energy: The energy derived when subatomic particles are separated from the atom.

Potential energy: Energy stored in the form of gravity, chemical bonds, nuclear particles, and mechanical springs.

Reflection: The behavior of a wave when it reaches a nonabsorbent material. The wave reverses and is directed back toward the source.

Trough: The negative or lowest point on a wave.

Wave: In physics, a naturally occurring phenomenon in which energy is transmitted in the form of peaks (high points) and troughs (low points).

Wavelength: The distance between peaks in a complete wave cycle.

Electricity

Alternating current (AC): A type of electrical current in which electricity changes direction to complete its circuit.

Ampere: A unit measuring the amount of energy passing a given point in a stated period of time.

Circuit: The path of free electrons as they move through conductive material. In a *closed circuit,* the electrons proceed unhindered and electrical energy is maintained; in an *open circuit,* the path of the electrons is interrupted, which stops the flow of current.

Conductivity: The relative ability of a substance to transmit free electrons or electricity.

Cycle: In alternating current, electrons change direction in the path of the circuit. The cycle is one complete change.

Direct current (DC): A type of low voltage electrical current in which electrons flow in one direction to complete a circuit. Battery power uses direct current.

Electric generator: A device used to convert mechanical power into electricity. A generator consists of a rotating shaft covered with a coil of conductive material. This shaft is passed through a set of magnets, creating an electrical current.

Electrostatic discharge: The sudden release of electrical energy from surfaces where charged particles have accumulated because of friction.

Ground wire: In electrical circuits, the ground wire in a plug or receptacle captures current that has escaped from its intended pathway and discharges it into the ground.

Hot wire: In electrical circuits, the hot wire is the one that carries the electrical current.

Impedance: In direct current, impedance is the opposition or interruption of current.

Insulator: A substance that does not conduct electrical current and is used to prevent electricity from seeking an alternate path.

Magnetism: The natural attraction of unlike charges.

Ohm: Unit which represents electrical resistance.

Receptacle: An outlet in an electrical circuit that receives a plug containing live current, completing the circuit.

Resistance: In electricity, the measurement of a substance's ability to conduct electricity.

Static electricity: The buildup of charged particles on a surface.

Transformer: A device that steps up or steps down the voltage in an electrical circuit.

Voltage: The electrical force in a circuit, measured as the amount of force that passes a given point over a stated period. Voltage is measured in amperes (A).

Light

Coherent light waves: Light waves which are lined up so that the troughs and peaks are matched.

Concave lens: A type of lens that is thinner at the middle than at the edges. A concave lens bends light rays away from the center.

Convex lens: A ground segment of glass, plastic, or sapphire that is thicker at the middle than at the edges. A convex lens is used to focus light rays on a small area.

Focal point: The exact location where light rays converge after passing through a convex lens.

Photon: In physics, the name given to a light particle. The particle theory is disputed by many scientists, who believe that light is wave energy.

Refraction: In optics, the ability of light to pass through a substance.

Refractive index: A measurement of a substance's ability to absorb light waves. The refractive index is higher in substances that light can pass through easily (e.g., glass, plastics).

Serial lenses: An optical system in which several lenses are lined up to produce a clear, well-defined image. Surgical endoscopes use serial lenses.

Heat

Conduction: The transfer of heat from one substance to another by the natural movement of molecules, which sets other molecules in motion.

Convection: The displacement of cool air by warm air. Convection usually creates currents as the warm air rises and the cool air falls.

Radiation: The transfer of heat by electromagnetic waves.

Thermal conductivity: The ability of a substance to conduct heat. Different substances have different abilities to conduct or transmit heat.

Thermoregulation: A complex physiological process in which the body maintains a temperature that is optimal for survival.

Sound

Doppler effect: The effect perceived when the origin or receiver of sound waves moves. The perception is an increase in the frequency of the waves and corresponding pitch.

Doppler ultrasound: A medical device that uses the Doppler effect and ultrasonic waves to measure and record tissue density and shape.

Harmonics: The quality of sound related to the frequency of the sound waves.

Ultrasound: A technology that uses high-frequency wave energy to identify anatomical structures and anomalies. In ultrasound imaging, sound waves are transformed into visual images on a screen.

Computer Technology

Central processing unit (CPU) the component of a computer that contains the circuitry, memory, and power controls.

Cursor: The visual marker, in the form of an arrow or some other symbol, that indicates an entry point on the computer screen.

Data: Electronic information.

Database: In computer technology, a compilation of information, usually lists or numerical information, that can be manipulated or calculated.

External drive: Data storage device contained in external hardware connected to the computer.

Flaming: Sending an inflammatory message or statement by e-mail. Flaming is a violation of e-mail etiquette and is an inappropriate use of the technology.

Hard copy: In computer technology, the paper form of data, records, or reports.

Hard drive: The component of a computer's CPU where most of the data are stored, including information the computer uses to operate.

Hyperlinks: In computer technology, electronic links between files and the electronic addresses for data associated with those links. Hyperlinks allow data to be obtained electronically and quickly from another computer through a computer network.

Icon: A visual cue on the computer screen. The icon is a small picture or graphic that is linked or connected electronically to data in the computer.

Import: To transfer a document, image, or other data from one electronic location to another.

Input: Information entered on the computer.

Internal drive: Data storage device which is an integral part of the computer.

Internet: A network of computers that are connected by wires, fiber-optic cables, or satellite signals. Computers connected to this system can receive and transmit data to other computers in the system.

Intranet: A computer network within a facility or an organization that can be accessed only by those employed or affiliated with the organization.

LCD: Liquid crystal display; a type of computer monitor that is thin and flat.

Menu: In computer technology, a list of tasks displayed on the monitor. Tasks are selected and executed from the menu.

Monitor: The computer screen.

Operating system: the electronic controller of all the data the computer needs to perform tasks.

Output: Electronic information in any form (e.g, paper, sound, images) created by the computer.

Password: A code that each user types on the keyboard to start a computer session. Passwords are also used to enter programs or request data from a public or institutional computer.

Peripherals: Accessory equipment used with the computer.

RAM: Random access memory; the memory capacity of a computer.

Save (data): Data are stored on the computer after they are created and before the computer is turned off; this is called *saving data*.

Software: Computer programs or applications that allow the user to perform different kinds of function and tasks, such as data or word processing.

Task bar: In graphics-based computer platforms, a horizontal or vertical block that contains small pictures or menus that activate tasks.

Toolbar: Similar to a taskbar, a block or bar containing icons that represent packets of data.

Touch screen: A computer screen on which tasks or commands are executed by touching an image on the screen. Touch screens are commonly used in computer-assisted and robotic surgery.

Window: In graphics-based computer platforms, the basic visual image within which tasks are performed.

Word processing: A type of computer software in which documents can be created.

World Wide Web: In computer technology, a network of links to data via an Internet system. The Web uses a special computer language protocol and is only one of many types of systems for transmitting data through a computer network.

INTRODUCTION

The field of medicine encompasses both human and technological principles. Rapid advances in technology in the past decade have been applied in all fields of medicine. Advances in surgery have been so rapid in the past 10 years that entire systems and methods of working have been changed, requiring continuous training and retraining. The human body has not changed, but the approach to medical and surgical problems often focuses on speed, efficiency, complete accuracy, and economics. Successes in technology have led to more and more complex machines and materials, as well as the use of computer technology to perform, analyze, record, and document medical procedures.

As a result of this shift, surgical technology has developed into a complex field of study and practice that follows two paths simultaneously: the human and the mechanical or technological.

TECHNOLOGY AND MEDICINE

The nonhuman aspects of surgical technology draw most heavily from the field of mechanics. At a very basic level, **mechanics** is the study of motion and objects. Mechanics is involved in both the handheld retractor and the computerized system that tells the surgeon how to remodel the patient's facial bones. Mechanics also is involved in heat, light, sound, electricity, and all the other forms of energy used in medical technology.

The origins of mechanics are found in the laws of physics. Physics is the complex study of matter, time, energy, force, and space. Physics describes the natural behavior of these concepts using complex mathematics. For example, without the mathematical formulas, we must simply accept that when an object is dropped from a height, it accelerates through space as it falls. The value of studying physics is that it helps us to better understand how the physical world behaves and why. In turn, the study of mechanics allows us to put that understanding to practical use.

Modern surgical technologists must ensure the safe use of electrical equipment, assemble and troubleshoot complex devices, and assist in their use on the surgical field. Many different applications of the principles of mechanics and physics are required. Likewise, their study is no longer simple or straightforward. Many different subspecialties have developed (Table 18-1).

MATTER

ATOMIC STRUCTURE

The **atom** is the primary unit that makes up all physical matter. It behaves in very distinct and predictable ways. There are many types of **subatomic particles** (i.e., particles that are smaller than atoms). The ones discussed here are the proton and the neutron, which are located in the center (nucleus) of the atom, and electrons, which occupy the atom's outer regions (Figure 18-1).

The average diameter of an atom is about 10^{-8} cm. The relative distance between the nucleus and its electrons is extremely large, and the weight of the atom depends mainly on the number of particles in the nucleus. If we compare a golf ball to the nucleus of the atom, the distance from the nucleus to the electrons would be over 6.2 miles (10 km).

Nucleus

The nucleus of an atom contains two main particles, a neutron and a **proton**. A proton has a positive electrical charge and is the heaviest of the subatomic particles. A **neutron** has a neutral charge. The net charge of the nucleus is zero, because usually the number of protons and neutrons is the same. The nucleus is the center of the atom.

Electron

An **electron** is much smaller than a proton or neutron. Its weight is almost negligible compared with the nuclear particles. The number of electrons in the atom varies with the type of element. The electron has a negative charge and orbits the nucleus in discrete, three-dimensional energy levels. These

Table 18-1

Specialties in Mechanics and Physics

Area of Study	Applied Theories	Surgical Applications
Classical mechanics	Newton's laws of motion* Harmonic motion Gravity	• Any instrument or device that oscillates, rotates, flexes, pivots, bends, or flexes. • Work as it applies to potential energy in humans and devices. • The design of tools and instruments and its relationship to work (e.g., hinged instruments). • Any device or instrument that uses wave energy, such as light, heat, electricity, or sound.
Biomechanics	Various	The principles of mechanics are used to explain and improve the function of the human body.
Thermodynamics	Laws of thermodynamics The nature of heat transfer States of matter	• Devices that create heat or cold (e.g., fluid warmer, patient thermal devices, sterilizers). • Compressed gas–powered equipment.
Particle, atomic physics	Nuclear physics Particle theory Wave motion	• Any device that uses electromagnetic radiation in the form of heat, light or electricity (e.g., ultrasound diagnostic devices, radiography, fluoroscopy).
Optical physics	Optics Light	• Any device with lenses (e.g., operating microscopes, endoscopes, lasers). • Equipment that uses or emits light (e.g., fiberoptic light sources). • Devices that produce an optical (not electronic) image.

*These theories are not always "intuitive" and often require mathematical expression for clarification.

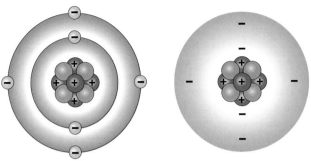

Figure 18-1 The atom. **A,** The nucleus contains positively charged protons and neutral neutrons. Negatively charged electrons surround the nucleus in energy "shells." **B,** Energy levels are not circular; rather, they resemble clouds. *(From Thibodeau G, Patton K: Anatomy and physiology, ed 6, St Louis, 2007, Mosby.)*

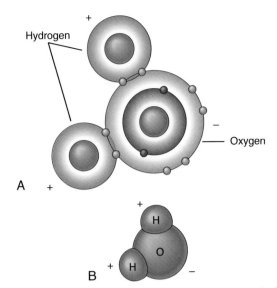

Figure 18-2 A molecule of water (H_2O) is composed of two elements: hydrogen (2 atoms) and oxygen (1 atom). *(From Thibodeau G, Patton K: Anatomy and physiology, ed 6, St Louis, 2007, Mosby.)*

energy levels are referred to as "clouds" because one electron moves randomly within its discrete or separate energy level, not in a linear path, as was thought to be the case when atomic structure was first studied. Atoms that have more than one electron have more energy levels. The more distant the energy level from the nucleus, the less energy is needed for an electron to separate from the nucleus. This is important to an understanding of electricity, which involves the movement of electrons from one atom to another.

Elements and Molecules

An **element** is a pure substance in which each atom has the same number of protons (this number is referred to as the **atomic number**). Regardless of the number of electrons and neutrons an atom has, the atomic number of the element remains the same. For example, the element iron has 26 protons, therefore the atomic number of iron is 26.

The **atomic weight** of an element is the sum of the weight of its protons and neutrons. An element can have a different number of neutrons. When this occurs, the substance is called an **isotope** of the element.

By international scientific convention, all known elements are classified and arranged on a standardized chart called the periodic table. The periodic table lists all known elements according to their mass and electronic behavior. The table, which was first developed in 1869 by Dimitri Mendeleev, has evolved as new elements have been discovered.

A **molecule** is two or more atoms held together (bonded) by chemical bonds (Figure 18-2). Just as atoms of a particular element have the same number of protons and neutrons, molecules of a substance are identified by the different elements that compose them. For example, a molecule of water always contains one hydrogen atom and two oxygen atoms (H_2O). *Organic compounds* are those in which one of the molecules contains the element carbon. These molecules are the basic structure of all living things.

STATES OF MATTER

We know from observing the physical world that substances take on different forms. These forms—liquid, solid, gas, and

plasma—are referred to as the **states of matter**. Most substances can exist in a variety of states. For example, when water is heated to 212° F (100° C), it becomes steam, its gaseous state. The state of the water has changed from liquid to gas, but it retains its molecular structure.

A **solid** is a substance in which the molecules are tightly bound in rigid formation. A **liquid** is formed when heat (energy) is applied to a solid. Common experience teaches us that some substances melt more readily than others. This is because the bonds of some molecules are stronger in some substances than in others. The point at which a substance turns from solid to liquid is called the melting point.

A substance assumes a gaseous state when the energy applied to it is greater than the energy bonds that hold the molecules together. When heated, the molecules move away from each other in random directions. Different substances become gas at different temperatures. This is referred to as the *boiling point* of the substance.

Plasma is gas in which the atom's electrons are separated from its nucleus. For this to happen, the temperature of the molecules must be very high. Plasma is found in the arc of incandescent light produced by a welding torch; it also is present in the gaseous areas surrounding stars.

MOTION

ELEMENTS OF MOTION

Motion is the result of energy and work. We can describe motion in mathematical or conceptual terms. **Newton's laws of motion** (Box 18-1) serve as the basis of many concepts of motion. Some important conceptual terms or qualities of motion are:

Box 18-1

Newton's Laws of Motion

Newton's First Law

An object at rest tends to stay at rest, and an object in motion tends to stay in motion at the same speed and in the same direction unless acted upon by an unbalanced force.

This means that an object that is not moving will remain stationary, and one that is moving will keep moving until a force acts upon it.

Newton's Second Law

The acceleration of an object is directly proportional to the net force acting upon the object and inversely proportional to the mass of the object.

This means that as an object falls, acceleration increases as the weight of the object increases.

Newton's Third Law

For every action there is an equal and opposite reaction.

This means that the amount of force needed to push an object equals the force needed to resist movement in the object being pushed.

- *Speed:* Speed is a description of how fast an object travels from one point to another. In mathematical terms, the *rate* is the time it takes to cover a certain distance, or time over distance. For example, a car traveling 70 miles per hour is another way of stating the rate of 70 m/1 hr. In surgical technology, we measure the speed of some powered cutting instruments in oscillations per second.

- *Distance and displacement:* Motion is the movement (displacement) of an object from one point to another or the return of the object to the point where it started. *Displacement,* therefore, describes how far the object went from its original position to its destination. *Distance,* a different concept, is the actual amount of space or ground the object covered during its period of motion.

- *Velocity:* Velocity is the speed of a moving object, measured as distance over time.

- **Momentum:** A mathematical relationship is used to describe the amount and weight of matter (called the *mass*) and the velocity of the mass. In this relationship, the greater the mass and velocity, the greater the momentum: Momentum = Mass × Velocity. In everyday terms, this means that the speed and mass of an object affect the amount of energy needed to change the momentum; that is, to stop it, change its direction, speed it up, or slow it down. Momentum is conserved in a closed system, in which no forces act upon the object.

- **Force:** In mechanics, force is the pulling or pushing of one object on another. Two conditions exist with regard to force: the objects touch, or they interact from a distance.

- *Vector:* A vector is an imaginary line with length and direction, or the path of displacement of an object. Length is measured in linear terms, such as meters.

CIRCULAR AND PROJECTILE MOTION

When an object travels in a circle, the distance of its path is called a **circumference**. Satellites and planets have a particular kind of circular motion. Within our solar system, the sun is the center of the planets. A satellite accelerates toward Earth because of the force of gravity. However, it does not crash into the Earth because of the curvature of the planet (gravity is the force that pulls all objects with mass towards each other).

When an object is thrown straight outward, it follows a curved path called **projectile motion**. This occurs because gravity pulls the object downward toward the ground.

ENERGY

All surgical devices and technologies depend on a form of **energy** for operation. The surgical technologist is required to have a fundamental understanding of these energy forms, especially as they relate to patient safety. The technologist must handle, assemble, and process the equipment in a way that protects it and prevents medical errors or malfunction. The first step in preventing accidents and errors with equipment understands the energy that powers the equipment or is emitted by it. Two types of energy are discussed, potential energy and electromagnetic energy. These classifications are used as an aid to comprehension. They are not rigid categorizations, but a general classification is helpful for learning about energy.

POTENTIAL ENERGY

Potential energy is also referred to as *stored energy.* Figure 18-3 illustrates the concept of stored energy.

GRAVITATIONAL ENERGY

Gravitational energy exists when a stationary mass or object is positioned such that gravity will cause it to move. A stationary rock on top of a cliff has potential gravitational energy because if pushed over the edge, it will fall. The **potential energy** of an object is measured by its mass (weight) and distance from the earth.

MECHANICAL ENERGY

Mechanical energy applies to springs or elastic material. When these are compressed and then allowed to resume a neutral position, they exert force and produce energy. When energy is applied to a spring to compress it, the spring travels a distance, returns to its original position (neutral), and then moves in the opposite direction. This movement is called an oscillation. If the force is applied to the spring only once, the spring continues to oscillate at lower and lower levels and then comes to rest. However, if the force is applied at a continuous rate and strength, the spring keeps moving (oscillating) the same distance in a negative and positive direction.

To understand mechanical energy, imagine an adult pushing a child on a swing. The person pushing the child

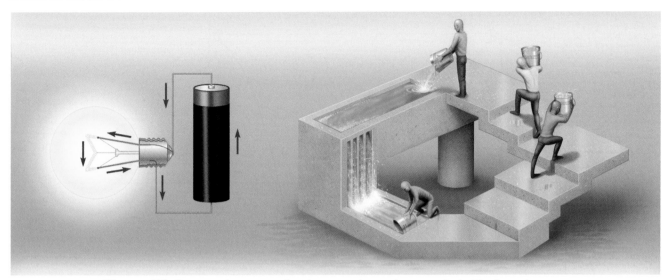

Figure 18-3 Potential energy. *Left,* A battery with stored energy. *Right,* The flow of water demonstrates the concept of potential energy. The potential energy is greatest at the top of the platform. *(From Giambattista A, et al: College physics, ed 2, New York, 2007, McGraw Hill. Reproduced with permission of the McGraw Hill Companies.)*

supplies the energy, and the weight on the swing is analogous to the spring. Each time the adult applies pressure (force) to the child, the swing moves forward and then back. These are equivalent to oscillations. The adult applies force on the swing just as the child reaches the limit of the backward (negative) motion of the swing. However, if the adult applies force when the swing has not reached the limit of backward motion, the adult will absorb the energy and be pushed backward. If the adult does not apply enough force to maintain the oscillations, the displacement will decrease.

CHEMICAL ENERGY

Molecules are bonded by several different kinds of forces. When these bonds are broken, energy is released. In physiology, energy is released when the bonds holding a molecule called *adenosine triphosphate (ATP)* is released from other molecules during the process called the *Krebs cycle.* The energy released during the Krebs cycle is used by the cell for physiological processes. This is an example of **chemical energy.**

Nuclear energy is contained in the bonds that hold the subparticles of the atomic nucleus together. Nuclear energy can be converted into electrical or electromagnetic energy.

ELECTROMAGNETIC ENERGY

Many devices used in surgery derive their energy from electromagnetic radiation. Most of the wave energy studied in this chapter is electromagnetic energy. Electromagnetic waves exist in a very large range of frequencies. It is important to remember that *the frequency of the wave determines the type of energy and its capabilities.* (Chapter 19 presents additional information on specific energy sources used in surgery.)

Electromagnetic energy exhibits wave behavior. The types of wave energy discussed in this chapter include:

- Electricity
- Light
- Heat
- Sound

WAVES

In simple terms, a **wave** can be described as a disturbance in a medium such as air, water, or a solid substance. Waves behave in predictable patterns, and their movements are measurable. Mechanical waves travel through a medium such as water or a solid. **Electromagnetic waves** move in the air or in a vacuum and are created by a vibrating electric charge.

Properties of Waves

Waves can be drawn, or plotted, as shown in Figure 18-4. As you can see, a wave has crests and troughs. The **crest** is the highest point of disturbance, and the **trough** is the negative or lowest point of disturbance. The resting point is the area of no disturbance or movement and is represented by the straight line.

Waves move out from their source. An example is a stone thrown into a pool of water. The water is energized by the force of the stone disturbing it. This creates concentric waves. When the stone sinks, the energy source is no longer present, and the waves begin to diminish in size and finally stop.

Wavelength is a measurement of one complete wave cycle; that is, the length from one crest to the next.

Amplitude is the point of greatest disturbance, or the height of an individual wave. This is measured in meters from the top of the crest to the point of rest.

Frequency is the number of waves that pass a point in 1 second. The unit of measurement for electromagnetic frequency is the hertz (Hz). As the frequency of a wave increases, the units of measurement change to reflect these numbers.

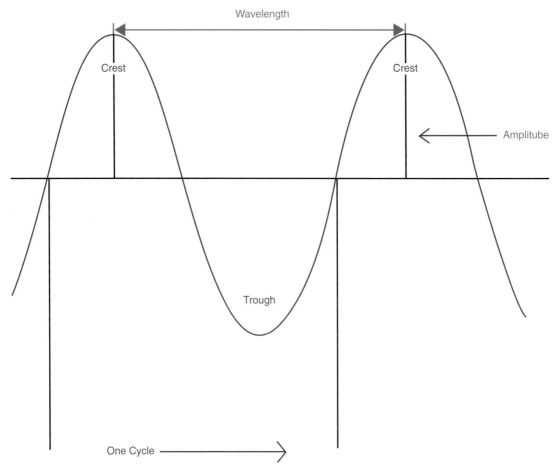

Figure 18-4 Wave characteristics.

Kilohertz (kHz) is thousands of hertz, and megahertz (MHz) is millions of hertz. Radio waves have the lowest frequency, at around 90 MHz.

The speed of a wave is measured in meters per second. The speed of a wave depends on whether the wave energy is mechanical or electromagnetic.

❖ *All electromagnetic waves travel at the same speed, regardless of the type of energy they produce.*

Reflection
When a wave reaches a boundary, it may pass through or be reflected back (**reflection**), depending on the nature of the boundary and the type of wave energy. For example, light can pass through a glass lens because the density of glass is low. Gamma rays used in medical radiographs do not penetrate the lead aprons worn by those who operate the equipment or other staff assisting in the process. Sound waves are reflected as an echo when they reach their boundary.

Interference
Waves that have the same wavelength and are propagated at the same time can be lined up exactly. In this case, we say that the waves are coherent. An example of coherent waves is laser

light. All the troughs and peaks match, and this creates a very intense white light. When waves are superimposed, the amplitude of the resulting wave is greater than any one of the individual waves. However, if the waves are not lined up (the troughs and peaks are out of synchrony), they will cancel each other out. Anyone who has seen waves on the shore has seen waves cancel each other when they come from different directions.

ELECTRICITY

APPLICATION IN SURGERY

Nearly all biomedical devices require electricity as their power source. Even optical instruments that use lenses, such as the endoscope and microscope, have imaging and power components that require electricity to move the equipment and provide light. Other complex devices, such as lasers, physiological monitoring equipment, diagnostic imaging equipment, and computer-assisted robotic systems, use complex circuits and high-voltage electricity.

Electricity is used directly to perform procedures in all forms of electrosurgery. Numerous risks and hazards are associated with electrosurgery. To ensure the safety of the patient and staff members, the surgical technologist and perioperative nurse are required to have more than a basic understanding of electricity. The following discussion of electricity forms the basis for a more advanced understanding of electrosurgery, which is discussed in later chapters.

NATURE OF ELECTRICITY

Recall that atoms contain positively charged protons, negatively charged electrons, and neutrons, which have no electric charge. The net charge on an atom is determined by the numbers of electrons and protons, which must be equal for the atom to be stable.

Electricity is created when electrons move from atom to atom. The movement of electrons and the energy this creates follow some basic laws, which are important to an understanding of electricity:

1. Opposite charges attract, and like charges repel.
2. Energy is never lost or destroyed, but it can be transformed from one form to another.

MAGNETISM AND ELECTRICITY

Some naturally occurring metals, such as iron, attract and repel charged particles. The two poles of an iron bar or magnet exhibit opposite forces. This produces a magnetic field, a three-dimensional force pattern created by the positive and negative charges of a polar magnet (Figure 18-5).

It is important to remember that **magnetism** is *not* electricity; however, the two are closely related. When one pole of a magnet is passed over a rotating coil of conductive material, such as a copper wire, electric current is induced through the wire. An **electromagnetic field** is created around the rotating coil, and the energy that results can be captured and controlled to do work.

CONDUCTIVITY

Recall that the atom's electrons move randomly within discrete energy levels around the atom. In certain types of substances, especially metals, electrons are easily displaced from the outer energy levels. They become free electrons. When an atom loses one of its electrons, the atom is left with a positive charge. Another free electron in the vicinity is attracted to this positively charged atom and attaches to it. An atom that has lost or gained an electron is called an **ion**. In some elements, electrons move from atom to atom, balancing and unbalancing the charges. The relative ability of a material to release free electrons is called **conductivity**.

Substances with low conductivity include rubber and glass, whereas metal has high conductivity. Temperature can alter the conductivity of a substance. For example, glass is nonconductive at a low temperature but conductive at a very high temperature.

It is important to remember that randomly moving free electrons are not the same as electricity. No work is being performed, and the net charge usually is neutral because the number of atoms losing electrons is equal to the number receiving them. Conductive material is simply the path through which the free electrons can be made to line up and move.

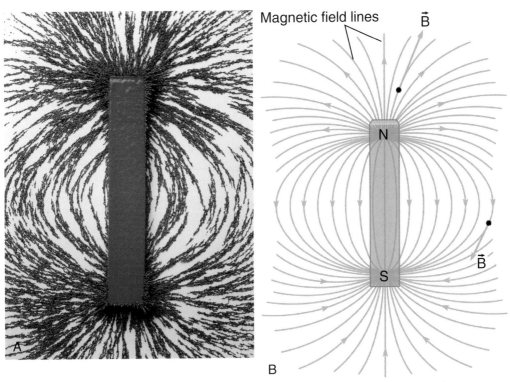

Figure 18-5 Force pattern of a bar magnet exhibited by iron filings. *(From Giambattista A, et al: College physics, ed 2, New York, 2007, McGraw Hill. Reproduced with permission of the McGraw Hill Companies.)*

INSULATORS

A substance with low or no conductivity is called an **insulator**. Examples of materials used in modern electrical insulation are polyethylene, polyvinyl chloride (PVC), and Teflon. Insulators are used to cover and provide a path for the electric current. Surgical instruments used in minimally invasive surgery have insulated sheaths to protect the patient from being burned by stray electricity.

The concept of conductivity is directly related to operational safety in electrosurgery. For this reason, it is important to think of conductivity as it relates to a substance and its environment. Box 18-2 describes conductive and insulating materials.

STATIC ELECTRICITY

Under certain circumstances, such as friction and low humidity, charged particles can accumulate on surfaces. If two surfaces have the same a net charge, they will repel each other. If the net charges are opposite, the surfaces will attract each other. This is called static electricity.

Electrostatic discharge occurs when the accumulation of charges on surfaces is so great that the air between the surfaces acts as a conductor. Air usually is not conductive; however, when the environment is very dry and sufficient friction exists between the materials, ions build up quickly and the air ignites. When a person's shoes accumulate static and the person then touches a conductive surface, such as a metal door handle, the charges are suddenly transmitted. This can cause a perceptible electrical shock.

Electrostatic discharge is a significant problem in industry and biomedical technology. The sudden, unexpected release of energy just described can be strong enough to ignite substances in the environment. In the past, when flammable anesthetic agents were commonly used, many precautions were taken to prevent static discharge. Although the phenomenon is less problematic now, with the regulated use of gases, static discharge is kept to a minimum with environmental controls such as low temperature and high humidity in the perioperative environment.

Box 18-2

Conductors and Insulators

Conductor	Insulator
Metal	Glass
Silver	Rubber
Copper	Fiberglass
Gold	Ceramic
Aluminum	Dry cotton
Iron	Wood
Steel	Plastic
Brass	Air
Other	Pure water
Water (with particles in solution)	
Concrete	

ELECTRIC GENERATORS

An **electric generator** converts mechanical energy into electricity. Generators provide the power to move electrical current through a conductive material. The generator does not produce the electrical current; it only provides the mechanical power to do the work. In simple terms, a generator is a coil of conductive material (usually metal wire) wound around a rotating shaft within a magnetic field. This creates electrical current.

ELECTRICAL CIRCUITS

Free electrons flow through conductive material in a continuous path, each electron "pushing" the one ahead of it; this is called a **circuit**. As long as the path is not interrupted, the electrons will continue to flow, much like water flows through a tube. Electrical current always seeks the path of least resistance. This is the basis of measures to provide electrical safety.

Direct Current DC

An electrical circuit that flows in one direction from one charged pole to the other is referred to as **direct current** (**DC**). A battery is an example of a DC power source. The battery has a negative and a positive pole. When a wire is attached from one pole to the other, electrons flow through the wire from one pole to the other (Figure 18-6). The circuit is closed, because there is no break in the flow. Battery-powered instruments use low-voltage direct current.

Alternating Current AC

With **alternating current** (**AC**), the direction of the flow changes back and forth within the circuit. The interval between directional changes is called a **cycle**. The rate at which the current changes directions is called the *frequency*. In the United States, the frequency of household power is 60 cycles per second.

AC is used for common municipal power and is the source of power for nearly every type of electrical device in medical technology. AC delivers high-voltage power. A clear understanding of alternating current paths, resistance, and conductivity is critical for all perioperative personnel. In this discussion, the basics of AC are explained. In Chapter 19, the use of electrosurgery and safety considerations are covered in detail.

Path of Alternating Current

Alternating current is brought into a facility such as a hospital or house from the municipal source through overhead or underground wires. The wires are assembled and redirected at the facility's electrical grid. This is a complex system where all electrical connections coming into the facility meet, are metered, and then are directed to the appropriate sections of the facility. This is also where electricity leaves the facility and returns to the municipal source, completing the electrical circuit. Figure 18-7 shows alternating current from high-voltage lines and its path through a household electrical system.

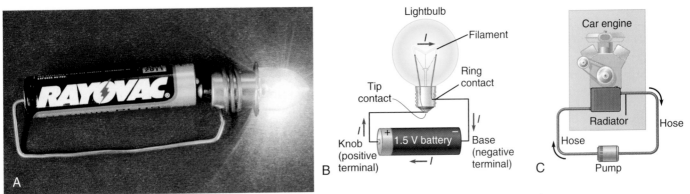

Figure 18-6 Direct current (DC). The battery has a negative pole and a positive pole. A wire attached to each end conducts electrons, which are condensed through a smaller wire filament, creating light. *(From Giambattista A, et al: College physics, ed 2, New York, 2007, McGraw Hill. Reproduced with permission of the McGraw Hill Companies.)*

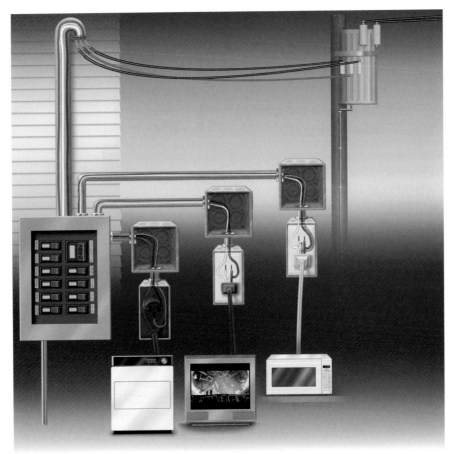

Figure 18-7 Household circuit using alternating current (AC) derived from a municipal electricity source. *(From Giambattista A, et al: College physics, ed 2, New York, 2007, McGraw Hill. Reproduced with permission of the McGraw Hill Companies.)*

Three wires make up the alternating current pathway as it is wired through a building, terminating at the **receptacle**, or electrical outlet. Each of the three wires has a different function. The **hot wire** is the power source from the power grid to the receptacle. This wire usually is covered in black, nonconductive material. The second wire, which usually is white, is called the *neutral wire*. It conducts electricity back to the grid and eventually out to the power pole or underground pathway.

The third wire, which usually is green, is called the *ground* or *ground wire*. The **ground wire** protects the circuit from a "short" or fault in the system, such as when the active and neutral wires come into direct contact. This causes sparking and heat. The ground wire receives the stray current and conducts it safely back to the facility's grid. A metal rod buried deep in the ground connects the grid to the ground, where electricity disperses and is rendered harmless.

Voltage

The force or power that pushes or drives electrons through the conductive material is called **voltage**. This is the potential energy expressed as units of charge. We measure the amount of charge that flows past a given point over a specific period. This unit of measurement is called an ampere or *Amp*. Voltage can be increased or decreased with a device called a **transformer**.

Resistance

In electricity, **resistance** is any interruption of current through the conductive material. Resistance depends on properties such as the type and thickness the material. Conductive materials are defined as having high or low resistance, depending on their ability to conduct electricity. Materials with low resistance have greater conductivity.

Resistance is used to transform one form of energy into another form. A common example is an incandescent light bulb. Current passes from a standard copper wire into the bulb's finer metal filament, which has a higher resistance than the wire conducting electricity to the bulb. Resistance at the filament causes it to become hot and glow. In this case, resistance is used purposefully to create a desired effect. The heating effect of the wire filament can be understood by comparing the electrons to water pressure. Water flowing through a hose remains at a constant pressure unless the diameter is decreased or increased. If you crimp the hose, reducing its diameter at that point, the pressure increases at the point of resistance. The point of resistance in an electrical circuit creates heat, which is analogous to the increased pressure in the hose.

Resistance is measured in units called ohms. We can measure the amount of resistance in conductive material with an ohm meter. In the perioperative environment, unintended resistance can result in injury to the patient. Electrical biomedical devices have self-monitoring capability, which stops the current when resistance exceeds a specific level. However, this does not prevent patient injury in all cases.

❖ *When resistance occurs, an electrical current may seek an unintended alternative path, which can terminate at patient tissue, causing severe burns.*

LIGHT

PROPERTIES OF VISIBLE LIGHT

Light is a form of electromagnetic radiation, but it also has properties of a particle. For this reason, scientists have debated whether light is a procession of particles or a wave structure. The particle theory attributes the name **photon** to a light particle.

Visible light is actually white light and is made up of different wavelengths. When separated, these distinct wavelengths are perceived as different colors. White light, which is transmitted through a prism, separates into distinct the wavelengths and its colors become visible. The same phenomenon takes place in a rainbow, in which the raindrops act as a prism.

Sight

We see an object because our eyes are able to interpret the image created when light encounters an object along our line of sight. The complexity of physiological interpretation is separate from the physical relationship between the object and light rays. We know intuitively that we can see objects directly only when they are "straight in front" of us. We can cause light rays to bend, such as in a fiberoptic cable, but under natural circumstances, the object must be within our line of sight to be seen.

Refraction

The ability to focus light through serial lenses, magnify the images, and transmit them to imaging systems is among the most important advances in modern surgical technology. Endoscopic minimally invasive surgery and microsurgery depend on these technologies, which include the manufacture of high quality optical systems.

Light rays passing through a medium such as glass or plastic bend because the speed of the rays is decreased; this is called **refraction**. The more dense the material, the slower the light will pass through it. The term **refractive index** refers to the speed at which waves (light or sound) pass through a medium. Glass, sapphire, and other transparent media have high refractive indices.

Reflection

Light waves exhibit a property called *reflection*. This means that when light rays encounter some surfaces, they can reverse direction. Reflection occurs when light rays encounter a mirror or other surface that does not fully absorb the light. The light rays are reflected at the same angle at which they contact the surface. Therefore, images seen in a mirror are those within the line of sight.

Coherence

As mentioned previously, coherence occurs when propagated waves are lined up so that their peaks and troughs match. Under natural circumstances, light is emitted from its source in all directions. However, light rays can be focused through a lens or propagated through a medium such as a gas. When light is passed through a lasing gas, it becomes coherent and intensive enough to cut through many different types of material, including tissue. This is the basis of laser energy, which is discussed in detail in Chapter 19.

LENSES

Lenses are made of highly refractive material. They are manufactured in such a way that light rays passing through a lens are focused on one point or spread out over a large area. When the rays are focused in a single area, the area is called the **focal point**. The shape of a lens determines how the light rays bend as they pass through it. A simple **convex lens** is thinner at the edges than at the middle. A **concave** lens is thinner at the middle than around the edges and causes the light to diverge or spread.

Lenses used in surgery and microscopy refract light rays so that they converge (come together) in one area to produce a magnified image. The eye focuses an image on the retina as light passes through the lens (Figure 18-8). Endoscopes use **serial lenses** to achieve a high level of clarity and brightness. In this lens system, several lenses are lined up inside the endoscopic telescope.

HEAT

Heat is a form of energy that is quantitative (measurable) and transferable. In physics, temperature is a characteristic of matter and is related to the movement of atoms and molecules. Recall that energy is never lost but can be changed from one form to another. For example, electricity can be transformed into thermal (heat) energy and used in electrosurgery.

HEAT TRANSFER

Heat transfer is important in patient care and safety in the perioperative environment. The body maintains a constant temperature to sustain life through a process called **thermoregulation**. However, illness, medications, and trauma (including surgery) can alter the body's natural ability to maintain the correct temperature. During surgery, the patient's core temperature may be dangerously lowered by anesthetic agents, blood loss, and tissue trauma.

Heat is transferred in three ways:
- Conduction
- Convection
- Radiation

Conduction

Heat **conduction** is caused by the natural vibrations of the molecules that make up a substance. Warmer substances have more movement than cold ones. When a warm substance comes in contact with a cooler substance, the molecules collide, which increases movement in the cooler material, raising its temperature. Some substances conduct heat more efficiently than others; this quality is called **thermal conductivity**.

An example of thermal conduction occurs when a saline irrigation solution is placed in a fluid warmer. The fluid warmer, which is an electrical heating element, comes in contact with the basin holding the saline solution. Energy is transferred to the basin, which causes molecular movement in the saline solution. The thermal energy of the saline solution dissipates to the cooler room air, but as long as the fluid warmer is sufficiently heated to overcome this energy transfer, the saline will remain warm.

The patient can lose heat by conduction when exposed to cold air in the environment. Children and older patients are particularly at risk for chilling. This can be prevented by using warming pads and tubular warm air blankets, which conduct heat at a controlled level.

Convection

Convection is heat transfer by the natural movement of heated air or water over a cooler surface. When air becomes warm, it rises, because the heated molecules become less dense and thus lighter. As the heated molecules rise, they carry energy.

An example of convection is seen when a radiator generates heat to the cool areas of a room. Warm air in the room is less dense and rises to the ceiling, where it displaces cooler air. A current occurs as the cooler room air sinks to the floor and the warm air rises. Figure 18-9 illustrates convection currents in the environment.

Radiation

Heat is given off from its source as electromagnetic energy; this is called **radiation**. This means that the energy behaves like all other waves. Some objects "glow" with heat, because these electromagnetic waves are within at the visible spectrum. The eye perceives the energy as light, because the wavelength of the object is perceptible. Objects that are hot but do not glow also have radiant qualities, but their wavelength is outside the visible range.

SOUND

PROPERTIES OF SOUND

Sound is a type of energy generated by the movement of waves through a substance such as air or water. Because sound is wave energy, it has many of the properties of other waves—

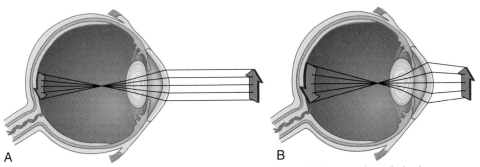

A   B

Figure 18-8 Focal points in the eye. Light converges inside the eye through the lens, which focuses the image on the retina. *(From Thibodeau G, Patton K: Anatomy and physiology, ed 6, St Louis, 2007, Mosby.)*

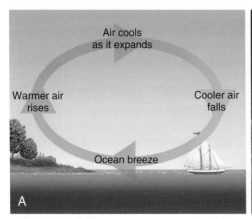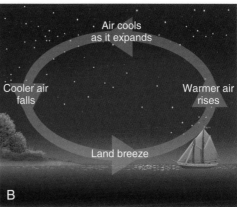

Figure 18-9 Convection currents in the environment. *(From Giambattista A, et al: College physics, ed 2, New York, 2007, McGraw Hill. Reproduced with permission of the McGraw Hill Companies.)*

loudness, which is subjective interpretation of the intensity, frequency (the number of waves that pass a given point in a given time), and amplitude (the intensity of the sound as measured in decibels [dB]), and pitch (our perception of the different frequencies). Sound is characterized as a disturbance in a medium. We perceive sound only when the vibrations are within the limits of the brain's ability to sense them.

Reflection

As wave energy, sound can be reflected, and this property is used in **ultrasound** technology, which is one of the most widely used diagnostic tools in medicine. In this process, sound waves with a frequency higher than those perceived by the human ear are transmitted through a medium, and the return signal is *transduced* (one energy form converted into another) into a visual image. The ultrasound wavelength is relatively short, which allows it to detect small targets. Advanced imaging techniques provide a concise picture of the ultrasound signal, which measures the density, size, and shape of the target anatomy. Electrocardiography uses ultrasound technology to produce an image of the heart (Figure 18-10). Extremely high energy sounds waves are used in surgical technology to separate molecules and remodel tissue. This technique is discussed more fully in Chapter 19.

Doppler Effect

Mechanical or electromagnetic waves are perceived by the human senses (vision and hearing) or by equipment that can track and display the wave forms as data. When we hear an ambulance siren, the sound waves seem to change pitch as they approach us. The pitch seems to get higher as the ambulance approaches and lower as it moves away. This change in pitch is due to a phenomenon called the *Doppler effect*. The siren does not actually change pitch or frequency as it moves away. The waves become wider and wider (or more "stretched") as they move outward from the source. When we are close to the source of the waves, the waves are more compressed and therefore higher in frequency; that is, more waves can fit into a smaller interval. The ear perceives these wide (or tight) intervals as high and low pitch. This is the **Doppler effect**.

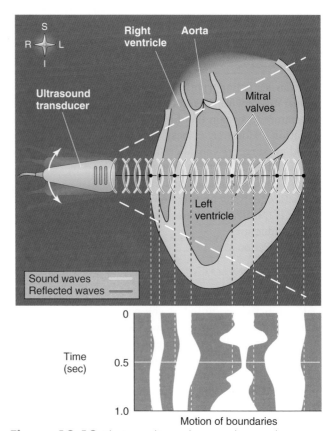

Figure 18-10 Electrocardiography uses ultrasound technology to produce an image of the heart. Sound waves are sent from a transducer to heart tissue, which reflects an accurate image. *(From Thibodeau G, Patton K: Anatomy and physiology, ed 6, St Louis, 2007, Mosby.)*

Doppler ultrasound uses both the Doppler effect and ultrasound waves to detect narrowing and obstructions in blood vessels. The Doppler equipment emits a signal that is reflected by the moving blood cells. The reflected sound is measured and transduced to a visual image. More advanced systems transduce signals into color images, which provide detailed information about the velocity and direction of blood flow.

For example, when force is applied to a string, the string oscillates back and forth (vibrates), creating wave energy as described previously. The oscillations of a string may be audible if their frequency is within hearing range. The quality of pitch is perceived as the oscillations move at greater or lesser frequency. The human voice is created by oscillations of the vocal cords, which are amplified by the larynx and other anatomical structures of the throat and mouth.

Harmonics

Sound exhibits a property called harmonics, which is related to the frequency of the wavelength. Although wave harmonics can be measured in other forms of **kinetic energy**, harmonics produces a particular quality of sound, which we distinguish in the human voice or in musical instruments.

COMPUTER TECHNOLOGY

COMPUTERS IN THE PERIOPERATIVE ENVIRONMENT

Computer technology is incorporated into many different types of equipment and biomedical devices used in the perioperative environment. Some of these include:

- Computer systems for recording patient information (patient charts) and other medical records.
- Preference cards for surgeons (indicates the surgeon's choice of equipment, supplies, positioning and other important information).
- Diagnostic imaging equipment (e.g., radiography, magnetic resonance imaging [MRI], computed tomography [CT], and fluoroscopy).
- Digital cameras and image output on monitors (screens) during surgical procedures.
- Robotic surgical systems.
- Computer tracking of hospital supplies, instruments, and equipment during reprocessing (disinfection and sterilization).
- Automatic patient billing systems for supplies used in surgery.
- Computerized operation of sterilizers and instrument decontamination equipment.

COMPUTER LEARNING TOOLS

As with any new skill, learning computer technology requires not only a basic understanding, but also time spent using the equipment and experiencing how it responds when commands are given (purposefully or accidentally). It is important and helpful to have someone who can coach the learner through the beginning phases of the learning process.

Many computer tasks are more easily understood by doing them rather than reading a description of them. Technology changes very rapidly, and information given in manuals and books can quickly become outdated. New technology commonly is developed and marketed within months.

Computer classes are offered at all community colleges, and more advanced skills can be developed after one or two introductory course. Once the learner is able to use the Internet, the best computer learning tools often are those that are an integral part of the computer platform or program. Interactive tutorials use audio, text, and graphic information to coach the learner from basic to advance skills. Tutorials are particularly useful for learning how to use programs such as word processing and spread sheets. The following discussion is an introduction to the basic concepts of computer use.

HOW COMPUTERS WORK

The computer's main function is to store data and retrieve them using electrical signals. Most people have seen computers on which information is viewed on a screen and data are entered on a keyboard. The data are stored on *chips,* or small electrical circuits that are not readily visible. The microprocessor is another type of computer technology. These extremely small chips contain information used by everything from mobile phones to complex industrial and medical equipment.

COMPUTER TERMS AND LANGUAGE

Computer technology uses a particular terminology and language to describe the following:

- What the computer *does* (e.g., displaying an e-mail)
- The *equipment* needed to perform the tasks (e.g., the keyboard or screen)
- The *process* used to make the equipment work (e.g., computer programs or the electrical signals that transmit information)

Computer terms mean very specific things. For example:

- Electronic information is called data.
- Pictures on a computer screen are called images.
- The process of entering information into the computer (by a human or another machine) is called inputting.
- Information received from the computer is called output. Output can be in any form, for example, a printed e-mail or an actual radiograph that has been taken and processed by a computerized radiographic machine.

❖ *Data are input into the computer and can be seen as an image on the screen or printed as paper output.*

Try to learn basic computer terms as you learn how to use a computer. These will help you and others communicate clearly as you work.

HARDWARE (PHYSICAL COMPONENTS)

The physical parts of a computer are is central core unit and peripherals. The core unit contains the wiring and complex circuits that run the computer and store data. The peripherals are other types of equipment that *interface* with (work with) the computer and are part of its operation, such as the computer screen, keyboard, and mouse.

Computer Core: The Central Processing Unit

The central processing unit, or **CPU**, is the computer's "thinking" equipment. The computer's memory is stored electronically inside this component. The switch for power on and off is located on the housing of the CPU.

Memory

The computer "remembers" the information programmed into its random access memory, or **RAM**. This is a physical part of the computer that connects with the main electrical circuits. These circuits, called the *motherboard,* perform all the different tasks needed to operate the computer. A portable type of RAM is called a *flash memory card* or just *memory card.* This is a solid state (no moving parts) storage device for RAM.

After data are input into the computer, RAM holds the information until the computer is switched off. To save the information so that it can be *retrieved* (brought back from the RAM), it must be encoded on some hardware. This hardware is called a *drive.*

Data Storage Devices
Disks and Drives

Data are stored in the computer or on portable hardware devices. The most common type of drive is called a disk. There are many different types of disks. The most common are The compact disk (CD), read-only CD (CD-ROM), and digital versatile disk (DVD) are "optical" disks that can store vast amounts of data and are extremely durable.

Disks interface with the computer through the drive. The two types of drives are the internal drive and the external drive. An internal drive is an integral part of the computer, such as the **hard drive**, where most of the computer's data are stored. The CD drive is also built into the computer, but it can be accessed from the outside through a small drawer or slot. This type of drive accepts CDs such as those that have music, photos, or information encoded on them.

An external drive is connected to the computer from the outside. This type of drive also stores data, but it can be easily removed (or unplugged) from the computer and taken to another computer for use. A flash drive, also known as a *thumb drive,* is 1½ to 2 inches (about 3.75 to 5 cm) long. It stores small amounts of data but is very portable and easy to use. Large, portable external drives can store significant amounts of data and are used to back up the internal hard drive or to expand the computer's storage capacity. A Zip drive is an external drive that is still available but seldom used because the data can be easily erased from it, and it holds a relatively small amount of data.

Drives used to be rigidly identified by a letter. This lettering system is no longer used in the way it was 10 years ago. The computer's hard drive usually is called the *C drive.* However, computers now have multiple drive capabilities, and these can be identified by any letter selected by the manufacturer of the device or the computer manufacturer.

Monitor

The **monitor** is the computer's screen, where data are viewed by the user. The screen is also called the *display* or *output display.* Several types of monitors are available, including the liquid crystal display (LCD) and the cathode ray tube (CRT). The **LCD** monitor is a flat screen (and sometimes is referred to by that name or as a *flat panel*). The monitor is operated from the keyboard or by touching the screen itself (**touch screen**).

Keyboard

The keyboard allows the user to type words, numbers, and symbols, which appear on the monitor or are identified as commands by the computer. The keyboard may be a separate component, or it may be integrated into the monitor and CPU as a single unit. Keyboards are available with letters and symbols in nearly every written language, including those that do not use the Roman (English) alphabet, such as Russian, Asian, and Arabic languages. Operations such as the on/off mode, Internet connection and audio commands may also be incorporated into the keyboard.

Mouse

The mouse is the user's "steering" component. It provides a means of selecting a visual cue on the monitor and signaling the computer to perform a task connected with that cue. The mouse rests on the table top, and the user places the hand in a comfortable position over the mouse. The mouse is synchronized to a pointer or other visual symbol that appears on the monitor. Buttons on the mouse are used to select and retrieve data displayed on the screen. Portable or compact computers have a touchpad built into the keyboard that performs the same tasks as a mouse.

Mice come in many styles and shapes. The mouse should fit the user's hand and should be comfortable to use. This is especially important for people who use the computer for many hours a day.

Speakers

Audio speakers produce audible output, or sound. The audio signals are transmitted from the computer drives to the speakers, which are built into the monitor or are attached.

Data Output

Data output is a visual or audible form of the information stored in the computer. Data output can be stored and reproduced in the form of a CD, digital video, paper printout, or sound that is transmitted through the computer's speakers. Older style disks have been replaced by compressed data in the form of a CD or DVD. Newer technologies are being developed to encode information in increasingly compressed forms. When the output is produced on paper or other physical readable form, it is called a **hard copy**. When the output is visible on the computer monitor or encoded on a disk or drive, it is called a soft copy.

A printer is the standard means of producing data output in paper form. Many types of printers are available for personal, commercial, industrial, and medical use. Printers produce hard copy, which can take the form of ordinary paper, a radiographic film, an electrocardiogram (ECG) strip, or some other type of readable material. A laser printer produces high quality output in color or black and white format. Other types of printers are the inkjet and solid ink types.

A scanner is a type of output printer used to copy paper data and place the information in the computer's memory. The scanner functions much like a plain paper copier. However, instead of producing a paper copy, it translates and compresses the data into computer language and stores it for later transmission or reproduction.

COMPUTER SOFTWARE

The term **software** is used to describe the electronic components of a computer. The computer needs information to perform the tasks that individuals program it to do. Unlike a mechanical device, which performs physical work, the computer sorts and computes information electronically. These tasks are made possible through the computer software.

To further define what software actually is, we need to know that the computer operates by reading a set of instructions that tell it what to do and how to do it. These instructions are contained in a code (called machine code), which is a series of billions of on-off switches. Combinations of on-off codes create endless possibilities for creating information (data) based on the on-off switch codes.

Data in the memory of the computer are organized into blocks of eight switches. Each switch is called a bit, and each block is called a byte. Computer programs (software) are described as having a certain number of bytes that operate in an exact way, giving the computer instructions to perform different tasks associated with that program.

Operating System

Computers are programmed to understand certain tasks through their operating system (OS). The OS is the electronic controller of all the data the computer needs to perform tasks. Several types of operating systems are commercially available. The most common are the Microsoft Windows, Macintosh, and Linux systems. In this discussion, the Microsoft system is used to describe basic functions and tasks.

Computer Programs

Computer applications, or programs, perform specific tasks. An application is used to produce text documents, calculate mathematical equations, play music, or display photographs. Many kinds of programs are available for home computing and professional tasks. The most common types are:

- **Word processing:** This program performs the functions of a typewriter with many additional features. Documents can be created and formatted into simple or complex styles. The most common commercially used programs are Microsoft Word and Word Perfect. An open source version is called OpenOffice. Word processing usually is the first application a new user learns.
- **Database** or *spreadsheet:* This type of program allows the user to enter complex data involving items, lists, and numerical or arithmetic information. Calculations and formulas associated with the data are also computed. Examples of databases are statistical analysis and bookkeeping programs.
- *Graphic design:* This type of program provides the computing tools needed to "draw" and manipulate figures or to create complex images based on quantitative data. Examples are programs for designing engineering or architectural structures.
- *Interactive educational programs:* These programs are designed to help the user learn subjects such as mathematics, languages, and physical sciences. Educational programs are available for nearly any subject.

Although commercially sold programs are the most popular, many computer users are switching to open source software. This type of software is noncommercial, and its intellectual property rights are in the public domain rather than belonging to a private corporation. These programs allow users to modify and openly share the processing information or language with others.

BASIC COMPUTER USE

Computer Motor Skills

To work on a computer, an individual must learn a number of motor skills. These are not difficult, but they require instruction and practice. Typing skills are required to enter data into the computer quickly and with a minimum of errors. Another important skill is operation of the mouse.

Pointing and Selecting with the Mouse

The mouse is used to select and manipulate data on the computer screen. The interface between the mouse and the screen is either a graphic arrow or an "I," which shows where the mouse is pointed. This is called a **cursor** or *pointer.* A command or icon is activated by setting the cursor on the icon or text and pressing one of the mouse buttons (right or left). This is called *clicking* on an item. When a screen feature is clicked, the computer understands that it has been selected for some action. For example, if you want to start a computer program, you first must click on the icon representing that program. One click selects the item, and two clicks open or retrieve the information associated with that item. The proper terms for the pressing the right and left buttons are *right click* and *left click.* A *double click* is two clicks of the same button.

Dragging

Dragging is a method of moving data icons and windows around on the monitor. To drag an item to a new location, place the cursor on the item. Left click and hold the button while moving the cursor, either by moving the mouse on the table top or with the mouse's track ball. When the item reaches the desired spot, release the button; this "drops" the item in the new location.

Elementary Operations

Start

To start the computer, it is necessary to locate the power button on the CPU or the keyboard. When the button is pressed, the computer begins to *boot up,* or start. The monitor lights up, and a logo appears on the screen. A password may be requested. If one is needed, a box appears on the screen asking for the password. The user must type the password in the box. Never share your password, and always *log off* after a computer session. This ensures that data are protected from manipulation by the next user (Box 18-3). When the computer accepts your password, another screen, will appear.

Desktop

In graphics-based platforms, the desktop is the background for all computer program work (Figure 18-11). It displays the visual cues needed to start programs and perform tasks. It also is the visual "home base" of the computer; that is, it

---

---

appears at the start and close of a computer session. The following sections discuss the items that appear on the desktop.

Note: The screen images and basic operations vary according to the year of publication for of the individual operating system and software.

Icon

An **icon** is a small picture or graphic cue associated with a program or data (see Figure 18-11). For example, particular information can be accessed through an icon that looks like a small file folder. Other examples of icons are those associated with documents, photographs, music, programs, Internet access, and power controls.

Start Menu

The Start menu is located at the bottom left corner of the desktop (Figure 18-12). This menu displays program icons and also a Help icon, where the user can access information on how to perform computer tasks. The Search icon is used to find data stored on the computer.

Task Bar

The **task bar**, located at the bottom of the screen, displays applications and documents that are active, or *running*.

Files and Folders

A file is an electronic location where data are stored. Files are also graphic images that appear on the desktop or hard disk. To access all the files of the computer:

Figure 18-11 Desktop.

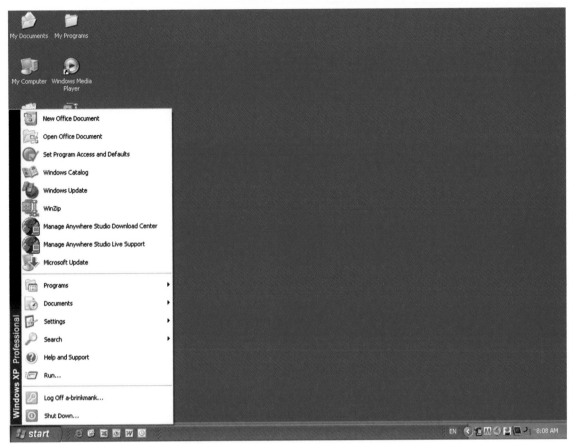

Figure 18-12 Start menu and task bar.

1. Right click on START.
2. Left click on EXPLORE.

This brings up a list of all the computer's files. Click on any file to select it. Double click to open the file and see the information. You can open a document inside the files by double clicking on it. To close a file, click on the small box with the X in the upper right corner of the document.

Windows

A **window** is a square frame that displays the boundaries of a document, graphic, or other image on the monitor. A window can be manipulated with the mouse. A window can be enlarged or reduced, or it can be moved around on the screen by dragging it with the mouse. To enlarge or reduce a window, look for three small boxes in the upper right corner. Left click on the middle box to reduce or enlarge the window. To change the size of a window, first reduce it and then drag the edges of the window to enlarge it. You can also change the window by dragging the lower right corner.

To remove the window from the screen while keeping it active (in use), click on the first (innermost) of the three boxes in the upper right corner. To restore the window to the screen, look for the tab associated with the window on the task bar and click on the tab.

Windows can be manipulated by clicking on one of the three boxes in the upper right corner. The far left box reduces the window. The middle box opens the window for viewing. The far right box will close the window and document completely. Do not close the window unless you have saved the document.

Toolbar

The **toolbar** is located at the top of a window (Figure 18-13). Many types of tool bars are available, each associated with specific programs. The toolbar displays icons and menus associated with tasks such as deleting text, saving documents to a file, computing a formula, and so on. To change the toolbar or to see different toolbar options, look for the toolbar menus at the top of the screen:

1. Left click on VIEW.
2. Left click on TOOLBARS.
3. Select a toolbar and left click on it.

To remove a toolbar, left click on the active toolbar from the VIEW menu.

Menu

A **menu** is a list of optional commands the user can select while viewing or manipulating data. The menu appears as a list from which the user can select and execute a command. Menus appear as part of a computer program, on the Internet, or as a component of the standard desktop. To use a menu, left click on a word in the menu such as WINDOW, FORMAT, or INSERT. A list of options immediately appears on the screen.

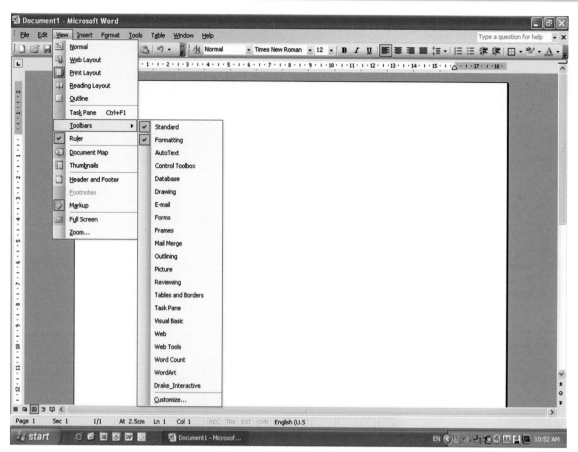

Figure 18-13 Toolbar.

To use an option, left click on it. This executes a task or opens a box with further options to select.

Scrolling

Scrolling is the method used to "turn pages" on the computer screen. Windows-based programs have a rectangular border on the right and bottom of the window. Inside these borders are arrows. To move through pages of a document, place the cursor on one of the arrows and left click or hold the mouse button down. This causes the document to move page by page. To stop scrolling, release the mouse button. You may also scroll through pages by dragging the square located within the borders.

Word Processing
Creating a Document

Word processing is a good way to learn how to use the computer. Many hundreds of options and formats are available on a word processing application. These can be learned over time with practice. The following are basic guidelines.

To start a new document in Microsoft Word, locate the WORD icon on the desktop or on the START menu. Click on this icon, and a new screen containing a blank "page" appears. The page is embedded inside a window (Figure 18-14). You can move the window around the screen by pointing and dragging it by the top of the frame.

Formatting Text

Text can be formatted and edited by using options on the STANDARD or FORMATTING toolbar (Figure 18-15).

Font

To change a font (typeface):
1. Select FORMAT/FONT. A list of fonts and sizes appears.
2. Click on the font you prefer and then confirm the command by clicking OK.

The font selected now is applied to the document. Another way to select the font is to click on the font menu displayed in the toolbar. To adjust the size of the font from the toolbar use, the menu located next to the font style. Select and click on the size desired.

Changing Case

Letter case (capital or small letter) is established using the keyboard Shift key. To change a case once it is entered on the screen:
1. Select FORMAT/CHANGE CASE.
2. Select and click on the appropriate case in the box that appears.

Indents and Spacing

To adjust the space between lines in the text:
1. Select FORMAT/PARAGRAPH from the toolbar.
2. Select the desired number of lines in LINE SPACING.

Figure 18-14 A window showing the boundaries of the document ready for typing and formatting.

To set the indent feature:
1. Select FORMAT/PARAGRAPH.
2. Choose the desired indentation feature from the menu displayed.

Page Numbers
To insert page numbers in the text:
1. Select INSERT/PAGE NUMBERS from the toolbar.

Selecting and Changing Text
To change the format or style of text that has already been entered in a document, you first must select the text with the mouse. This is done by positioning the cursor at the beginning of the word or sentence and then holding the left mouse button while moving the cursor over the text. Release the mouse button when all the desired text has been selected. Any format change will apply to the selected text. To *deselect* text, left click outside the selected area.

Editing Text
Delete, Move, and Paste Text
Sometimes text that has been entered must be deleted, or removed. To remove a word or small amount of text, place the cursor at the end of the area you want to delete and then backspace on the keyboard to remove. To remove large amounts of data, select the text with the mouse and press Delete or the backspace arrow on the keyboard. If you make a mistake in deleting text and you want to restore what was deleted, select EDIT and then UNDO TYPING from the toolbar.

To move text within a document:
1. Select the text.
2. Select EDIT/CUT from the toolbar.
3. Move the cursor to the desired location.
4. Left click.
5. Select EDIT/PASTE.

Spell Check
Spell check is a process in which the computer analyzes the spelling and grammar of the text and either suggests options for making corrections or makes them automatically. To use the spell check option:
1. Select TOOLS/SPELLING and GRAMMAR from the toolbar.

As the text is checked, a box with suggested corrections appears. To select one of the corrections, click on the option. The correction automatically replaces the error, and spell check continues until the entire text has been reviewed.

Graphics
Graphics are pictures used to enhance text documents. Pictures can be imbedded into the text from many different sources. Bringing an image from one electronic source to another is called importing. Most word processing programs include a set of standard or "stock" images that can be

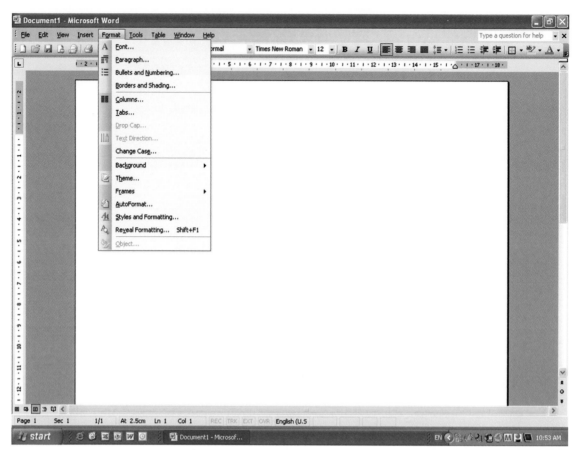

Figure 18-15 Formatting a document.

imported into a document. These are called *clip art,* and they do not require copyright permission. Images also can be imported from other documents or files you have stored in the computer. Images also can be obtained through the Internet or World Wide Web. However, these imported images must not be used indiscriminately. Professional and medical images may require formal permission from the owner of the image. Graphic images can also be "drawn" using a graphics program.

To import an image to text:

1. Place the cursor where you want the image to appear in the text.
2. Select INSERT from the toolbar.
3. Select PICTURE.
4. Select the source of the image and follow the prompts in the dialogue box.

Saving Data

The computer does not automatically preserve or **save data** that the user enters. If the computer is turned off while a document is open, data may be lost. Different computer platforms use various methods and commands for saving data before closing a session or turning off the computer. Data can be saved on the computer's hard drive (memory) or on external drives and disks.

Data should be saved frequently during computer work. Power surges, other technical problems, and human error can result in permanent loss of data. The most secure way to save data involves two operations: saving to the computer memory and backing up data on another drive or output, such as a CD, external drive, or paper. To save a document to the hard drive while using Microsoft Office:

1. Select FILE/SAVE AS.
2. When the dialogue window appears, select the file or drive where you want the document saved and click on it. Confirm the command by selecting SAVE.
3. After selecting the location for saving the document, you may select FILE/SAVE.

Printing Documents

Documents can be printed from the computer screen using a color or black and white printer. The printer is connected to the computer by cable and interfaces with it through its own software program. To print a document from the computer screen:

1. Select FILE on the toolbar.
2. Select PRINT. A dialogue box appears with options for style, paper size, and quality. Many other options become available by clicking on the PROPERTIES button. If no properties are selected, the computer reverts to its default settings.

Computer Networks

Types of Networks

The term computer network refers to two or more computers that are connected electronically. Networks allow the transfer of information from one computer to another.

The *Internet* is a vast computer network; it is *not* the same as the *World Wide Web*. The Web is a method of exchanging files, documents, graphics, and other discrete packets of information through the Internet. The method used to exchange and transfer the data is complex and beyond the scope of this discussion. However, it is important to understand that the Web is only one of many types of information systems that use computer networking.

An **intranet** is a system of multiple computers, in a facility or organization, that allows communication only within that system. Medical facilities often have their own intranet, which transmits useful information such as medical references, articles, and announcements about upcoming events. More important, hospital intranets publish the facility's policies and safety protocols so that everyone on the staff can continually update information about safety issues and patient care. E-mail is also part of the intranet system in most organizations. To access the intranet, you must use a password. When you log onto your employer's intranet server, always remember to log off before you quit the session. This prevents others from accessing information that you have entered.

Navigating the Internet and World Wide Web

Internet Research

Research on the Web is done through a search engine. This is a computer program accessed through the World Wide Web. The search engine allows the user to type in a topic or phrase, which is sent out through the network. The program then returns information in data blocks called *links*, which are listed by their Internet title and address. The user can open these links and access the material within. Examples of reliable search engines are Google and Lycos. To search Google for information on a topic, proceed as follows:

1. Open the Internet browser installed on the computer by clicking on it.
2. Look for the address bar in the Internet toolbar.
3. Enter http://www.google.com in the address bar and click *OK* or *Go* to confirm. The Google Web site will open.
4. Enter the search topic in the search box (Figure 18-16). A list of hyperlinks will appear. Click on any of these to access the information.

A vast amount of information is available on the Internet and World Wide Web. When these tools are used appropriately, research can be done quickly and efficiently. However, so much information is available that it sometimes is difficult to determine whether the source is reliable and the information is correct. Remember that anyone can post almost anything on the Internet, regardless of whether it is valid. It is up to the user to select information carefully.

Always scan your choices before you start opening files on the Internet. If you are doing professional research, use professional sites. If you want to buy a product or research products for sale (e.g., surgical equipment), use the commercial sites.

For academic research, it is wise first to locate an academic institution or professional association most appropriate to the topic and then search for the desired topic. For example, if you want to research a disease, instead of simply typing the name of the disease in the search box, try locating a medical or academic link first. Use organizations such as the Centers for Disease Control and Prevention (CDC), the American Medical Association (AMA), or the Mayo Clinic. These organizations' Web sites have extensive search engines that will give you accurate and authoritative information. If you do not know any professional organizations, use the Internet search engine to find one. Key terms such as *surgical organizations, infectious diseases,* or *medical reference* will also give you authoritative links. Look at the Internet address of the link before you randomly click on any of the choices. Educational institutions have "edu" in the address. Professional organizations have "org" in the address. If the address ends in "com," the site is a commercial one, with a focus on products to sell.

When researching a topic, try to be as concise as possible. For example, searching the word *surgery* in place of a specific type of surgery would return hundreds of thousands of documents, most of which would not be relevant. It is best to use combinations of words to research a topic. For example, use *orthopedic titanium knee* to obtain information about titanium implants used in orthopedic surgery of the knee.

Saving Internet Files

Information obtained through Internet searches can be saved on the computer in the same way that documents are saved. The best way to learn about saving and importing documents from the Internet is by studying and following the Internet tutorials, which are very easy to access on the toolbar. These tutorials and topical lists are designed to help both new learners and those who need more complex information. They are updated automatically by the Internet program itself and provide an excellent learning tool, especially when a more experienced person is available to answer questions that arise in the learning process.

E-Mail

Most people are familiar with e-mail, even if they do not use it regularly. This process allows individuals or groups to contact each other through e-mail programs on a network or the Internet and to send and receive messages, documents, and graphics electronically. When the user creates an e-mail and sends it through the Internet, it is first received by an e-mail server or agent, which processes and formats the data. The data are then sent electronically to the receiving agent, where the e-mail is directed to the receiver's Internet address. To learn how to compose and send e-mail, the new user should use the e-mail tutorial on the computer and consult another person who can demonstrate the process.

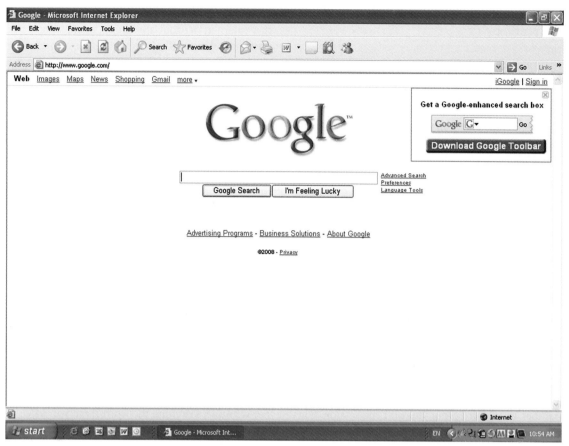

Figure 18-16 Google search engine and search box.

<u>Box 18-4</u>

E-Mail Etiquette

1. Always type in a subject heading so that the reader can identify the transmission.
2. It is appropriate in business or professional transmissions to begin the e-mail with a greeting, as in a letter, (i.e., Dear Dr. X, . . .).
3. Try to limit the transmission to one page. If a longer transmission is necessary, it should be formatted into a text document and sent as an attachment.
4. When one message is to be sent to more than four people, the names should be formatted as a group and the e-mail sent to the name of the group. This protects the confidentiality of the group members.
5. Attachments are documents, graphics, or other data sent as discrete and separate packets along with the e-mail. Large attachments often take a long time to transmit and can cause technical problems for the receiver. Large attachments, especially graphics, should be compressed before they are sent. Try to avoid sending large attachments to people who may not be interested in the information. Do not send attachments that contain information already stated in the body of the e-mail.
6. An e-mail in which the sender vents emotions or the text is inflammatory is called **flaming**. Flaming creates conflict and injures people. It is inappropriate and unacceptable. Examples of flaming are threats, inappropriate language, expletives, and emotional outbursts. Any words typed in upper case letters may be considered flaming if the context is negative.
7. Remember that an e-mail can be a legal document. What you say in an e-mail can be stored, retrieved, and used.
8. In professional correspondence, try to keep e-mails concise and to the point. Most people do not read an entire e-mail, especially if it is long. They read the first few lines and skim the remainder.
9. Always spell-check your e-mail before sending.
10. Include your name and contact information (if appropriate) at the end of the e-mail. Do not assume that the receiver knows who sent the e-mail.
11. Avoid saying things in an e-mail that you would not say to the receiver in person. Offensive and hurtful remarks in an e-mail are multiplied when the receiver cannot communicate body language or facial expressions, which are important methods of feedback that help us communicate with sensitivity and thoughtfulness.

Health care institutions often set up e-mail systems for their employees as a means of communicating messages and sending documents. New employees are instructed in how to access their mail and send messages within the system.

E-Mail Etiquette

E-mail is often casual in tone and can be sent and received almost instantaneously. The communicating parties are physically isolated from each other, and the transmissions can be anonymous. These qualities and human nature can result in improper use of e-mail. Within the last decade, a protocol for e-mail etiquette has been developed and accepted by the international Internet community. E-mail etiquette is followed in private and professional correspondence (Box 18-4).

CHAPTER SUMMARY

- Competence in surgical technology requires both the human element and technical expertise. The technical aspects of surgery draw most heavily from the field of mechanics.
- Mechanics is the study of motion and objects.
- The origins of mechanics are found in the laws of physics. Physics is the complex study of matter, time, energy, force, and space.
- The atom is the primary unit of matter that makes up all physical matter. The atom is composed of three primary particles: the proton, neutron, and electron.
- The nucleus, or center, of the atom contains two main particles, the neutron and the proton. The electron is much smaller than the proton and neutron and is negatively charged.
- Electrons occupy energy levels around the nucleus. When they are displaced, energy is released.
- A molecule is two or more atoms held together by chemical bonds. Atoms of a particular element have the same number of protons and neutrons; molecules of a substance are identified by the different elements of which they are composed.
- Matter can exist as a solid, liquid, or vapor (gas). These states do not change its chemical structure.
- Motion is the result of energy and work. The elements of motion are speed, displacement, distance, velocity, momentum, and force.
- When an object "moves" (or is moved), we say it is displaced.
- All surgical devices and technologies depend on some form of energy. Electricity is the most common form of energy used in medical devices.
- Mechanical energy is generated by compressing something that is elastic or springy. In its compressed form, it has potential energy.
- Chemical energy is derived from the different kinds of bonds that exist between molecules. When molecules are separated, the energy is released. Potential energy can be created when molecules bond.
- Electromagnetic energy, in the form of electricity, light, heat, and sound, is derived from electromagnetic radiation. All electromagnetic energy exhibits wave behavior.
- Wave behavior is predictable and measurable. The characteristics of waves are wavelength, frequency, and amplitude.
- Conductivity is the movement of electrons as they move from atom to atom. This movement follows the rule that opposite charges attract and like charges repel.
- Energy is never lost or destroyed, but it can be transformed from one form to another. Magnetism is not electricity, but the two are closely related. An electromagnetic field is created around a rotating coil, and the energy created can be captured and controlled to do work.
- A substance with low or no conductivity is called an insulator.
- Under certain circumstances, such as friction and low humidity, charged particles can accumulate on surfaces. If two surfaces have the same net charge, they will repel each other. If the net charges are opposite, the surfaces will attract each other. This is called static electricity.
- Free electrons flow through conductive material in a continuous path, each electron "pushing" the one ahead of it. This is called a circuit.
- An electrical circuit that flows in one direction from one charged pole to another is referred to as *direct current (DC)*. A battery is an example of a DC power source.
- In *alternating current (AC)*, the direction of the flow changes back and forth within the circuit.
- The force or power that pushes or drives electrons through a conductive material is called voltage.
- When the electricity flowing through a conductive material is made to flow through a more resistant one, heat or light is created.
- Unintended resistance in electrosurgery may cause current to seek an alternative path, causing severe burns on or in the patient.
- Light rays passing through a medium such as glass or plastic bend because the speed of the rays is decreased. This is called *refraction.*
- A lens can bend light rays according to the shape of the lens. A convex lens focuses light, whereas a concave lens spreads the rays.
- Heat can be transferred from one material to another by conduction, convection, and radiation.
- Sound is a type of energy generated by the movement of waves through a substance such as air or water. Ultrasound is used in diagnostic imaging. This technology is based on the reflective quality of waves.

- Computer technology now is used in nearly all types of complex medical devices.
- The computer's main function is to store data and retrieve it using electrical signals.
- A computer's *hardware* comprises its physical components. The electronic components of a computer are known as *software*.
- Computer applications or programs perform certain kinds of specific tasks.
- The most efficient way to learn basic computer skills is to do them with the help of a teacher or tutor.

- Computers are used for communication among staff members in health care institutions. Individual e-mail communication is password protected.
- All patient information kept on computers is strictly protected by data protection laws, in the same way that written and verbal information.
- Rules of etiquette for communication by e-mail have been adopted by an international community of electronic data users. These rules were created because of the improper use of e-mail.

REVIEW QUESTIONS

1. Surgical devices require energy sources to operate. What is the difference between mechanical energy and electromagnetic energy?
2. Define the properties of a wave.
3. Define conductivity.
4. What is insulation? How does it prevent the flow of electrons?
5. Why do electrons follow a conductive path?
6. What are the properties of visible light?
7. Describe three types of heat transfer. Give several examples of how heat transfer is directly related to patient safety.
8. Explain how ultrasound is used in diagnostic imaging.
9. How are data protected in institutional computers?
10. Why do we need rules for e-mail etiquette?

CASE STUDIES

1. In your hospital, you are part of the orthopedic team, which includes the surgical technologists who specialize in this field and a team leader. Your team leader needs to notify you of upcoming courses to be held at the health care facility. What is the best way to communicate this to all members of the team?
2. Discuss the ways in which you would prepare for and document a case, including tracking instruments, supplies, patient charges, charting, and communication without a computer.
3. The Doppler ultrasound creates images based on signals through the unobstructed interface between the hand-held transducer and the patient's skin. What might be the reasons for a distorted or incomplete image?
4. You are setting up for a case in which electrosurgery will be used. Your colleague asks you to prepare a patient grounding pad for use with the electrosurgery unit. You know that only bipolar energy will be used during the case, but you don't want to look unprepared. Should you prepare the grounding pad or not?
5. Discuss the importance of having knowledge in basic physics and computer technology as a surgical technologist.

BIBLIOGRAPHY

Association of periOperative Registered Nurses (AORN): *Standards, recommended practices and guidelines,* 2007 edition, Denver, 2007, AORN.

Bay Cities Public Schools: *Microsoft Office 2000 Tutorial*: 2000. Retrieved 8/12/08, at http://www.bcschools.net/staff/MicrosoftOffice.htm.

Halliday D, Resnick R, Walker J: *Fundamentals of physics,* ed 7, Danvers, Mass, 2005, John Wiley & Sons.

Henderson T: The physics classroom: 1996-2007. Retrieved 8/12/08, at www.physicsclassroom.com.

Medical Devices Agency: Clinical engineering device assessment and reporting: low/medium power electrosurgery review, 2002. March 2002: Retrieved 8/12/08, at http://www.wales.nhs.uk/sites3/docmetadata.cfm?

Medicines and Healthcare Products Regulatory Agency: MHRA evaluation 04080: high power electrosurgery review, 2004. September 2004: Retrieved 8/12/08 at www.NHSprocurement/CEP/surgicalequip/MHRA%2004080.pdf.

Microsoft Corporation: Using Microsoft 2000: 2007. Retrieved 8/12/08, at http://www.microsoft.com/education/o2ktutorial.mspx.

Stutz M: All about circuits, 1999-2000. Basic Concepts of Electricity. Retrieved 1/12/09, at http://www.allaboutcircuits.com.

Stutz M: All about circuits, 1999-2000. Volume I: AC. Retrieved 1/12/09, at http://www.allaboutcircuits.com.

Stutz M: All about circuits, 1999-2000. Volume I: DC. Retrieved 1/12/09, at www.allaboutcircuits.com.

Ulmar B: The ValleyLab Institute of Clinical Education electrosurgery continuing education module. July 2004. Retrieved 1/12/09, at www.valleylabeducation.org/pages/ed-esself/.html.

Energy Sources in Surgery

CHAPTER OUTLINE

LEARNING OBJECTIVES

After studying this chapter the reader will be able to:

- Describe how different energy sources are related to the electromagnetic spectrum
- Distinguish between monopolar and bipolar circuits used in electrosurgery
- Describe the use and components of electrosurgery
- Discuss the safe use of the patient return electrode
- List the primary hazards of electrosurgery and explain how to prevent accidents

- Distinguish between capacitive coupling and indirect coupling
- Explain how ultrasonic waves are used to perform surgery
- Discuss vessel sealing using radiofrequency energy
- Describe how lasers are used in surgery
- Recognize different types of laser media
- Discuss safety precautions used during laser surgery

TERMINOLOGY

Ablation: The complete destruction of tissue.

Active electrode: In electrosurgery, the point of the electrosurgical instrument that delivers current to tissue.

Active electrode monitoring (AEM): An electrosurgical instrument system that monitors the impedance of the instruments and stops the flow of electricity when it reaches a critical level.

Alternating current (AC): Electrical current that changes directions and transmits high-voltage electricity.

Amplification: In wave science, the phenomenon of increasing wave height by lining up the peaks and troughs of individual waves.

Argon: An inert gas used in electrosurgery to direct and shroud the electrical current.

Bipolar circuit: An electrosurgical circuit in which current travels from the power unit, through an instrument containing two opposite poles in contact with the tissue and then returns directly to the energy source.

Blended mode: In electrosurgery, a combination of intermediate frequency and intermediate wave intervals to produce a specific effect on tissue.

Capacitive coupling: A specific burn hazard of monopolar endoscopic surgery. It occurs when current passes unintentionally through instrument insulation and adjacent conductive material, into tissue.

Carbon dioxide: An inert gas used as a lasing medium during laser surgery.

Cauterization: The use of a hot object to burn tissue to achieve coagulation.

Circuit: The flow of electricity through a conductive medium.

Coagulum: A sticky, semiliquid substance that forms when tissue is altered by electrical or ultrasonic energy.

Coherency: A quality of laser light in which all light waves are lined up with troughs and peaks matching.

Conductive: The quality of a material to give up electrons easily and thus transmit electrical current.

Continuous wave lasers: Lasers that emit the laser light continuously rather that in pulses.

Cryoablation: A method of tissue destruction in which a probe is inserted into a tumor or tissue mass. High-pressure argon gas is injected into the probe, causing the surrounding tissue to freeze and eventually slough.

Cryosurgery: The use of extremely low temperature to destroy diseased tissue.

Current: The flow of electricity.

Current density: The concentration of current at any given point in the electrical circuit.

CUSA: Cavitron Ultrasonic Surgical Aspirator; this instrument destroys tumors through the use of high-frequency sound waves (ultrasound).

Cutting mode: In electrosurgery, the use of high voltage and relatively low frequency to cut through tissue.

Desiccation: The removal of water from tissue, causing it to die.

Direct coupling: The transfer of electrical current from an active electrode to another conductive instrument by accident or as part of the electrosurgical process.

Direct current (DC): A type of low-voltage current generated by battery.

Dispersive electrode: The part of the electrosurgical system that delivers current and heat directly to the tissue.

Duty cycle: In electrosurgery, the duration of current flow sometimes is referred to as the **duty cycle.** The duty cycle can intermittently be applied to produce the desired effect on tissue.

Electrosurgery: The direct use of electricity to cut and coagulate tissue.

Electrosurgical unit (ESU): The power generator and control source in the electrosurgical system.

Electrosurgical vessel sealing: A type of bipolar electrosurgery in which tissue is welded together using low voltage, low temperature, and a high-frequency current.

Electrosurgical waveforms: The transduced or actual waves generated when frequency, voltage, and power are delivered in different combinations during electrosurgery.

Eschar: Charred and burned tissue created by a high-voltage current.

Excimer: A type of lasing energy that is created when electrons are removed from the lasing medium.

Excitation source: In laser technology, the energy that causes the atoms of a lasing medium (gas or solid) to vibrate.

Frequency: In electricity, the periodicity of electromagnetic waves.

Fulguration: A process of tissue surface destruction used in electrosurgery.

Grounding pad: An alternate name for the patient return electrode.

Holmium:YAG: A solid crystal lasing medium that penetrates a wide variety of substances, including renal and biliary stones and soft tissue.

Impedance: The constriction of electrical current by a nonconductive material or an area of high density. This results in the transformation of electricity into thermal energy.

Implanted electronic device (IED): An electronic device that monitors and corrects physiological conditions. Electrosurgery may interfere with the function of such devices, which include pacemakers, internal defibrillators, deep brain stimulators, ventricular assist devices, and others.

Inactive electrode: An alternate term for the patient return electrode.

Insulate: To cover or surround a conductive substance with nonconductive material.

Isolated circuit: An electrical circuit that has no ground reference or method of conducting current into the ground at the site of use. Current is directed from the energy source, through the patient, and back to the source.

Laser: Acronym for light amplification by stimulated emission of radiation.

Laser classification: Industry and international system for grading laser energy according to its ability to cause injury.

Laser head: The component of the laser system that holds the lasing medium.

Laser medium: A solid or gas that is sensitive to atomic excitation by an energy source, which creates intense laser light and energy.

Lateral heat: The unintentional heating of tissue outside the direct area of electrosurgical application. Also called *thermal spread.*

Monochromatic: A characteristic of laser light in which the frequency of each wave is the same.

Monopolar circuit: In electrosurgery, a continuous path of electricity that flows from the electrosurgical unit to the active electrode, through the patient and the return electrode, back to the electrosurgical unit.

Neodymium:YAG: A solid lasing medium known for its attraction to protein and deep penetration into tissue.

Neutral electrode: An alternate term for the patient return electrode.

Nonconductive: The quality of a substance that resists the transfer of electrons and therefore electrical current.

Optical resonant cavity: The component of a laser system in which the lasing medium is contained and light is transformed.

Patient return electrode (PRE): A critical component of the monopolar electrosurgical circuit. The PRE is a conductive pad that captures electricity and shunts it safely out of the body and back to the electrosurgical unit.

Phacoemulsification: The destruction of cataracts using ultrasound technology.

Potassium-titanyl-phosphate (KTP): A low-power lasing medium that produces a very small diameter beam well-suited to microsurgery.

Pulsed wave lasers: Lasers that apply the laser light intermittently to the target tissue.

Q-switched lasers: An alternate name for pulsed wave lasers.

Radiant exposure: In laser technology, the combination of the concentration of laser energy and the length of time tissue is exposed to it.

Radiofrequency: Electromagnetic energy in which the frequency is in the area of radio transmission. In electrosurgery, radiofrequency electromagnetic waves are used to produce the desired surgical effect.

Radiofrequency ablation (RFA): The use of radiofrequency waves to destroy a tissue mass or surface.

Resistance: The restriction of electron flow in a direct current circuit.

Return electrode monitoring (REM): A safety system used in electrosurgery in which the PRE transmits continuous feedback on the quality of impedance in the electrode and stops the current when it becomes dangerously high.

Selective absorption: The absorption of a lasing medium into tissue being lased, according to its color and density.

Smoke plume: Toxic smoke emitted by tissue during electrosurgery and laser surgery.

Spray coagulation: An alternate term for fulguration.

Tunable dye laser: A type of laser formed by the combination of argon gas and specific dyes that alter tissue absorption of the lasing beam.

Ultrasonic energy: High-frequency energy created by vibration or excitation of molecules. This type of energy destroys tissue by breaking molecular bonds.

INTRODUCTION

Many forms of energy are used during surgery to cut tissue, coagulate blood vessels, and destroy diseased tissue. The most common forms are electrical, **radiofrequency**, kinetic (movement), sound (ultrasonic waves), thermal (temperature), and laser energy. Although electricity may be used to power these advanced medical devices, the energy used to perform the surgical procedure is not always electrical. For example, an instrument that generates ultrasonic waves is used to coagulate tissue. The instrument is powered by electricity, but the effect on the tissue is caused by vibration and friction.

Figure 19-1 shows the electromagnetic spectrum, which is the source of most energy. The importance of this figure is that it demonstrates the relationship between the frequency of electromagnetic waves and the energies they produce. The type of energy produced is directly related to the frequency of the waves. Some types of energy (e.g., light, color, and sound) can be perceived by the senses, whereas others are outside the range of human perception.

This chapter discusses common surgical devices that use electromagnetic energy and other types of energy. These devices are safe when used appropriately. However, they all carry the risk of serious injury. Surgical team members must understand the source of these risks to prevent serious accidents.

It is common practice for surgical personnel to identify a particular energy device by its proprietary name (company or trade name). However, these names do not identify the type of energy and, more important, the risks associated with them.

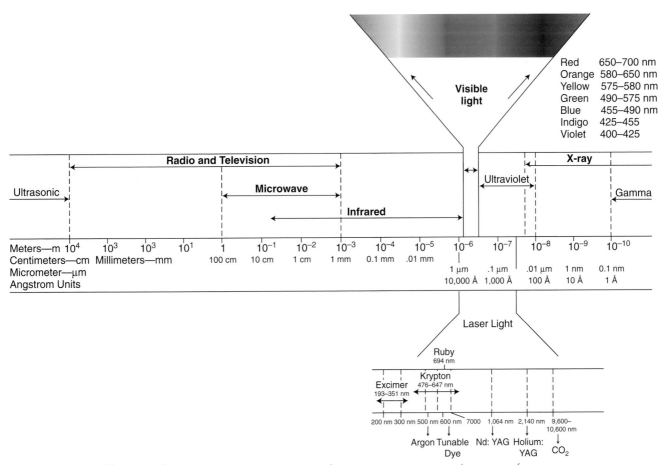

Figure 19-1 Electromagnetic spectrum. Electromagnetic waves are the source of most energy. The frequency of the wave determines the type of energy.

A clear understanding of this concept is very important in the prevention of injury to patients and personnel. The surgical technologist is responsible for knowing exactly what type (classification) of energy is being used so as to provide appropriate safety measures on the sterile field and while circulating.

ELECTRICAL ENERGY

REVIEW OF ELECTRICITY

Conduction

Electricity is the flow of electrons through a **conductive** medium; this is called **current**. Atoms of a conductive medium give up electrons easily, allowing them to flow through the circuit. **Nonconductive** material does not accept or give up electrons easily and is not a good pathway for electricity. Electricity is similar to the flow of water through a tube. The flow can be regulated, stopped, and started.

Current

The two types of electrical current are direct current and alternating current.

- **Direct current (DC)** flows in one direction only. This is the type of current found in low-voltage batteries.
- **Alternating current (AC)** switches direction at a constant rate (in the United States, this rate is 60 cycles per second). This type of current is generated by municipal power plants and produces high-voltage power.

Frequency

Because electricity is electromagnetic wave energy, it has a **frequency**, which is the number of wave cycles that occur in 1 second. High-frequency energy in the electromagnetic spectrum includes ultrasonic and radiofrequency waves. Recall from Chapter 18 that the frequency of all wave energy determines its type (e.g., visible light, electrical, radiation, radiofrequency, ultrasonic).

Impedance

The path of electricity from its origin to the destination is the **circuit**. When electricity is introduced through a conductive circuit, it continues to flow along an unimpeded path. When the path is interrupted by a less conductive medium, the current seeks a path around the **impedance**. If no alternate path is available, the electrical energy is transformed into heat or light. This heat is used to perform electrosurgery. Tissue impedance is the key to understanding electrosurgery.

Impedance to electricity is relative. A substance such as a copper wire can be very conductive, whereas glass and rubber are nonconductive. Nonconductive materials are used to **insulate** the conductive material carrying electricity to prevent injury and maintain the flow of electricity within its circuit. This is relevant to understanding how faults occur in electrosurgical devices and instruments that transmit electricity.

Electricity and the Body

The human body uses electrical energy to perform many vital functions, such as conduction in the heart to pump blood and impulses from one nerve cell to another. These are internal changes created by the movement of ions (charged molecules and elements).

When electricity is applied to the body externally, the tissue reacts according to the **voltage** and frequency. High voltage is potentially more damaging than low voltage. The frequency of the current also influences tissue effects. Table 19-1 shows the effects of electricity at different voltages and frequencies.

The body is very sensitive to low-frequency electricity. *As the frequency increases, the body's response decreases.* Wave energy at frequencies above 100,000 cycles (Hz) per second does not interfere with the body's normal bioelectrical activity. Tissue can be burned at these frequencies, but the heart and other bioelectrical mechanisms are not affected. However, frequencies at or below 100 kHz *do* interfere with the body's bioelectrical activity and can result in electrocution and cardiac arrest.

Electrosurgical units operate at extremely high frequencies (300,000 to 1 million Hz). At this level, tissue is can be burned, coagulated, and cut without risk of electrocution or cardiac arrest.

KEY CONCEPTS OF ELECTROSURGERY

Electrosurgery is the direct use of electrical energy to cut, coagulate, and weld tissue. The key concepts of electrosurgery are:

- Electrosurgery works by transmitting high-frequency electricity to tissue. The current is impeded at the point of contact with the tissue, and this creates heat.
- High-frequency current does not interfere with the body's normal functions, whereas a low-frequency current can cause electrocution or cardiac arrest. Elec-

Table 19-1

Effects of Electricity on the Body

Body Response	Direct Current	Alternating Current (60 Hz)	Alternating Current (10 kHz)
Slight perception	1 mA	0.4 mA	7 mA
Pain	5.2 mA	1.1 mA	55 mA
Severe pain and difficulty with respiration	90 mA	23 mA	94 mA
Fibrillation and possible cardiac arrest	500 mA	100 mA	—

mA, Milliampere; *Hz,* hertz; *kHz,* kilohertz.

trosurgery converts high-voltage, low-frequency electricity into very high frequency energy, which does not cause electrocution.

- Voltage and frequency can be safely manipulated at the power source to produce different tissue effects.
- Cautery is the application of a *hot object* to living tissue. The **electrosurgical unit (ESU)** delivers electrical energy, which meets impedance (loss of conductivity) in the tissue. Heat is created *in the tissue* at the point of **resistance**.

USES OF ELECTROSURGERY

EFFECTS OF ELECTRICAL CURRENT ON TISSUE

The way tissue reacts to electrosurgery depends on a number of variables:

- *Tissue type:* The amount of water and collagen in the tissue and its density.
- *Exposure time:* The duration of contact with the electrical current.
- **Current density:** As current density increases, tissue response also increases. Current density increases when voltage is forced through a small area.
- *Frequency and voltage of the electrosurgical wave:* Specific combinations of frequency and voltage produce different effects in tissue.

Direct application of hot implements to tissue has been used throughout history to stop hemorrhage and sterilize wounds; this procedure is called **cauterization**. Cauterization differs from electrosurgery, which uses high-frequency energy to cut and coagulate tissue. The term *cautery* often is used incorrectly to describe any kind of electrosurgery. In fact, cautery refers only to the application of a superheated object to tissue.

Some of the most common uses of electrosurgery include:

- Making an incision (cut) through tissue
- Coagulating blood vessels and stopping minor hemorrhage
- Destroying or removing diseased tissue
- Welding tissue together

COMPONENTS OF ELECTROSURGERY

POWER UNIT (GENERATOR)

The ESU power source (also called a *generator*) is the control and power unit (Figure 19-2). The modern power source is digitally controlled and has both monopolar and bipolar capability (explained later in the chapter). Power adjustments are programmable and controlled by push buttons on the screen panel. Digital waveforms showing the frequency, wavelength, amplitude, and other information is displayed on the screen. The ESU power source often is referred to as a *bovie*, which was the prototype ESU system introduced in the 1930s.

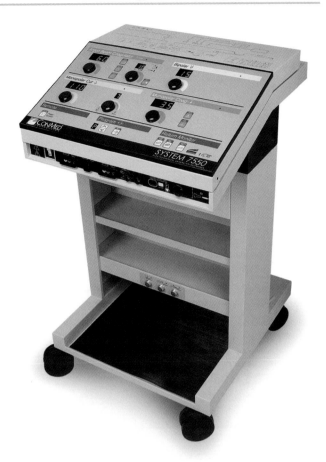

Figure 19-2 Electrosurgical power unit, also known as the *electrosurgical unit (ESU) generator. (Courtesy Conmed, Inc.)*

ACTIVE ELECTRODE

The **active electrode** is the actual contact point at the tissue. It is contained at the tip of the ESU handpiece, or "pencil" (Figure 19-3). The handpiece is connected to the power source by a lightweight cable. Many types of active electrode tips and instruments are available, because the devices are used in open surgery, minimally invasive surgery, and endoscopic procedures (Figure 19-4).

CONTROLS

The surgeon usually controls the ESU using a set of foot pedals. Some types of ESU pencils have switches on the handpiece.

PATIENT RETURN ELECTRODE (MONOPOLAR CIRCUIT ONLY)

The patient return electrode (or, simply, the return electrode) is a pad or thin plate that is placed close to the surgical wound site. It captures electrical current from the active electrode and transmits it back to the power unit (Figure 19-5). The return electrode is connected to the power source by a conductive cable fitted on the outside surface of the pad.

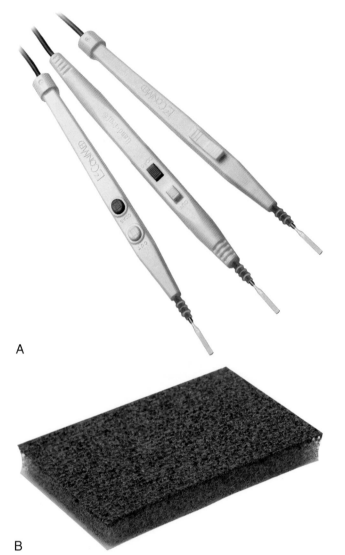

A

B

Figure 19-3 **A,** Monopolar active electrode pencil; also called the *bovie*. **B,** Cleaning pad for the electrosurgical unit (ESU) pencil. Accumulated tissue debris on the ESU pencil can serve as a source of burns and fire. The cleaning pad (also called a *scratch pad*) is used to wipe debris from the active electrode. *(Courtesy Conmed, Inc.)*

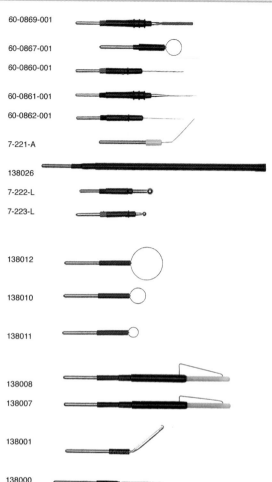

60-0869-001
60-0867-001
60-0860-001
60-0861-001
60-0862-001
7-221-A
138026
7-222-L
7-223-L

138012
138010
138011

138008
138007
138001
138000

Figure 19-4 Active electrode tips available for different types of monopolar electrosurgery. *1,* Flat tip—general cutting and coagulation. *2,* Loop—biopsy and cutting. *3,* Fine needle—precise desiccation. *4,* Coarse needle. *5,* Blunt needle. *6,* Angled needle. *7,* Flat tip with extension—deep tissue general use. *8,* Ball tip, regular—fulguration. *9,* Ball tip, long—deep tissue fulguration. *10* to *12,* Cutting loops, long. *13* and *14,* Conization loop—endocervical cutting and coagulation. *15* and *16,* Straight and angled long flat tips. *(Courtesy Conmed, Inc.)*

MONOPOLAR ELECTROSURGERY

Two types of circuits are used in electrosurgery: the **monopolar circuit** and the **bipolar circuit**. Both circuits use alternating current and require the power unit described previously.

In monopolar mode, electricity flows from the ESU through a power cable to the ESU pencil and active electrode. The active electrode transmits energy in the form of heat and electrical impulses.

❖ *When the electrode tip is activated, electrical current flows to the electrode tip. When the tip touches the body tissue, electricity is impeded. This creates intense heat and produces the desired surgical effect, such as cutting or coagulation.*

Monopolar electrosurgery uses high-voltage AC. The monopolar electrode is used primarily for cutting, coagulation, and desiccation.

PATIENT RETURN ELECTRODE

As mentioned previously, the **patient return electrode (PRE)** is a gel pad or thin plate with a conductive cable attached to its surface. The pad is placed on the patient before surgery whenever monopolar electrosurgery will be used. The PRE shunts electrical current dispersed from the active electrode back to the ESU power unit (Figure 19-6). The return electrode is known by a number of different names, such as the **dispersive electrode**, **inactive electrode**, **neutral electrode**, or **grounding pad**.

When properly applied to the patient, the PRE prevents burns, because it spreads the current at the point where it exits the body. However, if it is not applied correctly or if it becomes dislodged during surgery, the patient can suffer serious injury. Box 19-1 lists safety guidelines for use of the return electrode.

BIPOLAR ELECTROSURGERY

In **bipolar electrosurgery**, the surgeon uses a forceps or similar instrument that has two contact points (or a return point built into a single tip). Current leaves the power unit and travels from one pole to the other, passing only through the tissue between the contact points before returning to the ESU unit. The electrosurgical effect is restricted to this tissue, and current exits back through the instrument without dispersing through the patient's body. No PRE, or grounding pad, is used, because electrical current does not pass through the body. The voltage used in bipolar surgery is lower than that used for monopolar surgery, which makes the bipolar mode a safer technique with fewer risks for patient injury.

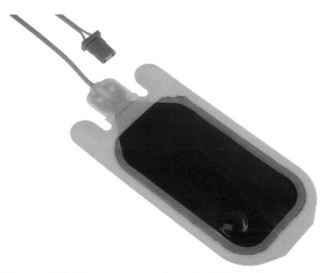

Figure 19-5 Patient return electrode (PRE) used in monopolar electrosurgery. The PRE is also known as a *patient grounding pad, dispersive electrode,* or *inactive electrode.* The purpose of the PRE is to provide a safe return path for electricity transmitted through the electrosurgical unit pencil and the patient's body. *(Courtesy Conmed, Inc.)*

Box 19-1

Safety Measures for Use of the Patient Return Electrode

- Always assess the patient's skin before and after applying the patient return electrode (PRE).
- The skin must be dry and free of hair. Moisture under the PRE can cause it to pull away from the skin. Shaving may be necessary for uniform contact with the skin.
- Use a PRE that has been stored in a sealed package only. The moisture content and quality of the conductive gel cannot be guaranteed with prolonged exposure to air.
- Inspect the PRE before applying it and check the expiration date on the package. The electroconductive gel must be moist and should have been stored at the temperature specified by the manufacturer.
- Use the correct size PRE for the patient's surface area. Operating room protocol determines the appropriate pad size.
- Pediatric size PREs are available. Never cut a PRE to fit the patient's size.
- The PRE must be placed close to the surgical site over a large muscle mass. Muscle has low impedance and is the best conductor. The PRE must not be placed over a prominent bony surface, scar, tattoo, hair, or fatty tissue; these increase impedance and can result in a burn.
- The PRE must be in complete contact with the skin, without tenting or buckling.
- Make sure the PRE cord has adequate slack to prevent pulling and displacement.
- Apply the PRE after final positioning to prevent dislodgement.
- Always check the PRE cable to make sure it is intact and undamaged. Check it from end to end, including the attachment clips and the plug or insertion point into the electrosurgical unit (ESU).
- Do not assume that single-use items are intact and free of damage. Inspect every device, every time.
- Do not use a PRE *if only bipolar electrosurgery* will be used.

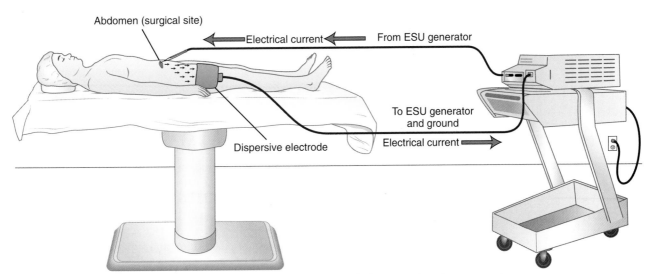

Figure 19-6 Monopolar electrosurgery circuit. With monopolar electrosurgical units, electrical current flows from the power source to the active electrode, through the patient's body, to the patient return electrode (PRE), which transmits it back to the power unit. This completes the circuit and prevents inadvertent patient burns.

The bipolar unit is used mainly on low impedance tissue because the low voltage is not strong enough to penetrate effectively through tissue such as bone or fat. An advantage of bipolar electrosurgery is that minimal heat is spread to surrounding tissues, which makes this technique safe for very delicate areas such as the brain and microvascular tissue. The bipolar unit delivers both cutting and coagulation modes and is especially useful for microsurgery, in which **lateral heat** spread would damage delicate nerves or blood vessels.

ELECTROSURGICAL WORKING MODES

The specific effects of electrosurgery (e.g., cutting, coagulation, and so on) are related to whether the electrical current is delivered continuously or intermittently. These modes are displayed on the power unit as **electrosurgical waveforms** (Figure 19-7). The modes are preset and programmable with guidance from the manufacturer's technical advisor. The waveform itself is simply a visual representation of current transmission.

The duration of current flow sometimes is referred to as the **duty cycle**. When the duty cycle is pulsed or intermittently applied, waves are connected by a continuous line, which represents a period when the current stops. Continuous repetition of high-frequency waves at low voltage is characteristic of the cutting mode. The coagulation mode appears as intermittent waves at low frequency and high voltage.

The **blended mode** provides a combination of intermediate frequency and intermediate wave intervals. Radiofrequency electrosurgery and microprocessor technology combine to allow the surgeon many choices of waveform blending, with safety features that prevent voltage spikes and accidental tissue injury.

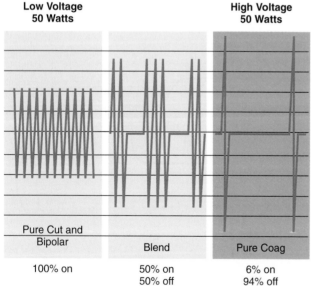

Figure 19-7 Electrosurgical waveforms. The effects of electrosurgery on tissue are related to voltage and whether current is delivered continuously or intermittently. *(From Rothrock J: Alexander's care of the patient in surgery, ed 17, St Louis, 2007, Mosby.)*

CUTTING

The **cutting mode** is produced by high-voltage energy. In this mode, the electrode is held above the tissue and does not make contact. The air between the electrode and the tissue acts as a conductor (called a *spark gap*), allowing the high-voltage current to flow between the tissue and the electrode.

The cutting mode causes tissue **desiccation** (burning with the loss of water content). When a thin, narrow active electrode is used, the current is very concentrated. The tissue heats rapidly, causing the water in the cells to explode. This releases steam and dissipates the heat. As the superheated tissue releases its water content, it quickly dries.

Cutting electrodes are available in many designs and configurations. These include the standard blade electrode and others such as wire loops, spatulas, and needle tips. The spatula electrode is most commonly used.

Microbipolar cutting is among the newer modes available in bipolar electrosurgery. Fine-needle electrodes are used to sever tissue safely, using blended frequency. Bipolar cutting probes are available in many designs, and bipolar scissors are also used to cut and coagulate tissue (see Figure 19-3).

COAGULATION

The voltage is lower in the coagulation mode than in the cutting mode. The electrode is held in contact with the tissue or slightly above it. During contact, the active electrode is held in brief or pulsed contact with the blood vessel. Heating is slower, which results in tissue "welding" that seals blood vessels. Lengthy contact results in the formation of **eschar**, or blackened, burned tissue. This can tear away from the surface and cause rebleeding. The buildup of eschar on the electrode increases impedance, which raises the temperature at the point of contact. Eschar also increases the risk of sparking at the point of tissue contact. Electrosurgical tips are coated with a protective substance such as Teflon or silicone to help prevent the formation of eschar.

The bipolar coagulation mode is safe for use on vessels when lateral spread is an important consideration, such as in microsurgery, vascular surgery, and neurosurgery. Bipolar forceps loops, probes, and hooks are used to cut and coagulate very delicate tissue.

FULGURATION

Fulguration, or **spray coagulation**, is performed on tissue with pulsed or intermittent application of the active electrode. In this technique the current is pulsed through the active electrode, which is held just above the tissue. The high voltage creates an arc of current that spreads over a relatively large area compared to direct contact techniques. The effect is a combination of coagulation and superficial tissue cutting.

ELECTROCAUTERY

As mentioned previously, electrocautery is the use of a heated element to occlude small blood vessels during surgery. A handheld electrocautery unit commonly is used during ophthalmological surgery. The unit is powered by double- or triple-A batteries. The active electrode is a fine metal filament that is controlled by a switch on the handpiece.

RADIOFREQUENCY ABLATION

Radiofrequency ablation (RFA) is the destruction of tissue using radiofrequency energy waves. This mode has numerous uses, including the destruction of tumors and endometrial tissue in gynecological surgery. During tumor ablation, an electrode is inserted directly into the diseased tissue. The high-frequency energy causes the molecules of the tissue to vibrate, which creates sufficient heat to destroy the tissue.

Bipolar RFA is used in conjunction with a conductive fluid medium to destroy diseased tissue. In this type of surgery, a hollow organ (e.g., the bladder or uterus) is filled with fluid, and the bipolar probe is used to destroy tissue in the fluid-filled cavity. RFA is also used to treat heart disease in which cellular damage creates irregular conduction patterns.

ELECTROSURGICAL VESSEL SEALING

Electrosurgical vessel sealing uses high-frequency, bipolar electrosurgery, low voltage, and physical pressure to create a weld in tissue. A number of vessel sealing systems are available, such as PK Technology (Figure 19-8), LigaSure, and Enseal. The elements of a vessel sealing system are:

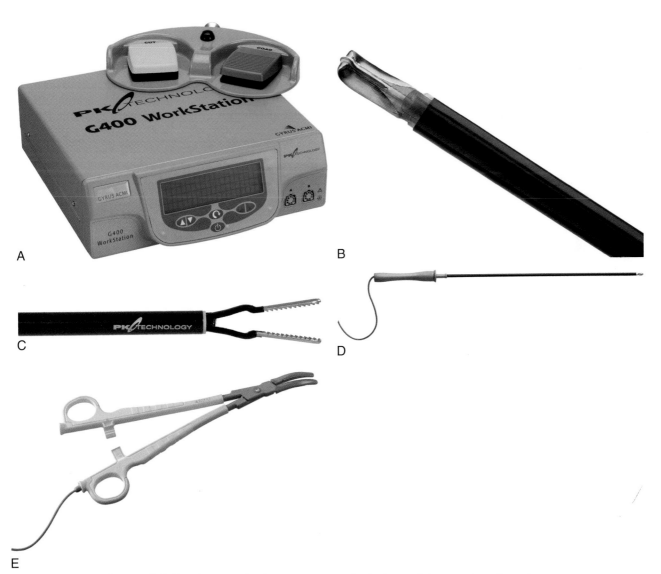

Figure 19-8 The PK Technology system provides high-speed, hemostatic cutting using bipolar energy. The system cuts, coagulates, and seals tissue while minimizing thermal spread. **A,** Power generator. **B,** Plasma J hook. **C,** Cutting tip. **D,** Plasma spatula. **E,** Open surgery forceps. *(Courtesy Gyrus ACMI, Inc.)*

- Transmission of radiofrequency waves to tissue through specialized grasping instruments
- Tissue impedance monitoring
- A microprocessor (programmable computer chip) that controls and programs the system
- An alarm system that automatically stops the current when the tissue seal is achieved

The vessel sealing system is used during resection procedures that traditionally require sequential clamping, suturing, and cutting. Whereas the traditional method of resection requires multiple instruments, the vessel sealing system accomplishes these tasks with only one instrument. This can reduce operating time and allow the surgeon to remain focused on the surgical site without the need for instrument exchange. The system is popular for selected patients in hysterectomy and some general surgery applications. A low temperature is used, which prevents charring and unintentional lateral heating. The instrument tip remains relatively cool, which prevents the tissue from tearing when the tips are released.

ARGON-ENHANCED ELECTROSURGERY

Argon gas is used in some procedures that use electrosurgical energy to focus the current during cutting and coagulation. Argon is inert and nonflammable but easily ionized. When a stream of argon gas is directed around the active electrode, it focuses the current and prevents sparking. Argon-enhanced electrosurgery also reduces smoke plume and displaces oxygen along its path. This increases the safety and efficiency of the procedure. It is particularly useful during long fulguration procedures that require extended electrosurgery.

ELECTROSURGERY SAFETY

Electrosurgery historically has posed one of the greatest risks in the operating room. Recent advances in technology have lowered but not removed the risk of patient burns. Patient fires and burns related to electrosurgical devices still occur because safety protocols are not followed or personnel fail to recognize the danger signs. All perioperative personnel are responsible for preventing these accidents. Surgical technologists must be familiar with the safe use of specific devices and equipment in their facility.

GENERATOR SAFETY

Modern generators now allow connections for both monopolar and bipolar functions. The system contains a self-check, which is activated before use. Power and blend settings can be preset and programmed into the unit. These features are convenient but may lead to safety risks when automatic settings are not appropriate for a specific tissue and impedance. During surgery, the perioperative team must suspect a problem if the surgeon repeatedly requests increases in power (voltage). This may indicate increased impedance, which can lead to fire or extensive burns.

Monopolar electrosurgery is performed through an **isolated circuit**. This means that the current travels only from the ESU generator, through the patient and the PRE, and back to the generator. There is no ground reference for discharge of electricity, as in older models of electrosurgery units.

Tissue impedance monitoring is available in many modern units. This safety feature provides automatic adjustments in voltage according to the impedance encountered in the tissue. Preprogramming of the automatic settings must ensure that the lowest power setting is used to achieve the desired surgical effect.

Generators must be used according to the manufacturer's specifications and within the guidelines of operating room policy. Written instructions and safety guidelines should be kept with the unit or close at hand to prevent misuse.

The surgeon is responsible for the direct use of active electrodes during surgery. However, if personnel have questions about power settings or other potentially harmful features, they must be able to participate in decision making from a firm knowledge base. This means that all staff members ultimately are responsible for the safe use of the ESU. Power settings must be used reasonably, and any alarms or other equipment warning systems require a response to prevent accident and injury. Alarm systems are designed to alert staff members to safety risks and should never be turned off or made barely audible. Loud music in the operating room has been identified as a barrier to hearing otherwise audible alarms. Box 19-2 presents safety guidelines for use of an ESU.

ACTIVE ELECTRODE SAFETY

Active electrode safety includes precautions to prevent accidental burns at the surgical site and electrical faults that occur between the electrode tip, handpiece, and connecting cord.

Box 19-2

Safety Guidelines for Use of an Electrosurgical Unit

1. Always inspect all power cords and cables before using the electrosurgical unit (ESU) generator.
2. Do not place items on top of the ESU generator. The unit's cooling system may not function properly, and this could result in overheating and malfunction.
3. Always allow the ESU to self-check, if this feature is available, before connecting cables.
4. Always ensure that the ESU generator is approved for the active electrodes and patient return electrodes in use. Do not attempt to use a return electrode monitoring system with a generator that does not recognize that feature.
5. Keep the generator away from other electronic and power sources, because they may cause electrical interference.
6. Keep fluids and fluid sources away from the generator. Never place fluid or solution containers on top of the generator, even if the containers are sealed.
7. Each generator is designed to operate with different waveforms and power settings.
8. Become familiar with your facility's equipment and its capabilities.

Recall that the active electrode is the metal tip of the instrument that conducts radiofrequency energy directly into the target tissue. In monopolar electrosurgery, the tip transmits high-voltage power with powerful cutting and coagulation properties. The tip is capable of severing dense tissue, including bone. It also can cause inadvertent burns to the patient and scrubbed team members when used improperly.

Before surgery, the active electrode and cord must be examined for integrity. The scrub is responsible for ensuring that no defects are present in the insulation of the instrument and that the active electrode is seated tightly into the hand-piece. Remember that disposable as well as reusable units can have defects. Do not connect the active electrode until the PRE is secure and connected to the ESU generator.

During surgery, the active electrode pencil must be kept in a nonconductive safety holster on the surgical field. The holster must be in plain sight of the team, and the ESU pencil must be replaced in it *after each use*. Never leave the pencil on top of the patient or drapes. Place the holster in a position that is convenient to the surgeon's reach so that the pencil can be easily stowed after each use. Do not attach the handpiece to the drapes by wrapping it around metal clamps or twisting the cord. Stray current can escape into the metal clamp. Twisting or tying the cord can break the conductive wires inside and put a strain on the insulation.

When eschar or **coagulum** (welded tissue) accumulates on the tip of the active electrode, the scrub should wipe it clean with a nonabrasive sponge. Abrasive materials or a scalpel blade should not be used to clean the electrode. Scraping the electrode causes abrasions and pitting, which make the tip more vulnerable to the buildup of tissue. Eschar creates increased impedance and heat, which causes sparking and lateral burns at the operative site. Combination suction-coagulation tips must also be kept free of debris. Always use water, not saline, to clear the inside of the suction tube, because water is nonconductive.

In some procedures the surgeon may want to use a hemostat or other clamp to conduct current from the active electrode to tissue. This is called "buzzing the hemostat." This practice is not recommended by safety agencies but occurs nevertheless. The risks associated with this use of electrosurgery are increased lateral heat and accidental burning of the person holding the hemostat.

HAZARDS IN MINIMALLY INVASIVE SURGERY

CAPACITIVE COUPLING

Capacitive coupling is a specific burn hazard of monopolar endoscopic surgery. It occurs when current passes inadvertently through instrument insulation and adjacent conductive material into tissue. Burns resulting from capacitive coupling are particularly dangerous in minimally invasive surgery, because the injury most often occurs outside the viewing area of the endoscope. The damage may go unnoticed until an infection develops at the burn site days later. Using only metal cannulas and active electrode monitoring (discussed later in the chapter) can prevent capacitive coupling.

DIRECTING COUPLING

Direct coupling is the flow of electricity from one conductive substance to another. This can occur when the insulation protecting the circuit has a defect or when an active electrode comes in contact with another conductive object. During minimally invasive surgery, direct coupling can occur when an active electrode touches the tip of another instrument in an instrument "collision." Direct coupling involving insulation failure can be more dangerous, because the resulting burn may not be detected immediately. In open surgery, direct coupling can occur whenever an active electrode insulator is inserted into a conductive metal sheath, such as a suction catheter. Direct coupling can be prevented by frequent inspection of insulation and proper care and handling of electrosurgical instruments. However, active electrode monitoring is the recommended method of preventing burns from insulation failure.

ACTIVE ELECTRODE MONITORING

Active electrode monitoring (AEM) is universally recommended by safety standard agencies to prevent accidental burns during electrosurgery. The system replaces nonmonitoring instruments with special AEM instruments designed to measure and react to impedance in the insulation. Recall that impedance along an electrical circuit results in heating. Defects in the insulation may cause current to escape through this pathway, but the flow is constricted or impeded, and this creates heat at the point of restriction. The AEM system measures impedance and immediately stops the flow of electricity when impedance reaches a critical level.

RETURN ELECTRODE MONITORING

Newer electrosurgical units use a safety feature that determines the impedance at the site of the PRE. The **return electrode monitoring (REM)** system, also known as the *return electrode contact quality monitoring system (RECQMS)*, automatically stops the flow of current when impedance reaches a preset level. An alarm system also alerts the user that impedance has exceeded a safe level. To function, the REM patient return electrode must be used with specific REM components.

PATIENTS WITH AN IMPLANTED ELECTRONIC DEVICE

A patient with an **implanted electronic device (IED)** requires special consideration when electrosurgery is planned. Implanted electronic devices include but are not limited to the following:

- Pacemaker
- Implanted cardiac defibrillator
- Deep brain stimulator

- Ventricular assist device (VAD)
- Spinal cord stimulator
- Programmable ventricular shunt
- Cochlear implant
- Auditory brainstem implant
- Bone conduction stimulator

These devices monitor and correct physiological dysfunctions and can be subject to interference from radiofrequency electromagnetic energy including electrosurgical equipment. The monopolar ESU poses particular risks for patients with IEDs, which can malfunction during use of the ESU.

To prevent patient injury related to IED interference, staff members must know the specifications for the type of IED and its location before surgery. In some cases the IED manufacturer must be notified to provide expert information on the specific device and potential interference. In some cases the manufacturer's representative may be present to help reprogram and test the device in the perioperative period.

All patients with an IED are monitored per hospital protocols, and standard procedures for ESU safety are followed.

SMOKE PLUME

During electrosurgery and laser surgery, tissue is destroyed or incised, and this process creates toxic smoke called **smoke plume**. Smoke plume contains about 95% water and 5% other products. The other products include chemicals, blood cells, and intact or fragmented bacteria and viruses. The potential hazards of these substances are infectious disease transmission, toxicity from chemicals, and allergy. The size of aerosol particles ranges from 0.1 to 0.8 μm. These droplets are capable of harboring much smaller viral and bacterial particles.

Smoke plume contains a number of toxic chemicals in concentrations that can potentially exceed those recommended by the Occupational Safety and Health Administration (OSHA). Among the chemicals found in smoke plume are toluene, acrolein, formaldehyde, and hydrogen cyanide. Both laser and electrosurgical plume contain living and dead cells. Disease transmission through smoke plume is a known risk to surgical personnel. Other transmissible biological particles, such as cancer cells, at laser and electrosurgical sites are an additional concern.

Risk Reduction

Smoke plume reduction or elimination is a mandatory process during electrosurgery and laser surgery. Normal room ventilation is not sufficient to capture chemical and biological particles from smoke plume. Two methods are used to prevent perioperative personnel from inhaling smoke: in-line room suction systems and commercial smoke evacuation devices. Room suction is designed to carry liquids, not smoke. These systems pull at a much lower rate than commercial smoke evaluation systems and must have in-line filters attached to be safe. Smoke evacuation systems are specifically designed to extract moist smoke plume from the surgical site.

Smoke Evacuation System

A smoke evacuation system contains a nozzle tip, suction tubing, filters, absorbers, and a vacuum pump. Smoke plume is evacuated at a rate of about 100 to 150 feet (30 to 46 m) per minute at the site of generation. It then is carried through a high-efficiency particulate air (HEPA) filter and trapped in absorbers. The filters are considered biohazardous waste and must be disposed of according to hospital policy. When a smoke evacuator is used, the nozzle tip must be within 2 inches (5 cm) of the surgical site to be effective. Fresh filters and tubing must be used for each patient. Some ESU systems now have intrinsic smoke evacuation systems.

KINETIC ENERGY

ULTRASONIC ENERGY

Ultrasonic energy is created when electricity is *transformed into mechanical energy* generated by high-frequency vibration and the forces of friction. The ultrasonic instrument simultaneously cuts and coagulates tissue by transmitting ultrasonic wave energy through specially designed forceps, scissors, or blades. The instrument vibrates at approximately 55,000 movements per second, and these vibrations cause protein molecules to rupture. One drawback of this type of energy is that it cannot cut tissue without coagulating it. When the instrument is applied, the tissue liquefies and forms coagulum, a sticky protein substance that congeals and welds the tissue in the same way that metal is melted to form solder.

Ultrasonic technology uses very a low temperature. Electrical current *does not* pass through the patient, therefore no grounding pad (inactive electrode) is required for this type of energy. Examples of ultrasonic energy systems are the SonoSurg (Olympus, Center Valley, Pennsylvania) and the Harmonic energy system (Ethicon, Somerville, New Jersey).

Although the ultrasonic scalpel does not transmit electrical current to the target tissue, the blades remain hot immediately after use. This is due to the vibration and friction produced by the instrument. The instrument must be held away from tissue during the cooling period to prevent accidental burns. The scrub should provide a moist towel on the surgical field where the instrument can be placed between applications.

ULTRASONIC ABLATION

Ultrasonic ablation is used as an alternative to electrosurgery. Tumor **ablation** is performed by inserting a series of needle probes directly into the tumor under direct fluoroscopic imaging. Other specialties that commonly use this technology are gynecology, endovascular surgery, neurological surgery, and ophthalmology. The **Cavitron Ultrasonic Surgical Aspirator (CUSA)** is commonly used for ultrasonic ablation and aspiration (suction) in tumor surgery. **Phacoemulsification** is a process which uses a delicate ophthalmological instrument (phacoemulsifier)that uses ultrasonic energy for the destruction of cataracts.

COLD THERMAL ENERGY

CRYOSURGERY

Cryosurgery is the use of an extremely cold instrument or substance to destroy tissue. Cryosurgery has been used for many years to treat small skin lesions. Liquid nitrogen is applied to tissue, which freezes almost immediately and eventually sloughs.

Cryoablation is a newer technique in which a probe is inserted into a tumor or tissue mass. High-pressure argon gas is injected into the probe, causing the surrounding tissue to freeze. The tissue is destroyed and eventually absorbed by the body. This surgical technique is often performed in the outpatient setting under guided fluoroscopy.

LASER ENERGY

Laser is an acronym for *light amplification by stimulated emission of radiation.* Laser surgery uses an intensely hot, precisely focused beam of light to cut and coagulate tissue. Electricity does not pass through the patient during laser surgery.

LASER STANDARDS AND REGULATIONS

The laser is a powerful instrument that has a variety of applications in manufacturing, engineering, biotechnology, and warfare. Laser technology has created a new field in medicine. However, lasers can also cause irreparable injury and destruction. Because of this, laser standards have been developed by governmental and private agencies. In health care, these standards are designed to protect both the patient and those who work with lasers. Some of the agencies involved in the regulation of laser safety are:

* The *American National Standards Institute (ANSI):* An organization of expert volunteers who develop the standards for laser use in specific professions.
* The *Center for Devices and Radiological Health (CDRH):* A regulatory agency of the U.S. Food and Drug Administration and the Department of Health and Human Services. This agency standardizes the performance safety criteria for manufactured laser products.
* The *Occupational Safety and Health Administration (OSHA):* A governmental regulatory body, OSHA follows accepted industry laser standards.
* The *Association of periOperative Registered Nurses (AORN):* The professional organization of perioperative nurses, which publishes a review and expert guidelines for use of lasers by perioperative professionals.

HOW LASERS WORK

Laser Light

Recall that light has both particle and wave characteristics. Ordinary light is made up of many wave lengths and colors.

When ordinary light is generated, the rays are transmitted from the source in infinite directions. However, laser light is unlike ordinary light. All the waves in the laser have exactly the same length and therefore are **monochromatic**. The waves are lined up so that their peaks and troughs are in exactly the same location, a quality called **coherency** (Figure 19-9).

The distinctive characteristics of laser energy are created when light is pumped into a sealed chamber and filled with a medium (i.e., a gas, solid, or liquid); this medium is called the **laser medium**. The chamber is called the **optical resonant cavity**. When photons of a specific energy enter the chamber, they stimulate the high-energy atoms in the chamber to vibrate or resonate in the same wave pattern. Mirrors in the laser system bounce the photons back and forth through the laser medium in the chamber. This increases the number of resonating parallel photons. This is called **amplification** (Figure 19-10).

Lasers are grouped into two categories according to the duration of the output waves:

* **Continuous wave lasers** produce a steady stream of light.
* **Q-switched lasers** (also called **pulsed wave lasers**) emit light in bursts or pulses.

Laser Components

The main components of the laser delivery system are:

* The *optical resonator* (also called the **laser head**): Contains the lasing medium and mirrors needed to amplify the light waves.
* The **excitation source**: Supplies the energy needed to increase the resonance of the lasing medium.

Monochromatic:
All waves have exactly the same wavelength (one color)

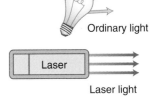

Ordinary light

Parallel:
All waves move in columns

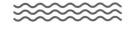

Laser light

Coherent:
All waves are exactly in step with each other (space and time)

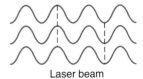

Laser beam

Figure 19-9 Comparison of normal and laser light. Ordinary light rays are transmitted in all directions. Laser waves are monochromatic, parallel, and coherent. They move in one direction and the waves are lined up, producing an extremely powerful source of energy.

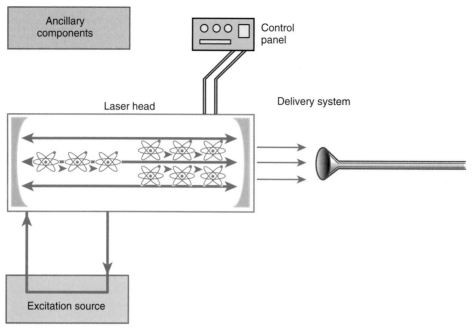

Figure 19-10 The characteristics of laser energy are created when light is pumped into a sealed chamber filled with a medium that excites the photons. *(From Rothrock J: Alexander's care of the patient in surgery, ed 17, St Louis, 2007, Mosby.)*

- The *delivery system:* The instruments or devices that transmits the lasing energy to the operative site. The system depends on the type of laser and surgery. A laser *fiber* (filament) is commonly used.
- The *control panel* and *touch screen:* Contain the control system for the laser functions and operations.
- *Accessory equipment:* Includes the cooling system and vacuum pump, if required by the laser type.

The modern laser is controlled by microprocessing technology. The optical resonator and control system are contained in a single unit, and accessory equipment is attached according to the needs of the surgery. The actual laser housing is contained within the laser unit, along with the cooling system and vacuum pump. The controls of the modern laser include a touch panel or screen on which surgical options can be selected and adjustments made.

Effects of Lasers

When laser light is directed at a surface, any of the following can occur:

- Absorption
- Reflection
- Scattering
- Transmission

Lasers are distinguished by the functional or biophysical reaction of the target tissue. The tissue reaction depends on the following:

- The laser wavelength
- The power setting
- The absorption quality of the cells (e.g., color, density, moisture content)

The quality of the laser energy depends on its density, which is determined by the voltage, the diameter of the beam, and the exposure time on the tissue. The sum of these is called the **radiant exposure**.

When certain types of laser light contact tissue, the cells become extremely hot. Just as in electrosurgery, a high temperature causes cell destruction through vaporization. Laser light can also weld tissue.

Selective absorption is an important characteristic of laser energy. This means that some cells absorb the lasing medium, whereas others do not. This characteristic prevents the spread of heat (and damage) outside the target tissue.

The type of gas or other substance used to create specific laser energy determines its absorption by the tissue. The moisture content and density of a particular tissue are important factors in the choice of laser medium.

LASER MEDIA

Lasers are distinguished by the medium or the element activated to transmit photons. These media include:

- Gases
- Solids
- Semiconductor
- Excimer
- Solid state
- Liquid Dye

Argon (Gas)

Argon gas lasers produce a visible blue-green beam that is absorbed by red-brown pigmented tissue such as hemoglobin.

The argon beam is not absorbed by clear or translucent tissue, therefore the beam can pass through the cornea, vitreous, and lens of the eye without burning these tissues. The argon beam is used for coagulation and for sealing or welding tissue.

The argon laser most often is used in dermatological and ophthalmological procedures. In dermatology, it is used to remove pigmented lesions because it is not readily absorbed by light tissue. In ophthalmology, it is used in surgery for retinal tears, glaucoma, macular degeneration, retinopathy, and retinal vein occlusion. The argon beam is delivered through a laser fiber in combination with the surgical microscope, slit lamp, or handpiece attached to an articulated (jointed) arm.

Carbon Dioxide (Gas)

The **carbon dioxide** laser is invisible to the human eye. The beam has a high affinity for water and functions at a superficial depth. A helium-neon laser beam that produces a red light is added to the carbon dioxide laser beam to make it visible. The helium-neon beam is sometimes called the "pilot light" because of its guiding function. The carbon dioxide laser is extremely versatile and is used in many surgical specialties, including microsurgery.

Holmium:YAG (Solid)

The holmium:yttrium-aluminum-garnet, or **holmium:YAG**, laser is a crystal containing holmium, thallium, and chromium. Its beam is outside the visible light range and able to penetrate all tissue types. This laser is used to cut, shave, contour, ablate, and coagulate tissue. It is extremely versatile and capable of ablating renal and biliary calculi as well as soft tissues. It has a low depth penetration, to a maximum of 0.4 mm. The holmium:YAG laser is used in urological; orthopedic; ear, nose, and throat (ENT); gynecological; gastrointestinal; and general surgery. It also is suitable for use in minimally invasive surgery.

Neodymium:YAG (Solid)

The **neodymium:YAG** (Nd:YAG) laser is created from a solid-state crystal or neodymium, yttrium, aluminum, and garget. As with the carbon dioxide laser, a helium-neon beam is used for visibility. The Nd:YAG laser beam has a high affinity for tissue protein but little for water. The beam is near the infrared region of the electromagnetic spectrum and has a penetration of 3 to 7 mm. Of all the laser types, the Nd:YAG has the greatest ability to coagulate blood vessels. Because of its deep penetration, it can coagulate vessels up to 4 mm in diameter. This laser can be used during endoscopic or flexible fiberoptic surgery. It is delivered through a laser fiber or probe in continuous or pulsed mode.

Potassium-Titanyl-Phosphate (Solid)

The **potassium-titanyl-phosphate** (KTP) laser is less powerful than the carbon dioxide or Nd:YAG laser, but it is capable of producing a minute beam that is well suited to microscopic surgery. The green laser light is readily absorbed by pigmented tissue and can be delivered by a number of different methods, including fiber, scanner, or microscope. The beam can also be transmitted through clear solutions. The KTP laser offers two wavelengths; this allows two separate sets of laser characteristics to be selected at any time. These provide hemostatic cutting and ablation as well as deep coagulation. The KTP laser is used in ENT, urological, gynecological, and general surgery and in dermatological procedures. KTP can also be combined with neodymium to double its frequency and increase versatility.

Excimer (Gas)

The **excimer** laser produces a cool beam by stripping electrons from the atoms of the medium in the chamber. This causes the energy bonds in the atom to break. The resulting shock waves stimulate short bursts of laser light. The light is delivered to the target tissue through fiberoptic bundles.

The beam of the excimer laser creates less heat than other laser types. This reduces damage to nearby tissues and also results in less carbonization of lased tissue. Specialized ultraviolet mirrors and optics are required to operate the laser safely. This laser is extremely precise and commonly is used in ophthalmological surgery and dermatology.

Tunable Dye (Solid)

The pulsed dye laser beam (**tunable dye laser**) is formed when fluorescent liquid or other dyes are exposed to argon laser light. The dye absorbs the light and produces a fluorescent broad-spectrum light. The spectrum of the light is then "tuned" to produce light of a particular wavelength (color). This provides versatility for a variety of tissue types and surgical specialties.

LASER SAFETY

Surgical lasers pose significant health and safety risks. These risks are manageable but require vigilance and attention to every detail of safety protocols. All perioperative personnel must know the protocols well and follow them carefully. The specific risks for patients and personnel are eye damage, tissue burns, fire, and smoke plume.

Laser classifications depend on the safety risks associated with their use:

- *Class 4:* Cause permanent eye damage if viewed directly or if viewed indirectly by reflection. These lasers can also ignite materials and cause skin burns. Most surgical lasers are class 4 lasers.
- *Class 3b:* Cause severe eye injury when viewed directly or by reflection. These lasers do not cause injury when the laser beam is diffused and do not normally present a fire hazard.
- *Class 3a:* Normally do not cause eye injury if viewed momentarily but present a hazard if viewed with collecting optics (e.g., fiberoptic cable, magnification loupe, or microscope.)
- *Class 2:* Emit radiation in the visible range of the electromagnetic spectrum. These lasers do not normally do harm when viewed briefly, although they can be hazardous when viewed for an extended period. Laser pointers and bar code scanners are class 2 lasers.

- *Class 1:* Are not hazardous for continuous viewing, are considered incapable of producing damaging radiation levels, and are exempt from control measures. Laser printers are in this category.

Note that class 3b and 4 lasers cause instantaneous retinal injury that may be irreparable. Class 4 lasers can penetrate the sclera and injure the retina. Turning the head away or turning away from the laser does not ensure protection because of the risk of scatter or reflection of the beam.

Recall the three specific characteristics of laser energy that distinguish it from ordinary white light: it is coherent (peaks and troughs match), monochromatic (all waves are of the same wavelength), and parallel (waves move in one direction only). These qualities make laser light extremely hazardous, because it can concentrate a tremendous amount of energy in one small area.

PRECAUTIONS AND GUIDELINES

- A laser safety officer is required to manage laser risks and define safety protocols.
- Lasers are key locked when not in use.
- Lasers are a potent source of ignition in the operating room. All fire safety precautions must be in place before the start of surgery.
- Only personnel trained in and proven knowledgeable about laser use and precautions are allowed to participate in laser surgery. All reflective surfaces in the laser environment are covered, made nonreflective, or removed from the environment.
- Laser warning signs must be placed on all entrances to areas where laser surgery is being performed (Figure 19-11).
- All personnel entering a room in which lasers are in use must wear protective eyewear (see the next section).
- Only flame-retardant drapes are used during laser surgery.

The two most common injuries associated with unintentional laser exposure are eye injury and skin burn. Lasers in the ultraviolet and infrared areas of the spectrum are the most damaging. They can penetrate the sclera and enter the lens, cornea, and retina. Eye injury can be permanent, especially if the retina is involved. Injuries range from corneal burns to blindness, especially when the retina is involved.

Heat generated by the lasing light beam is the major cause of tissue damage. Intentional use of the laser results in incision or dissection, tissue vaporization, and welding. Unintentional exposure can have the same effects. These range from reddening of the skin to third-degree burns. The following criteria determine the degree of thermal damage:

- The sensitivity of the irradiated tissue
- The amount of tissue affected
- The wavelength of the laser beam
- The energy level of the laser beam
- The length of time the tissue was exposed

Eye Safety and Skin Protection

The eye is the tissue most vulnerable to accidental laser exposure and injury. To protect the eyes during laser use, personnel must shield them from the *specific wavelength* of light. Protective eyewear of the correct optical density is required for various types of lasers. Eyewear must wrap completely around the eyes, covering the sides, top, and bottom so that no diffuse laser energy can reach the eye. Regular prescription eyeglasses do not offer protection. Only eyewear that is specifically approved for laser use can be used during laser surgery. Protective eyewear is available commercially, and manufacturers offer different styles and lens colors for each type of laser.

❖ *The color of the laser lenses is not an indication of the level of protection. The specific density of the lens, not the color, provides protection. There is no color code associated with laser type.*

The protective eyewear bears an inscription on the lens that details the optical density, and the eyewear must be labeled for the specific laser type. In addition to protective eyewear for staff members, other precautions must be followed to prevent eye injury. These include but are not limited to the following:

- Lens filters are placed over any endoscope viewing port.
- The patient's eyes are covered with wet eye pads or eye cups that are laser specific. Corneal eye shields are used for patients undergoing laser surgery of the eyelids.
- All patients undergoing surgery while awake wear protective eyewear.
- The windows to the operating room are covered, and warning signs are posted outside to caution against unprotected entry during laser procedures (see Figure 19-11).
- Appropriate protective eyewear is available on the outside of each entryway leading to a room in which lasers are being used.

Skin injuries result from direct contact with the laser beam. Environmental precautions are necessary to prevent these injuries. In addition, anyone entering a room in which lasers are in use must remove any metallic jewelry, which can reflect the laser beam or absorb heat. The patient's tissues are protected from inadvertent laser injury. Wet towels are placed around the operative site to prevent burns in the area.

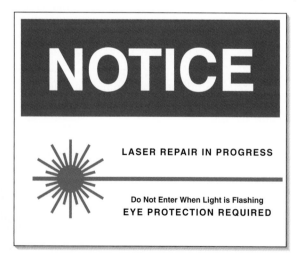

Figure 19-11 Laser warning sign.

Airway Protection

In addition to routine precautions against fire, particular attention is given to anesthesia equipment, especially during laser surgery involving the head and neck. Endotracheal tubes and other anesthesia equipment can easily ignite in the presence of laser energy and oxygen-rich anesthetic agents. To minimize the risk of an endotracheal fire, a special metallic foil is wrapped around the endotracheal tube before laser surgery. Oxygen flow is reduced to a minimum, and combustible gases are avoided.

Although an airway fire is a rare event, the possibility exists during laser surgery. When ignited, the endotracheal tube acts as a blowtorch, and flames may reach 5 to 10 inches (12.5 to 25 cm) within seconds. If a fire occurs, the tube may be removed or flushed with saline. The scrub and circulator should be prepared to offer emergency assistance to both the anesthesiologist and surgeons as needed.

CHAPTER SUMMARY

- Different forms of energy are used to perform surgery. The forms most commonly used are electrical, radiofrequency, kinetic (movement), sound (ultrasonic waves), thermal (temperature), and laser energy.
- Most energy is derived from electromagnetic waves. The frequency of the electromagnetic waves determines the type of energy produced.
- Electricity flows through a conductive medium following a path, or circuit.
- Direct current flows in one direction only. Alternating current switches directions (in the United States, at a rate of 60 cycles per second). Alternating current produces high-voltage energy.
- Electrosurgery uses high-frequency electromagnetic waves to cut, coagulate, and weld tissue.
- The way tissue reacts to electrosurgery depends on the type of tissue (i.e., the amount of water and collagen and the tissue's density), the exposure time, and the current density.
- Direct application of a hot object to tissue is called *cautery*. Cautery is not the same as electrosurgery.
- The components of electrosurgery are the power unit, active electrode, grounding pad or return electrode (monopolar only), and active electrode.
- Monopolar electrosurgery requires a return electrode to safely conduct current back to the generator after it passes through the body.
- Patient return electrode safety is a primary responsibility of everyone on the surgical team.
- In bipolar electrosurgery, the current does not travel through the patient's body before returning to the generator. The energy passes from the active electrode, through the tissue it contacts, and directly back to the active electrode and power generator.
- The specific effects of electrosurgery (e.g., cutting, coagulation) depend on whether the electrical current is delivered continuously or intermittently. These different modes are displayed on the power unit as electrosurgical waveforms.
- Continuous repetition of high-frequency waves at low voltage is characteristic of the cutting mode. The coagulation mode is manifested as intermittent waves at low frequency and high voltage.
- The blended mode provides a combination of intermediate frequency and intermediate wave intervals.

- Fulguration, or spray coagulation, is performed on tissue with pulsed or intermittent application of the active electrode. In this technique, the current is pulsed through the active electrode, which is held just above the tissue.
- Radiofrequency ablation is the destruction of tissue using radiofrequency energy waves. During tumor ablation, an electrode is inserted directly into the diseased tissue. The high-frequency energy causes the molecules of the tissue to vibrate, which creates sufficient heat to destroy the tissue.
- Argon gas is used in some electrosurgical procedures to focus the current during cutting and coagulation. A stream of argon gas directed around the active electrode focuses the current and prevents arcing (sparking). Argon-enhanced electrosurgery also reduces smoke plume and displaces oxygen along its path.
- Electrosurgery historically has been one of the greatest risks to patient safety in the operating room. Recent advances in technology have reduced but not removed the risk of patient burns.
- Monopolar electrosurgery is performed through an isolated circuit. This means that the current travels only from the ESU generator, through the patient and patient return electrode, and back to the generator.
- All team members must understand and respond to safety risks related to electrosurgery.
- Capacitive coupling is a specific burn hazard of monopolar endoscopic surgery. It occurs when current passes inadvertently through instrument insulation and adjacent conductive material into tissue.
- Direct coupling is the flow of electricity from one conductive substance to another. This can occur when the insulation protecting the circuit is defective or when an active electrode comes in contact with another conductive object.
- Active electrode monitoring is universally recommended by safety standard agencies to prevent accidental burns during electrosurgery.
- Return electrode monitoring, also known as *return electrode contact quality monitoring system (RECQMS)*, automatically stops the flow of current when impedance reaches a preset level.
- A patient with an implanted electronic device requires special consideration when electrosurgery is planned.

IEDs monitor and correct physiological dysfunctions and can be subject to interference from radiofrequency electromagnetic energy, including that produced by electrosurgical equipment.

- During electrosurgery and laser surgery, tissue is destroyed or incised, and this process creates smoke, called a *smoke plume,* which is known to be highly toxic. The two methods used to prevent perioperative personnel from inhaling smoke are in-line room suction systems and commercial smoke evacuation devices.
- Ultrasonic energy is created when electricity is transformed into mechanical energy as high-frequency vibration and friction.
- Ultrasonic technology uses a relatively low temperature. Electrical current *does not* pass through the patient, therefore no grounding pad (inactive electrode) is required for this type of energy.
- Vessel sealing systems use radiofrequency waves, low voltage, and physical pressure to create a weld in tissue bundles.
- Laser surgery uses an intensely hot, precisely focused light beam to cut, coagulate, and weld tissue.
- Laser light differs from ordinary light in that all the beams are focused in one direction and are exactly the same length.
- The distinctive characteristics of laser energy are created when light is pumped into a sealed chamber that is filled with a laser medium (a gas, solid, or liquid).

- Components of the laser delivery system are the optical resonator (laser head), excitation source, control panel, touch screen, and accessory equipment, including a cooling pump.
- When certain types of laser light contact tissue, the cells become extremely hot. Just as in electrosurgery, a high temperature causes cell destruction through vaporization.
- Selective absorption is an important characteristic of laser energy. This means that some cells absorb the lasing medium, and others do not.
- Lasers are distinguished by the medium or element that is activated to transmit the light. These include certain types of gases, solids, semiconductors, excimer, or dyes.
- Lasers can cause severe injury. The most common injuries are burns to the retina and skin and patient fire.
- Protective eyewear is required for different types of lasers. Each laser medium has its own required eyewear.
- Protective eyewear is not color dependent. The specific density of the lens, not the color, provides protection.
- Patient fires can occur when the laser light ignites the airway in an oxygen-rich environment. The patient's throat can become engulfed in flames within 1 second of ignition.
- The surgical technologist is responsible for correct action during a patient fire. The protocol is established by each health care facility.

REVIEW QUESTIONS

1. Discuss the difference between a bipolar circuit and a monopolar circuit.
2. Why do you place the patient return electrode over a large muscle mass?
3. What is active electrode monitoring (AEM)?
4. What kinds of electrosurgery require a patient return electrode?
5. Why doesn't the patient experience a cardiac arrest when electrosurgical procedures are used?
6. What is the effect of impedance of electricity as it flows through a conductive medium?
7. What is cryoablation?
8. Why does eschar on the active electrode create a hazard?
9. What does the acronym *laser* stand for?
10. What precautions are needed during laser surgery of the throat?
11. A colleague asks you why the laser goggles are not color coded. What would you say?

CASE STUDIES

Case 1

You are in a hurry to pass through a surgical suite where Nd:YAG laser surgery is in progress. You do not use protective eyewear, even though goggles are hanging on the door outside. You enter the room and turn your head away from the patient as you proceed to the other door. Just to be safe, you close your eyes for a few moments until you reach the door. Are you safe?

Case 2

You are asked to bring a 16-year-old from the holding area for surgery. When you arrive, you see that she has a metal ring through her lip. You explain to her that it is a hazard during electrosurgery. She tells you she cannot take it out because there is no way to remove it. How will you handle this situation?

Case 3

You are scrubbed during an emergency laparotomy in which monopolar electrosurgery is used extensively. Midway through the case, you notice that the power cord to the electrosurgical unit has been plugged into an extension cord to which the cardiac monitor is also connected. What should you do, if anything?

Case 4

You are at the scrub sink, preparing for an eye procedure in which laser surgery will be used. The surgeon's assistant is next to you at the sink. You notice that he is wearing a metal necklace. Can he tuck it into his scrub shirt?

Case 5

During a laparotomy, the assistant steps away from the field to answer a page. The surgeon asks you to hold a clamp that he has just placed over a vessel bundle. He proceeds to buzz the clamp. You suddenly feel a shock on the hand holding the clamp. What caused this? What should you do?

BIBLIOGRAPHY

Ball K: *Lasers: the perioperative challenge,* ed 3, Denver, 2004, the Association of periOperative Registered Nurses (AORN).

Fickling J, Loeffler C: Electrosurgical considerations for the patient with an implanted electronic device. *Clinical Information Hotline News.* Retrieved October 6, 2007, at www.valleylab.com/education/hotline/pds/hotline-0712.pdf.

Fickling J, Loeffler C: Using multiple accessories with one generator. *Clinical Information Hotline News.* Retrieved October 3, 2007, at www.valleylab.com/education/hotline/pdfs/hotline_0606.pdf.

Fickling J, Loeffler C: Valleylab electrosurgical generators: general cautions and warnings for patient and operating room safety. *Clinical Information Hotline News* 9(1), August, 2004. Retrieved October 3, 2007, at www.valleylab.com/education/hotline/pdfs/hotline_0408.pdf.

Fickling J, Loeffler C: Valleylab electrosurgical generators: general cautions and warnings for patient and operating room safety, *Clinical Information Hotline News* 10(1), January, 2005. Retrieved October 3, 2007, at www.valleylab.com/education/hotline/pdfs/hotline_0501.pdf.

Giesler C, Bowling M, Tobias D: Abdominal hysterectomy with the harmonic wave coagulating shears. *OB Management.* Retrieved October 5, 2007, at www.obgmanagement.com/pages.asp?id+5022.

Nagelhout J, Zaglaniczny K: *Nurse anesthesia,* ed 3, Philadelphia, 2005, Elsevier.

National Health Service: Report 06008: electrosurgical vessel sealing systems. Retrieved October 12, 2007, at www.wales.nhs.uk/sites3dometadata.cfrm?orgid=443&id=56037.

National Institutes of Health: Emerging local ablation techniques. Retrieved October 12, 2007, at www.cc.nih.gov/drd/sp/pdf/seminaris-2006wood.pdf.

National Institutes of Health Clinical Center: Overview for physicians: radiofrequency ablation. Retrieved October 20, 2007, at www.cc.hin.gov/drd/rfa/frame-doc.html.

Paschotta R: Encyclopedia of laser physics and technology. Retrieved October 25, 2007 at www.rp-photonics.com/encyclopedia.html.

Rothrock J: *Alexander's care of the patient in surgery,* ed 13, St Louis, 2007, Mosby.

Ulmer B: The Valleylab Institute of Clinical Education electrosurgery continuing education module: electrosurgery continuing education module, July 2004. Retrieved August 18, 2007 at http://www.valleylabeducation.org/esself/index.

Diagnostic and Assessment Procedures

LEARNING OBJECTIVES

After studying this chapter the reader will be able to:
- Describe the proper procedure for taking the patient's vital signs
- Accurately document vital sign measurements
- Describe the use of an electrocardiograph
- List and define commonly used imaging studies
- Describe common radiation therapy techniques
- Discuss basic blood and urine chemistry tests
- Describe different methods of tissue biopsy
- Describe the effects of malignancy on the body
- Discuss cancer screening

TERMINOLOGY

ABO blood groups: Inherited antigens found on the surface of an individual's red blood cells. These antigens identify the blood group (i.e., type A blood has type A antigens). Also known as blood types.

Acute illness: Sudden onset of disease or trauma or disease of short duration, usually 3 weeks or less.

Basic metabolic panel: Blood test commonly performed to measure metabolic markers such as electrolytes and other essential elements.

Benign: A term used to characterize a tumor that does not have the capability to spread to other parts of the body and usually is composed of tissue similar to its tissue of origin.

Biopsy: Removal of a sample of tissue for pathological analysis.

Brachytherapy: The implantation of small pellets of radioactive material to destroy tumors.

Chemistry test: Usually a blood or urine analysis that provides information on the metabolism and function of the body.

Chronic illness: An illness that has continued for months, weeks, or years.

Complete blood count (CBC): A blood test that measures specific components, including the hemoglobin, hematocrit, red blood cells, and white blood cells.

Computed tomography (CT): An imaging technique that allows physicians to obtain cross sectional radiographic views of the patient. The result is a CT scan or computed axial tomography (CAT) scan.

Contrast medium: A radiopaque fluid used in radiation studies to determine the shape and density of the anatomy.

Culture and sensitivity (C & S): A microbiological study in which cells or fluid are allowed to incubate and then are tested for infectivity and sensitivity to an antibacterial agent.

Diastolic pressure: The pressure exerted on the walls of the blood vessels during ventricular cardiac contraction.

Differential count: A test that determines the number of each type of white blood cell in a specimen of blood.

Doppler studies: A technique that uses ultrasonic waves to measure blood flow in a vessel.

Electrocardiogram (ECG): A noninvasive assessment of the heart's electrical activity. In the United States, electrocardiogram is abbreviated correctly as ECG. EKG is the European abbreviation.

Electrocardiograph machine: A medical device that receives electrical impulses transmitted by the heart through conductive pads and displays the activity on a graph in real time.

Electronic probe thermometer: A digital thermometer commonly used in the clinical setting.

Endoscopic procedures: Medical assessment of body cavities using a fiberoptic lensed instrument (endoscope).

Excisional biopsy: A section of tissue removed by cutting (excising) and submitted for pathological analysis.

Fibrin: A component of whole blood that promotes clotting.

Fluoroscopy: A radiological technique that provides real-time images of an anatomical region.

Frozen section: A process in which biopsy tissue is frozen, sliced, and examined microscopically.

Hematocrit (Hct): The ratio of red blood cells to plasma.

Hemoglobin (Hgb): The oxygen-carrying molecule found in red blood cells.

Hypocalcemia: An abnormally low serum calcium.

Hypokalemia: An abnormally low serum potassium.

Hyponatremia: An abnormally low serum sodium.

Imaging studies: Diagnostic tests that produce a picture or image.

Interstitial needle: A fine needle used to instill a radioactive isotope into a tumor.

Interventional radiology: Medical assessment procedures in which irradiation is used; usually requires invasive procedures combined with radiographic technology.

Invasive procedure: A medical or nursing procedure in which the skin is broken or a body cavity is entered.

Magnetic resonance imaging (MRI): A diagnostic technique that uses radiofrequency signals and magnetic energy to produce images.

Malignant: A term used to characterize tissue that shows disorganized, uncontrolled growth (cancer). Malignant tissue has the potential to spread locally or to distant areas of the body. It is then termed metastatic.

Mean arterial pressure (MAP): The average amount of pressure exerted throughout the cardiac cycle.

Metastasis: The spread of malignant or cancerous cells to a local or distant area of the body.

Neoplasm: A tumor, which may be benign or malignant.

Nuclear medicine: Medical procedures that use radioactive particles to track target tissue in the body.

Orthostatic (postural) blood pressure: A technique used to check the patient's blood pressure in the upright or recumbent position.

Palpating: Assessing a part of the body by feeling the outline, density, movement, or other attributes.

Partial thromboplastin time (PTT): A test of blood coagulation used in patients receiving heparin to determine the correct level of anticoagulation.

Phase change thermometer: A disposable adhesive strip impregnated with temperature-sensitive dots that indicate the surface temperature of skin.

Positron emission tomography (PET): A type of medical imaging that measures specific metabolic activity in the target tissue.

Prognosis: The outcome of a disease. For example, some types of cancer have a poor prognosis.

Prothrombin time (PT): A measurement of the time required for blood to clot.

Pulse pressure: A measurement of the difference between the systolic pressure and diastolic pressure. This can be a significant sign of metabolic disturbance.

Radioactive seeds: Small "seeds" of radioactive material that are implanted for cancer treatment.

Radionuclides or isotopes: In nuclear medicine, radioactive particles are directed at the nucleus of a selected element to create energy. These special elements are referred to as *radionuclides* or *isotopes*.

Radiopaque: A substance that is impenetrable by x-rays (gamma radiation).

Sphygmomanometer: An instrument used to measure blood pressure.

Staging (tumor staging): An international method of classifying tissue to determine the level of metastasis.

Sublingual: Under the tongue.

Systolic pressure: The pressure exerted by blood on the walls of vessels during the resting phase of the cardiac cycle.

TNM classification system: An international system for determining the extent of cancer spread and the level of cell differentiation, two attributes that determine treatment and prognosis.

Transcutaneous: Literally "through the skin"; it refers to a procedure in which a needle or other medical device is inserted from the outside of the body to the inside.

Tumor marker: An antigen present on the tumor cell, or a substance (protein, hormone, or other chemical) released by the cancer cells into the blood.

Tympanic membrane thermometer: A type of thermometer that measures the patient's core temperature by scanning the tympanic membrane.

Ultrasound energy: High-frequency sound waves used in many medical applications. Ultrasound imaging produces a picture of the target anatomy, which is shaded by tissue density.

Vital signs: Cardinal signs of well being: temperature, pulse, respiration, and blood pressure. These are measured to assess a patient's basic metabolic status.

INTRODUCTION

The first step in medical and surgical decision making is assessment, which provides clues and information about the nature of the patient's illness and the possible causes. Selection of the tests and procedures used to evaluate the patient's condition begins with a general assessment and proceeds to tests that are more complex. The assessment begins with a baseline history (described in detail in Chapter 12) and physical examination.

Diagnostic procedures and tests often are performed as part of an assessment to confirm or rule out a diagnosis. In some cases **invasive** procedures are required. An invasive procedure involves breaking intact skin or mucous membrane or inserting a medical device into a body cavity. Noninvasive procedures are limited to skin contact or no direct contact with the body. **Interventional** radiology procedures combine technologies such as radiology with invasive techniques.

Perioperative personnel often participate in selected invasive diagnostic and interventional procedures. These are performed in the surgical suite or in a designated specialty department. Routine tests such as blood analysis, urinalysis, and other **chemistry** studies are performed in the laboratory by technologists trained in that specialty. Conclusions about the result of a test or series of tests contribute to the diagnosis. Primary care providers and surgeons use advanced skills in patient assessment, interpretation of tests, and the disease process to make strategic decisions about treatment.

This chapter describes commonly performed metabolic tests and diagnostic procedures. Surgical technologists participate in selected invasive diagnostic procedures that are performed intraoperatively or in specialty departments. **Endoscopic procedures**, in which a fiberoptic instrument is passed through a body cavity for examination and biopsy, are described in Chapter 21 and in each procedural chapter according to specialty. Bacteriological and other tests required for investigation of infectious diseases are described in Chapter 7. Diagnostic tests associated with a particular medical specialty are described in the chapter associated with that specialty.

VITAL SIGNS

Taking a patient's **vital signs** allows an overall evaluation of the person's well-being. This is the most basic form of assessment. In some facilities, the surgical technologist may measure the patient's vital signs. These are documented and reported to the registered nurse or surgeon. The surgical technologist is not expected to interpret the measurements or make a diagnosis based on the results. However, *accurate measurement* is always required. The vital signs include:

- Temperature
- Pulse
- Respiration
- Blood pressure

A change in the vital signs can be an early warning of an **acute illness** (one that comes on suddenly) or a sign of a **chronic illness** (long-term disease). Vital signs are measured whenever a patient requires medical assessment. During general anesthesia or deep sedation, vital signs are measured with complex biomedical devices. In simple procedures performed with a local anesthetic, noninvasive techniques are used. The person measuring the vital signs must report immediately any variation from the *baseline values* (i.e., those taken at the beginning of an assessment period). The baseline values may vary from "normal" limits. Upward or downward trends and deviations from the baseline values are an indication of important changes in the patient's condition.

TEMPERATURE

The body requires a core (deep) temperature of approximately 99° F (37.2° C). The core temperature is regulated by the hypothalamus through a complex feedback system that balances the core temperature with environmental factors. However, when environmental factors or disease exceed the body's ability to adjust, vital functions deteriorate, and this can result in serious tissue injury or death.

Temperature is recorded and documented in degrees Celsius. The formula for conversion from the two systems is:

Fahrenheit → Celsius $C = \frac{5}{9}(°F - 32)$
Celsius   → Fahrenheit $F = (\frac{9}{5} \times °C) + 32$

Methods of Measuring Temperature

The site where the temperature is measured affects the reading that results.

- The oral temperature is measured under the tongue (**sublingual**), which is highly vascular and accurately reflects the core temperature. The normal oral temperature in a person at rest is 98.6° F (37° C). The range is 96.4° to 99.1° F (35.8° to 37.3° C).
- The *tympanic* temperature accurately assesses core temperature through the external auditory canal.
- The *rectal* temperature varies from 0.7° to 1° F (0.4° to 0.5° C) higher than the oral value.
- The *axillary* temperature is measured at the axilla. Readings are 0.5° to 1° F (0.3° to 0.6° C) lower than the oral value.
- The forehead, or *skin*, temperature varies with environmental changes.

Use of Thermometers

Always wash your hands before and after taking a patient's temperature. Thermometers can easily spread infection. Dispose of device covers in the appropriate container, because these are contaminated items. Do not use a unit that is grossly soiled. Use gloves and clean the device with disinfectant as recommended by the manufacturer. Probe and tympanic thermometers can harbor an infectious biofilm that may not be visible.

The **electronic probe thermometer** is commonly used in clinical assessment. This thermometer consists of a sensing probe connected to a handheld reader with a light-emitting diode (LED) or liquid crystal display (LCD) format. This type of thermometer is used primarily for oral and axillary measurement. Only a designated rectal probe thermometer is used for measuring the rectal temperature.

A clean probe cover must be used on each patient to prevent the spread of infection. The measurement is displayed after about 30 seconds.

To use the electronic thermometer, make sure the batteries are charged and the unit is clean. Insert the tip into a new disposable probe cover and press gently. This attaches the cover to the probe. Then proceed as follows:

- *Oral temperature:* Gently insert the probe under the patient's tongue.
- *Axillary temperature:* When the thermometer is used in the axilla, make sure the tip of the probe does not extend outside the body. In children, it is best to hold the upper arm in contact with the body to ensure an accurate reading. Stabilize the probe until the reading is obtained.
- *Rectal temperature:* Have the patient lie on his or her side with the uppermost knee flexed. The probe tip should be lubricated after the probe cover is applied. Spread the buttocks with one hand and gently insert the probe approximately 1½ inches (3.75 cm). If stool is

encountered during insertion, remove the probe, replace the cover, and begin again. Stabilize the probe until the reading is completed. The risk of puncturing the rectal mucosa and musculature exists when a rectal probe is used. This method is used *only when no other method is available*. The tympanic method is preferred over the rectal method.

Remove the probe and dispose of the cover in a hazardous waste container. Wash your hands thoroughly and record the measurement.

The **tympanic membrane thermometer** may be used on conscious or unconscious patients. It is the preferred method of temperature assessment in the clinical setting. The tympanic thermometer receives infrared signals from the eardrum. It provides an accurate reading of core temperature, because the tympanic membrane shares its blood supply with the carotid artery. The instrument is shaped like an otoscope, and disposable head covers are used to prevent cross-contamination among patients. *Never use a tympanic thermometer without a cover.*

To use the thermometer, first check the tip for soil or debris. Clean the probe using a soft alcohol wipe. Place a disposable cover over the tip. Direct the tip into the external ear canal. You may rotate the thermometer slightly to seat it into the ear canal and retract the skin in front of the ear to seat the tip. Release the skin before taking the reading. Remember that the infrared beam must "see" the tympanic membrane for an accurate reading. Press the activate button and wait for an audible beep from the thermometer. Remove the earpiece gently and dispose of the cover. Wash your hands and record the measurement.

The **phase change thermometer** is a disposable strip that is placed directly over tissue, usually the skin. The forehead or axilla may be used in the clinical setting. The reading is made in 2 to 3 minutes after application. This type of thermometer is affected by the environmental temperature and may not be accurate enough for some procedures.

Glass thermometers, which contain a colored solution, have been replaced by electronic or digital instruments. Mercury is no longer used in the manufacture of glass thermometers because of concerns with environmental safety. Health care workers occasionally may be required to use a glass thermometer, which first must be briskly shaken to lower the liquid column.

MEASURING THE PULSE

The pulse is a reflection of the stroke volume (amount of blood pumped through the heart) of each beat. The pulse is felt in the artery as it expands with each heartbeat. The normal heart rate varies according to age, condition, and metabolic level. Disease or injury alters the metabolic level and affects the heart rate, rhythm, and strength. Box 20-1 lists normal resting pulse rates by age. The normal pulse rate for an adult is 60 to 100 beats per minute.

The heart rhythm normally is regular. However, in younger adults and children, the rate may decrease with respiratory inspiration (inhaling). The *strength* of the peripheral pulse can

Box 20-1

Normal Pulse and Respiratory Rates by Age*

Age (Years)	Normal Pulse Rate (Range) (Beats per Minute)	Normal Respiration (Breaths per Minute)
0	120 (70–190)	30–40
1	120 (80–190)	20–40
2	110 (80–130)	25–32
4	110 (80–120)	23–30
6	100 (75–115)	21–26
8	100 (70–110)	20–26
10	90 (70–110)	20–26
12	90 (70–110)	18–22
14	85 (65–105)	18–22
16	85 (60–100)	16–20
18	75 (55–95)	12–20
Adult	75 (60–100)	10–20
Athlete	50–60 (50–100)	10–20

*Male children may have slightly lower values.

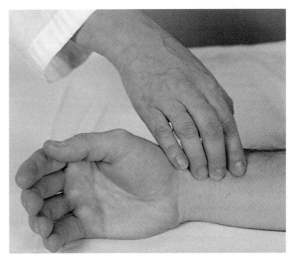

Figure 20-1 Measuring the radial pulse. *(From Jarvis C: Physical examination and health assessment, ed 5, Philadelphia, 2008, WB Saunders.)*

vary with changes in metabolism, disease, or injury. A normal pulse feels elastic and has moderate strength. A "bounding" pulse is one that feels exceptionally strong, whereas a weak pulse may be barely palpable or "thready." A three- or four-point scale is used to report the strength of the pulse:

- Bounding: 3+
- Normal: 2+
- Weak 1+
- Absent: 0

The pulse is measured by **palpating** (feeling) an artery. In a routine assessment, the radial artery is used. This is located along the radius on the inner side of the wrist (Figure 20-1). You may need to position your fingers in several locations to

Box 20-2

Location and Method of Palpating Major Arteries

- The *temporal artery* is located between the ear and outer eye in the depression above the cheek bone.
- The *carotid artery* is located in the depression between the sternocleidomastoid muscle and the trachea, at the side of the neck midway between the clavicle and the jaw.
- The *brachial artery* can be felt in the groove that runs along the side of the biceps muscle on the inside (medial aspect) of the upper arm. To locate this artery, flex the biceps to locate the groove and then relax the muscle to palpate. This pulse can also be felt in the antecubital fossa behind the elbow. This is the artery used to measure the patient's blood pressure.
- The *radial artery* is most often used to assess a patient's pulse in the clinical setting because it is easily accessible. Palpate this artery by placing the fingers on the radial bone and sliding them slightly toward the inner wrist so that they rest in the groove next to the bone.
- The *femoral artery* is very important in surgery. This artery is most often used to cannulate the larger vessels of the trunk for an angiogram (arteriography) and for placement of stents. To palpate the artery, place your fingers in the deepest furrow of the groin where the upper leg joins the pelvis. You may have to press firmly, because the femoral artery lies deep in the fascia and muscle.
- The *popliteal artery* is an extension of the femoral artery. It can be felt at the back of the knee in the depression at the top of the tibia, behind the patella.
- The *dorsalis pedis* branches from the popliteal artery and is located over the front of the foot in the depression between the great and second toe.
- The *posterior tibial artery* lies in the furrow between the Achilles tendon and the tibial process (ankle bone).

find the pulse. Always use the pads of your first three fingers to measure the pulse, because the thumb has its own pulse, which may be confused with the patient's pulse. Also, applying excessive pressure depresses the artery and stops circulation. Although the radial artery normally is used to measure the patient's pulse, any other artery can be used. Box 20-2 describes the location and method of palpating major arteries.

When you have located the pulse, count the number of beats in 30 seconds and multiply by 2 to get the beats per minute. If the pulse is irregular, you must count for 60 full seconds. Keep in mind that an irregular pulse or a missed beat may result in a difference of 4 or 5 beats per minute in your assessment measurement.

RESPIRATION

The respiratory rate is an objective assessment of the number of breaths per minute. The respiratory rate is altered by exertion, metabolic stress, strong emotion, and the effect of specific drugs, which can depress or stimulate the autonomic nervous system.

The respiratory rate is measured by observing the patient's thorax and recording the breaths per minute. It is measured when the patient is unaware, because people often alter their breathing pattern when under observation. The respiratory rate can be counted while the pulse rate is obtained. To measure the respiratory rate, count the number of breaths in 30 seconds and multiply by 2. Normal respiratory rates are listed in Box 20-1.

NOTE: Medical assessment of breath sounds, such as tone, pitch, pattern, and rhythm, is required for complex assessment of respiratory disease.

BLOOD PRESSURE

Blood pressure is the force exerted on the vessels walls. Vascular pressure changes during the cardiac cycle (filling of the heart chambers and shunting of blood through the heart). When the blood is forcefully pumped through the left ventricle, pressure is at its greatest. This is called the **systolic pressure**. As the heart muscle relaxes between contractions, blood pressure is lowered. This is called the **diastolic pressure**. The **mean arterial pressure (MAP)** is the average amount of pressure exerted throughout the cardiac cycle. When blood pressure is assessed, the difference between the diastolic and systolic pressures can be a significant sign. This is called the **pulse pressure**. Figure 20-2 shows changes in pressure that occur throughout the cardiac cycle. Many diseases cause changes in blood pressure. It also is important to understand how normal physiological processes can affect blood pressure.

Factors that Affect Blood Pressure

Normal blood pressure for an adult is 120/80 mm Hg. Pressure varies by age and is affected by various other normal physiological conditions, including:

- Weight
- Exertion
- Stress
- Strong emotion

Gender is another factor; blood pressure tends to be lower in adult women than in men. Important normal physiological factors that influence blood pressure include:

- *Cardiac output:* The total amount of blood pumped through the heart in 1 minute.
- *Stroke volume:* The amount of blood pumped during ventricular contraction. Total blood volume alters cardiac output.
- *Peripheral vascular resistance:* The static pressure of the blood vessels against the flow of blood. As blood vessels contract and relax, peripheral vascular resistance changes. Vessel obstruction also increases vascular resistance.
- *Resilience of the cardiac and vascular systems:* The elasticity of the vessels and heart muscle directly affects vascular pressure.

Procedure for Taking Blood Pressure

A simple blood pressure assessment requires both the diastolic and systolic measurements.

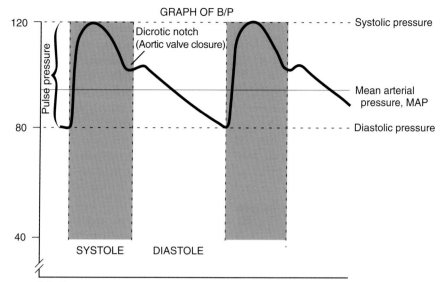

Figure 20-2 Graph of the cardiac cycle. *(From Jarvis C: Physical examination and health assessment, ed 5, Philadelphia, 2008, WB Saunders.)*

Blood pressure is measured with an electronic (digital) or manual **sphygmomanometer**, which requires the use of a stethoscope. The stethoscope method provides a more thorough assessment.

The method used to take the blood pressure is critical to obtaining a correct reading. Box 20-3 lists common errors in blood pressure measurement. A sphygmomanometer has three components: the cuff, the pump, and the gauge. A manual blood pressure apparatus has a round gauge with numerical values and a pointer. Electronic blood pressure devices display the measurement on an LED or LCD panel attached to the control unit. The blood pressure cuff is an inflatable bladder covered with fabric that is secured to the patient's limb with Velcro.

Blood pressure can be measured in several locations on an arm or a leg. For adults, the most common location is the upper arm (i.e., the brachial artery). The cuff should be no larger than 40% of the circumference of the person's upper arm. Cuffs are available in many sizes, from pediatric to extra large. An incorrectly sized cuff is a common error in blood pressure measurement (Box 20-3). This can lead to a falsely high or low reading.

The patient should be sitting or lying in a relaxed position. The arm must be at the level of the heart, and it should be supported on a surface. The person taking the reading may also support the arm, but it must be at heart level. Wrap the cuff around the patient's upper arm so that the air tubes are in line with the inner arm and brachial artery (Figure 20-3).

How to Use a Manual Sphygmomanometer

1. Before taking a reading, you must locate the general systolic pressure. Palpate the brachial artery, which is just above the antecubital fossa. Center the cuff above the fossa. Do not allow the cuff to slide down, because this obscures the measurement.

Box 20-3
Common Errors in Blood Pressure Measurement

Result of Measurement	Cause of Inaccuracy
False high systolic and diastolic pressures	• Blood pressure taken when patient is upset or anxious • Measurement taken after exertion • Wrong size cuff (too narrow) • Cuff too loose or unevenly wrapped • Arm below heart level
False low systolic and diastolic pressures	• Arm above heart level • Failure to inflate cuff sufficiently
False low systolic pressure	• Failure to inflate cuff sufficiently • Cuff deflated too quickly
False low diastolic pressure	• Stethoscope pressed too hard on artery
False high diastolic pressure	• Cuff deflated too slowly • Stopping deflation and reinflating • Failing to wait longer than 2 minutes between readings
Any type of error	• Working too fast • Faulty technique • Defective equipment

2. With your fingers over the brachial artery, inflate the cuff until the arterial pulse is no longer palpable. Continue to inflate another 25 to 30 mm above this point.

3. Release the cuff and wait 10 to 15 seconds. This allows blood to return to the artery.

4. Place the bell end of the stethoscope over the artery and inflate the cuff to the level you previously measured.

5. Slowly deflate the cuff and listen for the first sound of the pulse. Observe the correct level on the gauge or liquid column. *This is the systolic reading.*

6. Continue to deflate until you hear a muffled pulse and then the disappearance of the pulse. The diastolic measurement is *the point where the pulse was no longer audible.*

7. If the difference between the muffled sound and no sound is greater than 10 mm Hg, you must document all three

measurements. In some facilities, the middle sound is always documented.

8. To document the blood pressure, write the systolic pressure over the diastolic pressure (e.g., 140/70). If you document the middle sound, it is written between the diastolic and systolic pressures (e.g., 140/97/70).

Figure 20-4 shows the relationship between auscultatory sounds and pressure.

If the patient is to be assessed for **orthostatic (postural) blood pressure**, the pulse and blood pressure are measured with the patient in the recumbent position and again while the individual is sitting or standing. The patient's posture for each reading must be indicated in the documentation.

NOTE: A simple digital (automatic) sphygmomanometer provides the pulse rate, systolic pressure, diastolic pressure, and MAP. However, it does not measure important anomalies in the auscultatory sounds, and readings may be inaccurate, depending on the quality of the instrument and its maintenance.

ELECTROCARDIOGRAPHY

The **electrocardiograph machine** measures the electrical activity of the heart and displays it on a graph, known as an **electrocardiogram (ECG)**, for evaluation. To obtain the readings, electrodes are placed at strategic locations on the chest wall and extremities. These coincide with the heart's conductivity pattern. A 12-lead ECG is used for a complete assessment; a simple assessment can be made with a 3-lead ECG (Figure 20-5). ECG monitoring is a routine procedure for any patient undergoing general anesthesia or sedation, in the postoperative period, and for selective high-risk patients.

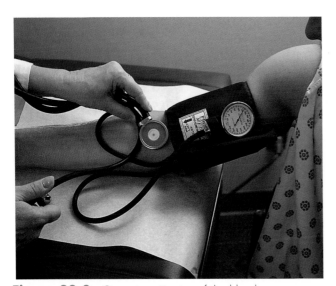

Figure 20-3 Correct positioning of the blood pressure cuff. *(From Jarvis C: Physical examination and health assessment, ed 5, Philadelphia, 2008, WB Saunders.)*

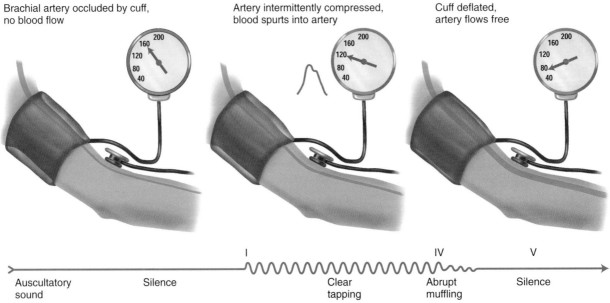

Figure 20-4 Korotkoff sounds and blood pressure. Taking the blood pressure with a sphygmomanometer and stethoscope provides a detailed assessment of the sounds. *(From Jarvis C: Physical examination and health assessment, ed 5, Philadelphia, 2008, WB Saunders.)*

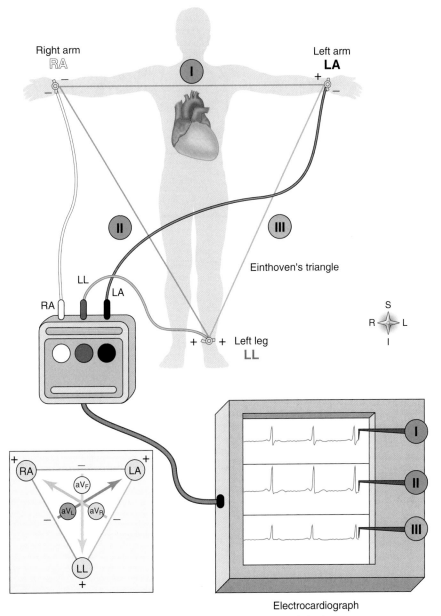

Figure 20-5 Three-lead electrocardiogram (ECG). *(From Thibodeau G, Patton K: Anatomy and physiology, ed 6, St Louis, 2007, Mosby.)*

The ECG machine has a console with a roll of paper that feeds automatically when the leads are in place and the machine is activated. Electrical activity through the heart is graphed by time and strength of impulse. This produces characteristic patterns indicating normal or abnormal conduction, which are recognizable to trained personnel.

As a diagnostic tool, an ECG provides detailed information about heart conduction. Each phase of the cardiac conduction system is represented on the graph. The waveforms correspond to the impulses that stimulate heart action, which pushes the blood through the chambers and valves. One complete heart cycle is represented by a series of waves, which have characteristic peaks, troughs, and duration. This is called a *QRS wave* (Figure 20-6). Certain kinds of patterns and variations indicate disturbances in the conduction system.

IMAGING STUDIES

As the name implies, **imaging studies** involve a "picture" of the patient's anatomy. Imaging studies provide information about the function and shape of regional anatomy. Selected studies are performed in the perioperative environment during surgery or in a separate department of the facility (Figure 20-7).

RADIOLOGY

X-rays are electromagnetic particles with a relatively short wavelength. A radiographic (x-ray) image is created when radiation passes through structures and strikes a medium (e.g., radiographic film) positioned in line with the

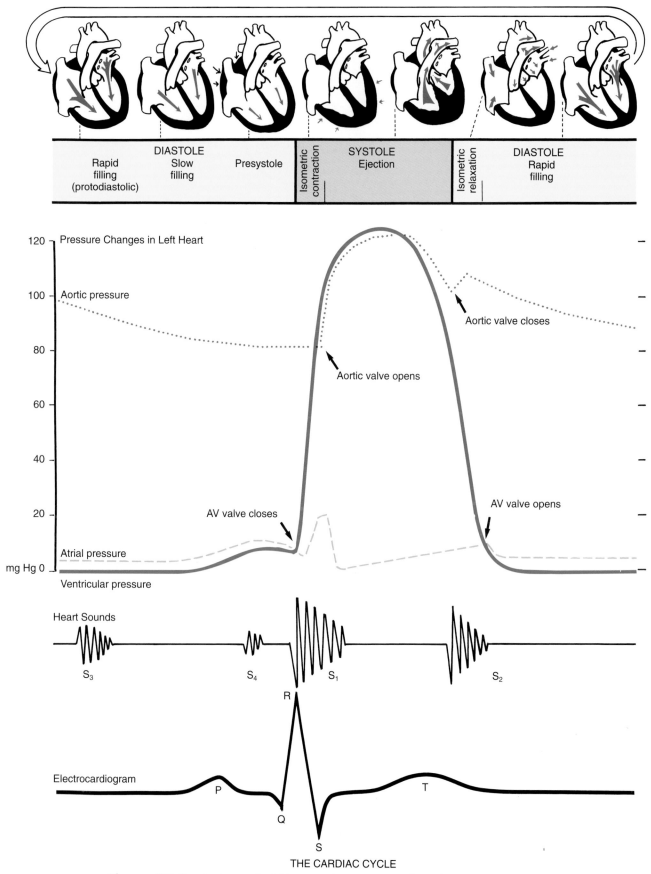

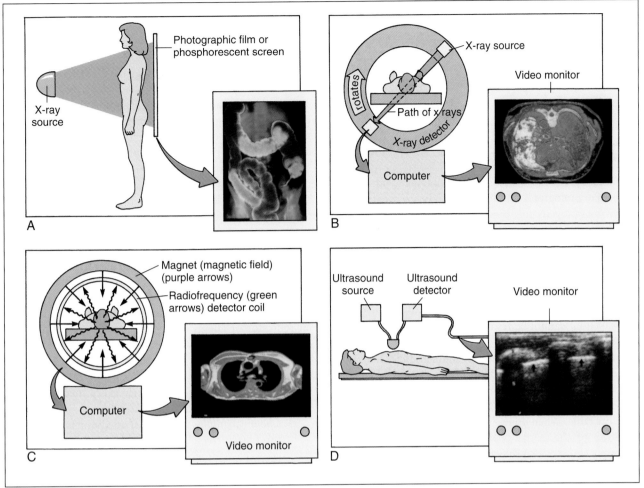

Figure 20-7 Types of imaging studies. **A,** Radiography. **B,** Computed tomography (CT). **C,** Magnetic resonance imaging (MRI). **D,** Ultrasonography (US). *(From Thibodeau G, Patton K: Anatomy and physiology, ed 6, St Louis, 2007, Mosby.)*

penetrating rays. X-rays penetrate body tissue at different rates according to density. Some materials and tissue do not allow full penetration of the x-rays (Figure 20-8). Radiographic images are recorded, and the output is available as electronic data or film. Historically all radiographs were recorded onto film. This method has been replaced by digital images, which can be stored on disks and transferred electronically.

❖ *Because radiographs use gamma radiation, all personnel must wear protective attire that prevents the penetration of radiation. (Safety precautions and protection against gamma radiation in the perioperative environment were discussed in detail in Chapter 15.)*

The images formed by x-rays display contrasts in density. An extremely dense substance produces a white image, whereas air produces a black image. Contours and outlines of organs, systems, and tissue are displayed as a combination of white, black, and grays. Images are taken from different angles and positions in order to visualize the structures from all sides and aid in assessment. These are interpreted by the radiologist who reports to the surgeon or other physician ordering the tests.

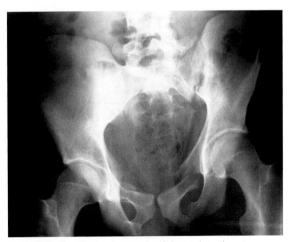

Figure 20-8 Flat radiograph of the pelvis showing dislocation of the left hip. *(From Garden O, Bradbury A, Forsythe J, Parks R: Principles and practice of surgery, ed 5, Edinburgh, 2007, Churchill Livingstone/Elsevier.)*

Diagnostic x-rays are often used to confirm a condition or to provide baseline studies for comparison following a surgical procedure. Baseline x-rays are taken in the radiology department as part of the preoperative preparation of the patient. Many different forms of x-ray imaging are used in modern diagnostic medicine. X-ray is also used in combination with other imaging techniques such as computed tomography and fluoroscopy.

STANDARD RADIOGRAPHY

The standard x-ray film (radiograph) is obtained with a fixed or portable radiograph machine. Both types are used in modern operating rooms; however, the portable radiograph machine is more common. This machine is transported to the operating room on an "on call" basis so that images can be obtained during surgery as needed. Many types of radiographic procedures can be done intraoperatively. They are most commonly used during orthopedic surgery, biliary procedures, and vascular surgery. A radiograph is also taken when a surgical count cannot be resolved and the risk exists that an item was left in the patient.

Intraoperative anterior-posterior radiographic films are obtained with the use of a Bucky platform. This is a Plexiglas or carbon platform mounted on the operating bed frame. The technician slides the film into the platform from the head or foot of the table. When done properly, this does not risk contamination of the sterile field. However, the target of the radiograph must be protected from contamination by the overhead tube. The machine is brought into position at the sterile field only after the area is protected with sterile drapes (Figure 20-9). A draped, portable radiographic film stand is used when other views are required. In these cases,

the scrub protects the sterile field, including instrument tables and other draped equipment, from contamination by the overhead radiograph machine.

CONTRAST RADIOGRAPHY

The term **radiopaque** refers to substances that x-rays cannot penetrate. In diagnostic medicine, a drug called a **contrast medium** is injected, instilled, or ingested to outline hollow organs or vessels before radiographs are obtained. The liquid contrast medium produces a solid white field in the area of the medium. Crevices, deviations, and the shape of a hollow structure can be clearly viewed on radiographs or fluoroscopy. (contrast media are discussed in Chapter 13.)

Contrast radiography carries a risk of allergy to the radiopaque medium, especially when the agent is injected. A careful patient history is used to determine whether the patient has had any previous reaction to contrast media. Allergy to iodine or agents containing iodophor may indicate sensitivity to contrast media. At one time, shellfish allergy was used as an indicator of allergy to contrast media. However, no evidence substantiates this in the medical literature.

Specific details for intraoperative contrast studies are described in the surgical procedure chapter for that specialty. Contrast studies are used in nearly every medical specialty. The most commonly performed are:

- *Cholangiography:* A contrast medium is injected into the biliary tree. This outlines the ducts of the biliary system for suspected stones, tumor, or dilation (Figure 20-10).
- *Angiography:* A contrast medium is injected into the cardiovascular system to determine areas of stricture or other anomalies of blood flow in vessels (Figure 20-11).

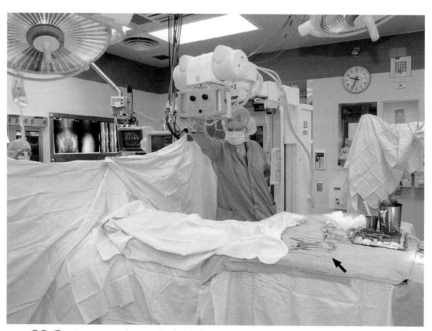

Figure 20-9 Protecting the sterile field during portable radiography. *(From Ballinger PW, Fra ED: Merrill's atlas of radiographic positions and radiologic procedures, vol 3, ed 10, St Louis, 2003, Mosby.)*

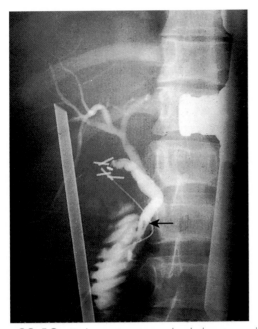

Figure 20-10 Endoscopic retrograde cholangiography showing the biliary tree. Note the surgical staples and endoscopic ports on the left. *(From Garden O, Bradbury A, Forsythe J, Parks R: Principles and practice of surgery, ed 5, Edinburgh, 2007, Churchill Livingstone/Elsevier.)*

- *Myelography:* A contrast medium is injected into the subarachnoid space for visualization of the spinal cord and nerve roots.
- *Retrograde pyelography:* A contrast medium is instilled into the urinary tract for visualization of the bladder, ureters, and kidney. This procedure is used to identify stones, strictures, tumor, or other anomalies of the urinary system.
- *Gastrointestinal studies:* In studies of the gastrointestinal system, barium, a radiopaque element, is used to fill and outline the structures. An upper gastrointestinal (GI) study is used to identify problems in the esophagus, stomach, and small intestine. For a study of the large intestine, barium is instilled into the distal colon and rectum (Figure 20-12).

FLUOROSCOPY

Fluoroscopy combines radiography with an image intensifier that is visible in normal lighting. A digital monitor allows the moving images to be seen in real time. Fluoroscopy is used diagnostically and intraoperatively during procedures using contrast media or during implantation of a biomedical device.

MOBILE C-ARM

The mobile C-arm fluoroscope is used in surgery for real-time imaging (Figure 20-13). The head of the fluoroscope is directed through the body onto an image intensifier on the underside of the C. The C-arm can be moved into place so that the operating bed is centered between the tube and the

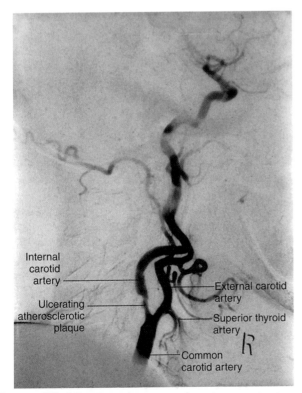

Figure 20-11 Carotid angiography using a contrast medium injected intravenously. *(From Garden O, Bradbury A, Forsythe J, Parks R: Principles and practice of surgery, ed 5, Edinburgh, 2007, Churchill Livingstone/Elsevier.)*

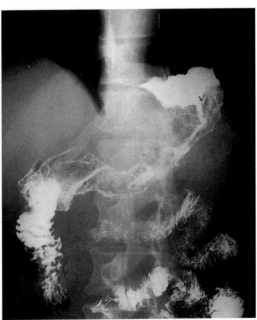

Figure 20-12 Barium study of the stomach showing extensive gastric carcinoma. *(From Garden O, Bradbury A, Forsythe J, Parks R: Principles and practice of surgery, ed 5, Edinburgh, 2007, Churchill Livingstone/Elsevier.)*

intensifier. Multiple images can be taken by moving the machine along the axis of the operating table. The C-arm is draped before positioning to allow freedom of movement along the sterile field and has replaced portable x-ray machines in many hospitals.

COMPUTED TOMOGRAPHY

In **computed tomography (CT)**, radiographic and computer technologies are combined to produce high-contrast cross sectional images. This technique allows precise tissue differ-

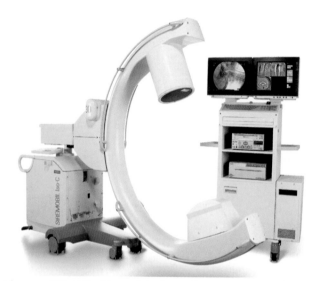

Figure 20-13 The mobile C-arm fluoroscope is used in surgery for real-time imaging. *(From Ballinger PW, Fra ED: Merrill's atlas of radiographic positions and radiologic procedures, vol 3, ed 10, St Louis, 2003, Mosby.)*

entiation and determination of the dimensions of anatomical structures. CT is enhanced with contrast media to assess structures such as ducts, blood vessels, and the gastrointestinal system.

MAGNETIC RESONANCE IMAGING

Magnetic resonance imaging (MRI) uses radiofrequency signals and multiple magnetic fields to produce a high-definition image (Figure 20-14). In this process, the patient is exposed to electromagnetic energy, which is emitted inside a closed body tube or an open platform. MRI produces two- or three-dimensional digital images in cross section and is used mainly to detect structural abnormalities, including tumors (Figure 20-15). Because the process involves a high level of electromagnetic energy, any metal in range of the device may be drawn toward the source of emission. This poses a genuine risk for injury to the patient and personnel working in the area. Images can also be distorted by the presence of metallic substances in the tissue. These include biomedical devices such as a pacemaker, vascular clips, and tattoos. MRI is performed in the interventional medicine or radiology department and occasionally intraoperatively in facilities that have a dedicated surgical suite.

POSITRON EMISSION TOMOGRAPHY

Positron emission tomography (PET) uses the combined technologies of computed tomography and radioactive scanning. PET is performed to produce an image not of a structure, but rather of a metabolic process. In this technique, a biological substance to be followed in the body is "labeled" with radioactive atoms. The labeling is performed by injec-

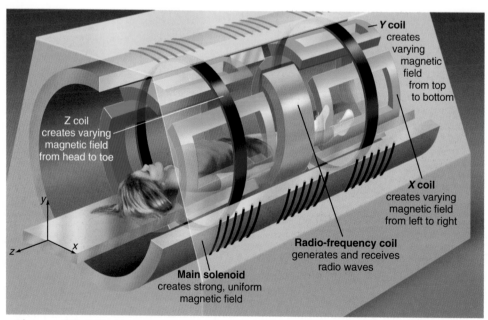

Figure 20-14 Magnetic resonance imaging (MRI) apparatus. *(From Giambattista A, et al: College physics, ed 2, New York, 2007, McGraw Hill. Reproduced wtih the permission of the McGraw Hill Companies.)*

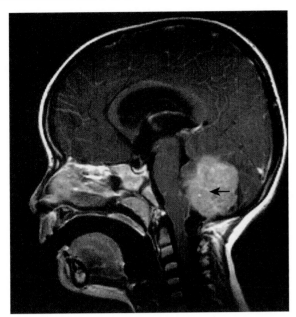

Figure 20-15 Magnetic resonance imaging of a tumor filling the fourth ventricle *(arrow)*. MRI uses radiofrequency signals and magnetic energy to produce high-resolution images. *(From Garden O, Bradbury A, Forsythe J, Parks R: Principles and practice of surgery, ed 5, Edinburgh, 2007, Churchill Livingstone/Elsevier.)*

tion. During PET, the radioactive particles emitted by the atoms are traced and computed to provide an image of the physiology and biochemical properties of tissue. These are displayed in three-dimensional color representations of the structure, such as the brain or heart.

ULTRASOUND

Ultrasound energy is generated by high-frequency sound waves. As a diagnostic tool, the sound waves are directed at tissue, which reflects the waves back to produce a real-time image. The images are digitalized for viewing, storage, and reproduction. Ultrasonic waves can be clearly traced through liquid or semiliquid substances. When the ultrasound probe is applied to skin or mucous membrane for deep tissue assessment, a gel coating is used as an interface because the high-frequency waves cannot be precisely tracked through air.

Ultrasound has many applications both intraoperatively and outside surgery. It is commonly used to obtain images of abdominal viscera and for pregnancy assessment. Images represent tissue density. The outline and internal density are identified by shades of black, white, or gray. When combined with the Doppler technique, ultrasound is used in vascular surgery to track the movement of blood and provide a screen image of velocity and viscosity. An intraoperative ultrasound probe is used to assess vascular structures and tissue density. Echocardiography is used in the same way to demonstrate motion of the heart.

Doppler studies use ultrasound for specific measurement of vascular flow. The Doppler probe, or transducer, provides

transcutaneous (through the skin) measurement of vascular obstruction. The sounds reproduced by the Doppler technique differ in pitch and quality and correspond to the movement of blood through a vessel. Doppler sounds can be directly interpreted, or they may be transmitted as wave signals and displayed on a digital screen for interpretation.

BLOOD TESTS

Blood tests routinely are done to assess the blood's chemistry, function, structure, and composition. The structure and type of blood cells present are also important assessment findings. Many hundreds of blood tests can be done and are routinely performed in the health care setting. The most basic tests are the complete blood count, tests for coagulation, overall blood chemistry, and verification of blood type. The arterial blood gas (ABG) test usually is performed in critical care situations.

COMPLETE BLOOD COUNT

The **complete blood count (CBC)** is a basic test used to evaluate the type and percentage of normal components in the blood (Box 20-4). A blood sample is drawn from the vein and centrifuged. This separates it into cellular and liquid components for evaluation. The CBC is a basic blood test used for screening medical, infections, and many other types of disease. When formulating a diagnosis, physicians always consider variations in normal blood values along with other signs and symptoms; they are never considered in isolation.

The blood components measured are:
- **Hemoglobin (Hgb):** The oxygen-carrying protein attached to red blood cells (erythrocytes).
- *Red blood cell count:* Erythrocytes make up most of the volume in peripheral blood. They are produced in red bone marrow and live for about 120 days. Their main function is to deliver oxygen to cells.

Box 20-4
Components of the Complete Blood Count

Component	Abbreviation
Hematocrit	HCT
Hemoglobin	HGB
Red blood cells	RBCs
Mean cell hemoglobin	MCH
Mean cell hemoglobin concentration	MCHC
White blood cells	WBC

Differential White Blood Cells

Segmented neutrophils	Segs
Band neutrophils	Bands
Eosinophils	Eos
Basophils	Basos
Monocytes	Monos
Lymphocytes	Lymphs
Platelets	Plt

- **Hematocrit (Hct):** The percentage of red blood cells in the blood (by volume). *Platelet count:* Platelets have important functions in the blood clotting mechanism, including clot retraction and activation of coagulation factor.
- *Differential leukocyte count:* White blood cells (leukocytes) are essential to the immune process. The **differential count** measures the number of each type of leukocyte by volume of blood. These are *monocytes, macrophages, band neutrophils, eosinophils, basophils,* and *lymphocytes,*

METABOLIC PANEL

The metabolic panel includes a number of tests to determine serum levels of substances that are crucial for metabolism. Many types of metabolic panels can be done. The **basic metabolic panel** includes blood glucose, carbon dioxide, creatinine, urea nitrogen, bicarbonate, and several important electrolytes. The exact tests included in any metabolic panel are determined by health care regulatory agencies and may change with reimbursement regulations.

COAGULATION TESTS

A number of blood studies may be performed to determine coagulation, which is a critical factor for the surgical patient. The tests are used to assess disease states and to monitor patients who are receiving antiplatelet drugs for a clotting disorder.

The mechanism of blood clotting is an extremely complex physiological activity that is divided into two processes, the *intrinsic pathway* and the *extrinsic pathway.* The extrinsic pathway occurs at the tissue level, and the intrinsic pathway occurs in the vascular system. Both systems activate a chemical called *factor X* and the formation of **fibrin** for clotting. The chain reaction of physiological events in the coagulation process is controlled by many chemicals, called *factors,* which are identified by Roman numerals. These are released in specific order, and if one is missing, the clotting mechanism is altered.

The prothrombin time (PT) and partial prothromboplastin time (PTT) are performed to evaluate the extrinsic coagulation system. They are also used for screening congenital deficiencies of factors II, V, VII, and X.

The prothrombin time (PT) is a measurement of coagulation time. The PT generally is used to monitor the patient on long-term anticoagulant therapy.

The **partial thromboplastin time (PTT)** or activated partial thromboplastin time (APTT) is commonly performed to assess the functional ability of the coagulation sequence. In this test, partial prothrombin is added to coagulated blood. The test is most commonly used to determine the effects of heparin therapy or to screen for clotting disorders.

ARTERIAL BLOOD GASES

Blood pH is regulated by an increase or decrease in specific ions (acid and base). A measurement of these ions (bicarbonate [HCO_3] and carbonic acid [H_2CO_3]) provides a snapshot of this balancing mechanism. The partial pressures of carbon dioxide (CO_2) and oxygen (O_2) are also measured and provide an assessment of the patient's ventilatory capacity. Oxygen saturation (O_2Sat) is the amount of oxygen attached to hemoglobin and available to the cells. Blood drawn for ABG testing is usually taken from the atrial artery and must be kept cold during transport, because temperature affects the accuracy of the results.

ABO GROUPS

A person's blood type or ABO blood group, is based on inherited antigens found on the surface of an individual's red blood cells. The *Rh type* refers to whether a specific antigen called *Rh* is present. An individual is typed as Rh positive or Rh negative according to whether this antigen is present.

The four significant ABO antigens are A, B, O, and AB. Individuals who lack A and B antigens are typed as *O.* Those who have type A antigens are typed as *A.* Those with B antigens are typed as *B* and those with both A and B are typed as *AB.*

An individual develops antibodies to the antigen he or she does not have. For example, a person with type A antigens develops antibodies to type B antigens. In the case of a transfusion, the antigen reaction is predictable when the ABO group is known.

The significance of the ABO grouping is that a transfusion of blood containing antibodies to the specific antigens of the blood group can cause a transfusion reaction. This can be a mild allergic reaction or a life-threatening condition. Blood incompatibility can lead to a hemolytic reaction in which the recipient's blood cells are destroyed. For this reason, any patient receiving blood products must be tested for blood grouping before transfusion is performed.

ELECTROLYTES

Body fluids contain both organic and inorganic substances. These substances are essential for homeostasis. Molecules of inorganic substances are capable of splitting to yield a charged particle or substance, called an *electrolyte.* Positively charged electrolytes are called *cations,* and those that are negatively charged are called *anions* (Box 20-5). Cations function mainly in the transmission of nerve impulses to muscles. The highest percentage of positive ions is found in the blood, the cells, intercellular spaces, and the gastrointestinal tract. Electrolyte imbalance can result in severe physiological disturbances. The cations potassium, sodium, calcium, and magnesium are rou-

---

Box 20-5

Electrolytes

Cations	Anions
Sodium (Na^+)	Chloride (Cl^-)
Potassium (K^+)	Phosphate (PO_4^-)
Magnesium (Mg^{++})	Bicarbonate (HCO_3^-)
Calcium (Ca^{++})	Sulfate (SO_4^-)

tinely measured in blood. Several anions are measured directly (such as "ion gap"). For more complex information on this topic, a blood chemistry or pathophysiology text should be consulted.

Potassium

Potassium is found mainly in the cells. It is necessary for the transmission of nerve impulses to skeletal, smooth, and cardiac muscle. It also functions in the conversion of carbohydrates for cellular energy and is critical in maintaining osmolality in the cells. **Hypokalemia** (decreased serum potassium) can result from persistent and severe vomiting and diarrhea, extensive tissue trauma, or shock. Certain drugs can also cause a drop in potassium.

Sodium

Sodium is the most plentiful electrolyte found outside the cell. It is responsible for regulation of body and cellular fluids and plays a critical role in the transport of substances into and out of the cell. It binds with specific negatively charged electrolytes to maintain the blood pH. **Hyponatremia** (low sodium) is caused by prolonged vomiting and diarrhea, use of certain diuretics, and surgery.

Calcium

Calcium is found in the cells and also in the extracellular fluid. It is most important in promoting myocardial contraction and in the conversion of thrombin to prothrombin, which is part of the blood clotting mechanism. Calcium contributes to cell permeability and is necessary for the development and maintenance of bone tissue. **Hypocalcemia** can result from parathyroid disease, vitamin D deficiency, and specific drugs such as corticosteroids and some diuretics.

Magnesium

Magnesium is important in the neurotransmission of all muscles but especially the myocardium. Like calcium, it contributes to cell permeability and also protein and carbohydrate metabolism. Magnesium is necessary for the transport of sodium and potassium through the cell membrane. Hypomagnesemia can be caused by drugs such as corticosteroids, laxatives, and some diuretics.

URINALYSIS

Standard urinalysis is performed to assess the body's overall health, with particular focus on the urinary tract. Simple screening is performed with a dipstick coated with reagents that register the levels of different substances in the urine. These substances are:

- Albumen
- Bilirubin
- Glucose
- Ketones
- Leukocytes
- Blood nitrite
- Urobilinogen

The pH and specific gravity are also assessed. The color, clarity, and odor of the urine are interpreted in the overall assessment. The sample is centrifuged to create sediment, which is examined for microorganisms, crystals, cells, and casts. Urine culture is performed to determine the exact organism associated with a urinary tract infection.

MICROBIOLOGICAL STUDIES

Tissue specimens and fluid suspected of being infected are analyzed to determine the presence and type of microorganisms. Samples that are suspected or known to be contaminated are taken intraoperatively in selected procedures. This is based on evidence of pus, inflammation, or devitalized tissue. A sample confirms the diagnosis and aids treatment decisions. One of the tests used to detect infection is **culture and sensitivity (C & S)**. In this test, a sample is allowed to incubate on a culture medium. After colonization, a number of tests are performed on the colonies to identify the exact microorganism. The sensitivity test exposes the cultured microorganisms to a variety of antibiotic substances during incubation. This determines which of the substances interferes with growth. (The handling of culture and sensitivity specimens during surgery is described in chapters 7 and 16.)

PATHOLOGICAL EXAMINATION OF TISSUE

Pathology is the study of diseases. Tissue pathology is the examination of tissue for the presence of disease. In surgery, pathology specimens are routinely obtained and sent to the pathology department for analysis. Each type of tissue requires special care to ensure that the cells are not damaged.

TISSUE BIOPSY

Biopsy is the removal of tissue for analysis and diagnosis. Protocols for tissue preservation vary according to the type of tissue, whether it will be examined immediately, and how it is to be analyzed. The protocol for handling specimens is developed by the facility's pathology department and is available for all perioperative personnel to study. (Chapter 16 presents information on the handling of specimens.) Biopsy specimens can be obtained in a number of ways:

- *Excision:* The surgical removal of a small portion of tissue. Excision usually refers to removal by cutting (also called **excisional biopsy**).
- *Needle* or *trocar biopsy:* The removal of tissue with a hollow needle or trocar, which is inserted into the tissue. A core sample of the tissue is removed in one or more locations of the suspected area. The needle can be inserted through the skin (percutaneously) or into tissue exposed during surgery. A hollow trocar may be used to remove a large core of tissue such as the bone marrow.
- *Brush biopsy:* A biopsy brush, a very small, cylindrical brush, is used to sweep a hollow lumen or cavity for cells. This technique is commonly used in diagnostic procedures of the larynx, throat, esophagus, and intestine during an endoscopic procedure. The procedure

removes only superficial cells and does not cut into the tissue. After biopsy, the brush is withdrawn and immediately swished in liquid preservative or saline to prevent drying.

- *Aspiration biopsy:* Fluid for pathological exam may be removed from semi-solid tissue by aspirating the fluid (removal with a syringe). The term centesis refers to aspiration of fluid.
- *Smear:* A smear is obtained by passing a swab or small brush over superficial tissue. The swab is passed over a glass microscope slide, which is sprayed with a cell fixative. The specimen can then be examined microscopically by the pathologist.
- *Frozen section:* Immediate microscopic and gross (without aid of the microscope) examination of suspect tissue is performed by **frozen section**. In this procedure, the tissue is removed and immediately placed in liquid nitrogen. This freezes the sample. It is then sliced into single-cell sections and analyzed microscopically. A surgical procedure is purposefully scheduled with a frozen section to determine the need for radical or more extensive excision of a tumor. A permanent section fixes the tissue slices on slides for preservation. (Chapter 16 presents a complete discussion of the intraoperative care of frozen section tissue.)

CANCER TERMS AND CONCEPTS

Surgery commonly is performed to diagnose or treat cancer Terms related to cancer treatment, classification, and diagnosis are used in the perioperative setting. A basic understanding of these terms and their origin is an important aspect of surgical practice.

DEFINITIONS

A **neoplasm**, or tumor, is an abnormal growth. A tumor is classified as **malignant** or **benign**. A malignant tumor is composed of disorganized tissue that exhibits uncontrolled growth. Malignant tissue has the potential to spread from the original site (called the *primary tumor*) to other parts of the body. A benign growth is composed of cells belonging to a single tissue type and does not spread to distant regions of the body. Any word with the ending—*oma* refers to a tumor (e.g., osteoma, leiomyoma, and lymphoma).

COMPARISON OF MALIGNANT AND BENIGN TUMORS

A benign tumor often resembles the tissue in which it originates. It does not undergo histological change (changes in the tissue type) but remains consistent during growth. These tumors usually are encapsulated or confined and do not infiltrate the tissue bed. A benign tumor may continue to grow but does not "take over" the functions of the original tissue. In contrast, a malignant tumor develops a disorganized vascular system and usually contains different types of cells or tissue. It invades the tissue of origin and captures its nutrients

and often its blood flow. Malignant cells release toxins that kill normal cells, and the tumor grows quickly and invasively. Cells from the malignancy break off and enter the lymph system, where they are transported to other areas of the body. New tumors may develop from these "seed" cells; this is called **metastasis**. Eventually the tumor disrupts or halts the normal function of vital organs. Malignancy usually results in death unless it is treated early.

A benign tumor may impinge upon nearby tissue or organs. This can interrupt blood supply, cause pain, or alter the function of healthy tissue. However, the tumor grows slowly compared to malignant tissue, and the benign tissue does not invade the healthy tissue or deplete its nutrients.

EFFECTS OF MALIGNANCY ON THE BODY

Malignancy causes specific injury to the body:

- The risk of thrombosis (blood clot) is increased as a result of inappropriate production of clotting factors by the tumor itself. The tumor may also block blood vessels, resulting in clotting.
- Pain is caused by direct injury to tissue or by pain mediators released by the tumor. As the tumor impinges on healthy tissue, the tissue dies, resulting in severe pain.
- Cachexia (tissue and body wasting) is characteristic of malignancy. As the tumor destroys tissue, the patient's metabolism is altered. Nutrients normally received by healthy tissue for growth and repair are captured by the malignant tissue, which continues to grow and spread.
- Anemia occurs as a result of internal bleeding and the body's inability to replace red blood cells.
- As the malignancy spreads, changes occur in the function of the target tissue. This results in many different disease conditions, depending on the organ or tissue function.

DIAGNOSTIC METHODS

Several tests commonly are performed to screen for suspected cancer. The exact type of test depends on the affected tissue.

Tumor Markers

A **tumor marker** is an antigen present on the tumor cell or a other substance (protein, hormone, or other chemical) released by the cells into the blood. Some markers are specific for certain types of cancer cells. Markers are not always reliable for diagnosing malignancy, because some benign tumors can also release markers. Tests for tumor markers are most useful in patients undergoing treatment when a comparison provides information during the course of therapy. An assessment tool for the detection of prostate cancer is measurement of the tumor marker prostate-specific antigen (PSA). Another common assessment marker is CA 125, which is present in some types of ovarian cancer.

Biopsy

A tissue biopsy is a sample of tissue, cells, or fluid that is removed from the body and examined for suspected disease.

Box 20-6

Box 20-6

Tumor-Node-Metastasis (TNM) Classification System

Tumor

Tx	The tumor cannot be assessed.
T0	No evidence of a primary tumor.
Tis	Carcinoma in situ.
T1-T4	Increasing tumor size or involvement of healthy tissue.

Nodes

Nx	Lymph nodes cannot be assessed.
N0	No evidence of lymph node involvement.
N1-3	Increasing involvement of regional lymph nodes.

Metastasis

Mx	Metastasis not assessed.
M10	No evidence of distant metastasis.
M1	Distant metastasis confirmed and site indicated.

A tissue biopsy can be a small segment of the suspected tissue, a cell washing, a smear, or a blood sample. The Pap smear (Papanicolaou test) is a familiar type of routine biopsy for cervical cancer. The frozen section specimen described previously is another type of biopsy.

Tumor Staging

Two methods are used to classify malignant tumors; this is called **staging**. One is by analysis of the cellular characteristics; the other is by the spread of cancer (i.e., the metastatic pattern). Staging provides a basis on which to select the most beneficial treatment. It also indicates the progress of treatment and the outcome, or **prognosis**. The staging process is an internationally used system called the **TNM classification system** (Box 20-6). *T* refers to the extent of the tumor, *N* refers to lymph node involvement, and *M* is the extent of metastasis. Tumors are also graded according to the level of cellular differentiation. Grades I through IV indicate decreasing levels of differentiation. Grade I cells show the most differentiation. Decreased differentiation indicate more serious disease, thus grade IV has increased risk of lethality than grade I.

NUCLEAR MEDICINE

Nuclear medicine involves the use of radioactive particles, which are directed at the nucleus of a selected element to create energy. These special elements are referred to as **radionuclides** or **isotopes**. Radionuclides emit gamma radiation and can be used for diagnosis and treatment. Administered intravenously, orally, or by direct deposition, they can be traced to reveal the structure and function of an organ, a system, a cavity, or a tissue.

RADIATION THERAPY

Tissue destruction by ionizing radiation is used in the treatment of a neoplasm. The delivery and implantation systems for radiation therapy include needles, seeds, and capsulated implants. Radiation therapy procedures are carried out in designated areas of the hospital or health facility by specially trained personnel. In addition to implantation procedures, intraoperative radiation therapy is used to deliver a single dose of radiation to a specific area of the body.

In needle delivery systems, cesium-137, a radioactive isotope, is enclosed in dose units and contained in special hollow needles for insertion into tissue. The needles are placed around the borders of the tumor. These are connected by heavy suture and secured to the patient's skin. The needles remain in place up to 7 days.

Radioactive seeds can be implanted directly into the tumor mass and may be left in the patient indefinitely. Cesium-137, iodine-125, and iridium-192 are used in this procedure. Seeds generally are used in tumors that cannot be removed by surgical resection because of precarious location or size. The procedure may be performed intraoperatively or in the interventional radiology department.

Short-acting radiotherapy in high doses can be delivered through **brachytherapy**. In this procedure, a capsule containing high-dose radiation is implanted using a special catheter. Radioactive pellets are inserted into the implanted catheter for several days and then removed. This treatment is used in breast and prostate cancer.

CANCER PREVENTION AND SCREENING

Many forms of cancer can be treated in the early stages of the disease. Public health promotion and screening procedures enable people to learn about cancer and protect themselves against some cancers. An updated review of screening recommendations can be found on the National Cancer Institute's Web site at http://www.cancer.gov.

CHAPTER SUMMARY

- The first step in medical and surgical decision making is assessment of the problem. The assessment begins with a baseline history and physical examination.
- An invasive procedure involves breaking intact skin or mucous membrane or inserting a medical device into a body cavity. Noninvasive procedures are limited to skin contact or no direct contact with the body.

- The vital signs are indicators of the patient's overall well-being. They are the most basic form of medical assessment. The vital signs include temperature, pulse, respiratory rate, and blood pressure, and in the care setting, a measurement of the patient's level of pain.
- The body requires a core (deep) temperature of approximately 99° F (37.2° C).

- Exertion, digestion of food, and disease increase the metabolic rate, and the environmental temperature can affect a person's core temperature. Variations in normal temperature are also affected by the location of the measurement and the patient's age and hormonal levels.
- A digital thermometer is used in most care settings. Glass thermometers are rarely used.
- The pulse is a reflection of the stroke volume (the amount of blood pumped through the heart) of each heartbeat. The pulse is felt in an artery as it expands with each heartbeat.
- The pulse is measured by palpating (feeling with the fingers) an artery. In routine assessment, the radial artery is used.
- The respiratory rate is a reflection of the patient's overall metabolic, cardiovascular, and neurological status. It is altered by exertion, metabolic stress, strong emotion, and the effects of specific drugs, which can depress or stimulate the autonomic nervous system.
- The respiratory rate is measured by observing the patient's thorax. It is recorded as breaths per minute. The respiratory rate is measured when the patient is unaware, because people often alter their breathing pattern under observation.
- Blood pressure is the force exerted on the vessels walls. Vascular pressure changes during the cardiac cycle (filling of the heart chambers and shunting of blood through the heart). This is called the *systolic pressure*. As the heart relaxes between contractions, the pressure decreases. This is called the *diastolic pressure*.
- The mean arterial pressure is the average amount of pressure exerted throughout the cardiac cycle.
- Pulse pressure is the difference between the diastolic and systolic pressures.
- Simple blood pressure assessment is done with an electronic or a manual sphygmomanometer and a stethoscope. The method used to take the blood pressure is critical to obtaining a correct reading.
- Blood pressure can be measured in several locations on a limb. The most common location for an adult is the upper arm (the brachial artery).
- If the patient is assessed for orthostatic (postural) blood pressure, the pulse and blood pressure are measured with the patient in the recumbent position and again while the individual is sitting or standing.
- An ECG machine measures the electrical activity of the heart and displays it on a graph for evaluation. To obtain the readings, electrodes are placed at strategic locations on the chest wall and extremities.
- An ECG provides detailed information about heart conduction. Each phase of the cardiac conduction system is represented on a graph generated by the ECG machine.
- X-rays are electromagnetic particles with a relatively short wavelength. An x-ray image (radiograph) is created when radiation passes through structures and strikes a medium (e.g., radiographic film) positioned in line with the penetrating rays.
- The images formed by x-rays display contrasts in density. An extremely dense substance produces a white image, whereas air produces a black image. Contours and outlines of organs, systems, and tissue are displayed as a combination of white, black, and grays.
- The term *radiopaque* refers to substances that x-rays cannot penetrate. In diagnostic medicine, liquid substances called *contrast media* are injected, instilled, or ingested to outline hollow organs or vessels before radiographs are taken.
- In surgery, the mobile C-arm fluoroscope is used for real-time imaging. The head of the fluoroscope is directed through the body onto an image intensifier on the underside of the C.
- In computed tomography, radiographic and computer technologies are combined to produce high-contrast cross-sectional images. Data collected during CT reflect the absorption coefficients of structures, which provide a method of exact measurement.
- Magnetic resonance imaging uses radiofrequency signals and magnetic energy to produce images. In this process, the patient is exposed to electromagnetic energy, which is emitted inside a closed body tube or an open platform.
- Positron emission tomography uses the combined technologies of CT and radioactive scanning. PET is performed to produce an image not of a structure, but rather of a metabolic process.
- During ultrasound imaging, high-frequency sound waves are directed at tissue. These are reflected back to produce an image of the tissue.
- Doppler studies use ultrasound to measure vascular flow. The reflected sound waves can be interpreted directly or transmitted as waveforms on a digital output monitor.
- The complete blood count is a basic test used to evaluate the type and percentage of normal components in the blood.
- A number of blood studies can be performed to determine coagulation, a critical factor for the surgical patient.
- The prothrombin time is a measurement of coagulation time. The PT generally is used to monitor a patient undergoing warfarin therapy or to screen a patient for a dysfunction of the extrinsic system. The partial thromboplastin time (or activated partial thromboplastin time) is done to assess the functional ability of the coagulation sequence.
- The ABO blood groups, also known as *blood types,* are categorizations based on inherited antigens found on the surface of an individual's red blood cells. The four significant ABO antigens are A, B, O, and AB. Individuals who lack A and B antigens are typed as *O.* Those who have type A antigens are typed as *A.* Those

with B antigens are typed as *B,* and those with both A and B are typed as *AB.*

- The significance of the ABO grouping is that a transfusion of blood containing antibodies to the specific antigens of the blood group can cause a transfusion reaction.
- Molecules of inorganic substances are capable of splitting to yield a charged particle or substance, called an *electrolyte.* Positively charged electrolytes are cations, and those that are negatively charged are anions.
- Electrolytes are vital for homeostasis and are responsible for nerve impulses, fluid balance, transport of substances into and out of the cell, and for balancing the blood pH. They also contribute to blood clotting, electrical activity in the cells, and energy conversion.
- Biopsy is the removal of tissue for analysis and diagnosis. The type of biopsy performed depends on the tissue, location, and previous assessment.
- Excision is the surgical removal of a small portion of tissue. Excision usually refers to removal by cutting (also called *excisional biopsy*).
- Needle or trocar biopsy is removal of tissue with a hollow needle or trocar, which is inserted into the tissue.
- Brush biopsy is performed with a very small, cylindrical brush used to sweep a hollow lumen or cavity for cells.
- In an aspiration biopsy, fluid for pathological examination is removed from semisolid tissue by aspirating fluid (removal with a syringe).
- A smear is obtained by passing a swab or small brush over superficial tissue. The swab then is passed over a glass microscope slide and sprayed with a cell fixative.
- A frozen section is removal of tissue for immediate pathological assessment. The tissue specimen is frozen and passed through a device that produces single-cell sections for examination.
- A neoplasm, or tumor, is excessive, disorganized growth of tissue.
- A malignant neoplasm consists of nondifferentiated cells that have the potential to break loose from the original site and spread to other parts of the body. A benign growth is composed of cells belonging to a single tissue type, and its cells are not released or spread to other parts of the body.
- Cells from the malignancy break off and enter the lymph system, where they are transported to other areas of the body. New tumors may develop from these "seed" cells. This is called *metastasis.*
- A tumor marker is an antigen present on the tumor cell or a substance (protein, hormone, or other chemical) released by the cells into the blood.
- Two methods are used to classify malignant tumors. This is called *staging.* One is by analysis of the cellular characteristics; the other is by the spread of the cancer, or metastatic pattern. Staging provides a basis for selecting the most beneficial treatment.
- Tissue destruction by ionizing radiation is used in the treatment of a neoplasm. The delivery and implantation systems for radiation therapy include needles, seeds, and capsulated implants.

REVIEW QUESTIONS

1. Describe the factors that can increase core temperature in the clinical setting.
2. Which methods of temperature assessment accurately reflect core temperature?
3. How do you correctly document the patient's vital signs? Give examples and explain what they mean.
4. What are the causes of a falsely high blood pressure reading?
5. What is "postural" blood pressure?
6. The peaks and troughs on the ECG reading correspond to what?
7. What is the purpose of a contrast medium?
8. Define radiotherapy.
9. What is the differential leukocyte count?
10. Compare the main differences between a malignant and a benign tumor.
11. What is a tumor marker?
12. Why do you think people do not take advantage of screening procedures for cancer?

BIBLIOGRAPHY

Chernecky C, Berger B: *Laboratory tests and diagnostic procedures,* ed 2, St Louis, 2008, Elsevier/Mosby.

McPhee S, Papdakis M, Tierney L: *Current medical diagnosis and treatment,* ed 46, 2007, McGraw Hill.

Porth C: *Pathophysiology concepts of altered health states,* ed 6, Philadelphia, 2007, Lippincott Williams & Wilkins.

CHAPTER 21

Minimally Invasive Endoscopic and Robotic-Assisted Surgery

CHAPTER OUTLINE

Introduction
Minimally Invasive Surgery
  Principles of Minimally Invasive Surgery
  Advantages of Minimally Invasive Surgery
  Potential Disadvantages of Minimally
    Invasive Surgery
  Risks Associated with Minimally Invasive
    Surgery
  Surgical Specialties
  Common Features
  Preoperative Preparation of the Patient
  Minimally Invasive Surgery Imaging
    System
  Operating Instruments Used in Minimally
    Invasive Surgery

Techniques Used in Minimally Invasive
  Surgery
Tissue Expansion at the Surgical Site
Hemostasis
Risks Associated with Electrosurgery
Specimen Retrieval
Endoscopic Setup
Flexible Endoscopy
Reprocessing Endoscopes and
  Instruments
Robotic Surgery
  Principles of Robotic Surgery
  Robotic Movement
  Classification of Robots
  da Vinci Surgical System

Advantages and Disadvantages of Robotic
  Surgery
Training for Robotics
Surgical Specialties and Robotics
Components of the Robotic System:
  Structure and Purpose
da Vinci Instruments
Surgeon's Console
Vision System
Setup and Sequence for Robotic
  Surgery
Special Roles of the Surgical Team

LEARNING OBJECTIVES

After studying this chapter the reader will be able to:

- Discuss the advantages and constraints of minimally invasive surgery (MIS)
- Describe the preparation of the patient for MIS
- Describe the function of each component of the imaging equipment used in MIS
- Discuss the care of a rigid endoscope
- Describe the surgical technique used for insufflation in laparoscopy
- List the risks associated with insufflation
- Describe the trocar-cannula system used in all MIS
- Explain how specimens are collected and retrieved during MIS
- Describe the specific electrosurgical risks of direct and capacitative coupling

- Describe the structure and function of a flexible endoscope
- Discuss the proper protocol for processing rigid and flexible endoscopes
- Describe the principles of robotic surgery
- Discuss the concept of cartesian geometry as it applies to robot design
- Describe robotic movements and classification
- Discuss training resources for robotic surgery
- List the three main components of robotic surgery and describe their function
- Identify possible methods of decontaminating and reprocessing robotic instruments
- Describe the roles of team members during robotic surgery

TERMINOLOGY

Abdominal adhesions: Bands of scar tissue on the outer membranes of the abdomen and the abdominal wall.
Active electrode monitoring (AEM): A method of reducing the risk of patient burns during monopolar electrosurgery. AEM systems stop the electrical current whenever resistance is high anywhere in the circuit.
Arthroscopy: Endoscopic surgery of a joint
Articulated: A jointed structure. In mechanics, an articulated arm is one with joints to allow movement of the structure.

Auxiliary water channel: A channel in the flexible endoscope used to deliver irrigation fluid at the tip.
Balloon dissector: A balloon device used to separate tissue planes during minimally invasive surgery.
Biopsy channel: A channel that extends the full length of a flexible endoscope and is used to retrieve biopsy tissue.
Camera control unit (CCU): The main control source for the video camera. The unit captures video signals from the camera head and processes them for display on the monitor.

Cannula: In minimally invasive surgery, a cannula is a slender tube inserted through the body wall and used to receive and stabilize telescopic instruments.

Capacitative coupling: In minimally invasive surgery, the unintended transmission of electricity from the active electrode to an adjacent conductive pathway, sometimes resulting in a patient burn.

Capacitor: A point in an electrical circuit where energy (usually heat or light) builds up or is stored between insulators.

Control head: The proximal section of a flexible endoscope where the controls are located.

Diagnostic endoscopy: A diagnostic procedure in which a long, flexible, fiberoptic tube is inserted into a body cavity for viewing and diagnosis.

Digital output recorder: During video-assisted surgery, digital signals are captured from the video camera and transmitted to a monitor. The digital output recorder processes these signals.

Direct coupling: In minimally invasive surgery, the transmission of electricity directly from one conductive path to another, such as from the active electrode to a conductive instrument.

Docking: In robotic surgery, the process of positioning the robotic instruments in the exact location over the patient so that instruments can be safely attached from their ports in the body cavity.

Elevator channel: A channel that extends the full length of a flexible endoscope and receives biopsy forceps or other instruments.

Endocoupler: A device that connects the endoscope to the camera.

Endoscope: A telescopic instrument with serial lenses that is used to view anatomical structures inside the body.

Extracorporeal: A term meaning "outside the body." In minimally invasive surgery, it refers to a technique for placing sutures in which the knots are formed outside the body and then tightened after they have been introduced into the surgical wound.

Eyepiece: The proximal portion of the endoscopic lens.

Focus ring: A device fitted on the endoscopic camera to focus the image seen through the lens system.

Gain: In electronics, the intensity of the signal.

Haptic feedback: Tactile feedback, conveyed from tissue to the hand when a hand instrument is used. Robotic instruments do not provide any tactile feedback.

High definition (HD): In video technology, the clarity of an image based on the number of signals (pixels) emitted by the camera. A high-definition format displays 1280×721 pixels in a rectangular image.

Imaging system: The combined components of the endoscopic system, which create the image captured in the focal view of the endoscope.

Insertion tube: The long, narrow portion of the flexible endoscope that is inserted into the body.

Instrument channel: A channel that extends the full length of a flexible endoscope and receives instruments during flexible endoscopy.

Insufflation: In minimally invasive surgery, inflation of the abdominal or thoracic cavity with carbon dioxide gas.

Insufflation unit: A device that regulates the flow and amount of carbon dioxide gas during insufflation.

Intracorporeal: A term meaning "inside the body." In minimally invasive surgery, it refers to a suture technique in which sutures are knotted and secured inside the patient.

Intravasation: The unintended absorption of irrigation fluids into the body.

Knot pusher: A device used to secure suture knots during minimally invasive surgery.

Laparoscopy: Minimally invasive surgery of the abdomen.

Ligation loop: A commercially prepared suture loop used to secure structures during minimally invasive surgery.

Light cable: The fiberoptic light cable that transmits light from the source to the endoscopic instrument. Sometimes called a *light guide.*

Light source: A device that controls and emits light for endoscopic procedures.

Master controllers: In robotic surgery, the nonsterile hand controls that manipulate surgical instruments.

Minimally invasive surgery (MIS): Surgery performed through small incisions using telescopic instruments.

Morcellization: A surgical technique in which tissue is fragmented to permit removal through an endoscopic cannula.

Nephroscopy: Endoscopic surgery of the kidney.

Open surgery: Standard surgery in which an incision is made and standard instruments are used.

Optical angle: The angle at which light is transmitted at the distal end of a fiberoptic or video endoscope.

Pixel: An element within each silicone chip contained within a device which produces electronic images such as those seen on a surgical monitor used in minimally invasive surgery. One pixel is represented as a signal. As the number of signals (pixels) increases, the quality of the image is enhanced.

Pneumoperitoneum: An abdomen insufflated or distended with carbon dioxide gas during laparoscopy.

Resectoscope: A surgical endoscope that has the capability of morcellization, or tissue fragmentation.

Robot: A mechanical device that can be programmed to perform tasks.

Standard definition (SD): A type of video format. The clarity of an image is based on the number of signals (pixels) emitted by the camera. A standard definition format displays 640×480 pixels in a rectangular image.

Stereoscopic viewer: In robotic surgery, the binocular lens system of the surgeon console.

Surgeon console: In robotic surgery, the nonsterile control unit used by the surgeon to manipulate instruments.

Telescopic instruments: Long, narrow instruments used during endoscopic surgery.

Telesurgery: A type of robotic surgery in which surgery is performed from a nearby location through computer-mediated instruments. In telesurgery, no direct physical contact with the instruments occurs.

Thoracoscopy: Endoscopic surgery of the thoracic cavity.

Trocar: A sharp, rod-shaped instrument used to puncture the body wall.

Veress needle: A spring-loaded needle used to deliver carbon dioxide gas during insufflation.

Video cable: In video-assisted endoscopy, the cable that transmits digital data from the camera head to the camera control unit and from the monitor to the output recorder.

Video printer: A device that stores and prints output data viewed through the video endoscope.

White balance: A procedure for adjusting the light color of the video camera to other components of the system.

INTRODUCTION

Endoscopic or minimally invasive surgery is performed by inserting instruments into the body through small, narrow incisions or a natural body orifice. Although this technique has been available for several decades, the advances in biotechnology of the past 10 years have enabled this surgical technique to be used in many surgical specialties.

Two types of endoscopic systems are discussed in this chapter:

*   **Minimally invasive surgery (MIS)** is performed using a rigid lensed telescope and long instruments, which are introduced into small incisions at the operative site. In this technique, the operative space may be enlarged with fluid or carbon dioxide. The goal of the minimally invasive technique is primarily surgical rather than diagnostic (Figure 21-1).
*   **Diagnostic endoscopy** and operative endoscopy usually are performed with a flexible, semirigid, or rigid endoscope that is inserted into an anatomical opening in the body. The lens system, channels for introducing small instruments, and light system are contained in one long tube. The endoscope usually is inserted into a body cavity through a natural orifice or small incision. Flexible endoscopy is used to assess the regional anatomy, to obtain tissue biopsies, and to perform minor surgical procedures (Figure 21-2). The rigid endoscope is used

to perform a surgical assessment and operative procedures, such as transurethral resection of the prostate and transcervical resection of a uterine fibroid tumor.

Terminology in the field of MIS and endoscopy is evolving along with the rapid technological advances in systems and instruments. In general, the term **telescopic instruments** refers to the rigid, lensed instrument used in MIS. The term **endoscope** is used to describe the flexible lensed instrument that is passed through a natural orifice for assessment or surgery of a hollow organ, duct, or vessel.

MINIMALLY INVASIVE SURGERY

PRINCIPLES OF MINIMALLY INVASIVE SURGERY

Minimally invasive surgery is a technique in which telescopic (long, narrow) instruments are inserted into the body through two or more small incisions. Narrow tubes called **cannulas** are inserted into each incision. These remain in place throughout the surgery and receive the telescopic surgical instruments. The cannulas protect the body wall and also maintain a seal between the inside of the body and the outside environment. To perform surgery inside the body, the surgeon inserts a slender optical telescope through one of the cannulas. The image seen through the endoscope is projected and enlarged onto one or more flat screen monitors. Surgery is performed by adjusting the endoscope to obtain different views and by manipulating the telescopic instruments as they appear on the monitor.

ADVANTAGES OF MINIMALLY INVASIVE SURGERY

MIS has many advantages over open surgery. Powerful high quality optical systems allow the surgeon to perform delicate procedures while viewing the surgical site on a video monitor, which enlarges the field of view and allows all members of the team to view the operative area. Telescopic instruments used

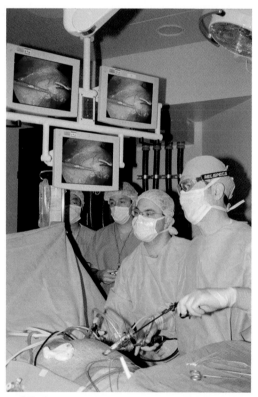

Figure 21-1 Minimally invasive surgery of the abdomen (laparoscopy). A lensed telescope with camera and long instruments are introduced into small incisions. The camera image is projected to a central monitor. *(Courtesy © Karl Storz Endoscopy America, Inc.)*

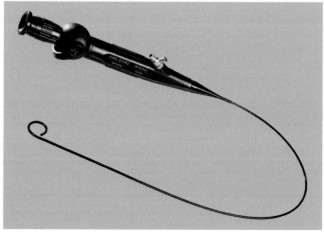

Figure 21-2 Flexible endoscopy. *(Courtesy © Karl Storz Endoscopy America, Inc.)*

in MIS are very small and capable of powerful hemostatic and cutting modalities. Most of these instruments can perform the same tasks as standard instruments. Open surgery generally requires a longer healing time than MIS because of the increased tissue trauma involved in entering the operative site. Patients undergoing MIS are able to resume normal activities sooner, and the hospital stay is shorter. Many types of MIS are performed in the outpatient setting, which is convenient and often less costly.

In summary, the advantages are:
* Reduced tissue trauma
* Less blood loss
* Less pain
* Faster recovery and return to normal activities
* Can be done as outpatient surgery in many cases
* Reduced postoperative pain
* Increased patient satisfaction
* Less costly

POTENTIAL DISADVANTAGES OF MINIMALLY INVASIVE SURGERY

Patients who have undergone previous abdominal procedures have a high risk of **abdominal adhesions** (scarring of organs that causes adherence to the peritoneal wall). This presents a risk of perforation during use of a **trocar**, a sharp, rodlike instrument that must be placed into the body wall to facilitate insertion of endoscopic instruments.

The technique used in MIS requires long, delicate instruments. Consequently, leverage is reduced, and the tactile feedback is different from that with standard instruments. Endoscopic instruments are limited in their range of motion. Withdrawing and inserting them into body cavities is sometimes awkward. The operating space is very small, which reduces maneuverability and may lengthen the duration of a procedure.

The image seen through the telescope is projected onto a monitor. Although the technologies used in MIS provide high resolution and excellent color, they are subject to distortion either from an error in the electronic system or mechanical problems with the instruments. As with all medical devices, personnel must be familiar with the equipment used in MIS, including how it works and what to do in case of failure. A disadvantage of MIS is the need for advanced and continuous training for all perioperative staff members. Surgical technologists and perioperative nurses are required to keep up-to-date on advances in the technology to provide the safest environment for the patient.

In summary, the limitations of MIS are:
* Highly advanced technological features require steep learning curves for new perioperative staff members.
* Requires special equipment
* Vision system errors and failures can result in sudden surgical complications.
* MIS instruments and equipment are expensive to lease, purchase, and maintain.
* Instruments have limited range of motion.
* Some procedures take longer than open surgery

* The operative site is projected as a two-dimensional picture rather than the natural three-dimensional view of the eye.
* Certain complications can be masked during MIS.

RISKS ASSOCIATED WITH MINIMALLY INVASIVE SURGERY

Not all patients are suitable for MIS. Some patients cannot tolerate the effects of *insufflation* (inflation of the abdominal cavity; discussed later in the chapter), which is routinely performed during **laparoscopy**. Endoscopic MIS is routinely performed, and the risks have been greatly reduced with advanced technology and staff training. Risk management for MIS is broad and comprehensive. It involves appropriate actions by medical, nursing, and assistive personnel. Current data show that the risks of MIS are probably no greater or less than those with open surgery, except in some experimental procedures.

All surgical risks depend on the condition of the patient at the time of surgery. Very sick patients are at greater risk of physiological problems, including those associated with positioning, abdominal insufflation, and the use of fluids to expand body cavities.

Blackout or distortion of the digital image is a specific risk during MIS. Troubleshooting capability and familiarity with the vision system are required of the perioperative staff. Every manufacturer of video endoscopic equipment provides training and written information on its systems. However, advanced technology in electronic data transmission and video-enhanced surgery cannot be learned by reading alone. The technologist must study procedure manuals and apply the knowledge directly to the equipment in real time before use in surgery. An emergency is not the time to learn how to troubleshoot the system.

SURGICAL SPECIALTIES

Advanced optical and digital technology has expanded the use of minimally invasive techniques to many surgical specialties. The principles of minimally invasive surgery are the same across all specialties. Common techniques are discussed briefly in this chapter and in more detail in the chapters on surgical procedures. Box 21-1 lists commonly performed minimally invasive surgical procedures by specialty.

COMMON FEATURES

MIS requires telescopic instruments and an imaging system. As mentioned previously, instruments are inserted through small incisions directly or through a cannula. Because the operative site is not exposed through an incision in the skin, an **imaging system** is required in all types of endoscopy and MIS. The components of the system include the telescope, fiberoptic light source and cables, monitor, data capturing system, and data output recorder. Video technology is now the accepted modality for transmitting images from the telescope to the monitor.

Box 21-1

Common Minimally Invasive Surgery Procedures by Specialty

General Surgery and Gastroenterology
Adrenalectomy
Appendectomy
Esophagectomy
Gallbladder procedures
Gastrectomy
Gastric reflux procedures
Hernia repair
Intestinal resection
Lymph node biopsy
Pancreatectomy
Parathyroidectomy
Pyloromyotomy
Splenectomy

Gynecology
Excision of fibroids
Exploratory laparotomy
Hysterectomy
Ovarian cystectomy
Radical hysterectomy for uterine cancer
Removal of fibroids
Repair of vesicle vaginal fistula
Tubal ligation
Uterine artery embolization for fibroids

Orthopedic Surgery
Ablation of bone tumor
Arthroscopy
Carpel tunnel release
Endoscopic spine surgery
Fracture of the pelvis
Periarticular and intraarticular fractures of the extremities
Rotator cuff repair
Shoulder instability repair
Spinal decompression
Spinal fixation
Total hip replacement

Unicompartmental knee replacement
Vertebroplasty

Thoracic Surgery
Fundoplication for gastroesophageal reflux
Lung procedures
Myotomy for achalasia
Repair of hiatal hernia
Thoracic sympathectomy

Cardiac Procedures
Atrial septal defect
Coronary artery bypass graft (CABG)
Mitral and tricuspid valve procedures
CABG (off pump)
Patent foramen ovale

Otorhinolaryngology
Removal of nasal and sinus tumors
Sentinel lymph node biopsy for head and neck tumors
Sinus surgery
Transcatheter laser treatment of vascular malformations
Transoral laser resection of peripharyngeal/laryngeal tumors

Vascular Surgery
Ablation of varicose veins
Balloon angioplasty and carotid stenting
Renal and peripheral artery stenting
Repair of abdominal and thoracic aortic aneurysms

Urology
Cystic decortication
Diagnosis and removal of kidney stones
Endoscopic exploration of the urinary tract
Endoscopic tumor biopsy
Nephrectomy
Pyeloplasty
Treatment for strictures and tumors of the urinary tract

Exposure of the surgical site differs according to the specialty. Because instruments are located deep in the body or within tightly enclosed tissue planes, a method of expanding body spaces or tissue planes is needed to safely operate and allow a thorough view of the anatomy. For example, in laparoscopy, the abdomen is filled with carbon dioxide (insufflation). In **arthroscopy** (MIS of the joint spaces), the anatomical space is filled with irrigation fluid. Hollow organs, such as the bladder, are filled with saline or other isotonic fluids during endoscopy. In some anatomical regions, such as the inguinal area, a balloon dissector is used to separate dense tissue planes without causing trauma.

Many MIS procedures require electrosurgery or other energies, such as high-frequency cutting and coagulation devices, for hemostasis and tissue dissection. Electrosurgical techniques and the risks associated with them are described in this chapter and in Chapter 19.

Preoperative preparation, including routine laboratory work and patient education, are performed for MIS. The physiological preparation is the same as for open surgery, and the exact preparation depends on the type and location of the surgery.

PREOPERATIVE PREPARATION OF THE PATIENT

Patients undergoing endoscopic MIS are prepared according to the anatomical location of the surgery. Preoperative preparation for an MIS procedure follows the same or similar protocols as open surgery.

Patient Positioning

The positions used for MIS procedures depend on the surgical site and the patient's physiological condition. In general, patient positioning for MIS is identical to that for open surgery. (See Chapter 10 for a more detailed discussion of patient positioning.)

- *Upper abdomen or lower esophagus:* The patient will may be tipped into reverse Trendelenburg position to displace abdominal viscera. A padded footboard is used to prevent the patient from sliding downward, but the footboard must be used with caution. Substantial padding is required to prevent nerve and vascular damage. Changes in table position require immediate attention to patient safety. The scrub must adjust the Mayo stand or other overhead tables. The circulator must ensure that the new position does not create pressure points between the patient and operating table.
- *Pelvic or lower abdominal procedures:* The patient is placed in the Trendelenburg position. This can compromise the patient's lung capacity and cause hypotension from increased pressure on the vena cava. A gynecological patient is placed in the lithotomy position, which exposes the patient to risks associated with popliteal nerve and vessel injury. Patients with limited range of motion require careful manipulation during positioning.
- ***Thoracoscopy*** and ***nephroscopy:*** Procedures of the lungs, bronchi, and upper urinary tract are performed with the patient in the lateral position.
- *Laryngoscopy, bronchoscopy, esophagoscopy, and mediastinoscopy:* Procedures of the upper airway, upper gastrointestinal tract, and mediastinum are performed with the patient in supine position, although a conscious patient undergoing bronchoscopy may be placed in the Fowler position.

Skin Prep and Draping

The skin prep and draping techniques used for minimally invasive procedures allow for the possibility of conversion to an open case. This is particularly true for laparoscopic, retroperitoneal, and thoracoscopic surgery, which are more likely to be converted than other types of surgery. Draping is extended to match the prep area needed for an open incision, as discussed in Chapter 11.

MINIMALLY INVASIVE SURGERY IMAGING SYSTEM

Endoscopic MIS is dependent on the collective functioning of the imaging components (Figure 21-3). A malfunction in any one component affects the others and may reduce patient safety. As imaging technology becomes increasingly complex, perioperative staff members have a responsibility to maintain current knowledge and skills.

The components of the imaging system include:
- Light source
- Light cable
- Surgical telescope (or endoscope)
- Camera head
- Camera control unit (CCU)
- Video cables
- Monitor
- Image management system

Light Source and Fiberoptic Cable

The **light source** transmits light to the fiberoptic **light cable** and telescope (Figure 21-4). The light source control panel is used to adjust the modes and light intensity. The light is transmitted from bulbs, which are fitted inside the unit. The control panel permits variable adjustments in light intensity, and an infrared filtering system allows the use of lower watt bulbs. The automatic mode of the light source controls the brightness of the image. However if more light is required, the **gain** (the signal intensity) is increased rather than light intensity.

High-resolution video endoscopy requires very intense white light. Xenon lamps therefore are preferred. Many types and models of light sources are available, but most are similar in design and operation.

The light emitted from the telescope is cool as long as the light cable is attached to the telescope. *Light rays emitted from the end of the cable when it is detached from the telescope are extremely hot.* The lighted end of a cable can ignite drapes, sponges, and other materials, especially in the presence of flammable or ignitable liquids such as alcohol.

> ❖ *Always turn the light source to its lowest or standby mode before disconnecting it from the telescope or light cable.*

The fiberoptic light cable (Figure 21-5) transmits light from the light source to the camera head or telescope. The cable is composed of many thousands of glass or plastic fibers, which are aligned in parallel longitudinal bundles. These fiberoptic bundles are delicate and easily broken by sharp impact or overflexing of the cable. The fiberoptic cable is securely attached to the light source on the control panel. Because cables of one manufacturer or model are often used with a different model light source, an adaptor may be needed at the connecting point. Adaptors must be available and in place before surgery.

Care and Safety

The care of fiberoptic cables is illustrated in Figure 21-6.
- Handle fiberoptic cables gently. When storing or transporting the cable, coil it loosely. Do not hang the cable; instead, store it in a flat position.
- Do not allow the cable to strike a hard surface. This can cause the fiberoptic bundles to fracture. Internal fractures are not visible from the outside.
- Inspect cables for exterior damage before using them.
- Power off the light source before connecting or disconnecting the cable. This prevents inadvertent contact between the beam and ignitable materials.
- Do not handle light source bulbs with bare skin. Skin oils can reduce the life span of the bulb.
- Attach the light cable with care. The cable may require an adaptor to fit the light source.
- Keep bulb replacements for the power source on hand. Xenon light sources have bulbs that have a finite life, and replacements must be immediately available during surgery.
- Clean and reprocess the cable according to the manufacturer's directions.

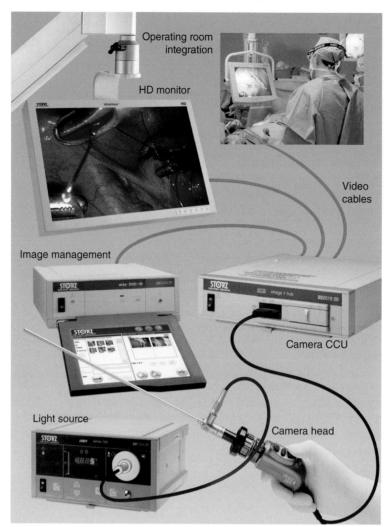

Operating room integration

HD monitor

Video cables

Image management

Camera CCU

Light source

Camera head

Figure 21-3 Imaging components used in minimally invasive surgery. Imaging begins with the telescope; the xenon light source is connected to the endoscope by a fiberoptic cable. The camera head reads the images and transmits them to the camera control unit (CCU). From there the images are transmitted to an image management unit, which can produce digital files of the images. The CCU also transmits digital images to the high-definition monitor, which is necessary to view the operative field. Further imaging is provided to other monitors or information systems through an integrated operating room system. *(Courtesy © Karl Storz Endoscopy America, Inc.)*

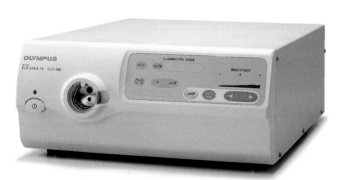

Figure 21-4 Fiberoptic light source. The xenon light source provides light to the telescope via a fiberoptic cable. *(Courtesy © Karl Storz Endoscopy America, Inc.)*

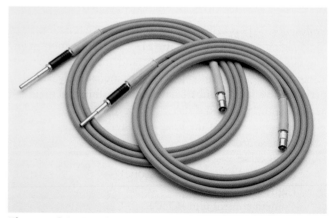

Figure 21-5 Fiberoptic cable connecting the light source to the endoscope. *(Courtesy © Karl Storz Endoscopy America, Inc.)*

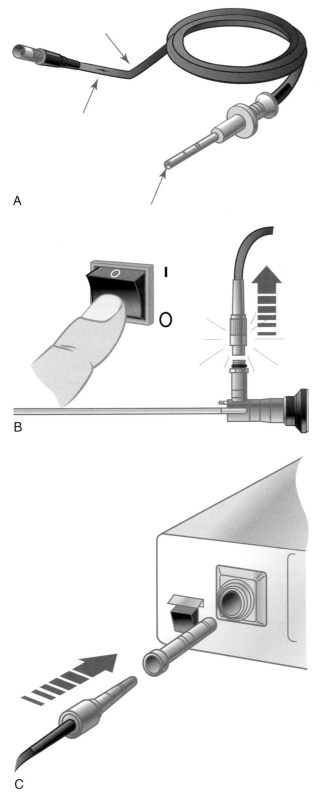

White Balance

All cameras must be **white-balanced** before each procedure. This is a procedure to adjust the light color to the other components in the system. To white-balance the camera: connect the light cable to the telescope, and power on the light on high (or according to the manufacturer's specification). Direct the lens of the telescope at a solid white object, such as the paper backing of a sterile drape (do not use porous or woven material, such as a surgical sponge, because this can cause shadows on the image). The white balance usually is registered automatically by the light source.

Rigid Telescope

The telescope contains the serial lens system, which captures the images illuminated at the tip. Light is transmitted to the telescope through the fiberoptic cable, which attaches near the **eyepiece** (Figure 21-7).

The optical features and dimensions of the telescopes are:

- **Optical angle:** The direction in which lenses are focused on the image. This is measured in degrees, usually 0, 30, and 45 degrees.
- *Diameter:* The diameter of the telescope shaft, measured in millimeters (mm).
- *Length:* The length of the telescope shaft, measured in millimeters (mm).

Care

Telescopes are delicate and expensive. Malfunction or damage to the instrument can cause patient injury and increased surgical time, resulting in a prolonged recovery.

The surgical technologist is responsible for handling and maintaining the telescope in a manner that prevents these errors. The following recommendations are guidelines only. The manufacturer's manual should be consulted for specific detailed care.

Guidelines for Handling Telescopes

- *Always hold the telescope by its head (heavier) end, never by the tip or shaft.* When the telescope is held by the lighter end, the weight of the headpiece can bend the shaft and damage the instrument.
- *Take care to prevent scratches or dents in the shaft of the telescope.* Contact with heavy instruments or sharps can easily damage the delicate optical system and insulation.
- *Use only lint-free, soft material to wipe the telescope.* Some woven materials can cause minute scratches on the lens and surface of the instrument. These can lead to blurring and distortion of the transmitted image. Do not allow oils to come in contact with the lens surface.
- *Never assume that the telescope has been checked for damage by others.* Everyone who handles endoscopic equipment, from reprocessing to end-user stage, has an equal responsibility to ensure the integrity of the instruments. It is the particular duty of the scrub to deliver a safe, properly working telescope to the surgeon (Figure 21-8).

Figure 21-6 Care of the fiberoptic cable and light source. **A,** Fiberoptic light cable: Do not use a cable that is damaged. Look for cuts, nicks, and indentations in the insulation. Make sure the appropriate adaptor tip is used. **B,** Power off the light source: Make sure the power switch is OFF before connecting or disconnecting the light cable. **C,** Cable adaptor and plug: Make sure the proper adaptor is used when attaching the cable plug to the power source. *(Courtesy of © Olympus, America, Inc.)*

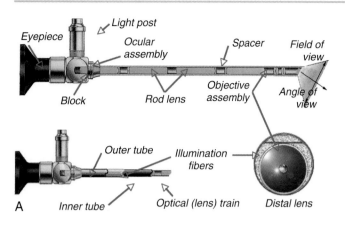

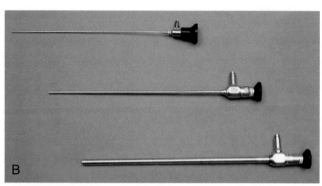

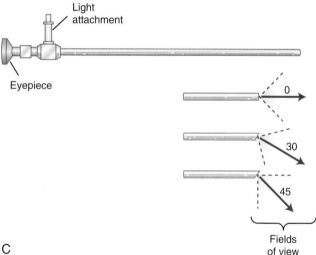

Figure 21-7 **A,** Inner lenses of a rigid endoscope. **B,** Endoscope length: 2 mm, 5 mm, and 10 mm. **C,** Lens angles are available at 0 degrees, 30 degrees, and 45 degrees. (**A** courtesy © Karl Storz Endoscopy America, Inc; **B** from Goldberg JM, Falcone T: Atlas of endoscopic techniques in gynecology, Philadelphia, 2001, WB Saunders; and **C** redrawn from Phillips N: Berry and Kohn's operating room technique, ed 10, St Louis, 2004, Mosby.)

• *Prevent lens fogging during surgery.* When the telescope is introduced into the body, the temperature difference creates fogging on the telescope lens. To prevent fogging, the telescope may be maintained in a warm water bath before use. Defogging agents may also be used on the lens before use.

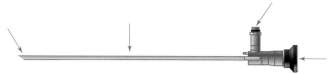

Figure 21-8 Care of the endoscope. Always inspect the endoscope for any nicks or dents. The shaft must be straight to prevent damage to the internal lenses on insertion. (Courtesy of © Olympus, America, Inc.)

Video Camera

The video camera receives visual data from the telescope and allows the surgeon to view structures without looking directly into the telescope. Modern surgical video cameras contain one or three solid-state silicon chips, which produce electrical signals that are amplified and displayed on a digital monitor. Three-chip cameras produce natural color images, which is important to the identification of pathology. Video chips are located in the camera head or, in some newer models, they may be located at the tip of the telescope. Each silicon element in the chip represents one **pixel**. The clarity of the image depends on the number of pixels (signals) or silicon units the chip contains. The more units, the clearer the image appears.

Image quality is derived from the quality of the optics, the lighting source, and the electronic capabilities of the system. The circuit used in video endoscopy is called a *charge-coupled device* (CCD). This allows the electrical charges (signals) to be converted into pixels or picture elements. These are related to colors, and each pixel is stored and recovered separately. Some CCD systems can support more than 65,000 colors. Systems that process a higher number of pixels have excellent resolution even when lighting is very dim.

The video format is the manner in which a video signal transmits information. Individual cameras can use specific formats, and this information is important to the camera's compatibility with other components in the system. Always check the compatibility of the camera with the video system when connecting them.

An important aspect of the video format is the horizontal to vertical ratio of the pixels. This contributes to the clarity and resolution of objects transmitted to the monitor. The **standard definition (SD)** format has an aspect ratio of 4 to 3, which represents 640 × 480 pixels per vertical line. The **high definition (HD)** format has a 16 to 9 aspect ratio, which is 7 times greater than SD.

Components of the Camera Head

Numerous styles of camera heads are available, but most have common components (Figure 21-9). The telescope mount or coupler connects to the telescope through a coupler, lever, or slide control. The **focus ring** clarifies the endoscopic image. The camera head may have other options, such as white balancing and VCR controls. The **endocoupler** connects the camera to the telescope and is specific to the type of camera

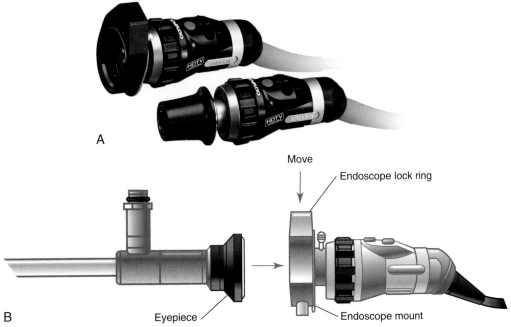

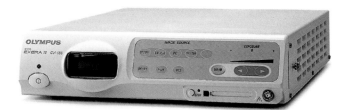

Figure 21-9 **A,** Camera heads. Note the couplers, which connect the camera to the endoscope. **B,** Camera head with endocoupler. *(Courtesy of © Olympus, America, Inc.)*

and scope in use. Some telescopes allow direct viewing without a coupler. Options for viewing the surgical site include monitor only or a combination of viewing through the telescope with projection to a monitor.

Care of the Camera Head

The camera head is delicate and must be handled with care. Always follow the manufacturer's instructions for assembly, reprocessing, and compatibility with other components of the vision system. Following some basic guidelines can help prolong the life of the camera and prevent breakdown during surgery:

- Hold the camera firmly when transporting it.
- When connecting and disconnecting the camera head, make sure the lock ring is disengaged. Also make sure the camera is firmly attached to the lock ring after engaging.
- When connecting the eyepiece, make sure it is firmly engaged. Never try to force or twist these connections together. They should connect smoothly and easily.
- Connect the camera and video plug only when the system is powered off. Do not disengage these plugs with power on.
- When connecting the camera head to the camera control center, do not bend or twist the camera cable. All connections must be dry before connection.
- Disconnect the camera cable by grasping the plug, not the cable.
- After connecting the camera head to the telescope and camera control unit, make sure the light is clearly emitted and is not flickering.

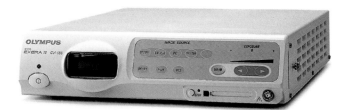

Figure 21-10 Camera control unit. *(Courtesy of © Olympus, America, Inc.)*

- Focus adjustment is made before surgery. Do not repeatedly turn the camera head, because this can cause damage. Make sure the mount is locked during focusing.

Camera Control Unit

The **camera control unit** (CCU) is the receptacle (socket)for the camera. It contains the controls for light intensity, white balance, and resolution (Figure 21-10). It also receives connections to the power mains and video output remote control. The unit captures video signals from the camera head and processes them for display on the monitor. A computer keyboard may be used in controlling the video display and other functions. The CCU should be able to convert SD to HD signals or vice versa so that images from one format can be viewed by another.

Video Cables

The **video cable** transmits digital data from the camera head to the CCU and from the monitor to the output recorder.

These high quality cables use fiberoptic systems, which are necessary for HD signals. Like all fiberoptic cables, the video cable can be easily damaged by rough handling or misuse, and the same care given to light cables should be applied to the video cable.

The video cables are patched into the system at the back of the CCU and have dedicated receptacles, which are clearly marked.

Digital Output Recorder

During video-assisted surgery, digital signals are captured from the video camera and transmitted to a monitor. The **digital output recorder** processes these signals. Data can also be transmitted to remote locations and input from other imaging processes integrated into the camera output.

The output recorder communicates with other components of the video system (camera, camera processor, and remote control) through cable connections. Integrated systems require specific knowledge about the compatibility of these devices and their connections.

The **video printer** records and stores images transmitted through the image system. Photographic images can be reproduced as paper or on a video disk. Newer systems use digital image technology with a standard personal computer (PC) card adapter. Moving or still images can be saved, catalogued, and recovered with greater storage capacity and transmission with a PC or other digital transmission system (Figure 21-11).

Monitor

The video monitor shows a projected image of the surgical site in real time. The monitor most commonly used is the flat panel (liquid crystal display [LCD]) monitor. New HD systems are displayed on a wide screen format. Although the image captured by the endoscopic video is circular, the wide screen covers the entire image by increasing the horizontal field of view and reducing the vertical field. This results in a full-screen image.

The monitor's resolution must be matched to the camera's capabilities to provide the clearest view. The 16 to 9 ratio monitor is best for displaying HD signals. Because the human eye has a wider horizontal view than vertical view, images displayed on the 16 to 9 monitor are more natural looking and less fatiguing for the eyes during surgery.

Equipment Cart

The equipment cart provides shelves for safe storage and transportation of video equipment. Carts are designed to provide power strips with dedicated receptacles for video components (Figure 21-12). Carts allow equipment to be moved safely and efficiently. An alternative design for equipment is suspension by overhead booms, which are commonly built into integrated operating rooms.

Specialty Telescopes

Specialty telescopes are designed to fit the anatomical and technical needs of surgical specialties, such as abdominal, orthopedic, thoracic, and gynecological surgery. Design features include length, diameter, channels for continuous irrigation, and electrosurgical capability.

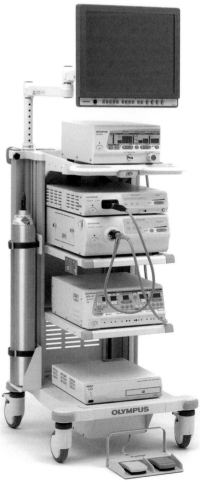

Figure 21-12 Equipment cart with monitor. *(Courtesy of © Olympus, America, Inc.)*

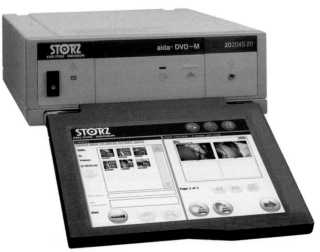

Figure 21-11 The digital output recorder processes signals from the video camera and produces printed or stored images. The recorder interfaces with other components through cable connections. *(Courtesy © Karl Storz Endoscopy America, Inc.)*

A **resectoscope** is a rigid telescope contained within a cutting and coagulating instrument; it is used in the sectional removal (resection) of tissue. The resectoscope commonly is used in genitourinary and gynecological surgery to remove tumors of the bladder and uterus and to resect the prostate. The resectoscope is fitted with a cutting tip that uses laser or electrosurgical energy to remove tissue. (Resectoscopic techniques are described in Chapters 24 and 25.)

Common specialty rigid telescopes include the following:
* *Laparoscope:* Abdominal and pelvic surgery
* *Arthroscope:* Joint surgery
* *Hysteroscope:* Surgery of the uterus
* *Thoracoscope:* Thoracic surgery
* *Nephroscope:* Kidney surgery
* *Cystourethroscope:* Surgery of the bladder and associated structures

Figure 21-13 shows common specialty telescopes and resectoscopes.

OPERATING INSTRUMENTS USED IN MINIMALLY INVASIVE SURGERY

Instrument Design

Endoscopic instruments are designed to perform a precise surgical task in a confined space. The handles and fulcrums are located at some distance from the working end. Hinges, springs, and valves are very small, and the success of the surgery depends on the efficiency of the mechanical design. A rotational design, such as that used in robotic surgery, allows the tip of the instrument to swivel in an arc, increasing the maneuverability of the instruments.

Instruments are supplied in reusable, disposable, and reposable types (only critical components, such as the tips, are disposable). The grip mechanism on endoscopic instruments is important to the ergonomics and precision of the tool. Long procedures require continued delicate control. This is enhanced by comfortable handles and good balance between the tips and handles.

The most common handle design is a transaxial type, which has two finger rings at a 90-degree angle to the long axis of the instrument. Because of the short fulcrum and flexibility of the instruments, the amount of applied force is greatly reduced in an endoscopic instrument. Examples of telescopic instruments are shown in Figures 21-14 through 21-16.

Types of Instruments and Their Uses

Retractors

Many retractor designs are available, but each uses the same principle as open surgery retractors. Because of the limited operating space, retractors extend from the tip of the shaft and flare out or curve at various angles. A probe (rod or hook) is often used to manipulate and retract tissue.

Scissors

Endoscopic scissors are available in straight, curved, and hooked configurations. In open surgery, dissection of tissue planes and cutting frequently are performed with scissors; in endoscopic procedures, they often are also performed using electrosurgery or ultrasonic shears.

Forceps

As are their open surgery counterparts, grasping instruments, including clamps and forceps, are commonly used in MIS. Some provide atraumatic grasping, whereas others penetrate the tissue. The working tips of endoscopic graspers match those of graspers for open surgery.

Suction and Irrigation Tips

Irrigation is used throughout the endoscopic procedure to keep the focal lens area clear of small bits of tissue and debris. These can fill the field and obscure the view because of the degree of magnification in the lens system. If hemorrhage occurs, the surgeon has no way to locate the bleeding vessel without pinpoint suction. The scrub should have irrigation and suction available at all times during the procedure. Irrigation is delivered through a single irrigation tip or a combination suction-irrigation system.

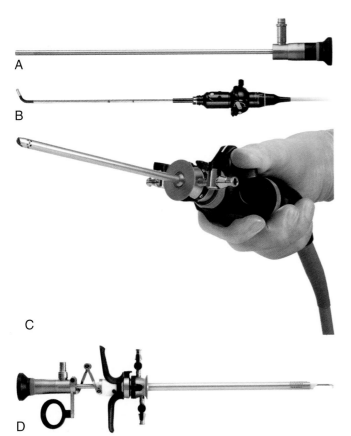

Figure 21-13 Endoscopes and resectoscopes. **A,** Rigid laparoscope. **B,** Deflectable tip video laparoscope. **C,** Arthroscope. **D,** Resectoscope. *(Courtesy of © Olympus, America, Inc.)*

Surgical Clips and Staples

The surgical clip appliers used in open surgery have counterparts in MIS. Disposable delivery systems are the most reli-

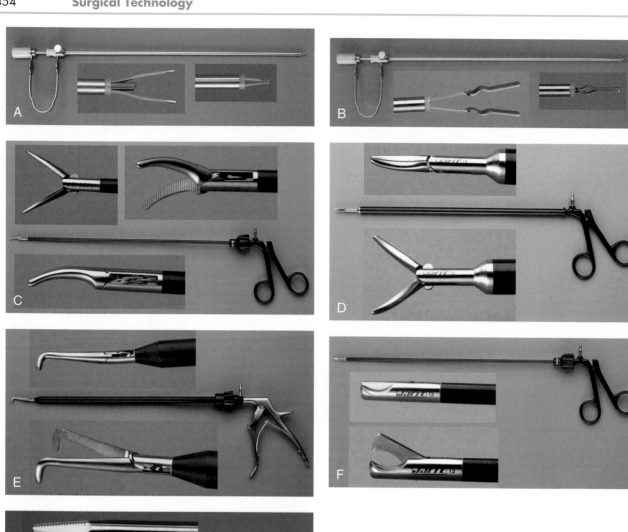

Figure 21-14 Endopolar and bipolar endoscopic instruments. **A** and **B,** Large bipolar forceps. **C,** Maryland forceps. **D,** Maryland dissecting forceps. **E,** Mixter forceps. **F,** Hook scissors. **G,** Jarit Supercut scissors. *(Courtesy Jarit Instruments, Hawthorne, NY.)*

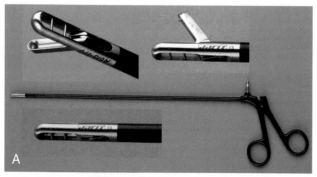

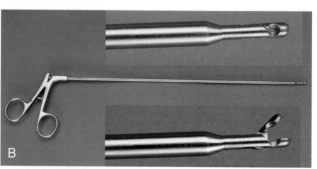

Figure 21-15 Biopsy forceps. **A,** Biopsy punch. **B,** Microbiopsy forceps. *(Courtesy Jarit Instruments, Hawthorne, NY.)*

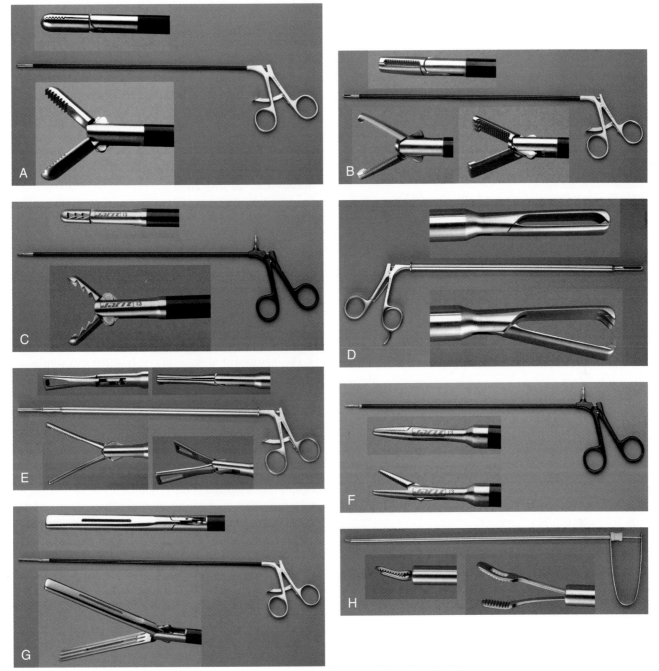

Figure 21-16 Endoscopic graspers. **A,** Grasper with ratchet. **B,** Allis grasper. **C,** Bipolar toothed grasper. **D,** Claw grasper and extracting forceps. **E,** Duval tip. **F,** Bipolar micrograsper. **G,** DeBakey forceps. **H,** Atrau forceps. *(Courtesy Jarit Instruments, Hawthorne, NY.)*

able, and these are commonly used for approximating tissue and resection. Clips are used in place of suture ligatures to occlude blood vessels or other types of hollow structures, such as the bile ducts. A disposable clip applier can deliver multiple clips in succession without reloading.

Stapling instruments are routinely used in open surgery (see Chapter 17). Endoscopic stapling instruments are most commonly used in laparoscopic and thoracoscopic surgery.

Care of Instruments Used for Minimally Invasive Surgery

The care of telescopes and other MIS instruments requires particular attention to the delicate nature of the instruments and the potential for patient injury. Equipment used in minimally invasive surgery represents a significant cost to the facility. Inferior instruments must never be used, and the chain of care starts before surgery and continues through the intraoperative and postoperative reprocessing periods.

Inspection

When to Inspect Instruments

1. Before use
2. During surgery
3. After the procedure
4. Immediately after decontamination
5. Before disinfection and sterilization

What to Look For

- Working ability (mechanical function)
- Surface defects
- Overall integrity (components are positioned correctly and connections are tight)
- Cleanliness (instruments must be free of debris and body fluids before use during surgery)

Check the working motion of the instrument. As with standard instruments, scissors must mesh smoothly. Grasping instruments are used heavily in endoscopic procedures and subject to wear. Make sure the jaws are even and meet in exact alignment at the tips. Any instrument with a spring mechanism must compress easily and return to neutral position smoothly. Check hinge pins and other mechanical attachments to make sure they are secure. Check for straightness. Sight the shanks and shafts of the instrument while rotating it to make sure no bends are present. Inspect sharp instruments, such as reusable trocars and Veress needles, for burrs or dullness. Remove damaged sharps from service.

Carefully examine the surface of all instruments for defects such as scratches, dents, or nicks (Figure 21-17, *A*). The long shafts of instruments are particularly vulnerable to defects from normal wear. Loss of integrity to the instrument insulation creates a risk for patient burns. Never deliver a damaged instrument to the sterile field.

Pay particular attention to the lens system, coupling fittings, and shaft (Figure 21-17, *B*). Inspect the distal lens and eyepiece for debris by observing them under indirect light. Look for scratches, chips, and fingerprints.

Look through the eyepiece to check for lens clarity. Rotate the telescope shaft to check all surfaces. If any obstruction appears, the lens may be damaged. Fogging may be caused by moisture trapped between the lens and seal, an indication of leakage. Check for straightness by observing the telescope end to end.

Electrosurgical instruments must be checked to make sure no breaks in the insulation are present. Even a small defect may transmit stray current and cause an unintentional burn (Figure 21-17, *C*).

Intraoperative Care

During surgery, instruments should be kept as clean as possible. Use a damp sponge to wipe the tips and instrument shafts. Suction tips should be flushed frequently to prevent clogging. Use only sterile water to clean instruments because it is hemolytic and does not erode instruments.

As instruments are used, replace them in a specific location on the instrument table or in a specialized instrument rack. Do not stack endoscopic instruments in a basin, because this can damage them. An orderly instrument table protects and preserves instruments.

The rigid telescope should be protected by placing it on a lint-free towel or in a warm water bath when not in use. Do not allow the lens to come in contact with oil. Keep the tip and shaft away from sharp objects and heavy instruments. To prevent the telescope from dropping from the sterile field, make sure cables and tubing are slack. Disconnect cables and

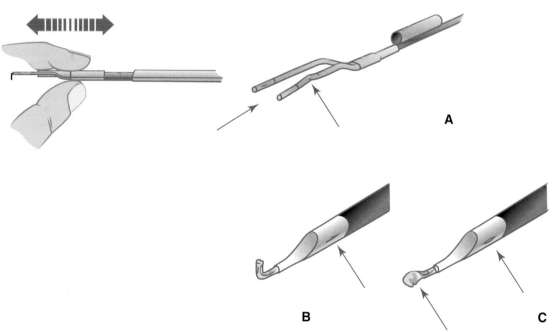

Figure 21-17   Care of endoscopic instruments. **A,** Examine the surface of the telescope.
B, Pay particular attention to the lens system, couplings, and shaft. **C,** Electrosurgical instruments must be inspected to ensure that there are no breaks in the insulation. *(Courtesy of © Olympus, America, Inc.)*

tubing when transferring the instruments from the operative field to the instrument table.

When surgery is complete, endoscopic instruments are processed according to the manufacturer's guidelines and hospital policy. All instruments must pass through a cleaning and terminal decontamination or sterilization process immediately after use.

TECHNIQUES USED IN MINIMALLY INVASIVE SURGERY

Trocar-Cannula System

A trocar and cannula system is used to create ports or channels through the body wall for insertion of MIS instruments. This system is most commonly used during laparoscopic abdominal surgery and thoracic MIS. The trocar is a solid rod with a tapered or sharp end that fits inside the hollow-tube cannula. The trocar and cannula are assembled by the surgical technologist before insertion into the patient. When assembled, the point of the trocar protrudes slightly beyond the end of the cannula (Figure 21-18). To insert the trocar and cannula, the surgeon makes a small incision in the body wall and advances the unit through the tissue. When the trocar is in the correct position, the surgeon withdraws it, leaving the hollow cannula in place. The cannula is to receive endoscopic instruments.

Features

Trocar-cannula systems can be disposable, reusable, or reposable. Single-use trocars are commonly used and bladeless trocars are also available. Cannulas are available in the following ranges:
1. Pediatric: 5 to 8 mm
2. Adult: 5 to 10 mm L
3. Large and special purpose (e.g., specimen retrieval) 10 to 15 mm.

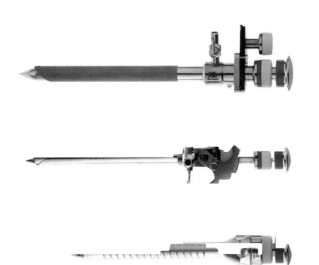

Figure 21-18 Trocar-cannula systems. The unit is inserted into a body cavity, and the trocar is withdrawn. The cannula remains in place to receive instruments during surgery. *(Courtesy © Karl Storz Endoscopy America, Inc.)*

It is important that the cannula remain stable during surgery. Therefore all cannulas are designed to provide a snug interface and a system for retention in surrounding tissue.

To prevent injury on insertion and provide a seal once they are in place, trocar-cannula systems have the following features:
- An expanding or dilating tip that provides a seal between the cannula and tissue
- Blunt trocar tips, which do not penetrate tissue but push it aside during entry
- Threaded trocar design to help guide the trocar on insertion
- Perforations or flanges to permit anchor sutures at the proximal end of the cannula
- Fabric or foam interface between the cannula and the body wall
- Optical trocars, which allow the passage of the viewing telescope as the cannula is advanced

Many cannula systems have a reducer ring at the proximal end. This allows a smaller diameter instrument to be passed through a larger cannula. Variable diameter seals are also available.

Trocar Placement

Abdominal surgery usually requires at least three trocars. These are placed according to the type of surgery to be performed. The video telescope usually is placed near the midline, approximately 10 inches (25 cm) above the pubic symphysis. This allows a broad view of the abdominal and pelvic contents. Other trocars are placed at strategic positions right or left of the midline.

TISSUE EXPANSION AT THE SURGICAL SITE

MIS is performed in a small space with restricted visualization of the surgical anatomy. This can lead to inadvertent injury to tissues outside the focal area of the telescope. Various methods are used to expand tissue planes atraumatically and create space at the surgical site:
- *Insufflation* of the abdominal cavity, which expands the abdominal wall and allows clear viewing of the abdominal viscera.
- *Continuous irrigation* or fluid distension of a cavity or joint space.
- *Balloon expansion* of tissue planes, such as the preperitoneal space and inguinal area.

Insufflation

Insufflation is a process in which the abdominal and sometimes the thoracic cavity are filled with carbon dioxide (CO_2) gas. This provides a clear view of the anatomy and permits safe entry of the rigid telescope and other instruments during the procedure. CO_2 gas is used because it is nontoxic, readily absorbed by the body, and nonflammable. The CO_2 gas is warmed before insufflation. This maintains the patient's core temperature and prevents fogging of the telescope lens.

Carbon dioxide is delivered to the patient from a tank reservoir via clear tubing. The **insufflation unit** is the control console for delivering the correct amount, temperature, and pressure of CO_2.

Safety Features of the Insufflation Unit

- High-flow and low-flow pressure control settings
- Effective leakage compensation
- Gas warming capacity (expanding CO_2 gas is rapidly cooling)
- Fluid sensor and filter guard to prevent infectious bacteria from entering the system and being shunted into the patient
- Audible and visual warning signals to indicate when pressure exceeds the programmed amount.

To create a **pneumoperitoneum**, the surgeon inflates the abdomen with CO_2 through a large-bore needle called a **Veress needle**. Before the Veress needle is used, the technologist should check its spring action. The spring is designed to retract the needle when resistance is met at the tip; this alerts the surgeon to possible obstruction during placement.

Before inserting the needle into the abdominal cavity, the surgeon places a penetrating clamp on each side of the umbilicus. The clamps are used to lift the abdominal wall upward, creating a space between it and the viscera. The surgeon makes a small stab incision in the superficial tissues at the umbilicus. The needle is then pushed through the abdominal wall at an angle to prevent injury of structures below.

A saline test often is done to verify the position of the Veress needle in the abdominal cavity. A 10-mL syringe filled with normal saline is attached to the hub of the Veress needle. If needle placement is correct, the saline drains by negative pressure into the abdominal cavity. After position verification, the insufflation tubing is attached to the needle (Figure 21-19).

> ❖ *Before it is attached, the tubing is flushed with CO_2 gas to purge any air from the tube and prevent air embolism.*

The control console is adjusted to deliver a steady level of gas through the tubing. The pressure usually is maintained at 12 to 18 mm Hg.

The risks and precautions associated with pneumoperitoneum are listed in Box 21-2. Many of these are the responsibility of the professional nursing staff. However, the surgical technologist must be aware of the risks to ensure the patient's safety at all times.

Continuous Irrigation and Fluid Distention

Continuous irrigation is a technique used in arthroscopic MIS, hysteroscopy, and cystoscopy. Fluid is instilled into a body cavity or space to expand it and provide continuous flushing of small tissue fragments and blood generated during tissue remodeling. These can obscure the view of the telescope.

Only nonconductive, salt-free fluids are used for continuous irrigation. This eliminates the risk of electrical conduction and fluid imbalance.

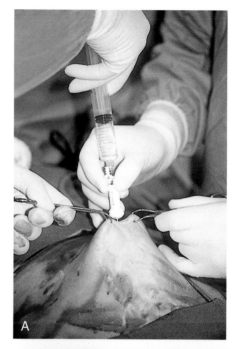

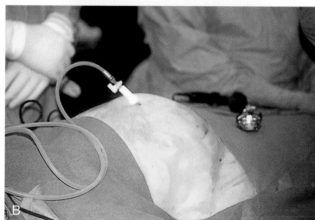

Figure 21-19 Insufflation of the abdomen for laparoscopy. **A,** The Veress needle has been inserted in the abdominal cavity. A syringe is attached to the hub of the needle to check for negative pressure. **B,** The insufflation tubing is attached to the Veress needle, and carbon dioxide is allowed to flow into the abdomen. *(From Nagle GM: Genitourinary surgery, St. Louis, 1997, Mosby.)*

Fluids Used for Continuous Irrigation

- Glycine
- Isotonic electrolytic solution (e.g., normal saline or Ringer's lactate)
- Mannitol
- Sorbitol
- Normal saline

Risks

When a body cavity or organ is filled with fluid during surgery, the risk exists that it will be absorbed into the vascular system; this is called **intravasation**. Injury is caused when the pressure of the irrigation fluid exceeds a safe level, causing fluid to enter the vascular system and thereby increasing blood pressure.

Risks and Precautions with Pneumoperitoneum

Risks

Insufflation presents a number of significant safety risks for the patient.

- Excess pressure can force carbon dioxide (CO_2) into the blood or cause decreased respirations and cardiac output.
- CO_2 can be irritating to nerves and cause severe postoperative pain in the shoulder region.
- Infectious organisms can enter the body from CO_2 tanks.
- Pneumoperitoneum can result in venous system embolism, which can cause death.
- Free gas may obstruct cerebrovascular flow, resulting in cerebrovascular accident (CVA).

Preventing Patient Injury during Insufflation

- Use only medical grade CO_2 for insufflation (tanks are labeled).
- Replace gas tank cylinders and check levels before the surgical procedure. Extra tanks must be kept on hand during surgery.
- Monitor the insufflator pressure at all times during surgery.
- Position the insufflator above the level of the surgical cavity.
- Always purge tubing of air before insufflation. Air in the tubing can result in a fatal air embolism.
- Replace the gas cylinder before the level is low. This prevents cross-contamination with particles from the tank via the insufflation tubing.
- Before inserting the Veress needle, check the spring action at the proximal end.
- Do not put pressure on the abdominal wall during or after insufflation. Leaning on the patient can create displacement of carbon dioxide and increase intraabdominal pressure.
- Always fit the patient with compression stockings or a sequential compression device before surgery (see the section on preparation of the patient in Chapter 11). These help prevent embolism.

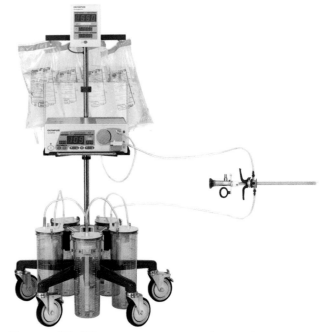

Figure 21-20 Continuous irrigation for use during minimally invasive surgery. Fluid is controlled by a pressure monitor, which should be used when the resectoscope is used (shown). *(Courtesy of © Olympus, America, Inc.)*

The circulating nurse and surgeon monitor fluid pressure during fluid distension procedures. Fluid is instilled by a pump or by a gravity system in which irrigation liquid flows into and out of the space through sterile tubing (Figure 21-20). An automated pump system is advantageous for controlling and maintaining a specific pressure, because as the pressure reaches a specified level, fluid is released from the cavity, preventing injury. The circulating nurse and scrubbed surgical technologist share responsibility for keeping track of the amount of fluid used and the amount of runoff during the procedure.

Balloon Dissection

Many balloon dissection devices are available that can create anatomical space in tissue planes. The **balloon dissector** is used in reconstructive plastic surgery and in vascular and abdominal wall procedures. These devices have a telescopic tube with an elastic balloon at the tip or long axis of the tube.

The tube is inserted into the tissue plane, and the balloon is inflated with air. This pushes the surrounding tissues aside without causing trauma and provides an anatomical space for the telescope and other instruments (Figure 21-21).

HEMOSTASIS

Hemostasis in MIS is achieved with electrosurgery (including bipolar radiofrequency energy), sutures, ligation clips, and ultrasonic technology. Instruments commonly used for electrosurgery in MIS include the probe, J-hook, and scissors. (The principles of electrosurgery are discussed in detail in Chapter 19.)

RISKS ASSOCIATED WITH ELECTROSURGERY

Specific risks are associated with electrosurgical techniques used during MIS. Patient burns can be caused by electrosurgical devices that coagulate and cut tissue. Instrument collisions and inadvertent tissue contact with the active electrode can result in severe injury to the patient. During minimally invasive surgery, instruments frequently are outside the view of the endoscopic lens. Burns may not be noticed or diagnosed until the signs and symptoms have burned or perforated of viscera, leading to infection and peritonitis.

Insulation Failure

All MIS instruments are insulated with materials that do not conduct electricity. However, insulation can be damaged, and poor quality manufacturing may produce an inferior instru-

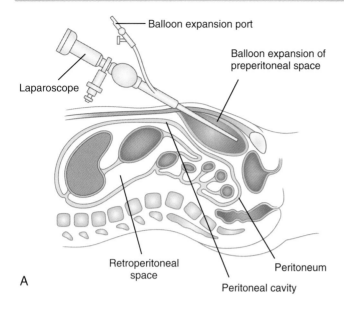

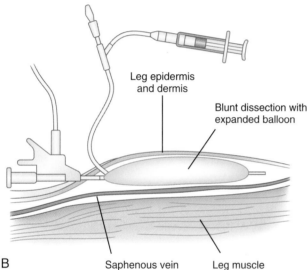

Figure 21-21 Balloon expansion. A balloon expander may be used to create a space for the insertion of minimally invasive instruments. **A,** Expansion of the preperitoneal space, commonly performed in hernia repair. **B,** Balloon expansion for removal of the saphenous vein for transplantation. *(Redrawn from Rothrock JC: Alexander's care of the patient in surgery, ed 12, St Louis, 2003, Mosby.)*

ment that is dangerous to use. Insulation failure can lead to patient burns when stray electrosurgical energy seeks a circuit and jumps to an alternative conductive path (i.e., the break in insulation).

Direct Coupling and Capacitative Coupling

In **direct coupling**, the active electrode comes in contact with another instrument capable of conducting electricity, causing the tissue in contact with the instrument to be burned. This effect is used deliberately when the surgeon grasps tissue with a conductive clamp and then touches the active electrode to the clamp. This transmits electrosurgical energy through the clamp and into tissue within the grasp of the instrument.

Unintentional direct coupling is a different matter. Electrosurgical energy can be transmitted from the tip of the active electrode to nearby instruments when they are accidentally touched or are close to each other, causing accidental burns.

Capacitative coupling occurs when stray electrical current is transmitted from an electrosurgical instrument or other conductive material to tissue, even though no break in the insulation may be apparent. Stray current, the cause of capacitive coupling, can be caused by a number of instrument configurations:

- The active electrode is threaded through a metal cannula.
- The active electrode is an integral part of the operating laparoscope.
- The active electrode is threaded through a metal suction-irrigation tube.

In these cases, as mentioned previously, the stray current causes the problem. In MIS, the tubular cannula or the housing of a telescope can act as a capacitor. A **capacitor** is a point in an electrical circuit where energy is built up or stored between insulators. Energy from the active electrode can travel through the cannula or other capacitative areas near the electrode. With a metal cannula, the energy is dispersed over a wide area and may not cause a problem. However, plastic cannula anchors can insulate the cannula from the body wall. In this configuration, electricity passes down the cannula and can cause a burn on contact with deep body tissue.

Risk Reduction and Prevention

The risk of patient burns from electrosurgery and MIS can be reduced or eliminated. All perioperative personnel must be alert to potential risks and take an active role in preventing injury.

Risk Reduction Measures

- The most effective means of preventing burns is **active electrode monitoring (AEM)**, a system in which the instruments are self-monitoring during use (e.g., AEM products [Encision, Boulder, Colorado]).
- Continually check instruments and surgical telescopes for damage, especially along the insulated areas and shafts.
- All-metal cannulas are the safest type. Never use hybrid cannulas (those constructed of plastic and metal).
- A continual need to increase the power setting may indicate a problem in the system. Check first before continuing to increase the power.
- Reprocess all instruments, including telescopes, according to the manufacturer's specifications to prevent damage, which can lead to patient injury.
- Always follow established hospital guidelines for handling and setting up endoscopic and minimally invasive equipment.
- Do not place electrical cords and fiberoptic cables across traffic areas in the operating room.
- Do not allow kinks and knots to develop; any cord that appears damaged must be immediately removed from service.
- Never allow electrical cords to come in contact with wet surfaces.

Ultrasonic Energy

Ultrasonic technology is used during MIS for coagulation and cutting (see Chapter 19). Ultrasonic energy coagulates tissue by creating a cool coagulum at the cellular level. No electrical energy and very little heat are involved. Ultrasonic systems include the SonoSurg (Olympus America, Center Valley, Pennsylvania) and Harmonic Scalpel (Johnson & Johnson, New Brunswick, New Jersey).

High-Frequency Bipolar Electrosurgery

High-frequency bipolar electrosurgery is used to coagulate and cut through tissue. Bipolar energy can be an effective method of hemostasis when the combination of low power and high frequency is used. High-frequency energy is transmitted from a power source unit connected to the specialty instruments by a cord, similar to monopolar electrosurgery. Some power sources are capable of producing both bipolar and monopolar energy. However, high-frequency units use a separate, dedicated power source. The PK Technology system (ACMI, Southborough, Mass.) is an example this type of high frequency/low temperature instrumentation. A hook probe most commonly is used to simultaneously cut and coagulate tissue. Scissors and grasping instruments are also available. PK Technology is also used in the Intuitive robotic system (described later in this chapter).

Laser

Laser technology is used in conjunction with some types of minimally invasive and endoscopic surgery. In these procedures, the lasing fiber is introduced through the cannula or flexible telescope and applied to tissue. Advances in digital technology have greatly increased the precision and efficacy of laser endoscopy. (See Chapter 19 for a complete discussion of laser surgery, including patient and user safety.)

Sutures and Ligation Devices

Ligation in endoscopic procedures is performed with many different devices and techniques. Electrosurgical and ultrasound modalities are have replaced traditional suture in many procedures. However, needles and sutures remain in use. Various instruments have been designed to tie knots, snug knots, and suture tissue within a confined space. Three types of methods are commonly used: extracorporeal technique, intracorporeal technique, and the pretied surgical loop. The pretied loop and Surgiwip (Covidien, Norwalk, Conn.) device are shown in Figure 21-22.

In the **extracorporeal** suture technique, the knot is tied outside the body cavity and then pushed into place with a **knot pusher** using the following technique: A swaged suture-needle combination is grasped with a needle holder and passed through the endoscopic cannula to the inside of the body. The needle is pushed through the tissue with the aid of an additional grasping instrument via a separate cannula. The suture-needle combination is withdrawn, and the needle removed outside the wound. The knots can then be formed without tightening outside the body and introduced back into the body via the cannula. They are then tightened with the knot pusher.

In the **intracorporeal** technique, the suture is knotted and tightened inside the body with two grasping instrument inserted into two separate cannula ports.

The suture or pretied **ligation loop** such as the Surgiwip is used when a tissue structure requires ligation rather than suturing. A loop of suture contained in a carrier, similar to a snare, is delivered through the laparoscopic and looped around the tissue, such as the appendix. The loop then is tightened, the suture ends cut, and the carrier removed.

SPECIMEN RETRIEVAL

Morcellization

For tissue specimens or remnants to be retrieved from the body during MIS, they must be small enough to fit through the cannula opening. Large specimens and dense tissue are reduced to small pieces by a process called **morcellization**. The morcellator reduces tissue to pulp, which can be suctioned from the wound.

A tissue *shaver* commonly is used in endoscopic nasal and orthopedic procedures. In endoscopic nasal sinus surgery, it is used to remove masses, polyps, and redundant tissue from the endothelial surface. The shaver suctions soft tissue into the cutting channel, where a spiral burr shaves it into small pieces. In orthopedic and neurosurgery, soft tissue, cartilage, and small bone fragments may also be reduced using this technique.

Large tissue specimens are retrieved through the abdominal wall through a retractable tissue bag inserted into a large port (cannula). The surgeon captures the organ into the bag and retracts the open portion to secure the contents. The bag then is withdrawn through the port. For extremely large specimens, an 18-mm port may be required for extraction.

ENDOSCOPIC SETUP

During surgery, the scrub should keep endoscopic instruments in a rack on the instrument table. This maintains them safely and helps the scrub identify them quickly. Always separate endoscopic instruments to protect them from damage by heavier equipment. Telescopes in particular should be maintained on a towel or other soft surface to prevent them from rolling off the table. If a warm water thermos is used for prewarming, it should be kept in an area of the instrument table where it will not be jarred or knocked over.

Nonpenetrating clamps must be used to secure cords and tubing to drapes. This prevents damage to fiberoptic and camera cables. Always allow sufficient slack on cord attachments and be alert to changes in table position, which can cause cords to be dragged.

Cable and cord connections differ according to the type of endoscopic equipment used. *The scrub should be familiar with the facility's equipment before participating as a solo scrub.* A dry run of equipment is a necessary part of learning endoscopic and MIS procedures.

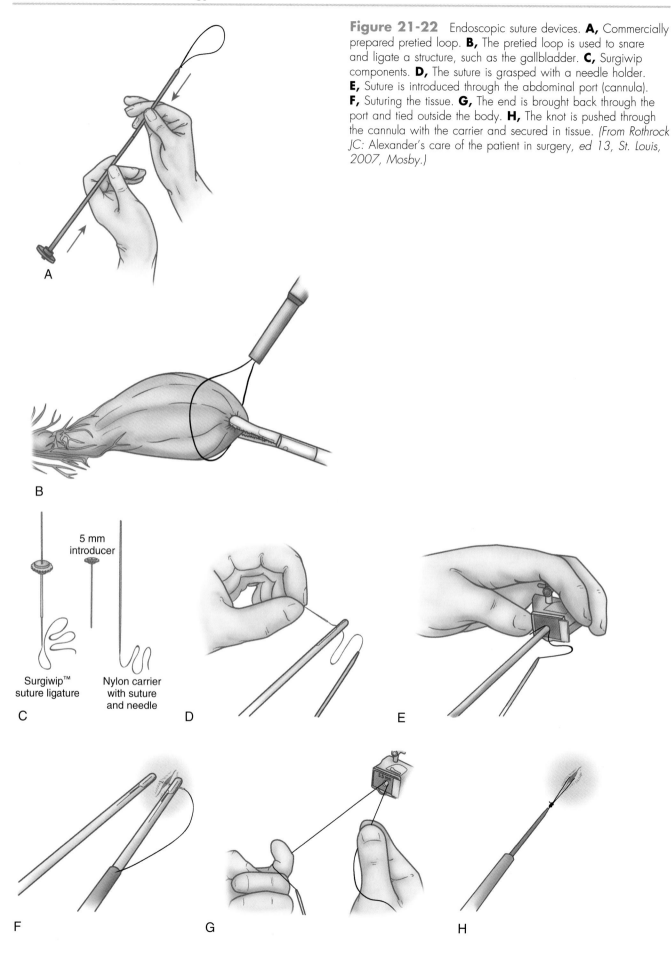

Figure 21-22 Endoscopic suture devices. **A,** Commercially prepared pretied loop. **B,** The pretied loop is used to snare and ligate a structure, such as the gallbladder. **C,** Surgiwip components. **D,** The suture is grasped with a needle holder. **E,** Suture is introduced through the abdominal port (cannula). **F,** Suturing the tissue. **G,** The end is brought back through the port and tied outside the body. **H,** The knot is pushed through the cannula with the carrier and secured in tissue. *(From Rothrock JC: Alexander's care of the patient in surgery, ed 13, St. Louis, 2007, Mosby.)*

A

B

5 mm introducer

Surgiwip™ suture ligature

Nylon carrier with suture and needle

C

D

E

F

G

H

When passing an instrument to the surgeon, always orient the instrument so that the working tip points downward. The scrub may help position the instrument into a cannula. In robotic-assisted MIS, the scrub helps lock the instrument into the robotic arm.

During MIS, the room lights usually are dimmed or powered off. One of the operating lights should be positioned over the instrument table to help the scrub identify and prepare instruments and supplies. This prevents errors and accidents.

Conversion to an Open Case

Any minimally invasive procedure has the potential to become an open case. In MIS involving body cavities (e.g., laparoscopy and pelvic and thoracic surgery), preparations are made to include the possibility of **open surgery**. Operative permits are signed with this consideration, and any equipment needed to convert to an open case must be prepared and made immediately available. Some surgeries are scheduled and planned to include both MIS and open stages.

Regardless of whether the conversion is an emergency, it is performed very rapidly. Preoperative planning reduces the risk of accident. When the MIS procedure is planned, the scrub and circulator consult the surgeon's preference card for an open procedure. Sterile supplies are collected and located where they can be retrieved and opened within minutes of the decision to convert to an open case. Accidents with equipment occur when personnel rush through the procedure without previous planning.

During conversion to an open case, the scrub must communicate directly with the circulator to make sure all cords and tubing are free. Camera cords and fiberoptic cables must be protected from injury during the conversion to an open case. These can become tangled in the drapes or fall to the floor when disconnected. Deliberate and purposeful actions help protect equipment during the conversion.

Instruments are quickly exchanged and endoscopic instruments carefully put aside. Standard operating instruments are delivered to the surgical table, and the scrub prepares for immediate incision while receiving other equipment from the circulator. Suction, electrosurgical instruments, and sharps are delivered first so that the open procedure can begin without delay. Sponges, instruments, and sharps are counted as distributed as in all cases.

FLEXIBLE ENDOSCOPY

Principles

Flexible (and semirigid) endoscopy is a method of viewing the inside of body passages and hollow organs, such as the gastrointestinal system, urinary bladder, uterus, nasal sinuses, bronchial tree, and larynx. During flexible endoscopy, the surgical endoscope is introduced through a natural opening in the body, such as the mouth, nose, or cervix. The scope is carefully advanced, and the interior tissues are examined with video-assisted technology or directly through the instrument's lens system. The surgeon can remove tissue for biopsy or take cell brushings through the flexible endoscope. Diagnosis is also made by visual examination of the tissues as they appear on the monitor at the time of the procedure.

The flexible endoscope most often is used for examination, visual exploration, and biopsy. Some procedures and specialties use a semirigid scope, which is a hybrid form of the rigid endoscope discussed later in the chapter.

Equipment Used in Flexible Endoscopy
Flexible Endoscope

The flexible endoscope has two main sections, the head and the insertion tube (Figure 21-23). The endoscope **control head** connects with the digital camera, optical system control handles, suction, and irrigation. Endoscopes that do not have a video camera also have an eyepiece on the control head. The fiberoptic light cable inserts into the control head to provide illumination. The control head also has the dials that operate the flexing mechanism at the distal end of the tube. The **insertion tube** is the component of the endoscope that enters the patient's body. The interior of the insertion tube contains the fiberoptic light channel, which terminates at the tip of the instrument.

Inside the endoscope are the optical components and channels for irrigation, air, and instruments. The **instrument channel** receives biopsy forceps, brushes, and other instruments used to remove tissue specimens. This channel is the largest one. The **biopsy channel** port is located near the junction of the control head and the insertion tube.

Some endoscopes may have an **auxiliary water channel** and an **elevator channel**. The water channel is used to clear blood and tissue debris from the lens. The elevator channel is used to manipulate instruments and remove tissue specimens. An air channel is used to insufflate the lumen of the gastrointestinal tract to create space in the same way as in a pneumoperitoneum. The tip of the insertion tube is operated at the control head to obtain rotational views of the anatomy within the focal area of the lens.

Imaging System

The vision system of the flexible endoscope is very similar to that used for MIS. A camera control unit and digital output recorder perform the same functions outlined previously. Video output is viewed on the LCD or plasma monitor, as in rigid endoscopy.

MIS may be assisted with a flexible endoscope for increased visibility of the anatomy. In these procedures, the flexible endoscope is managed by a separate team performing MIS through the rigid endoscope. Combined procedures of the abdomen and gastrointestinal tract are enhanced with the use of both technologies.

Technique

Flexible endoscopy usually is performed in an outpatient setting. The procedures are relatively short compared with MIS or open surgery. Ambulatory outpatients usually are discharged as soon as they have recovered from the effects of sedation.

After the patient has been sedated and positioned, the endoscopist introduces the insertion tube, examining tissue

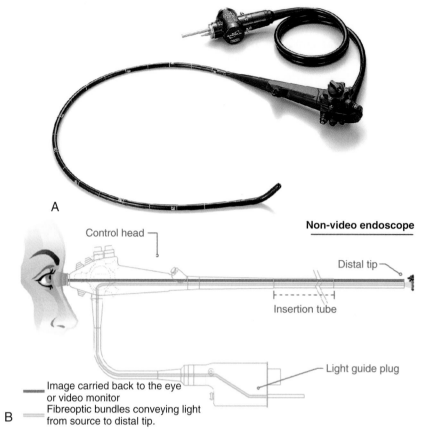

Figure 21-23 **A,** Fiberoptic gastroscope. **B,** Schematic of endoscope design. (*Courtesy of © Olympus, America, Inc.*)

and recording digital or camera images. Biopsies are taken with the aid of forceps, graspers, or biopsy brushes.

The surgeon is assisted by the scrub, who helps position the patient and prepares equipment and instruments. During the procedure, the scrub maintains suction and irrigation devices and helps place biopsy instruments into the endoscope. The scrub also receives specimens as they are withdrawn from the endoscope and properly preserves and documents them.

The scrub may also provide direct patient care after the procedure. This individual helps transport the patient to the recovery area and may be required to take the person's vital signs and record them on the patient's record.

REPROCESSING ENDOSCOPES AND INSTRUMENTS

Disassembly and proper reassembly is critical to safe reprocessing (cleaning, disinfection, sterilization). Reprocessing is discussed in this chapter rather than in Chapter 8 which covers disinfection and sterilization of so that the learner can easily refer to discussions and definitions of instrument components within this chapter.

Protocols and Standards
The endoscope is a complex instrument with channels, valves, spring fittings, and stopcocks. The endoscope and other instruments often come in contact with areas of the body that have a high level of bioburden. Debris can become trapped in the mechanisms and harbor infectious material. For these reasons, a systematic cleaning process that follows an established protocol is necessary to ensure the patient's safety.

Hospital policy for reprocessing endoscopes follows guidelines established by the Occupational Safety and Health Administration (OSHA), an agency of the U.S. Department of Labor, and every manufacturer of surgical endoscopes provides detailed instructions on the specific care of its equipment. A general overview of reprocessing is presented here.

Precleaning of Rigid Endoscopes
All immersible instruments and rigid endoscopes must be precleaned immediately after use in surgery. Endoscopes and accessories should be disassembled according to the manufacturer's instructions. Manual cleaning removes much of the tissue and body fluid trapped in crevices and fittings. This is done with enzymatic cleaner, a clean cloth, and a soft brush. Endoscopic instruments can be soaked briefly in an enzymatic detergent bath before precleaning.

Guidelines for Precleaning Instruments
1. Instruments are best transported in a covered container from the point of use to the cleaning area. They can be transported wet or dry. However, immediate soaking (transport in a wet bath) aids more complete cleaning.

Do not soak instruments for longer than 1 hour or as directed by the instrument manufacturer.

2. Before cleaning instruments, make sure to open all stopcocks, ports, and channels.
3. Separate the telescopes from other instruments for individual processing.
4. Follow the manufacturer's instructions for a compatible enzymatic bath. Do not exceed the recommended water temperature.
5. While cleaning, look for defects in the surface of the instrument. Look for any sign that the instrument housing and insulation are damaged. Remember that even small nicks or scratches can create a pathway for stray electricity and cause burns.
6. Use a long brush to clean the inside of tubes and lumens. Irrigate these with large amounts of enzymatic fluid. Reusable brushes must be terminally disinfected and sterilized between uses.
7. Clean air and water channels with forced air or as recommended by the manufacturer.
8. Do not submerge or allow any fluid to enter electrical connections or units! These should be wiped clean with an approved surface disinfectant.
9. Flush all ports with enzymatic solution and make sure all surfaces have been cleaned. Some types of stopcocks may be disassembled for cleaning. Always verify before attempting disassembly.
10. After cleaning, rinse all surfaces and channels of the instruments with deionized or sterile water. Make sure that every part of the instrument is rinsed to remove detergent and debris loosened during cleaning.
11. Drain the instruments and dry them.

Precleaning Optical Parts and Lenses

Disassemble the adapter from the light cable. Then proceed as follows:

1. If the endoscope has an eyepiece cap, remove it.
2. Clean the lens surface with a lint-free cloth and ethanol or isopropanol, or as directed by the manufacturer.
3. When cleaning lenses and optical surfaces, take care not to abrade or scrape the lenses. Do not use a brush to clean the optical surfaces.
4. Check the lenses of the endoscope. Look for any cloudiness or discoloration. Cloudiness is a sign of leakage. If you suspect the lens fitting has leaked, remove it from service after decontamination and sterilization according to manufacturer's specifications.

Ultrasonic cleaning is commonly used for stainless steel instruments. However, many instruments are not approved for this type of system, and the process may damage them. Always read and follow the manufacturer's written protocol regarding ultrasound cleaning. For endoscopic equipment that can be cleaned in this fashion, use caution when processing the instruments in the ultrasound cleaner.

Flexible Endoscope Processing

Flexible endoscopes are particularly difficult to clean. The ports and long tube channels trap debris, and determining how much has been removed during cleaning is difficult. An automatic reprocessor therefore is used (Figure 21-24). Read and follow protocols when using this type of system.

Before disinfection in an automatic reprocessor, several steps must be carried out to ensure patient safety.

1. Precleaning is performed as soon as possible after the procedure. The insertion tube is thoroughly cleaned with detergent solution. Detergent solution then is flushed through the air-water and auxiliary channels and removed with air suction.
2. The endoscope must be leak tested after precleaning. This is done to prevent water from entering the system during the remaining steps of reprocessing. The manufacturer's instructions for leak testing must be followed, and the leak testing equipment used must be compatible with the individual endoscope.
3. After the leak test, the endoscope is cleaned manually. This is done by submerging the instrument in detergent solution and cleaning all surfaces with a soft cloth. A suction pump and syringe are used to flush detergent through the instrument channels and ports, and a soft brush is inserted to clean any debris.
4. After detergent cleaning, complete rinsing is necessary to remove all traces of detergent and debris.
5. All water is removed from the instrument's channels and exterior. The endoscope may then be processed in an automated endoscope reprocessor according to the manufacturer's specifications.

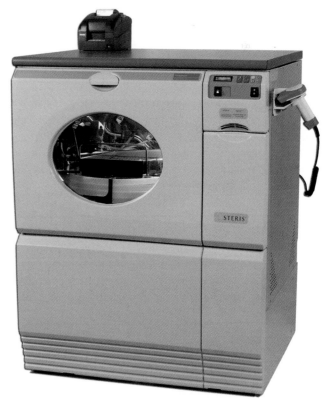

Figure 21-24 Automatic endoscope reprocessor. Automatic systems are used after terminal disinfection. (© 2008 STERIS Corporation. All rights reserved.)

Disinfection and Sterilization

After instruments have been thoroughly cleaned, they must be disinfected. High level disinfection kills 100% of *Mycobacterium tuberculosis.* The process of disinfection is specified by the manufacturer of the equipment.

Sterilization methods for endoscopic instruments vary with the type of equipment and the manufacturer's specifications. Instruments used in sterile areas of the body, including the vascular system, require sterilization before reuse. Some equipment, including cameras, may be steam sterilized, whereas others require ethylene oxide gas or other methods. Equipment that is sterilized by a method other than that specified by the manufacturer may be damaged, increasing the risk of patient injury. (Chapter 8 presents a complete discussion of disinfection and sterilization practices.)

ROBOTIC SURGERY

PRINCIPLES OF ROBOTIC SURGERY

A robot is a mechanical device that can be programmed to perform tasks. Robotic surgery combines the techniques of MIS with computer-guided instruments that are controlled remotely through a nonsterile interface system.

ROBOTIC MOVEMENT

The overall design of the surgical robotic system provides movements that closely resemble the coordinated actions of the human body, particularly the shoulders, arms, and hands. The robotic arm, which is an extension of the control unit, has degrees of "freedom" that allow pivoting, turning, and flexing motions. These motions are enabled by articulated (jointed) sections of the arm and instruments.

In robotic engineering, cartesian coordinate geometry is used to design and replicate these movements. In the cartesian system of geometry, the robotic arm moves in particular spatial dimensions: vertical, horizontal, and pivotal. The degree of rotation is the ability to turn, or *pivot* (perform rotational turns) on a 360-degree axis. The vertical and horizontal axes allow the arm to move up, down, side to side, and back and forth.

CLASSIFICATION OF ROBOTS

OSHA has published classifications of industrial robots. In this system, robots are classified according to their design and "reaching space" or *working envelope,* which is the actual space in which they move. The design configuration of the robot determines the types of movements it can perform. The robotic design allows pivoting, vertical, horizontal, and circular movements. Joints or articulations on a robotic arm provide many of these movements.

The robot's movement within its working envelope is controlled from a distance or through its sensing devices. These sensing devices react to the environment and respond according to the preprogrammed commands. A servo-controlled robot responds through its sensors. A non-servo-controlled robot has no sensing or feedback ability. The movement of these robots is through physical stops and switches, which are triggered by the presence of a physical barrier such as a wall or object in the path of the robot.

DA VINCI SURGICAL SYSTEM

The da Vinci surgical system (Intuitive Surgical, Sunnyvale, California) is used in many specialties and currently is the only system marketed for telesurgery, which is surgery performed through a type of videoconferencing in which the surgeons and operating room setup are located at one audiovisual terminal, and a trainer or group of students is able to watch at another. The da Vinci system enhances the surgeon's skills by scaling down and refining hand movements as the surgeon manipulates the instruments through the computer-mediated robotic system.

During MIS, trocars and cannulas are inserted at strategic anatomical locations at the operative site. The telescopic instruments and rigid endoscope are threaded through the cannulas, and surgery is performed through the cannulas. In robotic **telesurgery**, instruments are inserted manually or with electronic assistance but are controlled through a remote, nonsterile console near the sterile field. The computer-mediated instruments have the same flexion and rotational ability as the human hand. However, instead of being directly manipulated, they are controlled by the surgeon through the remote console.

The surgeon sits at the nonsterile console a few feet from the patient. The surgical field is viewed on a three-dimensional console screen, and the surgeon operates the instruments and camera by manipulating the hand and foot controllers of the console. The controllers simulate the hand-eye and instrument coordination of open surgery, but there is no direct physical contact between the controllers and the instruments.

The images transmitted by the digital endoscopic camera are refined and highly magnified on both the console screen and the image system screen. The images can be manipulated (sized, rotated, and integrated with other imaging data) and recorded as permanent or real-time data.

Robotic systems have tremendous accuracy, but they also are very complex; as do all medical technologies, they present a risk of malfunction and failure. Many of the skills and much of the knowledge acquired during robotics training is dedicated to preventing or minimizing the effects of malfunction. The purpose of this discussion is to provide an overview of the robotics system and to highlight safety considerations. Perioperative staff members learn how to operate the robotic system and deliver safe patient care through the manufacturer's training program and other resources available through their facility's robotics coordinator and in-service instructors.

ADVANTAGES AND DISADVANTAGES OF ROBOTIC SURGERY

When comparing robot with human capabilities, it is important to remember that robots cannot replace the human ability to make judgments or to make sense of and use qualitative information for the patient's benefit.

Because telesurgery surgery is always used in conjunction with minimally invasive techniques, robotics is compared with traditional MIS.

Advantages

- *Robotic endoscopic images are three dimensional.* Standard endoscopes transmit a two-dimensional view. During robotic surgery, the endoscopic image is captured and processed by stereoscopic viewer of the surgeon's console. This view closely approximates what the eye would perceive during open surgery. The advantages over the two-dimensional view are greater depth perception and increased precision.
- *Tremor and movement scaling are reduced.* The robotic system scales the surgeon's hand movements so that the effects of tremor are greatly reduced or removed. Hand tremor prevents safe and accurate movements in delicate surgery. This innovation allows surgeons to perform procedures that were seldom performed in the past.
- *Robotic instruments closely replicate human movement.* Standard endoscopic instruments have limited range of movement. This is because the surgeon's hand operates the instrument outside the channel of the endoscopic cannulas. Instruments used in robotic surgery can rotate in a full circle and perform many more pivoting movements compared with standard MIS techniques. These movements more accurately replicate the range of movement in the human hand and wrist than those of standard endoscopic equipment.

Disadvantages

- *The robotic system is expensive and uses valuable resources.* The robotic system requires a substantial investment both in money and time spent learning, coordinating, and managing the system. Robotic instruments cost thousands of dollars and must be discarded after limited use. These instruments contain electronic components and expensive raw materials that may never be recycled or recovered. Hospitals may never regain the initial cost of implementing a robotic system, and the relative human need for such systems is still the subject of debate.
- *Robotic systems require a specialist on-site coordinator.* Even though ample training opportunities are available for perioperative staff, the complexity of the system requires an on-site robotics coordinator. This individual receives extensive training in the operation and safety of the system and usually is responsible for training and orienting staff members new to the system. This requires planning and time allocation, as well as advanced management skills. Staff shortages can make this a disadvantage for startup and continuing education.
- *Surgeons must be trained to operate at the nonsterile console.* Training for robotics surgery is readily available. However, surgeons must relearn techniques as they apply to remote instrument manipulation. Among the new skills that surgeons must learn is the lost of **haptic feedback**. This is the

tactile sensation, or "feel," of the instruments during surgery. During robotic telesurgery, the surgeon must rely on vision alone while manipulating the hand and foot controllers. There is no feedback on the tension of an instrument or the feel of a suture knot on tissue. With time, these techniques can be mastered. However, a steep learning curve usually is required while the surgeon learns to operate without "touch" sensation on the tissues and instruments.

TRAINING FOR ROBOTICS

The robotic telesurgery system is complex and requires special training for all members of the surgical team. Training for the da Vinci system is available from the manufacturer at various teaching locations. During training, surgeons and other perioperative professionals have the opportunity for hands-on learning as well as didactic lectures on the system and how it works.

Robotic Training Topics and Methods

- System preparation and management
- Inanimate labs and skills development
- Surgical procedure training at various institutions using robotic systems already in use at those hospitals
- Dry runs on setup and procedure
- Video podcast and live teaching through the Internet

The surgical technologist should have access to both off-site and on-site learning opportunities. In addition to the manufacturer's training, other resources are available:

- In-service programs provided by the robotics nurse manager/supervisor
- In-service with visiting specialists, including the manufacturer's trainers
- Observation in scrub and circulating roles
- Dry runs
- Practice under direct supervision
- Continuous mentoring and feedback

As robotics technology is modified and refined, technologists must continue to advance their skills and knowledge. Opportunities outside the perioperative environment, including conferences and special training programs, are excellent resources for continuing education. Information on these resources is available from the robotics in-service coordinator and through the manufacturer of the system.

SURGICAL SPECIALTIES AND ROBOTICS

Robotic-assisted MIS is performed in a variety of specialties. Because robotics is a rapidly evolving technology, new procedures are in development. The examples below are the most common.

- Orthopedic surgery: Joint replacement procedures
- Cardiothoracic surgery: Valve repair, lung resection
- General surgery: Gastrointestinal resection, biliary surgery, removal of tumors
- Gynecological surgery: Hysterectomy, myomectomy, sacrocolpopexy

- Urological surgery: Prostatectomy, cystectomy
- Neurosurgery: Tumor resection

COMPONENTS OF THE ROBOTIC SYSTEM: STRUCTURE AND PURPOSE

The da Vinci system is commonly used in the United States and is described in this chapter. *This discussion is not intended to replace the formal training required to operate the system safely.* Specific information on the troubleshooting of components and the care and handling of instruments and other delicate part is readily available in formal training provided by the manufacturer.

Three main components make up the robotic system (Figure 21-25):

- The patient cart
- The surgeon's console
- The imaging (vision) system

The components are connected by cables, which relay information needed to operate the system and provide immediate feedback from one component to another. In this way,

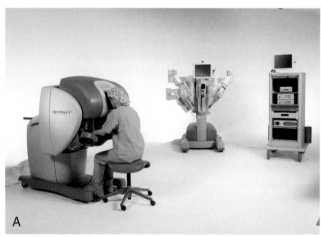

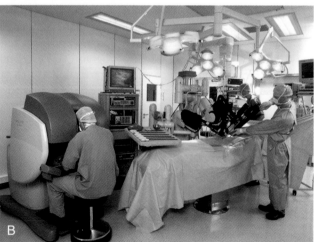

Figure 21-25 **A,** Components of the robotic system. *Left to right:* Image system, patient cart, surgeon's console. **B,** Operating room setup for robotic surgery. Note that the surgeon controls the instruments remotely while seated at the nonsterile console. *(Courtesy of Intuitive Surgical, Inc., 2007.)*

each component "talks" to the others so that commands given at any point can be immediately integrated into the system. The components have their own override features to prevent errors.

Patient Cart

The patient cart consists of a central column, vertical arms with movable joints, and a large base that contains a motor drive. A digital touch screen is located on the central column. Robotic arms convey the instruments and camera to the endoscopic cannulas. The cart is part of the sterile field and is draped before it is positioned over the sterile field.

Base and Power Drive

The cart is driven and steered by a manual or power-drive motor, which is operated from the back of the cart base, similar to a portable radiograph machine. A set of switches and a throttle are used to operate the motor drive. In the da Vinci system, these controls are located near the drive handles. Feedback information about the throttle and power status is clearly visible to the operator, who is positioned at the back of the unit. In the event of a power failure, manual controls are used to move and position the cart safely.

Setup Joints

Movable *setup joints* extend directly from the central column and are used to change the position of the component arms, which hold the instruments. An electronic clutch system powers the movement of the joints. Feedback on their position and status is provided through LED signals. The setup joints are movable in both the vertical and horizontal directions.

Patient Cart Arms

The patient cart arms move around a remote center on the patient cart. The remote center is a fixed location that facilitates optimum alignment and positioning of the cart arms.

The da Vinci system has two or three instrument arms and one camera arm (Figure 21-26). The arms function as the instrument "holders" and the interface with the surgeon's console. The arms have a wide range of motion to assist in correct alignment of instruments and the cannulas into which they are inserted. The instrument and camera arms are moved with the aid of an electronic clutch system, which allows the instruments to pivot at the cannula ports.

Although the instruments are controlled by the surgeon at the nonsterile console, the surgical assistant and scrub assist in loading them into the instrument arms. Just as in standard MIS, the scrub also maintains the sterile robotic instruments and passes them to the field as needed.

Monitor

The monitor, or touch screen, receives electronic signals from the camera head and controller and transmits them as digital output. The monitor can also display output from other forms of diagnostic imaging, such as ultrasound and magnetic resonance imaging (MRI). These images are controlled and posi-

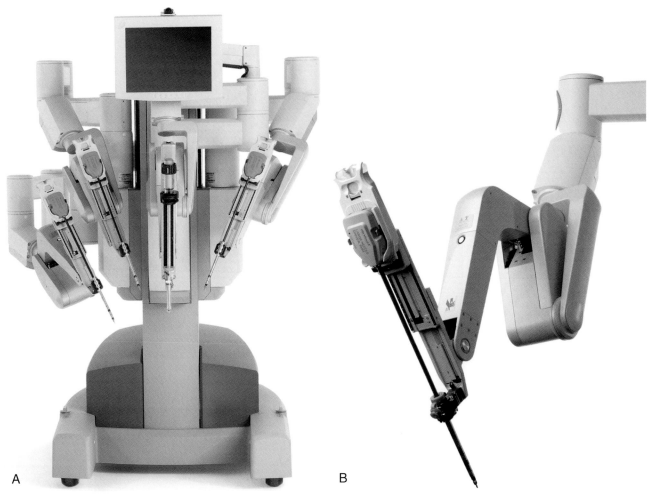

Figure 21-26 A, Close-up of the patient cart for the da Vinci robotic surgical system showing three instrument arms. The touch screen monitor is at the top of the patient cart. **B,** The underside of the instrument arm showing the instrument in place. Instruments are changed as needed by guiding them into the arm. A digital clutch system locks the instrument in place. (*Courtesy of Intuitive Surgical, Inc., 2007.*)

tioned at the surgeon's console and can also be manipulated on the draped touch screen by scrubbed personnel.

DA VINCI INSTRUMENTS

Instrument Design and Type

The da Vinci instruments are complex, computer-programmed tools. The programmed movements of the tips and articulated joints of the patient cart arms are controlled by the system's software. The instruments are loaded into the patient cart arms as needed during surgery. This task is performed by the surgical assistant and qualified scrub. Instruments are designed with a limited life span. Each insertion into the patient represents one "use" of the instrument. After the instruments have reached their maximum number of uses (the average is about 10 uses), they must be discarded. At the time of this writing, each instrument costs about $2,500.

The da Vinci instruments provide full rotational tips with flexion on all axes. A variety of instrument types is available.

Classification of Robotic Instruments

- Scissors
- Grasper
- Knife
- Probe
- Needle holder
- Ultrasonic energy instruments
- Electrosurgical instruments (monopolar and bipolar)
  Examples of these instruments are shown in Figure 21-27.

Reprocessing

As mentioned, instruments in the da Vinci system have a predetermined life span based on the number of actual uses or procedures. The instruments are sterilized between patients until they reach their predetermined life span (approximately 10 uses). Instrument heads and electronic components are cleaned, disinfected, and sterilized according to a specific set of protocols. The technologist or nurse should consult the manufacturer for detailed information and training in the care of robotic instruments. This ensures that the methodol-

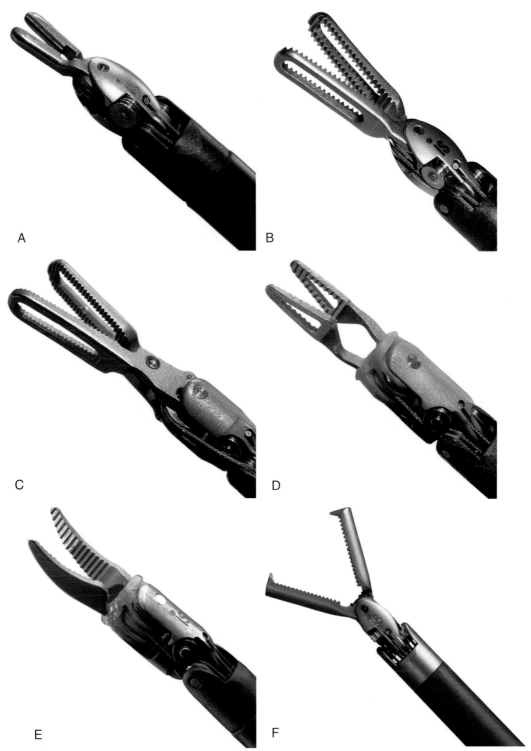

Figure 21-27 **A,** DeBakey forceps. **B,** Cardiere forceps. **C,** Prograsp forceps.
D, Precise bipolar forceps. **E,** Maryland bipolar forceps. **F,** Toothed forceps.

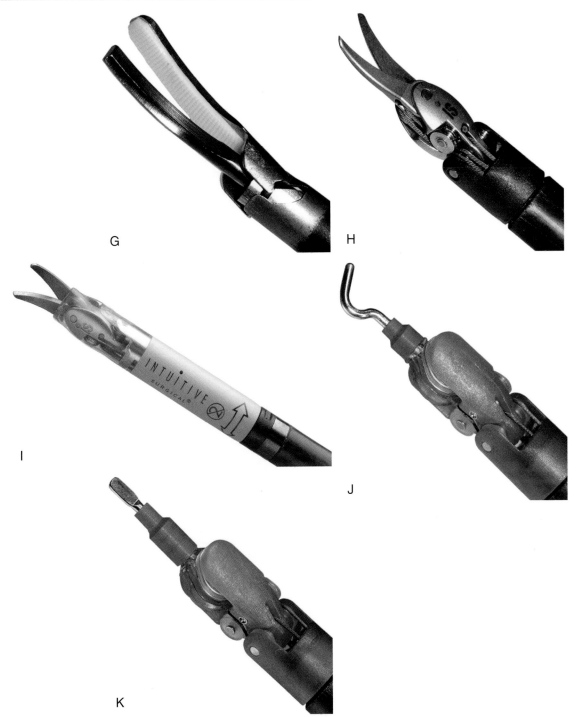

Figure 21-27, cont'd **G,** Harmonic shears. **H,** Curved scissors. **I,** Fine dissecting scissors. **J,** Cautery hook. **K,** Cautery spatula. *(Courtesy of Intuitive Surgical, Inc., 2007.)*

ogy is safe and up-to-date with any changes in technology, a likely occurrence in this rapidly evolving area of robotic biotechnology.

SURGEON'S CONSOLE

The surgeon's console contains the remote nonsterile controls. In standard MIS, the surgeon is a scrubbed member of the team. In robotic-assisted surgery, the surgeon is not scrubbed; he or she sits at the console and manipulates the instruments and other equipment using hand and foot controllers. The surgeon's console is placed outside the sterile field but close enough for effective communication between the surgeon and other members of the team.

The **stereoscopic viewer** provides three-dimensional images of the surgical site (Figure 21-28). Digital images are transmitted to the viewer from the endoscope. Before surgery, the surgeon makes adjustments to the seating, optical viewer, and intercom while his or her head is outside the viewer. The system is engaged when the surgeon places the head in the viewer. The screen displays icons that are status indicators for all components and diagnostic imaging. The intercom controls are also located in the viewer. The control pads of the console allow the surgeon to control the interface between components of the system. The **master controllers** and foot switch panel allow the surgeon to manipulate the surgical instruments and endoscope. Electrosurgery controls are also located in the foot switch panel (Figure 21-29).

VISION SYSTEM

Components

The vision components of the robotic system provide a high quality image of the surgical site. The digital image is picked up from the endoscope and transmitted through the camera control unit to the display and monitor on the surgeon's console. The endoscope has two optical channels, which project a three-dimensional image on the monitor and console screen.

The components of the da Vinci robotic vision system include:

- Endoscope
- Camera and camera cable assembly
- Camera control unit
- Illuminator (light source)

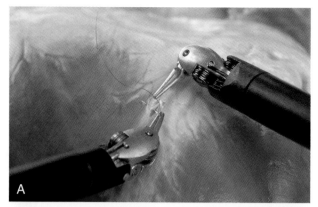

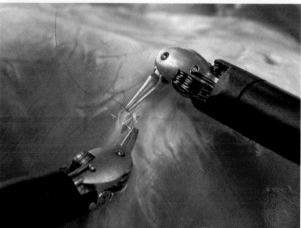

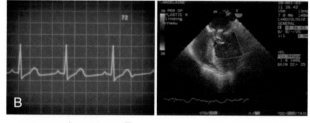

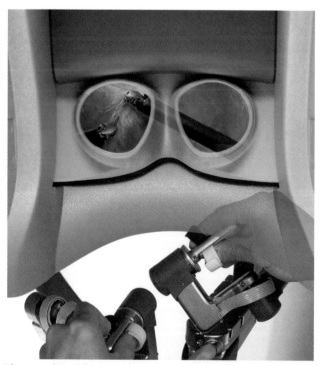

Figure 21-28 Surgical site through the three-dimensional viewer. Instruments are controlled with the master controllers (hand devices) and foot switches. *(Courtesy of Intuitive Surgical, Inc., 2007.)*

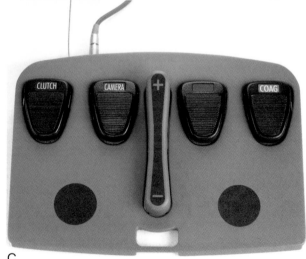

Figure 21-29 **A,** Surgeon's view through the three-dimensional viewer. **B,** Patient monitoring and diagnostic images are transmitted in real time to the surgeon's console. **C,** Foot controls. Note that the electrosurgical unit is also controlled by a foot switch. *(Courtesy of Intuitive Surgical, Inc., 2007.)*

- Video processing unit
- Monitor (touch screen)
- Stereo viewer

Components of the robotic vision system are comparable to the high quality digital vision systems used in MIS. The da Vinci system uses adaptors and connecting cables that are compatible with its system. HD or SD systems are available.

Endoscopes are available with straight or angled tips and in various sizes. The most commonly used are 5 mm and 12 mm. The camera and camera cable are attached to the endoscope at the sterile field and are available in HD or SD formats. The endoscope assembly contains the cable, CCD, camera body, sterile adaptor, and telescope.

The touch screen, CCU, focus controller, and illuminator are part of the vision cart. The cart also has shelves and storage compartments for accessory equipment such as gas tanks and adaptors.

SETUP AND SEQUENCE FOR ROBOTIC SURGERY

Room Setup

Robotic surgery requires that components be positioned in a way that optimizes safety and communication among team members during the intraoperative phase. The robotic components should be positioned according to the type of surgery and the configuration of nonmovable equipment in the room (Figure 21-30). All component cables must lie flat on the floor

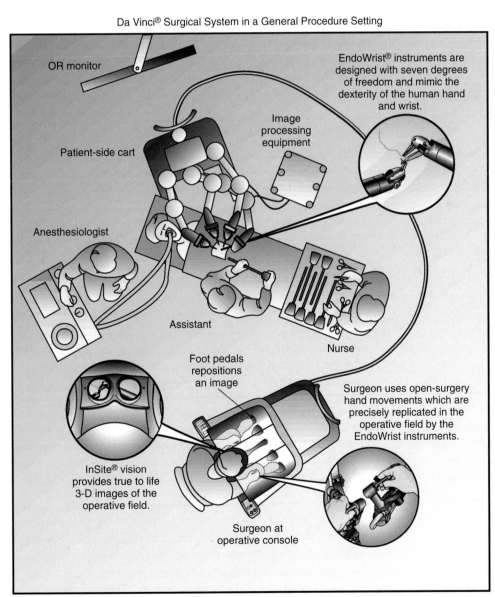

Da Vinci® Surgical System in a General Procedure Setting

Figure 21-30 Room setup for robotic-assisted surgery. *(Courtesy of Intuitive Surgical, Inc., 2007.)*

and in alignment. When the components are positioned, the following must be considered:

- Traffic into, out of, and around the operating room can dictate where the components are placed. Remember that the sterile field includes the patient and operating table, instrument tables, and draped equipment, including the patient cart. Position the equipment in a manner that protects the field from contamination by personnel moving about the room and nonsterile equipment.
- Robotic components are connected by dedicated cables. Position equipment in a way that facilitates safe connections. Do not suspend cables or drape them over equipment. Dedicated power receptacles are recommended for each component, which must be within reach of the receptacle.
- Communication is critical during robotic-assisted surgery. Make sure the surgeon can see and talk to the surgical assistant. Remember that the surgeon is seated at the surgeon's console, and this component is stationed outside the sterile field.
- The patient cart, on which the instrument arms are mounted, is part of the sterile field. It is positioned directly over the patient in the proper location for the type of surgery to be performed (e.g., laparoscopic, urogenital, or thoracic procedure). It is positioned after it has been draped and the instrument cannulas have been placed.

Sequence of Operation

The operative setup must be preplanned so that anesthesia time is not used for tasks that can and should take place before surgery. The robotic system requires many adjustments and selections of options. Documentation of these adjustments and information pertaining to surgeon's preference must be available before every setup.

Before surgery, the surgeon adjusts the components of the console so that the seat and optical viewer are at the correct position. All other options regarding instrument selection and manipulation are made at this time. Nonsterile connections, except those required after the patient cart is in its sterile position, can be made before surgery. This includes setting the correct location of the patient arms with respect to the central column (**docking**). System connections include mains power, system cables, auxiliary devices, video patch, and recording unit. All nonsterile equipment is checked to ensure that adaptors and cables are available and ready for operation.

During the sterile setup, the scrub assembles the sterile portion of the vision system and sets up the instruments in order of use. Drapes for the patient cart and camera are prepared in proper sequence.

As previously mentioned, the robotic cart is brought to the sterile field after the patient prep, draping, and placement of cannulas for surgery. The patient cart and arms and the camera cable are draped during the routine sterile setup or just before use. The cart is then protected from contamination until it is brought into position.

Before docking, nonsterile personnel must position the patient arm remote center at the correct distance from the cart tower to allow the instruments complete range of motion. After this is done, the cart can be docked. This procedure requires two people, one to position the cart physically and the other to provide instructions at the sterile field.

Once the sterile patient cart is in position, the instruments are docked into the patient cart arms and robotic surgery can proceed.

SPECIAL ROLES OF THE SURGICAL TEAM

Surgeon

Even though the surgeon participates as a nonsterile team member from the surgeon's console, the role of the surgeon during robotics procedures is the same as for any surgery. The surgeon directs the flow of the procedure and is responsible for coordinating the activities of everyone on the team.

Surgical Assistant

The surgical assistant is a scrubbed team member. In robotic surgery, the assistant performs other specific tasks at the sterile field. These include exchanging instruments on the sterile robotic arms and managing any instruments that are outside the control of the robotic system. For example, in gynecological surgery, the first or second assistant controls the uterine manipulator. The assistant works closely with the scrub to maintain a clean, safe operative field. Instrument exchanges and management of the sterile robotic components is the dual responsibility of the surgical assistant and the scrub.

Scrub

During surgery, the scrub performs routine tasks associated with all procedures at all stages, preoperative, intraoperative, and postoperative. Tasks specific to robotics are mainly associated with preparation of the equipment, adjustments, and instrument exchange.

In addition to working closely with the surgeon's assistant, the scrub maintains the robotic instruments during surgery and assists or directs the draping procedures. After the cannulas have been placed, the scrub may direct the positioning of the patient cart. The scrub is familiar with the operation of all electronic and vision components, assisting in registration and white and black balance.

As instruments are exchanged into the robotic arms, the scrub interprets the LED signals indicating the status of the instruments and protects them during insertion. The scrub may be required to operate the clutch system that operates the instrument arms while the instruments are outside the patient's body. The scrub also must be familiar with the touch screen options and assists in sterile adjustments at the monitor.

At the close of surgery, the scrub assists in retraction of the instrument and patient cart arms after the instruments have been withdrawn from the cannulas. At this point, the robotic system is disengaged and routine closure is performed. In the postoperative stage, the scrub prepares the instruments and equipment for cleaning and decontamination and assists the circulator in shutdown and stowing of the robotic system.

Circulator and Robotics Coordinator

The circulating nurse and nonscrubbed personnel perform all routine tasks required for safe patient care. The robotics coordinator circulates or directs other scrubbed and nonsterile staff during surgery. In robotic surgery, the circulator is required to maintain a safe environment while troubleshooting the system. This individual must be familiar with the operation of the system's components and assists in positioning, registration, and distribution of supplies and equipment. Two circulators can share the nonsterile duties of both patient care and assistance with the robotic system. The certified surgical technologist (CST) coordinator manages the technological aspects of robotic safety and ensures that equipment and instruments are properly managed and stored. This individual may also coordinate the robotics system with its commercial and educational representative and ensure that safety stand.

CHAPTER SUMMARY

- Operative MIS involves less tissue trauma and postoperative pain and a shorter recovery time compared with open surgery.
- MIS patients must be carefully screened, because not all patients are good candidates.
- MIS involves complex electronic and imaging systems. All team members must study the technologies involved and remain current with new developments in the specialty.
- The operative principle of MIS is that surgery is performed on internal organs from outside the body using telescopic instruments and an operative telescope, which projects the surgical site onto a monitor.
- The components of the MIS imaging system must be compatible.
- Risks associated with MIS include complications resulting from insufflation, extravasation, and unsafe electrosurgical technique.
- Preoperative preparation of the patient for MIS is the same as for open surgery, because as there is always the possibility that the case will convert to an open procedure if an emergency arises.
- MIS is performed in a dimmed operating room to enhance viewing on the video monitor. A dedicated light must be positioned over the instrument table to prevent accidents and errors.
- MIS instruments are extremely delicate and expensive. Care and handling require attention to detail and a knowledge of instrument design.
- MIS is practiced in nearly every surgical specialty. The most common applications are in abdominal, gynecological, orthopedic, thoracic, and genitourinary surgery.
- Reprocessing of MIS instruments is performed according to the manufacturer's instructions. Most instruments can be steam sterilized but require careful cleaning and decontamination before sterilization.
- Because MIS is performed in limited anatomical spaces, various techniques are used to open these tissue planes. Insufflation and fluid expansion are the two most common methods.
- Electrosurgery during MIS can increase the risk of patient burns because the instruments are not always under direct vision of the lensed telescope. Extra caution and vigilance are necessary to prevent patient injury.
- During flexible endoscopy, a flexible tube is inserted into a body cavity for diagnostic assessment, biopsy, and minor surgery.
- The rigid endoscope is used for resection of tumors and more complex surgery of the genitourinary tract and in gynecological procedures.
- Flexible endoscopes are available for many surgical specialties.
- Reprocessing of the flexible endoscope is a primary issue in infection control. This is because the endoscopes are used in semicritical areas of the body and may have a heavy bioburden.
- The protocol for reprocessing of endoscopes is established by health care organizations, guided by safety and accrediting agencies.
- Surgical robotics is a method of performing telesurgery. This is surgery performed from a remote location through the medium of a programmable machine.
- In the United States, only one surgical robotics system, the da Vinci system, has been approved for use in telesurgery.
- Robotic surgery requires extensive training and a considerable investment by the health care institution.
- The da Vinci system does not replace the surgeon and is always used in conjunction with MIS techniques.
- The main advantages of telesurgery are that it scales down the surgeon's hand movements to remove any tremor, and it greatly magnifies the surgical site.
- At this time there are no conclusive studies to show that robotic procedures provide better overall patient outcome than those obtained with traditional minimally invasive procedures.

REVIEW QUESTIONS

1. What patients would not be good candidates for minimally invasive laparoscopic surgery?

2. Explain how abdominal adhesions can cause injury during MIS.

3. How can the surgical technologist prevent patient injury during MIS?

4. Explain how the surgical site is transmitted to the monitor during video-assisted endoscopic surgery.

5. What would the effect be on a fiberoptic light if some of the fibers were broken?

6. In what ways are the physical aspects of minimally invasive instruments different from standard instruments used in open surgery?

7. What do you think might be the reasons for converting from an endoscopic surgery to open surgery?

8. What are the physiological risks to the patient during insufflation?

9. Compare the risks of stainless steel trocars and plastic or nonconductive trocars.

10. Explain the difference between capacitative coupling and direct coupling.

11. What is the role of the surgical technologist in preventing patient burns during the use of electrosurgery in MIS?

12. Explain some of the differences in processing a rigid endoscope and a flexible endoscope.

13. What are the advantages of robotic surgery?

14. What are some of the resources available for learning the techniques of robotic surgery?

15. Why is room setup so important during robotic surgery?

16. What role does the technologist have in patient safety during robotic surgery?

BIBLIOGRAPHY

American Society for Gastrointestinal Endoscopy: Multi-society guideline for reprocessing flexible gastrointestinal endoscopes, *Gastrointestinal Endoscopy* 62:1, 2003.

Association of periOperative Registered Nurses (AORN): *Standards, recommended practices and guidelines,* 2007 edition, Denver, 2007, AORN 2007.

Brown University: Robotic surgery. Retrieved January 16, 2009 at http://biomed.brown.edu/Courses/B11082105Groups/04/index.html.

Catalone B, Koos G: Flexible endoscopes avoiding reprocessing errors critical for infection prevention and control, *Managing Infection Control* June 2005, page 80. Retrieved 1/16/09 at http://www.olympusamerica.com/msg_section/files/mic0605p74.pdfl. Catalone C, Fickenscher K: Emerging technologies in the OR and their effect on perioperative professionals, *AORN Journal* 86:6, December 2007 pages 958-969.

Francis P: The evolution of robotics in surgery and implementing a perioperative robotics nurse specialist role, *AORN Journal* 83:3, July 7, 2006.

Intuitive Surgical: *da Vinci S surgical system interactive training tool: facilitator's guide,* Sunnyvale, Calif, 2005, Intuitive Surgical.

Intuitive Surgical: *da Vinci S surgical system user's manual,* Sunnyvale, Calif, 2007, Intuitive Surgical.

Khraim F: The wider scope of video-assisted thoracoscopic surgery, *AORN Journal* 85:6, June 2007. Olympus America: *Reprocessing Olympus GI endoscopes.* Training video 140/160/180 series, Center Valley, Pa, Olympus America. http//www.olympusamerica.com/msg_section/cds/cds_videos.asp. Retrieved Jan 16, 2009.

Rigdon J: Robotic-assisted laparoscopic radical prostatectomy, *AORN Journal* 84:5 pages 759-770.

Talamini M, Hanly E: Technology in the operating suite, *Journal of the American Medical Association* 293:7, 2005.

US Department of Labor: *OSHA technical manual: industrial and robot system safety.* Retrieved November 29, 2007, at http://www.osha.gov/dts/shta/otm/otm_iv_4.html.

Vangie D: Advancing patient safety in laparoscopy: the active electrode monitoring system, *Patient Safety & Quality Healthcare* May/June 2005. http://www.psqh.com/jayjune05/aems.html. Retrieved January 16, 2009.

Surgical Instruments

CHAPTER OUTLINE

LEARNING OBJECTIVES

After studying this chapter the reader will be able to:
- Differentiate types of instruments by their function
- Identify the different types of finishes on surgical instruments

- Describe the care and handling of instruments
- Describe several methods of learning about instruments
- Develop a personal plan for learning instruments

TERMINOLOGY

Bifurcation: A tube, duct, or other hollow structure that forms a Y split.

Boggy: Soft, doughy; a characteristic of diseased tissue.

Box lock: The hinge point of many surgical instruments.

Chisel: An orthopedic instrument used to slice bone; one side is straight and the other is beveled.

Clamp: An instrument designed to occlude or to hold tissue, objects, or fabric between its jaws.

Curettage: The removal of tissue by scraping with a surgical curette.

Cutting instruments: Instruments with a sharp edge that is used to cut and dissect tissue. This group includes scissors, scalpels, osteotomes, curettes, chisels, biopsy punches, saws, drills, and needles.

Dilators: Graduated, smooth instruments that are used to increase the diameter of an anatomical opening in tissue.

Double-action rongeur: A cutting instrument with two hinges in the middle. This provides greater leverage and cutting strength than a single-action instrument. Usually used to describe an orthopedic rongeur.

Elevator: A nonhinged sharp or dull-tipped instrument. An elevator is used to separate tissues or to bluntly remodel tissue.

Floor grade instruments: Surgical instruments manufactured from inferior metal that can bend and break easily. Fittings and joints are poorly constructed and fittings are poor quality.

Friable: Tearing or fragmenting easily when handled (tissue characteristic).

Fulcrum: The area on an instrument where the lever moves.

Gouge: A V-shaped bone chisel.

Hemostat: A surgical clamp most often used to occlude a blood vessel.

Histology: The study of the structure of tissue.

Honed: Sharpened.

Mixter clamp: A type of hemostat with a straight shank and a right-angle tip.

Points: The tips of a surgical instrument.

Rongeur: A hinged instrument with sharp, cup-shaped tips that is used to extract pieces of bone or other connective tissue.

Serosa: The delicate outer layer of tissue of most organs.

Shank: The area of a surgical instrument between the box lock and the finger ring

Single action rongeur: A cutting instrument that has one hinge.

Tenaculum: A grasping instrument with sharp pointed tips, generally used to manipulate or grasp tissue such as the thyroid or cervix.

Transect: To divide an organ by sharp dissection.

Undermine: To separate tissues layers on a vertical plane using dissecting scissors.

INTRODUCTION

Expertise in surgical instrumentation is among the most important roles of the surgical technologist. Familiarity with instruments, their names (sometimes different from one health facility to another), is *also one of the most difficult* learning curves for students of surgical technology.

The purpose of this chapter is not to provide a basis of memorization of instrument names. This skill comes with practice, experience, and patience. The purpose of this chapter is to provide the basis of understanding about how instruments work, why they are used on a particular type of tissue, and their general application, and to provide an appreciation of the surgeon's tools. A discussion on the types of tissue encountered in surgery is very important to the student's ability to think critically rather than by rote learning. Classification of instruments in groups according to their function assists in the eventual mastery of instrument names. Examples of common instruments are provided and should be accompanied by an instrument reference book, in much the same way that medical and nursing students carry a pharmacological reference with them in the early years of practice. To follow the analogy, medical students and doctors do not try to memorize all the drugs listed in a reference text. They learn by looking up the details of new drugs as they are encountered in their practice. Review and familiarity with real patients and situations re-enforce the learning process.

Like learning a foreign language, instrument names are best learned within a specific context or situation. That situation is usually the surgical procedure itself. It does take time and requires the patience of all who work with students. Most of all, it requires the patience of the learner.

SKILLS FOR KNOWLEDGE AND PRACTICE

The knowledge base for instrumentation includes:
1. The classification of instruments (e.g., retracting, cutting, crushing, clamping).
2. The relationship between the design of an instrument and the instrument's use in the body.
3. The care of instruments (i.e., preparation, handling, troubleshooting, and processing).
4. The correlation between a specific surgical procedure or task and the instrument required to perform it. This combines a knowledge of surgical procedures and anatomy with a knowledge of instruments.
5. The ability to recognize high quality instruments over those that malfunction, are a hazard by design, require repair, or are poorly manufactured.

Manual skills necessary for surgery include the ability to sort, arrange, and retrieve instruments with as little motion as possible. Skilled surgical technologists appreciate order and are able to handle hundreds of instruments and supply items in a limited space. They can remember where everything is on the instrument table and retrieve each item quickly. A level of mechanical ability is needed to correctly assemble instruments and supplies. This is enhanced by a person's desire to understand how things work and how they are put together. An appreciation of the craftsmanship and expertise involved in the manufacture of surgical instruments is an important attribute in anyone handling surgical instruments.

Most surgical instrument used in the modern operating room were invented and developed to overcome a technical problem in surgery. The scrub can anticipate and assist in instrumentation (selecting the correct instrument for the task at hand) through increased familiarity with specific surgical procedures and by learning which instruments are used on a particular tissue. This approach is based not only on knowledge of the procedure, but also on specific knowledge of anatomy and the nature of different types of tissues.

CRITICAL THINKING AND SURGICAL INSTRUMENTATION

Throughout this text, the surgical technologist is encouraged to apply critical thinking skills to all roles and tasks required in his or her work. Critical thinking as it applies to surgical instrumentation means applying knowledge of an instrument's capabilities, structure, design, size, and type to the surgical task at hand. A particular set of instruments is selected prior to surgery. During surgery the technologist must plan the set up and arrangement of instruments so that as the surgery progresses, needed instruments are immediately available on the instrument (Mayo) stand. Other are kept ready as the surgery progresses. Instruments are continually swapped from the Mayo stand to the back table as needed.

In order to anticipate which instruments are needed, the scrub has studied the procedure (or has previous experience) watches the progress of the surgery, is familiar with basic anatomical structures and the nature of the *tissues.*

WORKING WITH INSTRUMENTS

Instrument trays are assembled according to the particular surgical specialty. One of the best ways to learn the names of instruments is to set up instrument trays and handle the instruments. This creates an association of one instrument with others in the same specialty and permits examination of the instrument. Above all, associating one instrument with others in a group cues the brain to categorize them. This is a valuable learning aid.

As you set up a case and work with a preceptor, ask the name and function of any instrument you do not know. You may not remember all the names, but you will have established an association between that instrument and the surgical procedure in which it was used. As you pass the instrument, think of its name at the same time. This creates another associative cue.

Always try to associate the instrument with a surgery, tissue type or other cue. Simply looking at pictures or flash cards of instruments is not particularly efficient for learning. Without some associative cue, memorization is tedious and difficult. Memory is developed through association. The neural pathway to memory is linked with other information and events that occurred with the memory. That is why simply reading study material repeatedly does not ensure recall. To remember a picture, design, or object such as an instrument, you must associate it with something that becomes a cue. The cue might be some structural aspect of the instrument or a particular case on which you scrubbed. The name may remind you of some object or person. Memorization is personal because association is personal. Cues are a powerful tool for any kind of memorization. Speed of recall comes only after the cue is in place.

INSTRUMENT MANUFACTURING
AND DESIGN

MANUFACTURING

Surgical instruments represent a large investment for every operating room. There are two different grades of instruments—floor grade and surgical grade.

Floor-grade instruments are made from inferior metals and are imprecisely constructed. They tend to bend and break easily and often show pitting and staining within the first few sterilization processes. Floor-grade instruments are intended for use in less critical applications, such as suture and suture-removal kits in the emergency department. These instruments often are classified as single-use items.

Surgical-grade instruments are constructed of high quality stainless steel and other metal alloys, such as carbon and chromium, that resist bending, pitting, scratching, and dulling. Stainless steel is the most common metal used in surgical instruments but is also subject to corrosion. A manufacturing process called passivisation removes manufacturing impurities and coats the instruments to protect from corrosion. Repeated exposure to ultrasonic cleaning and harsh chemicals removes this coating and hastens corrosion and staining which is prevented by lubrication after cleaning. Instruments discussed in this chapter and textbook are surgical-grade instruments.

Three types of finishes are used on metal instruments. A bright, or mirror, finish is highly polished, reflects light, and may cause glare in the surgical field, affecting the surgeon's vision. A satin, finish on instruments reduces glare and light reflection which can lead to eye fatigue. However, satin finish instruments tend to stain more easily from the effects of detergents and low water quality. Ebony is a black chromium finish used for laser surgery. The dull black finish prevents laser beams from reflecting or bouncing off the instruments, which could injure or destroy nearby tissues.

Many instruments have expensive tungsten carbide inserts to maintain a sharp edge in scissors and gripping ability in needle holders. Instruments with tungsten carbide inserts usually are manufactured with gold-plated or black handles. These features allow precision work but are very expensive. Care of instruments is one of the primary responsibilities of the surgical technologist.

INSTRUMENT DESIGN

All instruments are balanced to fit the surgeon's hand. The distribution of weight between the handle (and finger rings) and the **fulcrum** is measured and tested for optimum performance. The hinges are perfectly **honed** to create a seamless surface when the instrument is closed. Ratchets are calculated to create the correct amount of spring and ease of opening without sticking or forcing.

Scissors must be particularly well balanced and precise. The blades are designed to slide over each other without interference. **Points** often are honed by hand to ensure that they have no burrs and that the tips come together precisely.

A microsurgical instrument used on the eye costs hundreds of dollars, and it can be ruined in an instant if it is dropped or a heavy object is placed on top of it. Using hemostats to pry open metal caps or to grasp metal sutures puts the jaws out of alignment, often permanently.

Instruments are designed to match their use and the type of tissue on which they are used. For example, blood vessels are never handled with an instrument that might puncture or bruise the tissue. However, fibrous tissue is very resilient and requires toothed instruments to maintain grasp.

Some important instrument design features are:
- Heavy or delicate
- Long or short
- Cutting or blunt tipped
- Narrow or wide
- Angled or straight
- Completely or partly occluding
- Traumatic or nontraumatic to tissue (toothed or smooth)

Although each instrument has a specific name, many surgeons ask for the instrument by its function rather than its name. For example, rather than ask for a "Weitlaner self-retaining retractor," the surgeon more often requests a "self-retainer." When asking for a **clamp**, the surgeon expects to receive the appropriate type of clamp used for that particular tissue.

TYPES OF INSTRUMENTS BY FUNCTION

GRASPING AND HOLDING INSTRUMENTS

Locking Clamp

A locking box lock clamp (also called a **box lock**) has one or more ratchets that remain closed after they are set. The locking clamp is a design used in many instruments refer to Figure 22-1 for example). Microsurgical instruments use a spring lock mechanism, which is used in the design of needle holders, shown below.

Thumb Forceps

Thumb forceps are used for grasping—usually during suturing for handling tissue during surgery. For example, during suturing, the surgeon holds the forceps in one hand and the needle holder in the other. Thumb forceps often are called "pickups." Toothed forceps have one or more teeth in the jaws. These are used to grasp skin or other connective tissue. Toothed forceps are named according to the number and type of teeth. For example, 1×2 forceps have one tooth and two slots; 2×3 forceps have two teeth and three slots. Examples

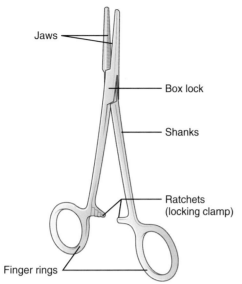

Figure 22-1   Parts of a box lock instrument.

Jaws

Box lock

Shanks

Ratchets
(locking clamp)

Finger rings

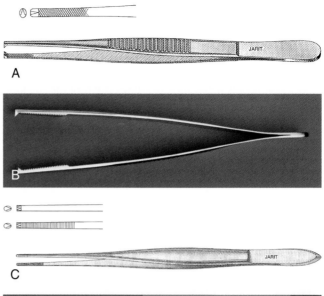

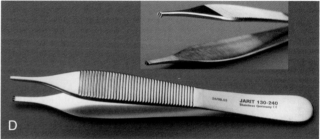

Figure 22-2   Tissue forceps. **A** and **B,** Single-toothed forceps. **C,** Cushing forceps. **D,** Adson tissue forceps. *(Courtesy Jarit Instruments, Hawthorne, NY.)*

of toothed forceps include Adson forceps with teeth, thumb tissue forceps with teeth, Bonney tissue forceps, and Cushing forceps.

Smooth forceps (no teeth) are used on delicate tissue such as serosa, bowel, blood vessels, or ducts. Examples include smooth thumb forceps, smooth Adson forceps, DeBakey forceps, and smooth Cushing forceps. Some forceps are serrated or have small, rounded teeth. Examples include Martin forceps and Russian forceps. Bayonet forceps are angled and typically are used in neurosurgical and nasal procedures. Figures 22-2 and 22-3 show common tissue forceps.

Biting Clamps

A biting clamp has teeth or sharp serrations in the jaws. An example of this type of instrument is the Kocher clamp. The toothed, or biting, clamp is used on avascular fibrous tissue, bone (i.e., tissue that has little blood supply) or on tissue that will be removed as part of the procedure. A bone clamp is serrated and designed to hold large bone fragments together. An example of a bone clamp is the Lane bone-holding clamp.

A **tenaculum** has one or more teeth in jaws that can be delicate or heavy. This instrument penetrates the tissue rather than just holding it with pressure on the outside surface. It generally is used in fibrous tissue, such as the cervix. A bone clamp, such as a Lewin clamp, is inserted into a bone for manipulation. Although similar in design to a towel clamp, the Lewin is manufactured with the weight and strength to withstand penetration through bone tissue. Examples of biting clamps used in different specialties are shown in Figure 22-4.

CLAMPING AND OCCLUDING INSTRUMENTS

Atraumatic Clamp

An atraumatic clamp usually has locking ratchets, but the tips do not close tightly over the tissue (Figure 22-5). This type of

clamp is used on delicate tissue that is highly vascular or easily injured. An example is the Duval lung clamp. The Babcock clamp is an atraumatic, noncrushing clamp usually used on the bowel or fallopian tubes. Other types of atraumatic bowel clamps have different kinds of jaw patterns. The jaws have flexible blades that occlude but do not crush the tissue. Examples include the Bainbridge intestinal clamp and the Doyen intestinal clamp. Whenever a long clamp, such as a vascular clamp is placed across a tissue structure, at an approximate right angle, this is called **cross clamping**. Cross clamping is frequently used in vascular surgery, and in intestinal surgery. For example *the surgeon places two "cross clamps" across the aorta.*

Occluding Clamp (Hemostat)

A **hemostat** blocks the flow of blood. The Kelly, Crile, and mosquito hemostats (Figure 22-6) are used to completely occlude a blood vessel while it is tied or sealed with the electrosurgical unit (ESU). Right-angled clamps, such as the **Mixter clamp**, are used for dissection and occlusion in deep wounds.

Vascular Clamp

A semioccluding vascular clamp is capable of varying low levels of compression between its jaws. These clamps are

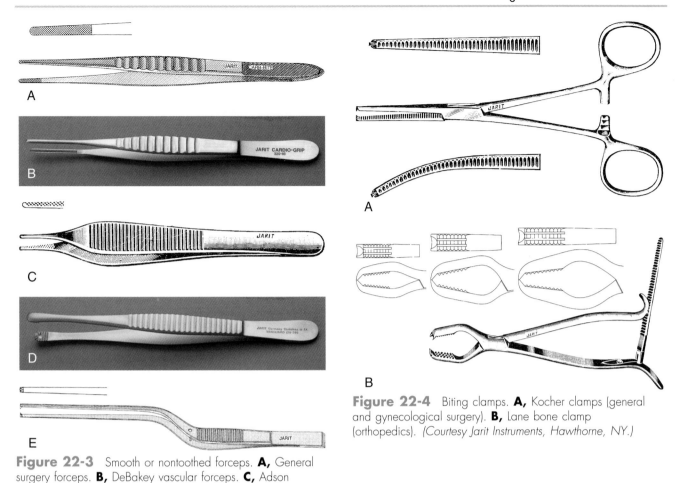

Figure 22-3 Smooth or nontoothed forceps. **A,** General surgery forceps. **B,** DeBakey vascular forceps. **C,** Adson forceps. **D,** Russian forceps. **E,** Bayonet forceps. *(Courtesy Jarit Instruments, Hawthorne, NY.)*

Figure 22-4 Biting clamps. **A,** Kocher clamps (general and gynecological surgery). **B,** Lane bone clamp (orthopedics). *(Courtesy Jarit Instruments, Hawthorne, NY.)*

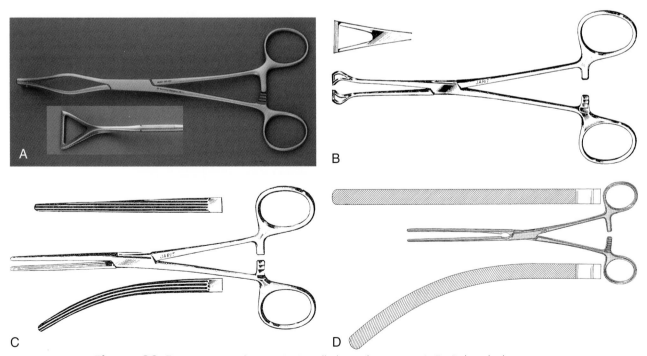

Figure 22-5 Atraumatic clamps. **A,** Duvall clamp (lung surgery). **B,** Babcock clamp (fallopian tubes, intestines). **C,** Bainbridge clamp (intestine). **D,** Doyen clamp (intestine). *(Courtesy Jarit Instruments, Hawthorne, NY.)*

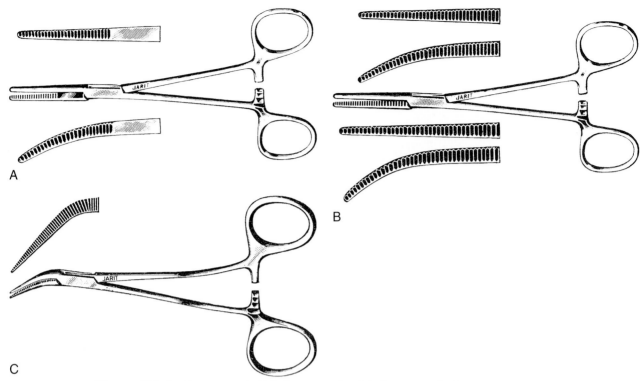

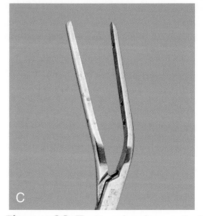

Figure 22-6 Hemostats. **A,** Kelly hemostats. **B,** Crile hemostats. **C,** Mosquito hemostats. *(Courtesy Jarit Instruments, Hawthorne, NY.)*

angled to allow access to blood vessels. Examples of vascular clamps include bulldog, Satinsky, Fogarty, Crafoord, and Cooley clamps (Figure 22-7).

CUTTING AND DISSECTING INSTRUMENTS

Scalpel

The common surgical scalpel (commonly called "the knife") is used whenever razor-sharp cutting is required for tissue dissection. A scalpel blade is detachable from the knife handle. Scalpel blades are numbered consistently among manufacturers, and the number indicates the shape and size (Figure 22-8).

Scalpel blades fit specific handles as follows:

- Scalpel handles: 3, 3 L, 7, 9   Blades: 10, 11, 12, 15
- Scalpel handles: 4, 4 L   Blades: 18 to 25

Another type of scalpel handle with interchangeable, disposable blades is called a *Beaver blade handle,* which uses Beaver blades (Figure 22-9). These usually are used in surgery of the eye and ear.

Examples of one-piece specialty knives are meniscus knives (Smillie knives) and those used in ear surgery (sickle knives) (Figure 22-10).

Scissors

Scissors are among the most frequently used and important instruments in surgery. Careful handling and processing of scissors is necessary to maintain sharpness, blade alignment, and sharp points. Tissue scissors are used to sever tissue and should never be used on other materials or surgical supplies, including suture material.

High quality surgical scissors are distinctive by the sharpness of the cutting edges, balance, metal composition, and the

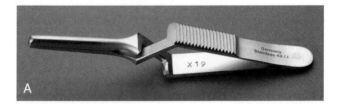

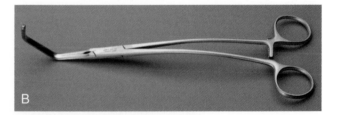

Figure 22-7 Vascular clamps. **A,** Bulldog clamp (actual size, 2 inches [5 cm]). **B,** Satinsky vena cava clamp. **C,** Fogarty clamp. *(A courtesy Jarit Instruments, Hawthorne, NY; B courtesy Codman & Shurtleff, Raynham, Mass; C from Tighe S: Surgical instrumentation, ed 7, St Louis, 2007, Mosby.)*

design of the point. Scissors with extremely sharp points are intended to sever extremely small points of tissue during dissection. If the points do not meet or are bent, this function is lost. The blades of the high quality scissor are coated with tungsten or other hardened alloy to maintain sharpness. Pitting and corrosion along the edge of the blade are signs of instrument abuse or poor quality.

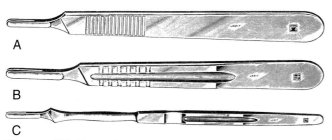

Figure 22-8 Scalpel handles and blades. Handles *(top to bottom)*: #3, #4, and #7. *(Courtesy Jarit Instruments, Hawthorne, NY.)*

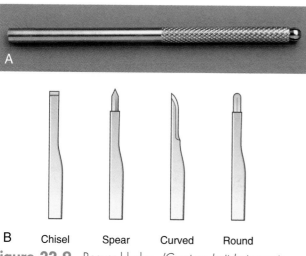

Figure 22-9 Beaver blades. *(Courtesy Jarit Instruments, Hawthorne, NY.)*

Surgical scissors are available in a wide variety of sizes and types (Figure 22-11).

- Small, sharp-tipped scissors, such as tenotomy scissors, are used for extremely fine dissection in plastic surgery.
- Castroviejo scissors are commonly used in microsurgery.
- Round-tipped, light dissecting scissors, such as Metzenbaum scissors, are used extensively on delicate tissue in general surgery.
- Fibrous connective tissue requires heavier scissors, such as the curved Mayo scissors. Dissecting scissors often are used to **undermine** tissue. In this technique, the scissors are inserted between two tissue planes and opened. The outside (dull) edge of the scissor separates the layers rather than cutting them apart, which would cause bleeding.
- Straight Mayo scissors are used for cutting suture. Scissors designed to cut tissue should never be used to cut suture, because this dulls the blades.

Rongeur

A **rongeur** is used to cut and extract tissue (Figure 22-12). The tips are cupped, and the edges of the cups are sharp. Rongeurs may have finger rings or may resemble household pliers. A rongeur may have a single hinge, as do scissors (**single-action** rongeur), or it may have two hinges (**double-action** rongeur). A double-action rongeur creates twice the leverage of a single-action rongeur. A heavier rongeur used in orthopedic and neurosurgical procedures is called a *Stille rongeur*. A long-handled rongeur, such as the Kerrison rongeur, often is used in spinal surgery. Long, fine-tipped rongeurs, such as the pituitary rongeur, are used to remove tissue in areas that are difficult to reach, such as the vertebral column and nasal sinus.

Many fine tipped rongeurs such as the *Kerrison* are categorized by the angle of their tips and described as either *upbiting* or *downbiting*. The angle of the rongeur tips allows the surgeon to cut and remove tissue in areas that may be difficult to reach.

During removal of tissue or bone with a small rongeur, the surgeon will point the tip of the instrument at the scrub so that the scrub can remove the tissue from the tips of the rongeur with a moistened sponge. The surgeon does not look away from the surgical wound. Do not pull the rongeur out of the surgeon's hand while cleaning the tip. Watch the field

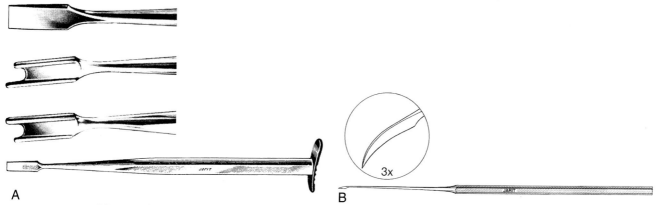

Figure 22-10 One-piece knives. **A,** Smillie cartilage knife (knee). **B,** House sickle knife (ear). *(Courtesy Jarit Instruments, Hawthorne, NY.)*

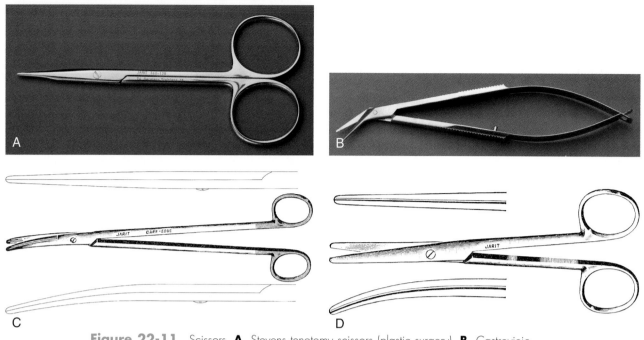

Figure 22-11 Scissors. **A,** Stevens tenotomy scissors (plastic surgery). **B,** Castroviejo scissors (eye and plastic surgery). **C,** Metzenbaum scissors. **D,** Mayo scissors (straight and curved shown). *(Courtesy Jarit Instruments, Hawthorne, NY.)*

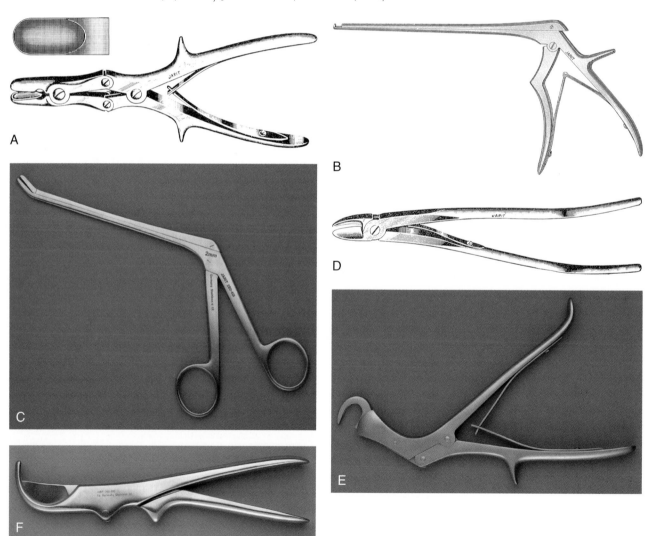

Figure 22-12 Rongeurs and bone shears. **A,** Stille-Luer rongeurs (orthopedics). **B,** Kerrison rongeurs (neurosurgery; ear, nose, and throat [ENT] surgery). **C,** Pituitary rongeurs (neurosurgery, ENT surgery). **D,** Bethune rib shears. **E,** Stile Giertz rib shears. **F,** Gluck rib shears. *(Courtesy Jarit Instruments, Hawthorne, NY.)*

carefully whenever a rongeur is used to keep up with the surgeon. As with any tissue specimen, all tissue must be retained in a small basin.

The distinction between a rongeur and a forcep is at times somewhat confusing. This is partly due to similar design and also the name of the instruments assigned by the manufacturer. For example, the "pituitary forcep" is sometimes referred to as a "pituitary rongeur." The basic design of this instrument is similar to the Kerrison rongeur in that the fulcrum is set close to the finger rings and tip is used for removing small bites of tissue from a confined space such as a vertebral disc or nasal sinus tissue. In general, the pituitary forcep is not designed to handle heavy fibrous tissue, whereas the Kerrison has the leverage and strength to remove bits of dense bone.

Shears

Shears are large **cutting instruments** used to cut bone. Some shears are designed so that the cutting edge is left or right of the hinge. As the name implies, side-cutting shears are designed to cut to the left or the right. Rongeurs and bone shears are shown in Figure 22-12.

Curette

The basic design of a curette is a small cup with a sharpened, serrated, or smooth rim at the end of a long handle. The curette is used in many specialties for scooping out tissue.

Very fine curettes are used in ear, paranasal, and spinal surgery. Larger, heavier curettes are used in orthopedic procedures. Soft tissue curettes are used in gynecological surgery for curettage of the endometrium. Sometimes curettes are used to remove very dense granulated (overgrown or scarred) soft tissue.

When asked for a curette during surgery, the technologist will usually be told which type is needed. In some cases, however, it will be apparent that only a sharp curette is required—for example, in orthopedic work, sharp curettes are required to scoop out portions of deceased or obstructing bone. In this case, a smooth rimmed curette would have no cutting effect.

Osteotome, Chisel, and Gouge

A **chisel** is an orthopedic cutting instrument that is used with a mallet (similarly used in sculpting or carpentry). Chisels are available in many widths and sizes that fit a particular specialty. For example, a chisel used in paranasal surgery is much more delicate than one designed for the tibia. An osteotome has two beveled sides, whereas a chisel blade is sloped on one side only. A large osteotome often is used to remove bone from the iliac crest for use as a graft elsewhere in the body. The chisel produces a straight-sided cut, similar to a notch. Both instruments' tips must be protected from damage. When the blade becomes pitted or chipped, it loses its precision and becomes a hazard. Both types of instruments should be kept in a metal rack where their blades cannot touch each other.

A **gouge** is a V-shaped bone chisel. Its cut looks like a small trough. Figure 22-13 shows the curette, chisel, osteotome, and gouge.

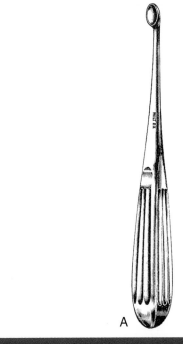
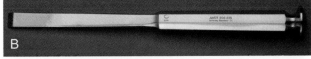
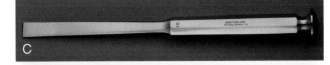
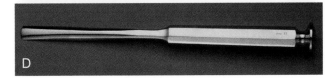

Figure 22-13 Curette, chisel, osteotome, and gouge. **A,** Curette. **B,** Chisel. **C,** Osteotome. **D,** Gouge. (**A** courtesy Miltex, York, Pa; **B** to **D** courtesy Jarit Instruments, Hawthorne, NY.)

Elevator

An **elevator** is used to separate or "elevate" tissue (Figure 22-14). The heavy, round cutting elevator, such as the Lambotte elevator, slices tissue as it elevates. The small, square-tipped Key elevator also has a sharp edge but is much more delicate. Very finely balanced elevators, such as the Penfield and Freer elevators, are used in soft tissue surgery. In vascular surgery, Penfield or Freer elevators are used to separate atherosclerotic plaque from the inside of a blood vessel. The elevator must be well balanced and light enough to convey feeling from the working end (the tip) to the surgeon's hand. The joker is a very commonly used elevator. Its short handle and strong tip make it ideal for separating connective tissue planes without causing bleeding.

Rasp

A rasp is used to remodel bone (Figure 22-15). Many sizes, shapes, and surfaces are available. Fine rasps are used in ENT

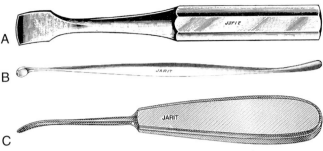

Figure 22-14   Elevators. **A,** Periosteal Key elevator. **B,** Penfield elevator (neurosurgery, ENT, plastic surgery). **C,** Joker elevator (multiple specialties). *(Courtesy Jarit Instruments, Hawthorne, NY.)*

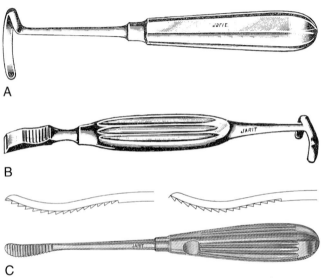

Figure 22-15   Rasps. **A,** Doyen rib stripper (used to remove periosteum). **B,** Matson elevator and stripper. **C,** Aufricht nasal rasp (ENT). *(Courtesy Jarit Instruments, Hawthorne, NY.)*

surgery for the delicate bones and surfaces of the nasal sinuses and ear. Heavy rasps are used to ream the medullary canal of long bones in preparation for an implant or to prepare the surface of the humerus before sutures are attached. A rib stripper is a type of rasp used to scrape tough connective tissue from the surface of a rib before it is cut with rib shears. Examples of rib strippers include Matson, Alexander, and Doyen rib rasps.

RETRACTING (EXPOSING) INSTRUMENTS

As the surgical wound is deepened, tissue layers and other structures such as blood vessels, nerves, organs, and other tissue must be gently moved away from the focal point of the operation. A retractor, which is almost always shaped in a modified right angle with the "blade" portion used as the retracting part, is used to perform this task. Retractors are described as:

- Handheld or self-retaining
- Deep or superficial
- Wide or narrow
- Malleable (bendable into any angle)
- Sharp or dull

Handheld vs Self Retaining Retractors

Handheld retractors range in size from the very fragile skin hook used in plastic surgery to the large, 4-inch (10 cm) wide Deaver retractor used in abdominal procedures. Other common retractors are the army-navy retractor (also called a U.S. retractor), the vein retractor, the Goelet retractor, the Richardson retractor, the ribbon retractor, and the Harrington retractor.

The rake retractor generally is used only for connective tissue. Sharp rakes or hooks are designed to grasp the undersurface of superficial tissues. Dull hooks and rakes are used in areas close to viable nerves or near blood vessels. Common handheld retractors are shown in Figure 22-16.

Self-retaining retractors hold tissue against the walls of the surgical wound by *mechanical action* (Figure 22-17). Self-retaining retractors can have many attachments suited to the needs of the surgery. The Thompson self-retaining, Bookwalter, and Balfour retractors are examples. Blades of various sizes and shapes can be attached to the frame to accommodate the specific needs of the procedure. Other examples include the Finochietto self-retaining retractor, which is used in cardiothoracic surgery, and the smaller Gelpi and Weitlaner retractors, which are used for superficial incisions, such as in the groin. The McPherson self-retaining lid speculum holds the eye open during ophthalmic surgery.

By definition, the self-retaining retractor works by some mechanical means to hold the blades in place in the surgical wound. This means the retractor is first positioned against the tissue to be retracted, and then opened manually or mechanically. From that point, it is not held in place by anyone on the sterile team. The potential for bruising, nerve, and vessel damage, and even serious injury, exists for any mechanical device used on living tissue. For this reason the retractor is placed carefully and may be cushioned using laparotomy (lap) sponges so that the bare blades do not press against the tissue. However, a sharp tipped or superficial self-retaining retractor such as a *Gelpi* or *sharp Weitlaner* is used without the aid of sponges as these would defeat their purpose of penetrating the tissue as it is retracted.

Selection of Retractors

The selection of a retractor is based on the length and depth of the incision. At the beginning of a procedure, superficial retractors are used, and as the incision is carried deeper, a longer blade or deeper retractor is required to create exposure. The *width* of the retractor blade is determined by the size of the incision and the tissue to be retracted. The retractor blade can be curved, right angled, or malleable (bendable to any angle).

DILATORS

Dilators are rounded tubular or tube-like instruments used to widen or stretch the inside diameter of a *lumen* (tissue with a hollow core). Cervical dilators are used to dilate the cervix so that instruments can be passed into the uterus. Urethral dilators are used to open strictures of the urethra. Dilators used within very narrow lumens may be designed with a small bullet-shaped tip attached to a slender catheter for more delicate vessels and ducts.

MEASURING INSTRUMENTS

Tissue and hollow structures are measured for many purposes. For example, the uterine sound is inserted into the cervix to measure the depth of the uterus from the cervix to the fundus. This is done to prevent perforation during **curettage**. Orthopedic calipers are used to prepare the bone for a joint implant. A depth gauge is used in orthopedic surgery to determine the length of screws to be implanted into bone.

A sizer is a trial, reusable replica of an implantable prosthesis. Rather than opening and contaminating many expensive implants, the sizer allows the surgeon to test a replica first. For example, before a cardiac valve is inserted, a sizer is used to determine the correct size. A surgeon may use a basic sterile ruler to measure tissue or specimen removed from the patient. Assorted measuring instruments are shown in Figure 22-18.

SUTURING INSTRUMENTS

A needle holder is used to grasp a curved needle during suturing (Figure 22-19). The length, weight, and type of tip must be matched to the suture and tissue. Using a heavy needle holder, such as a Heaney or Mayo-Hegar needle holder, to suture a small blood vessel is like manipulating a straight pin with a pipe wrench. Very fine sutures require fine needle holders. A sharp-tipped needle holder, such as the Sarot needle holder, is used for fine sutures (i.e., 4-0 and smaller). Many needle holders are serrated or slotted or have tungsten carbon inserts in the jaws for added durability and grip.

If the needle holder is too heavy, the surgeon will lose the "feel" of the needle. On the other hand, a lightweight or fine-tipped needle holder (e.g., the Webster needle holder) does not have enough surface area at the tip to grasp a heavy needle. A needle holder that is too delicate for the needle will cause the needle to twist during use. In any event, the surgeon will reject any needle holder and needle combination that is inappropriate.

Most needle holders are ratchet or spring locked. Always test the ratchets before the needle holder is used. If they do not mesh correctly, the needle holder may spring open unexpectedly. The smallest needle holders, such as the Castroviejo needle holder used in eye surgery and microsurgery, have a spring catch and may be locking or nonlocking. These are easily damaged if handled inappropriately. Only gentle pressure is needed to open and close a spring catch.

SUCTION TIPS

Suction (aspiration) is needed during a surgical procedure to clear blood, fluids, and small bits of tissue debris from the

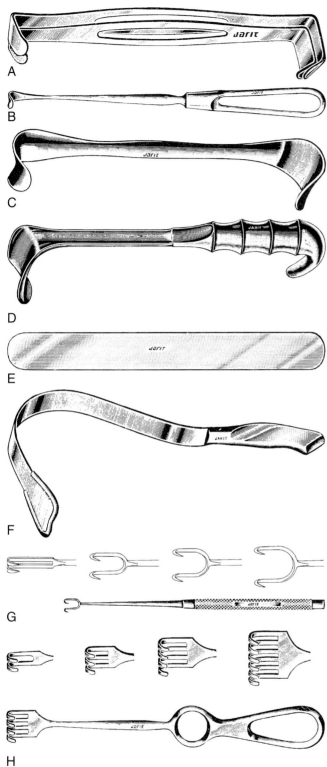

Figure 22-16 Handheld retractors. **A,** Army-Navy retractor (also called *U.S. retractor*). **B,** Vein retractor. **C,** Goelet retractor. **D,** Richardson retractor. **E,** Ribbon, or malleable, retractor. **F,** Harrington retractor (also called a *sweetheart retractor*). **G,** Skin hook. **H,** Rake. *(Courtesy Jarit Instruments, Hawthorne, NY.)*

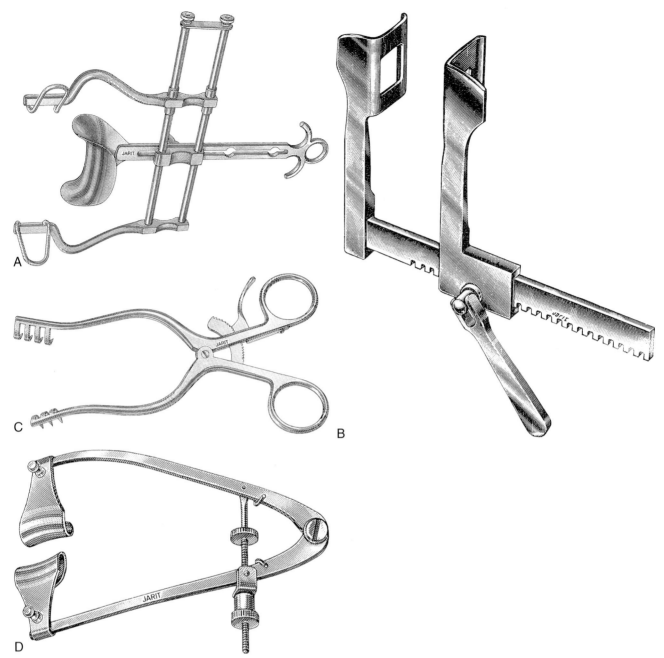

Figure 22-17 Self-retaining retractors. **A,** Balfour retractor (abdominal surgery).
B, Finochietto retractor (thoracic surgery). **C,** Weitlaner retractor (superficial surgery [e.g.,
inguinal area or limb]). **D,** McPherson eye speculum. *(Courtesy Jarit Instruments, Hawthorne,
NY.)*

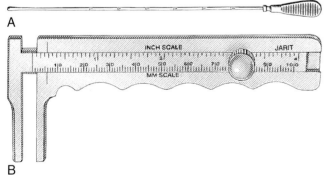

Figure 22-18 Measuring instruments. **A,** Uterine sound.
B, Caliper (orthopedics). *(Courtesy Jarit Instruments, Hawthorne,
NY.)*

surgical site and provide an unobstructed view of the anatomy.
Suction is provided using sterile plastic tubing, which attaches
to a suction tip (instrument) at one end and a closed suction
canister (non-sterile) at the other.

The instrument itself is varies in length and diameter to
very small (for eye and microsurgery) to larger tips for general
surgery and orthopedics. Tips are straight or angled and may
have a removable tip or shield that reduces the suction pressure. For example, the Poole suction tip is designed for
abdominal surgery and has a removable perforated guard that
protects bowel and intestinal organs from injury. The

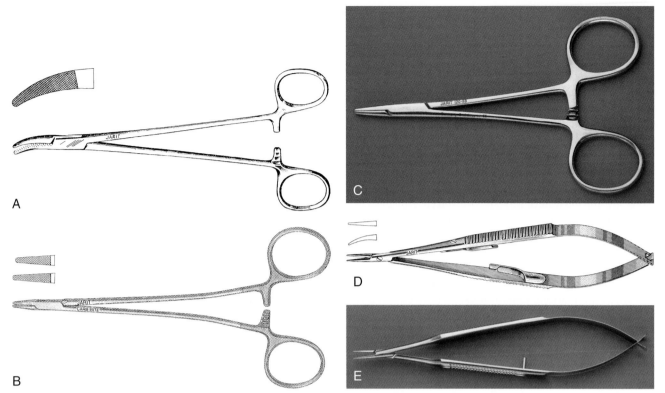

Figure 22-19 Commonly used needle holders. **A,** Heaney (broad tip) needle holder. **B,** Sarot (fine tip) needle holder. **C,** Webster needle holder (plastic surgery). **D,** Castroviejo needle holder with spring lock. **E,** Castroviejo needle holder without lock. *(Courtesy Jarit Instruments, Hawthorne, NY.)*

Yankauer or tonsil suction tip is designed to suction in the chest cavity and throat. The Frazier suction tip is designed to suction in superficial areas in the face, neck, and ear and in neurological and some peripheral vascular procedures.

Depending on the diameter of the lumen of the suction tip, the scrub may need to clear the suction tip periodically to remove clotted blood or debris, such as bone chips and dust. These are produced when orthopedic saws and drills are used. This can be done by dipping the suction tip in sterile water or by inserting a stylet (flexible wire) into the lumen. Three commonly used suction tips are shown in Figure 22-20.

TISSUE TYPES AND INSTRUMENT SELECTION

The selection of a particular surgical instrument is based on the tissue type, the depth of the surgical wound, the technical requirements of the instrument, and the surgeon's preference or experience. Normal tissues differ in texture, strength, elasticity, water, fat content, and permeability. If all body tissues were the same, far fewer instruments would be required. Normal tissue undergoes changes when diseased. Infection has a liquefying or fragmenting effect. Some tumors are extremely fibrous and tough. This information is important to both the surgeon and the scrub.

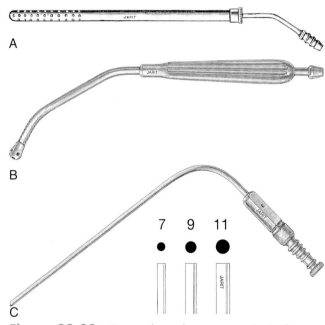

Figure 22-20 Commonly used suction tips. **A,** Poole suction tip. **B,** Yankauer suction tip. **C,** Frazier suction tip. *(Courtesy Jarit Instruments, Hawthorne, NY.)*

Visceral Serosa

The viscera, or organs of the body, are each covered by a fine membrane called the **serosa**. This membrane is easily punctured, and the underlying tissue layers can bleed profusely. Nontraumatic instruments are needed when handling this tissue. These includes non-penetrating forceps (smooth forceps), wide retractors which do not cut into the tissue, and suction tips which have a guard to decrease the aspirating pressure (level of "pull") on the tissue.

Friable Tissue

Tissue that is **friable** is very delicate, tends to bleed profusely, tears easily, and has little or no resilience. Infection or advanced age can cause normally strong tissue to become friable. Tissues such as the liver, spleen, and lung normally are friable. A strong membrane covers and protects these organs. However, these tissues must be handled by hand or with nontraumatic instruments. The liver and spleen can "break" or develop fissures when traumatized. Clamps must be nonoccluding and forceps nontoothed. When the spleen, liver, and intestines are retracted, the surface area of the retractor must be sufficiently wide to distribute the pressure. Edges must be protected with sponges to prevent the retractor edge from cutting into the tissue.

Intestine and Other Tubular Structures

Many anatomical structures with a lumen must be protected from puncture. These structures therefore usually are handled with smooth, nontraumatic instruments. Clamps used to *temporarily* occlude the intestine, fallopian tube, vas deferens, ureters, large blood vessels, and other ducts are only partly occlusive. That is, the jaws of the instruments do not meet in close approximation. Vascular clamps are designed to interrupt the flow of blood through a blood vessel without crushing the tissue. The jaws of a vascular clamp have fine ridges that prevent the clamp from slipping, yet do not crush or bruise the vessel.

The tips of the grasping instruments do not approximate as tightly as those of a hemostat. Examples are the Babcock clamp and the Allis clamp, which are commonly used on the intestine and the fallopian tubes.

Elastic Tissue

Elastic tissue is resilient and able to withstand a limited amount of stretching without injury. The peritoneal lining of body cavities, although elastic, can tear with extreme or repeated pressure. The vaginal vault and some glandular tissue, such as the tonsils, are elastic. These tissues can tolerate the amount of pressure exerted by a hemostat or low-compression biting clamps, such as an Allis clamp. Elastic tissue tends to heal rapidly unless diseased or infected.

Boggy Tissue

Tissue is described as **boggy** when it is heavy with fluid, inflamed, or diseased. Its normal resiliency is lost, and the organ becomes soft and doughy. Infected or edematous tissue is boggy and difficult to clamp and suture. In these cases the tissue is usually handled manually and non-occlusive clamps

such as the Babcock are used. In some cases, semi-liquid tissue must be suctioned or curetted out and the remaining raw surface treated with topical coagulant.

Fatty Tissue

Semisolid tissue has a high fat content. It does not compress well and tends to fragment into small pieces when clamped. Adipose tissue has few blood vessels compared with other types of tissue and may require a penetrating retractor, such as a sharp rake. The Allis clamp, which has fine serrations at the tip, often is used to clamp or grasp adipose tissue. The high fat content of this tissue may cause instruments to become slippery and difficult to handle. Forceps with teeth are required for suturing.

Bone

Bone tissue is resilient and somewhat springy when healthy. Large bones usually are manipulated with traction or leverage rather than direct pulling pressure. Notice that most bone retractors, such as the Bennett and Scoville retractors, have a toothed tip or a reverse curve that can be inserted under another bone for leverage (see Chapter 30).

Other Connective Tissues

Other types of connective tissues, such as cartilage and tendon, are extremely strong and resilient. Most joint surfaces are exposed to synovial fluid, which has an oily consistency. The tissue can be quite slippery, requiring toothed clamps or those with ridges to maintain hold. Tendons are also covered by a sheath that is relatively strong and smooth. Fascia often is grasped with Kocher clamps, which have one or two teeth at the tip. Cutting instruments, such as curved Mayo scissors, must be sharp and strong.

BODY PLANES AND STRUCTURE

Technical challenges arise during surgery because of the angles and depth of tissue planes. Instruments are needed that can reach around structures in all directions. The instruments' design and function allow the surgeon to penetrate, suture, extract, and ligate tissue in a variety of levels, planes, and spatial relationships. If the surgeon could flatten the body and work in a single dimensional plane, the procedure would be much easier. However, except in superficial surgery, this is not the case. Most procedures require the surgeon to work in a limited space in a small cavity. Some procedures require access to areas that are deep, restricted, and oblique (angled). An example is an abdominal approach to the esophagus or sigmoid colon. Familiarity with the body's tissue planes gives the scrub a greater appreciation of the surgical techniques required. More important, the scrub can see how the design of the instrument is critical in the performance of each step of the surgery.

An angled instrument has a tip that is curved or right angled. The function of this clamp is to reach underneath or around a structure. For example, blood vessels cannot be lifted out, therefore the instrument must accommodate the structure. The right-angle, clamp (sometimes referred to as a

Mixter clamp) is used along vertical planes of tissue, such as the sides of an incision. If the clamp were completely straight, it would have to be turned horizontally to clamp tissue along the wall of the incision. The right-angle clamp is perfectly suited for deep incisions, because it is used in its vertical position.

Right-angle scissors (e.g., Potts scissors) allow the surgeon to insert the scissor tip inside a vessel. The surgeon can aim the scissors straight down into the wound, but the tips follow the horizontal plane of the vessel.

The curves and **bifurcations** (areas where a tubular structure forms a Y) of hollow structures also present technical challenges. Flexible instruments have been developed to overcome this difficulty. Before the refinement of flexible endoscopes, lighted rigid scopes were used exclusively. Few areas of the body follow a straight path. A rigid, straight instrument is useful only when it can be manipulated at the tip. The technical advantage of the flexible endoscope is that the surgeon can directly view areas of the body that previously were not seen except through a surgical incision. The fiberoptic bundle can curve light and magnify the focal point at the tip of the scope.

When offering the surgeon instruments, the scrub should consider the body planes as well as the wound depth. The depth of the wound is one of the most important features in determining whether long or extra-long instruments will be needed. Recall from Chapter 16 that one of the technical goals of surgery is to handle tissue as little as possible. Surgical instruments are extensions of the surgeon's hands and allow the surgeon to manipulate tissue with minimal manual contact, which may cause unnecessary damage to the tissue. Long instruments allow the surgeon to place the hands at the margin of the wound while the tips of the instruments work deep inside. It is the scrub's responsibility to watch and anticipate the need for long instruments as the procedure progresses.

NOTE: Specialty instruments are discussed within each specialty surgery chapter.

CHAPTER SUMMARY

- Expertise in surgical instrumentation is among the most important roles of the surgical technologist. This role combines knowledge with excellent manual and observational skills.
- Critical thinking as it applies to surgical instrumentation means applying knowledge of an instrument's capabilities, structure, design, size, and type to the surgical task at hand.
- Surgical-grade instruments are high quality instruments constructed of stainless steel and other metal alloys, such as carbon and chromium, that resist marring, pitting, scratching, and dulling.
- Floor-grade instruments are intended for use in noncritical applications such as suture and suture-removal kits in the emergency department. These instruments are often classified single-use items.
- Burnished or satin-finished metal instruments prevent glare on the surgical field. Ebony is a black chromium finish used for laser surgery. The dull black finish prevents laser beams from reflecting or bouncing off the instruments, which could injure or destroy nearby tissues.
- The locking clamp (box lock) has one or more ratchets that remain closed after they are set.
- Thumb forceps are used to grasp tissue. For example, when suturing, the surgeon holds the forceps in one hand and the needle holder in the other.
- The biting clamp has teeth, cutting edges, or serrations in the jaws. An example of this type of instrument is the Kocher clamp. An atraumatic clamp usually has locking ratchets, but the tips do not close tightly over the tissue. This type of clamp is used on delicate tissue that is highly vascular or easily injured.

- An occluding clamp blocks the flow of blood. The hemostat is the most common example.
- A semioccluding vascular clamp is capable of varying low levels of compression between its jaws.
- A rongeur is used to cut and extract tissue. The tips are cupped and have sharp edges.
- Shears are large cutting instruments used to cut bone. Some shears are designed so that the cutting edge is left or right of the hinge.
- A curette is used in many different specialties for scooping out tissue.
- A chisel is an orthopedic cutting instrument that is used with a mallet (similarly used in sculpting or carpentry). An osteotome has two beveled sides, whereas the chisel blade is sloped on one side only.
- As the surgical wound is deepened, tissue layers and other structures (e.g., blood vessels, nerves, organs, and other tissue) must be gently moved away from the focal point of the operation. A retractor is used to perform this task.
- Dilators are used to widen or stretch the inside diameter of a lumen. A probe also is used for hollow tissue but is used to detect an obstruction or to follow a hollow tract.
- The selection of a surgical instrument is based on the tissue, the depth of the surgical wound, the technical requirements of the instrument, and the surgeon's preference or experience.
- The viscera (organs of the body) is covered by a fine membrane. Nontraumatic instruments are needed in the handling of this tissue.
- Tissues such as the liver, spleen, and lungs normally are friable. These tissues must be handled with nontraumatic instruments or with the hand.

- When the spleen, liver, and intestines are retracted, the surface area of the retractor must be sufficiently wide to distribute the pressure.
- Clamps used on the intestine, fallopian tubes, vas deferens, ureters, large blood vessels, and other ducts are only partly occlusive. The tips of the grasping instruments do not approximate tightly, as do those of a hemostat.

REVIEW QUESTIONS

1. What is the relationship between the characteristics of a particular type of tissue and the instruments that are used on that tissue?
2. On what types of tissue would you *not* use an instrument with teeth (one that punctures)?
3. What is the advantage of having a right-angled instrument?
4. What are the most efficient ways to learn the names of surgical instruments?
5. What types of tissue are friable?
6. Describe a tenaculum.
7. List the correct scalpel blade numbers and their handles.
8. How would you protect the cutting edges of instruments from damage during surgery?
9. What is the function of a self-retaining retractor?
10. Describe your personal plan for learning the names and uses of instruments.

CASE STUDIES

Case 1

As a student, you are scrubbed on a large case. Your preceptor has shown you which instruments will be needed during the case. As the preceptor names the instruments, you remember only a few of the names. To make matters more difficult, the preceptor does not tell you the technical name of the instruments but refers to them by the nicknames used at this hospital. How will you scrub on this case? What strategy might you use to pass the correct instrument even though you do not know the name?

Case 2

You are scrubbed on a large case. Loud music is playing, and it is difficult to hear the surgeon's requests for instruments. You know the instruments but have not had much experience with them. You make many mistakes, and the surgeon becomes irritated. What will you do?

Case 3

You have finished a case and are now preparing supplies to be taken to the decontamination area for processing. You have placed all instruments in appropriate containers for repro-cessing and discarded disposable and sharp items in the correct disposal containers. You are about to take your case cart to the decontamination area when the circulator asks whether you have a particular part for an instrument. You realize that you have discarded it in the sharps box, thinking it was disposable. What is the proper action?

Case 4

You have opened a case and are now scrubbed, preparing instruments for the start of surgery. Among the sterile goods is a complex instrument that you have not seen before. The instrument has been disassembled for sterilization, and you must now put it together. Little time is left, and you have 12 separate parts to assemble. What is the correct action? Consider the importance of not wasting operating time, the need for your attention at the sterile field, and prioritization of your time.

Case 5

The surgeon asks for a particular instrument during a stressful procedure. You pass the instrument she requested. She states, "Don't give me what I ask for, give me what I need here." What does this mean?

BIBLIOGRAPHY

Nilsen E: Managing equipment and instruments in the operating room, *AORN Journal* 81:349, 2005.

Spry C: *Care and handling of basic surgical instruments, AORN Journal* 86:S77, 2007.

Surgical Instrument Manufacturers and Catalogs
Aesculap Inc., USA at http://www.aesculapusa.com
C.R. Bard at http://www.bardurological.com
Codman & Shurtleff, Inc. at http://www.codman.com
Cook Medical at http://www.cookmedical.com
Gyrus ACMI at http://www.gyrusacmi.com
Jarit Instruments at http://www.jarit.com
Karl Storz Instruments at http://www.karlstorz.com
Katena Products, Inc. at http://www.katena.com
Medtronic, Inc. at http://www.medtronic.com
Olympus Surgical at http://www.olympussurgical.com
Sklar Instruments at http://www.sklarcorp.com
Snoden-Pencer at http://www.cardinalhealth.com
Storz at http://www.karlstorz.com
Stryker at http://www.stryker.com
V. Mueller at http://www.cardinal.com

CHAPTER 23

General Surgery

CHAPTER OUTLINE

SECTION I: ABDOMINAL WALL SURGERY

LEARNING OBJECTIVES

After studying this section the reader will be able to:

- Define the abdominal regions
- Recognize and name specific abdominal incisions
- Associate specific incisions with exposure to abdominal organs

- Describe the tissue layers of the anterior abdominal wall
- Differentiate between types of hernias
- Describe the operative principles of hernia repair

TERMINOLOGY: ABDOMINAL WALL SURGERY

Abdominal peritoneum: The serous membrane lining the walls of the abdominal cavity. The *retroperitoneum* is the posterior aspect. In surgical discussions, *abdominal* usually refers to the anterior aspect.

Direct inguinal hernia: A hernia that results from an acquired weakness in the inguinal floor.

Epigastric: A term referring to the region of the abdomen above the umbilicus.

Evisceration: Protrusion of the viscera outside the body as a result of trauma or wound disruption.

Fascia: In the abdomen, a tough, fibrous tissue layer between the parietal peritoneum and muscle layers.

Fistula: An abnormal tract or passage leading from one organ to another or from an organ to the skin; usually caused by infection.

Hernia: A protrusion of tissue under the skin through a weakened area of the body wall.

Hesselbach triangle: The area bounded by the rectus abdominis muscle, the inguinal ligament, and the inferior epigastric vessels. This region is most commonly associated with inguinal hernias.

Hypogastric: A term referring to the region of the abdomen below the stomach.

Incarcerated hernia: Herniated tissue that is trapped in an abdominal wall defect. Incarcerated tissue requires emergency surgery to prevent ischemia and tissue necrosis.

Incisional hernia: The postoperative herniation of tissue into the tissue layers around an abdominal incision. This may occur in the immediate postoperative period or later, after the incision has healed.

Indirect inguinal hernia: A hernia that protrudes into the membranous sac of the spermatic cord. This condition usually is due to a congenital defect in the abdominal wall.

Linea alba: A strip of avascular tissue that follows the midline and extends from the pubis to the xyphoid process.

McBurney incision: An incision in which the oblique right muscle is manually split to allow removal of the appendix.

Mesh: A pliable synthetic or biosynthetic material used to bridge the tissue edges of the abdominal wall. It is used during hernia repair.

Paramedian incision: An abdominal incision lying parallel to the midline.

Pelvic cavity: The lower abdominal cavity, which contains the bladder, uterus, and adnexa.

Pfannenstiel incision: A transverse incision below the umbilicus and just above the pubis; it generally is used for pelvic surgery.

Quadrants: Four designated regions of the abdomen.

Reduce: To replace or push herniated tissue back into its normal anatomical position.

Strangulated hernia: A hernia in which abdominal tissue has become trapped between the layers of an abdominal wall defect. The strangulated tissue usually becomes swollen as a result of venous congestion. Lack of blood supply can lead to tissue necrosis.

Subcostal: A term referring to the area of the abdomen that follows the slope of the tenth costal cartilage. A subcostal incision is made in this area.

Subcutaneous tissue: The fatty (adipose) tissue layer lying directly under the skin of the abdominal wall and other areas of the body.

Transverse incision: An incision that is perpendicular to the midline of the body.

Ventral hernia: A weakness in the abdominal wall, usually resulting in protrusion of abdominal viscera against the peritoneum and abdominal fascia.

Viscera: The organs or tissue of the abdominal cavity.

INTRODUCTION TO GENERAL SURGERY

The category of general surgery encompasses procedures of the abdomen and noncosmetic procedures of the breast. The organs and organ systems involved include the following:

- Abdominal wall
- Gastrointestinal system
- Biliary system (the gallbladder and associated structures)
- Spleen
- Pancreas
- Hepatic system
- Breast (noncosmetic procedures)

Although these regional systems remain in the category of general surgery, the trend increasingly is toward specialization. This is particularly true for bariatrics (the medical and surgical treatment of morbid obesity) and breast and gastrointestinal surgery.

General surgery also may include superficial procedures, which rarely extend deeper than the subcutaneous tissue, such as excision of common skin lesions (e.g., lipomas, sebaceous cysts) and other minor lesions.

INTRODUCTION TO THE ABDOMEN

The body is divided into semiclosed compartments, or cavities, that contain specific anatomical structures and organs (Figure 23-1, Table 23-1). The cavities are separated by membrane, muscle, and other connective tissue. The *abdominal cavity* contains the abdominal **viscera** (organs). The **pelvic cavity** contains structures of the reproductive, genitourinary, and lower gastrointestinal systems. The *retroperitoneal cavity* contains the kidneys, adrenal glands, and ureters. The anterior abdominal cavity is separated from the retroperitoneal cavity by the posterior abdominal peritoneum.

SURGICAL ANATOMY

ABDOMINAL QUADRANTS AND SECTIONS

The abdomen is divided into four major sections, or landmarks, called **quadrants** (Figure 23-2). Quadrants are often mentioned as the general location of a medical finding or anatomical structure. For example, a medical report may state, "The patient presented with tenderness in

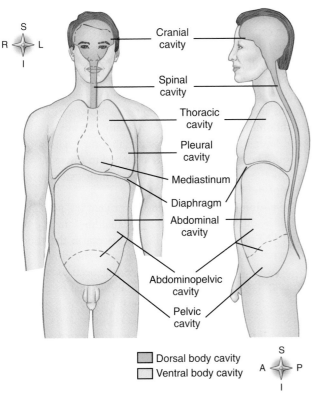

Figure 23-1 The major body cavities. (See Table 23-1 for the organs contained in individual cavities.) *(From Thibodeau G, Patton K: Anatomy and physiology, ed 6, St Louis, 2007, Mosby.)*

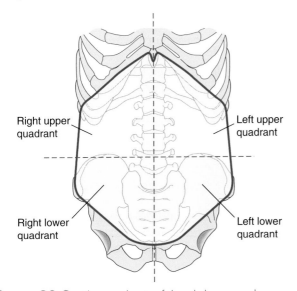

Figure 23-2 The quadrants of the abdomen and associated organs. *(From Garden O, Bradbury A, Forsythe J, Parks R: Principles and practice of surgery, ed 5, Edinburgh, 2007, Churchill Livingstone/Elsevier.)*

the right upper quadrant." The quadrants are named by location:

- Right upper quadrant (RUQ)
- Left upper quadrant (LUQ)
- Right lower quadrant (RLQ)
- Left lower quadrant (LLQ)

Table 23-1

Organs of the Ventral Body Cavities

Body Cavity	Organs
Thoracic cavity	
Right pleural cavity	Right lung
Mediastinum	Heart
	Trachea
	Right and left bronchi
	Esophagus
	Thymus gland
	Aortic arch and thoracic aorta
	Venae cavae
	Lymph nodes and thoracic duct
Left pleural cavity	Left lung
Abdominal cavity	
Right upper quadrant	Liver
	Gallbladder
	Colon
	Portions of the small intestine
Left upper quadrant	Stomach
	Pancreas
	Spleen
	Colon
	Portions of the small intestine
Retroperitoneal cavity	Kidneys
	Adrenal glands
	Descending aorta
	Ureters
Pelvic cavity	Ureters
	Uterus and adnexa (female)
	Prostate gland (male)
	Urethra
	Urinary bladder
	Sigmoid colon
	Rectum

The abdomen is divided into nine regions by an imaginary grid made by two vertical and two horizontal lines (Figure 23-3):

- Left and right hypochondriac regions: Rib area
- Left and right lumbar regions: Flank area
- Left and right iliac regions: Inguinal area
- **Epigastric** region: Upper abdomen (literally, "above the stomach")
- Umbilical region: Area near the umbilicus
- **Hypogastric** region: Lower abdomen ("below the stomach")

TISSUE LAYERS OF THE ABDOMINAL WALL

The abdominal wall encloses the ventral (front) part of the abdominal cavity and extends from the diaphragm to the pubis. It is composed of distinct tissue layers, which support the viscera; these layers comprise the following:

- Skin
- Subcutaneous fatty tissue (often called "sub-cu")
- **Fascia**

- Muscle
- Peritoneum

The fatty and skin layers are contiguous; the muscles cross each other and attach at different levels in the fascia. The *subcutaneous* layer lies directly under the skin. It is composed of lobulated adipose (fat), which varies in thickness from $\frac{1}{4}$ inch (0.63 cm) to more than 8 inches (20 cm).

The muscles and fascia of the abdominal wall protect the abdominal viscera. They move the upper body in flexion and rotation. The muscles also assist in respiration and in "bearing down" during defecation and childbirth. Two longitudinal

rectus muscles attach from the pubis to the fifth, sixth, and seventh *costal* (rib) cartilages. Lateral to the rectus muscles are the three flanking muscles: the transverse external oblique, internal oblique, and transverse abdominis muscles. These extend in several different directions, which increases support to the abdominal wall. The muscle groups are interrupted by tendons and surrounded by deep fascia, subserous fascia, and the abdominal peritoneum. The rectus sheath is a broad fascial layer that extends across the abdomen without interruption. The rectus muscles are attached to the rectus sheath close to the midline, or **linea alba,** which extends the full length of the midline (Figure 23-4).

The **abdominal peritoneum** (also called the *parietal peritoneum*) is a strong serous membrane that lines the abdominal cavity. The peritoneum protects the viscera in the abdomen and secretes serous fluid, which lubricates the viscera, allowing them to slide over each other easily. Sections of peritoneum fold back to connect the abdominal organs. The *mesentery* is an extension of the peritoneum that attaches to the posterior abdominal wall and fans out to cover the small intestine. The *greater omentum* is another extension of the serous membrane covering the stomach, duodenum, and part of the colon. These extensions are often referred to as *peritoneal reflections.*

INGUINAL REGION

The muscles, ligaments, and fasciae of the inguinal and femoral (groin) regions are more complex than those of the central and upper abdomen. A basic understanding of the tissue layers can best be acquired by studying the illustrations included here.

As the fascial layers continue into the pelvis, they pass in front of the two rectus muscles. Here the inguinal canal splits

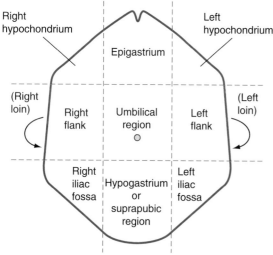

Figure 23-3   The nine regions of the abdomen. *(From Garden O, Bradbury A, Forsythe J, Parks R:* Principles and practice of surgery, *ed 5, Edinburgh, 2007, Churchill Livingstone/Elsevier.)*

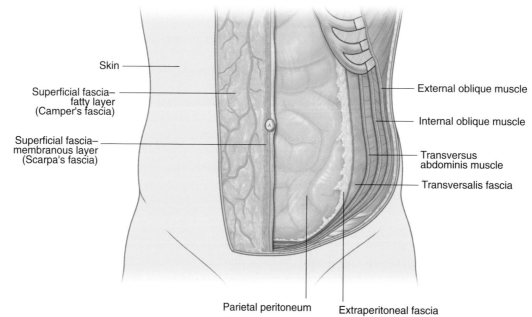

Figure 23-4   The layers of the abdominal wall. *(From Drake R, Vogel W, Mitchell A:* Gray's anatomy for students, *Edinburgh, 2004, Churchill Livingstone.)*

between the muscle layers near the inguinal ligament. The inguinal canal originates at an opening in the transversalis fascia at the deep inguinal ring and continues to the superficial inguinal ring. The *Hesselbach triangle* is the area bounded by the rectus abdominis muscle, the inguinal ligament, and the inferior epigastric vessels. This is the area associated with an inguinal hernia (Figure 23-5). The space is larger in the male than in the female, which corresponds to the higher incidence of inguinal hernias in males.

The spermatic cord in the male follows the inguinal canal and contains the following structures:
- Spermatic fascia
- Cremaster muscle
- Genitofemoral nerve
- Ductus deferens
- Lymph vessels
- Testicular vein and artery

ABDOMINAL INCISIONS

Abdominal incisions are named according to their anatomical location (Figure 23-6 and Table 23-2). Surgical technologists should become familiar with the following incisions and the abdominal structures associated with them:
- Midline incision
- **Paramedian incision**
- **Subcostal** incision
- Flank incision
- Inguinal incision
- **McBurney incision**
- Lower **transverse incision (Pfannenstiel incision)**

PATHOLOGY OF THE ABDOMINAL WALL

The most common pathology of the abdominal wall is a **hernia**. This is a protrusion of tissue through a defect or weakness in the abdominal wall. The weakness may be caused by a congenital anomaly, previous surgery, or injury. Hernias most often occur in the inguinal and femoral regions. A hernia

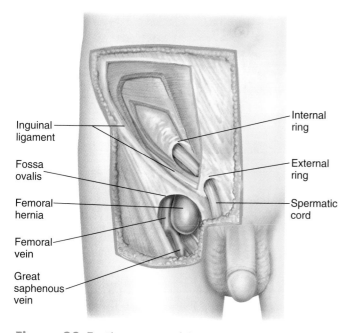

Figure 23-5   The anatomy of the inguinal region. *(From Seidel HM, Ball JW, Dains JE, Benedict GW: Mosby's guide to physical examination, ed 5, St Louis, 2002, Mosby.)*

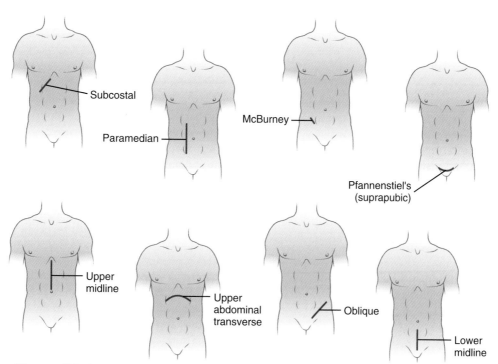

Figure 23-6   Incisions used in the abdominal wall. *(Modified from Rothrock JC: Alexander's care of the patient in surgery, ed 12, St Louis, 2003, Mosby.)*

Table 23-2

Types of Abdominal Incisions

Incision	Tissue Layers	Exposure	Details
Midline (upper and lower)	Skin Subcutaneous fat Fascia (linea alba) Abdominal peritoneum	Lower esophagus Stomach Small intestine Liver Biliary system Spleen Pancreas Proximal colon	A midline incision is made through the skin, subcutaneous fat, and the linea alba. This is the center of the fascial layer to which the rectus muscles attach; it is also an avascular area of the rectus sheath.
Paramedian (upper and lower)	Skin Subcutaneous fat Anterior rectus muscles Rectus fascia Abdominal peritoneum	*Right:* Biliary system Pancreas *Left:* Spleen Sigmoid colon	This is a muscle-splitting incision. It is less painful than a subcostal muscle-cutting incision for access to the upper quadrants.
Subcostal	Skin Subcutaneous fat Rectus muscles Fascia Abdominal peritoneum	*Right:* Biliary system Spleen Bilateral (chevron) Liver transplantation	This incision follows the lower rib margin in a semicurved shape; it is painful postoperatively.
McBurney	Skin Subcutaneous fat Fascia Oblique and transversalis muscles Abdominal peritoneum	Appendix	This incision is made on the right side, at an oblique angle, in the flank below the umbilicus; it is a muscle-splitting incision and offers only limited exposure.
Inguinal (oblique)	Skin Subcutaneous fat Fascia Muscle Ligaments Peritoneum	Muscles and fascia of the inguinal abdominal wall Spermatic cord Inguinal ring Abdominal ring Inferior epigastric artery and vein	This incision is used to gain access to the inguinal region for hernia repair; it also may be used for internal access to the spermatic cord.
Lower transverse abdominal (Pfannenstiel)	Skin Subcutaneous fat Rectus fascia Rectus muscles	Uterus Adnexa Bladder Access for cesarean section	This incision follows the natural skin folds to achieve cosmetic closure; it is very strong and offers good exposure to the pelvic contents.

may also occur along the linea alba, umbilicus, or an abdominal incision.

A hernia may require urgent surgical treatment when it causes pain or if the herniated tissue becomes trapped or strangulated by the surrounding tissue. This deprives the herniated tissue of its blood supply and may lead to necrosis. Table 23-3 lists common types of abdominal wall hernias.

DIAGNOSTIC PROCEDURES

Hernias are diagnosed through the findings of the physical examination, radiographs, ultrasound studies and in some cases CT scan.

PERIOPERATIVE CONSIDERATIONS

Surgery for repair of a hernia may be performed in the outpatient setting. Most patients arrive the day of surgery and can be discharged on the same day. Both open and minimally invasive surgical techniques are used.

The patient is placed in the supine position for procedures of the abdominal wall. Few procedures require a laparotomy. A retention Foley catheter may be inserted before surgery to decompress the bladder during repair of an inguinal or a femoral hernia. General or spinal anesthesia commonly is used.

INSTRUMENTS AND SUPPLIES

A laparotomy set is used for procedures involving the abdominal wall. Braided synthetic sutures and surgical mesh commonly are used to repair defects in the fascia. Monofilament suture may also be used. Most surgeons use a tapered needle, although surgical staples may also be used. Infected abdominal wounds generally are not closed beyond the fascial layer. However, heavy monofilament, synthetic retention sutures may be placed behind the line of incision.

Table 23-3

Pathology of the Abdominal Wall

Condition	Description	Considerations
Incisional hernia	Protrusion of abdominal tissue through one or more abdominal layers. This results from a previous abdominal incision which failed to heal completely or later broke down because of obesity, infection or disease.	May require mesh reinforcement to bridge and strengthen the tissue edges.
Strangulated hernia Incarcerated hernia	Tissue protruding from the hernia may become swollen and squeezed. This may result in local ischemia or other complications.	Strangulated hernia is an emergency condition requiring surgery to release the tissue and prevent ischemia and necrosis.
Indirect inguinal hernia	A hernia in which abdominal viscera slides into the inguinal canal from the deep inguinal ring. Herniated tissue may extend through the superficial ring in the spermatic cord into the scrotum or labia.	Usually caused by a congenital weakness in the inguinal ring. Surgery may be necessary.
Direct inguinal hernia	Protrusion of abdominal or inguinal tissue directly through the tranversalis fascia	The condition is usually acquired in older males.
Femoral hernia	A hernia arising from a weakness in the transversalis fascia below the inguinal ligament.	Occurs mainly in women and may require surgery to prevent incarceration.
Umbilical hernia	Abdominal wall defect occurring in the linea alba at the umbilical ring. Seen in infants and adults.	Rarely requires surgery. Incarceration is more common in obese adults.
Spigelian hernia	Rare hernia occurring between the transverse abdominis and rectus muscles.	Rarely diagnosed but seen occasionally during surgery for other reasons.

Surgical mesh is used for most hernia repairs (Figure 23-7). Biosynthetic mesh is made of synthetic material similar to suture (e.g., Prolene, Dacron, and Mersilene). The principle of mesh repair is to provide a bridge of strong material over the abdominal wall weakness and release tension on the tissue edges during repair and healing. During the remodeling phase of healing, scar tissue fills the spaces of the mesh in the same way that mesh fabric is used to hold new plant growth in bare soil.

Mesh is available in sheets or patches which are fitted at the edge of the defect (Figure 23-8). A patch usually is measured and cut during surgery, although precut patches are available.

SURGICAL PROCEDURES

OPEN REPAIR OF AN INDIRECT INGUINAL HERNIA

Surgical Goal

Open repair of an indirect inguinal hernia is performed to restore strength to the inguinal floor and prevent the abdominal viscera from entering the inguinal canal.

Pathology

An abdominal wall defect is an actual tear, an enlarged opening, or a weakened area in the abdominal wall. Defects can be congenital or acquired later in life. With an **indirect inguinal hernia,** the abdominal viscera protrude into the inguinal canal from the deep inguinal ring. In males, the herniated tissue can extend through the superficial ring, within the spermatic cord, and into the scrotum (male). In

females, the tissue can protrude into the labia. In both genders, the tissue can produce a bulge. Figure 23-9 shows the steps involved in the repair of an indirect inguinal hernia in a male.

Technique

1. A right or left inguinal incision is made.
2. The layers of the abdominal wall are incised, and the edges are retracted.
3. The spermatic cord is dissected from preperitoneal fat and other surrounding tissue.
4. The spermatic cord is retracted with a small Penrose drain.
5. The hernia sac is dissected from the cord and opened. The contents are pushed back into the abdomen.
6. The hernia sac is ligated with ties or a purse-string suture.
7. A synthetic mesh patch is sutured into place over the defect.
8. The abdominal wall is closed.

Discussion

The patient is placed in the supine position, prepped, and draped for a lower abdominal incision. The surgeon incises the skin over the groin using the skin knife. Both sharp and blunt dissection are used to separate the tissue layers and expose the hernia. Several hemostats can be placed on the edges of the fascia to retract it and expose the spermatic cord.

After identifying the cord, the surgeon carefully separates it from the hernia sac. Blunt dissection with a dry sponge is used to tease tissue from the surface of the cord. A small Penrose drain is used to retract the spermatic vessels and vas deferens (spermatic cord). The scrub should moisten the drain in saline before passing it to the surgeon. Dissection is

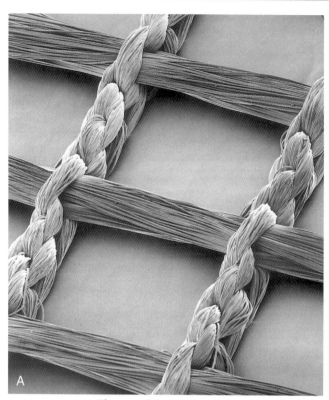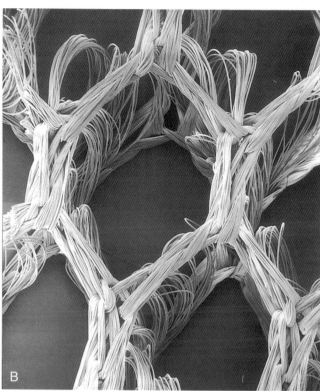

Figure 23-7 **A** and **B,** Enlarged view of mesh material. Newly formed tissue infiltrates through the weave to provide a strong bridge between layers of the abdominal wall. *(Copyright © 2008 Covidien. All rights reserved. Reprinted with the permission of Covidien.)*

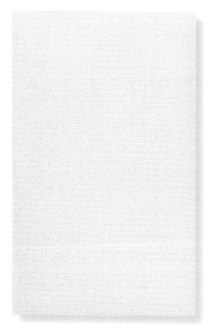

Figure 23-8 Fabric mesh for hernia repair. *(Copyright © 2008 Covidien. All rights reserved. Reprinted with the permission of Covidien.)*

continued to the level of the defect in the abdominal wall. The surgeon then uses Metzenbaum scissors to dissect the hernia sac away from the cord.

The hernia sac which opened, and the edges are grasped with hemostats. Using a finger or a dissector sponge mounted on forceps, the surgeon then pushes the contents of the sac back into the abdomen. If the defect is very small, it can be ligated. For large sacs, a purse-string suture of 2-0 synthetic absorbable material is placed around the neck of the sac. The excess neck tissue above the suture is cut away and removed as a specimen. An alternative method is to invert the sac imbricate (fold under) the edges with sutures.

If mesh is used to reinforce the defect, it is trimmed to match the size of the floor of the inguinal canal, and a small hole is made to allow the spermatic cord to emerge in its normal anatomical position. Precut mesh patches are also available. The edges of the mesh are secured with synthetic sutures or staples. The incision is then closed in multiple layers as follows:

1. *Fascia:* 2-0 nonabsorbable or absorbable synthetic suture
2. **Subcutaneous tissue:** 2-0 or 3-0 absorbable suture
3. *Skin:* Staples or 3-0 or 4-0 nonabsorbable suture

LAPAROSCOPIC REPAIR OF A DIRECT INGUINAL HERNIA

Two techniques are currently used for laparoscopic approach to a direct inguinal hernia:

- Transabdominal preperitoneal (TAPP) laparoscopy
- Total extraperitoneal (TEP) surgery

In the TAPP approach, a pneumoperitoneum is created, and the inguinal canal is entered via the abdominal cavity. In the TEP approach, instead of a pneumoperitoneum, the preperitoneal space is inflated with a balloon dissector, which expands the tissue planes (Figure 23-10).

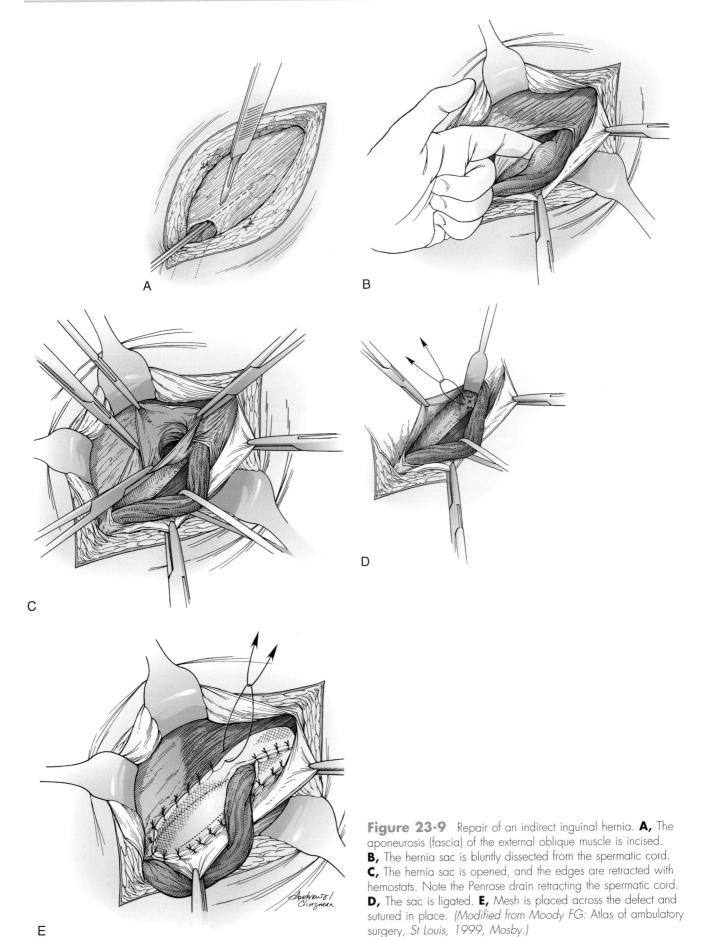

Figure 23-9 Repair of an indirect inguinal hernia. **A,** The aponeurosis (fascia) of the external oblique muscle is incised. **B,** The hernia sac is bluntly dissected from the spermatic cord. **C,** The hernia sac is opened, and the edges are retracted with hemostats. Note the Penrose drain retracting the spermatic cord. **D,** The sac is ligated. **E,** Mesh is placed across the defect and sutured in place. *(Modified from Moody FG: Atlas of ambulatory surgery, St Louis, 1999, Mosby.)*

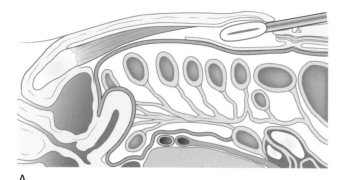

A

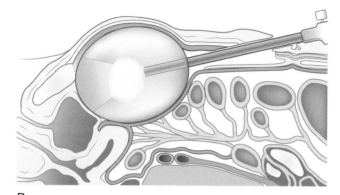

B

Figure 23-10 Repair of an inguinal hernia using a balloon expander. **A,** The expander is inserted into the extraperitoneal space. **B,** The balloon is expanded and the space maintained.

Surgical Goal

Laparoscopic direct hernia repair is the preferred technique to **reduce** herniated tissue and strengthen the inguinal floor. This procedure is less traumatic than open surgery and allows the patient to return to normal activity more quickly.

Pathology

A **direct inguinal hernia** arises from a defect behind the superficial inguinal ring in the inguinal floor, through the transversalis fascia. The defect is defined by an area called the **Hesselbach triangle,** which is bounded by the conjoint tendon, inguinal ligament, and inferior epigastric vessels. This is an acquired hernia that occurs most often in older men. Unlike with an indirect hernia, the protruding tissue rarely descends into the scrotum. The defect gradually becomes larger with age or obesity. Increased intraabdominal pressure ("bearing down") with heavy lifting or pulling can precipitate a large, painful direct hernia.

Technique

TAPP Procedure
1. Pneumoperitoneum is established, and trocars are inserted into the abdomen.
2. A transverse incision is made above the direct hernia space.
3. The weakened area in the pelvic floor is reinforced with mesh.
4. The peritoneum is closed.
5. Pneumoperitoneum is released, and the port incisions are closed.

Technique

TEP Procedure
1. A periumbilical incision is made through the rectus sheath.
2. Tissues are dissected manually and then retracted.
3. A balloon tissue expander is introduced.
4. The preperitoneal space is inflated, and the expander is removed.
5. A balloon trocar is inserted to seal the space.
6. Two additional 5-mm ports are created.
7. The direct or indirect hernia is reduced, and polypropylene mesh is secured over the defect.
8. The wounds are closed as for a transabdominal preperitoneal (TAPP) procedure.

Discussion

Transabdominal Preperitoneal Laparoscopy

For TAPP laparoscopy, pneumoperitoneum is established, and 5-mm ports are placed in the umbilicus and iliac regions. The laparoscope is inserted through the umbilical port.

The surgeon identifies the hernia and then grasps the hernia sac with endoscopic forceps or a grasper. A transverse (horizontal) incision is made in the peritoneum above the direct space with scissors, ESU, or an ultrasonic dissector. The peritoneum is retracted with right-angle retractors to expose the pelvic floor. Surgical mesh is introduced through the largest port. Surgical staples are used to attach the mesh to Cooper's ligament and to close the peritoneum. The pneumoperitoneum is released, and the fascial and skin layers are closed with 2-0 sutures or skin staples.

The technique for exposing a direct hernia is the same as for an indirect hernia. The hernia sac is incised or dissected from the spermatic cord with blunt dissection. Unlike in open surgical repairs, the sac is not ligated. Biosynthetic mesh is placed over the defect and stapled into place as for an indirect hernia. The pneumoperitoneum is released, and the wounds are closed with synthetic absorbable sutures and skin staples.

Total Extraperitoneal Surgery

For TEP surgery, the preparation of the patient is the same as for a TAPP procedure. However, pneumoperitoneum is not used in the TEP approach. Instead, the surgeon makes a small incision lateral to the midline, exposing the rectus muscle sheath. This opening is expanded with digital dissection. A balloon expander is inserted into the incision and inflated with air or normal saline. The balloon dissector is removed, and the space is maintained with gas insufflation.

Specially designed ports are available to seal the preperitoneal space. Two 5-mm trocars are inserted into the preperitoneal space. When all trocars are in place, the hernia is repaired as described previously.

OPEN REPAIR OF A FEMORAL HERNIA

Surgical Goal

Open repair of a femoral hernia is performed to reduces abdominal tissue (usually intestine) which has entered the femoral canal. The abdominal wall defect is closed to prevent recurrence.

Pathology

A femoral hernia arises from a defect in the transversalis fascia inferior to the inguinal ligament. The femoral ligament, artery, and nerve pass through the femoral canal which is usually tight enough to prevent abdominal viscera from entering this space. Multiple childbirth, obesity and inherent weakness in the abdominal wall can create a weakness in the fascia which can create herniation of abdominal tissue into the canal. It most often occurs in females and rarely in men.

Technique

1. The groin is incised on the affected side.
2. The hernia sac is identified and opened.
3. The sac is ligated and removed.
4. Synthetic mesh is secured over the defect.
5. The wound is closed in layers as for an inguinal hernia.

Discussion

The surgeon incises the groin and uses the ESU to extend the incision and control bleeding. Right-angle retractors are placed at each end of the wound. When the fascial layer has been incised, the outer membrane of the sac is elevated with curved hemostats, and a small incision is made with the scalpel or ESU. The incision then can be opened fully, allowing exploration of the sac. The contents of the sac are reduced.

The sac is then closed. The edges are grasped with small hemostats, and a purse-string suture is placed at the neck. The edges are trimmed and removed from the field as specimens, and the purse-string suture is then tightened. At this point, mesh may be sutured in place over the defect. All tissue layers are closed as described previously.

REPAIR OF AN INCISIONAL OR A VENTRAL HERNIA

Surgical Goal

The goal of **ventral hernia** repair is to remove a weak or infected scar in the abdominal wall and remodel the tissue with mesh bridge. Scar tissue lacks the organized blood supply of normal tissue and heals more slowly than normal tissue. Mesh may be used to repair a noninfected ventral hernia.

An **incisional hernia** sometimes develops if the wound becomes infected during the healing period. In advanced infection, a fistula may develop in the scar tissue. A **fistula** is a tract or tunnel through the tissue that develops a lining of epithelium. This is the same process that occurs in decorative body piercing (pierced ears or other skin). The constant drainage of pus prevents the fistula from healing, whereas newly injured tissue heals because fibrin and collagen cells at the site of injury join and weld the tissue together. Therefore the goal of fistula surgery is to remove the entire tract and its skin cells so that the newly "injured" tissue edges heal normally.

Pathology

A ventral hernia refers to any hernia occurring in the abdominal wall, excluding the groin or inguinal area. Ventral hernia often occurs as a result of previous abdominal surgery and is sometimes referred to as an incisional hernia. Abdominal wall weakness and herniation can be caused by

- Obesity with inherent weakness in the abdominal wall
- Previous or concurrent infection at the surgical site
- Extensive strain on the incision, often related to obesity
- Poor tissue healing as a result of metabolic disease, such as diabetes or alcoholism
- Repeat operations in the same location

If the tissue is infected at the time of primary closure, normal healing is delayed. When the incision does heal, the edges are not well integrated into the peripheral tissue, and the area becomes weak. Obesity or excessive strain on the incisional line pulls the weak tissue apart. As the incision line becomes weaker, the abdominal viscera are pushed through the defect. Small tracts containing fat and scar tissue are painful and can lead to further infection or strangulation. The bands of tissue are removed to prevent a recurring hernia.

If the abdominal wall ruptures (or is torn through trauma), the viscera can protrude outside the body. This condition is called an **evisceration.**

Technique

1. The abdominal scar is removed, and the edges of the previous incision are trimmed.
2. Old sutures are removed.
3. Abdominal adhesions are separated from the viscera and the interior abdominal wall.
4. Synthetic mesh is secured over the abdominal defect.
5. All layers of the abdominal wall are closed.

NOTE: If the wound and tissue edges are infected, the peritoneum and fascia can be closed and the remaining layers left to heal by secondary intention, from the base of the wound to the surface.

Discussion

To begin the surgery, the surgeon places several Allis clamps on the abdominal scar. These are used to apply countertraction on the scar while it is incised, first with a skin knife and then with the ESU. The scrub retains the scar as a specimen.

Sutures from previous surgery are removed with a straight hemostat and scissors or knife. A folded towel placed near the incision is convenient for the surgeon to wipe the suture remnants from the hemostat.

After the sutures have been removed, the surgeon may attempt to re-establish normal tissue planes by trimming and reducing superficial fascia and fatty tissue. The surgeon remodels the edges of the incision, which usually are ragged and poorly defined. In most cases it is not necessary to perform a laparotomy to repair an incisional hernia unless adhesions (scar tissue that binds the abdominal viscera) must be released or the hernia originates from the abdominal peritoneum. Generally only the fascia requires reinforcement and repair.

Once the wound edges have been trimmed and the tissue layers clearly defined, the incision can be closed. A mesh bridge often is sutured or stapled across the edges of the deep fascia. The tissue layers are then closed with interrupted sutures and skin staples. Tension on the wound can be relieved by using a heavy continuous suture (e.g., polydioxanone suture) through all layers or by using retention sutures with bolsters as discussed in Chapter 17.

UMBILICAL HERNIA REPAIR

Surgical Goal

Umbilical hernia repair is performed to repair an abdominal wall defect in the periumbilical region.

Pathology

An umbilical hernia is the result of a defect in the linea alba at the umbilical ring. This hernia is most common in children and usually disappears spontaneously by age 2. In adults, the hernia appears more frequently in individuals with a high body mass index. The sac of an umbilical hernia frequently has a small base, which increases the risk of tissue strangulation.

Technique

1. A periumbilical incision is made.
2. The linea alba defect is identified.
3. The defect is dissected free of any tissue, and the musculofascial margins are identified.
4. The defect is repaired with sutures or mesh.
5. The wound is closed

Discussion

See discussion of the repair of a ventral hernia.

SPIGELIAN HERNIA REPAIR

Surgical Goal

Spigelian hernia repair is performed to reduce the protrusion of a peritoneal sac, preperitoneal fat, or other abdominal viscera through a defect in the abdominal wall called the *spigelian zone.*

Pathology

The spigelian zone is the area of muscle attachment between the transverse abdominis muscle and the lateral edge of the rectus muscle. Spigelian hernias are very rare and occur mainly in individuals over age 60. The condition often is discovered during surgery for other reasons.

Technique

1. A skin incision is made.
2. The hernia sac is identified and resected.
3. The contents of the sac are reduced into the peritoneal cavity.
4. The defect is repaired as for an inguinal hernia.

Discussion

The patient is placed in the supine position. A skin incision is made 0.8 inch (2 cm) above the symphysis pubis and extended through the external and internal oblique muscles and the transversalis muscle. The hernia sac is identified. The sac's contents are examined closely for ischemia, the sac is resected, and the contents are reduced into the peritoneal cavity. The defect is repaired using the same techniques as for inguinal and ventral hernias. During resection and reduction, the surgeon must identify a direct or an indirect hernia. During repair, the hernia between the muscle layers is incorporated into the suture line. Biosynthetic mesh may be required for support of larger defects.

SECTION II: GASTROINTESTINAL SURGERY

LEARNING OBJECTIVES

After studying this section the reader will be able to:

- Describe the surgical anatomy of the gastrointestinal system
- Identify common open and endoscopic procedures of the GI system
- Use appropriate terminology to describe GI surgical techniques
- Describe basic resection and anastomosis of the GI system

TERMINOLOGY: GASTROINTESTINAL SURGERY

Anastomosis: A surgical procedure in which two hollow structures are joined (see Table 23-1).

Billroth I procedure: A gastroduodenostomy, or surgical anastomosis, of the stomach and the duodenum.

Billroth II procedure: A gastroduodenostomy, or surgical anastomosis, of the stomach and the jejunum.

Bowel technique: A method of preventing cross-contamination between the bowel contents and the abdominal cavity.

Decompression: A technique or process in which the stomach contents are continually drained into a collection device. Decompression is required after gastric surgery or disease.

Esophageal varices: Distended veins of the esophagus, caused by advanced liver disease. The condition occurs as a result of portal vein obstruction arising from fibrosis of the liver. Esophageal varices may bleed profusely.

Exploratory laparotomy: A laparotomy performed to examine the abdominal cavity when less invasive measures fail to confirm a diagnosis.

Gastroesophageal reflux disease (GERD): A condition in which the gastroesophageal sphincter allows gastric contents to back-flow (reflux) into the esophagus, causing irritation and mucosal burning and possibly leading to cancer of the esophagus.

Gastrostomy: A surgical opening through the stomach wall connecting to the outside of the body or another hollow anatomical structure.

Hiatus: An opening in the diaphragm where the esophagus passes from the abdominal cavity.

Laparotomy: A procedure in which the abdominal cavity is surgically opened. The techniques used for laparotomy are used for all open surgical procedures of the abdomen.

Mobilize: To surgically free up an organ or other structure by dissecting its attachments to other tissue. Most tissues of the body are attached by serous membranes or connective tissue. Whenever tissue is removed or remodeled, these attachments must be freed up. This often includes dividing and ligating attached blood vessels. This is called *tissue mobilization.*

Morbid obesity: A condition in which the patient's body mass index (BMI) is 40 or higher, and the individual is at least 100 pounds (45 kg) over the ideal weight despite aggressive attempts to lose weight.

Nasogastric (NG) tube: A flexible tube inserted through the nose and advanced into the stomach. The NG tube is used to decompress the stomach or to provide a means of feeding the patient liquid nutrients and medication.

-Ostomy: A suffix that refers to an opening between two hollow organs; for example, *gastroduodenostomy,* a surgical procedure that joins the stomach and duodenum.

Ostomy: A technique in which a new opening is made between a tubular structure such as the intestine or ureter and the outside of the body or another hollow structure or organ.

Percutaneous endoscopic gastrostomy (PEG): The insertion of a tube into the stomach for enteral feedings or gastric decompression.

Resection: Surgical removal of an organ (see Table 23-1).

Stoma: An opening created in a hollow organ and sutured to the skin to drain the organ's contents (e.g., an intestinal or ureteral stoma). A stoma may be a temporary or permanent method of bypass.

Stoma appliance: A two- or three-piece medical device used to collect drainage from a stoma. The appliance is attached to the patient's skin and completely covers the stoma. This allows free drainage into a collection device or bag.

INTRODUCTION

Gastrointestinal surgery includes procedures of the lower esophagus, stomach, small intestine, large intestine, rectum, and anus. Newer technologies and instruments now provide surgical interventions that are much less traumatic and more effective than in the past.

SURGICAL ANATOMY

ESOPHAGUS

The esophagus is a tubular structure that extends from the pharynx to the stomach. Food travels along its length by a combination of voluntary and involuntary muscle action. The esophagus enters the abdominal cavity at the level of the diaphragm. In the adult, it measures approximately 10 inches (25 cm).

STOMACH

The stomach is located just under the diaphragm in the left upper abdomen. The three contiguous anatomical sections of the stomach are the *fundus* (upper portion), the *body* (midsection), and the *antrum* (distal or lower portion).

The wall of the stomach contains an outer serosa, two inner layers of smooth (involuntary) muscles, and a submucosal lining. Two orifices (openings) provide continuity between the esophagus and the duodenum. These are the *cardia,* which communicates with the esophagus, and the *pylorus,* which opens into the duodenum.

A sheet of connective and vascular tissue, called *omentum,* attaches to the greater and lesser curvatures of the stomach. Whenever a portion of the stomach is removed or remodeled, the omentum must be divided from its attachments.

SMALL INTESTINE

The small intestine is the proximal portion of the intestinal tract. It extends from the pylorus of the stomach to the proximal end of the large intestine. The small intestine has three anatomical sections: the duodenum, the ileum, and the jejunum.

The duodenum is approximately 8 to 10 inches (20 to 25 cm) long. It receives *chyme* (liquefied food broken down by the stomach). The pancreatic duct (*duct of Wirsung*) and the common bile duct from the liver drain their contents into this section of the intestine.

The jejunum is approximately 9 feet (2.7 m) long. It connects with the ileum, which is approximately 13.5 feet (4 m) long. These sections are suspended from the abdominal wall by a sheet of vascular tissue called the *mesentery,* which supplies blood and lymph to the lower sections of the small intestine. During **resection** of the jejunum or the ileum, the mesentery must be clamped and divided from the intestine.

The tissue layers of the small intestine are similar to those of the stomach and large intestine. The inner surface of the small intestine has small, fingerlike projections called *villi,* which increase the surface area of the intestinal lumen and contain blood and lymphatic vessels. The small intestine terminates at the *cecum,* the first portion of the large intestine.

LARGE INTESTINE (COLON)

The large intestine extends from the distal ileum to the rectum and is divided into five distinct sections: the ascending colon, the transverse colon, the descending colon, the sigmoid colon, and the rectum. The colon measures about 5 feet (1.5 m) in the adult.

As mentioned previously, the first section of the large intestine is a blind pouch called the *cecum*. The terminal end of the cecum has a slender tube, called the *vermiform appendix*, which has no function and can become infected. The ascending colon extends upward behind the right lobe of the liver. The transverse colon then crosses the abdomen to the left, below the stomach. The descending colon extends downward on the left side of the abdomen and terminates at the sigmoid colon, which lies in the pelvic cavity. The sigmoid colon terminates at the rectum.

RECTUM AND ANUS

The distal 4 to 5 inches (10 to 12.5 cm) of the intestine is the *rectum,* which terminates at the *anal canal.* This section is lined with folded tissue. Two muscular sphincters in the anal canal control the release of feces to the outside of the body. The internal sphincter is composed of involuntary (smooth) muscle. The external sphincter is under voluntary control (striated muscle). The opening of the anal canal is called the *anus.*

Figure 23-11 illustrates the sections of the gastrointestinal system.

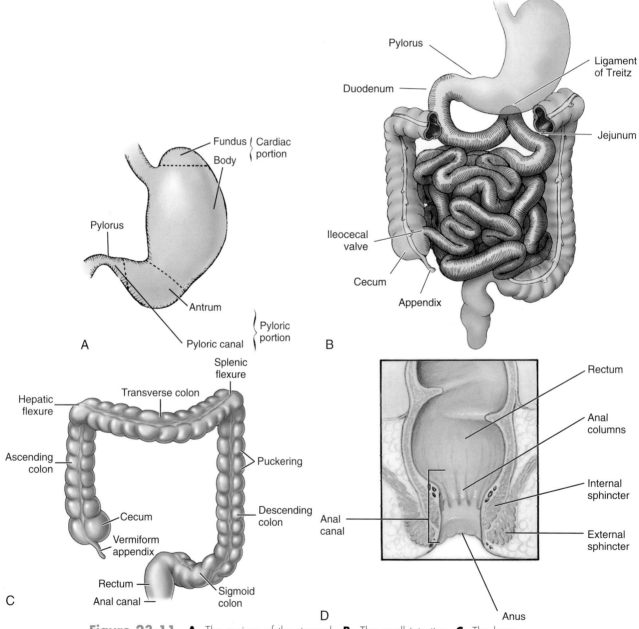

Figure 23-11 **A,** The regions of the stomach. **B,** The small intestine. **C,** The large intestine. **D,** The sigmoid colon, rectum, and anal canal. (**A** *and* **B** *modified from Rothrock JC: Alexander's care of the patient in surgery, ed 12, St Louis, 2003, Mosby;* **C** *modified from Herlihy B, Maebius NK: The human body in health and illness, ed 2, Philadelphia, 2003, WB Saunders; and* **D** *modified from Applegate EJ: The anatomy and physiology learning system, ed 2, Philadelphia, 2000, WB Saunders.)*

PATHOLOGY OF THE GASTROINTESTINAL SYSTEM

Table 23-4 describes various diseases and conditions that can affect the gastrointestinal system.

DIAGNOSTIC PROCEDURES

The presence of GI disease is confirmed primarily by imaging studies, blood and metabolic studies, and physical examination. Endoscopy (described later) often is performed before open or laparoscopic surgery. Biopsy and visual examination of the inner surface of the intestine and stomach are performed to rule out or confirm carcinoma and provide tissue for further tests. Contrast studies performed under fluoroscopy frequently are done to outline the GI structures. Other important imaging tools are magnetic resonance imaging (MRI), ultrasound, and computed tomography (CT).

CARE OF THE PATIENT

Positioning

During laparotomy and laparoscopy, patients are at high risk for hypothermia. Therefore thermoregulation is a high priority for patient safety during all abdominal procedures. A forced air warming system is used. Irrigation solutions are maintained in a solution warmer. Exposure of the patient is kept to a minimum in the perioperative period, and the patient is covered with warm blankets before and after surgery. Compression stockings or a sequential compression device is used during all lengthy laparotomy procedures to prevent deep vein thrombosis (DVT).

The patient is placed in the supine position for most laparoscopic and open surgery of the GI system. Exceptions are procedures that require perineal access, such as abdominoperineal resection. In these cases, the low lithotomy position may be used. The patient's arms are placed on armboards. The operating table is tilted into normal or reverse Trendelenburg position, depending on the anatomical exposure required during the procedure.

Patients undergoing surgery for morbid obesity require particular attention to safety during positioning. The operating table must be able to accommodate up to 800 pounds (360 kg). Extensions must be well padded, and great care must be taken in transferring the patient between the stretcher and the operating table.

Instruments

A basic laparotomy set is used for GI surgery. A separate GI set with clamps and grasping instruments is added; the clamps and graspers must be atraumatic and nonpenetrating (Figure 23-12). Vascular clamps may be required. Long instruments may be added, depending on the size of the patient.

Sharp dissection is performed with Metzenbaum scissors, an ESU, ultrasound shears (Harmonic system), and a high-frequency coagulator (LigaSure).

Babcock and Allis clamps are used to grasp intestinal tissue. Smooth or vascular forceps are used for suturing the mucosal layers. Resection of the bowel or stomach is performed with atraumatic clamps or with surgical stapling instruments. Atraumatic clamps do not close tightly over the tissue; rather, they leave a small amount of space to prevent crushing. Long intestinal clamps may be covered with soft rubber tubing to provide a snug seal on the tissue; these are generally referred to as *rubber-shod clamps*. Although they are not commonly used, some facilities may include them in a GI set.

When the bowel, omentum, and mesentery have been exposed, a Poole suction tip should be available. This tip has numerous openings, which prevents excess suction pressure on delicate tissue.

Surgical stapling instruments frequently are used in resection and **anastomosis.** These include systems that apply both linear and circumferential rows of staples.

Equipment and Supplies

Special equipment that might be required during GI surgery includes the following:

- High-frequency (HF) vessel-sealing system (e.g., LigaSure)
- Ultrasound scalpel
- Vessel loops for large vessel dissection
- Ultrasound probe
- Bowel bag (a plastic bag used to enclose the bowel during open surgery to prevent tissue dehydration)
- Temporary ostomy bag

Sutures

GI procedures require sutures or surgical staples for resection and anastomosis of the bowel, mesentery, and omentum. Suture closure usually is performed in two or three layers. Fine absorbable sutures (3-0 or 4-0) on a taper needle are used to close the mucosa and submucosa. The outer serosal layer can be closed with fine interrupted silk or synthetic material on a taper needle. Large vessels and vascular bundles are ligated with suture, surgical clips, or a vessel-sealing instrument (e.g., LigaSure). Large vessels of the omentum and mesentery often are secured with 0 or 2-0 suture ties.

TECHNIQUES IN GASTROINTESTINAL SURGERY

Many common techniques are used in gastrointestinal surgery. A surgical vocabulary has been developed that describes these (Table 23-5).

The GI system is a continuous "tube" attached to the abdominal and pelvic wall by a complex system of vascular membranes. These attachments limit the mobility of sections in the abdominal cavity and help prevent obstruction, especially in the intestine. To remodel a section of intestine or stomach, the surgeon must free up portions of these attachments (mesentery and omentum). This involves a technique of clamping the tissue, cutting it, and maintaining hemostasis. This called *mobilizing* the section (bowel or stomach).

The traditional method of mobilization involves clamping a section, ligating it with suture, and then incising it. Electro-

Table 23-4

Pathology of the Gastrointestinal System

Condition	Description	Considerations
Esophagus		
Cancer of the esophagus	Carcinoma of the esophagus often is related to combined alcohol and tobacco use or the diet. Esophageal cancer accounts for 6% of all gastrointestinal cancers.	Surgical resection of the esophagus is the most common treatment. Long-term survival rates are poor, because metastasis often occurs before the diagnosis is made. (See Transhiatal Esophagectomy.)
Diverticula	Diverticula are outpocketings (herniations) in the mucosa of the esophagus or intestine. This condition is acquired rather than congenital, and infection may result if substances are trapped in the pockets.	Esophageal diverticula, most commonly Zenker diverticula, may be treated surgically. (See Excision of an Esophageal Diverticulum.)
Esophageal varices	Esophageal varices are enlarged esophageal veins. In advanced disease, the veins may rupture, resulting in severe hemorrhage and death. The condition is caused by portal hypertension related to cirrhosis of the liver.	Severe cases may be treated with endoscopic injection of the veins with a sclerosing agent or a portal vein shunt.
Gastroesophageal reflux (GERD)	GERD is a backflow of gastric contents into the esophagus and throat, which results from a weak lower esophageal sphincter. It causes pain and eventual erosion of the esophageal mucosa.	Treatment is conservative in most cases unless the condition is severe. (See Transabdominal Hiatal Hernia Repair.)
Hiatal hernia	A hiatal hernia is a herniation of the stomach through an enlarged anatomical opening in the diaphragm. The defect causes the stomach to slide upward and may contribute to GERD.	Large hernias may be treated surgically. (See Transabdominal Repair of a Hiatal Hernia.)
Stomach		
Cancer	The risk of gastric carcinoma is increased by genetic predisposition and diet. Symptoms are usually absent until the disease is advanced.	Treatment is by subtotal or radical gastrectomy. (See Roux-en-Y Gastric Bypass.)
Omphalocele	An omphalocele is a congenital defect in which the abdominal contents are outside the body at birth.	See Chapter 34.
Helicobacter pylori infection	*H. pylori* infection is the most common cause of peptic ulcer, which is an erosion of the stomach mucosa and submucosa. *H. pylori* may be present in 50% of the population, but not all infections result in disease.	Antibiotics are effective for the treatment of *H. pylori* infection.
Noninfectious peptic ulcer	Peptic ulcers not caused by *H. pylori* are found in the stomach and duodenum. Erosion may penetrate to all layers of the tissue. Complications include obstruction, hemorrhage, and perforation.	The condition currently is treated medically with drugs that reduce the gastric acid content of the stomach. Surgical treatment is limited to emergencies involving hemorrhage or obstruction.
Trauma	Trauma of the stomach is extremely rare and usually is the result of intentional violence (e.g., knife wound or blunt trauma).	Surgical repair is indicated in laceration of the stomach.
Gastroschisis	Gastroschisis is a congenital defect that results in visceral herniation near the umbilicus.	See Chapter 34.
Small Intestine		
Crohn disease	Crohn disease is an inflammatory bowel disease that can occur anywhere in the gastrointestinal (GI) tract but is most common in the small intestine. Complications include ulceration, infection, fistula, and nutritional disorders.	Treatment is pharmacological and supportive, including nutritional therapy. Perforation or fistula requires routine bowel resection or repair.

Table 23-4

Pathology of the Gastrointestinal System—cont'd

Condition	Description	Considerations
Obstruction	*Obstruction* is a general term that encompasses a number of physical and chemical pathological conditions that prevent the intestinal contents from passing through the intestinal tract. Such conditions include volvulus, intussusception, and strangulation associated with a hernia.	Surgical treatment is required to prevent death of the intestinal tissue and peritonitis. (See Chapter 34 *Pediatrics*.)
Peptic ulcer	A peptic ulcer is an erosion and ulceration of the small intestine. It is commonly caused by *H. pylori* infection.	Medical treatment is successful for infection. If perforation occurs, emergency surgical intervention is necessary.
Trauma	Injury to the small intestine is rare; it usually is caused by intentional violence or by motor vehicle accidents.	Surgical repair of the intestine and surrounding attachments is performed as an emergency procedure. (See Laparotomy.)

Large Intestine, Rectum, and Anus

Condition	Description	Considerations
Colorectal cancer	Colorectal cancer is the second leading cause of cancer death in the United States. Carcinoma may be related to genetics, diet, or other environmental factors.	Prevention includes screening sigmoidoscopy and a test for occult fecal blood in adults over age 50.
Diverticular disease	Herniation of the intestinal mucosal layer through the muscularis layer. The disease most often occurs in the sigmoid colon and is almost certainly related to the diet found only in Western countries. It may cause infection or bowel perforation. Meckel's diverticulum occurs in the ileum as a rare congenital defect.	Treatment is conservative and involves attempts to change the diet. Severe cases of diverticulitis or those that result in perforation require bowel resection. The condition may be life threatening if perforation occurs. (See Partial Colectomy.)
Ulcerative colitis	Ulcerative colitis is a nonspecific inflammatory disease of the colon and rectum that is confined to this region. The disease creates deep crypts in the intestine, resulting in infection, bleeding, diarrhea, and pain. These patients are at high risk for bowel cancer.	The condition is treated with medications and management of symptoms. Surgery may be performed in severe cases. (See the discussion of abdominoperineal resection under Partial Colectomy.)
Intussusception	Intussusception is a rare condition that causes bowel obstruction, because one section of the intestine telescopes over another. It almost always occurs in children.	Emergency surgery is necessary to prevent bowel necrosis. (See Chapter 34.)
Hirschsprung disease	Hirschsprung disease is a congenital disease of the colon in which nerve tissue is absent. This results bowel obstruction in the neonate.	Surgical removal of the diseased bowel in the pediatric patient is indicated. (See Chapter 34.)
Polyps	Polyps are benign growths, found mainly in the rectosigmoid colon, that arise from the adenomatous tissue. They are caused by a defect in the growth pattern of normal tissue.	Polyps can be discovered on endoscopy and usually are removed for biopsy and to prevent progression to malignancy.
Hemorrhoids	Hemorrhoids are engorged veins of the rectal and sigmoid vascular plexus. The condition is related to increased venous pressure and genetic predisposition.	Surgery may be performed if conservative treatment fails to reduce the varicosities. (See Hemorrhoidectomy.)
Pilonidal cyst	A pilonidal cyst is a cyst of the sacrococcygeal area. The cause is unknown, but the condition may be related to improper development of hair follicles. Chronic infection of the cyst requires surgical treatment.	Surgical treatment includes excision and drainage of the cyst and removal of the fistulous tract. (See Excision of a Pilonidal Cyst.)

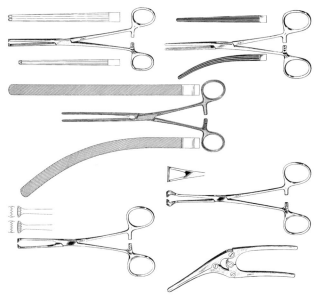

Figure 23-12 Gastrointestinal clamps. *Top, left to right:* Allen clamp, Bainbridge clamp. *Center:* Doyen clamp. *Bottom left:* Allis clamp. *Bottom right, top to bottom:* Babcock clamp, Payr clamp. *(Courtesy Jarit Instruments, Hawthorne, NY.)*

surgery commonly has been used to coagulate bleeders and to incise the tissue. However, newer energy modalities have replaced some of the traditional techniques. Ultrasonic technology is used to cut and coagulate tissue simultaneously. Vessel-sealing systems are used to coagulate tissue bundles and blood vessels (see Chapter 19). Surgical stapling devices are commonly used in GI surgery and often replace the clamping, cutting, and suturing techniques required in resection and mobilization (see Chapter 16).

ANASTOMOSIS

Anastomosis is the joining of two hollow structures by sutures, staples, or a combination of both. In GI surgery, anastomosis can be performed between any structures of the system. The suffix *–ostomy* means anastomosis. So, for example, a gastro-duodenostomy is an anastomosis between the stomach and duodenum. A duodenoduodenostomy is the removal of a section of duodenum and rejoining of the two limbs, or open ends of the duodenum. Ileostomy refers to an opening made between the ileum and the outside abdominal wall for drainage.

Anatomosis was historically performed using a technique in which two or even three layers of sutures were placed in a

Table 23-5

Surgical Techniques Used for the Gastrointestinal System

Term or Technique	Definition	Example
Resection (*verb:* resect)	A procedure in which a section of an organ is cut apart or removed.	A portion of the intestine is removed. If one of the free ends is surgically closed as a blind end, it is called a *stump*.
Anastomosis (*verb:* anastomose)	A procedure in which two hollow organs are joined surgically.	Placing sutures around the circumference of the two cut edges can join two hollow structures. This applies to portions of the gastrointestinal (GI) system and other hollow systems, such as blood vessels and organ ducts.
Division (*verb:* divide)	In surgery, a procedure in which one section of tissue is cut away from another. This differs from *resection*, in which a portion of the organ is removed.	Recall that the small intestine is attached to the mesentery, a loose connective tissue containing many major blood vessels. When a section of small intestine is removed, the mesentery must be divided from the intestine to free up the section.
Cross-clamp	To place one or more clamps at a right angle to a tube or vessel.	The "cross" simply refers to the angle of the clamp in relation to the organ or tissue.
Double-clamp	To place two clamps over a section of tissue to prevent bleeding when the tissue is severed.	Double-clamping is performed before a tissue that might bleed profusely is divided or cut. In the case of the GI structures, a section of intestine or stomach must be double-clamped before it is cut. This prevents hemorrhage and the release of fluids from the intestine or stomach.
Mobilization (*verb:* mobilize)	The freeing up of tissue from its attachments before anastomosis or resection.	No tissues in the body are free floating. Blood and lymph vessels, connective tissue, and membranes nourish and protect tissue. To remove tissue or to reconstruct the anatomy, the tissue must be removed from its normal attachments. Mobilization requires dissection or division.
Clamp and divide	To both double-clamp and divide tissue. Because the purpose of the clamps is to prevent bleeding, the tissue inside the jaws of the clamp must be sealed with the electrosurgical unit (ESU) or with suture ties.	During mobilization of the intestine, the surgeon repeatedly applies two hemostatic clamps, divides the tissue, and seals the tissue with the ESU or ties the cut ends. For the scrub, the tools needed are: • Two hemostats (e.g., Kelly, Mayo, Crile) • ESU or tissue scissors • Two ties (if the ESU is not used) • Suture scissors (if ties are used)

circumference around the two hollow structures in order to join them. Stomach or intestinal clamps were used to bring the two structures together while suturing took place. This technique is still used today, although surgical staples are used more frequently. These techniques are illustrated and described below in the surgical procedures sections. No matter which technique is used to perform an anastomosis, efforts are made to prevent spillage of the GI contents into the wound and maintain aseptic technique.

BOWEL TECHNIQUE

In all procedures involving the intestine, special precautions are taken to prevent contamination of instruments and supplies by the bowel contents; this is known as **bowel technique.** During bowel technique, also known as *isolation technique,* instruments and supplies used while the bowel is open are kept separate from all other sterile items. Contaminated supplies are confined to the Mayo stand and a designated basin. Instruments on the back table are kept "clean" (uncontaminated), and no items are exchanged between the back table and the Mayo stand while the bowel is open. After closure of the bowel, all contaminated instruments and supplies are removed from the field.

Before the abdomen is closed, the surgical team dons fresh gloves (and possibly also fresh gowns, depending on the facility's protocol). Fresh sterile drapes are placed over those used during the first part of the procedure. Fresh sterile sponges, sutures, ESU instruments, and suction tips are opened for use during closure. Many scrubs set up a separate closure stand with the needed suture materials and instruments.

NOTE: Isolation technique historically has been used during procedures involving resection of metastatic tumors.

SURGICAL PROCEDURES

DIAGNOSTIC AND OPERATIVE ENDOSCOPY

Perioperative Considerations

Endoscopy is an outpatient procedure, and the surgery is performed with the patient under sedation. This can be provided in a dedicated GI clinic or in a location near the postoperative care unit. High-risk patients who require extensive physiological monitoring may require an anesthesia care provider and an extended recovery. In all cases, physiological monitoring includes cardiac monitoring and monitoring of oxygen saturation, respiratory function, blood pressure, and level of consciousness. Although not usually painful, endoscopy can be uncomfortable. With light or moderate sedation, patients are able to respond to commands, and the airway is maintained without artificial support.

Preparation for endoscopy includes a period of fasting or dietary restriction, depending on the extent and type of endoscopic procedure. Upper GI studies require limitations on oral intake. Lower GI endoscopy requires dietary restrictions and an enema, which the patient can self-administer the day before the procedure.

❖ *A complete discussion of the technology, handling, and reprocessing of fiberoptic endoscopes is presented in Chapter 21.*

Gastrointestinal endoscopy is performed for the following purposes:
- To establish or confirm a diagnosis by direct visualization and biopsy
- To perform selected surgical procedures (these are restricted to surgery in which bleeding is minimal and the risk for technical complications is low)
- To allow postoperative inspection of the surgical site from within the lumen of the GI tract and for screening

ESOPHAGODUODENOSCOPY

Esophagoduodenoscopy (EGD), is diagnostic endoscopy of the esophagus, stomach, and proximal duodenum. Specific goals are:
- Direct diagnostic observation of the inside of the esophagus and duodenum, with biopsy.
- Treatment of varices (varices are prone to frequent bleeding and sometimes require emergency treatment).
- Sclerotherapy of **esophageal varices** (a method of reducing varices by injecting a sclerosing agent directly into the vein to shrink it).
- Polyp removal (polyps are small, benign mucosal outgrowths in the lumen of the esophagus).
- Endoscopic **gastrostomy** for insertion of a feeding tube.
- Placement of a stent for an esophageal stricture.

Technique

1. The patient is positioned and sedated.
2. The endoscope is coated with water-soluble gel.
3. The endoscope is inserted into the mouth.
4. The scope is advanced, and the tissues are examined.
5. Instruments are passed through the scope at the head of the endoscope.
6. Specimens are withdrawn and retained by the scrub.

Discussion

Before the procedure, the scrub should ensure that the endoscope, video equipment, and data storage devices are in working order and ready for use.

The patient is sedated and placed in the lateral position. A small amount of lubricating gel is put on the tip of the scope, and a bite block is inserted into the patient's mouth. Anesthetic spray is applied to the pharynx.

The insertion tube (the distal end of the endoscope) is advanced slowly, and the tissues are examined. Real-time digital imaging is performed to view the anatomy (Figure 23-13). If biopsy samples are taken, the scrub passes biopsy instruments to the surgeon and helps thread the tip into the instrument port. A number of procedures may be initiated at this point.
- *Injection of esophageal varices:* The scrub prepares the sclerosing agent, which is injected through the endoscope after needle placement in the varicosity.

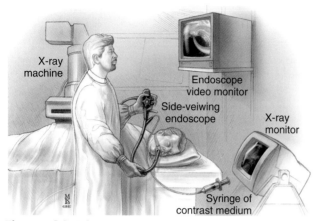

Figure 23-13 Esophagoduodenostomy with endoscopic retrograde pancreaticoduodenoscopy. *(Artwork is reproduced, with permission, from the Johns Hopkins Gastroenterology and Hepatology Resource Center. www.hopkins-gi.org, copyright 2008, Johns Hopkins University. All rights reserved.)*

- *Varicocele banding:* A special banding system is passed through the endoscope, and the varicosity is ligated.
- *Esophageal dilation:* Graduated dilators are introduced over a guide wire under fluoroscopy after endoscopic examination.
- *Insertion of an esophageal stent:* A self-expanding esophageal stent may be inserted to dilate and hold open a stricture caused by tumor. The stent is preloaded into an insertion device, which is threaded to the level of the stricture and released. It remains in place as a palliative measure.
- *Endoscopic laser therapy:* A neodymium-yttrium-aluminum garnet (Nd:YAG) laser may be used to debulk an esophageal tumor.

The scrub assists the surgeon by guiding long instruments into the endoscope and receiving them as they are withdrawn. Care must be taken to ensure that all specimens are immediately placed in the liquid specimen container, as directed by the surgeon. The specimen is cleaned from the biopsy forceps with a clean hypodermic needle or by swishing the tip in the specimen cup liquid.

If laser surgery is planned, all safety precautions are observed to prevent patient fires or burns (see Chapter 19).

At the close of the procedure, the scrub helps ensure that the patient is comfortable. Specimens are carefully labeled and recorded. Endoscopic equipment is cleaned and prepared for critical decontamination according to facility policy.

Postoperative considerations include monitoring for effective gag reflex, pain, and complete recovery from sedative drugs. The patient is taken to the postoperative recovery unit or a designated area of the outpatient area for observation and monitoring before discharge to home.

COLONOSCOPY

Colonoscopy, or "lower GI" endoscopy, is endoscopy of the large intestine. The procedure is used for diagnostic purposes and for minor surgery, such as:

- Removal of polyps
- Biopsy or removal of lesions that do not require resection
- Coagulation of small bleeding diverticula
- Laser treatment of small tumors
- Routine screening for colon cancer

Combined colonoscopy and laparoscopic surgery may be used during resection of the lower GI system.

Technique

1. The patient may or may not be sedated, depending on the procedure.
2. The patient is placed in the left lateral position.
3. The scope is lubricated and slowly advanced into the colon.
4. The colon is inflated with air to increase visualization of the tissues.
5. The colon is examined, and the intended procedure is performed.
6. The scope is withdrawn.

Discussion

Colonoscopy requires sedation of the patient. The procedure can be uncomfortable and embarrassing. The scrub should offer support throughout the procedure. The technique used to obtain biopsy samples and for other minor procedures is similar to EGD.

The patient is placed in the left lateral position. The individual should be covered with warm blankets, and only the lower back and buttocks should be exposed. A small protective drape can be placed over the pelvis to prevent soiling of bed linens.

The scope is lubricated with water-soluble gel and gently inserted into the anus. It is then advanced slowly. When the proximal colon is in view, the surgeon begins to withdraw the scope slowly while examining the mucosa. Air may be instilled into the colon with a pump attachment. This may cause the patient some discomfort, and the scrub should offer reassurance. As the scope is withdrawn, the length of the colon is examined for lesions and abnormalities. Digital photographs of any suspect tissue are taken. Suction and irrigation are controlled at the scope head. The scrub should make sure the irrigation reservoir remains full by refilling it as needed.

Cupped or brush biopsy forceps are guided through the scope. As tissue is withdrawn from the endoscope, the scrub receives the forceps and maintains control on the tip to ensure that the specimen is not lost. The specimen can be removed from the tip with a hypodermic needle or by swishing the tip in the specimen cup.

Postoperative considerations include observation for pain or bleeding and sensitivity to any medications given during the procedure. The patient is released from the outpatient department soon after the procedure.

SIGMOIDOSCOPY

Sigmoidoscopy is performed to examine tissue and/or obtain a biopsy specimen of the sigmoid colon and rectum. The patient is placed in the prone or lithotomy position, and the scope is introduced. Biopsy tissue can be obtained or rectal polyps can be removed with cup biopsy forceps.

LAPAROTOMY

Surgical Goal

A **laparotomy** is open surgery of the abdominal cavity for access to the abdominal organs. A laparotomy that is performed to confirm a diagnosis or to detect a specific pathological condition is called an **exploratory laparotomy**.

Technique

Opening the Abdomen

1. An incision is made through all layers of the abdominal wall.
2. The contents of the abdominal cavity are explored.
3. The edges of the wound are covered with moist laparotomy sponges, and a self-retaining retractor is put in place.
4. The intended procedure is initiated.
5. The wound is irrigated, and drains are inserted.
6. The abdominal layers are closed, and dressings are applied.

Discussion

The patient is placed in the supine position, prepped, and draped for a midline incision. When draping is completed, the scrub moves the Mayo stand up to the field below the wound site. The scrub may stand opposite the surgeon, with the Mayo stand positioned at the level of the patient's knees. This gives the surgeon room to work while allowing the exchange of instruments on the sterile field. The ESU and suction tubing are secured to the top drape. Two dry laparotomy sponges are placed on the field. When suction, the ESU pencil, and sponges are in place on the field, the skin incision is made. The skin knife is then removed from the field.

The skin incision exposes the subcutaneous layer that lies just under the skin. This layer usually is incised with the ESU pencil. Large bleeding vessels can be clamped with Kelly or Crile hemostats and ligated with fine suture ties or coagulated with the ESU (Figure 23-14).

The incision is carried through to the next layer, the fascia. At this level, the scrub should have small Richardson or U.S. retractors available for the assistant. The surgeon incises the layer with the scalpel deep knife or ESU and extends the incision as needed with the ESU or curved Mayo scissors. If the incision is not on the midline, the muscle layers are separated manually. The abdominal peritoneum is then visible. The scrub prepares several moist lap sponges and a self-retaining retractor.

All loose 4 × 4 sponges must be removed from the surgical field and only laparotomy sponges used. Any 4 × 4 sponges must be mounted on sponge forceps while the abdomen is open.

The peritoneum is lifted with hemostats, and a small incision is made with the deep knife or Metzenbaum scissors. The incision is carried deeper with scissors or the ESU.

The abdominal contents are then exposed. From this point on, only saline-moistened sponges are used. The scrub passes the moistened sponges to the surgeon, who covers the tissue edges to protect them from the self-retaining retractor. The self-retaining abdominal retractor is now placed in position by the surgeon and assistant. At this time, the surgeon explores the abdominal cavity for evidence of disease. When the area of disease has been located, the surgeon packs the abdominal contents away from the diseased area with several moistened lap sponges. A specific surgical procedure then can be initiated.

During the procedure, the scrub has the following duties:

- Keep the surgical field clear of instruments not in use.
- Keep the ESU tip free of tissue debris and in its holster.
- Exchange soiled sponges for clean ones.
- Keep loose items (e.g., needles, small dissecting sponges, suture wrappers) off the Mayo stand. Small dissecting sponges go on the field or Mayo tray only when mounted on the appropriate clamp. Needles must be mounted on a needle holder.
- Protect the field from contamination.
- Anticipate the needs of the surgeon.
- Receive and properly maintain any specimens.
- Notify the surgeon of any break in aseptic technique.
- Participate in sponge and item counts at the appropriate time.

Closure

After irrigation, the surgeon and assistant remove all sponges and instruments from the abdomen, the first count is initiated, and the wound is closed. The incision then is closed in layers. The choice of suture materials (absorbable, nonabsorbable, synthetic, or natural fiber) depends on the amount of tension on the incision, the wound classification, the size of the patient, and the surgeon's preference. The first count is done before the peritoneum is closed.

When all sponges and instruments have been removed from the abdomen, the surgeon's assistant grasps the edges of the peritoneum with several hemostats. The peritoneum usually is closed with a continuous suture using 0 or 2-0 absorbable suture with a taper needle. The fascia may be sutured with the peritoneum as a single layer, and a variety of materials, both synthetic and nonsynthetic, may be used. Nonsynthetic materials currently are favored for their strength and lack of reactivity in tissue. If the fascial layer is closed separately, 2-0 suture most often is used in patients who are not obese.

During closure of the fascia, the assistant retracts the skin and subcutaneous layer with U.S. or Richardson retractors. Toothed tissue forceps are used during closure of the abdominal wall.

Retention sutures may be placed before peritoneal closure in patients who are at risk of wound dehiscence. Size 0 or 1 retention sutures are placed approximately 1.2 inches (3 cm) behind the incision line, catching all layers of the abdominal wall. The suture is threaded through a short length of flexible tubing (bolster) before the knots are tied. This distributes the tension evenly along the retention suture and prevents it from tearing through the tissue (see Chapter 17).

The subcutaneous layer is closed with interrupted sutures of 3-0 Dexon, Vicryl, or chromic gut. Fine tapered needles are used. Skin closure often is performed with staples. Alternative methods, such as subcuticular or fine interrupted sutures, may be used in selected patients for a cosmetic closure. If staples are used, the assistant pulls the tissue edges together

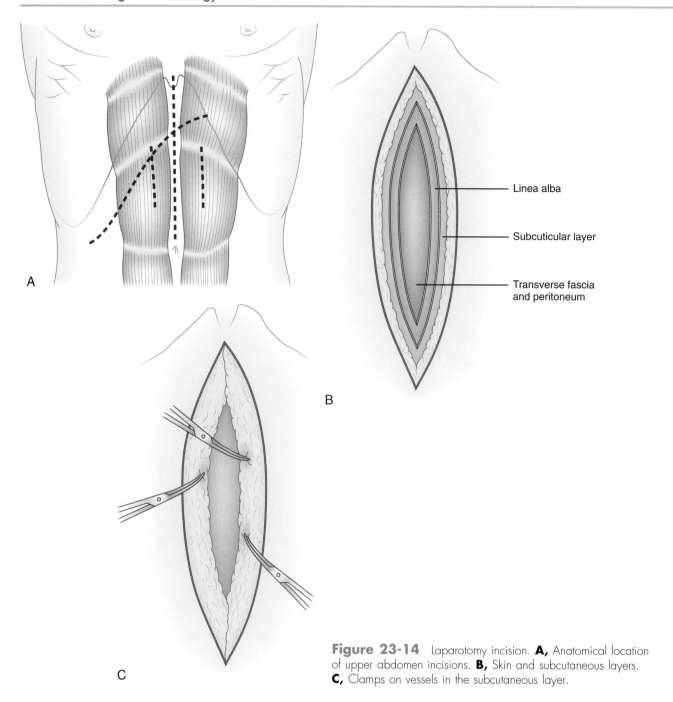

Figure 23-14 Laparotomy incision. **A,** Anatomical location of upper abdomen incisions. **B,** Skin and subcutaneous layers. **C,** Clamps on vessels in the subcutaneous layer.

with two Adson skin forceps while the surgeon places the staples across the incision. At the completion of skin closure, the scrub or surgeon places the dressings over the wound. The drapes are then removed, and tape is applied to the dressings by the circulator or surgeon.

EXCISION OF AN ESOPHAGEAL DIVERTICULUM (OPEN PROCEDURE)

Surgical Goal

In excision of an esophageal diverticulum, the esophageal diverticulum is removed and the wall of the esophagus is strengthened to prevent recurrence.

Pathology

A pharyngoesophageal diverticulum (sometimes called a *Zenker diverticulum*) is mucosa and submucosa that have herniated through the cricopharyngeal muscles. The condition, which occurs in patients over age 60, causes food particles to become temporarily trapped.

Technique

1. The patient is placed in the supine position with the head and neck turned and hyperextended to the patient's right.
2. An incision is made over the defect.
3. The diverticulum is dissected from the surrounding tissue.

4. The sac is ligated, and the stump is invaginated into the pharyngeal wall.
5. The pharyngeal muscle opening is closed with interrupted 2-0 absorbable sutures. The skin is closed with 4-0 absorbable, subcuticular suture.

Discussion

The patient is placed in the supine position with a shoulder roll under the affected side to hyperextend the neck. An incision is made over the area of the defect, usually extending from the inner border of the sternocleidomastoid muscle from the level of the hyoid bone to a point (0.8 inch) (2 cm) above the clavicle. The incision is carried through the skin and fine subcutaneous tissue. Bleeders are controlled with the ESU or fine suture ties. A spring-retractor thyroid retractor may be used to retain the superficial tissues. A small incision is made in the muscle with the ESU. The edges are then pulled aside with small right-angle retractors. The trachea is retracted separately, and the base of the diverticulum is dissected free. Dissection is performed with the ESU, smooth tissue forceps, and Metzenbaum scissors.

The diverticulum is grasped with a Babcock clamp and dissected free. When the base of the diverticulum is free of attachments, it may be resected with a right-angle surgical stapler (for sacs larger than 1.2 inches [3 cm]) or ligated at the base with 2-0 absorbable synthetic suture. If sutured, the stump of the sac is incorporated into the muscle fibers with fine sutures.

The wound is closed in layers with 3-0 absorbable sutures. The skin can be closed with surgical staples or nonabsorbable interrupted 4-0 sutures.

Postoperative Notes

Patients may require overnight observation in the hospital for postoperative bleeding or edema. A brief period of fasting may be required.

TRANSABDOMINAL REPAIR OF A HIATAL HERNIA

Surgical Goal

Nissen fundoplication commonly is performed to treat **gastroesophageal reflux disease (GERD)**. In this procedure, the upper stomach is wrapped around the esophagus below the **hiatus** to act as a sphincter. This prevents back-flow of the stomach contents into the esophagus.

Pathology

The gastric contents normally are prevented from entering the esophagus by the lower esophageal sphincter, which has sufficient pressure to prevent the backflow of stomach contents into the esophagus. Loss of pressure or tone in the lower esophageal sphincter allows the highly acidic stomach contents to wash into the esophagus, causing erosion of the esophageal mucosa. GERD causes pain, esophageal erosion, and respiratory irritation and can lead to esophageal cancer.

Technique

1. Pneumoperitoneum is established, and trocars are placed in the abdomen.
2. The liver is retracted upward.
3. The stomach is mobilized.
4. The phrenoesophageal membrane and crura are dissected free.
5. The lower esophagus is mobilized.
6. The hiatal hernia is repaired with sutures.
7. The upper portion of the fundus is wrapped around the distal esophagus and sutured in place.
8. The wound is irrigated.
9. The cannulas are removed, and pneumoperitoneum is released.
10. The trocar wounds are closed.

Discussion

Pneumoperitoneum is established, and three 5-mm trocars are placed. The liver is retracted upward to expose the lower esophagus as it passes through the diaphragm. A liver retractor or atraumatic forceps is used to lift the liver. Some surgeons wrap a Penrose drain around the stomach for retraction. The assistant may retract the stomach, which can then be divided from the omentum. A Harmonic scalpel frequently is used for dissection and coagulation.

The phrenoesophageal membrane and ligament, which adhere to the esophagus under the liver, then are divided with the Harmonic scalpel or fine scissors. This exposes the crura. If the patient has a hiatal hernia, it is repaired at this stage of the procedure. A gastric bougie is inserted orally by the anesthesia care provider, and the hiatus is sutured together with three or four nonabsorbable synthetic sutures. The bougie is then withdrawn.

Fundoplication

First, the surgeon must **mobilize** the upper stomach from its attachments to the omentum. The short gastric vessels are legated. The mobilized portion then is grasped with an atraumatic forceps and wrapped around the esophagus. The anesthesia care provider passes a gastric bougie (flexible tube) through the esophagus and into the stomach to gauge the diameter of the gastric sleeve. With the tube in place, the stomach wrap is secured with interrupted sutures through the seromuscular layers of the esophagus and stomach.

The sleeve is approximated with several interrupted sutures. Ethibond or a similar synthetic braided suture material is used for fundoplication. The gastric tube is then removed, and the gastric fold is inspected to ensure adequate constriction.

All cannulas are removed, the pneumoperitoneum is released, and the wounds are closed with absorbable sutures and skin staples or sutures (Figure 23-15).

Postoperative Considerations

Patients who had a laparoscopic procedure usually are discharged the same day as surgery. After a brief postoperative period, patients are normally symptom free.

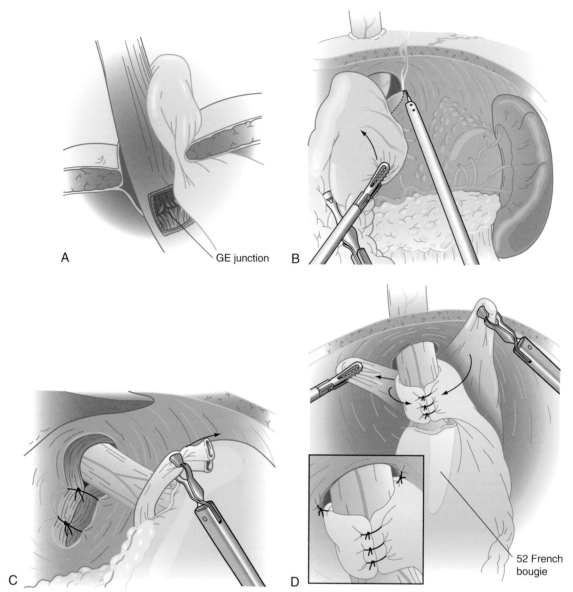

Figure 23-15 Transhiatal hernia repair (*Nissen fundoplication*). **A,** View of the gastroesophageal (GE) junction, with a portion of the stomach protruding through the hiatus. **B,** The crura is dissected to expose the hiatus. **C,** Sutures are placed through the crura to close the defect. **D,** Fundoplication (wrapping) of the stomach around the distal esophagus. An esophageal catheter (bougie) is inserted. *(From Townsend CM: Sabiston textbook of surgery, ed 17, Philadelphia, 2001, WB Saunders.)*

VAGOTOMY

Surgical Goal

Vagotomy is performed to reduce gastric enzymes by severing the nerves that control their release.

Pathology

Vagotomy is selective occlusion of portions of the vagus nerve as it branches over the stomach. This interrupts nerve transmission and reduces acidic secretions. Selective disruption of the vagus nerve traditionally has been used to control the release of stomach acid and treat peptic ulcer disease. Current knowledge about the mechanism of peptic ulcer and the relationship between ulcers and *Helicobacter pylori* as a causative

factor has significantly reduced the number of vagotomy procedures. If the procedure is performed through a small laparotomy incision or by laparoscopy, the nerve is ligated with surgical metal clips at one or more locations as it branches from the esophagus. This procedure is performed in conjunction with gastric resection.

Technique

1. A laparotomy is performed.
2. The esophagus is mobilized.
3. The left (posterior) and right (anterior) vagus nerves are resected.
4. The wound is closed.

Discussion

The abdomen already has been entered for gastric resection. The assistant retracts the liver upward using a Weinberg or wide Deaver retractor. Long Metzenbaum scissors and long fine tissue forceps are used to divide the esophagus from the attached peritoneal membrane. When the esophagus has been exposed, the surgeon retracts it using a long Penrose drain.

The surgeon retracts a portion of the vagus nerve with a long nerve hook. Two long right-angle clamps are placed across the nerve, which is divided, and the segment is passed off the field as a specimen. The right and left specimens are kept separate for pathological examination. The severed edges of the nerve are then clamped with ligation clips or ligatures. The procedure is repeated on the other side of the esophagus.

The wound is closed in layers as for gastric resection.

PERCUTANEOUS ENDOSCOPIC GASTROSTOMY

Surgical Goal

Percutaneous endoscopic gastrostomy (PEG) is a common method of providing access to the stomach through a flexible tube inserted through the abdominal wall.

Pathology

A gastrostomy tube is inserted to provide enteral feeding for patients who are unable to eat normally because of disease or trauma. Patients who require continuous gastric **decompression** after surgery are also candidates for insertion of a PEG tube.

Technique

1. A small (4- to 5-mm) upper midline or left upper paramedian incision is made through all layers of the abdominal wall. The anterior fundus of the stomach is picked up with two more atraumatic grasping clamps (Babcock or Allis clamps). Traction sutures may be inserted through the stomach wall to replace the clamps.
2. A purse-string suture is placed in the stomach wall at the location where the tube will be inserted.
3. The stomach is perforated with the electrosurgical unit (ESU) within the purse-string suture.
4. The stomach contents are immediately suctioned.
5. Small bleeding vessels in the stomach mucosa are coagulated with the ESU.
6. The stomach catheter is inserted into the perforation, the purse-string suture is tied, and a second purse-string suture is placed around the catheter.
7. The abdominal wall is secured to the stomach wall with sutures.
8. A second incision is made in the abdominal wall, and the catheter tip is brought out through this incision.
9. The catheter is secured to the skin, and dressings are applied.

Discussion

Open gastrostomy often is performed at the patient's bedside or in the interventional radiology department with the patient under conscious sedation. The PEG kit, which is prepackaged, includes the gastrostomy tube and accessories.

The surgeon enters the abdomen through a short left upper paramedian incision. The assistant retracts the wound edges with right-angle retractors while the surgeon identifies and grasps the stomach with two Babcock or Allis clamps. The surgeon brings a portion of the stomach into view through the incision.

If used, traction sutures are placed at this time. Two separate nonabsorbable sutures are placed through the stomach wall, and the ends are used for traction. When traction sutures are used, the clamps are removed.

A purse-string suture is placed through all layers of the stomach where the tube will be inserted. The surgeon makes a small perforation in the center of the purse-string suture with the ESU. The scrub should have suction immediately available as soon as the gastric incision is made, to prevent the spillage of gastric contents.

The feeding tube is then placed through the perforation, and the purse-string suture is tied. A second purse-string suture may be placed for added strength. The stomach is then sutured to the abdominal wall at the entry site.

The catheter tip is grasped with a large clamp, such as a Péan clamp, and pulled to the outside of the body through a second small incision. The tube is secured to the skin with sutures, and dressings are applied. A gastrostomy is shown in Figure 23-16.

Postoperative Considerations

Patients generally tolerate insertion of a PEG tube very well, and many are relieved to have an alternative to nasogastric intubation. The PEG tube is flushed before and after use. Residual stomach contents may be measured by aspiration with a 50-cc syringe.

PARTIAL GASTRECTOMY, BILLROTH I AND II (OPEN PROCEDURE)

Surgical Goal

In a partial gastrectomy, a diseased portion of the stomach is removed. The remaining portion is anastomosed to the duodenum or the jejunum.

Pathology

Partial gastrectomy usually is performed to treat gastric carcinoma, benign tumor, or chronic ulceration in which there is high risk of carcinoma.

Technique

1. A laparotomy is performed through an upper right or midline incision.
2. The stomach is mobilized from the omentum.
3. The gastrohepatic ligament is identified and divided.
4. The duodenum or jejunum is mobilized from the omentum.
5. The intestine is cross-clamped with two intestinal clamps, and the tissue is divided into two sections.
6. The intestinal stump is closed.

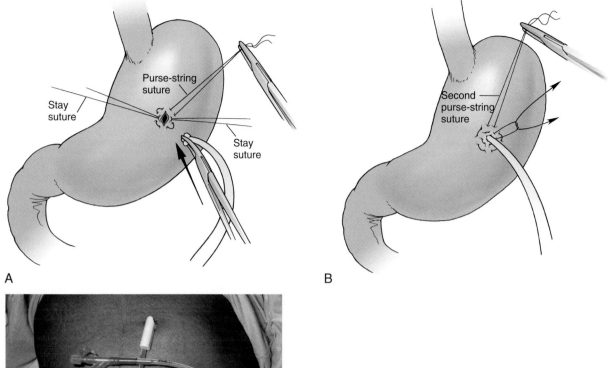

A

B

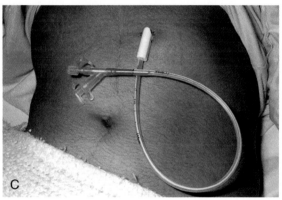

C

Figure 23-16 A, Gastrostomy. A purse-string suture is placed in the stomach wall with traction sutures. The tube is inserted through a small incision. **B,** The suture is tightened. **C,** The gastrostomy tube in place. (**B** from Moody FG: Atlas of ambulatory surgery, St Louis, 1999, Mosby; **C** from Garden O, Bradbury A, Forsythe J, Parks R: Principles and practice of surgery, ed 5, Edinburgh, 2007, Churchill Livingstone/Elsevier.)

---

7. The stomach is double-clamped and divided. The open stomach edges are sutured or stapled together.
8. The stomach is anastomosed to the duodenum or jejunum.
9. The abdomen is irrigated and closed in layers.

Discussion

Partial (subtotal) gastrectomy requires reconstruction of the stomach to maintain continuity of the GI tract. The method and location of anastomosis depend on the extent and type of pathology, the patient's overall condition and age, and the surgeon's preferred technique. The gastric pouch (the remainder of the stomach after resection) can be attached to the small intestine, or the divided end of the intestine can be attached directly into the stomach.

A laparotomy is performed through an upper midline incision. The surgeon examines the abdominal contents to determine the extent of disease and to select a site for anastomosis. The exact lines of resection are determined, and the stomach is mobilized from the ligaments, vessels, and omentum. The scrub should be prepared with many Mayo, Crile, or Kelly clamps, vessel clips, and suture ties. Suture liga-

tures are used on the major vessels of the stomach and omentum.

For the mobilization of the stomach, Allis or Babcock clamps are used to hold traction on the stomach while the omentum is divided from the greater curvature. After double-clamping the segments of omentum, the surgeon divides the tissue with dissecting scissors, the ESU, or an HF vessel-sealing system. The lesser curvature of the stomach is mobilized with the same technique.

When mobilization is completed, the surgeon places two intestinal cross-clamps (Kocher or Allen type) side by side across the duodenum (**Billroth I procedure**) or the jejunum (**Billroth II procedure**). An incision is then made between the two clamps. The duodenal or jejunal stump is closed with a stapling instrument or fine sutures. The stomach is cross-clamped and divided.

Hand-suturing and surgical stapling are the two techniques commonly used to join the stomach with the intestine. Although stapling instruments are commonly used, the scrub should also be familiar with the traditional two-layer suture closure. Stapling procedures involving the stomach and small intestine are discussed under Gastric Resection.

Hand-Suture Technique for Gastrointestinal Anastomosis

The intestine and stomach are made up of separate tissue layers, the outer serosa, smooth muscle, submucosa, and mucosa. Two suture lines are used to create the anastomosis. The inner suture catches the mucosa, submucosa, and muscle layers. The outer serosal layers of both structures are joined separately. Absorbable suture can be used for the inner closure, and absorbable or nonabsorbable sutures for the serosa.

To begin the anastomosis, the surgeon brings the cross-clamped sections close together. A traction suture is placed at each end. An outer row of sutures is placed, joining the two structures. Next, the surgeon makes two incisions, one on each side of the suture line. This exposes the inner lumen of the intestine (or stomach). The surgeon brings the inner layers together with continuous running or interrupted sutures. Finally, the outer layer is completed circumferentially with interrupted sutures. The double layer of sutures prevents leakage.

Stapling instruments have largely replaced traditional suturing techniques in GI anastomosis. If stapling instruments are preferred, the gastrointestinal anastomosis (GIA) and thoracoabdominal (TA) linear staplers are used to resect the stomach and intestine (see Chapter 17).

Gastrointestinal technique is observed, and any instruments or sponges in contact with the open tract are removed from the field. These are not used on the closed GI tract.

Before the surgical wound is closed, the abdomen is irrigated with antibacterial solution. A Penrose drain may be placed in the abdomen, and a PEG (percutaneous endoscopic gastrostomy) tube may be inserted for gastric decompression. If this is required, it is inserted before closure.

See Figures 23-17 and 23-18 for illustrations of Billroth I and Billroth II procedures.

Postoperative Considerations

After gastrectomy, patients may require continuous gastric decompression with a **nasogastric (NG) tube** or, for longer postoperative care, with a PEG tube. Patients are followed closely for signs of peritonitis.

LAPAROSCOPIC ADJUSTABLE BAND GASTROPLASTY FOR MORBID OBESITY

Surgical Goal

Band gastroplasty is performed for the treatment of morbid obesity. Nutritional intake is restricted by creating a small pouch in the proximal stomach. Food passes slowly into the stomach while creating a feeling of fullness.

The pouch is created by encircling the upper stomach with an inflatable band. The inner part of the band connects with a tube and saline reservoir implanted in the body wall. This allows the band to be filled from an external port imbedded in the subcutaneous tissue. Tension on the band is adjusted

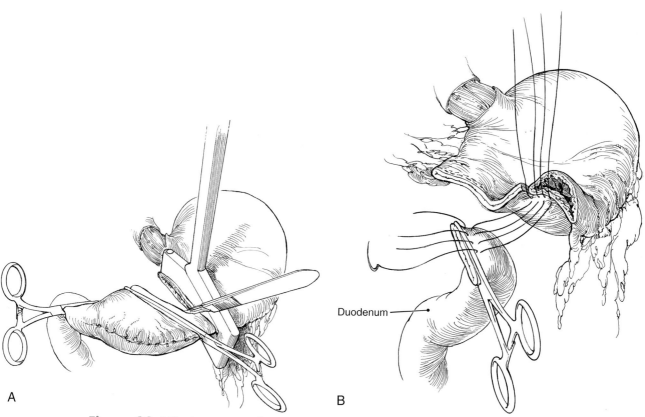

A   B

Figure 23-17 Anastomosis after gastrectomy: Billroth I procedure (end-to-end gastroduodenal anastomosis). *(From Economou SG, Economou TS: Atlas of surgical technique, ed 2, Philadelphia, 1996, WB Saunders.)*

Duodenum

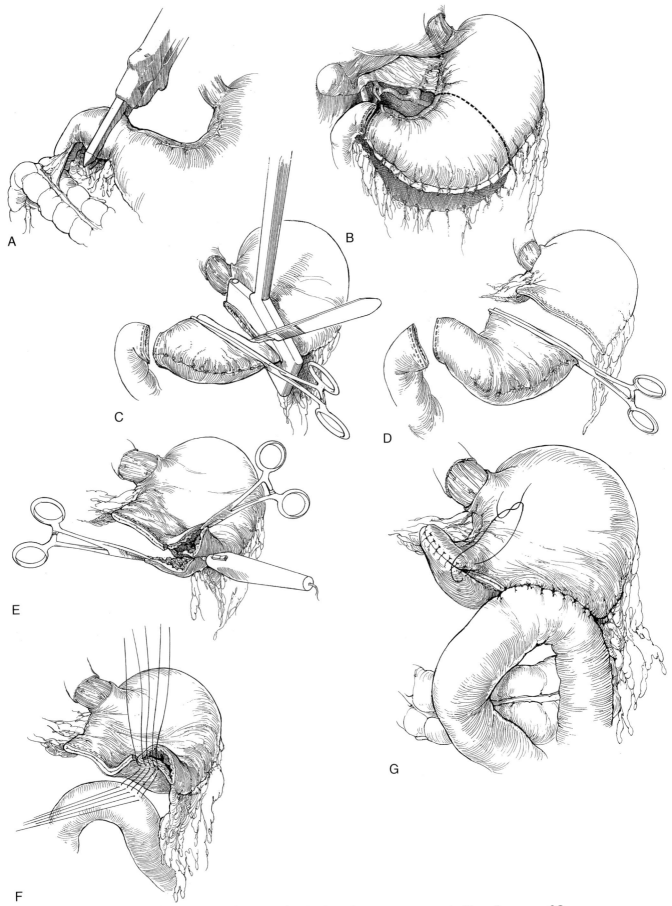

Figure 23-18 Billroth II procedure (end-to-side gastrojejunostomy). *(From Economou SG, Economou TS: Atlas of surgical technique, ed 2, Philadelphia, 1996, WB Saunders.)*

by adding or removing saline and thereby regulating the flow of food out of the pouch and into the stomach. Several different types of bands are available. The most commonly used is the Lap-Band, described here, although the more traditional Roux-en-Y procedure is also performed by some surgeons.

Pathology

Morbid obesity is a condition in which the patient's body mass index (BMI) is at least 40. The BMI is a ratio of the weight and height calculated by a specific formula: (weight in pounds)/(height in inches)^2 × 703. Obesity is an endemic health problem in the United States. It contributes to cardiovascular disease, cancers of the breast and large intestine, diabetes, stroke, urinary stress incontinence, and depression. Approximately 400,000 people die annually as a result of obesity in the United States. Society often regards morbid obesity as a moral failure in the patient, and there is strong social stigma associated with the disease.

Prospective patients are screened and usually are required to attempt conservative weight loss measures before surgical intervention. Criteria include:

- Motivation and commitment to weight loss
- Abstinence from alcohol and tobacco
- Absence of psychological factors that could hinder a successful outcome

Bariatric surgery has a long history of attempts to restrict food intake or cause poor nutrient absorption. Early radical gastric bypass procedures resulted in severe malabsorption and multiple medical problems related to nutrient deficiency. Other techniques, such as vertical band gastroplasty, have been abandoned because of failure to achieve the medical goal (patients alter their eating habits to include high-calorie liquids) or stenosis (narrowing) of the stomach outlet.

Adjustable gastric binding does not result in malabsorption, it is reversible, and it can be performed as minimally invasive surgery. Postoperatively the patient experiences rapid satiety after eating a small amount of food, which passes slowly from the pouch to the stomach. Patients must be screened preoperatively for suitability for the procedure.

Technique

1. Pneumoperitoneum is established, and trocars are placed through the abdominal wall.
2. The laparoscope and retracting and dissecting instruments are inserted.
3. The liver is retracted.
4. The peritoneum is divided between the top of the spleen and the esophagus.
5. A tunnel is created around the proximal stomach to accommodate the band.
6. The band is placed around the proximal stomach and secured.
7. The gastric wall is folded over the band and sutured in place.
8. The saline port and tubing are implanted and tested.
9. The wounds are closed.

Discussion

An operating table that can support up to 800 pounds (360 kg) must be available. Extensions and side attachments, including a footboard, are essential for patient safety. Long instruments (e.g., trocars) are required in most cases. A 15-mm trocar is required for insertion of the band. Two or three 5- or 10-mm trocars are also required.

Pneumoperitoneum is established, and trocars are placed at the xyphoid, umbilicus, and subcostal areas. The surgeon retracts the liver upward and uses an ESU hook or a Cavitron Ultrasonic Surgical Aspirator (CUSA) to separate or clear a space between the stomach and the omentum. Fatty tissue is also dissected away from the stomach.

A path for the band is created near the crura (the muscular junction between the stomach and the esophagus). This is done with a blunt dissector or forceps.

The scrub prepares the band by testing it for leaks. This is done by flushing it with normal saline. After flushing, 5 mL of saline is left in the band and tubing. The scrub should place a small knot at the distal end of the tubing or use a clamp to prevent saline from leaking from the tube.

The tube is inserted into the abdomen and fitted around the upper stomach.

To prevent the band from sliding up or down, it is secured to the fundus. A portion of the gastric wall is folded over the band and secured with several silk or Ethibond sutures. The tubing is brought out through the 15-mm trocar, and all the trocars are removed.

A trocar site is enlarged and carried to the fascia with sharp dissection. Heavy sutures are then placed in the fascia (Figure 23-19).

The tubing is cut, and saline is allowed to flow. The distal end is connected to the port, and the preplaced sutures are threaded through the port. The port and excess tubing are placed in the abdomen. The fascial sutures are then tied, and the abdominal incisions are closed and dressed with Steri-Strips.

Postoperative Considerations

Patients usually are discharged the same day they have laparoscopic surgery. The band is adjusted by injecting additional saline into the port percutaneously under fluoroscopy. In the first postoperative year, the band is adjusted three to four times; thereafter, it is adjusted yearly to ensure continued weight control.

ROUX-EN-Y GASTRIC BYPASS

Surgical Goal

The Roux-en-Y procedure is performed to bypass the distal stomach and re-establish continuity from the stomach to the jejunum. In this procedure, a large portion of the stomach is bypassed, and a gastric pouch is created. The anastomosis between the pouch and the jejunum substantially reduces the amount of food absorbed by the body.

Pathology

The Roux-en-Y procedure traditionally has been used to treat gastric ulcers and gastric carcinoma. It currently is also used to treat morbid obesity.

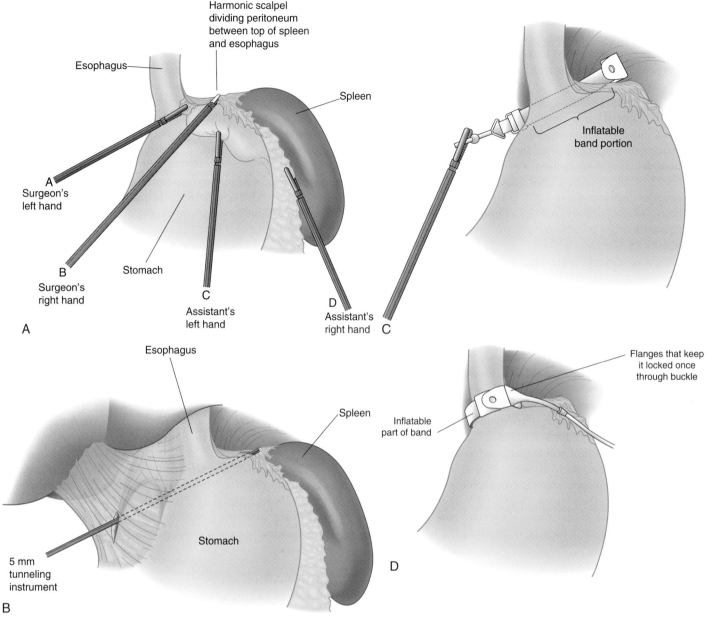

Harmonic scalpel dividing peritoneum between top of spleen and esophagus

Esophagus

Spleen

A Surgeon's left hand

B Surgeon's right hand

Stomach

C Assistant's left hand

D Assistant's right hand

A

Inflatable band portion

C

Esophagus

Spleen

Stomach

5 mm tunneling instrument

B

Flanges that keep it locked once through buckle

Inflatable part of band

D

Figure 23-19 Gastric banding procedure. **A,** The visceral peritoneum is divided at the antrum of the stomach (angle of His). **B,** A tunneling instrument is placed behind the stomach. **C,** An inflatable band is inserted through the tunnel. **D,** The band is locked in place. *(From Townsend CM: Sabiston textbook of surgery, ed 17, Philadelphia, 2001, WB Saunders.)*

Technique

1. The abdomen is entered.
2. The gastric pouch is created.
3. The jejunum is transected.
4. A gastrojejunostomy is created.
5. A jejunojejunostomy (Roux-en-Y anastomosis) is performed.
6. The wound is closed.

Discussion

After entering the abdomen, the surgeon makes a small hole in the lesser omentum at the level of the proposed partition. The TA 90 stapler is placed across the stomach at the partition site, and the staples are fired. A GIA stapler is used to close and transect the jejunum.

To create a new opening between the jejunum and the stomach, the surgeon makes two stab wounds to accommodate the forks of the GIA stapler. The stapler is inserted into the stab wounds, and the staples are fired. Silk sutures may be used to close the stab wounds. The Roux-en-Y (jejunojejunostomy) anastomosis is performed with the GIA instrument. The common opening between the two portions of jejunum is then closed with the TA 55 stapler. The wound is irrigated and closed in routine fashion (Figure 23-20).

Postoperative Notes

Weight loss is more rapid after Roux-en-Y surgery than with band gastroplasty. Patients who did not have the procedure

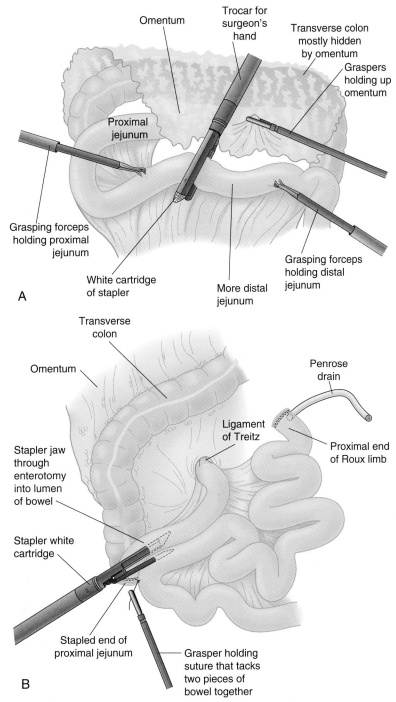

Figure 23-20 Roux-en-Y gastric bypass. **A,** The jejunum is divided with a surgical stapler. **B,** The stapler is placed for a side-to-side anastomosis.

Continued

for morbid obesity are followed carefully for adequate nutritional intake.

TRANSHIATAL ESOPHAGECTOMY

Adenocarcinoma and squamous cell carcinoma are the most common types of esophageal cancer. These cancers are treated surgically with esophagectomy in the early stage of the disease.

Transhiatal esophagectomy is performed through combined cervical and upper midline incisions. The esophagus is mobilized to the hiatus through the cervical incision, and the stomach is mobilized through the abdominal incision. The stomach is then brought upward, and an anastomosis is formed with the proximal esophagus. This approach is used to avoid a thoracotomy.

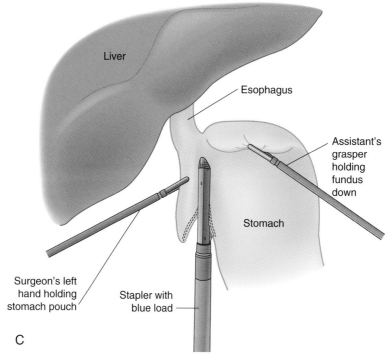

Liver

Esophagus

Assistant's grasper holding fundus down

Stomach

Surgeon's left hand holding stomach pouch

Stapler with blue load

C

Figure 23-20, cont'd C, The gastric pouch is created. *(From Townsend CM: Sabiston textbook of surgery, ed 17, Philadelphia, 2001, WB Saunders.)*

SEGMENTAL RESECTION OF THE SMALL INTESTINE

Surgical Goal

Resection of the small intestine is removal of a section followed by surgical anastomosis to maintain continuity of the intestinal tract.

Pathology

Resection of the small intestine is performed to treat obstruction, disease, or carcinoma.

Intestinal obstruction is a general term that encompasses a number of mechanical pathological conditions that can block the intestine and require emergency surgery. Obstruction can lead to perforation, necrosis resulting from ischemia, and peritonitis. The most common obstruction pathological conditions include:

- *Strangulation* of a loop of bowel by a defect in the abdominal wall (hernia).
- *Volvulus:* Twisting of the bowel on itself.
- *Intussusception:* Telescoping of the intestine (this occurs mainly in children and results in ischemia and necrosis of the bowel).
- *Paralytic ileus:* Paralysis of the ileum; this occurs most often as a postoperative complication or as a result of pelvic or back injury and peritonitis.

A *peptic ulcer* may lead to perforation of the duodenum and requires surgery to prevent peritonitis. A small ulcer may be repaired, or a short segmental resection may be required.

Technique

1. A laparotomy is performed through a midline incision.
2. The diseased tissue is identified.
3. The segment is mobilized.
4. The intestine is cross-clamped, and the intestine is divided into two sections.
5. A surgical stapling device can be used to resect the intestine, or the intestine can be divided and anastomosed with sutures.
6. The wound is closed in layers.

Discussion

The abdomen is entered through a midline incision. The abdomen is explored for disease and the intestine inspected. The intestine is mobilized from the omentum along the site of resection with Metzenbaum scissors, an ESU, or a vessel-sealing system. Larger mesenteric arteries are secured with surgical clips or suture ligatures.

Two methods of resection and anastamosis are used in current practice—surgical stapling and more traditional method of resection and anastamosis by suturing.

The bowel is cross-clamped with two intestinal clamps placed close together at each incision site in the bowel. The intestine is then incised between the clamps, and the diseased portion of intestine is removed as a specimen.

Resection and anastomosis can be performed using several techniques.

- *End-to-end:* The two intestinal "limbs" are sutured together circumferentially.

- *Side-to-end:* One limb is sutured closed, and the other is implanted in a longitudinal incision in the other limb.
- *Side-to-side:* Longitudinal incisions are made in each limb, and these are joined together.

When surgical stapling techniques are used, the site of bowel resection is identified and the peritoneal covering of the mesentery is incised on each side using the ESU or Metzenbaum scissors. The mesenteric vessels are dissected free, clamped, divided and ligated with size 3-0 sutures (silk has been traditionally used for this part of the procedure, although other non-absorbable materials are now replacing silk in some institutions). Alternatively large vascular staples can be used for ligation. Additional ligatures are often placed adjacent to the staples to ensure hemostasis.

The bowel is transected with a GIA-60 stapler and non-crushing intestinal clamps placed at each end of the stapled sections. The ends of the bowel can then be stapled or sutured by hand.

A layered suture anastomosis is performed by aligning the two ends of the intestine and rotating them outward. The inner layer is closed with a continuous or interrupted stitch of absorbable suture (e.g., chromic or Vicryl), and the outer serosa is closed with interrupted 3-0 or 4-0 sutures (e.g., Vicryl or silk).

The mucosa is closed with continuous or interrupted absorbable suture. The serosal layer can be sutured with interrupted absorbable or nonabsorbable sutures (Figure 23-21). The mesentery is repaired with interrupted absorbable sutures. The wound is irrigated, all bleeders are controlled, and the incision is closed in layers.

REMOVAL OF MECKEL'S DIVERTICULUM

Meckel's diverticulum occurs at the distal ileum. Surgical removal prevents ulceration and perforation. The condition arises from a congenital remnant of the umbilical duct. This procedure follows the technique of minor resection of the small intestine.

RESECTION OF THE COLON

Surgical Goal

In resection of the colon, a section of the large intestine is removed, and its continuity is restored by anastomosis or brought to the outside of the body as a colostomy.

Pathology

Resection of the colon is performed for treatment of carcinoma or ulcerative colitis or perforated or recurrent diverticula of the colon.

Technique

1. The abdomen is entered.
2. The diseased portion of the bowel is identified and isolated.
3. The bowel is cross-clamped and divided.
4. An end-to-end anastomosis is performed.
5. The wound is closed.

Discussion

The abdomen is entered through a midline incision. The surgeon explores loops of intestine to identify the portion to be removed. A wide margin of intestine on each side of the lesion also is removed if the lesion is cancerous. This often includes the distal ileum.

The intestine is mobilized from the mesentery with Metzenbaum scissors, an ESU or a vessel-sealing system. Larger mesenteric arteries are secured with surgical clips or suture ligatures.

When the colon is isolated, the selected segment is double-clamped at each end with intestinal clamps. The bowel is then divided between each set of clamps and passed off the field in a basin. At this point, the bowel is open and the risk of wound contamination exists. To help prevent this, the surgeon may place two lap sponges around the base of the intestinal stumps to isolate them.

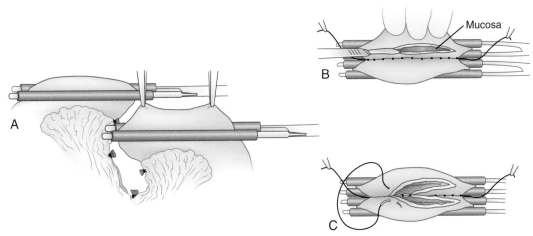

Figure 23-21   Anastomosis of the small intestine (end-to-end technique). Surgical staples are most commonly used, but some surgeons may prefer to use sutures. **A,** The clamped intestinal stumps are aligned. **B,** The mucosa is sutured. **C,** The muscle and serosal layers are sutured.

NOTE: Resection and anastomosis may be done with a surgical stapling device. If sutures are used for anastomosis, the first layer of interrupted sutures is placed in the serosa. Fine silk or synthetic absorbable suture-release (de-tach) needles are commonly used. The scrub should take care to place returned needles on a magnetic needle board or other such device as soon as the surgeon discards the needle. These needles are very small and may be easily lost in the rapid exchange between the surgeon and the scrub. The first and last sutures of the initial suture layer are left long to be used in traction.

After making double incisions in the bowel, the surgeon places a second layer of interrupted chromic gut 3-0 sutures swaged to a fine GI needle. The surgeon continues the interrupted sutures until the two intestinal lumens are joined. The intestinal clamps are removed, and a final reinforcing suture layer is placed.

NOTE: If resection and anatomosis is performed using surgical stapling techniques, the procedure for mobilizing omentum is the same as described above. The area of site of bowel transection is selected and small opening made in the mesentery using the ESU or Metzenbaum scissors. The ileum is then transected using a GIA-60 stapler. The colon is also transected after the stapler has been reloaded. The peritoneal covering of the mesentery are clamped, divided, and ligated in the area of the anatomosis. The anastomosis is performed by bringing the two limbs of the bowel in alignment and placing stay sutures at each end of the staple lines. Two openings is made in the bowel stumps to insert the forks of the GIA-60 instrument and one fork is positioned inside each bowel lumen. The GIA-60 is closed and fired, completing the anastomosis. The staple line is inspected and may be reinforced with sutures as needed. The TA-55 stapler is used to close the common opening which may also be sutured.

The final step in the procedure is closure of the mesentery. Interrupted 3-0 sutures of silk or chromic gut are used.

Bowel technique is now performed as described previously. After contaminated instruments and supplies have been removed from the field and sterile drapes positioned around the wound, the team dons fresh gowns and gloves. The wound is irrigated (in some operating rooms this is done before the changeover) and closed in routine fashion.

GASTROINTESTINAL STOMA

An **ostomy** is a procedure in which a portion of the intestine is divided and the open end is secured to the skin, draining the bowel contents outside the body. The opening is then called a **stoma.** A disposable ostomy pouch is used to collect intestinal fluid; this is a **stoma appliance.** The appliance system consists of an adherent skin wafer with an opening for the stoma and a collection reservoir that fits tightly into the skin wafer. The patient drains the collection reservoir as needed and changes it every few days. The appliance fits tightly over the stoma and adheres to the contours of the body to limit leakage and odor. After the disruption of the GI tract, the remaining part of the intestinal system becomes nonfunctional for digestion but is left intact. A small intestine stoma of the ileum is called an *ileostomy,* and a stoma of the large intestine is called a *colostomy* (Figure 23-22).

Before surgery, the surgeon and the ostomy nurse discuss the exact location of the ostomy, considering the patient's lifestyle and age and protection of the ostomy from the beltline. The site is drawn on the skin before surgery as a reference for the surgeon.

The location of an ostomy depends on the section of the intestine to be removed. An *end colostomy* is formed when the proximal end of the resected intestine is brought through the abdominal wall and sutured in place as described previously. A *double colostomy,* commonly called a loop colostomy, is one in which both sections of cut bowel are brought out through the abdominal wall. The double colostomy allows the bowel to remain nonfunctional for a period of healing. The two ends then are reconnected as a separate surgery.

A *loop colostomy* does not require resection and anastomosis. A loop of bowel is brought out and held in place with an appliance that prevents the loop from slipping back into the abdomen.

The patient's psychological and physical adjustments to an ostomy procedure depend on many factors. Body image at the time of surgery, developmental age, level of debilitation before the procedure, and family and professional support affect the patient's ability to accept the change.

Stoma care requires qualified patient teaching by a certified ostomy specialist. Patients require a period of adaptation while learning to care for the ostomy. The stoma nursing team provides psychological and social support, as well as technical assistance with stoma fit, cleansing, and emptying procedures. (For further information on the extensive postoperative care and nursing considerations, see the United Ostomy Associations of America Web site at http://www.uoaa.org)

Postoperative considerations for all colostomy patients include routine monitoring after the use of general anesthesia, with special attention to fluid and electrolyte balance. The ostomy site is monitored closely for ischemia, retraction, or prolapse.

LOOP COLOSTOMY

Surgical Goal

For a loop colostomy, a loop of large intestine is brought out through a small abdominal incision, sutured to the skin, and opened. The resulting colostomy serves as a temporary bypass for the evacuation of bowel contents.

Pathology

A colostomy is performed to give the bowel a rest after colon resection. The procedure also may be performed in the treatment of inflammatory disease or obstruction of the colon. The loop colostomy is closed when fecal diversion is no longer needed.

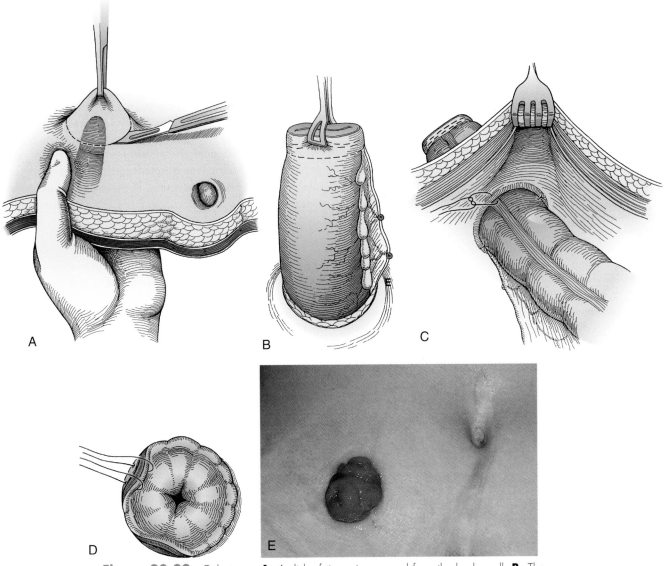

Figure 23-22 Colostomy. **A,** A disk of tissue is removed from the body wall. **B,** The intestinal stump is brought through the opening in the skin. **C,** The bowel may be sutured on the internal side. **D,** The bowel is everted and sutured to the skin. **E,** The healed stoma. (**D** modified from Bauer JJ: Colorectal surgery illustrated, St Louis, 1993, Mosby; **E** from Garden O, Bradbury A, Forsythe J, Parks R: Principles and practice of surgery, ed 5, Edinburgh, 2007, Churchill Livingstone/Elsevier.)

Technique

Opening

1. The abdomen is entered.
2. A small portion of the transverse colon is mobilized.
3. The mobilized bowel is brought out through the incision.
4. For a loop colostomy, a butterfly anchor or rod is inserted under the loop and anchored.
5. The wound is closed.
6. The loop is incised 24 to 48 hours after the procedure.

Closing

1. The skin edges around the colostomy are incised.
2. Dissection is carried to the peritoneum.
3. The colostomy edges are trimmed and sutured together.
4. The loop is allowed to retract into the abdomen.
5. The wound is closed.

Discussion

Opening

The abdomen is entered through a short transverse median or upper paramedian incision. The assistant retracts the abdominal wall with a right-angle retractor. Babcock clamps are used to grasp the loop of transverse colon.

The surgeon divides the bowel from its attachments to the omentum with Metzenbaum scissors and an ESU. An avascular area of the omentum is chosen for the mobilization. However, if blood vessels are encountered, these are clamped and ligated with fine sutures, surgical clips, or a vessel-sealing system.

When mobilization is complete, the loop of intestine is brought out of the abdomen, and a butterfly anchor or plastic colostomy rod is placed under the loop to prevent it from retracting into the abdomen. If a butterfly anchor is used, it is anchored through the needle ports with suture. The wound then is closed in standard fashion around the loop.

Closing the Stoma

After the patient has been prepped and draped, a gauze sponge is placed at the opening of the colostomy. This prevents gross contamination of the wound by fecal material. The surgeon then incises the skin around the edges of the colostomy. The incision is carried through the subcutaneous and fascial layers. The peritoneum is dissected free of the colostomy with Metzenbaum scissors. To prevent contamination of the peritoneal cavity, the colostomy is surrounded with one or two lap sponges. The surgeon then trims the skin from the edges of the colostomy.

The surgeon closes the colostomy by inserting two layers of suture through the colostomy edges. The first layer is closed with running or interrupted 3-0 absorbable (chromic) sutures swaged to a fine needle. A second layer of interrupted 3-0 or 4-0 silk sutures is placed over the chromic suture line. The bowel then is allowed to slide back into position in the peritoneal cavity, and the wound is closed in routine fashion.

PARTIAL COLECTOMY

Surgical Goal

A partial colectomy is performed to remove a section of diseased colon and restore continuity to the intestine.

Pathology

A colectomy is removal of part or all of the large intestine. The colon is removed to treat carcinoma, ulcerative colitis, diverticulitis, and intestinal obstruction.

Technique

1. A laparotomy is performed through a midline or left paramedian incision.
2. The colon is divided from retroperitoneal structures.
3. The mesentery between the duodenum and the right colon is dissected.
4. The omentum is divided.
5. The remaining mesentery, colon, and distal ileum are dissected free.
6. Atraumatic clamps are placed across the bowel at each end of the area to be resected.
7. An end-to-end anastomosis is made between the right colon and the proximal ileum.

Colostomy

8. An incision is made through the abdominal wall at the ostomy site.
9. The proximal end of the resected colon is brought through the abdominal wall and sutured in place.
10. The intestinal stump is closed.
11. The wound is closed in layers.

Discussion

Colectomy is the general term applied to removal of the large intestine. A specific term is used to identify the section that is resected (e.g., *transverse colectomy*). *Colectomy* can refer to complete removal or segmental resection. In this description, the sigmoid colon and rectum are not removed.

The surgeon performs a laparotomy through a midline or paramedian incision. If a colostomy is planned, the paramedian incision on the opposite side of the ostomy often is preferred to separate the stoma from the surgical incision and prevent contamination of the incision site. The area of resection is completely mobilized as described previously. Atraumatic Babcock and Allis clamps are used to grasp the bowel. Systematic dissection of the mesentery, major arteries, and peritoneal reflections is performed until all attachments are eliminated. An anastomosis then is performed as described previously.

Colostomy

If a colostomy is performed, the distal intestinal stump is closed in two or three layers. Surgical staples or sutures are used. The surgeon creates the stoma by making a circular incision through the skin and abdominal wall at the stoma site. The incision is carried to the peritoneum, and the proximal stump is brought through the abdominal wall. Small right-angle retractors are used to retract the wound edges. The bowel edges are then everted, and two layers of fine absorbable or silk sutures are placed; the deeper layer penetrates the full thickness of the severed ileum, and a more superficial layer is placed at the level of the skin. The epidermis itself is not sutured to the stoma.

Bowel technique is initiated as described previously. The wound is irrigated with antibacterial solution before closure. An ostomy bag may be fitted temporarily over the stoma.

Related Procedures

Ileotransverse Colostomy

An ileotransverse colostomy is the removal of a portion of the ileum and transverse colon with side-to-side anastomosis of the ileum and colon.

Postoperative Considerations

Patients are particularly monitored for signs of infection and of fluid and electrolyte imbalance related to loss of large sections of tissue. The stoma site is checked regularly for any signs of ischemia. The stoma is not fully functional for a number of days after surgery and may required suctioning. The stoma nurse consultant participates in postoperative care of the site and in patient support. As the stoma heals, changes are made in the type and configuration of the ostomy appliance.

ABDOMINOPERINEAL RESECTION

Surgical Goal

In abdominoperineal resection, the anus, rectum, and sigmoid colon are removed en bloc through combined abdominal and perineal incisions. The abdominal approach includes resection of the upper colon. A separate perineal exposure is used to mobilize the anus, rectum, and sigmoid colon, allowing removal of the specimen. The normal anatomy of the rectum is shown in Figure 23-23, *A*.

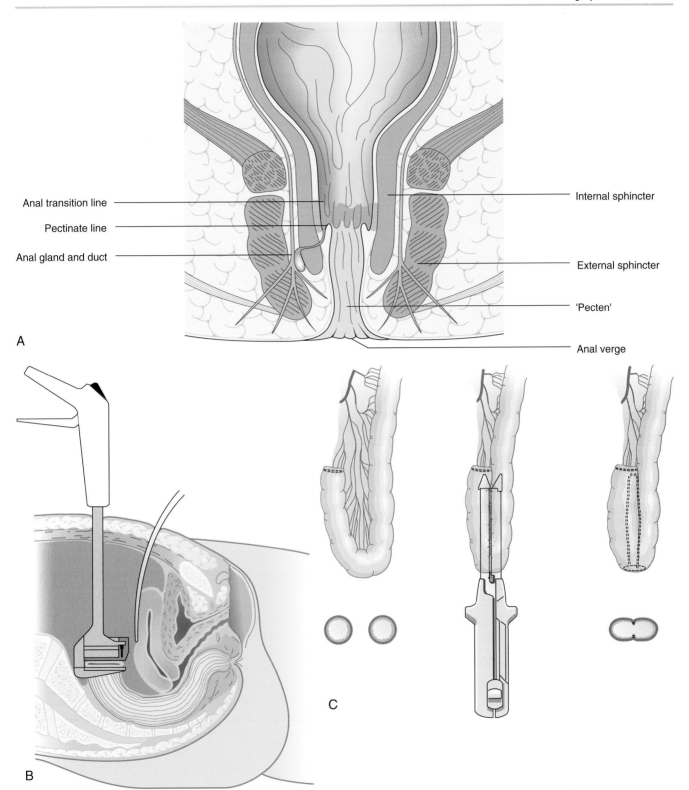

Anal transition line

Pectinate line

Anal gland and duct

Internal sphincter

External sphincter

'Pecten'

Anal verge

A

B

C

Figure 23-23 **A,** The normal anatomy of the anorectal canal. **B,** The thoracoabdominal (TA) stapler is used to close the rectal stump after resection of the abdominal colon. **C,** The gastrointestinal anastomosis (GIA) stapler is used to form an anal pouch from the ileum. The EEA stapler is used to bring the stapled ileal pouch into position. It can then be hand-sutured in place. (**A** from Garden O, Bradbury A, Forsythe J, Parks R: Principles and practice of surgery, ed 5, Edinburgh 2007, Churchill Livingstone/Elsevier; **C** from Townsend CM: Sabiston textbook of surgery, ed 17, Philadelphia, 2001, WB Saunders.)

Pathology

Abdominoperineal resection is the complete removal of the rectum and anus with pelvic dissection and removal of a portion of the colon for the treatment of cancer of the rectum.

Technique

1. The abdomen is entered.
2. The lesion is located, and the bowel is mobilized.
3. The colon is divided in an area proximal to the lesion.
4. A colostomy is performed, and the abdomen is closed.
5. The lower sigmoid colon, rectum, and anus are mobilized and removed.
6. The perineal incision is closed.

Discussion

Abdominoperineal resection requires two incisions and two anatomical approaches or surgical sites. The two surgical fields (one pelvic and one perineal) can be performed as one continuous procedure or two simultaneous procedures, with one team operating on the pelvic portion and a second at the perineal field. Two setups are needed for either technique. Two scrubs are needed for simultaneous procedures.

When the operation is performed with two teams working simultaneously, the patient is placed in the lithotomy position. Because the abdominal team has restricted space in which to work, the scrub on this team must stand slightly behind the assistant rather than in the usual position (standing next to the assistant). The scrub must take special care to prevent contamination while working in this awkward position.

During simultaneous procedures, the scrub on the lower team stands next to the surgeon, as for vaginal procedures. The surgeon usually performs the procedure while sitting. Both scrubs must remember that usually only one circulator is available to assist both teams. The scrubs should anticipate needed equipment before the procedure begins. This prevents confusion when the two surgical teams are working with one circulator between them. The procedure is discussed here as if performed by one team.

The surgeon enters the abdomen through a long midline incision. The surgeon then examines the colon and determines the line of resection. Mobilization of the colon includes isolation of the mesenteric tissue and omentum that contain diseased lymph nodes. The surgeon frees the colon from its attachments by double-clamping the tissue with Mayo clamps. The tissue between the clamps is divided with Metzenbaum scissors or an ESU, and the sections are ligated with silk, Vicryl, or Dexon ties. As mobilization continues, longer instruments are needed. The scrub must have an ample supply of Péan clamps, long right-angle clamps, and small sponge dissectors. Large blood vessels are clamped with right-angle or Péan clamps and ligated with suture ligatures. The scrub should have one or two suture ligatures ready at all times during the dissection.

Mobilization of the colon proceeds to the level of the levator muscles. At this point the abdominal dissection may be halted, if the remaining dissection cannot be performed through the pelvic approach. The surgeon places two intesti-

nal clamps across the bowel at the proximal end of the mobilized area. The proximal end of the divided bowel may be ligated temporarily with heavy sutures. To provide continuity of the bowel, an anastomosis is created between the descending colon and the rectum using the EEA circular stapler. To reconstruct the pelvic floor, the surgeon may suture a portion of the omentum to it.

To prepare a site for the colostomy, the surgeon incises a small circle in the abdomen using the skin knife and carries the incision through the abdominal wall with the ESU. The small disk of tissue is then passed to the scrub as a specimen. The proximal end of the bowel is brought through the circular incision and temporarily clamped in place while the abdominal incision is closed in routine fashion.

To create the colostomy, the surgeon everts the edges of the bowel stoma and sutures the edges of the skin using interrupted sutures of 3-0 chromic gut on a fine cutting needle.

Surgery from the perineal end begins as the surgeon places a heavy silk purse-string suture through the anus to occlude it. The perineum is incised, and rectal dissection is performed with the ESU and scissors. Large bleeding vessels are double-clamped and ligated with silk or Dexon. As the incision becomes deeper, Péan clamps are used to grasp the bowel attachments, as described in the abdominal portion of the procedure.

Dissection is continued until the surgeon reaches the previously mobilized area of the bowel. The entire specimen is delivered through the perineal incision. The surgeon then irrigates the wound. Interrupted sutures are used to close the tissue planes and avoid "dead space," which can lead to infection. One or two Penrose or a suction drain is placed in the wound, which is then closed with size 0 chromic gut, Vicryl, or Dexon. The skin is approximated with the surgeon's choice of nonabsorbable material and dressed with a bulky abdominal pad and gauze sponges. Illustrations for the procedure are shown in Figure 23-23, *B* and *C*.

Related Procedure

Proctocolectomy with an Ileal Pouch

Proctocolectomy with an ileal pouch involves the creation of an ileal pouch and anal anastomosis to provide fecal continuity and conserve the sphincter.

Postoperative Considerations

Radical surgery in which large portions of tissue are removed requires meticulous critical care observation and methodologies. This care begins in the postanesthesia care unit (PACU) and continues well into the postoperative recovery after the patient has been discharged to the intensive care unit or ward. Detailed care plans, which include hemostasis, fluid and electrolyte balance, thermoregulation, and monitoring for infection, are implemented by members of the critical care nursing and medical staffs.

APPENDECTOMY

Surgical Goal

An appendectomy is the removal of the appendix, a blind, narrow, elongated pouch that is attached to the cecum.

Pathology

The appendix is removed during acute infection to prevent rupture and treat peritonitis. The procedure may be performed as a prophylactic (preventive) measure when surgery is performed in the abdomen for other reasons. The procedure then is called an *incidental appendectomy.*

Technique

1. The abdomen is entered.
2. The appendix is isolated from the mesoappendix.
3. The appendix is ligated and removed.
4. A purse-string suture is placed around the stump of the appendix.
5. The wound is closed.

Discussion

There are two approaches to appendectomy—open and laparoscopic technique. Open technique is used in cases where perforation has occurred, there is significant risk of perforation or an abdominal mass has been discovered during preoperative assessment. Laparoscopic technique is indicated for most other cases. Both approaches are described in the following sections.

Open Technique

The abdomen is entered through a McBurney incision. The muscle layers are manually separated and the peritoneum entered. The assistant retracts the wound edges with a right-angle retractor. The surgeon then grasps the appendix with Babcock clamps and delivers it into the wound site.

The appendix is isolated from its attachments (mesoappendix) to the bowel with Metzenbaum scissors and the ESU. Portions are ligated it with free ties of 3-0 nonabsorbable suture until the appendix is completely mobilized.

A Babcock clamp is placed on the body of the appendix, which the assistant elevates. The surgeon then places a straight Kelly clamp at the base to compress the tissue. A ligature of 3-0 nonabsorbable suture is tied over the compressed base. The assistant then places a straight Kelly clamp above the knot.

A purse-string suture is placed around the base, and the suture ends are left long. The appendix now can be removed. The scrub should place a small basin on the field. A lap sponge is placed around the base of the appendix. The surgeon severs the appendix with the deep knife and places it along with the specimen in the basin, which is now contaminated and removed from the field.

The assistant buries the appendix stump in the cecum while the surgeon ties the purse-string suture. The wound is irrigated with warm saline solution, and the abdomen is closed in routine fashion.

Postoperative Considerations

Routine postoperative care is provided in the PACU. Particular attention is given to signs of infection related to possible spillage of bowel contents during the procedure. Pediatric patients generally recover very quickly from appendectomy.

Laparoscopic Technique

Surgical Goal

The appendix commonly is removed using a laparoscopic technique. Both open and laparoscopic approaches are shown in Figure 23-24.

Technique

1. Pneumoperitoneum is established.
2. Trocars are placed.
3. The appendix is divided from the mesoappendix.
4. A ligature is placed at the base of the appendix.
5. The appendix is severed and removed through a 10-mm cannula.
6. The appendix stump is sealed.
7. Pneumoperitoneum is released, and the trocars are removed.
8. The wounds are closed.

Discussion

Pneumoperitoneum is established, and a 10-mm trocar is placed near the umbilicus. In cases of acute appendicitis, a second, larger trocar is inserted into the midline below the suprapubic line. A third port is placed in the upper right quadrant.

The patient is placed in the Trendelenburg position. The surgeon then locates the appendix by systematically moving aside the large intestine with an atraumatic endoscopic grasper, such as a Babcock clamp, until the cecum is found.

After inspecting the abdominal cavity, the surgeon mobilizes the appendix. The tip of the appendix is retracted upward to produce traction. The mesoappendix is divided with scissors or the ESU and ligated with vessel clips or a surgical stapler.

After the appendix has been mobilized, it can be amputated from the cecum. Two ties are placed around the appendix between the lines of amputation, one at the base of the appendix and the other just above it. The appendix then is transected with the ESU, scissors, or GIA surgical stapler. The specimen is brought out through the 10-mm port using a specimen retrieval bag.

The stump of the appendix may be inverted and a purse-string suture placed at the base. This is done to contain the stump and prevent contamination of the abdominal cavity. If signs of contamination are noted, the surgeon takes a culture swab from the free fluid in the abdomen.

The wound is irrigated with antibacterial solution, and the pneumoperitoneum is released. A soft rubber drain may be placed if the risk of postoperative infection or excessive drainage exists.

HEMORRHOIDECTOMY

Surgical Goal

Hemorrhoids are removed for pain management and to prevent bleeding and infection.

Pathology

The venous plexus of the anal canal may become congested or distended, causing pain, bleeding, and prolapse outside the

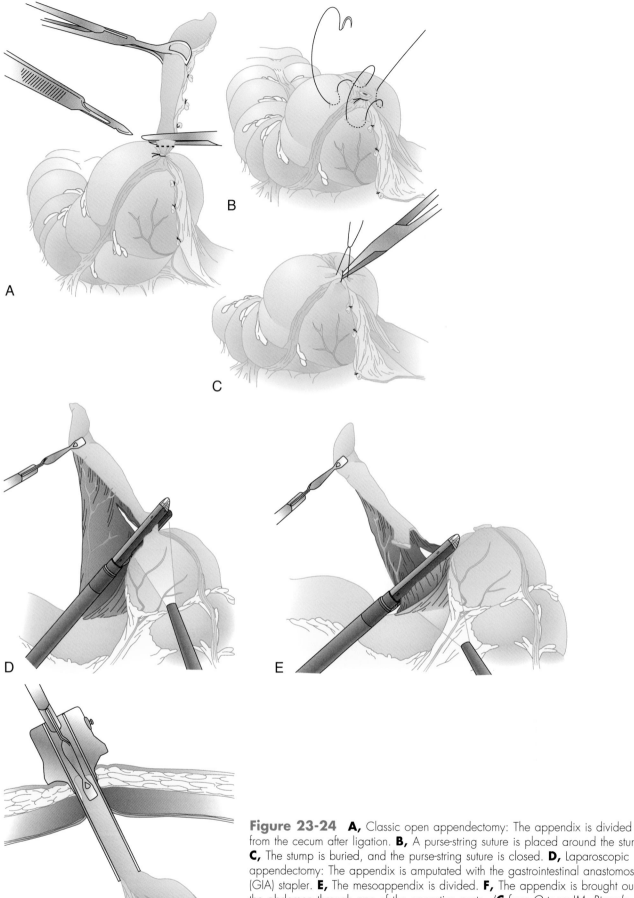

Figure 23-24 **A,** Classic open appendectomy: The appendix is divided from the cecum after ligation. **B,** A purse-string suture is placed around the stump. **C,** The stump is buried, and the purse-string suture is closed. **D,** Laparoscopic appendectomy: The appendix is amputated with the gastrointestinal anastomosis (GIA) stapler. **E,** The mesoappendix is divided. **F,** The appendix is brought out of the abdomen through one of the operative ports. (**C** *from Ortega JM, Ricardo AE: Surgery of the appendix and colon. In Moody FG: Atlas of ambulatory surgery, Philadelphia, 1999, WB Saunders;* **F** *from Moody FG: Atlas of ambulatory surgery, Philadelphia, 1999, WB Saunders.*)

anal canal. Venous distention most often is caused by pregnancy and obesity. A genetic predisposition may also influence the incidence in certain individuals. People whose occupations require constant sitting or standing are also at high risk for symptomatic hemorrhoids. Stage IV hemorrhoids remain outside the anal canal, causing frequent bleeding and severe pain. These are treated surgically.

Discussion

Hemorrhoidectomy most often is performed using one of the following methods:

- Ligation with an elastic ring to constrict and shrink the vein
- Laser treatment
- Removal with the ultrasound scalpel

These procedures may be performed in the outpatient setting with the patient receiving a local anesthetic; only in rare cases is hospitalization required. The application of elastic O rings currently is the most common procedure. The patient is placed in the prone or lithotomy position. The buttocks may be taped to expose the anus, which is dilated to allow access to the base of the hemorrhoids. The hemorrhoid is grasped with the McGivney ligator or a similar device, which discharges a Silastic O ring over the vein. No dressings are applied.

EXCISION OF A PILONIDAL CYST

Surgical Goal

Excision of a pilonidal cyst is performed to remove a pilonidal cyst.

Pathology

A pilonidal cyst is a congenital defect in which epithelial tissue develops below the surface of the skin in the area of the sacrum and coccyx. The cyst is removed when it causes recurrent infection in the area. A *sinus tract* (a channel leading to an abscess) often is present.

Technique

1. The extent of the fistula is determined.
2. The tract is incised around its circumference.

Discussion

If a sinus tract is present, the surgeon begins the procedure by inserting a probe into the tract. The probe identifies the exact location of the sinus and the cyst itself. The surgeon may want to inject dye into the sinus tract. If so, the scrub should have a blunt needle, syringe, and methylene blue dye available.

The area around the sinus is incised with the skin knife. The scrub must retract the skin with rake retractors as the surgeon deepens the incision. Using the cautery or a deep knife, the surgeon incises the subcutaneous layer. The incised tissue mass then is grasped with a Kocher or an Allis clamp for traction. The dissection continues until the sacrum is exposed and the en bloc tissue can be removed. Bleeding vessels are controlled with the ESU or ties of 3-0 Vicryl, Dexon, or gut.

The wound may be left open to heal. In this case, it is packed with iodophor gauze. Primary closure is performed if no infection is present at the site of the wound. The subcutaneous tissue is closed with 3-0 absorbable suture. The skin is closed with interrupted nonabsorbent sutures.

EXCISION OF AN ANORECTAL FISTULA

Surgical Goal

A fistula is excised to promote approximation of tissue edges and close the tract.

Pathology

A fistula is a tract or tunnel in normal or infected tissue. The tract remains open because of the constant drainage of pus or because the tissue lining the tract does not contain cells that normally initiate wound healing. Circumferential excision of the tract removes scar tissue and promotes closure and healing. An anal or a rectal fistula often arises from an infected fissure in the anal sphincter (Figure 23-25).

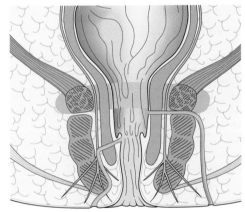

Low intersphincteric fistula   Trans-sphincteric fistula

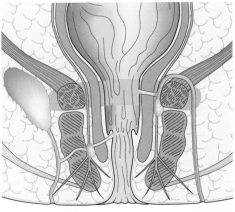

Ischiorectal fistula   Suprasphincteric fistula

Figure 23-25 An anal fistula involving the sphincter. *(From Garden O, Bradbury A, Forsythe J, Parks R: Principles and practice of surgery, ed 5, Edinburgh, 2007, Churchill Livingstone/Elsevier.)*

Discussion

The patient is placed in the prone position, and the buttocks are taped to expose the anus. The surgeon dilates the rectum and inserts a rectal retractor. A malleable probe is then inserted into the fistula to determine its depth. When the extent of the fistula has been determined, the surgeon makes a circular incision around the fistula where it communicates with the skin. The incision is carried along the length of the fistula with the ESU. The incised tissue is removed as a specimen.

The wound is not sutured; rather, it is dressed with iodophor plain packing.

SECTION III: SURGERY OF THE BILIARY SYSTEM, LIVER, PANCREAS, AND SPLEEN

LEARNING OBJECTIVES

After studying this section the reader will be able to:

- Describe the structures of the biliary system, liver, pancreas, and spleen
- Recognize instruments required for biliary, hepatic, pancreatic, and splenic surgery
- Describe the relationship of the liver and the portal vein in cirrhosis of the liver

- Identify the need for insertion of a T-tube (biliary system)
- Describe methods of hemostasis used during liver and spleen surgery
- Identify and describe priorities for an emergency procedure (splenectomy)

TERMINOLOGY: SURGERY OF THE LIVER, BILIARY SYSTEM, PANCREAS, AND SPLEEN

Bifurcation: A Y-junction in an anatomical structure such as a blood vessel or duct.

Bile: A digestive substance produced by the liver. Its main function is to emulsify fats (i.e., break them into small particles) so that the body can digest them.

Biliary system: The organ system that includes the gallbladder, hepatic ducts, common bile duct, and cystic duct.

Cirrhosis: A disease of the liver in which the tissue hardens and the venous drainage becomes blocked. It usually is caused by chronic alcoholism but may result from other disease conditions.

Common bile duct exploration (CBDE): A procedure to detect stones or strictures in the common bile duct. It usually is performed endoscopically before surgery.

Friable: A descriptive term for tissue that means fragile, easily torn, and may bleed profusely. Some disease states produce friable tissue. The liver and spleen normally are friable.

Lobectomy: Surgical removal of one or more anatomical sections of the liver.

Segmental resection: An anatomical resection of the liver in which segments divided by specific blood vessels and biliary ducts are removed.

Skeletonization: Surgical dissection to separate vessels or other small structures from the surrounding connective tissue attachments.

Subphrenic area: The area under or below the liver.

Transect: To surgically divide or cut into sections of tissue or an organ.

Trisegmentectomy: In hepatic surgery, the removal of the right lobe of the liver and a portion of the left. In practice, this is a multiple segmental resection.

Tumor margins: The edges of a tumor between the tumor mass and healthy tissue. When the surgical goal is to completely remove a tumor, the margins must be clear of any cancer cells in order to prevent recurrence of the tumor.

INTRODUCTION

Surgical procedures of the liver, biliary system, pancreas, and spleen are grouped together because of the proximity of these organs in the abdominal cavity. The gallbladder and liver share important drainage ducts, and the pancreas may be affected by disease of the other organ systems. The spleen shares the upper abdominal cavity with the other systems. Instrumentation, surgical exposure, equipment, and patient preparation are the same for all four systems.

SURGICAL ANATOMY

LIVER

The liver, gallbladder, spleen, and pancreas are located in the midabdominal cavity. The spleen lies in the upper left quadrant, beneath the diaphragm and posterior to the stomach. The liver occupies most of the upper right abdominal space and a portion of the left upper quadrant.

The liver is a large, vascular organ that aids digestion and the filtration of toxic substances from the body. It is divided into two major sections, or lobes, the right lobe and the left lobe, which are separated by the falciform ligament. These sections are identified by the **bifurcation** (Y-shaped division of a hollow anatomical structure) of the portal vein with right and left bile ducts. The vascular supply of the liver is derived from the hepatic artery and the hepatic portal vein. The liver is drained by the hepatic veins, which connect to the inferior vena cava.

The two lobes of the liver are further divided into eight subsections, according to their blood supply. The blood supply to each section is carried in a pedicle containing a bile duct, a hepatic artery, and a branch of the portal vein. Because each section is connected to its own pedicle, resection of an entire lobe requires dissection of the pedicle from the lobe and secure ligation of the pedicle, including the specific portion of the hepatic vein.

The liver is encapsulated by a thick, fibrous sheath called the *Glisson capsule*. Fibrous sheaths cover and protect the blood vessels and biliary ducts. These sheaths are continuous with the abdominal peritoneum and must be carefully dissected and mobilized before liver resection or anastomosis of the biliary system to another abdominal structure.

The anterior surface of the liver, which is in contact with the diaphragm, is referred to as the *right* and *left subphrenic spaces*. The *subhepatic space* lies between the peritoneal covering on the liver and the right kidney. These spaces are clinically significant. The subphrenic spaces are common sites of abscesses, and the subhepatic space can trap intestinal contents after a rupture of the appendix and become infected.

BILIARY SYSTEM

The **biliary system** includes the gallbladder, hepatic ducts, common bile duct, and cystic duct. The gallbladder is a small sac located under the right lobe (ventral side) of the liver. It is composed of smooth muscle and has an inner surface of absorptive cells.

The function of the biliary system is to produce, store, and release **bile,** which is composed of bile salts, pigments, cholesterol, lecithin, mucin (a glycoprotein), and other organic substances. Bile is necessary for the breakdown of cholesterol and helps stimulate peristalsis in the small intestine during digestion. It is formed in the liver and stored in the gallbladder.

Bile formed in the liver is released from the right and left hepatic ducts. These ducts converge to form the common hepatic duct. From the common hepatic duct, bile flows into the gallbladder through the cystic duct. When food enters the stomach, the gallbladder contracts, releasing stored bile into the common bile duct. Bile then enters the duodenum through an opening called the *ampulla of Vater*. This opening into the duodenum is shared by the pancreatic duct, which allows the release of pancreatic enzymes. The release of both bile and pancreatic enzymes is controlled by a sphincter at the ampulla called the *sphincter of Oddi*.

The hepatic and biliary anatomy is shown in Figure 23-26.

PANCREAS

The pancreas is an elongated, lobulated gland that lies inferior to the liver, behind the stomach. This organ has two landmarks, the head and the tail. The head, which is the broader portion of the gland, lies in the curve of the duodenum and is connected to the duodenal portion of the small intestine. The pancreatic duct (duct of Wirsung), which is the central duct of the pancreas, communicates with the duodenum at the ampulla of Vater, a location shared with the common bile duct. The tail of the pancreas lies near the hilus of the spleen. The pancreas produces insulin and glucagon, which aid in the digestion of carbohydrates.

SPLEEN

The spleen is a kidney-shaped organ that is extremely vascular and relatively soft. It lies under the diaphragm in the left upper abdomen (Figure 23-27). This organ destroys aged red blood cells, stores blood, filters microorganisms from the blood, and plays a major role in the immune system of the body. Because of its vascularity and location, vehicular and sports accidents often cause traumatic injury of the spleen. The spleen can be removed safely, without harming the body's ability to function, and this procedure is indicated whenever splenic hemorrhage becomes life-threatening. This is because hemorrhage is difficult to control without clamping the splenic arteries, and removal has little or no long-term medical consequence for most patients.

PATHOLOGY OF THE LIVER, BILIARY SYSTEM, PANCREAS, AND SPLEEN

Table 23-6 presents various diseases and conditions that can affect the liver, biliary system, pancreas, and spleen.

DIAGNOSTIC PROCEDURES

Diseases of the liver, biliary system, pancreas, and spleen have direct consequences on metabolism, digestion, the production of blood cells, and blood clotting. The symptoms of disease often are dramatic, and the diagnostic process is initiated when a patient presents with symptoms of pain, jaundice, diabetic pathology, or generalized weakness.

Blood tests can detect substances normally filtered by the liver and pancreas. Liver function tests measure liver enzymes and other chemicals. The liver is responsible for hundreds of physiological processes in the body. Specific blood tests are performed according to the presenting symptoms.

Imaging studies, including those that use contrast media, are done to outline organs and observe the movement of bile through the biliary system. Pancreatic imaging is used to detect stones and tumors, and the ducts may also be revealed if a contrast medium is used. Endoscopic retrograde pancreaticoduodenoscopy is performed to explore the ducts visually and for simple endoscopic procedures.

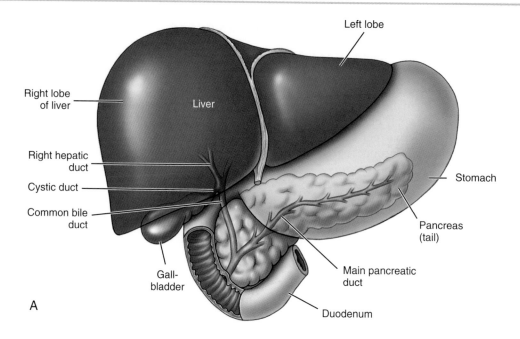

A

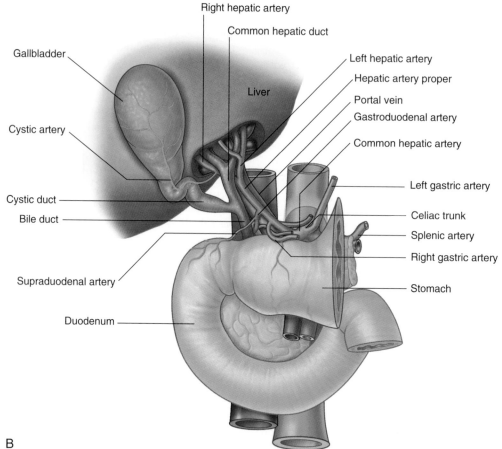

B

Figure 23-26 A, The biliary and hepatic anatomy. Note the position of the spleen and the main pancreatic duct (duct of Wirsung). **B,** Details of the biliary system. (**A** *modified from Herlihy B, Maebius NK: The human body in health and illness, ed 2, Philadelphia, 2003, WB Saunders; **B** from Drake R, Vogl W, Mitchell A: Gray's anatomy for students, Edinburgh, 2004, Churchill Livingstone.)*

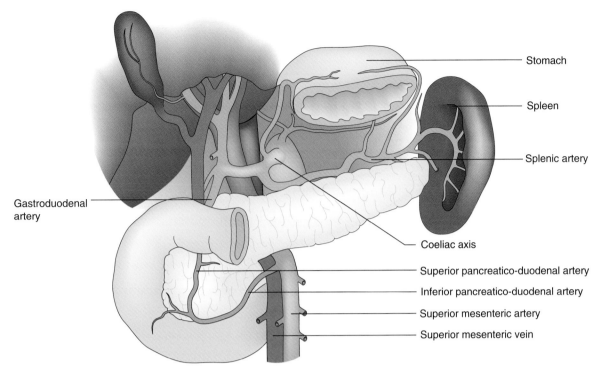

Figure 23-27 Anatomical relationship of the spleen and arterial system. *(From Garden O, Bradbury A, Forsythe J, Parks R: Principles and practice of surgery, ed 5, Edinburgh, 2007, Churchill Livingstone/Elsevier.)*

PERIOPERATIVE CONSIDERATIONS

PATIENT SAFETY

Patient safety considerations during surgery of the liver, biliary system, pancreas, and spleen are the same as for all laparotomy cases, with some additions. The organs of these systems are **friable** (delicate), and any tear or rupture can result in profuse bleeding that sometimes is difficult to control.

INSTRUMENTS

Procedures of the liver, biliary system, pancreas, and spleen require basic laparotomy instruments. Vascular instruments are needed for major resection procedures and for major hepatic surgery.

Because these accessory organs contain many ducts and blood vessels, right-angle clamps should be available with all procedures. These clamps allow the surgeon to reach underneath and around the blood vessels, ducts, and connective tissue attachments of the organs.

Procedures of the biliary system and pancreas, including choledochoscopy and endoscopic retrograde cholangiopancreatography (ERCP), sometimes require intraoperative use of flexible fiberoptic endoscopes. These scopes are inserted into the small ducts of the accessory organs to locate stones, tumors, or benign lesions.

SPECIAL EQUIPMENT AND SUPPLIES

Hemostasis is a major technical concern during surgery of the liver or spleen. Hemostatic techniques must include individual blood vessels and capillary bleeding. The ultrasonic scalpel and ESU may be used to cut and coagulate the tissue. **Skeletonization** (the removal of parenchyma and other connective tissues around a structure) of the hepatic and biliary system requires meticulous care to prevent hemorrhage and to preserve the essential blood supply to the organs. This is performed with dissecting scissors or an ultrasonic system. Vessel loops and surgical clips frequently are used to retract and ligate vessels. A HF vessel-sealing system (e.g., LigaSure) also is used.

Hemostatic agents used in surgery include the following:
- Microfibrillar collagen (Avitene, Instat)
- Oxidized cellulose (Surgicel)
- Topical thrombin
- Absorbable gelatin (Gelfoam)

Supplies required for intraoperative cholangiography include:
- Contrast medium (Diazotrite)
- Injectable saline
- 50- and 30-cc syringes
- Stopcock
- Cholangiocatheter

SURGICAL PROCEDURES

ENDOSCOPIC RETROGRADE CHOLANGIOPANCREATOGRAPHY

Selected patients can benefit from endoscopic procedures, such as ERCP, before biliary, hepatic, and pancreatic surgery. The procedure is performed in the outpatient setting in the

Table 23-6

Pathology of the Liver, Biliary System, Pancreas, and Spleen

Condition	Description	Considerations
Liver		
Alcoholic liver disease	Chronic alcohol abuse can lead to cirrhosis, hepatitis, and fatty liver disease.	Most deaths result from liver failure, bleeding varices, or kidney failure.
Cirrhosis and portal hypertension	End-stage alcoholic liver disease is characterized by fibrosis of the liver, which prevent the flow of blood and bile. Blood backs up into the portal vein, causing congestion and rupture of the esophageal venous plexus.	Palliative treatment includes endoscopic banding of esophageal varices and a portal vein stent. (See Transhiatal Esophagectomy.)
Cancer	Primary tumors of the liver are rare. Metastatic carcinoma arises from cancer of the breast, lung, and colon. Viral hepatitis B, C, and D often is implicated in liver cancer.	Surgical treatment can include hepatic resection. Treatment for metastatic disease is palliative. (See Segmental Resection of the Liver.)
Biliary System		
Cholecystitis	Cholecystitis is inflammation of the gallbladder related to obstruction of the bile ducts by stones and an increased concentration of bile in the bile ducts and gallbladder.	Symptomatic acute and chronic cholecystitis is usually treated by surgery. (See Laparoscopic Cholecystectomy.)
Cholelithiasis	Gallstones occur as a result of an increased concentration of bile, cholecystitis, and a change in the composition of bile. Cholesterol is a primary cause.	Symptomatic gallstones are removed surgically. (See Operative Cholangiography.)
Cancer	Cancer of the gallbladder often occurs in association with chronic cholecystitis. The prognosis is poor, with a 3% 5-year survival rate. Spillage of bile during surgery is implicated in dissemination of cancer cells and spread of the disease.	Early stage cancer of the gallbladder (T1) is surgically treated by cholecystectomy. Advanced stage cancer is palliative and may be treated by radical biliary resection.
Pancreas		
Pancreatitis	Pancreatitis is an inflammatory disease of the pancreas and peripancreatic fat that often results in tissue fibrosis and necrosis. Chronic pancreatitis is most commonly associated with alcohol abuse or biliary disease.	Treatment focuses on medical management of complex symptoms and associated conditions. Late stage conditions requiring management include renal failure, vascular collapse, respiratory failure, and gastrointestinal bleeding.
Cancer	Pancreatic cancer most often occurs as adenocarcinoma of the pancreatic head. This cancer progresses rapidly and has a low survival rate. The disease is associated with tobacco use and diet.	Surgical treatment includes pancreatectomy, splenectomy, and removal of associated structures. (See Pancreaticoduodenectomy [Whipple procedure].)
Spleen		
Trauma	Traumatic injury to the spleen is related to its location in the abdomen and highly vascular structure. Rupture of the spleen requires emergency surgery.	See Splenectomy.

interventional radiology department, and conscious sedation is used. The endoscope is inserted through the upper GI tract and guided into the duodenum and ampulla of Vater. A contrast medium is injected into the biliary and pancreatic ducts. Biopsy samples may be taken from the ducts and stones removed (see the section on EGD).

LAPAROSCOPIC CHOLECYSTECTOMY

Two common diseases of the biliary system are *cholelithiasis* (the presence of gallstones) and *cholecystitis* (inflammation of the gallbladder). The main components of gallstones are cholesterol and bilirubin. High blood cholesterol and obesity con-

tribute to the formation of gallstones, which can lead to blockage of the bile ducts. Obstruction increases the concentration of bile and results in swelling, pain, and infection. Obstructive jaundice occurs in biliary disease. Bilirubin, a normal byproduct of the breakdown of hemoglobin, is absorbed into normal bile. Biliary obstruction causes increased serum levels of bilirubin, resulting in toxicity.

Technique

Cholecystectomy
1. Pneumoperitoneum is established, and trocars are placed in the abdomen.
2. The gallbladder is retracted upward with a grasper.

3. The cystic duct, cystic artery, and common bile duct are dissected free.
4. The cystic duct and artery are occluded.

Intraoperative Choledochoscopy
5. An incision is made into the cystic duct.
6. The cystic duct is dilated.
7. The choledochoscope or ureteroscope is inserted, and stones are removed with a stone basket.
8. A second set of radiographs may be taken.

Completion of Cholecystectomy
9. The gallbladder is dissected from the underside of the liver with the electrosurgical unit (ESU) probe, hook, or scissors.
10. A grasper is used to remove the gallbladder from the abdomen through a 10-mm trocar site.
11. The abdominal cavity is irrigated.
12. A T-tube may be inserted for continuous postoperative drainage.
13. Individual trocar wounds are closed.
14. If used, the T-tube is attached to a drainage bag.

Discussion

Laparoscopic cholecystectomy now is commonly performed as an ambulatory procedure with rapid recovery. In the past, **common bile duct exploration (CBDE)** was performed during cholecystectomy. CBDE now is frequently performed before surgery as an endoscopic procedure.

The patient is placed in the supine position, and the abdomen is prepped and draped for a laparoscopy. In this procedure, four trocars are placed: an umbilical 10-mm trocar, an additional 10-mm trocar at the midline, and two 5-mm trocars at the axillary line. This procedure usually requires a 30-degree telescope to view the gallbladder, which lies high in the abdominal cavity.

The laparoscope is inserted through a 10-mm port. A straight locking grasper is inserted through one axillary trocar and used to apply upward traction on the gallbladder. The assistant maintains retraction on the gallbladder. The patient then may be repositioned into the reverse Trendelenburg position as the dissection continues. An additional grasper may be placed on the gallbladder.

The cystic duct and artery are exposed. Sharp dissection with scissors, an additional grasper, and an ESU hook may be used to separate the cystic duct and artery. After the cystic duct and artery have been isolated, surgical clips are used to ligate both structures. An additional clip may be placed over the cystic duct at the base of the gallbladder. The duct and artery are then divided. Operative cholangiography usually is performed at this stage of the procedure.

Common Bile Duct Exploration

Intraoperative CBDE and stone removal have been largely replaced by preoperative endoscopic procedures in which stones are removed before surgery. However, this part of the procedure is performed in some health facilities.

If stones are present, the surgeon extends the exploration by dilating the cystic duct with a balloon catheter. This is done by threading a guide wire through the cystic duct and into the common duct. The balloon catheter is inserted over the guide wire and slowly inflated with saline solution. The surgeon can remove single stones by slowly withdrawing the catheter. Common duct stones also can be flushed out with a high-pressure irrigation device. Any stones that fall into the abdominal cavity are retrieved with an endoscopic grasper. Stones also may be retrieved through the fiberoptic choledochoscope or ureteroscope as described in the following section.

Intraoperative Choledochoscopy

If a choledochoscopy is to be performed, an additional camera and monitor must be available. A small incision is made in the common bile duct, and the fiberoptic choledochoscope or ureteroscope can be inserted over the guide wire. Stones are retrieved with a stone basket.

The scrub receives all stones in a dry container. Any stones that are inadvertently dropped into the abdominal cavity are retrieved with grasping forceps. When all stones have been removed, a second cholangiogram may be taken.

Completion of Cholecystectomy

The gallbladder is dissected free of the underside of the liver (liver bed). Upward traction is maintained, because this puts some tension on the gallbladder and the tissue plane directly underneath and facilitates dissection. The surgeon uses the ESU hook, scissors, or Harmonic shears to separate the connecting tissues and free the gallbladder from the liver completely. A large grasper is inserted into the 10-mm subxyphoid (uppermost) port. The smaller graspers are used to "hand" the gallbladder to the larger grasper. The gallbladder is then extracted through the 10-mm trocar.

The scrub should receive the gallbladder in a small basin, taking care not to allow its contents to spill onto the surgical field.

A T-tube may be inserted at this time to produce continuous postoperative drainage of the common bile duct. The limbs of the T-tube are trimmed, and the tube is inserted through the uppermost trocar. The limbs of the tube are threaded into the common bile duct, and the long end is pulled through the trocar. The common bile duct is closed with endoscopic sutures. The abdominal cavity then is irrigated, and each trocar incision is closed with absorbable sutures and skin staples. The T-tube is secured to a drainage bag.

Postoperative Considerations
Patients may be discharged within 24 hours of surgery.

CHOLECYSTECTOMY AND OPERATIVE CHOLANGIOGRAPHY (OPEN TECHNIQUE)

Surgical Goal
A *cholecystectomy* is the removal of a diseased gallbladder. *Operative cholangiography* comprises imaging studies in which a contrast medium is injected into the biliary ducts to detect gallstones or a stricture.

Operative cholangiography is seldom performed, because significant evidence indicates that it does not improve the patient's outcome, and it increases the risk of injury to the common bile duct. In current practice, preoperative retrograde endoscopy is used to detect stones and for lithotomy. Laparoscopic surgery is the preferred technique for cholecystectomy.

Technique

1. The abdomen is entered through an upper midline or right subcostal incision.
2. The liver is retracted, exposing the gallbladder.
3. The gallbladder is grasped for retraction and manipulation.
4. The gallbladder is drained of bile.
5. The bile ducts are identified and isolated.
6. The cystic artery is ligated.
7. The cystic duct is clamped.
8. The gallbladder is mobilized from the liver bed.
9. Cholangiography is performed.
10. Stones are removed.
11. A T-tube may be inserted.
12. The wound is closed.

Discussion

Open cholecystectomy and CBDE have been replaced almost completely by laparoscopic techniques. A small number of patients require open surgery.

The abdomen is incised, and a self-retaining retractor is put in position. A Deaver or Harrington retractor is used to retract the liver and expose the gallbladder. Hemostasis is maintained with the ESU. If the gallbladder is distended with bile, the surgeon may drain it with a trocar fitted to the suction tubing or with a large-bore needle and syringe. After the trocar has been withdrawn, a Mayo clamp is used to seal the hole.

To start the dissection of the gallbladder, ducts, and vessels, a Péan or similar clamp is placed across the body of the gallbladder, which then is retracted upward. The peritoneal membrane. which covers the cystic duct, artery, and common bile duct, is incised with a scalpel or Metzenbaum scissors. The dissection is continued with scissors, fine-toothed forceps, and small sponge dissectors. When the cystic artery has been fully exposed, it is occluded with right-angle clamps and ligated with vessel clips.

Dissection and ligation of bleeding vessels is completed with scissors and right-angle clamps until the cystic and common bile ducts are exposed and dissected free. Operative cholangiography is performed at this stage of the procedure.

Operative Cholangiography

To begin operative cholangiography, the surgeon places two traction sutures of 3-0 silk through the wall of the cystic duct. An incision then is made between the sutures with a #11 scalpel blade or Potts scissors.

The scrub should have a cholangiocatheter, contrast medium, stopcock, and 30- or 50-cc syringe available. The contrast medium is prepared before the cholangiography:

1. The circulator distributes the contrast medium and injectable saline to the scrub. The contrast medium is diluted according to the surgeon's order. At least 30 mL of contrast medium solution should be prepared. The

solution is aspirated into the syringe, which is attached to a stopcock and cholangiocatheter.
2. All air bubbles are removed from both the syringe and the catheter (these appear as solid white spots on radiographs and can be interpreted as stones).
3. The scrub places a clamp across the catheter near its tip to prevent air from backing up into the syringe. The syringe, cholangiocatheter, and its attaching clamp are then passed to the surgeon.

The surgeon threads the tips of the cholangiocatheter through the incision in the cystic duct and advances it into the common bile duct. The catheter may be secured with a suture tie or vessel clip. All instruments and radiopaque sponges must be removed from the field, and a sterile drape is placed over the sterile field and the incision.

The C-arm then is brought into position, and the surgeon injects the contrast medium. Stones are removed under fluoroscopy. A balloon biliary catheter often is used to remove stones. The catheter probe is advanced beyond the level of the stone, the balloon is inflated, and the catheter is withdrawn, bringing the stones with it. Stones are also removed with gallbladder dilators, scoops, or a stone basket catheter. As the stones are removed, the scrub receives them as specimens.

Closure

When all stones have been removed, the cystic duct is ligated and the gallbladder is removed. The liver bed may be closed with fine absorbable sutures. If postoperative drainage is required, a T-tube is inserted into the common duct at this time. The ductal incision then is closed with 3-0 or 4-0 absorbable suture on a fine tapered needle. The long end of the T-tube is brought out of the wound and later attached to a collection bag. Penrose drains are inserted into the abdominal cavity, and the ends are brought through a stab wound near the main incision. The wound is irrigated with warm saline solution and closed in layers.

CHOLEDOCHODUODENOSTOMY/ CHOLEDOCHOJEJUNOSTOMY

Choledochoduodenostomy (anastomosis between the common bile duct and duodenum) and choledochojejunostomy (anastomosis between the common bile duct and jejunum) are rarely performed in modern surgical practice. Endoscopic stone retrieval now is the gold standard for the treatment of obstruction of the distal common bile duct (CBD), an indication for bypass of the CBD.

SPLENECTOMY

Surgical Goal

The spleen is removed surgically to stop hemorrhage caused by trauma or to treat disease.

Pathology

The spleen is vulnerable to rupture and extensive hemorrhage as a result of abdominal trauma. Splenic tissue is delicate and easily torn and has a rich vascular system. Its location in the abdomen makes it vulnerable to injury caused by the steering wheel in a motor vehicle accident. Injury during a contact sport is another common cause of splenic rupture.

The spleen also is removed to treat selected immune and blood disorders and cancer.

Technique

1. A laparotomy is performed.
2. Blood and clots are immediately removed from the abdomen.
3. The splenic artery and vein are digitally compressed to control bleeding.
4. An intestinal or a vascular clamp is placed across the major vessels.
5. The extent of injury is assessed.
6. If total splenectomy is to be performed, the splenic artery and vein are cross-clamped, occluded, and divided.
7. The lienorenal ligament is divided by sharp dissection.
8. The peritoneum is dissected from the spleen with sharp and blunt dissection.
9. The gastric vessels are divided, clamped, and ligated.
10. The gastrosplenic ligament is divided.
11. A suction drain is placed in the wound.
12. Hemostasis is secured, and the wound is closed in layers.

Discussion

Severe splenic trauma may be a life-threatening condition that requires immediate operative intervention. However, more conservative treatment is adequate for low grade trauma cases. CT scanning and ultrasound are now used to grade splenic injury. Conservative nonsurgical therapy is adequate for injuries that do not affect hemodynamic stability. Because multiple injuries may be involved in traumatic accidents, there is no definitive method of determining the exact cause of instability. In these cases, emergency surgery is indicated when systolic pressure falls below 90 mm Hg with no response to intravascular resuscitation.

In preparation for the surgery, the scrub should have a major laparotomy set, vascular clamps, and kidney pedicle clamps, depending on the surgeon's preference.

The type of sutures is specified. They usually include silk or synthetic nonabsorbable sutures to ligate the splenic artery and vein and the gastrosplenic vessels. Surgical clips are used throughout the procedure to secure small bleeders as they are encountered during the dissection.

Remember that during emergency surgery for acute hemorrhage of any kind, four major requirements must be met to stop the bleeding:

1. *Access:* The surgeon must have access to the hemorrhage site. This starts with a rapid laparotomy.
2. *Visualization* (ability to see structures directly): Retraction, either manual or self-retaining, must be established quickly. Suction must be available immediately to clear blood and clots. The scrub may be required to assist in suctioning and evacuating blood clots while passing other needed instruments.
3. *Good lighting:* Excellent lighting is required to locate and stop the hemorrhage. This is the collaborative duty of the scrub and the circulator. Remember to angle the surgical light toward the proximal end of the wound.
4. *Clamps:* Clamps are required to occlude the bleeding vessels. The scrub must have vascular, pedicle, and other hemostatic clamps immediately available on the field.

Two suctions must be available as soon as the abdomen is opened. These are used to evacuate the blood and clots from the abdomen so that the splenic vessels can be located and manually compressed. The scrub should have a large basin available to evacuate and remove large blood clots from the abdominal cavity as soon as the abdomen is opened. Laparotomy sponges are used in rapid succession as the bleeding is controlled.

The surgeon's assistant evacuates the blood clots and places a self-retaining retractor while the surgeon locates the splenic artery and vein. Even though the procedure moves quickly, safety techniques are still observed. The scrub must watch the wound, have equipment available, and use methodical, smooth movements in assisting.

A blood recovery system (e.g., Cell Saver) may be used immediately to replace blood. As soon as the splenic vessels are located, they are clamped with a pedicle or vascular clamp. When the vascular supply to the spleen has been controlled, the wound can be more carefully cleared of blood and the extent of damage ascertained. The splenic artery and vein may be ligated at this time. Heavy silk or synthetic suture ligatures are used to secure the vessels. Two or more ligatures may be used.

The wound is explored for other areas of trauma. The abdominal retractors may be repositioned at this time. Sharp and blunt dissection with Metzenbaum scissors and sponge dissectors is used to separate the lienorenal ligament from the body of the spleen. The gastric vessels are clamped or clipped and divided in the usual manner. The gastrosplenic ligament is then separated with Metzenbaum scissors, and the spleen is delivered from the wound.

If the spleen is to be repaired rather than removed, absorbable sutures are used to oversew the tear. Hemostatic agents (e.g., Gelfoam, Avitene, or Surgicel) are used to coagulate areas of capillary bleeding.

The surgeon examines the abdominal cavity again to ensure that all hemorrhage has been controlled and to locate any other areas of abdominal trauma. The wound then is irrigated with antibacterial solution. One or more drains are placed in the vicinity of the splenic pedicle, and the wound is closed in layers.

PANCREATICODUODENECTOMY (WHIPPLE PROCEDURE)

Surgical Goal

In the Whipple procedure, the head of the pancreas and duodenum and a portion of the jejunum, distal stomach, and distal section of the common bile duct are removed. The biliary system, pancreatic system, and GI tract are reconstructed.

Pathology

The Whipple procedure is performed for curative or palliative treatment of pancreatic cancer.

Technique

1. A laparotomy is performed through a bilateral or inverted V (bilateral subcostal) incision.
2. The duodenum is mobilized with blunt and sharp dissection. All vessels in the area of the proposed anastomosis are double-clamped, ligated, and divided.
3. The gastrocolic ligament and omentum are mobilized as in step 2.
4. The distal stomach is mobilized and transected.
5. The common bile duct is clamped and separated from the duodenum.
6. Vascular attachments to the jejunum are divided.
7. The jejunum is cross-clamped and divided.
8. The pancreas is transected.
9. The specimen is removed.
10. The gastrointestinal, biliary, and pancreatic systems are reconstructed.

Discussion

Pancreaticoduodenectomy is a radical operation that requires 5 to 8 hours to complete. Because the procedure includes elements of pancreatic, biliary, intestinal, and gastric procedures, the scrub should prepare all instruments normally used in these specialties. Most are included in a major laparotomy set. Vascular instruments should be added to the sterile setup in case vessel repair is required. Extra suction and two ESU sets sometimes are needed. Long instruments and wide retractors (e.g., wide Deaver and Harrington retractors) should also be available. Right-angle clamps are used throughout the procedure.

Much of the procedure includes meticulous dissection, management of bleeding, and anastomosis. The surgeon's preferred sutures are made available but should be distributed to the sterile field economically. Additional sutures and other equipment, such as sponges, vessel loops, and scalpel blades, should be held in reserve. Extra surgical towels and half-sheet drapes should be available to keep the operative site orderly and clean. The risk of infection increases with the duration of the procedure. Recall that increased handling of instruments and equipment also increases the risk of contamination.

Sterile irrigation and water to soak instruments must be kept fresh during a long procedure. The scrub should attempt to keep instruments clean and free of tissue debris. Extra gloves for the team should be readily available but not opened onto the sterile field.

To understand the techniques used in this procedure, the surgical technologist should review procedures learned previously. These resection procedures are performed in succession, and the essential ducts and hollow organs are reconnected to restore function. The reconstruction phase of the procedure can be performed with surgical staples, sutures, or a combination of the two techniques. Variations on the Whipple procedure can be done, and the exact resection depends on the pathological condition. The procedure commonly includes resection of the head of the pancreas, a distal portion of the stomach, the duodenum, gallbladder, and common bile duct. Reconstruction procedures include:

- Gastric resection and gastrojejunostomy (in some procedures the stomach is not resected)
- Intestinal resection and anastomosis
- Choledochojejunostomy or choledochoduodenostomy
- Pancreatojejunostomy

Table 23-7 describes the areas of resection.

The patient is placed in the supine position, prepped from the nipple line to midthigh, and draped for a laparotomy. The abdomen is entered through a long midline incision. The surgeon explores the bowel and other organs for evidence of metastasis and extension of the tumor. This will determine if resection is achievable. The wound is packed with moistened lap sponges, and a self-retaining retractor is placed in the usual manner. Accessory retractors or a self-retaining retractor fitted with attachments (Thompson or Bookwalter) is used.

The procedure begins with mobilization of the duodenum, which is attached to the peritoneal reflection (an extension of the abdominal peritoneum). The surgeon separates loose connective tissue from the duodenum with the ESU. The lower third of the stomach is separated from the omentum in the proposed area of resection.

Table 23-7

Reconstruction Using the Whipple Procedure

Normal Anatomical Structure	Postreconstruction Configuration
The duodenum is continuous from the distal stomach to the jejunum.	The duodenum and a portion of the jejunum are removed. A portion of the proximal jejunum is removed.
The distal stomach is continuous with the duodenum.	The gastric omentum attachments are divided, and the distal (lower) third of the stomach is removed. The remaining gastric section is attached to the jejunum with a side-to-side technique.
The common bile duct is an extension of the common hepatic duct and communicates directly into the duodenum at the ampulla of Vater.	The common bile duct is divided just below the Y-junction of the cystic and hepatic ducts. The common bile duct is anastomosed to the jejunum with an end-to-side technique.
The pancreatic duct communicates with the duodenum at the ampulla of Vater.	The head of the pancreas is removed, and the remaining portion is anastomosed to the jejunum with an end-to-end or side-to-side technique.

The stomach then is resected from the jejunum and the two structures. A side-to-side anastomosis is performed. The surgeon performs this step using a surgical stapling instrument or by clamping the stomach with Payr or Allen clamps and performing a traditional two-layer closure. Absorbable and silk 2-0 and 3-0 sutures are used for the anastomosis.

The duodenum is retracted, and the common bile duct is exposed and divided. The common bile duct is anastomosed to the jejunum. Anastomosis of the GI tract is performed as described in Table 23-5. The cystic duct is attached to the jejunum (choledochojejunostomy) later in the procedure. The junction of the duodenum and jejunum (duodenojejunal flexure) is divided.

The pancreas is resected with both sharp and blunt dissection. The pancreatic duct must be identified and preserved for attachment to the jejunum. When all bleeding has been controlled and attachments have been divided between the accessory organs, the specimen is removed. The scrub should receive it in a basin.

Reconstruction of the GI tract continues with an end-to-end pancreatojejunostomy. An end-to-side, single-layer choledochojejunostomy is then performed. Individual sponge and needle counts must be performed before the anastomosis of the stomach and intestine.

After the reconstruction is complete, the surgeon irrigates the wound with antibacterial solution and inspects each anastomosis for leakage. When hemostasis has been completely secured, one or more abdominal drains are placed in the abdomen. The wound is then closed. Figure 23-28 shows the completed anastomoses.

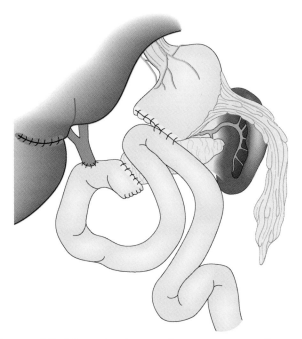

Figure 23-28 Whipple procedure anastomoses. *(From Garden O, Bradbury A, Forsythe J, Parks R: Principles and practice of surgery, ed 5, Edinburgh, 2007, Churchill Livingstone/Elsevier.)*

Postoperative Considerations

After radical surgery, the patient recovers in the PACU and may be taken to the intensive care unit (ICU) for observation. Complex physiological monitoring is performed throughout the initial phases of postoperative recovery. As normal homeostasis returns, the patient is still monitored for metabolic and renal function, infection, and fluid and electrolyte balance.

LAPAROSCOPIC DISTAL PANCREATECTOMY

Surgical Goal
In a laparoscopic distal pancreatectomy, a portion of the tail of the pancreas is removed for palliative treatment of a malignant tumor or to remove a benign lesion. Splenectomy may be performed during the procedure.

Pathology
Cancer of the pancreas usually is well advanced at the time of diagnosis. The survival rate is less than 3% in 5 years. Alcoholism and biliary reflux are common causes of pancreatitis that leads to pancreatic adenocarcinoma. Pancreatic resection may be performed if the tumor is localized in one area. Partial pancreatectomy offers palliative treatment for metastasis.

Technique
1. Pneumoperitoneum is established.
2. Four abdominal ports are created.
3. The gastric arteries and branches are ligated.
4. The splenocolic ligament is incised.
5. The spleen is mobilized.
6. The pancreas is retracted upward.
7. The splenic artery and vein are exposed and ligated.
8. A linear surgical stapler is used to transect the tail of the pancreas.
9. The specimen is removed with a specimen retrieval bag.
10. A 15-mm port is extended by at least 2 mm.
11. The spleen is divided into sections and brought out of the abdominal cavity through the retrieval bag.
12. An abdominal drain is placed.
13. Trocars are removed, and pneumoperitoneum is released.
14. The wounds are closed.

Discussion
Pneumoperitoneum is established, and four trocars are placed in the abdomen. A 12-mm port is placed above the umbilicus for the laparoscope. A 15-mm port is inserted below the left costal margin, and a 5-mm port is placed at the left costal margin. The fourth port is inserted into the subxyphoid area.

After examining the abdominal cavity, the surgeon incises the gastrocolic ligament using blunt dissection or a Harmonic scalpel. This creates access to the gastric arteries and branches. These vessels are ligated with surgical clips and divided or coagulated with the ESU. The splenocolic ligament and peritoneal attachment to the spleen are then incised.

The pancreas is freed from the retroperitoneum and elevated with an atraumatic retractor to gain access to the splenic vein and artery. These are clamped and divided. When the spleen has been freed from its vascular attachments, the surgeon must **transect** the pancreas with a linear stapler (e.g., the GIA II). Bleeding from the severed surface of the pancreas is controlled with the ESU The pancreas is placed in a specimen retrieval bag and removed. The spleen then is divided into small pieces and delivered from the wound through the 15-mm port.

A small abdominal drain may be placed in the wound, which is then irrigated. All instruments are removed from the abdomen, and the pneumoperitoneum is released.

Individual ports are sutured with absorbable suture and skin staples.

SEGMENTAL RESECTION OF THE LIVER

Surgical Goal

Hepatic resection is performed to remove a portion of the liver to treat a benign or malignant tumor. Segmental resection or lobectomy is the usual approach for tumor removal. **Segmental resection** involves the removal of one or more of the nine liver segments. **Lobectomy** is the removal of one or more of the major lobes of the liver: the right lobe, the left lobe, or the entire right lobe and a portion of the left (called *right hepatic* **trisegmentectomy**).

Pathology

The most common indication for liver resection is a malignant liver tumor. The tumor may be primary (the original source of the cancer) or metastatic (cancer that has spread from another location in the body). The most common type of liver tumor is metastatic, especially those that arise from primary tumors in which the blood supply is drained by the portal vein. Primary liver tumors are rare. Cancer of the liver usually is well advanced by the time it is diagnosed. Less common indications for liver resection include parasitic disease, infection, and laceration or trauma of the liver.

Technique

1. A laparotomy is performed through a subcostal, median, or paramedian incision. The surgeon explores the abdominal cavity to evaluate the extent and location of diseased tissue. Intraoperative ultrasound may be used to identify segments associated with the diseased tissue.
2. Moist laparotomy sponges are used to pack the abdominal viscera away from the liver. Additional laparotomy sponges are placed between the diaphragm and the liver.
3. A self-retaining retractor is placed in the abdomen.
4. The abdominal cavity is examined for evidence of disease.
5. The pedicle segment is identified, and individual vessels and ducts (bile duct, hepatic artery, and portal vein branch) are dissected free.
6. Ultrasound may be used, or methylene blue dye may be injected into the pedicle to stain the segment and identify the exact anatomical boundaries.
7. The pedicle structures are clamped and ligated.
8. The liver segment is resected.
9. Hemostasis is secured.
10. An abdominal drain is placed in the wound.
11. The wound is closed in layers.

Discussion

Liver resection follows diagnostic studies, including percutaneous needle biopsy performed under MRI or ultrasound guidance in an outpatient setting.

A laparotomy is performed through a right subcostal, midline, or paramedian incision. After entering the abdomen, the surgeon examines the liver and adjacent viscera. This may be done before or after a self-retaining retractor is placed in the wound. Because of the size of the liver and the wide exposure required, a self-retaining retractor with accessory attachments often is used. Before placing the retractor, the surgeon places moist laparotomy sponges over accessory organs surrounding the liver and between the liver and the diaphragm.

One of the areas in which sponges often are retained is the **subphrenic area** (under the diaphragm). The scrub counts all sponges placed in the wound, taking special care to note those placed in this area of the abdomen.

After all retractors have been placed, the surgeon examines the diseased segment. A sterile ultrasound Doppler probe may be needed to determine the segmental location of the tumor. Removal of liver segments requires identification and dissection of veins, arteries, and ducts that branch into each segment. The scrub must watch the field and observe the progress of the dissection, passing the appropriate instruments to the surgeon as needed.

To begin the resection, the surgeon dissects the attachments between the liver and abdominal wall, such as the falciform ligament. To perform a segmental resection, the surgeon must locate the correct segment pedicle. These two steps of the procedure are performed with the standard dissecting instruments. The surgeon may need to place an additional retractor at the top of the incision to displace the liver upward. A Harrington retractor or wide Deaver retractor may be used here. The surgeon protects the liver with a moist laparotomy sponge and uses the hand to expose the ligaments that attach the liver to the posterior wall of the abdomen. The ultrasonic scalpel and aspirator (CUSA) may be used to expose the pedicle where it branches into the parenchyma.

At this stage, the surgeon must identify the exact borders of the segment. If multiple segments are to be removed, all ligament attachments are transected during the procedure. A common method is to begin dissection at the pedicle (at the hilum of the liver) and follow the structures into the parenchyma, using the ultrasonic scalpel or ESU to resect the liver tissue. If this approach is used, the surgeon temporarily stops the vascular supply to the segment by applying vascular clamps across the vessels that supply that segment. This prevents excess bleeding during the dissection.

An alternative method is to first identify the pedicle structures and then inject methylene blue dye into the pedicle. The methylene blue dye enters the pedicle structures and stains the segment that includes the tumor. If this technique is used, the scrub should have methylene blue dye, a 10-mL syringe, and the surgeon's preferred needle for injection. A small Silastic catheter may be attached to the hub of the needle and syringe.

When the portal (branches of the portal vein) and pedicle structures and appropriate segment have been identified, the pedicle structures are individually clamped, ligated, and transected. The pedicle and portal structures are ligated with silk, synthetic nonabsorbable suture, or surgical staples.

The liver segment can be resected at this point. The surgeon scores the segment using the ESU. Complete resection is performed with the ESU, CUSA, or Harmonic scalpel or by finger fracture (the surgeon uses the hand to "break" the parenchyma along the lines of resection). At the completion of the resection, the liver bed and raw surfaces must be free of hemorrhage. The argon beam coagulator and ESU l typically are used to secure hemostasis. An abdominal drain (e.g., Jackson-Pratt or Penrose drain) is placed in the wound, which is closed in layers as for a laparotomy.

LIVER TRANSPLANTATION

Surgical Goal

The goal of transplantation is to replace a diseased liver with a donor organ.

Pathology

In adults, liver transplantation is performed in selected cases for conditions that result in end-stage liver disease (ESLD), such as **cirrhosis** not related to bile stasis, autoimmune disorder, and neoplasms.

Transplantation Considerations

Transplantation is a joint effort that involves the organ procurement agency and the host hospital. (Chapter 3 presents a more complete discussion of the role of each of these organizations.) The procedures for both donor and recipient are complex. Protocols for the technical as well as the medicolegal aspects of the process require many individuals and professional coordination. The basic considerations and technical points are presented here as a basis for advanced practice.

The donor procedure involves multiple organ procurement from a *heart-beating donor* as described in Chapter 3. The procedure is carried out by the procurement agency under the supervision of a transplant coordinator. The liver is removed with all accessory arteries, including the celiac artery, portal vein, vena cava, and common bile duct. After procurement, the liver is transported to the recipient facility by the procurement agency. The time between organ procurement and transplantation usually is about 10 hours.

The setup for transplantation requires extensive patient care equipment, similar to that required for cardiac surgery. This equipment includes devices for complex physiological monitoring, patient warming, a blood warmer, cold slush basins, physiological fluids, and a crash cart (defibrillator and emergency drugs).

Liver transplantation is a complex procedure that requires advanced surgical nursing and technology.

Technique

Recipient Procedure

1. Midline and bilateral subcostal incisions are made.
2. The liver is mobilized with sharp and blunt dissection.
3. The vena cava is mobilized.
4. The hepatic artery, portal vein, and common bile duct are mobilized and clamped.
5. The liver is removed.
6. The donor liver is positioned in the right upper quadrant.
7. The vena cava and portal vein are anastomosed from the recipient to the donor liver.
8. Clamps on the vena cava and portal vein are released to allow the flow of blood.
9. Bleeding is controlled, and the anastomosis sites are monitored for leakage.
10. When hemostasis is achieved and the blood supply to the liver has been measured, the hepatic artery is anastomosed to the donor artery.
11. The common bile duct is anastomosed to the duodenum or jejunum
12. The wound and all incision sites are examined carefully for leakage, and liver profusion is checked.
13. The wound is irrigated, and drains are placed.
14. The incision is closed.

SECTION IV: BREAST SURGERY

LEARNING OBJECTIVES

After studying this section the reader will be able to:
- Describe the structure of the breast
- Discuss supportive communication with the patient undergoing breast surgery
- List and compare diagnostic tests for breast cancer
- Recognize and identify instruments required for breast surgery
- Describe techniques used in breast surgery to remove a tissue mass
- Describe techniques used in tissue-conserving breast surgery

TERMINOLOGY: BREAST SURGERY

Body image: In psychology, the way a person sees himself or herself through the eyes of others. A negative body image can severely affect a patient's sense of identity and social and personal interactions.

Excisional biopsy: The removal of a tissue mass for pathological examination.

Frozen section: A technique used to examine biopsy tissue in which the tissue is frozen in liquid nitrogen and then processed through a microtome. The microtome cuts the mass into microscopic slices for examination under the microscope. Frozen section is performed during surgery so that the surgeon can determine whether immediate radical surgery is needed.

Hook wire: A device used to pinpoint the exact location of a non-palpable mass detected during a mammogram. A fine needle is inserted into the mass during the examination, and the tissue around the needle is removed for pathological examination and definitive diagnosis.

Mastectomy: A procedure in which breast tissue, including the skin, areola, and nipple, is removed, but the lymph nodes are not removed. Also called a *simple mastectomy.*

Modified radical mastectomy: A procedure in which the entire breast, nipple, and areolar region are removed. The lymph nodes also are usually removed.

Sentinel lymph node biopsy (SLNB): A procedure in which one or more lymph nodes are removed to determine whether a tumor has metastasized. Other lymph nodes may be removed periodically to determine whether metastasis has occurred.

Skin flap: A flap that is created by incising the skin and cutting it away from the underlying tissue to which it is attached. The flap can be increased in size or "raised" as it is enlarged by dissection.

Staging: A complex method of determining the severity of a malignant tumor. Lymph node involvement and the tumor's size, location, and type are considered.

Subcutaneous mastectomy: A procedure in which the breast is removed, but the skin, nipple, and areola are left intact. Also called a **lumpectomy**.

Technetium-99: A radioactive substance used to identify sentinel lymph nodes.

Wire localization biopsy: A procedure in which a hooked wire is inserted under fluroscopy into tissue suspected of being cancerous. The tissue surrounding a hook wire is removed.

INTRODUCTION

Most noncosmetic surgical procedures of the breast are performed for the treatment of cancer. Breast cancer diagnosis and treatment is a surgical specialty that has advanced greatly in the past two decades. Procedures that were common 10 years ago may never be performed in most clinical facilities. However, the psychological and social consequences of a cancer diagnosis have not changed. This aspect of patient care remains a critical concern of those caring for a patient undergoing breast surgery.

SURGICAL ANATOMY

The breasts lie within the fascia of the anterior chest wall from the second to the sixth ribs. The breast is composed of glandular, connective, and fat tissue contained within extensions of fibrous ligaments that radiate from the nipple to the periphery of the breast. Membranes or septal ligaments separate each of these radial sections. Each breast has about 15 to 25 separate sections. The glandular tissue forms clusters or small lobes, which are interspersed with alveoli that contain the secretory cells that form milk (Figure 23-29).

The intralobar ducts communicate from the glandular lobes. These ducts lead to the lactiferous ducts and reservoir and then open at the nipple. The nipple contains glandular, vascular, nerve, and epithelial tissue and is centered in the *areola,* a circular area of darkened skin. Small nodes in the areola contain sebaceous glands. Estrogen and progesterone, secreted cyclically and during pregnancy, cause the areola to darken.

The breast tissue changes with development of the individual, hormonal changes, pregnancy status, and nutritional state. The release of breast milk and other secretions from the nipple is controlled by complex hormonal changes.

The upper thoracic lymph drains to the axillary lymph nodes. This is an important anatomical feature, because cancer staging and diagnostic surgery often require biopsy of one or more axillary lymph nodes. The type and extent of change in the lymph nodes is a primary determinant of the disease outcome and survival rate.

PATHOLOGY OF THE BREAST

Table 23-8 presents various diseases and conditions that can affect the breast.

BREAST CANCER

Breast cancer is the leading cause of death in women age 20 to 59 in the United States. Improvements in diagnostic technology and aggressive public health campaigns in the United States have increased the reported number of cases of cancer in the last 10 years. This is due to early detection. Invasive ductal carcinoma is the most common type of breast cancer. Risk factors include a family history of breast cancer, benign breast disease, and hormonal conditions that result in late menarche or menopause. Breast cancer in men accounts for 0.8% of all breast cancers. The annual mortality rate for male breast cancer averages 400, compared with 400,000 in women.

Cancer **staging** is used to determine the possible outcome and options for treatment. However, the final decision rests with the patient, in consultation with the primary health care specialist, surgeon and oncologist. (Chapter 20 for a description of the cancer staging process.)

Breast cancer treatment has changed radically over the past 20 years, with a tendency toward less radical surgery. Early detection combined with improved chemotherapy and radiological treatment now provide an equal or better outcome than the radical mastectomy performed routinely several decades ago.

A range of procedures is available for surgical management of a breast tumor. These include:
- *Needle aspiration biopsy,* which usually is performed in the physician's office to confirm a cystic mass.
- *Fine needle insertion* into the suspect mass, with immediate surgical excision and **frozen section.** This is followed by breast-conserving surgery (**lumpectomy** or segmental resection), with or without lymph node excision.
- *Sentinel node detection and biopsy* followed by breast-conserving surgery and axillary node dissection.

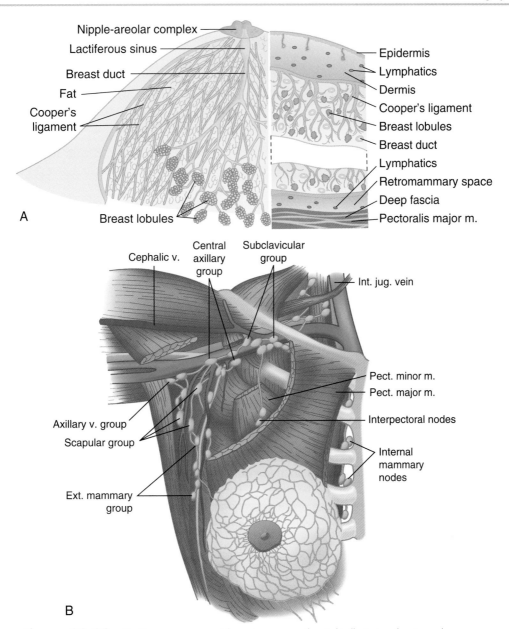

Figure 23-29   A, Breast anatomy. The cutaway on the right illustrates the tissue layers. The breast is supported by deep fascia and muscle. **B,** The axillary anatomy, showing lymph node drainage and the vascular supply. *(From Donegan WL, Spratt JS: Cancer of the breast, Philadelphia, 1988, WB Saunders.)*

Table 23-8

Pathology of the Breast

Condition	Description	Considerations
Cancer	Common types include intraductal, ductal, and inflammatory carcinoma.	Tumor staging and lymph node involvement determine the prognosis.
Fibrocystic disease	This disease is common in women age 30 to 50. It produces a noncancerous breast mass that can be detected on palpation or by a mammogram.	Treatment is symptomatic for pain. The differential diagnosis can be made after mammography with needle aspiration or a biopsy.
Mastitis	A condition involving inflammation and infection of the breast tissue, usually during lactation.	Late presentation may require incision and drainage.

- *Breasts conserving procedures,* such as lumpectomy and segmental resection.
- *Mastectomy (preplanned)* for advanced metastatic cancer or as a prophylactic procedure in high-risk patients.

Breast-conserving surgery with sentinel node biopsy is now the choice of most oncologists unless the cancer is advanced at the time of presentation. The prognosis is influenced more by the extent of lymph node involvement than by the size of the breast tumor.

DIAGNOSTIC PROCEDURES

Table 23-9 presents diagnostic procedures of the breast.

PERIOPERATIVE CONSIDERATIONS

PSYCHOLOGICAL CONSIDERATIONS

For most women, the breast reflects reproductive ability and **body image** and secures feminine identity. Surgery of the breast threatens these images and can produce anxiety and depression. Increased public awareness of breast cancer and advanced technology for early detection have increased women's ability to take an active part in breast health. Breast tumors also can occur in men, but the incidence is very low.

Although early detection is an important advance in breast medicine, the prospect of surgery remains an emotional and difficult issue for the patient. The patient's need for emotional support requires health care professionals to listen to the patient and support and acknowledge her feelings. The clinician's most important role in providing support is to provide a calm presence and to convey respect for the patient's feelings.

Reconstructive breast surgery may be done immediately after a mastectomy or as a separate procedure at a later date. The patient may enter a deep grieving period after such radical surgery. Psychological support at this time is critical in restoring the patient's positive self-image.

POSITION AND DRAPING

Breast surgery is performed with the patient in the supine position. A pad may be placed under the affected side at the level of the back to elevate the affected area. The affected arm is prepped and draped free in most cases, except for a simple lumpectomy without axillary node dissection.

If the arm is draped free, an armboard is used as in limb surgery. This allows the surgeon to manipulate the arm for exposure to the axilla at various angles. Care must be taken not to allow the arm to drop off the armboard during surgery.

INSTRUMENTS AND SUPPLIES

Surgery of the breast requires general surgery instruments and a plastic surgery set. Senn, vein, and other small retractors are needed for breast biopsy. Surgical clips, absorbable and non-absorbable sutures, and an ESU are used for hemostasis. Vessel loops are needed for retraction of deep veins, arteries, and nerves. Wound drains include the Jackson-Pratt, Hemovac, and simpler gravity drains, such as the Penrose drain. The ESU is used extensively in radical breast surgery. The surgeon may require a nerve stimulator to differentiate blood vessels from small nerves during dissection of the chest wall and axilla.

Table 23-9

Diagnostic Procedures of the Breast

Type	Description	Considerations
Breast self-examination (BSE)	Women and men are taught how to perform BSE by a primary care professional. The procedure for BSE involves systematic palpation of the breast and axillary region and visual examination, starting at age 20.	The patient should be instructed by a qualified health professional who can answer questions and make sure the patient understands the procedure and its importance.
Clinical examination	The clinical examination involves palpation and visual examination of the breasts by a qualified health professional.	Women in their 20s and 30s should have a clinical examination every 3 years.
Mammogram	A mammogram is a radiological examination of the breasts for detection of masses or other lesions.	Mammography is the only screening method effective for the detection of nonpalpable lesions. A yearly mammogram is recommended for women age 40 or older.
Fine-needle aspiration (FNA)	A fine-gauge needle is inserted into a suspect breast mass, and tissue (cells and fluid) is withdrawn for examination and diagnosis.	This procedure may be performed in the physician's office.
Stereotactic biopsy	The patient lies prone on the mammography table with the breast isolated. A computer-assisted needle is guided into the suspect mass, and a core sample is withdrawn.	This procedure is less invasive than surgical biopsy. Stereotactic technology provides accurate placement of the needle and has a 96% accuracy for detecting cancer.

WIRE LOCALIZATION AND BREAST BIOPSY

Surgical Goal

Wire localization is the insertion of a fine wire into a breast mass during fluoroscopy. The wire is taped in place, and surgical biopsy is performed at the site of the wire. This is a specific technique used to identify the site of a suspected mass whereas needle biopsy is used to withdraw a small amount of fluid and cells for pathological analysis.

Technique

1. During mammography, the patient is prepped and a local anesthetic is administered in the area of the mass.
2. A hook wire assembly is inserted into the mass.
3. The wire is secured to the patient's skin with tape.
4. The patient is transferred to the operating room.
5. Additional prep solution may be applied gently around the site of the needle.
6. The patient is draped for an excisional biopsy of the breast.
7. The needle is located, and an elliptical incision is made that includes the needle and a margin of skin.
8. The incision is continued through the subcutaneous and breast tissue, including a 1- to 2-cm margin. Small rake retractors are placed in the wound edge.
9. The needle and tissue are removed, and the tissue is examined by the pathologist for clear margins.
10. If the tissue is malignant or if the tumor margins are not clear of cancer cells, a more extensive procedure may be initiated, or the surgery may be deferred for 24 hours.
11. The breast tissue is closed with 3-0 absorbable suture.
12. The skin is closed with sterile adhesive strips.

Discussion

The patient is admitted for surgery immediately after placement of a hook needle during mammography or ultrasound. After administration of an anesthetic, the breast is gently prepped to avoid dislodging the needle. A fenestrated body drape is then applied. Care must be taken not to displace the needle during the prep and draping.

The surgeon begins the procedure by making an elliptical skin incision around the **hook wire.** The surgeon then uses Metzenbaum scissors to increase the depth of the incision. Senn retractors or small rakes are placed at the wound edges. Scissors rather than an ESU are used to complete the dissection to avoid distorting the margins of the mass. Allis clamps may be used to grasp the tissue during dissection. The specimen, with identification needle intact, is delivered to the pathologist for examination. If the margins of the specimen are *not* clear of tumor, additional tissue is removed and examined. When the margins include a clear area of 0.4 to 0.8 inch (1 to 2 cm), the wound is closed.

The excision site is irrigated with warm saline and closed with several subcutaneous, interrupted sutures of absorbable synthetic material. The skin usually is closed with sterile strips or a subcuticular suture.

SENTINEL LYMPH NODE BIOPSY

Surgical Goal

The procedure for **sentinel lymph node biopsy (SLNB)** involves injection of isosulfan blue dye, radioactive material (**technetium-99**), or both directly into the breast mass or nearby. Both materials may be used to track the lymph nodes visually (dye) and by gamma ray emission (technetium-99). The technetium then is tracked with a device similar to a Geiger counter.

If radioactive material is used, it may be injected 2 hours or longer before surgery in the nuclear medicine department. Isosulfan is injected at the time of surgery to provide greater visibility of the nodes. Surgery for node excision then follows.

NOTE: Isosulfan blue may cause anaphylactic shock in some patients. When used in conjunction with SLNB, the patient is monitored carefully throughout the procedure. A crash cart must be immediately available in these cases.

Pathology

Sentinel lymph nodes are usually located at the proximal axillary lymph chain. A metastatic tumor in the breast drains (theoretically) first to these nodes. Excision of the sentinel nodes is an alternative procedure to axillary lymph node dissection, in which 10 or more nodes are removed for preventive treatment. Sentinel node excision may be appropriate only in selected patients with a low risk of metastasis.

Technique

1. The breast mass or biopsy site from previous surgery is injected with technetium-99.
2. A gamma ray detecting probe is used to determine which lymph nodes are affected.
3. The affected nodes are marked with a dye pen.
4. The patient is prepped and draped for excisional biopsy.
5. Isosulfan is injected into or near the breast mass.
6. The sentinel nodes are removed.

Discussion

Excisional biopsy of sentinel nodes follows the techniques used for superficial axillary exploration. Only nodes identified by gamma ray emission are removed by superficial surgery. This may precede excision of the breast mass. The scrub must provide a separate container for each node and ensure that they are identified appropriately.

BREAST-CONSERVING SURGERY FOR A MASS (LUMPECTOMY, SEGMENTAL MASTECTOMY)

Surgical Goal

A breast mass is removed to confirm a diagnosis or to treat malignancy. The mass is excised ensuring that the margins are completely free of cancer cells. Axillary dissection to remove a group of lymph nodes or removal of selective sentinel lymph nodes may be performed during the same procedure. Analysis of the mass by frozen section is done during surgery; this determines the extent of the excision discussed and planned with the patient before surgery. Figure 23-30 shows the possible incisions for an excision procedure.

In a skin-sparing (subcutaneous) mastectomy, the overlying skin tissue, the areola, and the nipple are not removed. An implant may be placed immediately after the procedure.

Pathology

Both malignancy and some benign breast neoplasms generally present as a mass that is visible with imaging studies or that can be detected by palpation. A mass smaller than 0.4 inch (1 cm) usually is not palpable and is detected with routine mammography or other imaging techniques. Gynecomastia, which is excess breast tissue in the male, is caused by a hormonal imbalance and usually is treated medically. Mastectomy may be required if the condition does not respond to medical treatment.

Technique

1. An incision is made at the border of the areola or directly over the tumor mass.
2. The mass is grasped with one or more Allis clamps and excised using sharp dissection.
3. Hemostasis is maintained with fine sutures or an electrosurgical unit (ESU) needle.
4. The specimen may be marked with sutures for orientation and then removed for pathological examination.
5. After the pathology report is received, the wound is extended to include a greater portion of the breast.
6. Sentinel lymph node biopsy may be performed through a separate incision.
7. The wound is irrigated.
8. Drains are placed in the wound.
9. The wound is closed.

Discussion

The skin incision is made along skin lines drawn preoperatively. This incision is carried through the subcutaneous and breast tissue with Metzenbaum or Mayo scissors. Small bleeders are coagulated with a needle-point ESU tip. A spatula ESU tip generally is not used for en bloc removal of a suspect mass, because this may obliterate the tissue margins and obscure a diagnosis.

The surgeon grasps the subcutaneous and breast tissue with two or more Allis clamps. The scrub should have retractors available as the incision is extended to deep tissue. Small rake or Senn retractors can be used for shallow retraction, and right-angle retractors (small Richardson or Deaver retractors) are needed for deeper excision. Hemostasis is maintained with fine absorbable sutures and electrosurgical needle.

As the excision is extended, Raytec sponges should be removed from the field and replaced with laparotomy sponges. A Raytec sponge can be easily lost inside the breast wound, especially if the excision is deep.

The specimen is removed in one piece. The surgeon may place one or more sutures on the periphery for identification of the margins. These must be carefully preserved. The breast wound may be closed at this time, or closure may be delayed until axillary dissection is completed.

Axillary Dissection

Axillary lymph nodes, which drain the breast, can include cancer cells from a malignant tumor. To gain access to the axillary nodes, the surgeon makes an incision just below the upper axillary fold. This tissue plane includes the subcutaneous and fascia layers. The lower flap is tapered toward the chest wall.

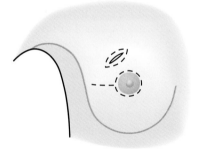

Lateral extension can increase axillary exposure

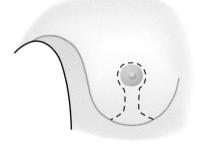

Wise pattern

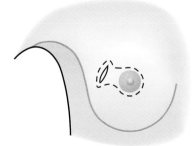

Incision when biopsy site near areola

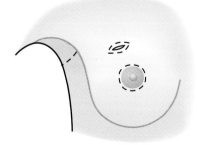

Incision when biopsy site remote from areola with axillary incision for lymphadenectomy

Figure 23-30 Incisions for a skin-sparing biopsy. *(From Townsend CM: Sabiston textbook of surgery, ed 17, Philadelphia, 2001, WB Saunders.)*

After the flaps have been created, right-angle retractors are placed along the edges. The pectoralis muscles are then retracted to expose the axillary vein and its small branches. These are clamped and divided. The axillary vein is ligated with silk sutures. Small branches may require fine suture ligation or surgical clips. The surgeon continues to dissect the axillary tissue to expose the two major nerves in this area (thoracic and intercostobrachial nerves). These nerves must be preserved during node dissection. Vessel loops are placed under the nerves with a right-angle clamp. Axillary tissue containing the nodes is then dissected away from the underlying muscle.

Before closing the axilla, the surgeon may place a Jackson-Pratt or Penrose drain in the wound. If a closed suction drain is used, the end is brought out through a small stab incision near the main incision. The drain is secured with one or two nonabsorbable sutures. The wounds are closed in two layers. The axilla and subcutaneous breast tissue are closed with interrupted absorbable sutures. The skin is closed with a running subcuticular suture of the surgeon's choice.

MASTECTOMY

Surgical Goal
The goal of mastectomy is to remove the entire breast. The extent of axillary dissection depends on the cancer stage and other factors.

- In a **total** (or **simple**) **mastectomy,** the entire breast is removed. The axillary lymph nodes are not removed, and the muscles of the chest wall are preserved.
- In a **modified radical mastectomy,** the entire breast is removed, and complete axillary dissection with excision of nodes is performed.
- In a *radical mastectomy* (rarely performed) the entire breast, all axillary nodes, and the chest wall muscles are removed.

Pathology
Subcutaneous mastectomy is performed for primary tumors with clear margins.

Technique

1. The skin and subcutaneous tissue are incised in an elliptical pattern.
2. The skin flaps are raised to the previously marked areas and retracted with skin hooks.
3. Lateral edges of the flaps are carried to the edge of the latissimus dorsi muscle.
4. Large perforating blood vessels are ligated and secured.
5. The breast and deep fascia are dissected away from the pectoralis muscle.
6. The specimen is dissected free from the lateral chest wall and axilla.
7. Intercostal arteries and veins are ligated and divided.
8. The axillary flap is raised, preserving the axillary vein and nerves.
9. The axillary tissues are further dissected from the surrounding muscles and ligaments
10. The specimen is removed.
11. Hemostasis is maintained.
12. Two suction drains are placed in the wound.
13. The ends of the pectoralis minor muscle are sutured together.
14. The flaps are closed with skin staples, subcuticular suture, and sterile adhesive strips.
15. A soft, bulky dressing is placed over the wound.

Discussion
Historically, a radical mastectomy (i.e., removal of the breast and chest wall muscles and fascia, as well as complete axillary excision) was the only treatment available for a malignant breast mass. This procedure now is rarely performed. Radical mastectomy has been modified, and it is indicated only for late presentation of chest wall metastasis arising from a primary breast tumor.

To begin the procedure, the surgeon marks both the incision and the extent of the skin flaps. Incising the skin and creating a space between the skin and the underlying tissue creates a **skin flap.** This is called *raising a skin flap.* In this procedure, the skin flaps include subcutaneous tissue. The superior and anterior flaps are extended to the previously marked lines on the skin. Skin hooks are used to elevate the flaps and extend the dissection.

The surgeon uses sharp dissection to carry the flaps deeper to the edge of the latissimus dorsi muscle. The scrub should have two ESU units available so that one can be cleaned while the other is in use. As large blood vessels are encountered, they are ligated with surgical clips and divided or clamped and secured with silk ties. The surgeon separates the breast and fascial tissue from the pectoralis major muscle. The skin flaps are retracted gently to preserve their blood supply and to prevent bruising and ischemia at the edges.

Axillary dissection is a continuous part of this procedure. Rake or Richardson retractors are placed over the axillary edge of the incision. Blunt rakes are preferred to prevent puncturing of the skin in this area. An additional right-angle retractor or narrow Deaver or Richardson retractors may be needed for the medial side of the incision.

Tributaries of the axillary vein are exposed and cross-clamped with right-angle clamps; they are then divided, and clipped or ligated. For level III node dissection, the surgeon must sever the pectoralis minor muscle with the ESU. Retraction of the pectoralis muscles with right-angle retractors exposes the axillary tissues. The specimen is dissected from the chest wall and muscles. The apex may be marked with a suture for pathological identification.

The surgeon then may pass the specimen to the scrub, who receives it in a small basin. Before closing the wound, the surgeon places two suction drains in the axilla and brings the ends out at the lateral chest wall. The ends of the pectoralis minor muscle are sutured together with absorbable sutures.

The wound is irrigated with antibacterial solution and closed in layers. Absorbable subcutaneous sutures are placed. The skin is closed with a running subcuticular suture or skin staples, depending on the surgeon's preference.

CHAPTER SUMMARY

- The body is divided into semiclosed compartments or cavities that contain specific anatomical structures and organs. The cavities are separated by membrane, muscle, and other connective tissue.
- The abdomen is divided into four major sections, or landmarks, called *quadrants.*
- The Hesselbach triangle is the area bounded by the rectus abdominis, inguinal ligament, and inferior epigastric vessels. This is the area associated with inguinal hernias.
- Abdominal incisions are named according to their anatomical location, specifically: midline, paramedian, subcostal, flank, inguinal, and lower transverse incisions.
- A McBurney incision is a short, right transverse incision used in appendectomies.
- Surgery of the abdominal wall is performed to repair a hernia, which is an acquired or a congenital defect in the fascia, muscle, or other tissues.
- A hernia requires urgent surgical treatment if the trapped (incarcerated) viscera becomes strangulated (deprived of blood).
- An indirect inguinal hernia arises from the internal inguinal ring. Herniated tissue protrudes into the spermatic cord and sometimes descends into the scrotum. A direct hernia is related to a weakness in the abdominal wall; herniated tissue protrudes through the transversalis fascia in the posterior wall of the inguinal canal.
- Surgical mesh is used for most hernia repairs. Biosynthetic mesh is made of synthetic material similar to suture (e.g., Prolene, Dacron, and Mersilene).
- An incarcerated hernia is one in which the abdominal viscera are trapped between tissue layers and deprived of blood.
- During repair of an inguinal hernia, protruding tissue is pushed back into the abdominal cavity, and the defect is closed with sutures or surgical staples.
- A femoral hernia is more common in women than in men and results from a weakness in the transversalis fascia.
- A ventral hernia usually is caused by incomplete healing of a previous abdominal wall incision and often is related to obesity.
- Gastrointestinal (GI) surgery includes procedures of the lower esophagus, stomach, small intestine, large intestine, rectum, and anus.
- A laparotomy is a procedure in which the abdomen is opened surgically.
- A surgical vocabulary has developed that describes techniques commonly used in gastrointestinal surgery.
- During bowel technique, also known as *isolation technique,* instruments and supplies used while the bowel is open are kept separate from all other sterile items. This prevents prevent contamination of the surgical wound and of "clean" instruments by the bowel contents.
- Esophagoduodenoscopy is diagnostic endoscopy of the esophagus, stomach, and proximal duodenum. The procedure often is called an "upper GI."
- Colonoscopy is endoscopy of the large intestine; it is referred to as "lower GI" endoscopy.
- During all endoscopic procedures, the scrub assists the surgeon by guiding the long instruments into the endoscope and handling them when they are withdrawn.
- During a laparotomy, all loose 4×4 sponges must be removed from the surgical field. Only those mounted on sponge forceps are used while the abdomen is open.
- Nissen fundoplication is commonly performed to treat gastroesophageal reflux disease. In this procedure, the upper stomach is wrapped around the esophagus below the hiatus to act as a sphincter.
- Subtotal gastrectomy requires reconstruction of the stomach to maintain continuity of the GI tract. In a Billroth I procedure, the stomach is anastomosed to the duodenum. In a Billroth II procedure, the stomach is anastomosed to the jejunum.
- Hand-suturing and surgical stapling are the two techniques commonly used to join the stomach with the intestine.
- Obesity is an endemic health problem in the United States. It contributes to cardiovascular disease, cancers of the breast and large intestine, diabetes, stroke, urinary stress incontinence, and depression. Approximately 400,000 people in the United States die annually as a result of obesity.
- Band gastroplasty is performed to treat morbid obesity. A small pouch is created in the proximal stomach, restricting nutritional intake.
- The Roux-en-Y procedure is performed to bypass the stomach and re-establish continuity from the stomach to the jejunum. In this procedure, a large portion of the stomach is bypassed and a new gastric pouch is created.
- Resection of the small intestine is performed to treat an obstruction, an ulcer, or a carcinoma.
- *Intestinal obstruction* is a general term encompassing a number of mechanical pathologies that block the intestine and require emergency surgery.
- An ostomy is a procedure in which a portion of the intestine is divided and the open end is secured to the skin, draining the bowel contents outside the body. The opening is then called a *stoma.*
- A temporary stoma is created when a section of the bowel is made nonfunctional during the healing process.
- Stoma care requires qualified patient teaching by a certified ostomy specialist. Patients require a period of adaptation while learning to care for the ostomy.

- When a patient with a stoma is prepped for surgery, the stoma itself is prepped last to prevent contamination of the site.
- In abdominoperineal resection, the anus, rectum, and sigmoid colon are removed en bloc through combined abdominal and perineal incisions. Two teams may operate simultaneously.
- An appendectomy is the removal of the appendix, a blind, narrow, elongated pouch attached to the cecum. A McBurney incision is used to approach the appendix.
- The venous plexus of the anal canal may become congested or distended, causing pain, bleeding, and prolapse outside the anal canal. These lesions are called *hemorrhoids.*
- A hemorrhoidectomy most often is performed using elastic ring ligation, laser techniques, or an ultrasound scalpel.
- A pilonidal cyst is a congenital defect in which epithelial tissue develops below the surface of the skin in the area of the sacrum and coccyx. The cyst is removed when it causes recurrent infection of the area. A sinus tract (a channel leading to an abscess) often is present.
- End-stage alcoholic liver disease is characterized by fibrosis of the liver, which prevents the flow of blood and bile. Blood backs up into the portal vein, causing congestion and rupture of the esophageal venous plexus.
- Traumatic injury to the spleen is related to the organ's location in the abdomen and its highly vascular structure. Rupture of the spleen requires emergency surgery.
- Procedures of the biliary system and pancreas, including choledochoscopy and endoscopic retrograde cholangiopancreatography, sometimes require intraoperative use of flexible fiberoptic endoscopes. These scopes are inserted into the small ducts of the accessory organs to locate stones, tumors, or benign lesions.
- During endoscopic retrograde cholangiopancreatography, a fiberoptic endoscope is inserted through the upper GI tract and guided into the duodenum and ampulla of Vater. Biopsies may be taken from the ducts, and stones may be removed.
- Two common diseases of the biliary system are cholelithiasis (the presence of gallstones) and cholecystitis (inflammation of the gallbladder). High blood cholesterol and obesity contribute to the formation gallstones, which can block the bile ducts.
- Choledochoscopy is endoscopic examination of the bile ducts. It may be performed as a diagnostic procedure or to remove gallstones.

- A cholecystectomy commonly is performed to treat chronic inflammation of the gallbladder and to prevent infection.
- Gallstones must be kept dry after they are received as specimens during surgery.
- The spleen is removed surgically to stop hemorrhage from trauma or to treat disease. Splenic tissue is delicate and easily torn and has a rich vascular system. Its location in the abdomen makes it vulnerable to injury caused by the steering wheel during motor vehicle accidents.
- Trauma to the spleen is a life-threatening condition that requires immediate operative intervention. Because of its highly vascular structure, the spleen can suffer extensive blood loss in a short time.
- The Whipple procedure is performed for palliative treatment of pancreatic cancer. In this procedure, the head of the pancreas and duodenum, and a portion of the jejunum, distal stomach, and distal section of the common bile duct are removed. The biliary system, pancreatic system, and GI tract are reconstructed.
- In the segmental approach, one or more of the nine liver segments are removed.
- In a liver lobectomy, one or more of the major lobes of the liver (right, left, or the entire right lobe and a portion of the left) are removed. The most common indication for liver resection is a malignant liver tumor.
- Most noncosmetic surgical procedures of the breast are performed for the treatment of cancer. In the United States, breast cancer is the leading cause of death in women age 20 to 59.
- Wire localization is the insertion of a fine wire into a breast mass during fluoroscopy. The wire is taped in place, and surgical biopsy is performed at the site of the needle.
- Sentinel lymph nodes occur at the proximal axillary lymph chain. A metastatic tumor in the breast drains (theoretically) first to these nodes. The purpose of sentinel node biopsy is to diagnose metastasis.
- In a skin-sparing mastectomy, the overlying skin tissue, the areola, and the nipple are not removed (subcutaneous mastectomy).
- In a total or simple mastectomy, the entire breast is removed. The axillary lymph nodes are not removed, and the chest wall muscles are preserved.
- In a modified radical mastectomy, the entire breast is removed, and complete axillary dissection with excision of nodes is performed.
- In a radical mastectomy (rarely performed), the entire breast, all axillary nodes, and the chest wall muscles are removed.

REVIEW QUESTIONS

Section I: Abdominal Wall Surgery

1. Discuss the importance of knowing the names of the abdominal regions.
2. What is the significance of the linea alba?
3. What are the primary tissues of the abdominal wall?
4. Name five abdominal incisions and the organs associated with them.
5. What is the principle involved in hernia repair with biosynthetic mesh?
6. What is the difference between a direct inguinal hernia and an indirect inguinal hernia?
7. Describe an incarcerated hernia. What causes this condition?
8. Describe how you would dress an infected incisional hernia. List the supplies and briefly state why you would use them.

Section II: Gastrointestinal Surgery

1. Why are compression stockings used during lengthy procedures?
2. What stapling instruments would you include on a setup for a gastric resection?
3. Describe bowel technique and why it is used.
4. When a patient is positioned for bariatric surgery, what special safety precautions are practiced?
5. What is the principle of Nissen fundoplication surgery?
6. Study the bowel instruments listed in this chapter. What are the common design features of grasping and clamping instruments?
7. Define *anastomosis*, *resection*, and *mobilization*. List several instruments used in these techniques.
8. What is a bowel obstruction?
9. What is a stoma?

Section III: Surgery of the Biliary System, Liver, Pancreas, and Spleen

1. Why is the spleen removed rather than repaired after severe trauma?
2. Why do esophageal varices form in advanced cirrhosis?
3. What structure drains bile after a cholecystectomy?
4. What procedure has replaced operative cholangiography in modern surgical practice?
5. What are the surgical priorities in emergency surgery for a ruptured spleen?
6. Review and explain the preparation of Avitene, Surgicel, and Gelfoam for use in a surgical wound.
7. Which handheld retractors might be used to retract the liver during gallbladder surgery?
8. Why is it dangerous for bile to spill into the abdominal cavity during gallbladder surgery?

Section IV: Breast Surgery

1. Why do women have more options for breast cancer surgery now than they did 20 years ago?
2. What is BSE?
3. What is the difference between needle aspiration and stereotactic biopsy?
4. Why is dye used during sentinel node biopsy?
5. Why is the arm of the affected side draped free during many breast procedures?
6. Describe how you would handle and maintain a breast biopsy sample for frozen section.
7. What is the principle of sentinel node biopsy?
8. What retractors should be available for tissue-sparing mastectomy?
9. Why isn't the ESU used for dissection of a breast tumor?

BIBLIOGRAPHY

Bland KI, Copeland EM: *The breast: comprehensive management of benign and malignant disorders,* ed 3, Philadelphia, 2004, WB Saunders.

Murray SS, McKinney ES, Gorrie TM: *Foundations of maternal-newborn nursing,* ed 3, Philadelphia, 2002, WB Saunders.

Porth CM, Kunert MP: *Pathophysiology: concepts of altered health states,* ed 6, Philadelphia, 2002, Lippincott Williams & Williams.

Rothrock JC: *Alexander's care of the patient in surgery,* ed 13, St Louis, 2007, Mosby.

Thibodeau G, Patton K: *Anatomy and physiology,* ed 6, St Louis, 2007, Mosby.

Townsend C: *Sabiston textbook of surgery,* ed 17, Philadelphia, 2004, WB Saunders.

CHAPTER 24

Gynecological and Obstetrical Surgery

CHAPTER OUTLINE

SECTION I: GYNECOLOGICAL AND REPRODUCTIVE SURGERY

LEARNING OBJECTIVES

After studying this section the reader will be able to:

- Describe the primary features of reproductive anatomy
- Discuss common gynecological diseases and conditions that may require surgery
- Identify gynecological instruments and equipment
- Identify common diagnostic procedures in reproductive medicine
- Describe the principles and technique of hysteroscopy

- Explain the rationale for using electrolytic or nonelectrolytic distention fluid in hysteroscopy
- Explain the importance of maintaining aseptic technique during vaginal procedures
- Apply the principles and techniques of gynecological surgery during a variety of procedures
- Describe the appropriate psychological support of a patient undergoing an obstetrical or a gynecological procedure

TERMINOLOGY

Ablate: To remove or destroy tissue.

Adnexa: A collective term for the ovaries, fallopian tubes, and their connective and vascular attachments.

Bladder flap: A peritoneal fold between the bladder and the uterus.

Coitus: Sexual intercourse.

Colposcopy: Microscopic examination of the cervix.

Cystocele: A herniation of the bladder into the vaginal wall.

Dermoid cyst: A mass arising from the germ layers of the embryo that contains tissue remnants, including hair and teeth.

Dilation: Opening of the cervix during labor (measured in centimeters).

Electrolytic media: Fluids that contain electrolytes and therefore can transmit an electrical current.

En bloc: A term meaning "in one piece." In surgery, it describes the technique of removing tissue.

Endometriosis: The growth of endometrial tissue outside the uterine cavity.

Episiotomy: A perineal incision made during the second stage of labor to prevent the tearing of tissue.

Extravasation: The absorption of the fluid into the vascular system, leading to increased blood pressure and possible death related to fluid overload. This occurs during surgery when distension fluid used during endoscopic procedures is absorbed through large blood vessels in the bladder or uterus.

Fibroid: See Leiomyoma.

Hyperplasia: An excessive proliferation of tissue.

Hyponaturemia: Low serum sodium. Severe hyponaturemia and death can result from the use of hypotonic distension fluids used during hysteroscopy.

Hysteroscopy: The use of a special endoscope for diagnostic procedures and interventional surgery of the uterus.

Incomplete abortion: The demise of the embryo or fetus and expulsion of the tissue.

LEEP: Loop electrode excision procedure. In this technique, an electrosurgical loop is used to remove a core of tissue from the cervical canal.

Leiomyoma: A fibrous, benign tumor of the uterus that usually arises from the myometrium.

Menarche: Menstruation, menses.

Menorrhagia: Excessive bleeding during menses.

Missed abortion: An abortion in which the products of conception are no longer viable but are retained in the uterus.

Obturator: A blunt-nosed instrument that is inserted through the sheath of a rigid endoscope or hysteroscope to protect the tissue as the instrument is advanced.

Oophorectomy: Removal of the ovary.

Papanicolaou (PAP) test: A diagnostic test in which epithelial cells are taken from the endocervical canal and examined for abnormalities that can lead to cervical cancer.

Parturition: Birth.

Patency: The condition of being open; an unobstructed passageway (e.g., a patent fallopian tube).

Perineum: The anatomical area between the posterior vestibule and the anus.

PID: Pelvic inflammatory disease; PID is caused by a sexually transmitted disease or some other source of infection. It causes scarring of the fallopian tubes and adhesions in the abdominal and pelvic cavity.

Rectocele: A bulging of intestinal tissue into a weakened posterior vaginal wall.

Transcervical: Literally, "through the cervix." In surgery, a transcervical approach means that surgery is performed by passing instruments through the cervix.

INTRODUCTION

Obstetrical and gynecological surgery (OB-GYN) is a combined medical-surgical specialty. Gynecology focuses on the treatment and prevention of diseases affecting the female reproductive system. Fertility medicine combines gynecology and endocrinology to achieve and maintain pregnancy. Obstetrics relates to the process of pregnancy and birth (**parturition**).

In addition to providing routine surgical assistance in gynecological procedures, surgical technologists are employed in the obstetrical department or freestanding childbirth center. This specialty requires a high level of knowledge not only about anatomy and physiology, but also about important psychosocial factors that influence the process of childbirth. Normal childbirth is included in this chapter as an introduction to this specialty.

SURGICAL ANATOMY

UTERUS

The uterus and associated organs of the female reproductive system are located in the anterior female pelvic cavity. The uterus is roughly pear shaped, approximately 3 inches (7.5 cm) long, and 2 inches (5 cm) deep. It houses and protects the fetus during pregnancy. It is composed of thick muscular tissue and is suspended in the pelvic cavity by ligaments that completely enclose the organ (Figure 24-1). Two fallopian tubes communicate directly with the interior of the uterus at each lateral "horn" of the uterus. The superior (upper) portion of the uterus, which lies above the insertion of the fallopian tubes, is called the *fundus*. The middle portion is called the *body*, and the lower portion is the *cervix* (Figure 24-2). The uterus normally tilts forward in the pelvic cavity, with the fundus closest to the anterior abdominal wall. However, variations occur and usually are not significant. The cervix is approximately 0.8 to 1.2 inches (2 to 3 cm) long and communicates directly with the vagina through a small orifice called the *external os*. During labor and childbirth, the os dilates as the cervix thins (*effaces*) to provide an opening for the fetus to emerge.

Structure

The endometrium, which lines the uterus, changes under hormonal influence and with pregnancy. It is continuous with the lining of the fallopian tubes and the vagina. The myometrium is a thick muscular layer that is continuous with the muscles of the vagina and the fallopian tubes. The myometrium contracts during childbirth and menses. The perimetrium, or outer serous layer of the uterus, is a reflection (folding back)

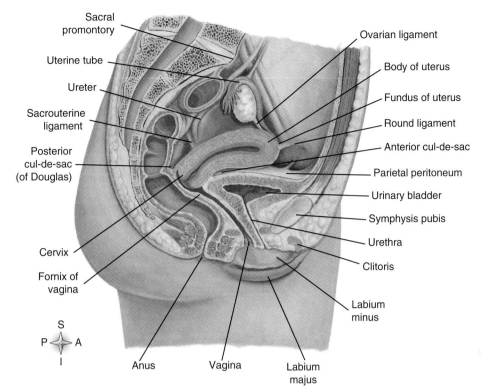

Figure 24-1 The pelvic cavity. Note the position of the urinary structures in relation to the uterus. *(From Thibodeau G, Patton K: Anatomy and physiology, ed 6, St Louis, 2007, Mosby.)*

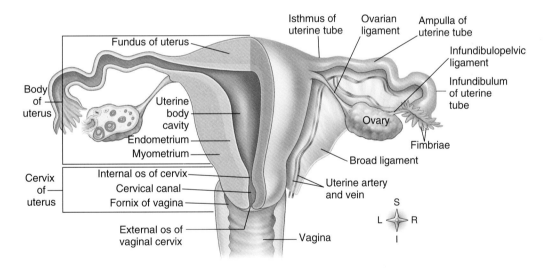

Figure 24-2 The uterus and adnexa. *(From Thibodeau G, Patton K: Anatomy and physiology, ed 6, St Louis, 2007, Mosby.)*

of the abdominal peritoneum over the bladder. This forms a pouch called the *cul-de-sac*; the fold is called the *bladder flap*.

The *cervix* is the lower neck of the uterus. It extends into the vaginal vault. The opening of the cervix is called the *cervical os*. The os is dilated for **transcervical** procedures, or it may dilate naturally under hormonal influence during childbirth. The os has two anatomical sections, the external os and the internal opening. These two openings communicate by means of a short canal.

Uterine Ligaments

The uterine ligaments sometimes are difficult to picture and understand. The broad ligaments suspend the uterus from the pelvic wall. Above the broad ligaments, near the fallopian tubes, lie the round ligaments, which help suspend the uterus anteriorly. The cardinal ligaments lie below the broad ligaments and provide the primary support for the uterus. The uterosacral ligaments curve along the bottom of the uterus and attach it to the sacrum.

FALLOPIAN TUBES

The two fallopian tubes attach directly to the uterus, one on each side. Each fallopian tube has four sections: the *interstitial section,* which connects to the uterus; the narrow *isthmus* in the midportion; the *ampulla,* which is the widened portion of the tube; and the *infundibulum,* the terminal end of the tube. The *fimbriae* are small projections that extend from the end of the tube. These direct the ovum toward the infundibulum during ovulation. The fallopian tube is very narrow (3 to 5 mm wide). It is not connected to the ovary, but is suspended from the upper margin of the pelvis by the infundibulopelvic ligament. The lower margin is suspended by the mesosalpinx. Surgery of the fallopian tube usually requires dissection of the mesosalpinx, which frees the tube from its attachments. The fallopian tube, the ovaries, and their ligaments are collectively called the *adnexa.*

OVARIES

The ovaries secrete the female hormones. They lie on each side of the uterus in the upper portion of the pelvic cavity. The ovaries are suspended by the mesovarium, or peritoneal tissue attached to the uterus by ovarian ligaments. The ovary is oval and approximately 1.5 inches (3.75 cm) long. Each ovary contains approximately 1 million eggs, which are present at birth.

The fibrous outer layer of the ovary, called the *cortex,* contains follicles that hold ova in different stages of maturity. The inner core of the ovary, the *medulla,* is composed of connective and vascular tissue. Vesicles in the medulla hold the immature ova, which are stimulated to mature after puberty. The development and release of the ova are influenced by the pituitary gland, which stimulates the gonadotropic hormones luteinizing hormone (LH) and follicle-stimulating hormone (FSH). Ova remain in hormone-secreting follicles and develop in stages until they are released from the ovary. A complete cycle is called the *ovarian cycle.*

VAGINA

The vagina, or vaginal vault, is a muscular passageway that shares a thick fibrous wall with the rectum on the posterior side and the bladder on the anterior side. The vagina extends from the vestibule, or introitus (opening to the outside of the body), to the uterine cervix, which protrudes at the upper vagina. The recessed areas around the cervix are referred to as *fornices.* The function of the vagina is to enable sexual intercourse (**coitus**) and delivery of the fetus during childbirth.

The vaginal lining is composed of thick connective tissue covered with epithelium. The lining has numerous folds, called *rugae,* that can distend during childbirth. The tone, lubrication, and elasticity of the vaginal mucosa are influenced by the level of female sex hormones, especially estrogen. After menopause (cessation of ovulation), a decrease in hormonal levels results in loss of elasticity, changes in the vaginal pH, and dryness.

VULVA

The structures that together make up the external genitalia are called the *vulva* (Figure 24-3).

Mons Pubis

The mons pubis is a raised mound of tissue that protects the symphysis pubis. It is covered with skin and contains connective and fatty tissue that is continuous with the lower pelvic wall. It is covered with somewhat coarse hair that develops at puberty.

LABIA MAJORA

The labia majora are two external folds of adipose tissue that envelope the perineal area. They are extensions of the anterior mons pubis. They encircle the vestibule and protect the external genitalia.

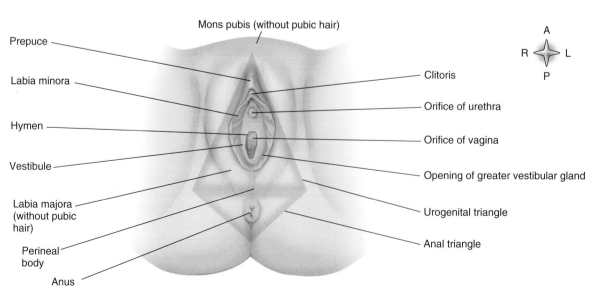

Figure 24-3   Structures of the vulva. *(From Thibodeau G, Patton K: Anatomy and physiology, ed 6, St Louis, 2007, Mosby.)*

LABIA MINORA

The labia minora are bisectional (composed of two sections) and lie directly beneath the labia majora. The two sections come together anteriorly, where they are attached by the frenulum. Anteriorly, they meet just in front of the clitoris to form the prepuce (hood) and are continuous with the vaginal mucosa.

CLITORIS

The clitoris is a highly vascular organ that contains sensitive erectile tissue. It projects slightly from the anterior folds of the labia minora. A fold of skin, called the *prepuce* or hood, covers the clitoris and is formed by the superior juncture of the labia minora. The clitoris, which is protected by the folds of the labia majora, becomes engorged and highly sensitive during sexual excitation.

VESTIBULE

The term *vestibule* refers collectively to all the structures located within the labia minora. The vestibular glands collectively include the *Skenes* glands (paraurethral glands) and the Bartholin glands. The Skene glands are two small, paired glands that lie beneath the floor of the urethra, which terminates at the urethral meatus within the vestibule. The Bartholin glands lie on both sides of the vestibule and secrete mucus during sexual intercourse. These glands are homologous to the bulbourethral glands in the male.

HYMEN

The hymen is a thin vascular fold of tissue that attaches around the entrance of the vagina. The hymen separates the vagina from the vestibule. In the young female, the membrane is usually but not always intact. The membrane generally is torn during coitus and then remains as a notched membrane, which may be further reduced during childbearing.

Perineum

The *perineum* is located between the posterior vaginal wall and the anus. Incision into the perineum exposes the strong connective tissue and muscles of the pelvic floor. The perineum may be incised during the second stage of labor to prevent tearing when the baby's head emerges through the birth canal. This is referred to as an **episiotomy.**

OVARIAN (MENSTRUAL) CYCLE

The ovarian cycle is characterized by hormonal and physical changes that occur regularly from the onset of **menarche** (menstrual periods) until menopause (cessation of natural childbearing). The cycle is controlled by a complex feedback system involving hormones of the pituitary, hypothalamus, and ovaries. The ovarian cycle is approximately 28 days long, with normal variation. The cycle occurs in distinct phases:

1. *Follicular phase:* This phase lasts from day 1 to day 14. In this phase, the levels of FSH and LH rise, and a small number of graafian follicles containing the immature ova begin to develop. The fastest growing follicle secretes estrogen, which blocks FSH and stops continued development of the other follicles. When more than one follicle reaches maturity simultaneously, a multiple pregnancy can occur.

2. *Ovulatory phase:* This phase begins approximately 14 days from the start of the cycle and lasts from 16 to 32 hours. The estrogen level falls, and progesterone is secreted by the follicle (the corpus luteum [CL]). This causes the release of the ovum, which leaves a small, blisterlike structure on the surface of the ovary. The ovum is picked up by the fimbriae of the fallopian tubes to enable fertilization.

3. *Luteal phase:* The luteal phase begins approximately on day 16 and lasts approximately 12 days. After ovulation, the corpus luteum secretes estrogen and progesterone. This triggers changes in the endometrium in preparation for implantation of a fertilized ovum. If fertilization does not occur, the FSH and LH levels fall, the CL regresses, and the endometrial lining is shed (menstruation occurs).

PATHOLOGY OF THE FEMALE REPRODUCTIVE SYSTEM

Common pathology of the female reproductive system include functional abnormalities caused by multiple factors, infectious disease, and cancer. Significant diseases are listed in Table 24-1.

DIAGNOSTIC PROCEDURES

PATIENT HISTORY AND PHYSICAL EXAMINATION

Diagnosis of a gynecological condition begins with a history and physical examination. These are completed well before any surgical decisions are made. The physical examination includes a complete review of systems (ROS) with a manual internal (vaginal) examination. Information for evidenced-based medical assessment is derived from the following:

- *Menstrual history:* The year of menarche, the start of menopause, and the history of any diseases or abnormal menstruation. It also includes the duration and amount of monthly flow, characteristics of blood (clots and size), pain, or other symptoms.

- *Obstetrical history:* The number of pregnancies and the course of each pregnancy; the number of successful pregnancies, fetal deaths, and full-term and premature births; and the number of hours in labor and the weights of infants at birth.

- *Use of contraceptives:* The type used, whether the patient feels confident with that technology, and whether barrier protection was used against sexually transmitted diseases (STDs).

Table 24-1

Pathology of the Female Reproductive System

Condition	Description	Considerations
Bartholin gland abscess	Infection of a Bartholin gland may occur if the gland is obstructed.	Infection of a Bartholin gland is extremely painful. Incision and drainage of a cyst or abscess usually is required. (See Removal of a Cystic Bartholin Gland.)
Cancer of the vulva	Squamous cell carcinoma is the most common type of vulvar cancer. High-risk strains of the human papilloma virus (HPV) are associated with an increased risk of vulvar cancer.	Surgical treatment varies according to staging. Metastasis spreads to the inguinal, femoral, and iliac lymph nodes. (See Vulvectomy.)
Cervical cancer	The most common and easily treated cancer of the reproductive tract with early diagnosis; may be associated with HPV types 16, 18, 31, and 33.	Early detection is done with a Pap smear, cervicography, and culposcopy. Surgical treatment is effective in most noninvasive cases. Advanced stage cancer may require hysterectomy. (See Loop Electrosurgical Excision Procedure (LEEP).
Endometrial cancer	Unrelated to cervical cancer, endometrial cancer is associated with obesity and high levels of circulating estrogen.	Definitive diagnosis is made by curettage and histological examination of the endometrium. (See Dilation and Curettage.) The condition is treated with total abdominal hysterectomy with lymph node excision and peritoneal washing. (See Total Abdominal Hysterectomy.)
Endometriosis	A condition in which endometrial tissue develops anywhere outside the uterus, most often on the abdominal viscera. The tissue remains responsive to hormonal changes and causes pain, bleeding, and scarring. The cause of endometriosis is unknown.	Endometriosis can occur anywhere in the abdomen. Conservative treatment focuses on pain management and hormone therapy. Surgery may be necessary to remove endometrial tissue.
Menorrhagia	A condition of excessive menstrual bleeding.	Menorrhagia is conservatively treated with hormonal therapy. Surgical endometrial ablation is performed to destroy the tissue. (See Hysteroscopic Endometrial Ablation.)
Leiomyoma	Also called *fibroid tumor*, a benign neoplasm arising from the uterine smooth muscle tissue. The tumor is attached to the uterine body and develops in any of the tissue layers. The condition may cause excessive or irregular bleeding, obstruction, and infarct.	Conservative treatment is medical. Large or pedunculated fibroid tumors may require surgical removal or hysterectomy. Uterine artery embolization can be performed to manage excessive bleeding. (See Myomectomy.)
Ovarian cyst	A persistent or bleeding ovarian follicle that fails to regress after ovulation can become cystic. Polycystic ovary syndrome (PCOS) is diagnosed in women with persistent multiple cystic follicles. The condition is associated with obesity, diabetes, or other forms of insulin resistance.	Conservative treatment involves hormonal or insulin-sensitizing therapy. Laparoscopic surgery may be performed to remove persistent follicles and release abdominal adhesions. (See Laparoscopic Management of an Ovarian Mass.)
Ovarian cancer	The three types of primary ovarian malignancy are epithelial cancer (90% of cases), germ cell cancer, and gonadal stroma. Ovarian cancer is among the most lethal cancers. Metastasis generally occurs before a diagnosis is made.	Exploratory laparotomy or laparoscopy is required for definitive diagnosis with staging. Cytological washing with tumor debulking may provide palliative treatment.
Cystocele Rectocele Enterocele	Conditions caused by herniation of the rectum (rectocele) or bladder (cystocele) into the vaginal wall. An enterocele occurs when a weakness of the uterosacral ligaments allow the intestine to bulge into the vaginal vault.	In severe cases, surgery is performed to strengthen the vaginal wall. (See Repair of a Cystocele and a Rectocele [Anterior and Posterior Repair].)
Uterine prolapse	Weakness and stretching of the cardinal ligaments results in uterine prolapse. The uterus bulges into the vagina, causing discomfort. In severe cases, the uterus can protrude outside the vagina, leading to desiccation, infection, and an increased risk of cancer.	Conservative treatment involves nonsurgical insertion of a pessary (retention ring) at the proximal vagina. The goal of surgical treatment is to reduce the uterine ligaments and increase their strength. (See Repair of a Cystocele and a Rectocele [Anterior and Posterior Repair].)
Ectopic (extrauterine) pregnancy	Implantation of the embryo outside the intrauterine cavity is an emergency that requires immediate surgical intervention to prevent rupture and hemorrhage. Ectopic pregnancy may be related to previous pelvic infections.	Very early ectopic pregnancy can be treated with methotrexate. Surgery is required to remove midstage or advanced stage pregnancy. (See surgical techniques for ectopic pregnancy and salpingectomy.)

- *History of previous infection:* The type of infection, treatment, and possible or known exposure to the human immunodeficiency virus (HIV).
- *Signs and symptoms:* Abnormal bleeding, such as postcoital bleeding, spotting between periods, **menorrhagia** (excessive bleeding during menstruation), and dyspareunia (painful intercourse). Abdominal or genital pain, vaginal discharge, color, odor, and amount. Signs of prolapse or uterine hernia (e.g., pressure on the vaginal wall and irritation).
- *Current medications and allergies:* Current over-the-counter (OTC) medicines, prescription drugs, current or past allergies, and history of substance abuse.
- *Family history:* Family members with cancer, gynecological disease, obstetrical problems, fetal demise, or fetal abnormalities.
- *Social history:* Living situation, stability in the family unit, physical or emotional abuse in the social or family environment, and access to social support.

PREOPERATIVE MALIGNANCY SCREENING

Preoperative testing for malignancy involves a combination of tests, which may include routine blood tests and a serum CA-125 test (tumor marker blood test). These combined assessment tools provide substantial data for estimating the risk of malignancy before surgical intervention. Laparoscopy provides a further means of assessment.

IMAGING TECHNIQUES

Ultrasound and Sonohysterography

Pelvic or transvaginal ultrasound is commonly used to assess the reproductive system and the stages of pregnancy. Ultrasound is also used during pregnancy to detect fetal abnormalities, gender, and gestational age.

A newer technique, called *sonohysterography,* provides greater clarity of ultrasonic images. In this process, normal saline, lactated Ringer solution, or 1.5% glycine is injected into the uterine cavity through a small transcervical catheter before ultrasound testing. This procedure is replacing hysterosalpingography, because it is safer, painless, and does not require exposure to radiation.

Hysterosalpingography

In hysterosalpingography (HSG), a radiological contrast medium is injected into the uterus and fallopian tubes. Fluoroscopy is then used to visualize the uterus and tubes. The procedure is performed under light sedation.

Magnetic Resonance Imaging

Magnetic resonance imaging (MRI) is a more precise tool for diagnosis than ultrasonography or sonohysterography. MRI reveals the exact location and size of tumors. It can determine the extent of tumor invasion into the myometrium. Congenital anomalies in the reproductive track are extremely clear with MRI, and the images assist preoperative planning for reconstructive surgery.

CERVICAL AND ENDOMETRIAL BIOPSY

The **Papanicolaou (Pap) test** is used to screen for cervical cancer. Superficial endocervical (epithelial) cells are collected from the internal cervical os with a delicate plastic "brush." The brush then is swirled in prep solution, which is used to prepare a series of microscope slides. Abnormal epithelial cells can indicate early stage cancer or precancerous tissue changes.

Culture of the endocervical and vaginal environment is performed to isolate specific nonresident organisms such as chlamydia, herpes, and *Trichomonas vaginalis.* A test for beta-hemolytic streptococci also is done during pregnancy. Screening for the human papilloma virus (HPV) can be performed during routine cervical cancer screening. Evidence of abnormal epithelial cells or a positive test result for high-risk HPV strains is followed by **colposcopy**, which is the microscopic examination and biopsy of the cervix. During culposcopy, the cervix is painted with acetic acid, which causes preinvasive cells to appear white. These areas are biopsied with forceps.

Cone Biopsy of the Cervix

Epithelial carcinoma of the cervix or severe dysplasia (abnormal cells) may be treated with cone biopsy. This involves the removal of a circumferential core of tissue around the cervical canal. The cone biopsy encompasses the abnormal cells for a conclusive diagnosis of invasive carcinoma. Conization most often is performed using a local anesthetic and an electrosurgical loop filament. The technique is referred to as a *loop electrosurgical excision procedure* (**LEEP**). A LEEP can be done during culposcopy in the outpatient setting. Laser energy may also used to perform conization.

HYSTEROSCOPY

During hysteroscopy, a semirigid or rigid hysteroscope is used to examine the interior of the uterus and to perform selected operative procedures. The uterus is filled with a clear fluid to increase visibility (see Hysteroscopy later in the chapter).

PSYCHOSOCIAL CONSIDERATIONS

Psychosocial considerations for the obstetrical or gynecological patient concern reproductive ability and social, cultural, family, and community expectations. In many women, body image and identity are closely linked with the patient's ability to reproduce and to care for her children.

The patient's developmental age is an important aspect of clinical care. Younger patients often associate genital surgery with extreme violations of privacy and social taboos. In the perioperative experience, the child is encouraged to yield to examination and touch that she has been culturally and socially trained to resist. Exposure of and focus on the genitals can create feelings of embarrassment, confusion, fear, and uncertainty, all of which require great tact, patience, and empathy on the part of the caregiver. Respect for the patient's modesty is an obvious prerequisite in all cases. Each step of the surgical preparation should be explained to the patient in terms she can understand. Reassurance from the primary caregiver before surgery can ease the fear of surgery.

Patients of childbearing age can be very fearful of reproductive surgery, seeing it as a threat to their reproductive ability. Other patients may feel relieved that long-term medical problems will be resolved. Surgery may also hold the promise of reproductive ability, and patients undergoing procedures to restore reproductive function can experience emotional fluctuations of hope and worry.

Cancer surgery creates feelings of fear and grief. Women of childbearing age may be particularly vulnerable to grieving and depression related to the loss of reproductive ability.

POSITIONING

Most gynecological procedures are performed with the patient in the supine or lithotomy position (Figure 24-4). Patient safety considerations for the lithotomy position are fully discussed in Chapter 10. Critical safety considerations for the lithotomy position are as follows:

1. Protect the patient's modesty and dignity at all times, even when the patient is anesthetized.
2. All patients must wear antiembolism stockings or a sequential pressure device.
3. When the patient is placed in the lithotomy position, raise both legs simultaneously and slowly into the stirrups—this requires two people. No exceptions can be made.
4. When raising the legs into the stirrups, make sure the hips are slightly externally rotated. At no time should the knees or hips be allowed to drop laterally, because this can dislocate the knees or avulse the hip joint.
5. Raise or lower the patient's legs only after the anesthesia care provider has advised that it is safe. Placing the

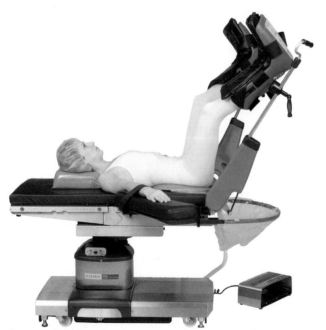

Figure 24-4 Lithotomy position for transvaginal or transcervical procedures. (© 2008 by STERIS Corporation. All rights reserved.)

patient in the lithotomy position may cause changes in blood pressure.
6. When operating the lower table break, make sure the patient's hands are not near the break.
7. When lowering the legs from the stirrups, follow the same procedure as for raising them: two people are required, and the move must be performed slowly to prevent injury.

TEAM POSITIONING

The surgeon may operate from either side of the patient during open procedures. During abdominal procedures, a right-handed surgeon stands at the patient's left side. This allows the best access to the pelvis. The scrub should stand to the patient's right unless otherwise directed. During laparoscopic procedures, the patient is placed in the low lithotomy position, and one assistant is positioned at the foot of the table. A pregnant patient usually is positioned in modified left lateral position to prevent hypotension from pressure on the vena cava by the fetus.

During vaginal procedures, the scrub is in an awkward position, with the back table placed at the foot of the patient, behind the surgeon or at the side. This requires the scrub either to reach across the front of the surgeon and assistants or pass equipment between them. Neither option is entirely satisfactory; the scrub must take care to prevent contamination of the field in either position.

SKIN PREP AND DRAPING

Gynecological procedures are performed with the patient in the supine or lithotomy position. Skin prepping usually includes both abdominal and vaginal prep with insertion of a Foley catheter. A uterine manipulator (internal cervical retractor) is inserted after the vaginal prep for selected laparoscopic procedures.

The order of prepping for a combined abdominal/vaginal prep is as follows:

1. The perineal prep is performed first. The rationale for this is to prevent possible contamination of the abdomen from splashed droplets during the perineal prep.
2. Always prepare the two sites sequentially, *not simultaneously.*
3. A separate prep kit and gloves are required for each site.

Chapter 11 presents a complete discussion of the surgical skin prep.

INSTRUMENTS

Tissue of the reproductive system varies from extremely delicate to very strong and fibrous. Procedures of the fallopian tubes require atraumatic graspers and delicate dissecting instruments. A bipolar electrosurgical unit (ESU) is used rather than a monopolar type, which produces more heat and is less precise. Microinstruments are used to anastomose the fallopian tubes.

The fibrous ligaments that surround the uterus are capable of suspending the pregnant uterus and several quarts of amniotic fluid for many months. These tissues are richly supplied with large blood vessels, which require tight, strong clamps that do not slip during surgery. The uterus itself is composed of strong, thick muscle fibers that require heavy dissecting scissors and toothed or grooved clamps (e.g., Heaney or Kocher clamps) for resection. Laparoscopic instruments are specialized for reproductive structures; they include Babcock or other atraumatic forceps, Harmonic shears, a monopolar hook dissector, graspers, and a vessel-sealing system.

Figures 24-5 through 24-7 show common gynecological instruments. Open gynecological procedures of the pelvic cavity require a general surgery setup with uterine clamps, plus additional atraumatic clamps (e.g., Babcock forceps and vascular forceps) for handling the fallopian tubes, ovaries, and bowel. Long instruments are needed for patients who are deep bodied and for deep pelvic procedures. Harmonic shears and a high-frequency (HF) vessel-sealing system often are used during uterine surgery. Hysterectomy and resection of uterine neoplasms often are performed with a combination of cutting and coagulating technologies.

Transvaginal pelvic procedures require vaginal speculums and long instruments, including uterine clamps and heavy dissecting scissors. Instruments can easily slip off the surgical field onto the floor during transvaginal surgery. Unlike in abdominal surgery, in which the surgical field is flat and contiguous with the instrument tables, during vaginal procedures there is an open gap between the patient (the operative site) and the sterile instrument table. Because of this, various clips, pockets, and instrument holders and magnetic pads are attached to the lithotomy drape to prevent instruments from dropping to the floor. These are helpful, but it is best to have extra sterile instruments (especially forceps and dissecting scissors) and ESU pencils available.

Transcervical procedures require graduated cervical dilators, uterine sounds, forceps, sharp and smooth curettes, and an ample supply of sponges. Suction and a monopolar ESU or HF bipolar electrosurgical unit are needed for all procedures. A variety of active electrode tips are required for selected procedures, such as endometrial ablation or removal of intrauterine lesions.

Procedures of the external genitalia require small (7- to 9-inch [17.5- to 22.5-cm]) plastic surgery instruments, as well as regular dissecting scissors, fine-tipped hemostats, forceps, ESU, and 4 × 4 sponges. Fine scalpel blades (e.g., #15 and #11) are also used.

EQUIPMENT AND SUPPLIES

Equipment for obstetrical and gynecological surgery is divided into categories by type and approach to the procedure. Most abdominal procedures are performed using minimally invasive techniques. Laparoscopic equipment includes the appropriate-size telescopes, trocars, imaging equipment, and carbon dioxide insufflation unit. (This technology is described fully in Chapter 21, which describes minimally invasive surgery and techniques used during basic laparoscopy.)

Transvaginal access to the uterine cavity requires a hysteroscope and components, such as tubing, imaging equipment, and distention fluid pump. Other specialty equipment that

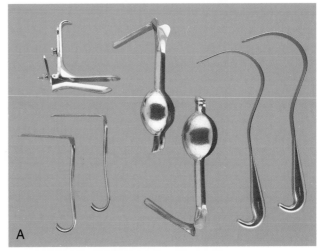

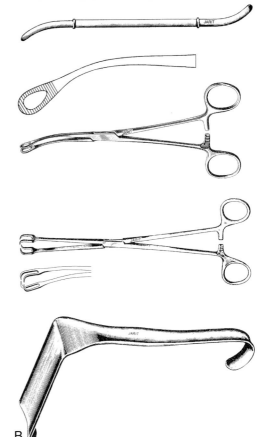

Figure 24-5 Vaginal instruments. **A,** Speculums and retractors. **B,** *Top to bottom:* Hanks cervical dilator, sponge forceps, cervical tenaculum, Sims retractor. *Right,* Uterine curettes. (**A** *from Tighe SM: Instrumentation for the operating room, ed 6, St Louis, 1999, Mosby;* **B** *courtesy Jarit Instruments, Hawthorne, NY.)*

might be needed during hysteroscopy includes cutting loops, a suction curette, or a vaporization electrode.

DRUGS

A variety of drugs are used during reproductive diagnosis, surgery, and labor. Many reproductive drugs are available to control fertility, hormonal dysfunction, and diseases of the reproductive system. Relatively few are used in the intraopera-

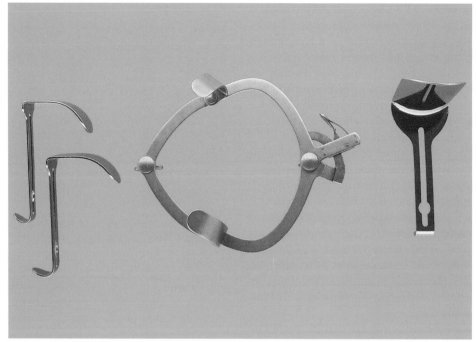

Figure 24-6   Pelvic retractors. O'Sullivan, O'Conner retractor with bladder blade. *(From Tighe SM: Instrumentation for the operating room, ed 6, St Louis, 2003, Mosby.)*

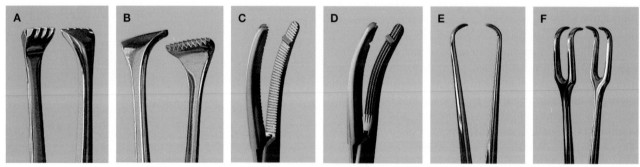

Figure 24-7   Uterine tissue clamps. **A,** Allis clamp. **B,** Allis-Adair clamp. **C** and **D,** Heaney clamps. **E,** Single-toothed tenaculum. **F,** Double-toothed tenaculum. *(From Tighe SM: Instrumentation for the operating room, ed 6, St Louis, 2003, Mosby.)*

tive period or during labor. (Anesthetics and pain medications are discussed in Chapter 12.) Other drugs not classified specifically for use in obstetrical or gynecological surgery may be administered for conditions that arise during labor, and delivery (e.g., hypotensive drugs or electrolyte replacement fluids).

Dyes and Stains

Colored dyes are used to identify and trace anatomical structures during assessment. Methylene blue dye is used during a hysterosalpingogram to verify the patency of the fallopian tubes. Acetic acid (Monsel solution) is used during culposcopy to reveal areas of abnormal cervical tissue. Lugol solution is also used during culposcopy for staining the cervix during the Schiller test.

Vasoconstrictors

The drug vasopressin (Pitressin) causes construction of blood vessels when injected. This drug, which is used in emergency

cardiac response, may be injected into the uterus during hysterectomy or into a benign uterine tumor to prevent bleeding during removal.

Uterotropic Drugs

Drugs that enhance uterine contractility are given during labor and after cesarean section and abortion. Oxytocin (Pitocin) is administered after delivery of the fetus and placenta to prevent postpartum hemorrhage. The drug Pitressin must not be confused with Pitocin. Methylergonovine (Methergine) is an ergot alkaline that is administered after abortion to enhance uterine contractions and control uterine bleeding.

SUTURES

Gynecological surgery involves many types of tissue. The following sutures are commonly used:

- *Uterine ligaments and vessels:* Absorbable synthetic 0 to 2-0 taper needle

- *Bladder reflection:* Absorbable synthetic 2-0 to 3-0 small taper needle
- *Ovary:* Absorbable synthetic 3-0 to 4-0 small taper needle
- *Fallopian tube repair/anastomosis:* Inert monofilament or braided 5-0 to 7-0
- *Vaginal vault:* Absorbable synthetic 2-0 to 3-0 medium curved needle
- *Plastic procedures of the vulva:* Nylon, Prolene, or other monofilament, 3-0, 4-0; $^3/_8$ cutting needle

SURGICAL TECHNIQUES IN GYNECOLOGICAL AND REPRODUCTIVE SURGERY

LAPAROSCOPY

Many abdominal procedures of the reproductive system are performed as laparoscopic surgery. Chapter 21 presents a complete description of minimally invasive surgery (MIS) techniques, including equipment, approach, special safety considerations, and perioperative patient care. The scrub should be familiar with these before approaching the gynecological specialty. A general review of techniques includes:

1. The laparoscope (its use and handling)
2. Imaging systems used in laparoscopy (components and how to use them)
3. Instruments (their use and care)
4. Carbon dioxide (CO_2) insufflation (techniques and patient safety)
5. Safe use of a monopolar and a HF bipolar ESU in laparoscopy
6. Use of vessel-sealing systems (e.g., LigaSure)
7. Ultrasonic cutting and coagulating systems (e.g., Sono-Surg, Harmonic shears)

The principles of laparoscopic surgery apply to the pelvic and combined vaginal-pelvic procedures discussed in this chapter. During laparoscopic pelvic surgery, the uterus is retracted with a uterine manipulator. This instrument is placed through the cervical os after the complete abdominal and vaginal prep and immediately before surgery. The handpiece of the manipulator is accessible outside the perineum, where it is grasped (usually by the assistant) under the guidance of the surgeon.

ABDOMINAL PROCEDURES

LAPAROSCOPY: GENERAL TECHNIQUE

Surgical Goal

Many abdominal and pelvic procedures now can be performed using MIS techniques. (Chapter 21 presents a complete discussion of the techniques and equipment used in laparoscopy Table 24-2.)

Pathology

Gynecological surgery now is routinely performed laparoscopically for medical conditions that previously required laparotomy.

Table 24-2

Laparoscopic Gynecological Instruments

Instrument	Use
10-mm Allis clamp	Grasping the myometrium, large myomas, and large ovarian cysts after drainage
	Removing specimens from the abdominal cavity
Hook scissors	Cutting through very dense tissue
Metzenbaum scissors with monopolar capability	Dissection
	Cutting
	Simultaneous coagulation and cutting
Bowel grasper	Manipulation of the bowel
	Retraction
Monopolar hook	Incising and coagulating
Biopsy forceps	Removing peritoneal or ovarian specimens
Maryland dissector	Blunt dissection
Standard grasper	Tissue handling
	Manipulation
Suction-irrigation probe with Poole sleeve. The probe connects to a handle with trumpet valves for separate suction and irrigation. Irrigation is introduced through a plastic tube connected to irrigation fluid.	Hydrodissection
	Aspiration of fluids and clots
	Irrigation
Aspiration needle (14 gauge)	Withdrawal of fluid from cysts
Alligator grasper	Grasping myoma tissue
	Retrieving specimens

Technique

1. Vaginal and abdominal preps are performed.
2. A Foley retention catheter is inserted into the bladder.
3. Dilation and curettage may be performed.
4. A uterine manipulator is inserted into the cervix.
5. The patient is draped for exposure to the perineum and pelvis.
6. Pneumoperitoneum is established, and the laparoscope is introduced into the abdomen (Figure 24-8).
7. Additional trocars are placed, depending on the surgical objectives.
8. The uterus, adnexa, and abdominal wall are examined.
9. A specific procedure is performed.
10. The trocars are removed, and pneumoperitoneum is released.
11. If a uterine manipulator has been used, it is removed, and the cervix is inspected for injury.
12. The perineum is dressed with a pad.

Discussion

The abdomen, perineum, and vagina are prepped for a combined procedure. A dilation and curettage (D & C) often is performed in conjunction with a laparoscopy (discussed

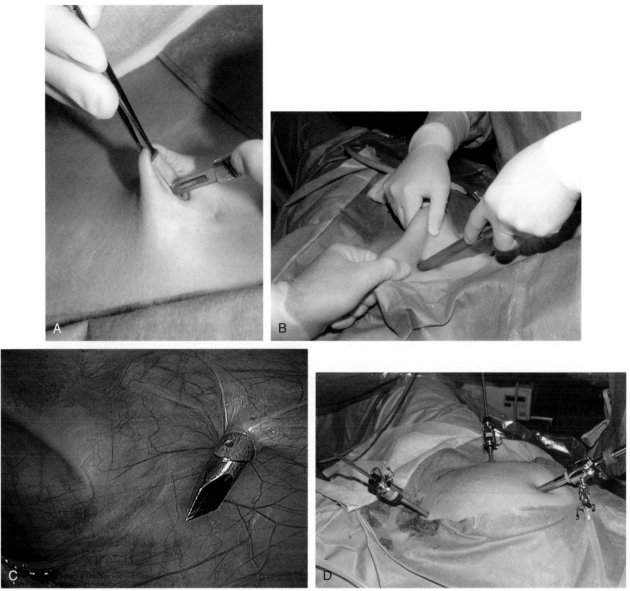

Figure 24-8 Laparoscopy. **A,** Vertical infraumbilical incision. **B,** A trocar is inserted through the incision. **C,** The trocar is inserted under direct vision of the telescope. **D,** Three ports are placed in the abdomen. Note the insufflation tube *(lower right)*. *(From Goldberg JM, Falcone T:* Atlas of endoscopic techniques in gynecology, *Philadelphia, 2001, WB Saunders.)*

later). After the D & C, a uterine manipulator is inserted into the cervix. The manipulator provides a means of retracting the uterus from the perineum while laparoscopy is ongoing. Once the manipulator is in place, the patient can be draped using routine techniques.

To start the procedure, the surgeon elevates the abdominal wall manually by inserting two sharp towel clips on either side of the umbilicus. This lifts the wall away from the retroperitoneal vessels. A nick is made in the periumbilical region with the scalpel. A Veress needle then is inserted into the periumbilical incision, and saline is injected into the needle port. Negative pressure in the abdomen pulls the saline into the abdomen. This demonstrates that the needle has cleared any viscera or vessels. The needle is attached to insufflation tubing to start a controlled pneumoperitoneum. An alternative technique is to insert the trocars without using the Veress needle.

The first port is used to receive the laparoscope. Secondary trocars are inserted as needed.

❖ *The dangers and risks of pneumoperitoneum are thoroughly described in Chapter 21. The scrub must review these safety features before participating in a laparoscopic procedure.*

When the surgery is complete, the trocars are removed. The pneumoperitoneum is released, and the umbilical port is removed. Trocar sites are closed with fine absorbable suture on a cutting needle. The sites may be dressed with Steri-Strips.

Postoperative Considerations

After laparoscopy, patients are closely observed for signs of embolism, infarct, and hemorrhage in the immediate postoperative period. Patients experience shoulder pain for several days postoperatively as a result of the pneumoperitoneum and referred pain from the diaphragm.

LAPAROSCOPIC TUBAL LIGATION

Surgical Goal

Tubal ligation is performed to block the passage of ova through the tube and prevent implantation in the uterus. Tube-sparing techniques may be performed to facilitate reversal.

Pathology

The fallopian tube receives the female ovum after its release from the ovary. The ovum is moved along the tube, is fertilized there, and eventually implants in the uterine lining. Surgical blockage prevents implantation (pregnancy) and development of a fetus.

Technique

Many techniques for tubal ligation have been developed in recent years. The most popular are application of Silastic bands and clips.
1. Pneumoperitoneum is established.
2. *Coagulation:* Using a single laparoscopic port with operating channel, the surgeon can use bipolar forceps to coagulate the fallopian tube.
3. After coagulation, the fallopian tube may be transected.
4. *Fallope ring method:* A loop of the fallopian tube is drawn into a ring applicator. A Silastic O ring is released over the loop, and the loop is then released. The ring causes necrosis of the loop.
5. *Filshie clip:* A clip is applied over the fallopian tube.
6. The ports are withdrawn, and the wounds are closed.

Discussion

Tubal ligation was the first procedure to be performed with the laparoscope. Three methods commonly used are described in the following sections. The patient is placed in the low lithotomy position and prepped for abdominoperineal access. The uterine manipulator is inserted before surgery. One or two trocars are placed in the abdomen after pneumoperitoneum has been established. The assistant may retract the uterus using the uterine manipulator; this brings the tubes into laparoscopic view. Atraumatic forceps (e.g., Babcock forceps) are used to elevate the tubes, which are then occluded by one of the three methods discussed next. The trocars are withdrawn, and the pneumoperitoneum is released. The trocar sites are closed with synthetic absorbable suture and Steri-Strips. The uterine manipulator is carefully withdrawn.

Transection and Coagulation

The fallopian tube is grasped with a Babcock forceps or endoscopic grasper. The HF bipolar unit is used to sever the tube and coagulate the free ends.

Fallope Ring

For the Fallope ring method, the scrub loads a small Silastic O ring into a ring applicator. The surgeon inserts the applicator into the trocar site and withdraws a loop of the fallopian tube into the applicator. The Silastic ring is ejected over the loop, which is then released back into the pelvis (Figure 24-9). The loop causes local ischemia and eventual necrosis of the loop of tissue.

Filshie Clip

For the Filshie clip procedure, the Filshie applicator is inserted through the single port. The clip is applied over the fallopian tube and clamped in place (Figure 24-10). After the procedure, instruments are withdrawn, and the pneumoperitoneum is released. One or two deep sutures are inserted, and the skin is closed.

Open tubal ligation through a minilaparotomy incision or after cesarean section may be performed with the Irving or Pomeroy technique. In this procedure, the fallopian tube is severed and ligated. The proximal stump buried in the uterine serosa with several absorbable sutures. The Irving technique is shown in Figure 24-11.

LAPAROSCOPIC MANAGEMENT OF AN OVARIAN MASS

Surgical Goal

Exploratory laparoscopy is performed to confirm the pathology of an ovarian mass. Preoperative evaluation of a mass is routine in all procedures. Ovarian cysts are removed to determine their pathology and for cancer staging as explained in Chapter 20. **Oophorectomy** (removal of the ovary) or ovarian cystectomy (removal of an ovarian cyst) may be performed during laparoscopy. The scrub should also be prepared for transition to an open case.

Pathology

Functional Ovarian Cyst

Normally during the ovarian cycle, several ovarian follicles begin to mature. The dominant follicle continues to form, whereas the others rupture spontaneously; these are referred to as *functional ovarian cysts.* Occasionally these form benign fluid- or blood-filled cysts, which regress normally. Persistent cysts may be removed surgically.

Teratoma

A teratoma (also called a **dermoid cyst**) is a common ovarian tumor that arises from one of the germ layers of the developing embryo. The tumor persists throughout development and may contain hair, teeth, sebaceous material, and skin, which are normal components of the germ layer. A teratoma may be malignant but seldom causes symptoms. Most are found incidentally during ultrasound or surgery for other reasons.

Benign Ovarian Tumor

Benign ovarian tumors include cystadenomas and mucinous cystadenomas. These tumors are rarely malignant, but they can become quite large, requiring removal of the ovary.

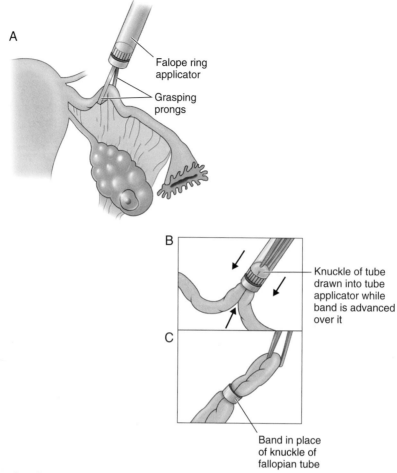

Figure 24-9   Fallope ring tubal ligation. The Silastic ring applicator is used to grasp the tube, retract it, and apply the O ring. *(From Falcone T, Hurd W: Clinical reproductive medicine and surgery, Philadelphia, 2007, Mosby.)*

Technique

1. Pneumoperitoneum is established.
2. The abdomen is explored, and surgical staging is performed.
3. A cyst is identified, and the outer membrane (cortex) is incised.
4. The edge of the cyst cortex is grasped, and the dissection is started.
5. The cortex is everted, and dissection is continued until the cyst is completely mobilized.
6. The cyst or mass is brought out of the abdomen through a retrieval bag or vaginal incision.
7. The surgeon examines the cystic bed and controls bleeding with the electrosurgical unit (ESU).
8. If the cyst ruptures, the abdomen is irrigated with copious amounts of lactated Ringer solution.

Discussion

Laparoscopic management of ovarian cysts depends on the size and type of cyst and the risk of malignancy. Spillage of a potentially malignant cyst is always avoided to prevent the spread of cancerous cells (seeding). A large cyst can be removed through a specimen retrieval bag and a 10-mm trocar port.

The patient is placed in the low lithotomy position, prepped, and draped for a laparoscopic procedure. After pneumoperitoneum has been established, the surgeon examines the abdominal contents. Cancer staging and pelvic washing may be performed at this point. Pelvic washing provides a medium for the collection of cells, which can be evaluated postoperatively. For pelvic washing, 50 to 100 mL of normal saline is introduced into the abdomen, and the fluid is then aspirated and retained as a specimen.

To remove a cyst, the surgeon incises the cortex (outer covering) of the cyst without rupturing it. The incision is made with fine scissors or the ESU pencil. The cortex is removed using blunt dissection. An atraumatic grasper may be used at this point to facilitate removal. A suction-irrigator may be used to separate the cyst from the cortex. Bleeders are controlled with the bipolar ESU.

The specimen is protected from rupture and placed in a specimen retrieval bag. The bag is delivered through a 10-mm trocar port, with the bag opening advanced ahead of the speci-

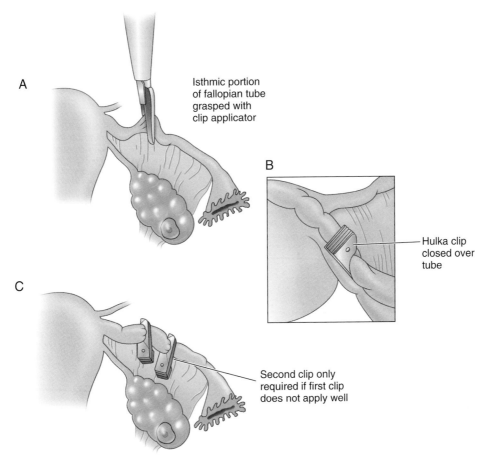

A
Isthmic portion
of fallopian tube
grasped with
clip applicator

B
Hulka clip
closed over
tube

C
Second clip only
required if first clip
does not apply well

Figure 24-10 Filshie clip method of tubal ligation. *(From Falcone T, Hurd W: Clinical reproductive medicine and surgery, Philadelphia, 2007, Mosby.)*

men. The cyst contents can then be safely aspirated (Figure 24-12). If the specimen is too large for retraction, it can be reduced with a morcellator and the pieces can be brought out through the bag opening. An alternative method of removing large specimens is to make an incision in the uterine cul-de-sac and deliver the cyst through the vagina. The peritoneal reflection (bladder flap) is then repaired with absorbable sutures.

A teratoma is removed intact by sharp dissection and extracted through a specimen retrieval bag using the technique described previously. If rupture occurs, the abdominal cavity is thoroughly irrigated with normal saline. A frozen section may be performed at the time of laparoscopy to determine the need for more radical surgery.

In some cases, complete removal of the ovary may be indicated after laparoscopic assessment and staging. The technique used requires dissection of the ovarian ligaments. This is performed with the ultrasonic scalpel, fine dissecting scissors, and probe. Ovarian vessels are occluded with fine staples, the bipolar ESU, a vessel-sealing system, or absorbable ligature loops. Once the ligaments have been released and bleeding controlled, the ovary can be withdrawn from the abdominal cavity through a large port and specimen retrieval bag. The ports are removed, and the pneumoperitoneum is released.

Individual wounds are closed with absorbable sutures and skin staples.

MICROSURGICAL TUBAL ANASTOMOSIS

Surgical Goal

Tubal anastomosis is performed to restore continuity to the fallopian tube, whether to reverse tubal ligation or to treat another condition.

Pathology

Obstruction of the fallopian tube frequency occurs as a result of an infection that spreads from the lower genital tract to the uterus, fallopian tubes, and ovaries. According to the Centers for Disease Control and Prevention (CDC), approximately 1 million women per year acquire pelvic inflammatory disease (**PID**) as a result of genital tract infections. Of these, 100,000 women become infertile and 150 die[1]. The causal organism usually is *Chlamydia trachomatis* or *Neisseria gonorrhoeae,* which cause scarring and loss of fertility. Reconstruction and tubal anastomosis are performed to restore function after infection or to reverse a previous tubal ligation. The following technique is used to reconstruct the fallopian tube with occlusion at the uterine junction.

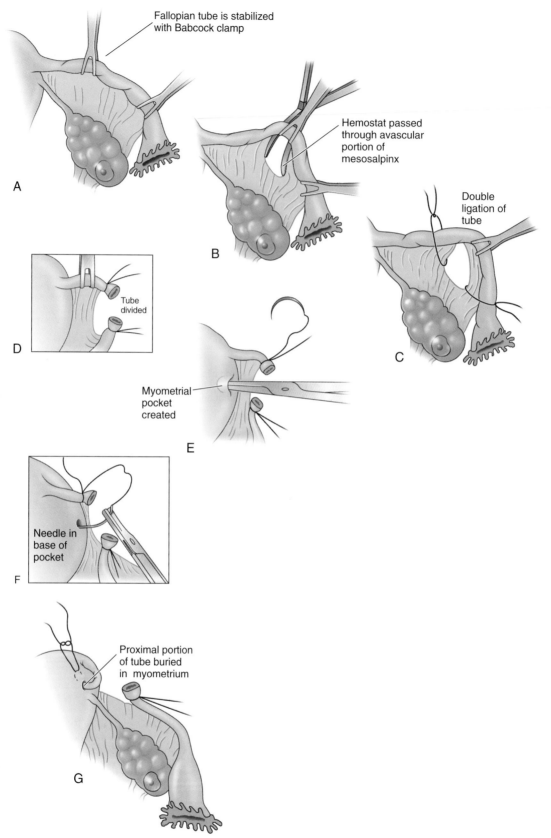

Fallopian tube is stabilized with Babcock clamp

Hemostat passed through avascular portion of mesosalpinx

Double ligation of tube

Tube divided

Myometrial pocket created

Needle in base of pocket

Proximal portion of tube buried in myometrium

A

B

C

D

E

F

G

Figure 24-11   Classic Irving technique of open tubal ligation. *(From Falcone T, Hurd W: Clinical reproductive medicine and surgery, Philadelphia, 2007, Mosby.)*

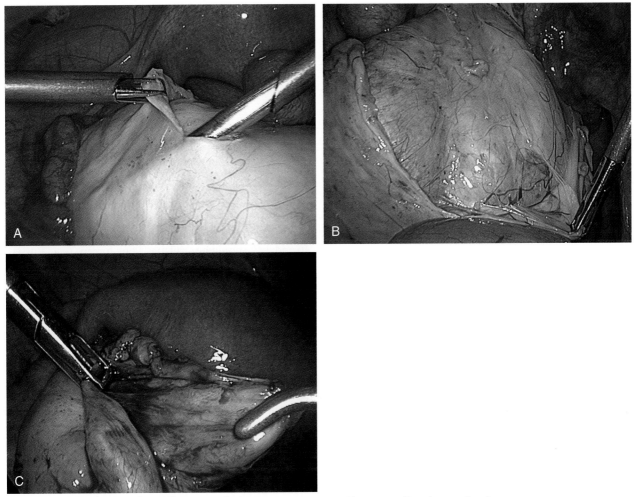

Figure 24-12 Removal of an ovarian cyst. **A,** The cyst wall is dissected with a hydrodissector. **B,** Dissection of the cyst wall is nearly complete. **C,** The body of the cyst is grasped and removed from the ovary. *(From Goldberg JM, Falcone T: Atlas of endoscopic techniques in gynecology, Philadelphia, 2001, WB Saunders.)*

Technique

1. A pelvic laparotomy is performed.
2. The proximal fallopian tube is excised.
3. The proximal tube is transected until patency can be demonstrated with indigo carmine dye.
4. The distal tube is transected and tested as in step 3.
5. Stay sutures are inserted to bring the two tube segments into exact alignment.
6. An inner layer of sutures is placed circumferentially in the tube.
7. The tubal serosa is anastomosed.
8. The mesosalpinx is sutured together.
9. The tube is again infused with dye to confirm patency.

Discussion

Surgery to restore **patency** (an unobstructed passageway) to the fallopian tube is performed with the operating microscope. The procedure frequently is performed laparoscopically.

The exact technique required for tubal anastomosis depends on the pathological condition. If the tube is diseased or if the two segments to be joined differ greatly in size, the procedure becomes more complex, because the larger segment must be reduced to fit the smaller end.

The patient is placed in the low lithotomy position for access to the cervix and intrauterine cavity during surgery. The abdomen is entered through a transverse pelvic incision. A self-retaining O'Connor or O'Sullivan retractor is placed in the wound, and the bowel is packed away from the uterus with moist laparotomy sponges. The patient may be placed in a slight Trendelenburg position to allow gravitational displacement of the abdominal organs.

The surgeon retracts the uterus with a tenaculum and locates the fallopian tube, mesosalpinx, ureter, and uterine ligaments. Before beginning the procedure, the surgeon may inject the fundus of the myometrium with vasopressin to control hemorrhage. Continuous irrigation may be used to locate microscopic bleeders. A solution of glycine or lactated Ringer solution is used.

The proximal end of the occluded area is grasped with toothed forceps, and the serosa of the tube is incised with an ESU needle. The incision is carried through the tube with the microdissecting rod. Small bleeders are controlled with the microbipolar forceps.

The tube then is fully transected with iris scissors or some other fine-tipped, sharp scissors. The proximal side is lifted, and the peritoneal serosa is excised at the uterine body. This incision is carried deeper with scissors. If patency is not evident, the dissection is repeated proximally.

Indigo carmine or methylene blue dye is instilled transcervically to establish patency of the tube where it communicates with the uterus.

The distal segment of the tube is then dissected from the mesosalpinx, and the outer (peritoneal) tissue of the tube is incised with the bipolar ESU. The segment is divided with iris scissors or other fine-tipped, sharp scissors, using the same technique as for the proximal segment. The surgeon then irrigates the distal segment with indigo carmine dye using a Stangel cannula. The appearance of the dye at the severed end indicates patency.

The two segments are then anastomosed. Stay sutures are placed and tagged with fine, small hemostats. Nylon or polypropylene 8-0 or 9-0 suture with a tapered needle is used for the anastomosis. A two-layered anastomosis is performed. If the uterine myometrium has been incised, it is repaired with 6-0 sutures.

The serosa and mesosalpinx of the tube are closed with interrupted 8-0 sutures. Indigo carmine dye is instilled into the tube to confirm that it is patent. The abdominal wound is irrigated and closed in layers.

Microsurgical tubal anastomosis is shown in Figure 24-13.

LAPAROSCOPIC-ASSISTED VAGINAL HYSTERECTOMY

Surgical Goal

Laparoscopic-assisted vaginal hysterectomy (LAVH) is the removal of the uterus by a combined laparoscopic and vaginal approach. It is the most common approach to hysterectomy. The uterine ligaments, adhesions, and any other attachments are released through the abdominal portion of the procedure. The vaginal cul-de-sac is opened, and the specimen is removed vaginally.

Pathology

The LAVH approach for hysterectomy can be performed for benign tumors, **endometriosis**, and early stage uterine malignancy

Technique

1. The patient is placed in a low lithotomy position, prepped, and draped for a combined abdominal-vaginal approach.
2. Pneumoperitoneum is established, and three or four trocars placed.
3. The pelvic cavity is assessed for disease and anatomical anomalies.
4. The uterine ligaments are divided.
5. The bladder is dissected from the uterus.
6. The uterine arteries may be dissected at this stage or deferred to the vaginal portion of the procedure.

7. The posterior cul-de-sac is incised.
8. Surgery is shifted to the vaginal approach.
9. The uterine vessels are ligated and the specimen removed vaginally.
10. The vaginal cuff is oversewn and laparoscopic incisions closed.

Discussion

LAVH requires two setups, one for the laparoscopic portion and one for the vaginal approach. The setup for the vaginal approach includes a vaginal hysterectomy set, ESU, and sutures for ligation and bladder flap closure. Synthetic sutures (0 and 2-0) should be available. Long forceps (e.g., Russian or toothed forceps) are needed for closing the bladder flap. Sponge forceps and 4 × 4 sponges are used until the bladder flap is closed.

The patient is placed in the lithotomy position, prepped, and draped for a combined abdominal-perineal approach. Pneumoperitoneum is established, and three or four trocars are placed in the lower abdominal cavity. The pelvis is examined carefully to determine the extent of disease. Adhesions are released with the bipolar ESU during exploration to open up the pelvic space for thorough exploration and to prepare for uterine dissection.

The scrub should have Harmonic shears, a vessel-sealing system, suction, and irrigation available during exploration. Endoscopic instruments (e.g., uterine clamps, probe, HF bipolar ESU, and monopolar ESU) should be available. Preformed suture ligatures may be required if the uterine vessels are secured by the laparoscopic approach.

The surgeon divides the uterine ligaments and incises the uterovesical peritoneum. If the uterine arteries are to be divided at this stage, this is performed by ligation with heavy synthetic sutures, radiofrequency vessel sealing system (see Chapter 19) or surgical staples. The vessel bundles are then severed to free the uterus. Note that it is more common for the vessels to be ligated from the vaginal incision. Before shifting to the vaginal portion of the procedure, the surgeon incises the posterior cul-de-sac, creating communication between the pelvic cavity and the proximal vaginal vault.

The surgeon then shifts to the vaginal approach. The uterine vessels are ligated and severed, and the specimen is delivered through the cul-de-sac. Small bleeders are controlled with the ESU, and the bladder flap is closed with a running suture of 2-0 or 3-0 absorbable synthetic material.

The laparoscope and trocars are removed, the pneumoperitoneum is released, and the abdominal incisions are closed with absorbable suture.

❖ A laparoscopic hysterectomy is performed using the steps just described, except that the procedure is completed laparoscopically. The uterus is removed through a large trocar and specimen retrieval bag.

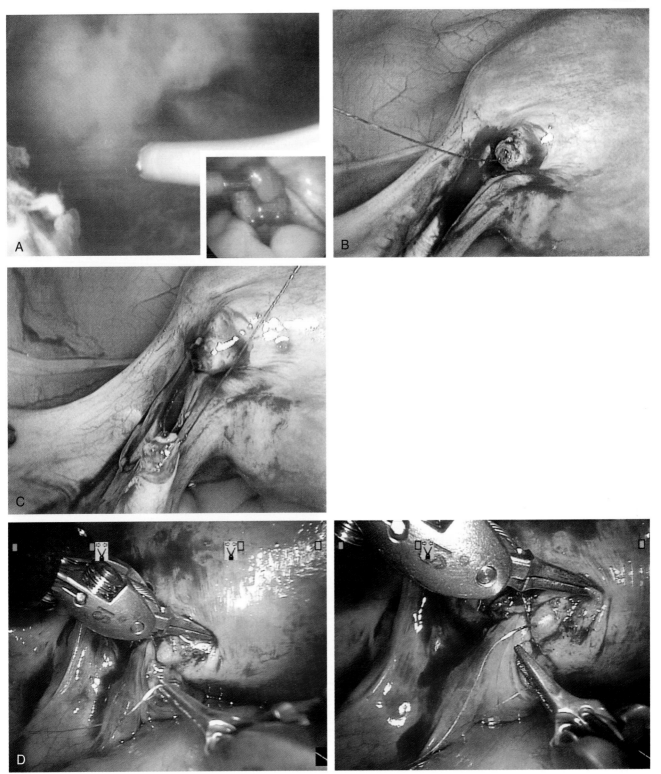

Figure 24-13   Microsurgical tubal anastomosis. **A,** The fallopian tube has been infused with methylene blue dye and incised sagittally. This creates an anastomosis site free of adhesions. **B,** Traction sutures are placed on the outer edge of the tube. **C,** The tubal portions are approximated. **D,** Anastomosis is performed with the da Vinci robotic system. *(From Falcone T, Hurd W: Clinical reproductive medicine and surgery, Philadelphia, 2007, Mosby.)*

TOTAL ABDOMINAL HYSTERECTOMY

Surgical Goal

In a total abdominal hysterectomy (TAH), the uterus is surgically removed through a pelvic incision.

Pathology

In the past, open abdominal hysterectomy was the only method available for removal of the uterus. Laparoscopic hysterectomy now is commonly performed. However, open hysterectomy remains an option for selected patients for the treatment of endometriosis, large fibroid tumors, dysfunctional uterine bleeding, and uterine prolapse. TAH includes removal of the uterus and cervix.

Technique

1. The abdomen is entered through a transverse pelvic incision.
2. The round ligament is clamped, divided, and ligated.
3. The incision is carried anteriorly to the peritoneal bladder reflection.
4. The bladder is dissected from the lower uterine segment, creating a bladder flap.
5. Dissection of the uterine ligaments and arteries is carried to the vaginal cuff.
6. The cervix is incised circumferentially and amputated from the vaginal cuff.
7. The uterus is removed, and the specimen is passed from the surgical field.
8. The vaginal cuff is grasped with clamps and sutured.
9. The previously dissected bladder flap is reattached.
10. The abdominal wound is irrigated and closed in layers.

Discussion

The patient is placed in the supine position. After a routine abdominal and vaginal prep, a Foley catheter is inserted for continuous urinary drainage. A lower midline or Pfannenstiel incision can be used for a hysterectomy. The incision traverses the lower abdomen approximately 3 to 4 inches (7.5 to 10 cm) above the symphysis pubis.

To begin the surgery, the surgeon makes a transverse skin incision and extends it through the subcutaneous tissue with the ESU. The next layer, the fascia, is entered with the scalpel, and the incision is lengthened with curved Mayo scissors. The surgeon then grasps one edge of the fascial margin with two or more Kocher clamps. Using blunt dissection, the surgeon separates the fascia from the underlying muscle.

This procedure is repeated on the lower fascial margin. The muscle layer is then divided manually. The peritoneum is incised with the scalpel, and the incision is lengthened with Metzenbaum scissors. A self-retaining retractor (e.g., O'Sullivan, O'Connor, or Balfour retractor) is placed in the wound. The surgeon packs the bowel away from the uterus with moist lap sponges.

The surgeon isolates the uterus by severing it from the uterine ligaments, ovaries, and fallopian tubes. Beginning with the round ligaments, the surgeon double-clamps, divides, and ligates each attachment with suture ligatures. Heaney, Heaney-Ballentine, or Masterson forceps usually are used for this part of the procedure. The scrub should have at least four of these clamps available on the Mayo stand.

Absorbable suture is used to ligate the ligaments. Chromic gut or absorbable synthetic suture on large tapered needles is used. To divide the ligaments, the surgeon uses curved Mayo scissors or the scalpel. Long instruments should be available if the patient has a deep pelvis.

The surgeon mobilizes the uterus to the level of the bladder. At this point, the bladder is continuous with the uterus; both organs are attached by a peritoneal covering. Using Metzenbaum scissors and long tissue forceps, the surgeon separates the two structures by dissecting the peritoneal covering away from the bladder. When the bladder has been separated from the uterus, mobilization is continued.

At the level of the cervix, long Allis or Kocher clamps are placed around the edge of the cervix, and it is divided from the vagina. The surgeon uses long scissors or the long scalpel to divide the tissue. This maneuver completely frees the uterus, which is passed to the scrub. All instruments that have come in contact with the cervix or vagina must be kept separate from the rest of the setup. The specimen and isolated instruments should be received in a basin.

To close the wound, the surgeon first closes the vaginal vault where it was separated from the cervix. Absorbable sutures of the same type used on the uterine ligaments are used. The muscular layer of the vagina is closed with figure-of-eight sutures. After closing the vagina, the surgeon uses 2-0 or 3-0 suture on a small tapered needle to reattach the bladder flap.

The abdominal wound is irrigated with warm saline and checked for bleeders. To close the abdomen, the surgeon grasps the edges of the peritoneum with several Mayo clamps. The peritoneum is closed with a running suture of size 0 absorbable suture swaged to a tapered needle. The muscle tissue may be loosely approximated with three or four interrupted absorbable sutures. The fascial layer is closed with a wide variety of sutures, absorbable or nonabsorbable, usually size 0 or 2-0. The subcutaneous tissue usually is approximated with 3-0 interrupted absorbable sutures. The skin is closed with staples or a subcuticular running suture.

The process of an abdominal hysterectomy is shown in Figure 24-14.

RADICAL HYSTERECTOMY

Surgical Goal

A radical hysterectomy involves dissection and wide removal of the uterus, tubes, ovaries, supporting ligaments, upper vagina, and pelvic lymph node chains.

Pathology

A radical hysterectomy is performed to treat pelvic malignancy. Endometrial cancer is the most common type of cancer in the female reproductive tract. It occurs most often in women 55 to 65 years of age and rarely in those younger than 40. Risk factors for endometrial cancer include endometrial **hyperplasia** (excess proliferation of tissue) related to prolonged estrogen stimulation, obesity, diabetes mellitus, hyper-

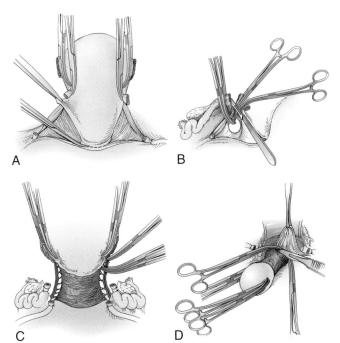

A

B

C

D

Figure 24-14 Abdominal hysterectomy. **A,** The anterior ligaments have been clamped, cut, and tied, allowing access to the broad ligament. Size 0 absorbable sutures are used for ligation. **B,** The fallopian tube and ovarian ligament are clamped and divided. Heavy suture ligatures are placed through the vascular bundles. **C,** The uterine vessels are clamped and divided at the level of the cervix. **D,** The uterus can now completely divided. The peritoneal closure is made with interrupted or running sutures of absorbable synthetic material. *(Modified from Gershenson DM, DeCherney AH, Curry SL, Brubaker LC: Operative gynecology, ed 2, Philadelphia, 2001, WB Saunders.)*

tension, or polycystic ovary syndrome (PCOS). It is a slow-growing cancer, and painless bleeding is the primary symptom. The diagnosis is made by dilation and curettage (D & C).

Technique

1. The abdomen is opened through a lower midline incision.
2. The retroperitoneal space is entered, and retractors are placed.
3. The round and infundibulopelvic ligaments are clamped and ligated.
4. The ureter is identified and retracted with a vein retractor.
5. The iliac artery, obturator fossa, and ureter are dissected of lymph and connective tissue.
6. A lymph gland dissection is performed bilaterally.
7. The uterine artery and vein are clamped, cut, and double-ligated.
8. The peritoneal reflection of the bladder is dissected from the cervix and vagina.
9. The cul-de-sac is opened, and the uterosacral and cardinal ligaments are resected and ligated.
10. The upper vagina is mobilized, and the paraurethral tissues are removed.

11. The upper vagina is cross-clamped and divided, and the specimen is removed.
12. The vagina is closed with a running locked suture.
13. The pelvic incision is closed.
14. Sump or gravity drains may be placed in the wound.
15. The abdominal wound is closed in layers and dressed.
16. Vaginal packing may be used.
17. A perineal pad is placed.

Discussion

In a radical hysterectomy, the uterus, tubes, and ovaries, together with most of the parametrial tissues and the upper portion of the vagina, are removed **en bloc**. The ureters are dissected from the paracervical structures so that the ligaments supporting the uterus and vagina can be removed leaving the uterus intact. The procedure is similar in technical aspects to pelvic exenteration (described later). The scrub should be prepared for extensive dissection and resection of pelvic structures. The dissection progresses from the pelvis to the upper vagina.

The patient is prepared for a lengthy surgery. Compression stockings or a sequential compression device is applied before surgery. A warm air mattress is prepared, and the temperature and fittings are carefully monitored throughout the procedure. A Foley retention catheter is inserted before surgery, and the urinary output is assessed during the perioperative period. Blood loss is calculated by weighing sponges and measuring suction waste compared with irrigation solution used intraoperatively.

The patient is placed in the low lithotomy position and prepped for access to the abdomen and perineum. A vaginal prep is performed before the abdominal prep, according to standard aseptic practice.

Long dissecting instruments (e.g., right-angle clamps, long Metzenbaum scissors, toothed forceps, and long, curved hemostats) are used intermittently with the ESU. Suture ligatures of size 0 and 2-0 synthetic absorbable material are needed to secure large vessels during dissection. As the dissection progresses, individual lymph nodes may be dissected and removed. The scrub should keep these separate and according to the surgeon's orders.

Deep pelvic procedures require particular attention to sponge and instrument counts, because items can easily be lost in the wound. In addition to routine counts, the scrub should keep track of lap sponges placed in the wound. Throughout a long procedure, the scrub should maintain a clean work space and ensure that instrument tips are free of tissue debris. A basin of water used for maintaining instruments intraoperatively must be kept fresh.

A midline abdominal incision is made, and the tissue layers are divided in the usual manner. An O'Sullivan, O'Connor, or similar self-retaining retractor is positioned. The abdomen is packed with moist laparotomy sponges, and the retroperitoneum is incised. Handheld right-angle retractors may be used at this stage. Tissue planes are then developed around the bladder, rectum, uterine ligaments, and ureters. The peritoneal reflection of the bladder is incised with long

Metzenbaum scissors or the ESU. Vein retractors or narrow Penrose drains may be requested to retract the ureters once they are isolated. The large vessels of the uterus are resected and ligated. A vessel-sealing system may be used to secure hemostasis. The uterosacral ligaments are then transected along the sacrum in the space between the posterior vagina and the rectum. Posterior and lateral dissection continues to the level of the upper vagina, which frees the specimen. The scrub should have a basin available in the field to receive the specimen.

Wound closure includes the vaginal cuff, retroperitoneum, peritoneum, and abdominal wall. The wound is irrigated, and hemostasis is secured as layers are closed. A count is performed before each layer is sutured.

The vaginal cuff (proximal vagina) is closed with size 0 synthetic absorbable suture. The retroperitoneum is sutured with 2-0 suture of the same material. The abdominal wall is then routinely closed. A suprapubic catheter may be put in place to ensure urinary function. A Penrose or sump drain may be inserted before the abdomen is closed and the wound is dressed with gauze squares.

Postoperative Considerations

After radical abdominal or pelvic surgery, the patient is closely monitored for urinary output, hemorrhage, and infection. The patient may recover in the postanesthesia care unit (PACU), or she may be taken directly to the intensive care unit (ICU), depending on her physiological status at the close of surgery.

PELVIC EXENTERATION

Surgical Goal

Pelvic exenteration is performed to treat metastatic cancer. It involves the complete removal of the rectum, the distal sigmoid colon, the urinary bladder and distal ureters, and the internal iliac vessels and their lateral branches. All pelvic reproductive organs and lymph nodes, as well as the entire pelvic floor, pelvic peritoneum, levator muscles, and perineum, are removed. A partial anterior or posterior exenteration can be performed, depending on the origin and extent of the cancer.

Pathology

Pelvic exenteration is performed for metastatic carcinoma of the cervix, endometrium, ovary, or vagina when conservative treatments have failed.

Technique

1. The patient should be positioned with lithotomy stirrups and prepped for an abdominal/perianal approach. This position allows access without disruptive positioning changes.
2. A long midline incision is made from the symphysis pubis to the umbilicus, and the abdomen is opened.
3. A second incision is made within the perineum and encircling the vestibule and anus.

4. The peritoneal cavity is explored for metastasis to the liver, the nodes of the celiac axis, the superior mesenteric artery, and the paraaortic tissues.
5. The pelvis is explored for lymph node involvement. If negative findings are noted, retractors are placed and the small bowel is packed with moist lap sponges.
6. The sigmoid mesocolon is mobilized and sectioned with intestinal clamps, a scalpel, or a stapling device.
7. The proximal end of the sigmoid mesocolon is exteriorized through the left side of the abdomen; an intestinal clamp is left across the lumen for later use, when the permanent colostomy is secured to the skin.
8. The remaining sigmoid mesentery is clamped, cut, and ligated down to and including the superior hemorrhoid vessels. Long instruments and sutures are used to reach the deep pelvic sutures.
9. The distal sigmoid colon is closed with an inverting suture. The sigmoid colon and rectum are mobilized from the sacrococcygeal area by blunt and sharp dissection.
10. The lateral pelvic peritoneum is cut, and all vessels and ligaments are clamped, cut, and double-ligated.
11. The bladder is separated from the symphysis pubis down to the urethra.
12. The ureters are identified and divided; the proximal ends are left open for urinary drainage, and the distal ends are ligated.
13. The hypogastric artery, internal iliac vein, and superior and inferior gluteal vessels are exposed, clamped, double-ligated, and cut. The external iliac vein is retracted to allow evacuation of the obturator fossa contents, leaving the obturator nerve intact. Care must be taken to preserve the sacral plexus and sciatic nerve.
14. The internal pudendal vessels are identified, isolated, ligated with transfixion sutures, and cut. The remaining soft tissue attachments are clamped and cut. These steps are performed on the opposite sides of the patient.
15. A deep elliptical perineal incision is made.
16. The rectal coccygeal and lateral attachments of the levator muscles are severed.
17. The paravesical and paravaginal tissues are resected from the periosteum of the symphysis pubis and pubic rami.
18. The specimen is removed.
19. Hemostasis is secured, and the wound is closed in layers.
20. Abdominal hemostasis is secured.
21. The anastomosis is made between the ileal segment and the ureters.
22. An external ileal stoma is placed on the right side of the abdomen.
23. A gastrostomy tube is placed in the stomach.
24. The abdominal wound is closed in layers.
25. A colostomy is created.
26. The wounds are dressed, and drainage devices are applied to the colostomy and ileostomy stomas.

Discussion

Total pelvic exenteration is performed only after all other treatment options have failed. The procedure involves resection and reconstruction of all organs of the pelvic cavity. (These procedures are discussed separately in relevant chapters; resection of the bowel and bladder are described in Chapters 23 and 25.) Surgical preparation of the patient requires strict attention to physiological monitoring and homeostasis. The relative length of the surgery adds some technical difficulty for the scrub and circulating team. Care of the patient requires constant monitoring, and the technical needs for supplying ample sutures, sponges, and other items are demanding. The scrub must take care to keep an orderly setup, paying attention to setting priorities. Meticulous dissection, anastomosis, and hemostasis are performed throughout the procedure. (Refer to the techniques and patient care described under Radical Hysterectomy.)

TRANSCERVICAL PROCEDURES

HYSTEROSCOPY

Principles

During hysteroscopy, a fiberoptic hysteroscope is inserted through the cervix and into the uterus. This technique is used to assess the uterine cavity endocervix and the lower uterine segment and for selected operative procedures. Operative hysteroscopy is indicated for intrauterine pathology, such as polyps, leiomyoma, adhesions, and septal defects of the uterus. To obtain a clear view of the uterine wall, the surgeon distends the uterine cavity with fluid. This allows small blood clots and other tissue debris to be removed and maintains a clear view. Distention fluid enters through the hysteroscope via a monitored pump system. Waste fluid is released as fresh fluid enters, which provides continuous irrigation.

Examination, biopsy, and surgical procedures are performed through the hysteroscope and operating channels in the same way that cystoscopic surgery is performed through the bladder. Biopsy and resection using a variety of energy technologies (e.g., laser, HF bipolar electricity, and automated ablation) can be performed through the hysteroscope.

Uterine Distention

As mentioned, during hysteroscopy the uterine cavity must be distended. In the past, carbon dioxide gas or viscous fluid (Dextran 70) was used. *These methods are no longer considered safe.* Uterine insufflation with CO_2 poses the risk of death from gas embolism, because high pressure, low volume gas is forced into open vessels during an operative procedure. CO_2 insufflation is used only when no operative procedures are planned. When CO_2 is used, the Trendelenburg position is not used, because it increases the risk of embolism.

Dextran 70 was commonly used as a distention fluid in the past because its high viscosity created a crystal clear field and prevented leakage during surgery. *This distention fluid is rarely used today.* The primary reason is the risk of fluid extravasation, toxicity, and allergic reaction. Extravasation is absorption of the fluid into the vascular system, leading to increased blood pressure and possible death related to fluid overload. A toxic reaction to Dextran 70 can lead to disseminated intravascular coagulopathy (DIC), in which the body's clotting mechanism is greatly diminished. This may result in death from microvascular hemorrhage.

Safe Uterine Distention

Low viscosity fluids have largely replaced CO_2 and Dextran 70 as a means of uterine distention. An isotonic solution, such as normal saline, is used for all procedures *except those that require monopolar electrosurgery*.

❖ *Use of monopolar electrosurgery during hysteroscopy requires the use of a hypotonic, nonelectrolytic distention fluid. This is because the flow of current must travel directly from the point of contact (the active electrode) to the inactive electrode (the patient grounding pad) and back to the ESU control unit.*

If electrolytic solutions are used with the monopolar circuit, electricity would be dispersed throughout the fluid and might cause patient burns.

Extravasation and fluid overload are always risks during uterine distention. Hypotonic fluids create an additional risk of death from severe **hyponatremia** (low serum sodium level). Meticulous monitoring of fluid is required throughout hysteroscopy. The scrubbed and circulating teams are jointly responsible for tracking the amount used and the rate of flow during a procedure. Recovered fluid (that which is released from the uterine cavity as waste during the procedure) is constantly computed against fluid instilled to determine the potential amount absorbed by the body. If fluid overload occurs during surgery, the procedure may be terminated immediately and the patient treated.

Hysteroscope

The hysteroscope may be rigid or semirigid. A rigid scope incorporates a 12- to 30-degree angled lens at the distal tip. A 0-degree lens is also available, although less seldom used. The main components of the instrument are the sheath and operating channels. The operative scope has a large sheath to permit insertion of instruments and a channel for instilling the distention medium.

The hysteroscope is inserted into the uterus with the sheath in place. The main operating channel receives the telescope, and side channels, controlled by stopcocks, receive accessory instruments. The main channel is fitted with rubber gaskets that prevent the backflow of distention fluid. Both double-channel and single-channel sheaths are available. Some models have separate channels for the telescope and the liquid medium used to flush fluid and debris from the uterus while operating at the same time (Figure 24-15).

Imaging System

Fiberoptic light is used to illuminate the surgical site during hysteroscopy. Equipment includes a standard fiberoptic light cable and xenon light source. The digital imaging system, which is similar to the laparoscope, has video components, including a monitor, video cable, and image management system. (Chapter 21 presents a complete discussion of digital imaging.)

Operating Instruments

Most hysteroscopic procedures require 3-mm instruments, although 2-mm accessories are available for very fine tissue dissection. The instruments are the standard type, including

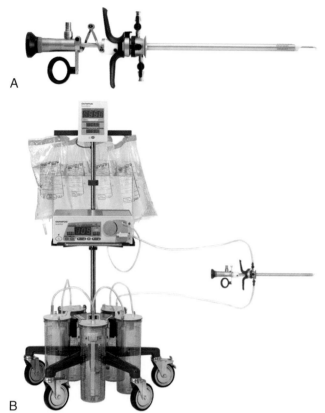

Figure 24-15 A, A resectoscope is used for therapeutic hysteroscopy. Note the cutting-coagulation loop on the distal end. **B,** A fluid distention system for use with the resectoscope. Note that the fluid pressure is regulated to prevent extravasation and subsequent fluid overload, which may cause serious patient injury. *(Courtesy Gyrus ACMI, Inc., Southborough, Mass.)*

scissors, graspers, biopsy forceps, and ESU and laser fibers. A variety of tips are available for HF bipolar and standard monopolar ESUs. These include the ball tip, spring tip, needle, and loop electrodes used for removing polyps and dense tumors.

Flexible instruments can be fitted into the deflector bridge. A suction cannula and flexible catheter are used to remove blood clots, debris, blood, and mucus and to inject the liquid medium. Rigid and semirigid instruments are inserted directly into the sheath.

Resectoscope

The intrauterine resectoscope is used to remove polyps, subcutaneous leiomyomas, and uterine adhesions.

The resectoscope has a 0- or 12-degree telescope inserted into a separate sheath. A spring-loaded handle retracts and exposes the loop-shaped electrode tip, which shaves and coagulates tissue when activated. As tissue is removed from the uterine wall, it remains free-floating in the liquid medium until it is flushed from the uterine cavity. The advantage of the loop resectoscope is that it can both shave and coagulate tissue bit by bit, so that bleeding can be easily controlled.

The resectoscope is constructed with an outer sheath that allows fluid outflow and an inner sheath for continuous irrigation. Specimens are morcellized and retrieved through the distention fluid.

HYSTEROSCOPIC ENDOMETRIAL ABLATION

Surgical Goal

The goal of endometrial ablation is the destruction and scarification of the endometrium to render it nonfunctional.

Pathology

The endometrium, which lines the uterine cavity, is made up of two layers. The functional layer lies over the basal layer and proliferates during the endometrial cycle under hormonal influence. It is sloughed off during menstruation and is replaced throughout the endometrial cycle. Abnormally heavy menses can result in anemia and abdominal pain.

NOTE: The term *dysfunctional uterine bleeding* has been replaced by the more precise term *abnormal uterine bleeding (AUB)*.

Women who no longer want to become pregnant and have attempted conservative treatment for excessive menstrual bleeding are offered endometrial ablation after conservative treatment has failed. Destruction of the endometrium prevents or reduces menses and is not reversible. The procedure is only performed in women who do not want a future pregnancy. The endometrial tissue is destroyed by the procedure thereby making normal implantation impossible.

Current gynecological practice offers a number of safe, effective methods of endometrial ablation. Three common procedures are rollerball ablation (electrocoagulation) and global (reaching all areas of the endometrium) endometrial ablation using an intrauterine device. Cryoablation and radiofrequency ablation are also available. Laser ablation is no longer routinely offered because of complications and injury. Other techniques have proven to be effective and less expensive without the risks associated with laser surgery.

Technique
Rollerball Ablation
1. The patient is prepared for hysteroscopy.
2. The cervix is dilated.
3. A dilation and curettage is performed
4. The endometrium is assessed for pathology with the hysteroscope.
5. The resectoscope with roller ball electrode is reinserted into the cervix.
6. Nonelectrolytic distention fluid is infused into the uterine cavity for use with a monopolar electrosurgical unit (ESU).
7. A rollerball electrode is used to ablate the endometrium.
8. The endometrium is again assessed.
9. The resectoscope is withdrawn.

Technique
Global Endometrial Ablation
1. Hysteroscopy is performed after cervical dilation.
2. The balloon ablation device is inserted into the uterine cavity and activated.
3. The uterine cavity is again assessed by hysteroscopy.

Discussion

The patient is placed in the lithotomy position, and a vaginal prep is performed. Hysteroscopic examination is performed before and after the ablations. Any lesions, such as polyps or other growths, are removed before ablation to ensure separate pathological assessment. A D & C often is performed before ablation to rule out endometrial cancer. Fluid distention of the uterus depends on the type of ablation planned. Monopolar electrosurgical instruments require **nonelectrolytic media** (e.g., glycine, mannitol, sorbitol) for distention. Bipolar HF electrosurgery requires **electrolytic media**, such as normal saline.

Roller ball ablation is performed with a ball-tip electrode and resectoscope. This is an electrosurgical procedure and therefore requires all safety precautions associated with electrosurgery. After assessing the uterus with the hysteroscope, the surgeon systematically applies a 3-mm roller ball tip to coagulate and desiccate the endometrial tissue. The surgeon begins with the lower uterine segments and proceeds to the cornual region.

In global endometrial ablation, most of the endometrial surface is affected by the ablation method. Global ablation procedures are "blind" (i.e., they are not done under direct visualization of the hysteroscope or resectoscope). A variety of methods can be used for global ablation:

- The NovaSure system consists of a radiofrequency controller, disposable ablater, CO_2 canister, desiccant, and operating system. This system delivers radiofrequency energy through the device, which is inserted into the uterine cavity. It measures impedance while delivering the energy to **ablate** the tissue. The device automatically stops when impedance reaches a dangerous level.
- ThermaChoice UBT system includes a silicone balloon catheter with impeller, umbilical cable, and controller, which monitors temperature and pressure. The balloon is inserted and filled with 5% dextrose in water. As the balloon is distended, it begins a warming cycle that reaches 188.6° F (87° C). At this temperature, the endometrium is destroyed within 8 minutes. Safety features of the system prevent overheating and overdistention.
- The Hydro ThermAblator uses a 0.9% sodium chloride solution and a rigid hysteroscope. A D & C is performed, and a rigid scope then is used to fill the uterine cavity with saline. The temperature is automatically raised and measured. The active ablation phase reaches 176° F (80° C) and remains at that temperature for 10 minutes. A cool-down period is then initiated, and the flushing phase is completed. The device is then withdrawn.
- HerOption Uterine Cryoablation uses a cryotherapy probe and compressed gas to achieve temperatures below 0° C to freeze the endometrium. The procedure is carried out under direct ultrasonography guidance. The probe is activated sequentially and followed by a short heating cycle.

Postoperative Considerations

Most methods of endometrial ablation are performed in an outpatient setting, and the patient is allowed to return home the same day. Severe cramping and watery discharge are expected for several days postoperatively. Patients are provided home care instructions on the danger signs of uterine perforation and infection. Few women experience complete amenorrhea after the procedure, and repeat treatment may be required.

MYOMECTOMY

Surgical Goal

Myomectomy is the removal of a benign leiomyoma (**fibroid**) of the myometrium to control bleeding and prevent pressure on other structures in the pelvis. Submucosal myomas can be removed with the resectoscope.

Pathology

A **leiomyoma** is a benign, smooth muscle tumor of the uterus (Figure 24-16). These tumors may cause abnormal uterine bleeding and lead to anemia, or they may impinge upon adjacent structures, causing pain or dysfunction.

Technique

1. The patient is prepared for hysteroscopy as described previously.
2. After cervical dilation, a double-sheath resectoscope is inserted.
3. The uterine cavity is irrigated and infused with distention fluid.
4. A resectoscope loop is used to shave and coagulate tumor tissue.
5. The outer sheath is removed to flush out the sectioned tumor pieces. Alternatively, the cervix may be further dilated and sponge forceps used to remove pieces of tumor.
6. The myoma is reduced until it is level with the endometrium.

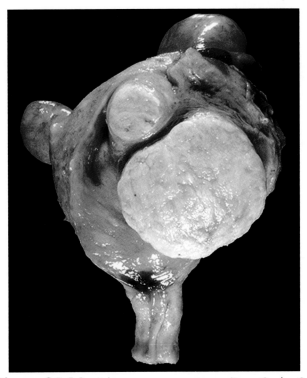

Figure 24-16 A large myoma specimen. *(From Canby C: Problem based anatomy, St Louis, 2007, WB Saunders.)*

Discussion

The patient is placed in the lithotomy position, prepped, and draped as for endometrial ablation.

The procedure begins as the surgeon dilates the cervix and inserts the resectoscope sheath with or without an **obturator**, which is a blunt-tipped rod that is advanced ahead of the sheath to protect the tissue from injury. If used, the obturator is removed after insertion of the sheath.

A resectoscope with a 0-degree or fore-oblique telescope is inserted into the cervix. The resectoscope is surrounded by an 8- or 9-mm sheath, which has an insulated tip to prevent contact between the active electrode and the outer sheath. The outer sheath provides inflow of the distention fluid. A bridge attachment allows entry of the electrodes.

As mentioned, the resectoscope has a spring-loaded handle that operates the active electrode loop. The surgeon removes sections or slices of tissue by repeatedly looping a small portion of tissue and drawing it into the resectoscope. This cuts and coagulates the tissue and releases it into the uterine cavity, where it is flushed out through the resectoscope sheath.

Bleeding can also be controlled by the ball electrode attachment of the resectoscope. The surgeon flushes irrigation fluid and tissue by removing the outer sheath and allowing the fluid to drop into the perineal drape.

The procedure is complete when the tumor is level with the endometrium. All specimen pieces must be retrieved and collected for pathological examination.

LOOP ELECTRODE EXCISION PROCEDURE

Surgical Goal

In the loop electrode excision procedure, a core of tissue is removed from the endocervix to remove cancerous or precancerous tissue.

Pathology

Squamous cell carcinoma is the most common cause of cervical cancer. A diagnosis is made after a positive Pap test with atypical cells is followed by culposcopy and tissue biopsy. During culposcopy, the cervix is examined microscopically with the aid of acetic acid. The acid causes the atypical cells to turn white, allowing clear identification and removal. If a biopsy shows invasion of atypical or precancerous cells, LEEP is indicated.

Technique

1. The surgeon grasps the cervix with a single-toothed tenaculum.
2. A local anesthetic is injected into the cervical canal.
3. A loop electrode is used to remove tissue from the cervix.
4. A ball electrode is used to control bleeding.

Discussion

The patient is placed in the lithotomy position, prepped, and draped for a vaginal procedure. The surgeon infuses the cervix with a local anesthetic. The anterior lip of the cervix is grasped with a tenaculum. A disposable loop electrode is then used to make a circumferential incision around the os. The specimen

is removed for pathological examination. The loop electrode is then replaced with a ball coagulator, which is used to coagulate the area of the excision. The cervical cone tissue is sectioned and examined carefully for the depth of cellular invasion. This determines the need for more radical surgery.

DILATION AND CURETTAGE

Surgical Goal

In dilation and curettage, sharp and smooth curettes are used to remove the surface of the endometrium through a transvaginal approach.

Pathology

A D & C may be performed for diagnostic purposes, to terminate a pregnancy, or to treat abnormal uterine bleeding.

Technique

1. The uterine depth is measured with a uterine sound.
2. The cervix is dilated with graduated dilators.
3. Curettes are used to remove endometrial tissue.

Discussion

The patient is placed in the lithotomy position. The bladder may be emptied with a straight catheter. The patient is then prepped and draped for a vaginal procedure. The surgeon stands or sits at the foot of the operating table. The scrub should stand next to the surgeon. To begin the procedure, the surgeon places an Auvard speculum in the vagina. The surgeon then grasps the anterior lip of the cervix with a tenaculum and retracts it slightly forward and downward.

A uterine sound is inserted into the cervix to measure its depth and position. This prevents accidental perforation during the procedure. The surgeon dilates the cervix with Hagar, Pratt, or Hank uterine dilators.

After cervical dilation, the surgeon places a Telfa dressing on the posterior edge of the vagina. The uterus is then gently curetted, and the specimen is collected on the Telfa. The technologist should have several types and sizes of curettes available, including smooth, sharp, and serrated. When curettage is complete, the Telfa is removed and passed to the scrub. Both the Telfa and specimen are placed in a container for pathological examination.

TERMINATION OF PREGNANCY (ABORTION)

Surgical Goal

Abortion is the termination of a viable pregnancy. The remains of a fetus are surgically removed from the uterus after fetal death.

Discussion

Termination of a pregnancy may be advised for medical reasons, or a woman may undergo elective abortion according to the restrictions of gestational age and the age of the mother, which vary according to state law. Medical abortion is performed when the pregnancy endangers the health or life of the

Table 24-3

Types of Spontaneous (noninduced) Abortion

Complete	Expulsion of all products of conception. Surgical intervention is not necessary.
Incomplete	A portion of the products of conception have been expelled. Medical intervention may be necessary to control hemorrhage.
Inevitable abortion	The cervix is dilated and there is rupture of the membranes or vaginal bleeding. The products of conception have not been expelled.
Missed abortion	Undiagnosed and undetected embryonic or fetal demise (death); the products of conception are not expelled.
Septic abortion	Severe uterine infection associated with abortion.
Threatened abortion	Uterine bleeding without cervical dilation occurring before 20 weeks gestation.

mother, when the fetus is likely to die, or when a pregnancy is the result of rape or incest. The reasons for elective abortion are defined by the woman. Surgical abortion by suction or extraction is performed between 4 and 24 weeks' gestation. A D & C may be performed at 4 to 12 weeks' gestation. Most surgical abortions are performed at 12 to 14 weeks' gestation. Preoperative counseling is provided in all cases. Terms related to spontaneous abortion are defined in Table 24-3.

The patient is placed in the lithotomy position and prepped for a vaginal procedure. Sedation and cervical block anesthesia or local infiltration of the cervix is administered. A D & C is performed as described previously, and the suction probe used to remove the contents of the uterus. The contents are documented as *products of conception* and retained as a tissue specimen. Complications of surgical abortion include perforation of the uterus and incomplete removal of the uterine contents, which can result in bleeding or infection.

TRANSVAGINAL AND VULVAR PROCEDURES

VAGINAL HYSTERECTOMY

Surgical Goal
For a vaginal hysterectomy, a transcervical approach is used to remove the uterus.

Pathology
See Total Abdominal Hysterectomy.

Technique

1. A circumferential incision is made in the vaginal mucosa at the base of the cervix.
2. The surgeon partly mobilizes the uterus by sequentially incising and ligating the uterine ligaments.

3. The peritoneal reflection of the bladder (bladder flap) is dissected from the uterus.
4. The uterus is completely mobilized and removed.
5. The bladder flap is reconstructed.
6. The peritoneum is closed.
7. The deep vaginal incision is closed.

Discussion
Transvaginal hysterectomy is selected as an approach in selected patients in which surgical access is adequate to perform surgery safely, and in those who are suitable for outpatient surgery or early discharge. Transvaginal approach is less painful and provides early return to normal activities unless there are postoperative complications.

The patient is placed in the lithotomy position, prepped, and draped for a vaginal procedure. A pocket drape should be attached to the perineal drape. The bladder is drained with a straight catheter during the prep.

The surgeon grasps the cervix with a uterine tenaculum. Using the scalpel or curved Mayo scissors, the surgeon makes a circumferential incision around the cervix, separating the vaginal mucosa and fascia from the body of the cervix. This incision exposes the first set of ligaments, which are double-clamped, divided, and ligated with suture ligatures of size 0 synthetic absorbable material on a tapered needle.

The posterior peritoneum is elevated with toothed tissue forceps and incised with the scalpel or scissors. With the peritoneal cavity open, the surgeon removes the peritoneal reflection of the bladder from the uterus using Metzenbaum scissors. The assistant retracts the bladder upward with a Sims or Heaney retractor. The scrub must have long tissue forceps and long dissecting scissors available as the mobilization is carried deep into the pelvis.

Mobilization of the uterus continues until it is completely free. The uterus then is removed as a specimen. Before closing the peritoneum, the surgeon closes the bladder flap with a running suture of 2-0 absorbable synthetic material on a small curved needle. The peritoneum is then closed with a running absorbable suture. A perineal pad is placed over the perineum to absorb any drainage from the wound.

REPAIR OF A CYSTOCELE AND RECTOCELE (ANTERIOR-POSTERIOR REPAIR)

Surgical Goal
Herniated tissue of the anterior and posterior vagina is reduced, and the vaginal walls are reconstructed.

Pathology
A **cystocele** (herniation of the bladder) and a **rectocele** (herniation of the rectum) occur when the musculature and connective tissues become weakened and prolapse against the anterior and posterior vaginal walls. The most common cause is pregnancy. The pelvic floor provides support to the intestinal and genitourinary structures, especially during pregnancy, when gravity pulls the fetus downward and stretches the ligaments and muscles. Repair and reconstruction of the

supportive structure restores normal function and relieves discomfort and pain.

Technique

1. The anterior vaginal mucosa is incised.
2. The surgeon grasps the incision edges with Allis clamps.
3. Blunt and sharp dissection is used to create a tissue plane between the vaginal mucosa and the submucosal connective tissue.
4. The dissection is continued to the bladder neck.
5. The vaginal wall is reconstructed with sutures.
6. The posterior vaginal wall is incised, and steps 2 and 3 are repeated.
7. The tissue plane is continued to the rectum.
8. Sutures are placed across the rectal musculature to reconstruct the pelvic floor.
9. The vaginal mucosa is sutured closed.

Discussion

Anterior Repair

The patient is placed in the lithotomy position, prepped, and draped for a vaginal procedure. The patient also is catheterized.

The surgeon inserts a weighted speculum into the vaginal outlet. The cervix is grasped with a tenaculum and retracted. Using the scalpel or curved Mayo scissors, the surgeon makes an incision in the anterior vaginal wall. The edges of the incision are grasped with several Allis clamps. These are fanned out to distend the tissue edges and delineate the plane between the mucosa and the connective tissue underneath.

With the tissue planes exposed, the surgeon uses a 4 × 4 sponge to push the connective tissue off the mucosa. This technique of blunt dissection effectively separates the two tissue layers and creates a flap (the vaginal mucosa) with a minimum of bleeding. The technologist should have ample sponges available. As the sponge becomes moist, its surface becomes smooth, and the sponge is less effective for dissection. The curved Mayo scissors are used alternately with sponges to continue the dissection to the level of the bladder.

During this portion of the procedure, the assistant or scrub may be required to retract the superior vaginal vault upward with a lateral (Heaney) right-angle retractor. This elevates the roof of the vagina and exposes the dissection plane.

❖ *During retraction, the scrub should exert gentle, even pressure on the retractor to prevent bruising and hematoma in the vaginal mucosa.*

When the dissection has reached the bladder neck, several sutures of size 0 chromic gut or synthetic absorbable sutures are placed through the fascia and pulled laterally. This tightens the tissue and prevents the bladder from bulging. The edge of the vaginal mucosa is measured over the repair, and the edges are trimmed. The mucosa is then approximated with running or interrupted sutures of absorbable material, usually of the same size as that used on the bladder repair.

Posterior Repair

To begin the posterior repair, the surgeon places two Allis clamps in the posterior vaginal wall and makes a small transverse incision between them. The assistant provides traction on the clamp as described in the anterior repair. The techniques used in anterior repair are repeated to the level of the rectum. The levator muscles and fascia then are brought together and tightened with absorbable interrupted sutures, and the vaginal mucosa is repaired. A self-retaining catheter may be inserted. Figure 24-17 shows the repair of a cystocele.

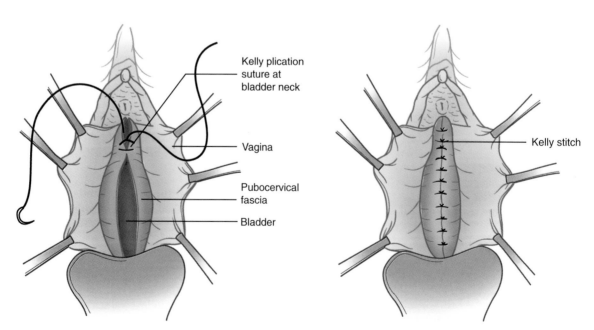

Kelly plication suture at bladder neck

Vagina

Pubocervical fascia

Bladder

Kelly stitch

Figure 24-17 Cystocele repair. Allis clamps are placed on the periphery of redundant tissue, and the vaginal wall is strengthened with interrupted sutures. *(From Seidel HM et al: Mosby's guide to physical examination, ed 5, St Louis, Mosby.)*

VAGINOPLASTY

Surgical Goal

Vaginoplasty is performed to create a functional vagina (neovagina) to facilitate sexual intercourse. Several different procedures currently are performed to achieve the surgical goal. The following procedure uses a vaginal mold and skin graft. Alternatives include peritoneal skin flap grafts or combination tissue grafts.

Pathology

A congenital abnormality of the mullerian ducts during fetal development can result in the absence of the vagina or uterus, a condition referred to as *mullerian agenesis*. Other defects occur with this anomaly, but the absence of the vagina and uterus is the most common presentation. Patients usually are diagnosed during puberty, because the onset of menarche is delayed. The external genitalia and hormonal levels are normal. Although normal childbirth is not possible, patients may undergo in vitro fertilization (IVF) and surrogate pregnancy. The cause of mullerian agenesis is unknown.

Technique

1. A split-thickness skin graft is obtained.
2. The graft is fitted around a vaginal mold.
3. An incision is made through the vaginal vestibule.
4. Subcutaneous connective tissue is dissected.
5. A vaginal space is created for the mold.
6. The mold and graft are fitted in the vaginal space, and the labia are sutured.
7. Approximately 1 week after surgery, the initial mold is removed.
8. A removable mold is used during the 6-month postoperative period.

Discussion

Before surgery, the patient is counseled to provide her with information about reproductive alternatives and to ensure that she understands the procedure and postoperative therapy. As mentioned, most patients are diagnosed during adolescence, and this developmental period is distinguished by a search for identity and strong peer approval. It is important for perioperative personnel to understand the emotional impact of the diagnosis and procedure and to offer appropriate support to the patient.

During the first stage of the procedure, a split-thickness skin graft is taken from the buttocks or thigh. The buttocks are a preferred site because of scarring. If the buttocks area is used, the patient is placed in the prone position. The area is prepped and draped. A sponge soaked in epinephrine solution may be applied to the graft site to produce local vasoconstriction. Mineral oil then is applied to the site, and a dermatome is used to remove the split-thickness graft. (This procedure is discussed fully in Chapter 29.) The donor site may be dressed with an Opsite. The patient may then be placed in the supine position for the vaginoplasty. The perineum, thighs, and abdomen are prepped, and a Foley catheter is inserted.

A small draped table may be useful for preparation of the graft. A dermatome, square basin, forceps, sponges, and vaginal mold should be available before the graft is taken. Immediately after harvesting, the skin graft is placed through a skin mesher. This removes blood clots and allows serous fluid to escape from the graft. The graft is then placed around the mold. The scrub should place the transplant in a square basin and place it in a protected area of the prep or back table. The graft is covered with sponges moistened with saline.

A perineal incision is made between the rectum and the urethra. The ESU is used to coagulate small bleeders. The scrub should have Hagar dilators available, according to the surgeon's preference. A tunnel is then made through the subcutaneous tissue with digital separation or dilators. Meticulous hemostasis is necessary to ensure uniform contact between the graft and the tunneled opening.

After the tunnel is created and hemostasis has been secured, the graft transplant is fitted in the opening and secured with several fine absorbent sutures. The labia are approximated with several 2-0 or 3-0 sutures of synthetic material on a cutting needle. The wound is dressed with absorbent gauze. This concludes the first stage of the procedure. The patient remains on bed rest during this period.

Approximately 1 week after the first procedure, the patient is returned to the operating room so that the vaginal mold can be removed. The patient is placed in the lithotomy position, and a perineal prep is performed. The surgeon may remove the sutures during the skin prep, and the used instruments must be removed from the field completely.

The mold is carefully removed and placed in a small sterile basin. The neovagina is then irrigated with warm saline and assessed for any signs of inflammation, infection, or blood clots. A soft adjustable mold is then fitted carefully into the space. The mold is not sutured.

Postoperative Considerations

The soft mold remains in place intermittently for the next 3 months after surgery; it is removed during defecation and urination to prevent expulsion. Approximately 6 months is required for complete healing and normal function. Complications, including infection, fistula, and constriction, may occur during the initial postoperative period. The steps of a vaginoplasty are shown in Figure 24-18.

REPAIR OF A VESICOVAGINAL FISTULA

Surgical Goal

A vesicovaginal fistula is a small, hollow tract that connects the bladder to the vagina. Fistulous tracts can be caused by infection or trauma. Chronic fistulous tracts are lined with epithelial tissue, which prevents the tract from closing. The surgical goal is to incise the length of the tract and remove this tissue. The fascial layer that separates the bladder from the vagina is approximated. Healing then can occur normally, and urine is prevented from draining into the vagina.

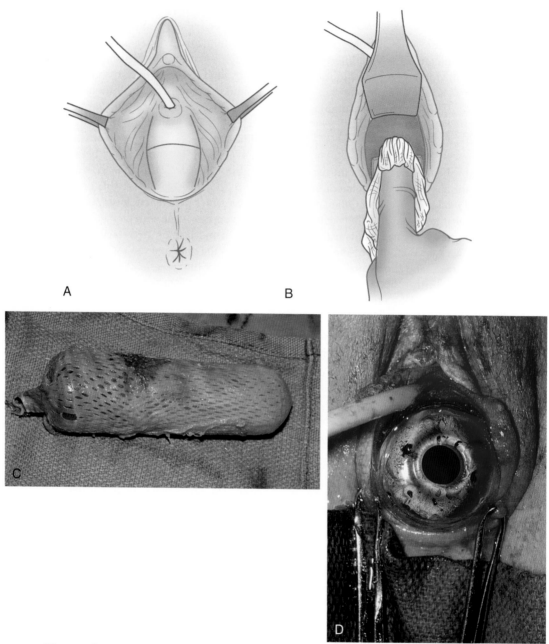

Figure 24-18 Vaginoplasty. **A,** A transverse incision is made in the vaginal vestibule. **B,** Blunt dissection is used to make a space is made for the vaginal implant. **C,** A skin graft covers the glass mold. **D,** The graft and implant in place. The implant is removed after the graft has integrated into the neovagina. (**B** from Rothrock J: Alexander's care of the patient in surgery, ed 7, St Louis, 2007, Mosby; From Falcone T, Hurd W: Clinical reproductive medicine and surgery, Philadelphia, 2007, Mosby.)

Pathology

A vesicovaginal fistula may be caused by a traumatic penetrating injury, infection, radiation therapy that thins and weakens the pelvic structures, vaginal birth, or chronic inflammation. Urine drains into the vagina, causing irritation and incontinence. The fistula may extend into the urethra. The repair may be approached through pelvic laparotomy or vaginally. A pelvic approach is required when the tract occurs in the proximal vaginal vault. A vaginal exposure is described here.

Technique

1. The surgeon grasps the edge of the tract with two or more Allis clamps.
2. A metal probe may be placed in the fistula to identify its course. Diagnostic procedures, including instillation of a contrast medium, may have preceded the surgery. Films obtained from the procedure show the route of the fistula.
3. The tissue around the fistula is sharply dissected.

4. A tissue plane is created between the bladder and the fistula with sharp and blunt dissection.
5. The mucosa is inverted, and sutures are placed through the smooth muscular layer and mucosa.
6. An internal layer of sutures is placed in the bladder.
7. The edges of the vaginal wall are repaired.
8. An indwelling Foley catheter is placed.

Discussion

The patient is placed in the lithotomy position, prepped, and draped for a perineal incision. The surgeon places an Auvard or Sims retractor in the vagina to expose the fistula. A malleable probe is inserted into the fistula. The surgeon then uses dissecting scissors to make a circular incision around the probe and fistula. The surgeon carries this incision the full length of the fistula with dissecting scissors until the anterior bladder wall is exposed. Two lateral retractors may be placed in the vagina for better exposure. The surgeon creates a tissue plane between the bladder and the fistula with sponge dissectors or by sharp dissection.

When the bladder mucosa and smooth muscle layer have been exposed, the surgeon inverts the bladder tissue layers and approximates the edges with double-layer, interrupted 3-0 sutures of absorbable material. The vaginal wall is repaired with size 0 or 2-0 sutures. A Foley catheter may be inserted into the bladder at the close of the procedure.

REPAIR OF A RECTOVAGINAL FISTULA

Surgical Goal

A rectovaginal fistula is a tract between the rectum and the vagina. Surgical repair closes the defect and prevents fecal material from draining into the vagina. A number of different procedures have been developed for repair of RV fistula, including patch grafts (allograft or porcine), flap and advancement grafts. In simple cases, excision of the fistula.

Pathology

A rectovaginal fistula may be caused by vaginal or rectal trauma, childbirth, Crohn's disease, radiation therapy, chronic inflammation, or infection. A fistulous tract allows fecal material to drain into the vagina, causing infection, emotional distress, and social isolation.

Technique

1. The fistula is exposed.
2. A tissue plane is created around the defect.
3. The vaginal wall is incised, exposing the deep layers of the rectum.
4. The plane is carried to the rectal outlet.
5. The fistula is completely excised and removed.
6. The levator muscle, mucosal defect, and vaginal wall are repaired.
7. A Foley catheter is inserted.

Discussion

The patient is placed in the lithotomy position for vaginal approach while jacknife position is preferred for rectal approach. Routine prepping and draping is performed according to the required position.

To begin the procedure for a vaginal approach, the surgeon places a weighted retractor in the vagina. A malleable probe is then used to define the extent of the fistula. The assistant grasps the posterior wall of the vagina with Allis clamps to produce traction across the fistula. A circular incision is then made around the fistula with the scalpel or dissecting scissors. Toothed tissue forceps are used to pick up the edge of the tissue as it is incised. Metzenbaum scissors are used to follow the tract and create a tissue plane between the tract and the deep tissue.

The vaginal wall is then grasped and incised with scissors, exposing the wall of the rectum. The surgeon incises the tissue around fistula along its length. If necessary, the perineal floor may require suture reinforcement to restore strength to the muscles. Interrupted sutures of synthetic absorbable material are used. Sutures are placed until the defect is closed and the repair is secure. A Foley catheter is placed at the close of the procedure.

More complex procedures are required for fistulas which are located in the distal anus or those that are subject to chronic infection. A diverting stoma may be required for selected patients during the healing period.

REMOVAL OF A CYSTIC BARTHOLIN GLAND

Surgical Goal

The procedure for removal of a cystic Bartholin gland removes a cyst and the associated Bartholin gland to prevent recurrence of the cyst and infection.

Pathology

The Bartholin glands are a common site of cyst formation. The cyst may become infected, and in such cases, surgical removal is indicated.

Technique

1. The labia minora are retracted and secured to the skin.
2. The mucosa overlying the cyst is incised.
3. The cyst and sometimes the gland are removed.
4. The wound edges are secured open with small sutures.

Discussion

The patient is placed in the lithotomy position, prepped, and draped for a perineal incision.

The surgeon may begin the procedure by securing the labia minora laterally with sutures or small skin staples. A curved incision is then made in the mucosa over the cystic gland. The incision is lengthened with Metzenbaum scissors. Small bleeders are coagulated with the ESU.

The gland and the cyst may be removed together, or the cyst may be dissected away from the gland with dissecting scissors. The wound edges are secured open with sutures to allow secondary closure, as in marsupialization. This procedure is illustrated in Figure 24-19.

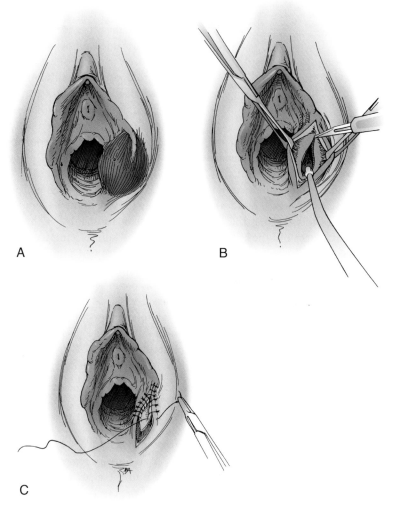

Figure 24-19 Bartholin gland cyst. **A,** An infected Bartholin gland may become cystic. **B,** An incision is made over the skin and wall of the cyst. **C,** The cyst wall may be everted and sutured to the skin to prevent recurrence. *(Modified from Gershenson DM, DeCherney AH, Curry SL, Brubaker LC: Operative gynecology, ed 2, Philadelphia, 2001, WB Saunders.)*

VULVECTOMY

Surgical Goal

Vulvectomy is surgical excision of the labia, clitoris, and inguinal and pelvic lymph nodes and is performed to treat cancer of the vulva.

Pathology

Cancer of the vulva represents about 5% of all genitourinary carcinomas. It is more common among women over the age of 60. Most invasive carcinoma that involves the lymph nodes is seen in this age group. Local vulvar cancer (vulvar intraepithelial neoplasm) appears to be associated with some strains of human papilloma virus (HPV).

Technique

1. The surgeon makes a wide incision around the vulva, extending laterally to include the labia majora.
2. A second incision is made on the interior edge of the first.

3. The incision is carried to subcutaneous and connective tissue.
4. The tissue specimen is retracted with Kocher and Allis clamps.
5. Hemorrhage is controlled with the ESU and suture ties.
6. The specimen is removed in one piece (**en bloc**).
7. An incision is made in the posterior vaginal wall.
8. The levator muscles are sutured.
9. Bilateral groin incisions are made.
10. Lymph nodes are removed.
11. Suction drains are placed.
12. All incisions are closed. A skin graft is placed as needed.
13. A Foley catheter is inserted into the urethra.

Discussion

Vulvectomy may be performed as a simple or radical procedure. In the past, simple vulvectomy was performed to remove only the lesion itself and a margin surrounding it. This procedure is rarely performed now because of the disfiguring results and increased incidence of cancer in younger patients. *Skinning vulvectomy,* in which only the skin of the vulva is removed, usually by laser surgery, is the preferred procedure for noninvasive lesions. Radical vulvectomy (described below) is a complex procedure involving groin exploration, lymph-node removal, and wide resection of the lesion and adjacent tissue.

The patient is placed in the lithotomy position, prepped, and draped for lower abdominal and perineal incisions. Instruments and equipment used in the perineal portion of the procedure are kept separate from those of the groin procedure. Two set-ups may be created to isolate the perineal equipment. Gloves and gowns are changed for the groin procedure, according to the surgeon's directions.

The surgeon begins the procedure by making a large elliptical incision around the vulva. The incision encompasses the labia minora, labia majora, and clitoris. A second incision is made superior to the urethral orifice and encompasses the vagina. The surgeon grasps the skin edges of the incision with Allis clamps and carries dissection through the subcutaneous and connective tissues of the vulva. The assistant provides traction on the tissue edges while the surgeon incises and coagulates the tissue, creating a block of tissue that will be removed.

Large bleeding vessels are clamped with small hemostats and ligated with fine absorbable sutures or coagulated with the ESU. The vulva is removed en bloc when the dissection and mobilization are complete. The specimen is isolated from the set-up that will be used on the groin dissection.

The assistant next inserts a right-angle retractor into the superior portion of the vagina. A Heaney lateral retractor is typically used. The surgeon then incises the posterior vaginal mucosa and uses interrupted sutures of absorbable material, size 0 or 2-0, to strengthen the connective tissues of the posterior pelvic floor. The mucosal incisions are closed with size 2-0 or 0 absorbable sutures. If the excision is narrow, the skin edges may be directly closed. Several subcutaneous sutures may be needed to prevent an open pocket between the tissue layers. The skin is closed with interrupted monofilament synthetic sutures.

The groin excision is carried out through bilateral inguinal incisions. After incising the skin, the surgeon extends the incision to the inguinal chain. Exposure to these lymph nodes follows a dissection similar to that of inguinal hernia. Lymph nodes are located within the connective tissue. The surgeon removes the nodes individually using sharp dissection and controls bleeding with the ESU and suture ties of absorbable material.

Wound closure is carefully performed to prevent seroma in the postoperative period. Penrose drains may be placed in the inguinal incisions. The wounds are closed in layers to obliterate "dead space" where fluid might collect. Interrupted sutures of 2-0 and 3-0 absorbable material are used to close deep tissue layers. The skin is closed with surgical staples and dressed with bulky gauze fluffs and an abdominal pad.

SECTION II: OPERATIVE OBSTETRICAL PROCEDURES

LEARNING OBJECTIVES

After studying this section the reader will be able to:
- Describe common complications of delivery
- Identify necessary actions for assisting in the management of obstetrical complications
- Recognize and name common instruments used to repair birth lacerations or an episiotomy

TERMINOLOGY

Amniotic fluid: Water around the fetus in the uterus.

Amniotic membranes: Two membranes that encase the fetus, amniotic fluid, and placenta during pregnancy.

APGAR score: Method of assessing neonate according to Respiratory rate, color, reflex response, heart rate, and body tone.

Birth canal: The maternal pelvis and soft structures through which the baby passes during birth.

Breech presentation: Presentation of the baby in which the buttocks or feet deliver first.

Cerclage: A procedure in which a suture ligature is placed around the cervix to prevent spontaneous abortion.

Eclampsia: A seizure during pregnancy, usually as a result of pregnancy-induced hypertension.

Ectopic pregnancy: Implantation of the fertilized ovum outside the uterus.

Epidural: A type of anesthesia in which the anesthetic is delivered through a small tube in the patient's back to relieve pain in labor. The patient usually is in bed and catheterized during labor in which this form of anesthesia is used.

Fetal demise: Death of the fetus.

Gestational age: The age of the baby as measured in the number of weeks from conception.

Hemorrhage: Continuous bleeding from a pathological cause.

Incompetent cervix: A condition in which previous cervical injury results in repeated spontaneous abortions.

Labor: The process of regular contraction of the uterine muscle that results in birth.

Meconium: A nearly sterile fecal waste that accumulates while the fetus is in the uterus. It is passed within the first few days after birth.

Normal spontaneous vaginal delivery (NSVD): A normal delivery of the fetus, without the need for medical intervention. The normal birth process.

Nuchal cord: A complication of pregnancy in which the umbilical cord is wrapped around the fetus' neck. This may lead to obstructed blood flow to the fetus.

Placenta: The organ that transfers selected nutrients to the baby during pregnancy.

Placenta abruption: Premature separation of the placenta from the uterine wall after 20 weeks' gestation and before the fetus is delivered.

Placenta previa: A complication of pregnancy in which the placenta implants completely or partly over the cervical os. In this position, the placenta begins to bleed as it separates from the cervix during labor.

Prenatal: The period of pregnancy before birth.

Presentation: A term that refers to the part of the baby that comes down the birth canal first.

Prolapsed cord: Complication of pregnancy in which the umbilical cord emerges from the uterus during labor and may be compressed against the material pelvis or the vagina. This can cause obstructed blood supply to the fetus.

Suprapubic pressure: Pressure that is applied downward on the patient's abdomen just above the pubic bone.

Uterus: The muscular organ that holds the baby and the placenta during pregnancy.

INTRODUCTION

Birth is a physiological process that seldom requires interventions for a healthy mother. Mother and baby are linked during pregnancy as the mother's body accommodates to the growing baby. Healthy mothers usually provide a nourishing environment that produces a healthy baby. The placenta plays a major role in the baby's health by allowing essential nutrients to pass from the mother's blood to the baby. Failure of the placenta to function, for any reason, can be life-threatening to the baby. Many medical and obstetrical problems are identified before birth. Unexpected problems that arise during **labor**, birth, or after birth can present as emergencies that threaten the life of the mother or the baby. Surgical technologists may be asked to assist in a variety of roles during emergency situations.

STAGES OF PREGNANCY

Development of the embryo and fetus occurs when the ovum is fertilized by sperm, which normally occurs in the fallopian tube. The combination of chromosomal material from each completes the fertilization process. The egg passes through early embryonic development as it moves into the **uterus** and implants in the endometrium, about 10 days after fertilization. As the embryo grows, distinct developmental changes occur. The embryonic stage ends at week 8, and the fetal period begins.

During development, fetal circulation begins shortly after conception. Changes in the endometrial cells provide nourishment and protection for the fetus. The **placenta** is a thick organ that adheres to the uterus on the maternal side. The fetal side contains large vessels within the structure's smooth membranes. The umbilical cord, which attaches to the placenta, contains the umbilical artery and vein and communicates directly with fetal circulation.

Fetal membranes surround the growing fetus and are filled with **amniotic fluid**. The two membranes, the *chorion* and the *amnion*, are very close together. The amnion is continuous with the umbilical cord. The fluid-filled sack in which the fetus develops protects it against physical injury and also maintains thermoregulation. The watery environment allows the fetus to move and develop without restriction (Figure 24-20).

Average normal gestation occurs over 40 weeks and is marked by predictable growth patterns that can be measured by ultrasound. **Prenatal** assessment is performed throughout gestation to ensure that fetal development progresses normally and to detect complications early. Abdominal ultrasound is routinely used to assess pregnancy (Figure 24-21).

COMPLICATIONS OF PREGNANCY

PLACENTAL ABRUPTION

The placenta is the organ that acts as a filter from mother to baby; it allows nutrients to pass from the mother's blood to the baby and rids the baby of waste products. It is essential to the life of the baby during the entire pregnancy. The placenta attaches to the uterine wall and grows during pregnancy to accommodate the baby's needs. **Placental abruption** is a premature separation of the placenta from the uterine wall after 20 weeks' gestation and before the fetus is delivered (Figure 24-22). A variety of conditions can cause abruption, such as abdominal trauma, abnormalities of the uterus, a short umbilical cord, and hypertension. Abruption of the placenta from the uterine wall can be partial or complete. Abruption of the placenta presents as vaginal bleeding and sometimes concealed bleeding. The baby has a good chance of surviving if half of the placenta remains attached to the uterus. **Fetal demise** results if the entire placenta separates from the uterus. If this happens during labor, fetal distress is evident during monitoring of the fetal heart. The woman may experience increased abdominal tenderness and back pain. If delivery is not imminent, a cesarean section is necessary.

PLACENTA PREVIA

During normal labor, the baby's head is pushed toward the cervix, and the cervix begins to thin. Eventually the cervix dilates to about 10 cm, thins out, and becomes part of the lower uterus. Normally the placenta implants on the uterine wall, far from the uterine opening (cervix). The location of the placenta usually is identified on routine ultrasound scans in the prenatal period. **Placenta previa** occurs when the placenta implants completely or partly over the cervical os (Figure 24-23). In this position, the placenta begins to bleed as it separates from the cervix during labor. The amount of bleeding is greater when the placenta covers the cervix completely. Sudden **hemorrhage** is life-threatening to both mother and baby. An immediate cesarean section is necessary to

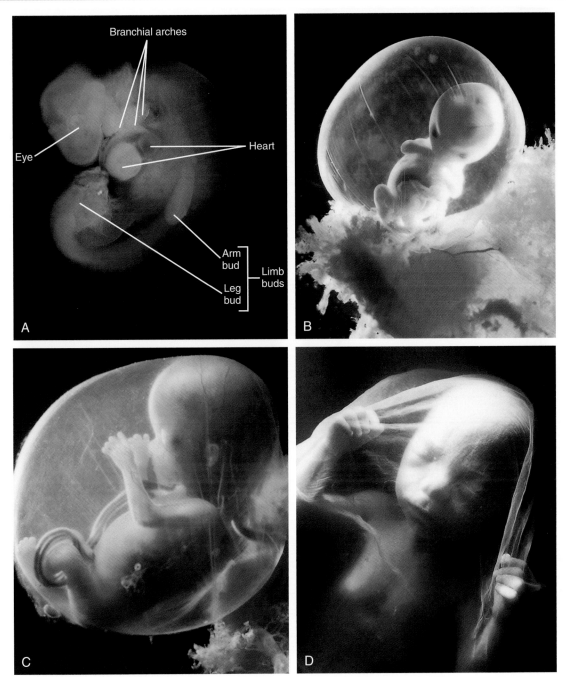

Figure 24-20 Embryonic life. **A,** 35 days. **B,** 49 days. **C,** 12 weeks. **D,** 16 weeks. *(From Thibodeau G, Patton K: Anatomy and physiology, ed 6, St Louis, 2007, Mosby.)*

prevent fetal death and maternal hemorrhage. Often hemorrhage can be prevented if a cesarean section is performed before labor begins.

PREGNANCY-INDUCED HYPERTENSION

Pregnancy-induced hypertension (PIH) is diagnosed as high blood pressure that occurs only during pregnancy after 20 weeks' gestation. PIH may be mild and monitored but not treated, or it may be severe and affect other systems, such as the kidneys (proteinuria), liver (elevated liver enzymes), and blood (low platelets). It also can lead to maternal seizure

(**eclampsia**). This disease process is also referred to as *toxemia* and *pre-eclampsia*. It usually occurs in the first pregnancy, but its cause is unknown. Hypertension can constrict blood flow to the placenta and baby, resulting in a small baby and placenta. If this occurs or if symptoms worsen, the labor is induced artificially with drugs. During the induction, the mother may receive medicines intravenously to reduce the risk of seizure, although this is rare if the mother is receiving preventive medication. If a seizure occurs, it usually lasts 60 seconds or less, but it may be life-threatening to the baby and mother. Airway maintenance is of primary importance during a seizure, therefore airways usually are within easy reach in

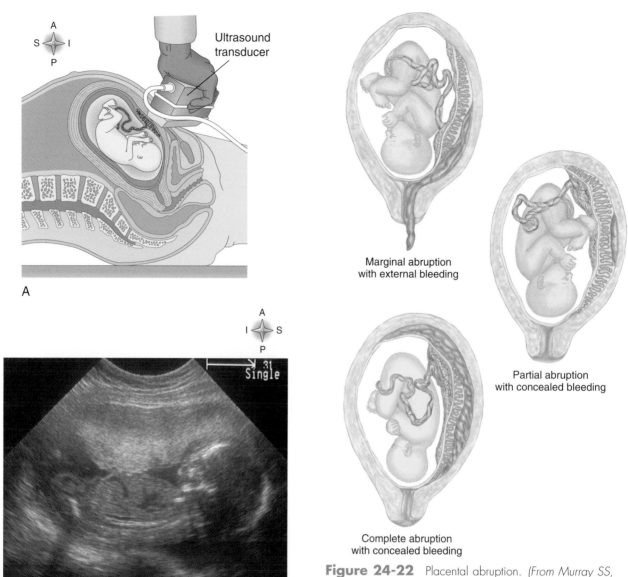

Figure 24-21   A, Ultrasound assessment of the fetus. **B,** Sonogram of the fetus. *(From Thibodeau G, Patton K: Anatomy and physiology, ed 6, St Louis, 2007, Mosby.)*

Figure 24-22   Placental abruption. *(From Murray SS, McKinney ES: Foundations of maternal–newborn nursing, ed 4, Philadelphia, 2006, WB Saunders.)*

each labor room. Once the mother's condition has stabilized after a seizure, a cesarean section can be performed.

NUCHAL CORD

An umbilical cord wrapped one or more times around the baby's neck is called a **nuchal cord**. This usually occurs with an active baby in the early months of pregnancy, when there is plenty of room for the baby to move. A nuchal cord is seldom diagnosed before labor, but it may be suspected if the baby's heart rate decreases markedly during contractions. If the nuchal cord is tight, blood flow through it will be constricted during contractions as the baby moves downward, causing the baby's heart rate to slow markedly. After this, the heart rate may return to a normal range. Usually babies

recover from this labor stress and are born with the cord around the neck. However, if the baby's heart continues to decrease markedly with every contraction and takes longer to recover to a normal rate, the baby may become too stressed to deliver vaginally. A cesarean section may be an option if delivery is still hours away. If the baby is delivered with a nuchal cord, it usually is not a problem to slip the cord over the head or, alternatively, clamp and cut it before the body is born.

LACK OF LABOR PROGRESS

During labor, the baby is expected to make steady progress through the **birth canal**, maneuvering into appropriate positions that provide the best fit for the baby's head and the maternal pelvis. Various problems can occur to impede this process. These include weak contractions, a fetal head that is not flexed sufficiently or is tilted to the side, or a fetal head

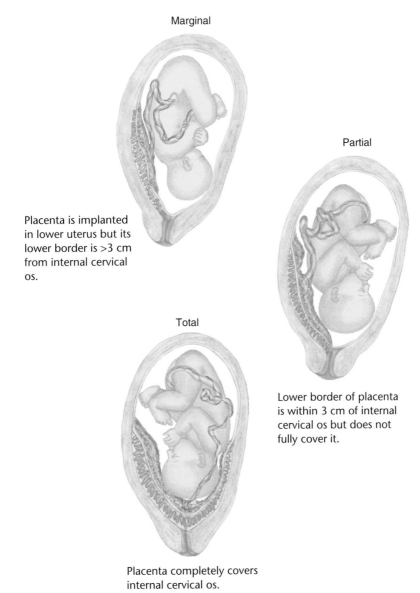

Marginal

Placenta is implanted in lower uterus but its lower border is >3 cm from internal cervical os.

Partial

Lower border of placenta is within 3 cm of internal cervical os but does not fully cover it.

Total

Placenta completely covers internal cervical os.

Figure 24-23 Placenta previa. *(From Murray SS, McKinney ES: Foundations of maternal–newborn nursing, ed 4, Philadelphia, 2006, WB Saunders.)*

that is too large to fit through a narrow maternal pelvis. Some positions of the baby's head require more room in the pelvis (e.g., babies who are "face up"). If diagnosed early in labor, maternal position changes or manual manipulations on the fetal head may help rotate the baby into a better position for descending through the birth canal. If this fails or if the baby is too large (or the mother's pelvis is too small), then progress is impeded and a cesarean section is needed.

CORD PROLAPSE

During pregnancy, membranes extending from the edge of the placenta encase the baby as it moves in a water-filled environment as described previously. Normally, the amniotic sac remains intact until labor. When the **amniotic membranes** break spontaneously or artificially, the amniotic fluid flows out of the vagina. If the fetal head is not low in the birth

canal and the membranes rupture, there is a chance the umbilical cord may be swept in front of the baby's head with the flow of water and may lodge in the vagina or even outside the vagina. When the cord precedes the fetal head, **cord prolapse** has occurred. This rarely happens before labor begins but can persist during labor. This condition is more likely with a breech **presentation** or an excess of amniotic fluid. When the cord precedes the baby in the birth canal, it can be compressed by the baby's head as it presses against the cervix and maternal pelvis. This reduces or stops the flow of oxygen to the baby. This condition requires an emergency cesarean section. In rare cases, the birth may occur vaginally if the cord prolapses suddenly along with the amniotic sac. The baby's head then follows with the next contraction. The nurse, midwife, or physician who discovers this problem puts counterpressure on the baby's head at the vaginal outlet to reduce cord pressure while the woman is quickly moved to the operating room. In case of a pending emergency, the operating room staff is notified and a setup prepared. However, there may be little time between the diagnosis of cord prolapse and the start of surgery.

BREECH PRESENTATION

A **breech presentation** occurs when the baby's feet, knees, or buttocks enter the birth canal before the head. This can be a difficult, long labor that stresses the baby and the mother. It usually is diagnosed before labor, but it may be missed. If this position is known in the prenatal period, attempts can be made to change the position so that the head presents first. Before 38 weeks' gestation, the woman can try positions at home to rotate the baby. If these fail, she is likely to be scheduled for a procedure to rotate the fetus. This is called a *version*. If attempts to change the baby's position fail, a cesarean section is scheduled. Few physicians or nurse-midwives conduct planned breech deliveries. Most breech deliveries are unplanned, imminent, or occur with a twin birth. If the fetus is not too large and contractions are consistent and strong, breech birth is possible. Dangers include a compressed umbilical cord, cord prolapse, and impinged fetal arms or head. Both physicians and nurse-midwives learn maneuvers to facilitate the breech birth, and extra hands may be called for to keep the baby's head flexed (**suprapubic pressure**), to position the bed or the mother, and to resuscitate the baby. Breech babies often are stressed and present with thick **meconium** at birth. Ideally, a good pediatric team is present to attend the birth, but if a delay occurs, assistance for suctioning the baby's airway may be requested.

DIAGNOSTIC TESTS

Pregnancy test: The pregnancy test detects the hormone human chorionic gonadotropin (HCG) either in the blood or the urine. HCG can be quantified in a blood test to assess whether the level is increasing at the expected rate in the first trimester. A pregnancy is confirmed most often by ultrasound or detection of a fetal heartbeat.

Ultrasound scans: Ultrasound is routinely used for a variety of tasks in pregnancy. It is useful for assessing fetal age if the last menses is unknown. Transvaginal ultrasound in the first trimester can determine the **gestational age** within 3 to 5 days. A diagnostic ultrasound performed at 18 weeks may be useful for identifying some types of fetal defects and confirming the gestational age. Ultrasound is commonly used in pregnancy for checking fetal growth, amniotic fluid volume, fetal position, and the location of the placenta.

Routine blood and urine tests: Routine blood and urine tests include tests that may affect the health of the present baby or of subsequent babies. These tests include:

- *Maternal blood type, Rh, and antibody screen:* These tests are important in the event transfusion is needed after hemorrhage. A negative Rh factor in the mother may induce her to make antibodies against her baby if she is exposed to the baby's Rh-positive blood (at birth or if bleeding during pregnancy). If the mother is Rh positive, she receives anti-D immunoglobulin at 28 weeks' gestation and again postpartum if her baby is Rh positive. This prevents the formation of antibodies against future Rh-positive babies during gestation. The antibody screen also confirms the presence of antibodies to other blood types.
- *RPR (rapid plasma reagin) syphilis antibody test:* Syphilis is a sexually transmitted infection that can be passed to the baby during pregnancy. It causes a variety of defects or miscarriage, depending on the maternal stage of the disease.
- *Rubella antibody testing:* Rubella can cause severe defects or miscarriage if contracted by the mother in the first 16 weeks of pregnancy.
- *Human immunodeficiency virus and acquired immunodeficiency syndrome (HIV/AIDS) screening:* HIV infection and AIDS can be transmitted to the baby during pregnancy, birth, or through breast milk.
- *Hepatitis B:* This disease can be transmitted to the baby during pregnancy or through breast milk and may cause liver cancer if left untreated in the newborn.
- *Screening for gonorrhea and chlamydia:* These diseases can be passed to the baby during its passage through the birth canal, resulting in respiratory or eye infections and blindness if left untreated after birth. The diagnosis is made by cytological examination of a cervical smear or by a urine test.
- *Complete blood count (CBC):* This test is performed to diagnose anemia, insufficient platelets, or an increased white blood cell count indicating infection.
- *Cervical cancer screening (Pap smear):* The Pap smear is routinely done during prenatal care. It detects abnormal cells and HPV, which can cause cervical cancer.
- *Maternal serum screen:* This blood test is done at 16 to 18 weeks' gestation to screen for three or four biochemical markers in the maternal blood that indicate the baby's risk for Down syndrome, spina bifida, and trisomy 18. If the test is positive, the woman may decide to undergo amniocentesis to confirm the diagnosis.
- *Urine culture:* This culture is routinely done on the first prenatal visit to detect a urinary tract infection. Asymptomatic urinary tract infection may occur during pregnancy, and an untreated infection can lead to pyelonephritis (kidney infection) and preterm labor.

NORMAL VAGINAL DELIVERY

As mentioned, the birth of a term baby is a normal event that seldom requires intervention. The event is called a *normal spontaneous vaginal delivery (NSVD)*. The birth usually occurs in a labor room with the mother's friends or relatives present as support. In many locations, the mother can chose her position for birth, especially if she is not medicated and able to position herself. More often, she may have an **epidural** to relieve pain that may prolong the pushing phase of labor.

As the baby's head emerges, the tissues around the vagina and perineum stretch. The period for this stretching is longer if this is the mother's first vaginal birth, and lacerations of the vagina, perineum, or labia may result. If the fetal heart rate remains below 100 beats a minute and the baby's head is near but not immediately delivering, the physician or nurse-midwife may incise the perineum to provide a wider opening and hasten delivery. This is called an *episiotomy,* and it requires sutures following delivery. Once the baby is born, has been dried, and the umbilical cord has been cut, the physician or nurse-midwife inspects the perineum for lacerations or extension of the episiotomy.

The placenta usually is delivered within 20 minutes after birth and may be assisted by gentle cord traction, the administration of oxytocic drug, a maternal squatting position, or breast-feeding. After delivery of the placenta, the perineum is repaired. Lacerations or extensions of the episiotomy rarely go through the entire vaginal tissue to the rectal mucosa (fourth-degree laceration) or into the rectal sphincter (third-degree laceration). It is very common to repair a laceration that involves the muscles between the vagina and rectum (second-degree laceration) or a laceration of the vaginal mucosa (first-degree laceration). Lacerations along the side of the vagina occur less often. Repairs are done with 3-0 absorbable suture (polyglycolic acid or chromic on a tapered needle) except for rectal mucosal and labial repairs, which are done with 4-0 absorbable suture.

The scrub should have a basic vaginal set and general surgery instruments. Right-angle retractors (e.g., Heaney or Sims lateral retractors) should be included. A simple closure kit includes Allis and Kelly or Crile clamps. Curved Heaney and Metzenbaum scissors, needle holders, Adson forceps, or single-toothed tissue forceps may be used for skin and subcutaneous repairs.

IMMEDIATE POSTPARTUM CARE

Postpartum care includes monitoring the status of the mother and baby during this immediate transition. During the first 2 hours, the mother's blood pressure, pulse, and respirations are assessed every 15 minutes and her temperature is taken hourly. During this time, the nurse also checks her bleeding by giving firm uterine massage. A firm uterus means that the muscles of the uterus are tight, squeezing the small blood vessels that fed the placenta during pregnancy and thus minimizing bleeding. The mother may receive IV medication to increase uterine tone, which prevents postpartum bleeding.

If the mother received an epidural anesthetic, she is monitored for return of sensation and ability to mobilize. Full mobility and ability to urinate is expected within 1 hour after discontinuation of the anesthetic. As soon as she is able, she may eat and drink normally.

NEWBORN CARE

The baby usually is dried and stimulated immediately after birth. If all is normal, and the mother agrees, the baby can remain on her abdomen. The baby is assessed according to the American Pediatric Gross Assessment Record, commonly known as the **APGAR score.** This includes the following assessment parameters:

- Respiratory rate
- Color
- Reflex response
- Heart rate
- Body tone at 1 and 5 minutes after birth

A score of 2, 1, or 0 is given for each parameter. A score of 7 to 10 is considered normal; a score of 4 to 6 indicates mild to moderate depression; and a score of 0 to 3 indicates severe depression. It is important that the baby maintain a temperature of about 98.6° F (37° C). This can be done by drying the baby and providing a warm environment (e.g., a baby warmer or skin-to-skin contact with the mother or father while keeping the baby covered). Respirations, heart rate, and temperature are monitored every 15 minutes in the first hour or two. The baby is most alert in the first hour after birth and eager to suck. Breast-feeding during this time has many benefits, such as augmenting uterine contractions and facilitating bonding between mother and baby. The baby's weight and length can be obtained once the baby is warm and stable.

The immediate postpartum period is an important time for both mother and baby as they transition into a new phase of life. Each health care facility has a set of guidelines for care. The mother's and father's preferences also should be taken into consideration. Hospital personnel can provide a supportive, calm, and private environment to assist the family while gathering critical assessments of the status of mother and baby.

OBSTETRICAL PROCEDURES

CESAREAN DELIVERY

Surgical Goal

A cesarean section (commonly called a *C-section*) is the surgical removal of the fetus through the abdomen.

Pathology

A cesarean section is medically necessary when the mother's life is in jeopardy and for obstetrical conditions that would result in fetal death. Some of these conditions are:

- Transverse, breech, or other malpresentation of the fetus
- Prolapsed umbilical cord
- Ruptured placenta (placental abruption)
- Delivery of the placenta ahead of the fetus (placenta previa)
- Active genital herpes infection
- Previous cesarean section
- Cephalopelvic disproportion (CPD) (the fetus cannot be delivered through the pelvis because of its shape)
- Failure to progress
- Prolapsed cord
- Toxemia
- Diabetes

Technique

1. A low transverse or midline incision is made to the level of the rectus muscles.
2. The muscles are separated manually.
3. The peritoneum is elevated with two hemostats, and a small hole is made between the clamps.
4. The peritoneum is divided with scissors.
5. Large bleeders are clamped but not ligated or coagulated.
6. The peritoneal reflection of the bladder (bladder flap) is divided from the uterus with Metzenbaum scissors.
7. A bladder retractor is placed on the lower edge of the incision, and the bladder is displaced downward.
8. A small transverse incision is made in the uterus with the scalpel.
9. The scrub brings the suction without metal tip, bulb syringe, and bandage scissors near the wound.
10. The uterine incision is extended with the bandage scissors.
11. Amniotic fluid is quickly suctioned from the open uterus.
12. The assistant applies pressure to the upper abdomen while the surgeon rotates the baby's head into view.
13. The baby's nose and mouth are immediately suctioned with the bulb syringe or a separate suction catheter (e.g., DeLee suction catheter).
14. The baby is removed from the uterus.
15. The umbilical cord is double-clamped and cut with bandage scissors. One clamp is released slightly to fill two blood collection tubes.
16. The baby is handed over to the infant resuscitation team for care.
17. The placenta is delivered, and the remaining fluid and blood are suctioned from the wound.
18. The uterus is closed in layers.
19. The abdomen is closed in layers.

Discussion

A cesarean section can be scheduled, or it may be done as an emergency procedure. If the procedure is scheduled (e.g., a repeat C-section), a spinal or an epidural anesthetic is administered and a regular setup can be done.

An emergency delivery occurs very quickly. If a general anesthetic is given, time is extremely critical to prevent fetal anesthesia and to correct the condition that caused the emergency. In emergency surgery, several instruments are used to start the procedure and safely deliver the baby. In many cases, lack of time may prevent a normal setup.

As soon as the technologist has scrubbed and donned gown and gloves, the following items, which are adequate to deliver the baby, should be prepared:

1. Laparotomy drape
2. Scalpel
3. Lap sponges
4. Mayo clamps (four to six)
5. Metzenbaum scissors
6. Bladder retractor (DeLee or the bladder blade from a Balfour retractor)
7. Hemostats (e.g., Kelly or Crile clamps)
8. Bandage scissors
9. Suction tubing
10. Bulb syringe

When the patient is brought into the operating room, an infant warming unit and personnel from the nursery and pediatrician must be available to receive and care for the baby immediately after delivery. The patient is placed on the operating table in the supine position. A cushioned pad may be placed under the patient's right side for elevation to prevent aortocaval compression by the fetus. Such compression can cause hypotension of the mother due to decreased return blood flow to the heart, and this may cause fetal hypoxia.

The patient is prepped and draped quickly after administration of an anesthetic, or prepping and draping may be done before a general anesthetic is administered.

The surgeon enters the abdomen through a midline or Pfannenstiel incision. The incision is carried to the muscles, which are divided by hand. Bleeders are clamped but are not ligated or coagulated, to save time, unless the hemostats obstruct the surgeon's view or are in the way. Before entering the peritoneum, the surgeon elevates it with two Mayo clamps. The surgeon then makes a small incision between the clamps.

The peritoneal incision is lengthened with Metzenbaum or Mayo scissors. The peritoneal reflection of the bladder then must be separated from the uterus. This is done with Metzenbaum scissors and blunt dissection. When the bladder flap has been removed, a bladder retractor is placed over the lower edge of the incision and the bladder is retracted downward, away from the uterus.

Just before the uterus is entered, the scrub must bring the suction tubing (without a tip), bulb syringe, bandage scissors, and scalpel to the surgical field. The surgeon makes a small incision in the uterus and deepens it with the bandage scissors. The blunt tip of the bandage scissors prevents injury to the fetus.

The scrub must remove the scalpel from the field immediately to prevent injury to the baby or a team member.

As soon as the uterus is opened, the scrub places the tip of the suction tubing at the edge of the incision to aspirate amniotic fluid. The assistant applies pressure to the upper abdomen while the surgeon grasps the baby's head and delivers it from the uterus. The bulb syringe is used immediately to suction the baby's nose and mouth. If a second suction is available, a flexible suction catheter is used to clear the baby's airway.

Extra laparotomy sponges should be available. The surgeon delivers the baby from the uterus and places the infant on the mother's abdomen. The surgeon clamps the umbilical cord with two Mayo clamps and severs it with bandage scissors. The scrub must have two blood specimen containers in hand to receive cord blood. The surgeon releases one of the Mayo clamps slightly to fill the containers. The scrub caps these and passes them to the circulator.

The baby is handed to the resuscitation team and placed in the warming unit. The baby is again suctioned and dried, oxygen is administered as needed, and the baby is assessed. The infant then may be taken to the nursery or ICU.

As the baby is handed over to the resuscitation team, attention again must be directed to the mother. The scrub places a large basin on the field to receive the placenta, which is delivered from the uterus.

The surgeon grasps the edges of the uterus with sponge forceps, Duval lung clamps, or Collin tongue clamps. These are atraumatic clamps that prevent maceration of the uterine incision during closure.

A count is required before the uterus is closed.

The uterine incision is closed with a two-layer size 0 running absorbable suture. The surgeon then may attend to any bleeders, which are coagulated with the ESU or ligated with suture ties. When the wound is clean and dry, the remaining layers are closed.

The bladder flap is closed with a running suture of 2-0 or 3-0 absorbable suture on a taper needle. The remaining layers are closed in routine fashion, and the wound is dressed with sterile dressings. A cesarean section is shown in Figure 24-24.

SURGICAL TREATMENT OF AN ECTOPIC PREGNANCY

Surgical Goal
In an **ectopic pregnancy**, the fertilized egg implants outside the uterus. The fallopian tube is a common site of ectopic implantation. Tubal rupture requires emergency surgery to control hemorrhage. The surgical goal is to control bleeding and remove the embryo. A laparoscopic or an open approach may be used, depending on the patient's condition and the surgeon's choice.

Pathology
Ectopic pregnancy occurs most often in the fallopian tube (tubal pregnancy). Risk factors include a previous history of PID, smoking (reduces tubal motility), previous tubal surgery, and a history of STD infection. Tubal rupture, hemorrhage, and hypovolemic shock can be rapidly fatal. Early tubal pregnancy may be treated with methotrexate, which causes embryonic death. As mentioned, the surgery may be performed laparoscopically or through open surgery. An open approach is discussed in the next section, although techniques are similar for both types of surgery.

Discussion
Two approaches may be utilized in the surgical treatment of an ectopic pregnancy: salpingectomy (complete removal of the affected fallopian tube) and salpingostomy (removal of the tubal contents with preservation of the tube).

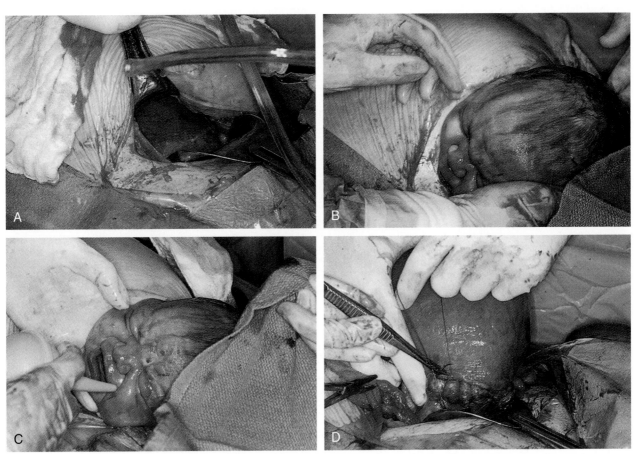

Figure 24-24 Cesarean section. **A,** The uterus is entered through a transverse incision. **B,** The fetal head is brought through the incision. **C,** Suction is used to clear the airways. **D,** Heavy sutures are used to close the uterus. (*From Murray SS, McKinney ES: Foundations of maternal–newborn nursing, ed 4, Philadelphia, 2006, WB Saunders.*)

The patient is placed in the supine position, prepped, and draped for a laparotomy. A Pfannenstiel incision is used to open the pelvic cavity. If the ectopic pregnancy has already ruptured, the scrub must be prepared for surgical hemorrhaging. The scrub should have suction and irrigation immediately available. Clots are removed manually, and the source of the bleeding is identified as quickly as possible. A basin should be placed on the field to receive the blood clots. A self-retaining retractor may or may not be inserted during this stage of the procedure. When the bleeding has been controlled, the embryo (or tube and embryo) can be removed. In all approaches, the scrub should have an ample supply of Mayo and Crile clamps available. Suture ligatures of fine absorbable synthetic material or surgical staples may also be required soon after the start of the procedure.

Salpingectomy

To control the bleeding, the surgeon may cross-clamp the fallopian tube and mesosalpinx with Mayo or Crile clamps. The tube then is resected with the HF bipolar ESU. Suture ligatures may also be used. (In laparoscopic surgery, Harmonic shears, staples, or pretied ligatures are used.)

Salpingostomy

Tube-preserving surgery requires incision of the tube and removal of the embryo, with irrigation and suction. Reconstruction of the tube is done at the time of surgery or deferred until a later date. The tube is grasped with Babcock forceps, and a small incision is made with a scalpel, needle electrode, or ultrasonic scalpel. The embryo is removed using irrigation and fine forceps. The ESU is used sparingly to prevent scarring. The tube is irrigated and may be left to heal by secondary intention.

The surgery is complete after the wound has been irrigated and carefully examined for any bleeding. The wound is then closed in layers. The skin is closed with staples or a subcuticular suture and Steri-Strips (Figure 24-25).

SURGICAL TREATMENT OF CERVICAL INSUFFICIENCY

Surgical Goal

Recurrent spontaneous abortion occurs when the cervix dilates spontaneously during the second or third trimester. Surgical intervention to prevent spontaneous abortion may be performed before or during pregnancy. In transabdominal **cerclage** (TAC) and transvaginal cerclage (TVC), a synthetic band or sutures may be placed around the cervix to prevent dilation.

Pathology

The cause of **incompetent cervix** has not been identified. It may be associated with cervical trauma, including conization of the cervix, laceration, and previous cerclage. *Cerclage remains controversial, because the data are insufficient data to prove that the procedure is effective.* The American College of Obstetricians and Gynecologists (ACOG) recommends cerclage only for patients with a history of three or four previous unexplained spontaneous abortions. ACOG further states that the procedure should be limited to pregnancies in which fetal viability has been achieved. *This is because of the fetal morbidity and fetal mortality associated with the procedures.*[2]

Traditional treatment for early spontaneous abortion historically led to the development of various types of cerclage.

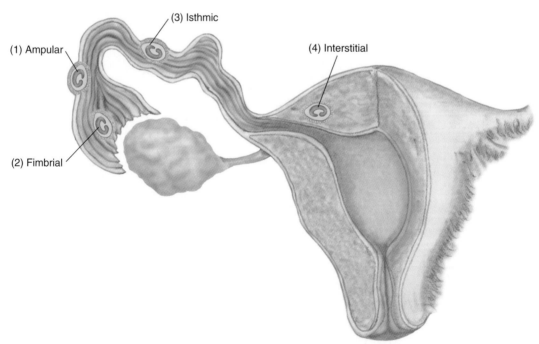

Figure 24-25 Ectopic pregnancy. *(From Murray SS, McKinney ES: Foundations of maternal–newborn nursing, ed 4, Philadelphia, 2006, WB Saunders.)*

The Shirodkar and McDonald procedures are just two of many types of cerclage in which a suture was placed around or through the cervix. These procedures have been modified many times over the decades, and cerclage is now identified by terms that are more exact. The proper terms are transabdominal, high transvaginal, or low transvaginal cerclage. The procedures are seldom performed because of the risks stated previously.

In TVC, a synthetic band is placed around the proximal cervix through a vaginal approach. In TAC, sutures are placed at the internal cervical os, which is approached through an abdominal incision. Delivery by cesarean section is required after TAC.

TVC is performed through a short suprapubic incision. The ureterovesical fold is incised and retracted, and a tunnel is made through the paracervical tissue. Several sutures of heavy Mersilene are then placed at the internal cervical os. The ureterovesical fold is closed with a running suture of size 0 or 2-0 absorbent synthetic suture, and the pelvic incision is closed in layers.

TAC is performed with the patient in the lithotomy position. The cervix is retracted with sponge forceps, and a circumferential incision is made at the highest (proximal) point of the cervix. A narrow strip of Mersilene tape is then placed around the cervix, and the paracervical tissue is closed with interrupted 2-0 or 3-0 synthetic absorbable sutures.

CHAPTER SUMMARY

- The uterus and associated organs of the female reproductive system are located in the anterior female pelvic cavity.
- The uterus is roughly pear shaped, approximately 3 inches (7.5 cm) long, and 2 inches (5 cm) deep. It houses and protects the fetus during pregnancy. It is composed of thick muscular tissue and is suspended in the pelvic cavity by ligaments that completely enclose the organ.
- The cervix is the lower neck of the uterus. It extends into the vaginal vault. The opening of the cervix is called the *cervical os.* The os is dilated for transcervical procedures, or it may dilate naturally under the influence of hormones during childbirth.
- The two fallopian tubes are attached directly to the uterus, one on each side. Each fallopian tube has four sections: the *interstitial section,* which connects to the uterus; the narrow *isthmus* in the midportion; the *ampulla,* which is the widened portion of the tube; and the *infundibulum,* the terminal end of the tube.
- The ovary is the female gonad, or sex gland. The two ovaries secrete the female hormones. They lie on each side of the uterus in the upper portion of the pelvic cavity.
- Ova are contained within hormone-secreting follicles and develop in stages until they are released from the ovary. A complete cycle is called the *ovarian cycle.*
- The vagina, or vaginal vault, is a muscular passageway that shares a thick fibrous wall with the rectum on the posterior side and the bladder on the anterior side. The vagina extends from the vestibule, or introitus (opening to the outside of the body), to the uterine cervix, which protrudes at the upper vagina.
- The structures that together make up the external genitalia are called the *vulva.*
- The mons pubis is a raised mound of tissue that protects the symphysis pubis from injury.
- The labia majora are two external folds of adipose tissue that envelope the perineal area. They are extensions of the anterior mons pubis, which encircle the vestibule and protect the external genitalia.
- The labia minora are bisectional (composed of two sections) and lie directly beneath the labia majora.
- The clitoris is a highly vascular organ that contains sensitive erectile tissue. It projects slightly from the anterior folds of the labia minora.
- The term *vestibule* refers collectively to all the structures located within the labia minora. The vestibular glands collectively include the Skene glands (paraurethral glands) and the Bartholin glands.
- The perineum is located between the posterior wall of the vagina and the anus. Incision into the perineum exposes the strong connective tissue and muscles of the pelvic floor.
- The ovarian cycle is characterized by hormonal and physical changes that occur regularly from the onset of menarche (menstrual periods) to menopause (cessation of natural childbearing). The cycle is controlled by a complex feedback system involving hormones of the pituitary, hypothalamus, and ovaries.
- The follicular phase extends from day 1 to day 14 of the ovarian cycle. The ovulatory phase begins approximately 14 days from the start of the cycle and lasts from 16 to 32 hours. The luteal phase lasts for about 12 days. The ovum is released during the ovulatory phase.
- Squamous cell carcinoma is the most common type of vulvar cancer. High-risk strains of the human papilloma virus (HPV) are associated with an increased risk of vulvar cancer.
- Endometriosis is a condition in which endometrial tissue develops anywhere outside the uterus, most often on the abdominal viscera. Surgery may be necessary to remove the tissue.
- Menorrhagia is excessive menstrual bleeding, which may be treated with endometrial ablation.
- A leiomyoma is a benign neoplasm of uterine muscle that is surgically removed when it causes uterine bleeding, pain, and impingement on other structures.
- Herniation of the rectum (rectocele) or bladder (cystocele) into the vaginal wall occurs when weakness of the uterosacral ligaments allows the intestine to bulge

into the vaginal vault. A surgical procedure called *anterior and posterior repair* is performed to correct the condition. In this procedure, herniated vaginal tissue is reduced and the vaginal wall is reconstructed.

- Implantation of the embryo outside the intrauterine cavity (ectopic pregnancy) is an emergency that requires surgical intervention to prevent rupture and hemorrhage.

- The Papanicolaou (Pap) test is used to screen for cervical cancer. For this test, superficial endocervical (epithelial) cells are collected from the internal cervical os.

- Epithelial carcinoma of the cervix and severe dysplasia (abnormal cells) are treated with cone biopsy, which involves removal of a circumferential core of tissue around the cervical canal.

- During hysteroscopy, a semirigid or rigid hysteroscope is used to examine the interior of the uterus and to perform selected operative procedures. The uterus is filled with a clear fluid to increase visibility.

- Psychosocial considerations for obstetrical and gynecological patients include reproductive ability and social, cultural, family, and community expectations.

- Gynecological procedures are performed with the patient in the supine or lithotomy position. Skin prepping usually includes both abdominal and vaginal prep, with insertion of a Foley catheter. A uterine manipulator (retractor) is inserted after the vaginal prep for selected laparoscopic procedures.

- Many gynecological surgical procedures are now routinely performed laparoscopically for conditions that previously required laparotomy.

- Tubal ligation is performed to block the passage of ova through the tube and prevent implantation in the uterus. Tube-sparing techniques may be performed to facilitate reversal.

- Laparoscopic management of ovarian cysts depends on the size and type of the cysts and the risk of malignancy. Spillage of a potentially malignant cyst is always avoided to prevent seeding. A large cyst can be removed through a specimen retrieval bag and 10-mm trocar port.

- Obstruction of the fallopian tube frequency occurs as a result of infection, which spreads from the lower genital tract to the uterus, fallopian tubes, and ovaries. According to the Centers for Disease Control and Prevention, approximately 1 million women a year in the United States develop a pelvic inflammatory disease as a result of genital tract infections. Of these, 100,000 women become infertile, and 150 die.

- Microscopic surgery to restore patency (an unobstructed passageway) to the fallopian tube is performed with the aid of the operating microscope. The procedure is frequently done laparoscopically.

- LAVH involves the removal of the uterus by a combined laparoscopic and vaginal approach. It is the technique most often used for a hysterectomy. This procedure requires two setups, one for the laparoscopic portion and one for the vaginal approach.

- TAH is the surgical removal of the uterus and cervix.

- A radical hysterectomy involves the dissection and wide removal of the uterus, tubes, ovaries, supporting ligaments, and upper vagina, as well as the pelvic lymph node chains.

- Pelvic exenteration is performed to treat metastatic cancer. It includes complete removal of the rectum, the distal sigmoid colon, the urinary bladder and distal ureters, and the internal iliac vessels and their lateral branches. All pelvic reproductive organs and lymph nodes and the entire pelvic floor pelvic peritoneum, levator muscles, and perineum are removed.

- During hysteroscopy, a fiberoptic hysteroscope is inserted through the cervix into the uterus. This technique is used to examine the uterine cavity endocervix and lower uterine segment and for selected operative procedures.

- To allow a clear view of the uterine wall during hysteroscopy, the uterine cavity is distended with fluid. This allows small blood clots and other tissue debris to be removed.

- Uterine distention poses a risk of extravasation (the absorption of hypotonic fluid through the open vessels of the uterus) during hysteroscopy. This can lead to a low serum sodium level and death.

- The scrubbed surgical technologist and the circulating team are jointly responsible for tracking the amount of fluid used and the rate of flow of uterine fluid during hysteroscopy.

- The use of monopolar electrosurgery during hysteroscopy requires the use of a hypotonic nonelectrolytic distention fluid. This is because current must flow directly from the point of contact (the active electrode) to the inactive electrode (patient "grounding pad") and back to the ESU control unit.

- Global endometrial ablation is performed "blind" (i.e., without the aid of a hysteroscope).

- The uterine resectoscope may be used to remove a benign smooth muscle tumor. The resectoscope shaves off small pieces of the tumor, which are flushed from the uterine cavity.

- During colposcopy, the cervix is examined microscopically. Acetic acid is applied to the tissue to identify tissue abnormalities.

- Endometrial ablation is the destruction of the endometrium. The goal of the procedure is destruction and scarification of the endometrium, which becomes nonfunctional.

- Three common techniques used in uterine ablation are roller ball ablation (electrocoagulation) and global (reaching all areas of the endometrium) endometrial ablation with an intrauterine device. Cryoablation and radiofrequency ablation are also available.

- Myomectomy is the removal of a benign tumor (fibroid) of the myometrium to control bleeding and prevent pressure on other structures in the pelvis. Submucosal myomas can be removed with the resectoscope.
- A loop electrode excision procedure is an electrosurgical technique that removes a core of tissue from the endocervix to remove cancerous or precancerous tissue.
- In dilation and curettage, the surface of the endometrium is removed with sharp and smooth curettes through a transvaginal approach.
- Termination of a pregnancy may be advised for medical reasons, or a woman may undergo elective abortion according to the restrictions of gestational age and the age of the mother, which vary according to state law.
- During a vaginal hysterectomy, the uterus is removed through a transvaginal approach.
- A congenital abnormality of the mullerian ducts during fetal development can result in the absence of the vagina or uterus, a condition referred to as *mullerian agenesis.*
- During vaginoplasty, a functional vagina is constructed using a skin or peritoneal graft.
- A rectovaginal fistula is a tract between the rectum and the vagina. Surgical repair closes the defect to prevent fecal material from draining into the vagina.
- The Bartholin glands are a common site of cyst formation. The cyst may become infected, and in such cases, surgical removal is indicated. The gland and the cyst may be removed together, or the cyst may be dissected away from the gland with dissecting scissors.
- Birth is a physiological process that seldom requires interventions for the healthy mother. Mother and baby are linked during pregnancy as the mother's body accommodates the growing baby.
- The placenta is a thick organ that adheres to the uterus on the maternal side. The fetal side contains large vessels that are contained within the structure's smooth membranes. The umbilical cord, which attaches to the placenta, contains the umbilical artery and vein and communicates directly with the fetal circulation.
- Development of the embryo and fetus occurs when the ovum is fertilized by sperm; this normally occurs in the fallopian tube. The combination of chromosomal material from the ovum and the sperm completes the fertilization process.
- The fetal membranes surround the growing fetus and are filled with amniotic fluid. The two membranes, the chorion and the amnion, are very close together.
- The average normal gestation occurs over 40 weeks and is marked by predictable growth patterns that can be measured by ultrasound.
- Placental abruption is premature separation of the placenta from the uterine wall after 20 weeks' gestation and before the fetus is delivered.
- Placenta previa occurs when the placenta implants completely or partly over the cervical os. In this position, the placenta begins to bleed as it separates from the cervix during labor.
- Pregnancy-induced hypertension (PIH) is diagnosed as high blood pressure that occurs only during pregnancy after 20 weeks' gestation.
- Hypertension can constrict blood flow to the placenta and baby, resulting in a small baby and placenta.
- An umbilical cord wrapped one or more times around the baby's neck is called a *nuchal cord.*
- When the cord precedes the fetal head, this is called *cord prolapse.* When the cord precedes the baby in the birth canal, it can be compressed by the baby's head as it presses against the cervix and maternal pelvis.
- Cord prolapse requires an emergency cesarean section. In case of a pending emergency, the operating room staff is notified and a setup is prepared. However, there may be little time between the diagnosis of cord prolapse and the start of surgery.
- When the baby's feet, knees, or buttocks enter the birth canal before the head, this is called a breech presentation. If attempts to change the baby's position fail, a cesarean section is scheduled.
- The birth of a term baby is a normal event that seldom requires intervention. The event is called a *normal spontaneous vaginal delivery.*
- An episiotomy is an incision made in the perineum during the last stage of delivery to provide a wider opening for the baby.
- The placenta usually is delivered within 20 minutes after birth. Its delivery may be assisted by gentle cord traction, medication in the intravenous line, maternal squatting position, and breast-feeding.
- Immediately after delivery, the baby is stimulated and dried. An APGAR score (respiratory rate, color, reflexes, heart rate, and body tone) is used to assess the baby.
- A cesarean section is the surgical removal of the fetus through the abdomen.
- A cesarean section is medically necessary when the mother's life is in jeopardy and for obstetrical conditions that would result in fetal death.
- A cesarean section may be planned, or it may be performed as an emergency. In emergencies, there often is little time between notification of the surgical staff and the start of surgery.
- An ectopic pregnancy is the implantation of the fertilized egg outside the uterus. The fallopian tube is a common site of ectopic implantation. Tubal rupture requires emergency surgery to control hemorrhage.
- Ectopic pregnancy occurs most often in the fallopian tube (tubal pregnancy). Risk factors include a previous history of pelvic inflammatory disease, smoking (decreases tubal motility), previous tubal surgery, and a history of sexually transmitted disease.
- In transabdominal cerclage and transvaginal cerclage, a synthetic band or sutures may be placed around the cervix to prevent dilation.

REVIEW QUESTIONS

1. What is the rationale for performing the perineal prep ahead of the abdominal prep in combined access procedures?

2. Discuss uterine distention solutions used for high-frequency bipolar surgery and monopolar surgery. What is the rationale for using nonelectrolytic versus electrolytic solutions in each case?

3. Why does uterine distention fluid have to be closely monitored during hysteroscopy?

4. List the risks of the lithotomy position and the precautions needed to prevent injury.

5. Review the imaging system components for laparoscopy found in Chapter 21. List the components and their basic use.

6. What is the risk of allowing an ovarian cyst to rupture into the pelvic cavity during surgery?

7. Babcock clamps usually are required for any surgery of the fallopian tubes. Why wouldn't a Kocher clamp be used instead?

8. During laparoscopy and removal of tissue, such as a morcellized tumor or an ovarian cyst, a specimen retrieval bag is used to remove the specimen from the abdomen. What size trocar is needed when a specimen retrieval bag is used?

9. Radical abdominal and pelvic procedures, such as pelvic exenteration and the Whipple procedure, are performed much less often now than they were a few years ago. What do you think are the reasons for this?

10. Consider a situation in which you are called to scrub for an emergency cesarean section. What is the minimum instrumentation and equipment you should have ready when the mother is brought into the operating room? Assume that your instrument tray is open and the Mayo stand is draped, but you have no instruments on the Mayo stand. The surgeon is ready to start; you have approximately 3 minutes to prepare for abdominal entry and removal of the baby.

REFERENCE

1. Centers for Disease Control and Prevention: Sexually Transmitted Diseases Surveillance, 2007 Chlamydia. Accessed January 16, 2009 at http://www.cdc.gov/std/stats07/chlamydia.htm

2. Ressel G: Practice guidelines: ACOG releases bulletin on managing cervical insufficiency. *Am Fam Physician* 69(2):436–439, 2004. Accessed Jan 16, 2009 at www.aafp.org/afp/20040115/practice.html

BIBLIOGRAPHY

Baggish MS, Barbot J, Valle RF: *Diagnostic and operative hysteroscopy: a text and atlas,* ed 2, St Louis, 1999, Mosby.

Economou SG, Economou TS: *Atlas of surgical technique,* ed 2, Philadelphia, 1996, WB Saunders.

Falcone T, Hurd W: *Clinical reproductive medicine and surgery,* Philadelphia, 2007, Mosby.

Gershenson DM, DeCherney AH, Curry SL, Brubaker LC: *Operative gynecology,* ed 2, Philadelphia, 2001, WB Saunders.

Goldberg JM, Falcone T: *Atlas of endoscopic techniques in gynecology,* Philadelphia, 2001, WB Saunders.

Greibel C, Halvorsen J, Golemon T, Day A: Management of spontaneous abortion, *AmFam Physician* 72(7):1243–1250, 2005. Accessed January 16, 2009 at http://www.aafp.org/afp/2005100/1243.html.

Hunt RB: *Text and atlas of female infertility surgery,* ed 3, St Louis, 1999, Mosby.

Moody FG: *Atlas of ambulatory surgery,* St Louis, 1999, Mosby.

Murray SS, McKinney ES, Gorrie TM: *Foundations of maternal–newborn nursing,* ed 3, Philadelphia, 2002, WB Saunders.

Porth CM: *Pathophysiology: concepts of altered health states,* ed 7, Philadelphia, 2004, Lippincott Williams & Williams.

Raz S: *Atlas of transvaginal surgery,* ed 2, Philadelphia, 2002, WB Saunders.

Genitourinary Surgery

CHAPTER OUTLINE

LEARNING OBJECTIVES

After studying this chapter the reader will be able to:
- Describe the functional anatomy of the genitourinary system
- Identify and describe common genitourinary procedures
- Describe common pathological conditions of the genitourinary system

- Distinguish between transurethral, endoscopic, and open genitourinary procedures
- Identify essential genitourinary instruments
- Describe the role of the surgical technologist in transurethral surgery

TERMINOLOGY

Arteriovenous fistula (or shunt [AV shunt]): Surgical creation of vascular access for patients undergoing hemodialysis.

Benign prostatic hyperplasia (BPH): Nonmalignant enlargement of the prostate gland, which occurs mainly in men over age 40.

Calculi: Stones caused by the precipitation of minerals, such as calcium, and other substances from the urine or kidney filtrate.

Circumcision: Removal of all or part of the prepuce (foreskin) of the penis.

Cystoscope: A fiberoptic instrument used to assess the lower genitourinary tract and in transurethral surgery. Also called a *cystourethroscope.*

Cystoscopy assistant: A trained surgical technologist or nurse whose primary specialty is transurethral surgery. The cystoscopy assistant functions in circulating and scrub roles.

Enucleation: The removal of tissue or an organ without previous fragmentation or dissection.

Epispadias: A rare congenital abnormality in which the opening of the urethra is on the dorsum of the penis. This anomaly does not usually occur in isolation but is part of a more complex set of defects of the urogenital system.

Extracorporeal shockwave lithotripsy (ESWL): A procedure in which ultrasonic sound waves are used to pulverize kidney or gallbladder stones.

Extravasation: The absorption of irrigation fluids into the vascular system, which causes fluid overload and can result in cardiac arrest.

Foley catheter: A retention catheter with an expandable balloon at the distal end.

Glomerular filtration rate (GFR): An indication of kidney function in which serum creatinum (normally filtered by the kidney) is measured.

Hematuria: Blood in the urine.

Hydronephrosis: Distension of the renal pelvis and proximal ureter caused by an obstruction in the ureter and reflux of kidney filtrate.

Hypospadias: A congenital abnormality in which the urethra opens inferior to its normal location. It is normally seen in males, when the urethra opens on the undersurface of the penis.

Hypothermia: An abnormally low core body temperature.

Indwelling catheter: A urethral or ureteral catheter that is left in place.

Lithotripsy: A procedure in which stones are crushed within a body cavity, such as the bladder.

Meatotomy: A procedure in which a small incision is made in the urethral meatus to relieve a stricture. A topical anesthetic is used.

Micturition: Urination.

Nonelectrolytic: Nonconductive; nonelectrolytic solutions must be used for bladder distension or continuous irrigation whenever the electrosurgical unit (ESU) is used.

Percutaneous: A term for a procedure that is performed "through the skin." For example, in percutaneous nephroscopy, the nephroscope is inserted into the kidney through a skin incision.

Pyeloplasty: Reconstruction of the ureter in the renal pelvis. This procedure usually is performed to repair a distended ureter caused by a ureteral obstruction and backward flow of urine.

Reflux: Backward (opposite of its normal direction) flow of a body fluid. Urinary reflux is backward flow of urine into the ureter or kidney.

Resectoscope: A cutting instrument used to remove and coagulate tissue piece by piece. It is used in conjunction with endoscopic procedures to remove tumors or other tissue, such as the prostate or endometrium.

Retrograde pyelography: Imaging studies of the renal pelvis in which a contrast medium is instilled through a transurethral catheter. *Retrograde* refers to flow, which is opposite (or backwards from) the normal direction.

Specific gravity: The ratio of the density of a fluid compared to water. The specific gravity of urine is an important diagnostic tool.

Staghorn stone: A large, jagged kidney stone that forms in the renal pelvis.

Stent: A supportive catheter that is placed in a duct or tube to allow fluids to pass through while the duct heals.

Straight catheter: A urinary catheter used for one-time drainage of the bladder. It may be called a "red Robinson" or simply a "Robinson" catheter.

Suprapubic catheter: A bladder catheter inserted through the skin in the suprapubic area of the abdomen.

Tamponade: An instrument or other device that puts pressure on tissue, usually to stop bleeding.

Torsion: Twisting of an organ or a structure on itself. Torsion may cause local ischemia and necrosis.

Transurethral: Surgical access through the urethral orifice. The term also may describe an instrument that enters the bladder through the urethral meatus.

Urethrotomy: A small incision made in the urethra to reduce scarring or relieve a stricture.

INTRODUCTION

Genitourinary (GU) surgery includes procedures of the urethra, bladder, ureters, and kidneys. It also includes surgery of the male reproductive system (i.e., the testicles, penis, and accessory structures). Three common approaches are used in GU surgery:

- **Transurethral surgery:** Surgery is performed through a flexible or rigid fiberoptic endoscope inserted through the external urethra. This provides direct visualization and access to the lower urinary tract, including the urethra, bladder, prostate gland, and ureters.
- *Open surgery:* Surgery that is performed through an open incision in the abdomen (including the retroperitoneum) or flank. Many procedures that were performed with the open technique can now be done using minimally invasive surgery.
- *Minimally invasive surgery:* Closed procedures that are performed using **percutaneous** (through the skin) endoscopic techniques, such as laparotomy and nephrotomy.

NOTE: GU procedures performed exclusively on newborns or infants are described in Chapter 34.

SURGICAL ANATOMY

RETROPERITONEAL CAVITY

The *retroperitoneal cavity* (also referred to as the retroperitoneal *space*) lies posterior to (behind) the peritoneal cavity. Unlike the viscera of the abdominal cavity, the organs in this space are embedded in dense muscle, fascia, and fatty tissue. This arrangement supports the structures and protects them from injury. The retroperitoneal space is covered on the anterior side by the *retroperitoneum*, a serous (fluid producing) membrane. Surgical access to the organs in the retroperitoneum is gained through the abdominal peritoneum, the flank, or the back.

KIDNEY

The kidneys are the primary organs for filtration of the blood. Two kidneys normally are located in the retroperitoneal cavity at the level of the twelfth thoracic vertebra (Figure 25-1). The right kidney usually sits lower than the left. The kidneys are supported by dense fascia and fatty tissue.

Two main tissue layers make up the kidney: the outer layer, the *cortex*, and the inner layer, the *medulla*. The cortex is covered with strong fibrous tissue and contains portions of the microscopic tubules that filter the blood. The medulla is composed of eight to 12 large collecting areas called the *renal pyramids*.

A notched area on the medial side of each kidney is called the *hilum*. The ureter, renal artery, and vein emerge from this area. At this point the ureter opens into the *renal pelvis* of the kidney, which branches into sections called *renal calyces* (Figure 25-2).

Nephron

Although the kidney appears as a dense, continuous tissue, the microscopic structure is extremely complex. Each kidney has about 1 million filtering units, called *nephrons*. Each nephron communicates directly with the vascular system through a capillary structure called the *glomerulus*. The glomerulus is composed of a vast system of microscopic tubules that communicate directly with the capillaries to filter the blood. The capillary network of each nephron is contained within a space called the *Bowman capsule* (Figure 25-3).

Blood flows into the capillary network through the efferent arteriole of the glomerulus. As the blood circulates through the microscopic capillaries, fluid (glomerular filtrate) moves selectively into the Bowman capsule. Proteins and cells remain in the blood, but other substances cross the arterial membrane and enter the capsule. The filtrate then moves into the nephron tubules. The glomerulus can filter about 125 mL per minute. This is referred to as the *glomerular filtration rate (GFR)*.

Filtrate is continually refined as it moves through the tubules. Each renal tubule has a parallel capillary. Substances are selectively moved from the blood into the tubules (a process called *secretion*) and from the tubules into the blood (called *absorption*) according to osmolality (solutes contained in the fluid) and membrane permeability. This is why diseases of the circulatory system, such as hypertension or arteriosclerosis, can affect the kidneys and damage this delicate transport system.

As filtrate moves through the tubules, electrolytes, nonorganic salts, and water, which the body needs to maintain homeostasis, are absorbed from the filtrate back into the circulatory system. The tubule system is divided into specific regions, which filter certain substances. These regions are

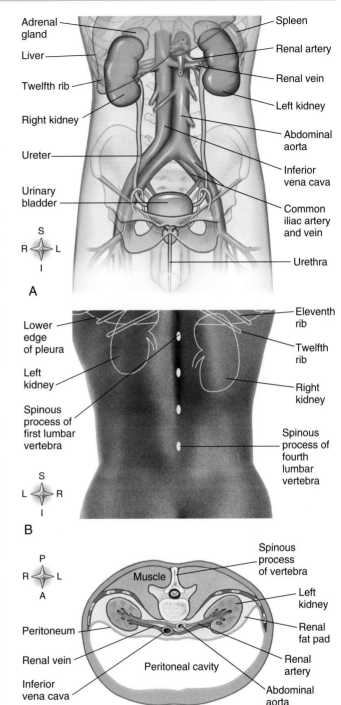

Figure 25-1 The kidneys, ureters, and associated blood vessels lie in the retroperitoneal cavity. *(From Abrahams P, Hutchings RT, Marks SC: McKinn's color atlas of human anatomy, ed 4, St. Louis, 1999, Mosby.)*

called the *proximal tubule*, the *loop of Henle*, and the *distal convoluted tubule*.

Note that some diuretics are called "potassium-sparing" drugs. This type of diuretic prevents excessive loss of potassium across the capillary membrane, which is an undesirable side effect of many diuretics.

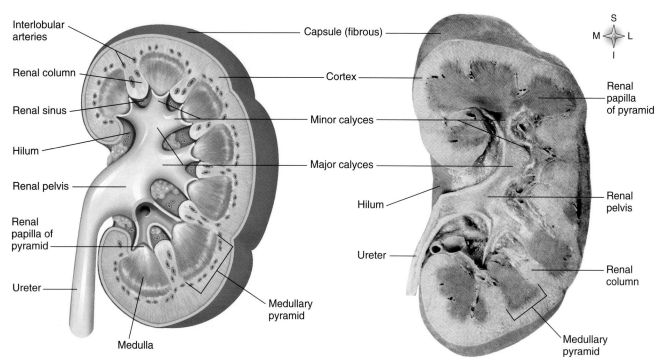

Figure 25-2 The kidney, showing the layers, pyramids and collecting tubules, and ureter. *(From Brundage DJ:* Renal disorders, *St Louis, 1992, Mosby.)*

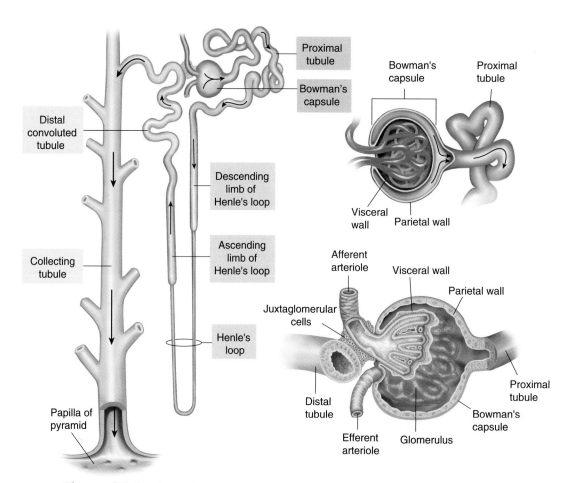

Figure 25-3 The nephron and Bowman capsule. *(From Brundage DJ:* Renal disorders, *St. Louis, 1992, Mosby.)*

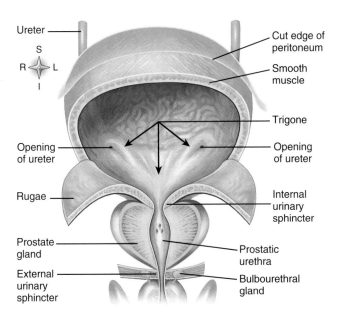

Figure 25-4 Urine formation. *(From Thibodeau G, Patton K: Anatomy and physiology, ed 6, St Louis, 2007, Mosby.)*

From the renal tubules, the filtrate enters the *renal calyces* (sing., calyx) and renal pelvis, which communicates directly with the *ureters*. The ureters are the collecting and transport areas for filtrate. Each ureter carries filtrate into the bladder. Once it enters the bladder, the filtrate is referred to as *urine*. Urine is, excreted from the body through the *urethra*. Filtrate and urine are sterile throughout the length of the system; they become *potentially* contaminated by the environment in the periurethral areas such as the distal urethral orifice (Figure 25-4).

Kidney Stones

Kidney stones (**calculi**) are formed by the precipitation of specific salts from the filtrate which becomes supersaturated. Stones can become lodged in the kidney itself or can migrate into the ureters. Stones rarely form in the bladder. The crystalline structure of stones is jagged and sharp, and they cause nearly unbearable pain and nausea in the patient. Most small stones pass through the urinary tract without treatment. However, stones in the upper urinary tract can cause obstruction and anuria (decreased or no urinary output), kidney abscess, and sepsis. Renal calculi can therefore be considered a medical emergency.

Kidney stones may be seen in many different diseases, including hyperparathyroidism, increased absorption of calcium in the intestine, chronic urinary tract infection, high protein intake, and the use of some drugs. Specific stone types are associated with each condition.

Calculi may be removed surgically or reduced with **extracorporeal shock wave lithotripsy (ESWL)**. A specific patient criterion for ESWL is individuals for whom spontaneous passage of a stone might present a danger to themselves or others (e.g., pilots and physicians); also, only specific types of stones are suitable for this type of treatment.

ADRENAL GLANDS

The *adrenal glands* are paired organs that lie on the medial side of the upper kidney. The gland has two layers: the outer cortex and the inner medulla. The adrenal glands secrete corticosteroids and hormones necessary for metabolism. Blood is supplied to each gland by the aorta and branches of the renal and inferior phrenic arteries. The adrenal glands are important in the production of norepinephrine and epinephrine, which are necessary for functions of the autonomic nervous system.

URETERS

In adults, each ureter is about 12 inches (30 cm) long and about 5 mm in diameter. The ureter is a three-layered tubular structure; it has an outer fibrous layer, a middle muscular layer, and an inner mucosal layer. Urine moves along the ureter by *peristalsis*, which is the segmental contraction and relaxation of the ureter's muscular layer.

Each ureter enters the bladder at the *ureterovesical junction*, which is located in the lower bladder.

BLADDER

The urinary bladder lies behind the symphysis pubis in the pelvic cavity. The wall of the bladder is composed of four tissue layers: the outer serosa, the muscular layer, the submucosa, and the inner mucosa. The distal portion of the bladder is called the *trigone*. This triangular region has both superficial and deep muscle layers. The superficial layer extends into the bladder neck of the female and into the proximal portion of the urethra in the male. The trigone has three corners that correspond with the two ureteral openings and one urethral opening (Figure 25-5).

Urine is excreted from the bladder by the process of **micturition** (urination), which is activated by sphincter muscles in the bladder neck. These muscles are controlled by the autonomic nervous system, which maintains retention or release of urine.

URETHRA

Female

The *urethra* communicates with the lower bladder to enable excretion of urine from the body. In the female, it leaves the bladder at the trigone and is embedded in the levator muscles of the pelvic floor. The urethral opening, the *meatus*, is located on the midline of the labia near the clitoris. The proximal urethra is composed primarily of smooth muscle tissue. The periurethral muscles on the pelvic floor support the distal urethra and aid in sphincter control. Two small, mucoussecreting glands (the *Skene's glands*) are located on each side of the urethra just inside the meatus.

Male

The male urethra exits the bladder and continues to the end of the penis, terminating at the urethral meatus. The male

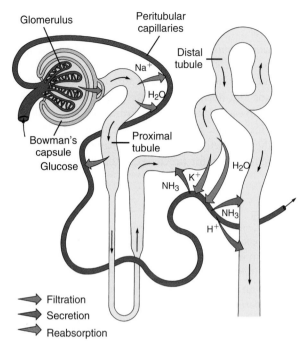

Filtration
Secretion
Reabsorption

Figure 25-5 The bladder and lower urinary tract in the male. *(From Thibodeau G, Patton K: Anatomy and physiology, ed 6, St Louis, 2007, Mosby.)*

urethra is divided into several distinct parts. The *prostatic urethra* begins at the bladder neck and passes through the center of the prostate gland, which surrounds the urethra distal to the bladder. The midportion is called the *membranous urethra*. The distal, or *cavernous, urethra* is the distal end, which extends the length of the penis.

REPRODUCTIVE STRUCTURES OF THE MALE

Scrotum and Testicles

The *scrotum* is a layered tissue sac that encases the testicles. The skin of the scrotum contains numerous folds, or *rugae*, and is continuous with the perineum. The inner layer of the scrotum is composed of fascia and dartos muscle. In cold environments, the dartos retracts the testicles closer to the body; it relaxes when the ambient temperature is warm. This temperature regulation system protects the *spermatozoa* (male reproductive cells) produced by the testicles.

The testicles are enclosed within a fibrous membrane called the *tunica vaginalis*. A septum in the scrotum separates the two testicles. The internal structure of the testicle is composed of tightly coiled tubules and ducts that produce sperm. The smallest units of this ductal system are the *seminiferous tubules*. Testosterone, the primary male sex hormone, is produced in these tubules, which communicate with the larger efferent ductules, epididymis, and vas deferens. The vas deferens exits the testicle at the superior end and joins the ejaculatory structures of the pelvis.

Epididymis

The *epididymis* is a convoluted duct that secretes seminal fluid, the liquid substance that gives sperm mobility through the male reproductive tract.

Vas Deferens

The *vas deferens* joins the epididymis with the ejaculatory duct. It passes through the inguinal canal in the abdominal wall at the level of the internal ring. At this level, it lies inside the spermatic cord, a strong tubular structure that includes nerves, blood vessels, and lymphatic tissue. The vas deferens continues across the bladder and ureter, where it meets the opening of the seminal vesicle and forms the ejaculatory duct. The paired ejaculatory ducts traverse the prostate gland and terminate at the urethra.

Seminal Vesicles

The seminal vesicles are paired structures situated close to the ejaculatory duct at the proximal end. These vesicles (saclike structures) secrete approximately 60% of the semen (the ejaculatory fluid containing sperm).

Prostate Gland

The *prostate gland* surrounds the urethra and secretes an alkaline fluid that contributes to seminal fluid. The gland is divided into six lobes covered by a fibrous *prostatic capsule*. The function of the prostate is production of some components of seminal fluid.

Bulbourethral Glands

The bulbourethral glands (also called *Cowper glands*) are paired structures that lie just below the prostate on each side of the urethra. These glands secrete mucus, which contributes to the total volume of the semen.

Penis

The penis is suspended at the pubic arch by fascia. The body of the penis is composed of several columns of tissue. Two dorsal columns, called the *corpora cavernosa*, (sing., corpus cavernosum) are composed of spongy vascular tissue. The columns are separated by a septum and bound together by a fibrous sheath. A third tissue column, called the *corpus spongiosum*, encloses the urethra. The distal portion of the corpus spongiosum forms the *glans penis*, which is covered by skin called the *prepuce* or *foreskin*. During **circumcision**, the foreskin is removed. The *corona* is the recessed tract at the base of the glans.

Figure 25-6 illustrates the male reproductive system.

PATHOLOGY OF THE GENITOURINARY SYSTEM

Table 25-1 discusses common genitourinary conditions. Figure 25-7 illustrates common GU pathology.

KIDNEY DIALYSIS

The kidneys normally remove waste products from the blood. Without this function, the body becomes quickly weakened by toxins produced during normal metabolism. Kidney dialysis is a procedure that performs this function in patients with chronic and end-stage renal disease (ESRD). The two types of kidney dialysis are *hemodialysis* and *peritoneal dialysis*. Dialy-

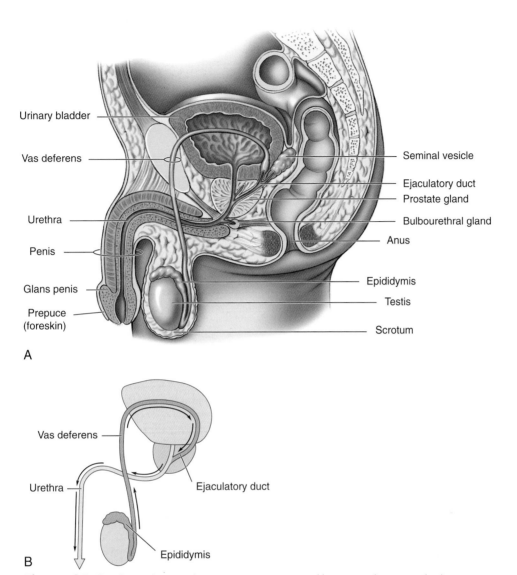

Figure 25-6 The male reproductive system. *(From Herlihy B, Maebius NK: The human body in health and disease, ed 2, Philadelphia, 2003, WB Saunders.)*

sis is performed regularly, or it can be done as an emergency procedure to remove ingested toxins from the blood that otherwise would lead to immediate kidney failure. Patients receiving dialysis treatment have a restricted lifestyle and frequently are facing a poor disease outcome. The extreme shortage of donor kidneys and the rigorous dialysis schedule, which determines the patient's quality of life, often lead to depression, which is particularly common in hemodialysis patients.

HEMODIALYSIS

During hemodialysis, the blood is shunted into a heparinized hemodialysis machine, where it passes through a series of membranes and a dialyzing solution that filter waste and return the blood to the body. Blood leaves the body through an artery and is returned through a vein. Electrolytes and other substances can be added to the blood during dialysis as needed. The process normally takes about 3 hours and is performed three or four times a week in a dialysis clinic or at home.

For access to the vascular system, an **arteriovenous fistula (or AV shunt)** is created surgically. In this procedure, a major vein and artery (usually the radial) are anastomosed, or an artificial graft is implanted to connect the artery and vein. The fistula or AV shunt is used to access the vascular system during dialysis. Hemodialysis patients are extremely careful of their AV access sites and need to take precautions to prevent injury at the site. (The procedure for an AV shunt or a fistula is performed by a vascular surgeon and is described in detail in Chapter 33.)

PERITONEAL DIALYSIS

During peritoneal dialysis, a Silastic tube is implanted in the suprapubic peritoneal space. Dialysis solution is instilled into the catheter. The solution remains in the peritoneal cavity and

Table 25-1

Pathology of the Genitourinary System

Condition	Description	Considerations
Kidneys, Adrenal Glands, and Ureters		
Calculi (stones)	Stones are formed by crystalline mineral and salts precipitated from filtrate produced in the kidney.	Conservative treatment is medical and dietary. Large stones are fragmented and allowed to pass naturally through the urinary system or removed surgically. (See Cystoscopy; Flexible and Rigid Ureteroscopy; and Kidney Stones.)
Cancer	Primary cancer of the kidney arises from the cortex and renal pelvis. The greatest risk factor is smoking.	Early detection by magnetic resonance imaging (MRI) and computed tomography (CT) scanning has improved diagnosis and cure rates in the last decade. Nephrectomy with regional lymph node removal may be performed for early treatment.
Cystic kidney disease	Renal cysts originate in the nephron as a result of obstruction. Fluid-filled cysts impinge on vascular structures, causing loss of kidney function. Cystic disease may be acquired or congenital. Polycystic disease is hereditary and has no treatment.	Treatment is palliative and symptomatic. End-stage disease causes renal failure, requiring dialysis.
End-stage renal disease (ESRD)	ESRD is renal failure that cannot be reversed. It has many causes, including diabetes, hypertension, systemic lupus, nephrotic syndrome, and infection (ingestion of *Escherichia coli* is a common cause of renal failure).	ESRD patients receive kidney dialysis and supportive medication. Kidney transplantation may be performed.
Glomerulonephritis	Kidney infection and autoimmune disorders may affect any part of the nephron and glomerulus. *Glomerulonephritis* is a general term rather than a specific disease.	Treatment depends on the disease and the functional level of the kidney. Renal failure occurs in advanced disease.
Hydronephrosis	Distention and loss of function of the ureter or renal pelvis related to urinary reflux (backward movement of urine) caused by an obstruction such as stricture, stone, or tumor.	Treatment is related to the cause of the reflux. Reconstruction of the renal pelvis may be necessary to restore function.
Trauma	Injury to the kidney is most commonly caused by a blow to the flank or back. This most commonly occurs during contact sports or as a result of intentional violence.	Treatment depends on the extent of the injury. Surgical intervention may be necessary for hemorrhage or reconstruction.
Wilms' tumor (nephroblastoma)	The most common tumors in children—arising in the kidney.	Refer to Chapter 34.
Addison disease	Addison disease is adrenal insufficiency. This is a rare disorder with many different causes, including autoimmune disease and certain tumors.	Treatment includes hormone replacement. Other therapy depends on the causes, which may be complex and rare.
Cushing syndrome	Cushing syndrome is overproduction of glucocorticoid, which is secreted by the adrenal glands; the condition can be related to several pathological conditions of the pituitary gland, an adrenal tumor, or other tumors.	Treatment depends on the exact cause.
Bladder and Urethra		
Cancer	Bladder cancer is the most common form of urinary tract cancer; tumors are derived from the bladder lining.	Treatment is surgical and palliative. (See Cystectomy.)
Neurogenic bladder disorder	*Neurogenic bladder disorder* is a general term that refers to pathogenic loss of bladder function related to neurological damage. Common causes are spinal cord injury, cerebrovascular accident, brain lesion, peripheral nerve disease, and infection.	Treatment is medical and depends on the cause.
Trauma	Traumatic injury to the bladder occurs most often in motor vehicle accidents and is related to pelvic fracture.	Treatment for bladder injury is surgical and medical.
Urinary incontinence	The most common cause of urinary incontinence is loss of sphincter control at the bladder neck. This may be related to multiple childbirths or advancing age. Hypertrophy of the prostate also causes involuntary loss of urine.	Conservative treatment includes hormone replacement therapy in women and specific exercises to increase the tone of the pelvic floor muscles. Surgical treatment is available for selected patients. See specific bladder procedures and resection of the prostate.
Urinary tract infection (UTI)	A UTI is an infection of the lower urinary tract. It is commonly caused by *E. coli* contamination of the distal urethra or by a sexually transmitted disease. Chronic UTIs may result in scarring of the urethra that requires surgery.	Treatment is medical for active infection. Release of a urethral stricture may be required. (See Cystoscopy.)

Table 25-1

Pathology of the Genitourinary System—cont'd

Condition	Description	Considerations
Male Reproductive System		
Benign prostatic hyperplasia (BPH)	Age-related enlargement of the prostate gland. This causes urethral constriction, leading to reflux and incontinence.	Conservative treatment is medical. Surgery is indicated in more severe cases. See specific procedures for resection of the prostate.
Cancer of the prostate	Adenocarcinoma is the most common type of prostate cancer. Increased screening and early detection account for the "rise" in incidence.	The diagnosis is made on the basis of the physical examination and the patient's history. The most common treatment is surgical or radiation therapy. (See the sections on prostatectomy.)
Cryptorchidism	Cryptorchidism is a congenital anomaly in which one or both testicles fail to descend into the scrotum in fetal life. The condition is associated with reduced fertility, tumor, and negative sexual and body image in the young male.	Treatment is surgical. The goal is to bring the testicles into anatomical position in the scrotum. (See Chapter 34.)
Epispadias	Epispadias is a rare congenital malposition of the urethra. The urethra may open on the top side of the penis or may be exposed along the full length; it most commonly occurs in association with a complex of defects, including extrophy of the bladder.	Correction of the defects requires extensive surgery. (See Chapter 34.)
Erectile dysfunction	Failure to achieve or maintain an erection in the male can be caused by one or more functional or physiological problems affecting the vascular, endocrine, or nervous system. Dysfunction may also be psychogenic.	Treatment depends on the cause. When conservative treatment and counseling fail, a penile implant may be surgically inserted. (See Insertion of a Penile Implant.)
Human papilloma virus (HPV)	HPV is a sexually transmitted disease that may lead to penile cancer. Specific strains are linked with cervical cancer. Most men are carriers.	Lesions caused by HPV may be found and removed from any mucous membrane of the body, but they are particularly common in the perianal area and the penis. They are removed chemically or with ESU or laser ablation.
Hydrocele	A hydrocele is a fluid-filled sac surrounding the testicle. In newborns, the condition arises from a defect of the spermatic cord. A hydrocele may also arise from injury or in association with an inguinal hernia.	Congenital hydrocele usually resolves without treatment. Surgery may be indicated for a persistent hydrocele or in conjunction with hernia repair.
Hypospadias	Hypospadias is a common congenital defect in which the urethra fails to develop fully. This results in urethral shortening and displacement of the urethral meatus.	The condition is corrected surgically in one or more stages, depending on the complexity.
Orchitis/ epididymitis	Inflammation and infection of the testicle and epididymis is commonly related to viral diseases (e.g., mumps) and to sexually transmitted diseases, such as chlamydia and gonorrhea.	Treatment is medical; the infected individual and his partner or partners are all treated.
Penile cancer	Penile cancer is a rare cancer that originates in the squamous cells of the glans or foreskin.	Treatment is surgical and involves wide excision of the tumor or penectomy (amputation of the penis).
Phimosis/ paraphimosis	Phimosis is a condition of the uncircumcised male in which the foreskin adheres to the glans and cannot be retracted.	Treatment is medical and surgical. (See Circumcision [Adult].)
Sexually transmitted diseases (STDs)	STDs are caused by specific pathogens and spread by sexual contact. STDs are a significant public health problem in the United States.	Treatment includes drug therapy. Prevention requires rigorous health education and barrier protection (condoms).
Testicular cancer	Testicular cancer is a rare cancer that arises from the germ cell (reproductive cells) of the testicle.	Early diagnosis has improved survival rates in the past 20 years. Treatment includes orchiectomy and radiation therapy. (See Orchiectomy.)
Testicular torsion	Rotation of the testicle is related to a congenital anomaly or occurs as a result of vigorous activity in young males. Torsion is a medical emergency, because the testicular blood vessels may be occluded, resulting in ischemia and necrosis of the testicle.	Treatment is immediate surgery to save the testicle. Orchiectomy may be required if the testicle is nonviable.
Varicocele	Varicocele is a condition of enlarged, dilated veins in the scrotum.	Treatment includes surgical removal of the affected veins or scleral treatment in which the vein is injected with an agent that shrinks the vessel. (See Varicocelectomy.)

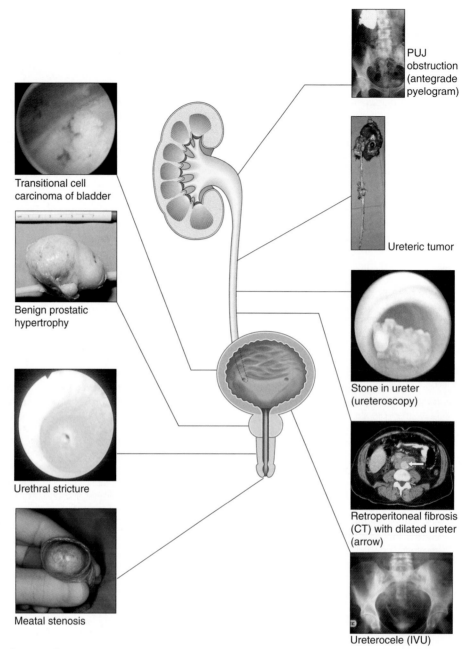

Figure 25-7 *Genitourinary pathology. (From Garden O, Bradbury A, Forsythe J, Parks R: Principles and practice of surgery, ed 5, Edinburgh, 2007, Churchill Livingstone/Elsevier.)*

slowly extracts metabolic wastes using the peritoneum as an osmotic filter. The fluid then is removed. The total dwell time may be 4 to 6 hours, and the entire process can be performed by the patient.

DIAGNOSTIC TESTS

The primary function of the urinary system is to filter metabolic waste from the blood. Therefore many laboratory tests in GU disease focus on the presence or absence of substances found in the blood and urine. Imaging tests are performed to outline the structures of the GU system, to observe its function, and to detect tumors.

URINALYSIS

In a healthy adult, the kidneys produce about 3.2 pints (1.5 L) of urine per day. The main components of urine are water (95%) and solutes (5%). Urinalysis is performed to detect specific substances, both normal and abnormal, in the urine. Filtrate can be sampled from any location in the upper urinary tract. This is often necessary to detect abnormalities caused by disease in a specific location within the kidney or ureter. Urine is obtained directly through a catheter inserted into the bladder or by collection as it passes from the body; the latter may be a single sample or the amount collected over 24 hours.

Simple urinalysis provides basic information about substances such as the blood, glucose, and white blood cells. The physical characteristics of urine are also important. Odor, color, density, and clarity have specific clinical significance, which can help confirm disease. Microscopic examination reveals the presence of blood cells, cell fragments, and other metabolic substances. Infection of the bladder or other locations in the urinary tract may be detected by the presence of protein or blood cells in the urine. A simple dipstick test can be used for screening purposes, and urine culture and sensitivity (discussed in Chapter 7) may be performed to confirm a diagnosis and determine the appropriate antimicrobial therapy.

The presence of protein in the urine is an important diagnostic sign. Albumen is a primary protein component of the blood. Normally, the glomerulus allows very little protein to cross the capillary system and into the filtrate. Therefore albumen in the urine may be a sign of glomerulus disease. Specific tests for urine albumen are routinely performed when kidney disease is suspected.

The **specific gravity** (the ratio of the density of urine compared to water) is an important indicator of the concentration of solutes in the urine. Dissolved solutes are present after filtration in the kidney. Therefore the specific gravity provides important information about the hydration of the body and also the kidney's ability to maintain fluid balance. The specific gravity is measured with a calibrated hydrometer or urinometer.

BLOOD TESTS

The presence or absence of specific substances in the blood reveals kidney function. Expected values of chemicals and metabolic products in the blood shift in kidney disease. An increase in certain substances can mean that harmful waste products are not filtered out of the blood; other tests and clinical studies must be performed to arrive at a proper diagnosis.

Glomerular Filtration Rate

The serum creatinine or **glomerular filtration rate (GFR)** measures the rate of creatinine clearance from the blood. Creatine is a metabolic byproduct of muscle metabolism that normally is filtered by the kidney tubules. However, it is not reabsorbed. The GFR is measured as the amount of creatinine filtered per minute. This is an important test of kidney function. Blood creatinine begins to rise when the GFR is about 50% of normal.

Blood Urea Nitrogen

Measurement of the blood urea nitrogen (BUN) is a test that assesses the elimination of urea from the liver. Urea is a waste product formed in the liver as a product of protein metabolism. Normally it is cleared by the kidneys. The blood urea value may indicate renal failure, but it is also influenced by protein intake, age, and hydration.

TISSUE BIOPSY

Biopsy samples of the kidney, bladder wall, or other tissues of the GU tract are removed for microscopic pathological testing.

IMAGING STUDIES

Imaging studies provide the basis of diagnosis for both functional and physiological disease. Imaging provides a permanent record of the shape, location, and density of structures. Selected studies also can detect stones or malformation of the tubes and ducts of the urinary system. The following imaging studies are commonly used:

- *Computed tomography (CT):* CT is the preferred method for imaging tumors of the kidney. Noncontrast helical CT is used to diagnose calculi.
- *Fluoroscopy:* C-arm fluoroscopy (real-time radiographs) is used in many imaging studies.
- *Intravenous urography:* This process involves radiographic studies using a contrast medium, which is injected intravenously to obtain serial radiographs of the renal pelvis and calyces. The rate of emptying and the size of the ureters are also measured.
- KUB: This is a radiograph of the kidney, ureters, and bladder. A KUB may be used to outline structures of the urinary system, including any stones larger than 2 mm. However, CT is now preferred for stone imaging, because stones of all types are visible, and even small stones can be seen.
- *Micturating cystourethrogram (MCU):* This study provides images of the bladder (cystography) while it is emptying. A contrast medium is instilled into the bladder via a catheter, and images are obtained during urination.
- *Magnetic resonance imaging (MRI):* MRI provides an extremely detailed assessment and is commonly used in the diagnosis of tumors.
- *Nuclear imaging:* Radioisotope scanning is used in GU studies to detect metastasis arising from a primary tumor of the prostate.
- *Retrograde ureteropyelogram:* **Retrograde** injections are made using a catheter inserted into the ureter. A contrast medium is instilled into the catheter and viewed with fluoroscopy.
- *Ultrasonography:* Ultrasound is one of the first-line imaging techniques used in GU medicine. It is used in the assessment of patients who are ineligible for CT or other forms of radiographic exposure.

POSITIONING

A number of patient positions are used in GU surgery, depending on the type of surgery and the techniques to be used. Rigid cystoscopy and ureteroscopy are always performed with the patient in the lithotomy position, although the supine position may be used for flexible cystoscopy. The supine position is used for open abdominal approaches to the bladder and for laparoscopic surgery of the prostate. The lateral position is the most common open approach for a flank incision, which provides exposure of the kidney and ureters. The prone position may be used for endoscopic nephroscopy. Prepping and draping routines follow standard procedures, as discussed in Chapter 11.

INSTRUMENTS FOR OPEN GENITOURINARY PROCEDURES

Open GU procedures require specialty and general surgery instruments. The ureters are extremely delicate and require atraumatic clamps, such as Babcock clamps. Right-angle and Schnitz (tonsil) clamps frequently are used to occlude vessels and for blunt dissection. Vessel loops made of Silastic or cotton are commonly used to retract blood vessels.

Kidney procedures may require kidney pedicle clamps, which have right-angle jaws for reaching around the back of the pedicle. Vascular clamps are required for procedures involving the renal arteries or whenever temporary interruption of the kidney's blood supply is necessary. Fine-tip needle holders are needed for both kidney and ureteral procedures, because the sutures are fine and the needles are very small.

Most prostate procedures are now performed using minimally invasive surgery (MIS). However, if open surgery is required, prostate retractors and grasping clamps are required, as are right-angle clamps and general surgery instruments. Instruments for open GU surgery are shown in Figures 25-8 and 25-9.

Surgery of the vas deferens and repair of penile anomalies require plastic surgery or microsurgical instruments. MIS instruments (Figure 25-10) are used in percutaneous nephroscopy, laparoscopy, and transurethral (cystoscopic) surgery.

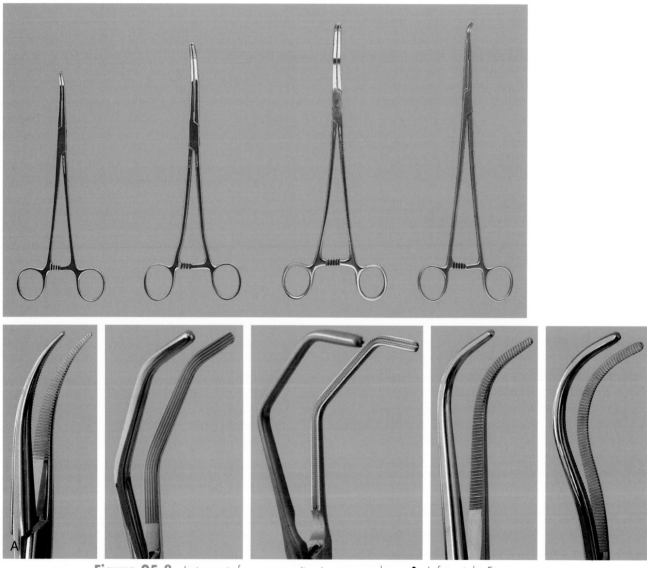

Figure 25-8   Instruments for open genitourinary procedures. **A**, *Left to right:* Fine hemostatic forceps; Satinsky clamp; Herrick kidney clamp; Satinsky vascular clamp; right-angle clamp; Mayo kidney clamp. *(From Tighe SM: Instrumentation for the operating room, ed 6, St. Louis, 2003, Mosby.)*

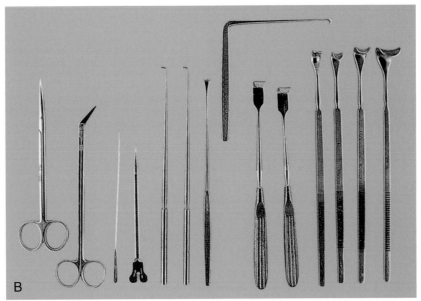

Figure 25-8, cont'd **B**, Nephrectomy and ureteroplasty instruments. *Left to right:* Metzenbaum scissors; Potts scissors; probe and grooved director; two nerve hooks; two Love nerve retractors (straight and right angle); two Little retractors; four vein retractors. *(From Tighe SM: Instrumentation for the operating room, ed 7, St Louis, 2007, Mosby.)*

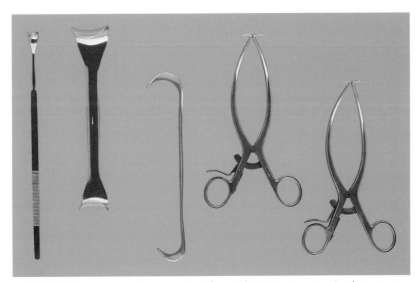

Figure 25-9 Prostatectomy instruments. *Left to right.* Vein retractor; Goulet retractor (two views); Gelpi retractors. *(From Tighe SM: Instrumentation for the operating room, ed 6, St Louis, 2003, Mosby.)*

ENDOSCOPIC INSTRUMENTS

RIGID CYSTOSCOPE

A rigid **cystoscope** is passed through the urethral meatus for diagnostic or operative procedures. The cystoscope is the precursor to the modern cystourethroscope. In this text, the term *cystoscope* is used to describe the modern transurethral scope. However, the surgical technologist should understand that the current scopes have more advanced technological and surgical capabilities than the cystoscope used in the past.

The optical system of the scope provides a number of angles of vision. The *direct forward scope* (0 degrees) is useful for viewing the urethra and for use with the *urethrotome* (an instrument used in sharp dissection of the urethra). The *right-angle scope* (pointing up or down 30 degrees) is used for viewing the entire bladder and for insertion of the ureteral catheters. A 45-degree scope is also available.

The cystoscope has many components for performing diagnostic and surgical procedures. The instrument is the optical portion of the scope. It contains the lenses, which magnify the target image.

The *Brown-Buerger* cystoscope ranges in size from 14 to 26 French (Fr). The most common size for adults is 21 Fr. This scope has two sheaths to accommodate a ureteral catheter and accessory instruments. The *McCarthy panendoscope* ranges in

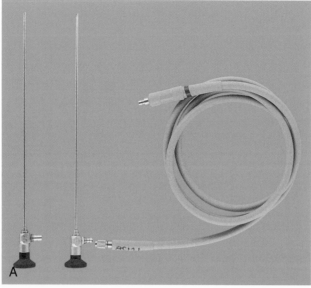

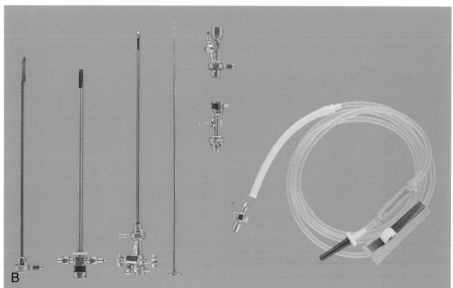

Figure 25-10 Endoscopic instruments. **A,** Cystourethroscope. **B,** Cystoscope and light guide, cystoscope sheath, deflector, obturator, bridges, and fluid tubing. *(From Tighe SM: Instrumentation for the operating room, ed 6, St Louis, 2003, Mosby.)*

size from 14 to 30 Fr. This scope is used with a fore-oblique telescope. The *Wappler* cystoscope combines the functions of the Brown-Buerger and McCarthy scopes. The sheath size ranges from 17 to 24 Fr. The scope accepts suction and irrigation accessories, and a ureteral scope can be passed through it.

SHEATH

The sheath is a hollow tube that serves as a passageway for the instruments used during cystoscopy and resection. The telescope is inserted into the sheath before it is passed into the urethra. The sheath allows the use of operative accessories, instruments, suction, and irrigation. The sheath has attachments that accept the instruments and irrigation tubing. The tip may be beveled or oblique. The main operating channel receives the telescope, and side channels, controlled by stop-

cocks, accept the accessory instruments. A *bridge* attaches to the head of the scope and accepts accessory tools.

OBTURATOR

Before the sheath is placed inside the urethra, a blunt, round-tip *obturator* is placed inside the sheath. The obturator tip advances ahead of the sheath and protects the wall of the urethra from abrasion during insertion. The obturator may be straight or deflecting (able to be turned to the side).

RESECTOSCOPE

A **resectoscope** is a transurethral, electrosurgical instrument used to remove small fragments of tissue. It consists of an endoscope, sheath, obturator, and electrosurgical loop, which cuts and coagulates target tissue inside the bladder. The handle of the resectoscope contains a spring mechanism that operates the retractable loop (active electrode) at the tip. During resection surgery, the instrument is inserted through the urethra and bladder to remove tumors or resect the prostate or other tissue in the bladder space. The loop is applied to tissue and retracts it into the instrument, simultaneously cutting and coagulating it.

Resectoscopes vary by operating mechanism. Most use a spring mechanism described previously. The most common type is the Iglesias resectoscope. The resectoscope uses electrosurgical energy to excise tissue from the bladder, urethra, or prostate. The sheath usually is a size 24 to 28 Fr and is made of fiberglass to prevent a short circuit and patient burns. The working element of the resectoscope, which is inserted through the sheath, has a channel for a telescope and cutting electrode. The cutting electrode cuts and coagulates the tissue. As with other electrosurgical (ESU) systems, a variety of tips are available. The loop electrode commonly is used during resection procedures. Figure 25-11 shows a resectoscope and accessories.

IMAGING SYSTEM

The imaging system used in GU endoscopy is the same as for other endoscopes (see Chapter 21). A fiberoptic light or liquid cable connects the cystoscope to the fiberoptic xenon light source. Other components of the imaging system are fully discussed in Chapter 21.

URINARY CATHETERS

A catheter is a hollow tube made of a flexible, synthetic material, such as Teflon-coated rubber. A variety of ureteral and urethral catheters may be used during GU procedures. The lumen, or bore, of the catheter is measured in French, and sizes range from 7 to 26 Fr. Catheters are designated by number, and as the number of a catheter decreases, the lumen diameter also decreases. The catheters most commonly used are in the 16 to 18 range. Retention catheters also have a retention balloon size, which is measured in cubic milliliters.

Urinary catheters are used for a variety of purposes, including:
- Short-term urinary drainage
- Continuous urinary drainage
- Hemostasis and evacuation of blood clots or blood
- Continuity of the urethra or ureters

URETHRAL CATHETERS

Two common types of catheters are the **indwelling (Foley) catheter**, which has a balloon or flange at the proximal tip, and the **straight catheter** (also called a *Robinson* catheter), which is used for temporary bladder drainage.

The *Foley* catheter is available in a variety of types and balloon sizes. The three-way balloon catheter is used for intermittent or continuous bladder irrigation. A large, 30-mL balloon catheter is used postoperatively as a **tamponade** (used to apply pressure against a tissue or opening). This type

is used after transurethral resection of the prostate to control bleeding.

The Foley catheter is the most common type of urinary catheter. It is retained in the bladder by an inflatable balloon at the end of the catheter. Sizes 8 through 30 Fr with a retention balloon of 5 to 30 mL are available. The smaller balloon is used for simple retention, and the larger retention balloon is used postoperatively to maintain hemostasis, as described previously. After it is placed in the bladder, the balloon is inflated with sterile water. The larger balloons may be inflated to as much as 120 mL for greater hemostatic efficiency.

The *Phillips* catheter is straight but differs from the straight catheter in that one end has a screw tip designed to accept a filiform (a small catheter advanced through a urethral stricture). The filiform has a smaller diameter than the catheter and is easily manipulated in the urethra.

The *coudé* catheter may be straight or may be a Foley retention type. This type of catheter has a firm rubber tip or beak that is used to facilitate its passage through a false urethral passage or past anatomical prominences in the urethra or in an enlarged prostate.

Urethral catheters are shown in Figure 25-12.

URETERAL CATHETERS

Assorted ureteral catheters are used for both open and closed procedures. General uses are:
- To provide a method of instilling a contrast medium into the ureter and kidney for retrograde **pyelography** radiographic studies.
- To provide immediate drainage of a ureter.
- To provide temporary drainage of a ureter after a procedure. In this case, the catheter may be left in place during healing. This type is called an indwelling catheter or **stent**. An indwelling catheter may be attached to a calibrated collection system to measure output.
- To keep the ureter open to allow a stone to pass.
- To bypass a stone or tumor.
- To block the ureteral opening during radiographic studies.
- To identify a structure during open procedures.
- To obtain urine specimens or renal washings from the kidney.

Ureteral catheters have graduated marks so that the surgeon can see how deeply the catheter is inserted.

The Braasch bulb or cone-tip catheter is used to occlude the ureteral orifice during imaging studies when a contrast medium is injected during retrograde pyelography.

Other commonly used catheters are the whistle-tip, round-tip, spiral-tip, and olive-tip catheters (Figure 25-13).

URETERAL STENT

A ureteral stent is a particular type of ureteral catheter. It is a thin, flexible tube that is threaded into the ureter temporarily or for a defined period to help urine drain from the kidney to the bladder or to an external collection system. A ureteral stent is placed in the ureter to provide continuous flow of

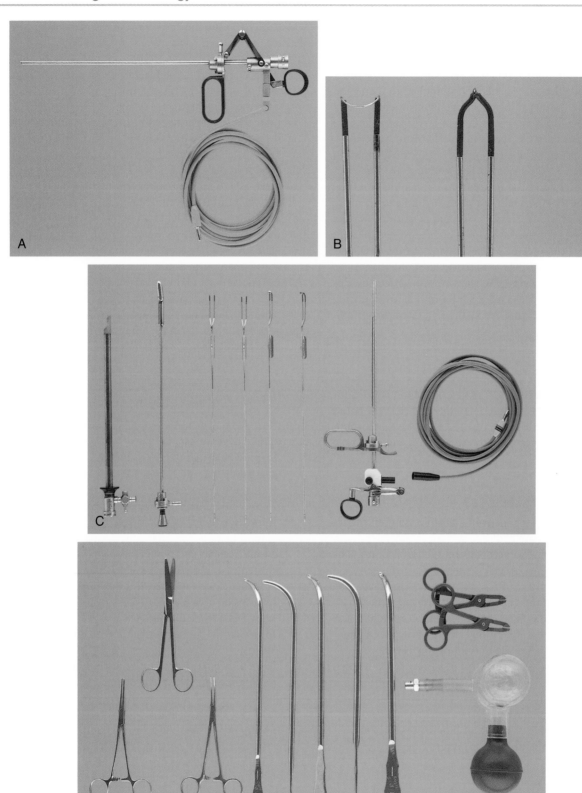

Figure 25-11   A, Resectoscope. **B,** Cutting tips. **C,** *Left to right:* Resecting sheath; deflecting sheath; resection loops with resectoscope and power cord. **D,** *Top left:* Mayo dissecting scissors. *Bottom left to right:* Crile hemostats; Van Buren urethral sounds; Ellik evacuator.

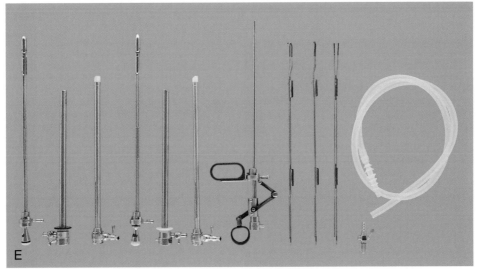

Figure 25-11, cont'd **E,** *Left to right:* Resectoscope, working elements and electrodes. *(From Tighe SM: Instrumentation for the operating room, ed 6, St Louis, 2003, Mosby.)*

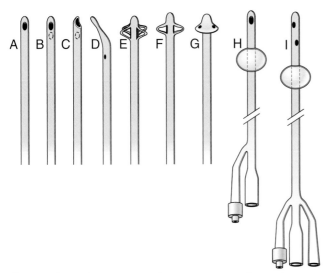

Figure 25-12 Urinary catheters. **A,** Conical-tip catheter. **B,** Robinson catheter. **C,** Whistle tip urethral catheter. **D,** Coudé olive-tip catheter. **E** and **F,** Malecot catheter. **G,** Pezzer catheter. **H,** Foley retention catheter. **I,** Three-way irrigation catheter. *(Modified from Walsh PC, Retik AB, Vaughan ED et al: Campbell's urology, ed 8, Philadelphia, 2002, WB Saunders.)*

urine to the bladder. Ureteral stents may be used in patients with an active kidney infection or with diseased bladders (e.g., as a result of cancer or radiation therapy). Alternatively, ureteral stents may be used during or after urinary tract surgical procedures to provide a mold around which healing can occur, to divert the urinary flow away from areas of leakage, to manipulate kidney stones or prevent stone migration before treatment, or to make the ureters more easily identifiable during difficult surgical procedures.

The stent may remain in place for the short term (days to weeks) or for the long term (weeks to months). The size, shape, and material of the ureteral stent to be used depend on

the patient's anatomy and the reason the stent is required. Most stents are 5 to 12 inches (12 to 30 cm) long and have a diameter of 1.5 to 6 mm.

Several types of stents are used. They can be made of durable and biocompatible silicone, polyurethane, or some other copolymer. The stent may have a collar, a double-J configuration, a pigtail, or a coil to minimize migration into the renal pelvis or bladder. During cystoscopy, the stent is passed through the cystoscope and over a guide wire into the ureter, where it remains fixed for internal urinary drainage. As described for ureteral catheters, some types of stents are used to identify ureters and provide external drainage intraoperatively.

The indwelling pigtail catheter is a type of J-stent; this refers to its ability to maintain the form and shape of the ureter. The catheter maintains patency in the ureter to allow a stone or urine to pass. During insertion, a guide wire is placed in the lumen of the catheter, which gives it some stiffness while guiding the catheter. Once the catheter is in place, the wire is removed, and the distal end forms a J or slight spiral, which holds it in place. The distal end may be sutured to the patient's skin to allow for a noninvasive removal. This type of catheter is also used during ESWL.

EQUIPMENT

ELECTROSURGICAL UNIT

Electrosurgery is used in both open and transurethral procedures. As in other specialties, electrosurgery in GU surgery is delivered through many types of instruments. The most common ESU devices are the "pencil," and bipolar cutting and coagulation instruments. The resectoscope, discussed in Chapter 24 is used in transurethral procedures and performed in the presence of continuous irrigation. Safety hazards are associated with the use of electrosurgical equipment in the

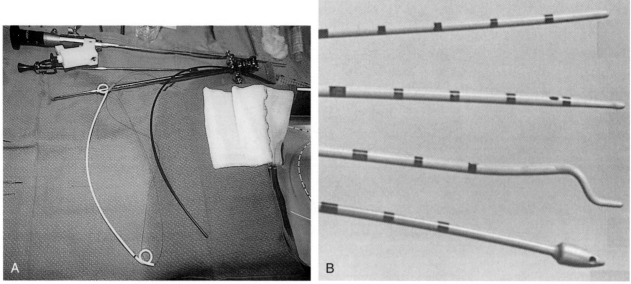

Figure 25-13 A, Ureteral catheters and stents. **B,** Ureteral catheters. *Top to bottom:* Round tip, olive tip, spiral tip, and conical or bulb tip. (**A** *from Nagle GM:* Genitourinary surgery: perioperative nursing series, *St Louis, 1997, Mosby;* **B** *from Walsh PC, Retik AB, Vaughan ED et al:* Campbell's urology, *ed 8, Philadelphia, 2002, WB Saunders.*)

presence of fluids. The cystoscopy assistant must understand these principles (see Continuous and Intermittent Irrigation).

The grounding plate may be placed on the patient's thigh or waist. It must be placed over a fleshy area and never over a bony prominence. The ESU should be placed on the lowest setting, which is increased gradually as directed by the urologist.

MICROSCOPE

An operative microscope is used during fine reconstructive surgery, laser ablation, and vaporization of lesions. The use and care of the microscope are described in Chapter 26.

LASER

The neodymium/yttrium-aluminum-garnet (Nd:YAG), carbon dioxide (CO_2), tunable dye, and argon lasers typically are used in GU surgery. Certain aspects of laser use are discussed in particular procedures in this chapter, but the reader should review all safety precautions discussed in Chapter 19.

TECHNIQUES IN TRANSURETHRAL SURGERY

Most procedures of the kidneys, ureters, bladder, and urethra are performed with a flexible or rigid endoscope. Two techniques are commonly used:

- *Cystoscopy:* A rigid or flexible cystoscope is used for transurethral assessment and procedures of the lower GU tract, including the urethra, bladder, and prostate gland.

- *Ureteroscopy:* A rigid or flexible ureteroscope is inserted through the urethra and advanced into the renal pelvis and ureter. Surgery is performed through the lumen of the scope.

Although cystoscopy is considered a clean contaminated procedure, most facilities ensure that all equipment is sterile to prevent cross-contamination. (Chapter 21 presents a discussion of endoscopic reprocessing, both sterile and clean contaminated).

CYSTOSCOPY ROOM

Transurethral procedures take place in a specialized cystoscopy ("cysto") room. This dedicated surgical suite has all the equipment needed to perform diagnostic or therapeutic procedures.

The cystoscopy table has accommodations for continuous drainage, intraoperative fluoroscopy, and radiography. The cystoscopy table differs from the standard operating table in that it is designed to maintain the patient in the lithotomy position, receive radiograph cassettes, and allow for drainage of irrigation fluid. The stirrups of the table are adjustable and removable, and radiograph cassettes are placed in a hollow space built into the table. Irrigation fluid is directed into a drainage tray at the foot of the table. The tray is covered with a wire mesh plate that can be sterilized for resection procedures when tissue specimens are evacuated with the irrigation solution.

More extensive and modern cystoscopy rooms include digital data recording and equipment for video-assisted transurethral and ureteroscopy surgery.

CYSTOSCOPY ASSISTANT

Most facilities employ a **cystoscopy (cysto) assistant**. This is a trained surgical technologist or nurse whose main duty is to work in this specialty. Other perioperative staff in the department may have little clinical time in the cystoscopy room and thus would not have the opportunity to learn about the specialty. The system is efficient as long as the cysto assistant is available at all times. However, if this person is absent, other staff members must take the individual's place. A written protocol should be available for all staff members.

The cysto assistant performs duties as a scrub and circulator. After donning sterile gloves, the assistant sets up the instrument table and all other sterile equipment. The urologist usually does not require a scrub, therefore after setting up the supplies, the assistant removes his or her gloves and functions as a circulator during the case.

During a cystoscopic procedure, the circulator has the following responsibilities:

1. Remain in the room at all times unless otherwise directed by the urologist.
2. Connect the nonsterile ends of the power cables or suction tubing.
3. Open sterile supplies for the urologist as needed.
4. Replace irrigation bottles as they empty and note the number of bottles used.
5. Receive any specimens from the urologist and label them properly.
6. Monitor the patient's vital signs every 15 minutes if a local anesthetic is used during the procedure.

After a cystoscopic procedure, the circulator has the following responsibilities:

1. Assist in transferring the patient from the cystoscopy table to the stretcher and accompany the urologist or anesthesiologist to the postanesthesia care unit (PACU).
2. Transfer any tissue or fluid specimens to the designated area and record them in the specimen log.
3. Put away nonsterile supplies used during the procedure.
4. Transfer soiled equipment to the workroom and carry out proper terminal sterilization or decontamination of the equipment.
5. The surgical technologist may be responsible for maintaining a current inventory of surgical supplies and for communicating with manufacturers' representatives.

POSITIONING

The patient is placed in the lithotomy or the supine position, depending on the type of endoscopy to be performed. Rigid endoscopy requires the lithotomy position, whereas the supine position can be used for flexible endoscopy. Patient safety in the cysto room is the same as for other procedures. However, many cysto patients are elderly, which requires extra care to prevent overabduction of the hips or rapid changes in position. Patients are helped to the cystoscopy table from the stretcher and given clear but gentle direction during the transfer.

All patients are moved gently and with consideration for their individual physical ability. The cystoscopy stirrups are a modified (lower) version of those used commonly in open procedures involving the lower genital and perianal area.

The lithotomy position is embarrassing for most patients. However, perioperative personnel help the patient by making the position as comfortable as possible. The patient's dignity should be protected, and the patient must not be exposed unless necessary. Talking to the patient often eases apprehension, and preparatory steps for the procedure should be explained in straightforward terms.

Temperatures in the cysto room are kept quite low, and safety procedures to maintain patient thermoregulation must be maintained. Warm blankets should be available as soon as the patient enters the room, and the patient's comfort should be maintained throughout the procedure

When the patient is positioned for cystoscopic procedures, the buttocks must be in line with or just over the table break with the legs supported by knee crutches or stirrups. Assistants must become familiar with the type of stirrup used in their facility. Stirrups must be padded correctly to prevent pressure on the peroneal nerve. Knee crutches are commonly used in many facilities. These place weight on the popliteal space (behind the knee) and can damage the nerves and blood vessels in this area. Ample padding, with the weight of the knee equally distributed, helps prevent injury. Foam or gel padding provides the safest cushioning.

PREPPING AND DRAPING

Skin prep for cystoscopic procedures includes the entire perineum, external genitalia, and pubis. A perineal drape with waterproof shield is used for procedures that require continuous bladder irrigation.

INTRAOPERATIVE IMAGING

Intraoperative imaging techniques, including radiographs and fluoroscopy, are commonly used during cystoscopy. The cystoscopy table is specially constructed to accommodate the C-arm, and most operating rooms now have permanent radiograph capability in the GU cystoscopy room.

Digital imaging of the operative site during endoscopy is performed through the camera head of the flexible endoscope. Imaging systems used in endoscopic GU surgery are similar to those used in other specialties. The components include the following:

- Light source and fiberoptic cable
- Camera head (endoscopes)
- Camera control unit
- Video cables
- Digital output recorder
- Monitor
- Equipment cart

These components are discussed in detail in Chapter 21.

CONTINUOUS AND INTERMITTENT IRRIGATION

During cystoscopic procedures, the bladder is distended with fluid to enhance visualization of the internal structures. Continuous irrigation flushes blood and tissue debris from the focal site during a procedure.

> ❖ *Whenever electrosurgical instruments are used, the irrigation fluid must be **nonelectrolytic** (containing no electrolytes). These fluids cannot transmit or disperse electricity.*

The electrosurgical instruments are used "under water" within the distension and irrigation fluid. Electrolytic solutions, which *do* contain electrolytes, cause electrical current to disperse throughout the fluid. This reduces the ESU's ability to cut and coagulate. The distention solutions most commonly used during electrosurgery are *sorbitol* and *glycine*.

Sterile distilled water may be used during assessment of the bladder and retrograde pyelography which do not require electrosurgery.

> ❖ *Water is not used during endoscopic resection procedures, because water causes hemolysis (rupture of red blood cells). During resection of the prostate, significant contact occurs between the irrigation solution and open veins of the prostate.*

Absorption of irrigation fluid (**extravasation**) may result in vascular overload. The assistant must accurately monitor the amount of fluid used and collected as runoff during a procedure to assess the amount absorbed.

Continuous irrigation is provided in 1- and 3L airtight plastic bags and closed-unit tubing. A pumping unit regulates the amount of flow. Pressure is regulated by a combination pump and pressure regulator or by gravity flow. The assistant is responsible for ensuring a continuous flow of fluid during the procedure.

The solutions used in surgery are stored in a fluid warmer. The warmer must be carefully maintained and checked frequently to ensure that the temperature is safe. Fluid warmers may contribute to increased hemorrhage, because the warm water suppresses or delays the body's natural clotting mechanism. Bladder spasm or **hypothermia** may occur when cold irrigation solutions are used. The assistant must verify the surgeon's orders for the solution type and temperature before a procedure.

ANESTHESIA

Most patients receive a local or topical anesthetic for diagnostic cystoscopy. In males, a local anesthetic in solution may be instilled into the bladder or penis. For females, cotton-tip applicators are dipped in an anesthetic and inserted into the urethral meatus. Lidocaine gel (1% or 2%) typically is used for this purpose. Monitored sedation or a spinal or general anesthetic may be used for complex procedures.

TRANSURETHRAL (CYSTOSCOPIC) PROCEDURES

CYSTOSCOPY

Description

Cystoscopy is surgery of the distal GU system performed with an operative cystourethroscope. Basic cystoscopy for visual assessment is performed at the start of any transurethral procedure.

Technique

1. The patient is placed in the supine position on the urology table. Low lithotomy stirrups or knee crutches are used to abduct and externally rotate the patient's legs.
2. The patient is prepped and draped for a perineal procedure.
3. A topical anesthetic or water-soluble anesthetic solution is instilled into the urethra.
4. Urethral dilation is performed as needed.
5. The sheath and telescope or obturator are lubricated and inserted into the urethra.
6. The obturator is removed.
7. The bladder is filled with a distension medium.
8. The surgeon examines the urethra and bladder from all angles.
9. Diagnostic and operative procedures are performed.

Discussion

The components of the basic setup for cystoscopy are listed in Box 25-1. The bladder is emptied with a straight catheter, and a sterile urine specimen is obtained. A rigid cystoscope is lubricated with water-soluble or lidocaine gel and inserted into the urethra (Figure 25-14).

Box 25-1

Basic Setup for Cystoscopy

Cystoscopy pack (gowns, towels, drapes)
Sterile gloves
Cystourethroscope
Cystoscopy irrigation tubing
Albarrán bridge
Catheter adapters
Lateral and fore-oblique telescope
ESU
Bugbee electrodes
Penile clamp
Luer-Lok stopcock
Water-soluble lubrication gel
Irrigation solution
Fiberoptic light source
Small prep basin with sponges
Specimen containers
Lead aprons
Laser units (if required)
Syringes
Assorted catheters

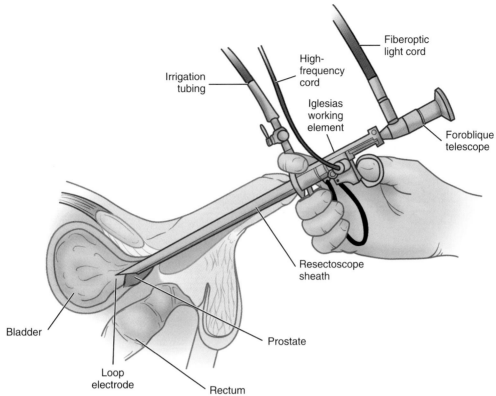

Figure 25-14 Cystourethroscope during operative cystoscopy. Note the connections for irrigation, high-frequency electrosurgery, and fiberoptic light. *(From Rothrock J: Alexander's care of the patient in surgery, ed 17, Philadelphia, 2007, Mosby.)*

The continuous irrigation fluid is instilled. The obturator is then removed, and any residual urine is collected in the specimen container. The urethra and bladder are examined. When this process is complete, the instruments are removed and the solution is drained from the bladder.

URETHRAL DILATION AND URETHROTOMY

Surgical Goal
In urethral dilation and urethrotomy, the urethra is dilated to relieve a stricture. Phillips filiforms and followers, graduated sounds (dilators), or balloon dilators may be used for this purpose. A **urethrotomy** is a small incision made in the internal urethra to release scar tissue or other stricture. Instruments used for dilation are shown in Figure 25-15.

Pathology
Urethral stricture other than that caused by an enlarged prostate gland may be caused by scarring from a previous trauma, infection of the urethra, or a congenital anomaly. If dilation is ineffective, a urethrotomy is performed.

Discussion
Dilation and urethrotomy precedes routine diagnostic cystoscopy. Stricture of the urethra is a common condition in GU disease, and dilation of the urethral stricture may be performed as an isolated procedure. Urethral dilation often is

necessary to allow instruments to pass through the urethra during surgery.

Many types of dilators are available. Filiforms are very small rods with a threaded distal end. The threaded portion accepts all sizes of followers, which are larger dilators in graduated sizes. Van Buren sounds are graduated metal rods. All sounds are first lubricated and then introduced slowly to avoid lacerating the urethra.

Urethrotomy is performed with the urethrotome, which is inserted to the point of stricture under direct visualization. A small incision is made into the structure, and a urethral catheter is inserted. The catheter is left in place during the initial healing period (3 to 5 days after surgery).

A related procedure is a **meatotomy** (meatoplasty), in which a small incision is made in the urethral meatus to relieve a stricture. As a stand-alone procedure, a meatotomy is performed on pediatric patients to release scar tissue. Infection or previous dilation of the urethral meatus can result in scarring and partial obstruction. A topical anesthetic is applied, and fine scissors are used to make a very small incision in the meatus. Healing occurs by secondary intention.

Tissue Biopsy
Tissue biopsy is performed with cup forceps or with a flat wire basket commonly used for ureteralscopic assessments. Cell biopsy can be taken from the bladder with the cytology brush. After the specimen is retrieved on the brush, the technologist

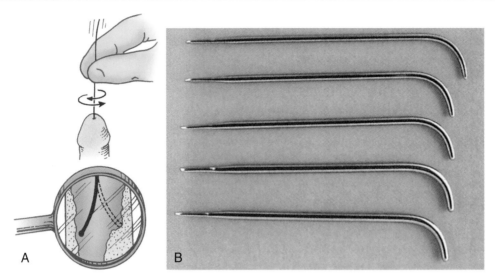

Figure 25-15   A, Use of a coudé catheter to release a urethral stricture. **B,** Urethral sounds. (**A** *From Rothrock J: Alexander's care of the patient in surgery, ed 17, Philadelphia, 2007, Mosby;* **B** *from Tighe SM: Instrumentation for the operating room, ed 7, St Louis, 2007, Mosby.)*

agitates the brush gently in normal saline to release the cells from the brush.

Postoperative Considerations

Bleeding and edema of the urethra are the most common complications of cystoscopic procedures. Urinary retention may occur as a result of pain or swelling. However, it generally is self-limiting and resolves spontaneously.

MANAGEMENT OF CALCULI

Surgical Goal

Calculi are removed from the ureter and urethra to relieve pain and restore continuity to the urinary tract.

Pathology

Renal stones are crystalline minerals and salts that precipitate from urine. The exact cause is unknown. They are the most common cause of urinary tract obstruction. The jagged structure of urinary calculi causes excruciating pain. Many types of calculi can occur, and each is composed of a different substance. Stones cause obstruction, pain, and infection and damage the urinary tract. Most calculi occur in the kidneys; they seldom form in the bladder.

Discussion

Bladder calculi, which do not pass through the urethra unaided, may be managed in several ways. Small stones may be grasped with stone-grasping forceps. A lithotrite is a specialized instrument that grasps and crushes the stone.

After routine cystoscopic assessment, the surgeon introduces the lithotrite into the scope. Under direct vision, the stone is crushed, and small pieces are flushed out of the bladder with an Ellik evacuator. Bleeders are coagulated with the Bugbee active electrode. Bladder stones must be retained in a dry container for pathological assessment.

TRANSURETHRAL RESECTION OF THE PROSTATE

Surgical Goal

In transurethral resection of the prostate (TURP), the prostate is removed with a resectoscope inserted through the urethra.

Pathology

Enlargement of the prostate generally is related to infection, a benign tumor, or malignancy. **Benign prostatic hyperplasia (BPH)** is nonmalignant enlargement of the prostate gland, which can occur in men over age 40. The prostate enlarges in two ways. In one type of growth, cells multiply around the urethra, causing obstruction. In the other type of growth, or middle-lobe prostate growth, cells grow into the urethra and the bladder outlet area. Obstructive disease may cause **reflux (backward flow)** of urine, infection, and difficulty voiding. BPH is commonly treated by resection.

Technique

1. The patient is positioned and prepped for a perineal procedure.
2. The bladder and bladder neck are assessed.
3. The urethra is dilated.
4. The resectoscope is inserted into the urethra.
5. The prostate is resected systematically.
6. Fragments are flushed from the bladder and collected as specimens.
7. The resectoscope is withdrawn, and a 30-mL Foley catheter is inserted.

Discussion

The patient is placed in the lithotomy position. A routine cystoscopy is performed with a 30-degree lens to evaluate the bladder and other structures. During resection, continuous irrigation or bladder distention with a nonelectrolytic solution (e.g., sorbitol or glycine) is used to maintain a clear surgical field and to evacuate small pieces of tissue.

Continuous irrigation permits clear visualization during resection. The resectoscope is constructed with an outer sheath that allows fluid to flow out of the instrument. Irrigation fluid must be maintained. As mentioned, a solution warmer is used to prevent hypothermia.

The surgeon lubricates the cystoscope and inserts it into the urethra. The obturator then can be removed, allowing the bladder to drain. The cysto assistant should be prepared to collect urine from this sample, because it will be submitted for analysis. Irrigation fluid is then instilled into the bladder. The bladder is assessed, and the cystoscope is removed.

The urethra is then dilated with van Buren sounds. The resectoscope is inserted, and resection begins at the middle and lateral lobes and continues in a systematic pattern. The small pieces of tissue that are released into the irrigation fluid may be evacuated with an Ellik evacuator or a Toomey syringe. The technologist must retain all pieces of specimen for pathological examination in a small basin.

After resection, a three-way Foley catheter is inserted, and the bladder is irrigated to ensure adequate flow and hemostasis. The catheter remains in place for 12 to 24 hours.

NOTE: Transurethral resection of a bladder tumor (TURBT) is performed in the same manner as TURP.

Other minimally invasive techniques used in prostatectomy include laser and transurethral needle ablation using ultrasound. TURP is illustrated in Figure 25-16.

Postoperative Considerations

After a TURP procedure, the patient may remain catheterized for several days to facilitate irrigation of the bladder. Possible postoperative complications include:

- Incontinence
- Impotence
- Infertility
- Passage of semen into the bladder instead of the urethra (retrograde ejaculation)
- Urethral stricture

FLEXIBLE AND RIGID URETEROSCOPY

Transurethral ureteroscopy is performed with a flexible or rigid ureteroscope. Ureteroscopy commonly is performed for the following:

- Diagnosis of congenital anomalies, disease, or trauma of the ureters and renal pelvis
- Management of renal calculi
- Tissue biopsy from the ureter or renal pelvis
- Management of ureteral stricture

A flexible ureteroscope ranges in size from 6.9 to 9 Fr. The flexible tip allows the scope to be positioned in the renal pelvis and advanced into the calyces. The ureteroscope has working channels for the insertion of instruments, suction, and irrigation.

A rigid ureteroscope is designed to accept accessory instruments, and the scope also has designated channels for suction, irrigation, and a telescope. A small-diameter, semirigid ureteroscope is narrower than 7.5 Fr. This allows dilation of the tip under direct vision. Rigid and flexible scopes often are used in the same surgery, each providing functions necessary to the procedure. For example, the rigid scope is used to dilate the lower ureter to allow passage of the flexible scope. The rigid scope is also used to implant catheters and stents (Figure 25-17). Instruments required for a ureteroscopy are listed in Box 25-2.

Irrigation

Irrigation fluid can be delivered through a pump or manually through the channel used for the working instruments. Sterile saline is used for most procedures that do not require the ESU. Sorbitol or glycine is used when electrosurgery is required. A contrast medium may be added to the irrigation fluid for a fluoroscopic examination.

Use of The Ureteroscope

The flexible ureteroscope is inserted with the aid of a guide wire made of Teflon-coated stainless steel. The guide wire is passed through the scope and advanced into the ureter and

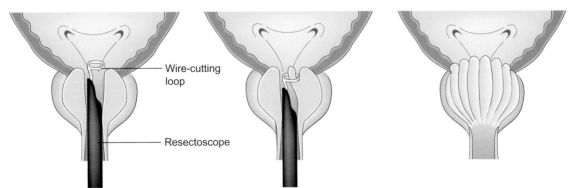

Figure 25-16   A, Transurethral resection of the prostate (TURP). An electrosurgical cutting loop is inserted through the urethra. **B,** The cutting loop is drawn back along the resectoscope sheath, cutting and coagulating the hypertrophied prostate. **C,** Prostatic capsule with prostate removed. *(From Garden O, Bradbury A, Forsythe J, Parks R: Principles and practice of surgery, ed 5, Edinburgh, 2007, Churchill Livingstone/Elsevier.)*

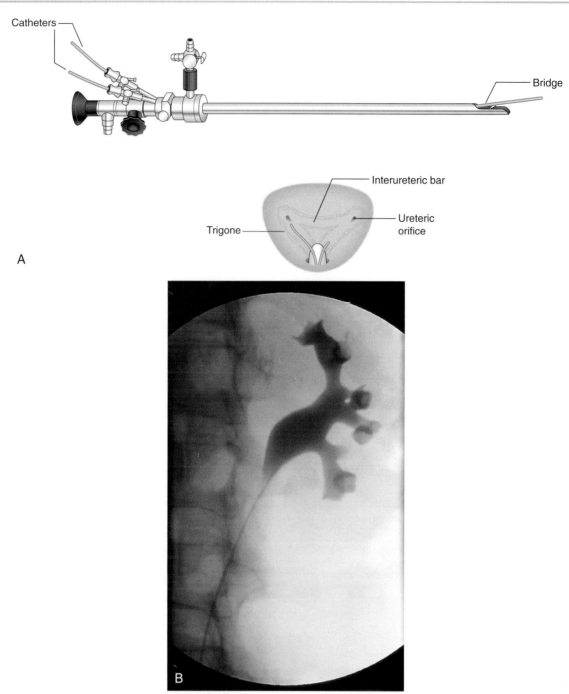

Catheters

Bridge

Interureteric bar

Trigone

Ureteric orifice

A

B

Figure 25-17 **A**, Cystourethroscope with bridge for insertion of urethral catheters. **B**, Retrograde ureteropyelography. The catheter is passed into the renal pelvis, and a contrast medium is injected. *(From Garden O, Bradbury A, Forsythe J, Parks R: Principles and practice of surgery, ed 5, Edinburgh, 2007, Churchill Livingstone/Elsevier.)*

renal pelvis under fluoroscopy. The ureteroscope is then advanced over the wire. The ureter may be dilated with a balloon dilator. After the scope is positioned in the renal pelvis, the flexible tip can be deflected to enter the renal calyces. Accessory instruments are threaded into the working channels to perform various types of procedures as described earlier.

Biopsy

Tissue biopsy is performed with cup forceps or with a flat wire basket. Cell biopsy can be taken with the cytology brush. After the specimen is retrieved on the brush, the technologist agitates the brush gently in a prepared specimen container holding normal saline to release the cells from the brush.

Box 25-2

Ureteroscopy Instruments

Ureteroscope
Guide wires
Cystoscope
Saline for irrigation
Connectors and tubing
Three-way stopcock
Syringes (20 and 50 cc)
Contrast media
Lithotriptor (as needed)
Grasper
Stone basket
Double-lumen catheter
Ureteral dilators
Active fulgurating electrode
Luer-Lok connectors
Specimen containers

Tumor Removal

Tumors can be removed by fulguration using the ESU or the holmium:YAG laser. Tumor tissue may also be removed in small increments using a resectoscope. In this case, tissue specimens must be retrieved and collected for pathological examination. (Chapter 19 presents a complete discussion of laser use and safety.)

Treatment For Calculi

The ureteroscope is used to remove or destroy stones in the renal pelvis or ureter. A rigid ureteroscope is inserted after the guide wire. Laser energy is delivered through a small quartz fiber (filament) to fragment the stone. An accessory such as a wire prong grasper or basket then can be used to extract fragments through the endoscope.

In flexible ureteroscopy, two guide wires are required. The first is a safety guide wire, and the second is used to facilitate insertion of the endoscope.

SURGERY OF THE MALE EXTERNAL GENITALIA

CIRCUMCISION (ADULT)

Surgical Goal

Circumcision is the removal of the prepuce (foreskin), which is done to improve hygiene and to abide by cultural and religious reasons.

Pathology

An uncircumcised male may develop a number of conditions that affect the glans and foreskin. Skin detritus can become trapped between the foreskin and glans, leading to infection and scarring. In these conditions the foreskin cannot be retracted from the glans (phimosis), or it adheres to the base of the glans and cannot be returned to its normal anatomical position (paraphimosis).

Some evidence indicates that uncircumcised males may be at risk for penile cancer related to repeated infection or exposure to human papilloma virus (HPV) (see Chapter 7). In general, circumcision is widely practiced. It may be a cultural practice, or it may be related to the perception that penile hygiene is enhanced by circumcision. Circumcision for adherence to religious tradition is practiced in the Jewish faith.

Technique

1. The foreskin is measured and marked.
2. The foreskin is pulled down over the glans with straight hemostats.
3. A dorsal incision is made in the skin and carried circumferentially.
4. The foreskin may be sutured to the corona and dressings applied.

Discussion

The patient is placed in the supine position, prepped, and draped with a small fenestrated sheet. The coronal ridge is outlined with a skin scribe to identify the incision. The surgeon places several Kelly, Crile, or mosquito hemostats on the edge of the prepuce. A longitudinal incision is made on the dorsal side of the foreskin with fine dissecting scissors. The incision is carried circumferentially around the prepuce, and small bleeders are controlled with the ESU.

The surgeon then sutures the wound edges to the corona with 4-0 or 5-0 interrupted absorbable sutures. The wound is dressed with petrolatum gauze.

Postoperative Considerations

Complications after circumcision are rare. However, bleeding and infection may occur. Infection is prevented with routine wound care and maintaining cleanliness of the site.

CHORDEE REPAIR

Surgical Goal

During chordee repair, constrictive penile tissue is released, allowing the penis to assume a normal (anatomical) position.

Pathology

Chordee is a congenital downward curvature of the penis caused by a band of connective tissue between the urethral opening and the glans. Chordee can be caused by a short urethra, fibrous tissues connecting the urethral opening, or both.

Discussion

A chordee may be surgically repaired anytime after 6 months of age. The goals of surgery are to improve the appearance and function of the penis.

If the chordee is the result of skin tightening, the doctor may shorten the dorsal foreskin and remove any fibrous tissue causing the curvature. If associated with hypospadias, chordee is corrected at the time of the hypospadias repair.

The patient is placed in the supine position and prepped and draped for a perineal procedure. A traction suture of 5-0 silk is placed through the glans. The planes on the shaft of the penis are dissected to the fascial layer.

The skin overlying the distal urethra is dissected free of its attachments to the urethra and the distal shaft. A 25-gauge butterfly needle is then inserted into the penile corpora, and normal saline is injected. This demonstrates any fibrous bands, which are dissected and released with fine tissue scissors. On completion of the release, the tissue is closed with 4-0 or 5-0 absorbable suture.

HYPOSPADIAS REPAIR

Surgical Goal

Hypospadias results in shortening of the urethra. The meatus can appear along the penile shaft or at the base of the scrotum.

Pathology

Hypospadias is a common congenital anomaly involving incomplete development of the distal urethra. This results in ventral shortening of the penis during erection and nonanatomical location of the urethral meatus. The defect has doubled in both incidence and severity in the past 15 years, with no apparent reason for the increase.

Discussion

Many procedures have been developed to treat hypospadias. The exact approach depends on the severity of the defect. Simple repair of the penis is performed in an outpatient setting, usually in one procedure. The principle of the technique is reconstruction of the urethra using a graft from the foreskin or buccal skin (the inside of the mouth). The urethra is thus extended, and the penile tissue is reconstructed around it. A urethral catheter is left in place during the initial postoperative period.

NOTE: **Epispadias** is a very rare condition in which the urethral meatus is located on the top side of the penis. This defect is associated with extrophy of the bladder and other developmental defects of the pelvis and GU system.

Figure 25-18 illustrates the procedure for hypospadias.

INSERTION OF A PENILE IMPLANT

Surgical Goal

A penile implant is surgically placed to treat impotence caused by organic disease. Two types of implants are available: a semirigid implant and an inflatable reservoir implant.

Pathology

A malfunction in the erectile system of the penis most often is caused by neurological disease, diabetes, vascular disease, or psychological issues. Patients for whom no organic cause can be found are carefully screened for this procedure.

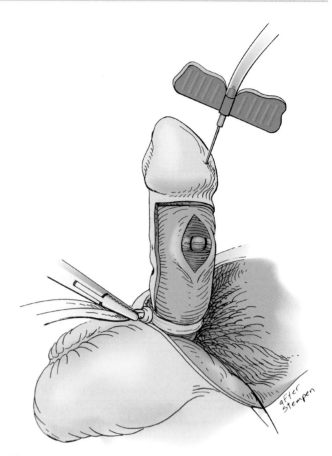

Figure 25-18 Hypospadias. *(From Walsh PC, Retik AB, Vaughan ED et al: Campbell's urology, ed 8, Philadelphia, 2002, WB Saunders.)*

Technique

1. A small incision is made at the base of the scrotum.
2. The tunica is incised to expose the corpus layer.
3. An implant inserter is positioned into the corporal tunnel, and the implant is put in place. This is repeated on each side of the penis.
4. A pocket is created in the scrotum for the pump.
5. A tunnel is made through the external ring to accommodate the reservoir.
6. The transversalis fascia is incised, and the reservoir is positioned.
7. The cylinders and pump are connected and tested.
8. The incisions are closed.

Discussion

Many types of inflatable penile implants are available. Each manufacturer provides detailed instructions on the tools and techniques used to place the implant. The technique described here uses an inflatable pump manufactured by American Medical Systems.

This surgery has three parts, and the system has three components. The cylinders are placed in the corpora cavernosa of the penis and can be inflated by the patient. The pump is placed surgically in the scrotum, and the reservoir, which contains the cylinder medium, is placed in the inguinal area.

The three-piece prosthesis has a fluid-filled reservoir that is placed into the abdominal wall. The pump release valve is located in the scrotum, and the two inflatable cylinders are located inside the penis.

The patient is placed in the supine or lithotomy position, prepped, and draped for a scrotal approach. The scrotum is incised, and the corpora cavernosa are exposed. The prosthesis cylinder is loaded onto a Furlow inserter and placed into the penile shaft. The pump is implanted in the scrotum, and the reservoir is inserted through the inguinal ring. Once the reservoir has been placed and inflated and the tubing has been connected, the device is tested in inflation and deflation. The incision is closed with a subcuticular suture and a supportive dressing is applied. The procedure is shown in Figure 25-19.

VARICOCELECTOMY

Surgical Goal

Varicocelectomy is ligation of the veins of the testes to reduce venous backflow of blood into the internal spermatic veins. It is done to improve spermatogenesis.

Pathology

A varicocele is a vascular abnormality in which the pampiniform venous plexus (veins of the spermatic cord) of the scrotum is dilated. The venous plexus can become twisted and dilated in the same manner as varicosity in the legs. The condition is associated with infertility, resulting in poor semen quality and sperm production. Varicocele may result in atrophy of the testis and is usually treated in adults.

Technique

1. An incision is made in the inguinal region below the external ring.
2. The fascia is divided, and the spermatic cord is isolated.
3. Varicose veins and tributaries are ligated with clips.
4. The incision is closed.

Discussion

Techniques for varicocelectomy include retroperitoneal, inguinal, and subinguinal varicocele repairs with and without magnification, laparoscopic repair, and percutaneous varicocelectomy with radiographic embolization of the internal spermatic veins.

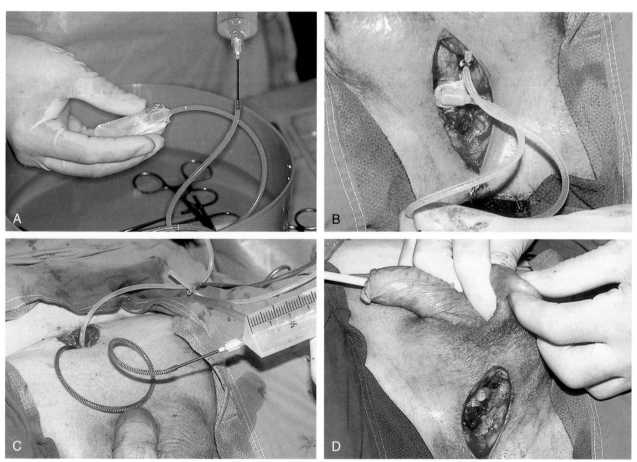

Figure 25-19 Penile implant. **A,** Preparation of the reservoir. **B,** Placement of the reservoir and cuff in the perineal incision. **C,** The reservoir and pump are filled with Hypaque to the appropriate volume. **D,** The pump is tested. *(Courtesy American Medical Systems, Minnetonka, Minn.)*

A 0.8- to 1.2-inch (2 to 3 cm) incision is made inferior to the level of the external ring. The incision is carried to the fascia. The spermatic cord is identified and then bluntly mobilized and grasped with a Babcock clamp. The cord is lifted to the level of the incision, and a Penrose is placed around it. At this stage the operating microscope may be introduced.

The spermatic fascia is incised and the testicular artery and veins identified. The veins are ligated with vessel clips or fine non absorbable suture.

Once all external spermatic veins have been divided, the cord is returned to the scrotum. The incision is closed with a 5-0 Monocryl subcuticular closure and reinforced with Steri-Strips.

HYDROCELECTOMY

Surgical Goal
A hydrocele is a benign, fluid-filled sac that develops in the anterior testis. It is drained and removed to prevent rupture and hemorrhage.

Pathology
A hydrocele may arise from trauma, infection, tumor, or as a result of peritoneal dialysis. It also may occur as a congenital condition related to failure of the internal ring to close in fetal life.

Technique
1. An incision is made in the scrotum over the hydrocele.
2. The hydrocele sac is brought out of the scrotum.
3. The sac is incised and emptied.
4. The incision is closed.

Discussion
The patient is placed in the supine position and prepped for a scrotal incision. The surgeon makes a small incision in the scrotum using the ESU. The hydrocele is delivered from the scrotum without rupturing it, and the ESU used to make a small incision in the sac membrane. The scrub should have suction immediately available to drain the sac, which is excised and removed. An alternative technique is to open the sac, evert the edges, and suture them to the surface of the testicle (Figure 25-20). The surgeon may insert a small Penrose drain in the wound, which then is closed in two layers with fine absorbable sutures. A bulky gauze dressing is applied.

Postoperative Considerations
Swelling and bleeding may occur in the immediate postoperative period.

ORCHIECTOMY

Surgical Goal
Orchiectomy is the surgical removal of one or both testicles.

Pathology
Removal of one testicle most often is performed in cases of testicular carcinoma or **torsion** (twisting of the testis, result-

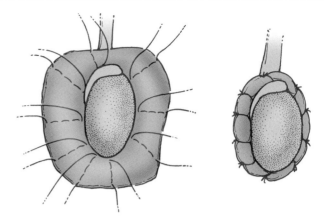

Figure 25-20 Hydrocele. The tunica vaginalis has been folded on itself and sutured in place to prevent recurrence. (From Rothrock J: Alexander's care of the patient in surgery, ed 17, St Louis, 2007, Mosby.)

ing in ischemia and necrosis). Bilateral orchiectomy may be performed to control metastatic carcinoma of the prostate.

Technique
1. An incision is made in the scrotum.
2. The testicle is mobilized using sharp and blunt dissection.
3. The spermatic vessels and vas deferens are clamped and divided.
4. The vascular structures and vas deferens are ligated.
5. The scrotum is closed.

Discussion
Testicular cancer usually arises from the germ (reproductive) cells of the male. It represents 1% of all cancers, but it is the most common cancer among young men. Early screening and vigorous public health campaigns have lowered the incidence in the past several decades.

Torsion of the testicle is rotation of the testicle around its proximal attachments. This causes interruption or complete cessation of the blood supply to the testicle, resulting partial or complete necrosis of the organ. The cause of torsion is related to a combination of weak (scrotal) fascial attachment and vigorous exercise. Orchiectomy is performed only when the testicle cannot be saved.

Orchiectomy can be performed using local anesthesia with sedation or with general anesthesia. The patient is placed in the supine position, prepped, and draped for a scrotal incision.

The surgeon makes a 1- to 1.2-inch (2.5- to 3-cm) midline incision into the anterior scrotal wall with a #15 blade. Using sponges and manual dissection, the surgeon separates the testicle from the fascia and subcutaneous tissue. This technique exposes the tunica vaginalis. The surgeon then delivers the testicle from the scrotal sac. Bleeders are controlled with the ESU.

The spermatic cord is identified, and the vas deferens is separated, doubled-clamped, cut, and ligated with 2-0 Vicryl ties. The testicular artery and veins are cross-clamped with Kelly or Mayo clamps. The tissue vessels are divided with the

ESU and ligated with size 0 absorbable synthetic suture ligatures.

The spermatic cord is replaced in anatomical position, and the septal layers are closed with a 3-0 Vicryl running suture. The wound is closed with an interrupted or subcuticular suture on a fine cutting needle. Antibiotic ointment may be applied to the incision. Dressing consists of gauze fluffs and a scrotal support. Testicular prosthetics may be inserted at the time of surgery or in a subsequent procedure.

Postoperative Considerations

Complications following orchiectomy may include those expected following cessation of testosterone production. These include loss of libido, fatigue, and tenderness of the breasts. Patients are prescribed testosterone postoperatively to prevent these symptoms. However, testosterone therapy may increase the risk of osteoporosis.

Patients undergoing orchiectomy require counseling both preoperatively and postoperatively. Loss of reproductive functions can result in depression, especially for young men.

VASECTOMY

Surgical Goal

Elective sterilization is performed by removing a section of the vas deferens and sealing the free ends. This prevents the movement of sperm through the ejaculatory ducts.

Technique

1. The scrotum is incised.
2. The vas deferens is isolated.
3. The duct is cross-clamped, and a section is removed.
4. The ends of the severed duct are coagulated.
5. The incision is closed.

Discussion

The patient is placed in the supine position, prepped, and draped for a scrotal incision. A local anesthetic (e.g., 1% or 2% lidocaine) is injected at the raphe with a 25- to 27-gauge needle.

The surgeon makes a small (0.4 inch [1 cm]) incision in the proximal scrotum over the vas deferens. Blunt and sharp dissection are used to isolate the vas tubule. Small bleeders are coagulated with the needle-point ESU.

The duct is cross-clamped, leaving a short section between the clamps. This surgeon transects and removes this section. The two severed ends of the vas deferens are coagulated with the ESU. The scrotum is closed with fine interrupted absorbable sutures. A bulky gauze dressing is applied.

The procedure for a vasectomy is illustrated in Figure 25-21.

VASOVASOSTOMY (REVERSAL OF A VASECTOMY)

Surgical Goal

Vasovasostomy is the surgical anastomosis of the vas deferens to restore continuity after vasectomy.

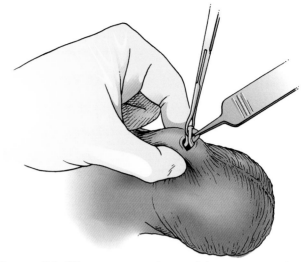

Figure 25-21 Vasectomy. The vas deferens is grasped with Babcock forceps through a scrotal incision. *(From Walsh PC, Retik AB, Vaughan ED et al: Campbell's urology, ed 8, Philadelphia, 2002, WB Saunders.)*

Pathology

Approximately 35,000 men per year undergo a vasectomy reversal in the United States. Anastomosis of the vas deferens is performed to restore fertility.

Technique

1. An incision is made over the vasectomy site.
2. The vas deferens is identified.
3. The operative microscope is brought to the field.
4. The ends of the vas deferens are prepared for anastomosis.
5. The anastomosis is performed.
6. The incision is closed.

Discussion

The patient is placed in the supine position and prepped for a groin incision. A vasovasostomy may be performed using a local block, epidural, spinal, or general anesthetic. The operating microscope is used for the anastomosis once the initial incision has been made.

A vertical scrotal incision is made directly over the site of the vasectomy, and the vas deferens is mobilized above and below the vasectomy site. The vas deferens is incised with a scalpel below and above the vasectomy site to provide clean edges for the anastomosis. A small amount of seminal fluid is expressed. This is preserved as a specimen to determine whether live sperm are present. The surgery continues even if the results are negative. The distal end of the vas is resected until a normal lumen is visible.

The two ends are placed closely together and held in place with an approximator clip. A two-layer anastomosis is used to close the duct. Anchoring sutures of 9-0 nylon suture are first placed through the muscular layer of the cut ends. The inner layer of the duct is identified, and an anastomosis is performed with 10-0 nylon suture. The second layer is anastomosed with 9-0 nonabsorbable interrupted sutures. The

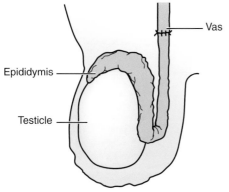

Figure 25-22 Reversal of a vasectomy. *(From Phillips N: Berry and Kohn's operating room technique, ed 10, St Louis, 2004, Mosby.)*

wound is closed in two layers with 3-0 and 4-0 absorbable suture.

Postoperative Considerations

Patients are monitored for postoperative swelling and possible hemorrhage. Severe injury to the spermatic artery during the procedure may lead to an atrophic testicle, although this is a rare complication. Reversal of a vasectomy is shown in Figure 25-22.

IMPLANTATION OF TESTICULAR PROSTHESES

Surgical Goal

Testicular prostheses are implanted after orchiectomy. A suprapubic approach is used to prevent postoperative infection.

Discussion

A 1.6- to 2-inch (4- to 5-cm) horizontal incision is made over the pubic symphysis. The ESU is used to extend the incision through the fascial layer. The spermatic cord is exposed and retracted with a Penrose drain. The testicular prosthesis is placed into the scrotal sac after hemostasis has been secured. A purse-string suture of 3-0 silk is used to close the neck of the scrotum. The fascia is closed with a 3-0 Vicryl, and the skin is closed with a 4-0 subcuticular suture. Steri-Strips and a gauze dressing are applied to the incision site.

SURGERY OF THE BLADDER AND URETERS

SUPRAPUBIC CYSTOSTOMY

Surgical Goal

Cystostomy is the insertion of a **suprapubic catheter** into the bladder for drainage. The catheter is inserted through a percutaneous or open approach.

Pathology

A suprapubic catheter is implanted to divert urine from the bladder directly to the outside of the body, bypassing the urethra. This done after surgery that requires urinary diversion (urethral or bladder surgery) and to eliminate the need for long-term urethral catheterization, which may lead to a urinary tract infection.

Technique

Open Procedure
1. A suprapubic incision is made.
2. The space of Retzius is entered.
3. The catheter is positioned in the bladder.
4. The bladder and wound are closed.

Discussion

The patient is placed in the supine position, prepped, and draped for a suprapubic incision. The incision passes through the skin, fatty subcutaneous layer, fascia, and muscle fibers. The peritoneal cavity is not entered, because the area lying between the bladder and the symphysis pubis (the space of Retzius, which is the operative site) is bounded superiorly (at the top) by the abdominal peritoneum. Because the muscle fibers are quite vascular and contain many large veins, the technologist should have an ample supply of lap sponges available. The surgeon makes the incision with the scalpel and carries it through to the bladder with the cautery pencil or dissecting scissors.

The surgeon places two Allis clamps on the bladder wall and makes a small incision between the clamps. A purse-string suture then is placed around the bladder incision, and the catheter is threaded into the bladder. A Malecot, Pezzer, or proprietary percutaneous catheter is used. The purse-string suture is tied snugly around the catheter, and the bladder incision is closed with size 0 or 2-0 interrupted sutures of chromic gut swaged to a tapered needle. The suprapubic incision then is closed in layers.

Percutaneous Approach

In an alternative method of suprapubic drainage, a Silastic catheter is placed in the bladder through a stab wound in the skin made over and through the bladder wall. A Cystocath catheter is commonly used. To insert the catheter, the surgeon uses a #11 knife blade to make the small stab incision. The Cystocath kit comes complete with a trocar and cannula, which are thrust through the stab incision. The trocar then is removed, and the catheter is inserted through the cannula. The surgeon removes the cannula and places a Silastic disk over the catheter and attaches it to the patient's skin with surgical adhesive. The wound is neither sutured nor dressed.

CYSTECTOMY

Surgical Goal

Cystectomy is the total or partial removal of the bladder. This procedure is performed most often to treat bladder cancer.

Pathology

Bladder cancer is the second most common cancer of the GU system (prostate cancer has the highest incidence). It arises most frequently from the transitional cells. The diagnosis is made by cystoscopy, which includes cytological brushing or bladder washing to collect cells for pathological assessment.

Total cystectomy is indicated for small, invasive tumors that penetrate the bladder wall. A more conservative partial cystectomy may be performed when cancer staging reveals no lymph node metastasis. After a cystectomy, a false bladder may be constructed using a portion of the ileum (see Ileal Conduit).

Technique

1. A lower midline incision is made and carried to the bladder.
2. The bladder is dissected, and major vessels are controlled.
3. The bladder is elevated to expose the cul-de-sac and peritoneum.
4. The bladder is dissected from the rectal wall.
5. The bladder pedicles are clamped and divided.
6. The broad ligament is incised, and the posterior vaginal wall, bladder neck, and proximal urethra are mobilized.
7. Males: The prostate and prostatic ligaments are mobilized and divided.
8. The urethra is cross-clamped and divided. The specimen is removed en bloc.
9. A urinary diversion procedure is initiated.

Discussion

If the patient is a male, prostatic instruments are required. A major laparotomy set is used for all cases. The scrub should have vessel loops, umbilical tapes, and a narrow, long Penrose drain available for retraction.

The patient is placed in the supine or low lithotomy position and prepped for a lower midline incision. A Foley catheter is inserted.

To begin the surgery, the surgeon makes a lower midline incision. The urachus (the fibromuscular attachment at the umbilicus) is clamped and divided. A self-retaining retractor (typically a Bookwalter retractor) is placed in the wound, and the bowel is packed away from the bladder with moist laparotomy sponges. If a lateral approach to the bladder is used, the duodenum and colon are packed to one side. The ureters are dissected and then transected from the bladder to increase mobilization.

The bladder is elevated, and each side (lateral pedicle) of the bladder is dissected separately. The internal iliac artery is identified, ligated, and divided. Branches also are ligated. Right-angle clamps often are used to pass suture ties under vessels during the dissection. The scrub should have a variety of sizes available. Heavy silk sutures or vascular clips typically are used to occlude the vessels. In the male, the vas deferens is divided with the urethra.

The bladder is retracted upward, and the peritoneum is incised. The anterior rectal wall is dissected free from the bladder. This exposes the seminal vesicles and prostate in the male, or the posterior vaginal wall in the female. The lateral pedicles of the bladder are mobilized, divided, and ligated with silk sutures or surgical clips. In the female, the broad ligament is excised to the level of the ovary and fallopian tubes. The surgeon separates the posterior vaginal wall from

the bladder using blunt dissection. The vaginal vault is closed after the excision.

The anterior dissection continues with dissection of the prostate away from the pubis. The ESU is used frequently to control small vessels that communicate with the prostate. The ESU tip must be kept clean. During the later stages of the dissection, the ESU is used often.

The urethra is isolated with a vessel loop or umbilical tape, clamped, and divided. The remaining fascial attachments are released, and the specimen is removed. A urinary diversion surgery is initiated. After a cystectomy, an ileal conduit or similar neobladder is created.

ILEAL CONDUIT

Surgical Goal

In an ileal conduit procedure, a functional bladder is constructed with a loop of bowel that is brought out of the abdominal wall. A stoma is created for urine drainage. This procedure has been widely successful for urinary diversion.

Pathology

Urinary diversion away from the bladder is performed before or after a radical cystectomy, in which the bladder and surrounding tissue have been removed as a treatment for cancer.

Technique

1. The bowel is mobilized to free a section of ileum.
2. The ileum is transected, and the proximal ileal segment and mesentery are closed.
3. The distal and proximal sections of the ileum are anastomosed.
4. The ureters are implanted into the ileal pouch.
5. A stoma is created in the abdomen.
6. A suction drain is placed in the incision, which is closed in layers.

Discussion

Many of the techniques used in this procedure are discussed as part of the bowel procedure (see Chapter 23). In preparation for the procedure, the scrub should have gastrointestinal and long instruments available.

The patient is placed in the supine position, and a Foley catheter is inserted. The patient then is prepped and draped for an abdominal incision (usually a low midline incision). To begin the procedure, the surgeon enters the abdomen and retroperitoneal cavity. A large self-retaining retractor is placed in the wound. A portion of the large intestine and adjoining ileum are mobilized, as for a bowel resection.

A linear stapling instrument may be used to resect the proximal limb of the ileum. The two severed ileal limbs are then anastomosed. When traditional suturing methods are used, four intestinal clamps are placed across a segment of the ileum, two at each end. The surgeon then divides the ileum in both locations, cutting between the sets of clamps with the ESU. The proximal end of the ileum is closed with a double layer of absorbable suture. The surgeon identifies the ureters and may place a small Penrose drain around them

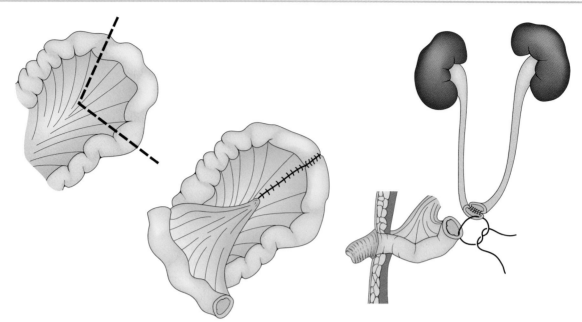

Figure 25-23 Ileal conduit. *(From Garden O, Bradbury A, Forsythe J, Parks R: Principles and practice of surgery, ed 5, Edinburgh, 2007, Churchill Livingstone/Elsevier.)*

for retraction. The ureters are divided from the bladder, and an end-to-side anastomosis is made between the ureters and the isolated segment of the ileum. The anastomosis is performed with 4-0 interrupted sutures of absorbable material.

Stoma Formation

To perform the ileostomy, the surgeon first incises the skin over the area of the proposed stoma, excising a small disk of tissue from the abdominal wall. Dissection is taken down to the rectus muscle. A Kelly clamp is passed bluntly through the rectus muscle. The open end of the ileal segment is then brought through the hole and everted. The edge of the stoma is sutured to the abdominal wall with 3-0 interrupted absorbable sutures. The wound is then irrigated, and a suction drain is placed in the abdomen. Closure is routine as described for a laparotomy. The approach used in ileal conduit is illustrated in Figure 25-23.

URINARY INCONTINENCE

Many procedures to correct urinary incontinence have been developed in recent years. Public demand for a rapid, relatively noninvasive procedure and interest among genitourinary surgeons have resulted in many experimental surgeries. Special devices and equipment have been quickly developed and marketed to meet the technical requirements of these procedures. Some have shown promise, whereas others have been discarded because of failure or technical difficulty and a steep learning curve for the surgeon.

No longitudinal studies have been performed to analyze the long-term success of these newer procedures, which are all based on the classic Marshall-Marchetti-Krantz and Burch

procedures. In all cases, the bladder neck and urethra are suspended from and anchored to the pubic symphysis or pubourethral ligaments with various devices, such as sutures, screws, needles, tape, mesh, or biological material. Laparoscopic and vaginal procedures are preferred over open retropubic techniques. Other procedures, such as implantable electronic devices that control the symptoms of incontinence and a synthetic sphincter, also have been approved in the United States.

The procedures in this section are limited to standard surgeries. The surgical technologist will be able to adapt these to implantation of devices and newer procedures that may or may not have technological longevity.

VESICOURETHRAL SUSPENSION (MARSHALL-MARCHETTI-KRANTZ PROCEDURE)

Surgical Goal

Vesicourethral suspension (Marshall-Marchetti-Krantz procedure) is a suspension of the bladder neck and urethra to the cartilage of the pubic symphysis to treat urinary stress incontinence in the female.

Pathology

Urinary incontinence is involuntary loss of urine. The condition has many causes, including multiple childbirths, prolonged or obstructed labor in childbirth, diabetes, neurological injury, and age. Stress incontinence occurs during exertion of the pelvic muscles, or "bearing down." Functional incontinence can be classified as a bladder or a urethral disorder. In most cases, loss of urethral support at the ureterovesical junction or proximal urethra is seen. Overflow incontinence is caused by an "overactive" detrusor muscle with a normal urethra.

Urinary incontinence is both a hygienic and a psychosocial problem. The number of new cases has increased as the population of aging adults has grown.

Technique

1. A lower midline or Pfannenstiel incision is made, and the space of Retzius is entered.
2. The bladder is retracted upward.
3. Several sutures are inserted into the bladder neck and attached to the back side of the symphysis pubis.
4. The wound is closed.

Discussion

The patient is placed in the low lithotomy position and prepped and draped for a combined suprapubic and perineal procedure. A vaginal prep is performed, and a Foley catheter is inserted.

The surgical technologist should have long instruments available, including long needle holders and long Allis clamps.

A suprapubic incision is made and carried through the space of Retzius. A wide Deaver or bladder blade retractor is placed over the bladder to retract it upward, exposing urethra; this is managed by the assistant.

The surgeon grasps the bladder neck with several long Allis clamps. Several 2-0 interrupted sutures of Dexon or Dacron, mounted on a small, stout, tapered needle, are then placed through the bladder neck and cartilage of the symphysis pubis. Several of these sutures are placed in succession. The sutures are left long.

The assistant lifts the urethra by applying transvaginal pressure on the urethra; this releases tension on the sutures to allow the sutures to be tied. After this maneuver, the scrub must reglove the assistant. This completes the procedure. A large Penrose drain is placed in the space of Retzius, and the wound is closed in routine fashion.

The Marshall-Marchetti-Krantz procedure is illustrated in Figure 25-24.

PUBOVAGINAL SLING

Surgical Goal

The bladder neck is held in suspension with a biosynthetic strip or fascia graft which is attached to the abdominal wall.

Technique

1. A low transverse incision is made to expose the rectus muscle.
2. The anterior vaginal mucosa is incised, and the incision is carried to the urethra and bladder neck.
3. An anterior vaginal wall flap is created, and dissection is carried to the pubic bone.
4. The graft is measured and positioned.
5. Cystoscopy is performed to assess tension on the graft.
6. The graft is secured.
7. A suprapubic catheter is inserted.
8. The wounds are closed.

Discussion

Material for the sling is taken from the rectus fascia, abdominal fascia, or fascia lata (requiring a separate small incision in the thigh). Biosynthetic materials include polypropylene mesh, Mersilene, Silastic, or Gore-Tex, which are marketed under various proprietary names. Commercially prepared sling systems may include accessory attachments and instruments for securing the sling.

The graft of fascia lata may be an allograft or an autograft. An autograft is fascia lata that has been removed from the

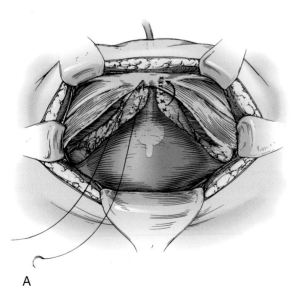

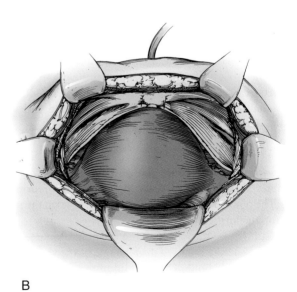

A   B

Figure 25-24 Marshall-Marchetti-Krantz procedure (vesicourethral suspension). **A,** Sutures are secured through the bladder neck. **B,** The vaginal wall is sutured to the symphysis. (Modified from Walsh PC, Retik AN, Vaughan ED et al: Campbell's urology, ed 8, Philadelphia, 2002, WB Saunders.)

patient's own fascia in one of two ways. In the abdominal approach, the rectus fascia is removed laterally from one iliac crest to the other through a Pfannenstiel incision. The fascia also may be removed in the lateral thigh through two vertical incisions midthigh and above the knee. The graft is dissected out through a tunnel created between the two incision sites.

An allograft may be freeze dried or fresh frozen fascia lata obtained from a cadaver. Fresh frozen fascia lata is the preferred material for repair, because it produces a stronger repair with minimal dissection and a faster recovery time than an autograft or synthetic material. If an allograft is used, the patient may have the procedure performed on an outpatient basis. If an autograft is used, the patient may need to be hospitalized for up to 3 days for postoperative pain management.

In the pubovaginal sling procedure, the graft is attached to the pubic bone, therefore in addition to the normal instrumentation required for cystoscopic and bladder-suspension procedures, the scrub must have a drill and an anchoring system available

The patient is anesthetized and placed in the lithotomy position with Allen stirrups. A lower abdominal and vaginal prep is performed. If a fascia lata autograft is to be obtained from the thigh, a separate setup for prepping, draping, and instrumentation is needed for the operative leg. The patient is draped with lithotomy drapes. Cystoscopy is performed, and a Foley catheter is inserted.

The labia majora may be sutured laterally for retraction. An Auvard weighted vaginal speculum is inserted, and a local anesthetic with epinephrine is injected into the lower abdominal incision site and the vaginal mucosa to maintain hemostasis.

A lower transverse incision is made just above the symphysis pubis. The tissue is spread by blunt dissection to expose the anterior rectus muscle. The incision is packed with sponges moistened with an antibiotic solution.

The vaginal portion of the procedure is then performed. The surgeon inserts a Foley catheter into the urethra and measures the length of the urethral meatus by placing the Foley catheter and inflating the balloon at the internal vesicle neck. The catheter is marked, deflated, and removed. The balloon on the catheter is then reinflated, measured, and again deflated. The catheter is reinserted into the patient.

To create space for the sling, the surgeon incises the anterior vaginal mucosa, raises the vaginal mucosal flap, and continues dissection to expose the pubic bone. The surgeon perforates the endopelvic fascia and enters the retropubic space. The power drill is used to create small holes in the pubic bone for anchoring the sutures.

The sutures are then anchored to the pubic bone.

A Stamey needle is passed through one of the vaginal incisions to the pubic bone. The free end of the suturing system is passed parallel to the posterior symphysis pubis. The needle is guided through the fascia and periurethral tissues along the bladder neck. The Foley catheter is again removed, and a cystoscope is used to check the position of the needle. The same process is followed at the other vaginal incision site.

The free end of the suture then is placed through the graft. The Stamey needle is used to pass the graft to the pubic site. The graft is sutured to the pubic bone or paraurethral fascia. The free end of the graft is passed between the urethra and vaginal mucosa. The surgeon places the free end of the graft into the opposite vaginal wound. The excess graft is excised, and the process is repeated for the other side.

The tension of the graft (ability to stop the urinary flow) is tested before the sling is sutured in place. The surgeon performs this step with the cystoscope and by inflating the bladder with fluid. The surgeon may directly visualize the flow of urine, and as the assistant applies tension and pulls the suture upward, the flow of urine should stop. The surgeon then sutures the graft in place. Testing is repeated on the opposite side of the graft before it is secured.

A suprapubic catheter is inserted while the bladder is still full of fluid. The abdominal incision is closed with an absorbable suture. The vaginal mucosa is closed with an absorbable suture, and a packing coated with sulfa cream is inserted into the vagina.

The pubovaginal sling procedure is illustrated in Figure 25-25.

Related Procedures

- Tension-free vaginal tape
- Needle urethropexy
- Inter-Stim implantation
- Artificial urethral sphincter

PROSTATE PROCEDURES

Prostatectomy traditionally has been performed by cystoscopic resection or open surgery using various perineal and suprapubic techniques. Modern prostatectomy is performed laparoscopically, robotically, or through an open approach (perineal or suprapubic) and by cystoscopic resection. Brachytherapy, which involves the implantation of radon seeds, and cryosurgery also are done to treat prostate cancer.

PERINEAL PROSTATECTOMY

Surgical Goal

Perineal prostatectomy is the removal of a prostatic adenoma through a perineal approach. In the past, prostatectomy often resulted in impotence and incontinence. Nerve-sparing procedures now are practiced to prevent these complications.

Pathology

Cancer of the prostate is a slow-growing cancer. There are about 230,000 cases and 40,000 deaths per year in the United States. A prostate-specific antigen (PSA) blood test and digital rectal examination are the initial tests. A percutaneous biopsy is performed if the results of these tests are abnormal. Surgical intervention is discussed with the patient, and all treatment options are provided in counseling.

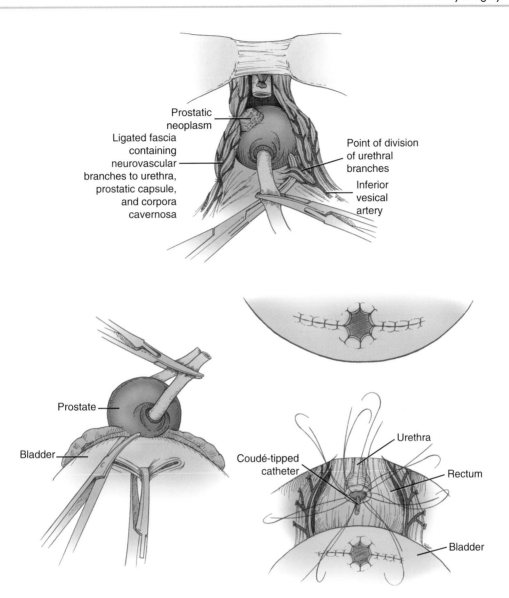

Figure 25-27, cont'd.

frozen section, and lymph node removal is performed at the time of prostate surgery. The results of the frozen section determine the need for wider pelvic excision.

Laparoscopic Prostatectomy

Laparoscopic prostatectomy is performed with the patient in the low lithotomy position. Three or four trocar ports are used, including an umbilical site for the camera port. After pneumoperitoneum has been established, the camera port is placed and the remaining trocars are inserted under direct vision.

The procedure follows anatomical dissection for the open prostate technique. The prostate is systematically dissected from the bladder, seminal vesicles, urethra, rectum, and vascular bundles. The ESU or LigaSure system is used to coagulate and to cut away the margins of the prostate, which contain the neurovascular supply necessary for erectile function. Endoscopic clips are used to ligate the two vascular bundles on either side of the prostate.

Once the dissection planes have been established and the prostate can be enucleated from the capsule, the urethra is divided as in an open procedure. The prostate is removed through an endoscopic collection sac.

Continuity of the urethra is re-established after insertion of a Foley catheter. Anastomosis of the urethra to the bladder is performed in two layers using continuous fine monofilament sutures. The Foley catheter remains in place.

Bleeding is controlled, and the wound is irrigated with warm saline. The ports are withdrawn, and the incisions are closed with one or two layers of absorbable synthetic suture and Steri-Strips.

Postoperative Considerations

With laparoscopic or robotic-assisted surgery (see the following section), the patient can be discharged from the hospital 1 or 2 days after surgery. The urethral catheter remains in place to allow the urethral anastomosis to heal. Patients experience some level of incontinence in the recovery period.

Nerve-sparing procedures provide a greater level of continence and erectile function.

ROBOTIC-ASSISTED PROSTATECTOMY

Robotic-assisted laparoscopic prostatectomy follows the surgical techniques used in the routine laparoscopic procedure, with some technical differences. The robotic arms are used to guide the instruments, and the monitor view is three-dimensional and magnified by 10.

The preparation of the patient is the same as for laparoscopy. The patient is placed in the low lithotomy position, and the robotic arms enter from between the patient's knees. The surgical technologist and the surgeon's assistant operate at the bedside.

The anatomical and surgical steps of the procedure are the same as those described for laparoscopy. The prostate is dissected from the bladder, urethra, rectum, seminal vesicles, and vascular bundles as described previously. An important difference in the robotic procedure is the ability to access smaller and more complex anatomical structures with the Endowrist graspers and scissors and the bipolar ESU. In the hands of an experienced surgeon, this provides a more complete dissection.

The roles of the surgical technologist in the procedure include those outlined in Chapter 21. The technologist assists in instrumentation, providing the correct instruments as requested. The technologist also is responsible for inserting instruments into the robotic locking device with the help of the surgical assistant. Other considerations for maintaining a sterile field and safe patient environment are the same as for all procedures. (Chapter 21 presents a more detailed discussion of the robotic setup and technique.)

SURGERY OF THE URETER AND KIDNEY

URETERAL DIVERSION

Surgical Goal

Injury, disease, or a congenital anomaly of the ureter may result in a distended, obstructed, or nonfunctional ureter. Ureteral diversion surgery is performed to restore continuity between the kidney and the bladder.

Pathology

Diseases that constrict the ureter result in **reflux** or a buildup of filtrate in the renal pelvis. This is referred to as **hydronephrosis**. Over time, the ureter or its proximal junction at the kidney becomes grossly distended and damaged. The term *vesicourethral reflux (VUR)* refers to conditions of backward flow from the bladder and the ureter. Examples of common obstructive pathological conditions include the following:

- Calculi that can constrict the ureters and cause injury
- Infection that results in ureteral scarring
- Prostatic hyperplasia
- Congenital abnormalities that result in stricture or malfunction

- Retroperitoneal or abdominal tumor that exerts severe pressure on the ureters
- Disease or a congenital defect that arises at the ureterovesical junction in the bladder

Discussion

Ureteral diversion surgeries vary according to the severity of disease in the ureter. The goal of surgery is to reimplant the ureter in a new location and provide continuity of urine flow.

The site of implantation determines the techniques and approach to surgery. Ureteral procedures, both open and laparoscopic techniques, use an approach from the flank or abdomen. Patient positioning, instruments, and equipment correspond to these approaches. General surgical instruments, including delicate dissection scissors, clamps, and forceps, are required. Vascular forceps often are used to prevent injury to the ureter.

The ureter itself is extremely small, and in all cases a ureteral stent is required at some point in the surgical and postoperative period. The ureter is anastomosed with 4-0 to 7-0 absorbable sutures. Traction sutures and Silastic vessel loops are used in all cases. A Penrose drain often is used for ureteral retraction. The muscles and fascia surrounding the ureters are dissected with standard instruments and small sponge dissectors.

The following are some of the terms used to describe ureteral surgery:

Pyeloplasty (Figure 25-28): *Pyelo* (renal pelvis) and *plasty* (reconstruction). Pyeloplasty is the reconstruction of the ureter at the level of the renal pelvis.

Uretero: Indicates a procedure of the ureter. (Do not confuse *uretero* with *urethro*, which pertains to the urethra.)

Ureteroplasty: Reconstruction of the ureter.

Ureterostomy: Anastomosis of the ureter with another hollow structure to provide continuity.

Transureteroureterostomy: Trans (across or joining), *uretero* (pertaining to the ureter), *ostomy* (joining two hollow or tubular structures). Transureteroureterostomy is the crossing of one ureter to another to create an anastomosis between the two ureters. This technique may also be called a *ureteroureterostomy*.

Vesicoureterostomy: Vesico (bladder), ureterostomy (anastomosis of the ureter). Vesicoureterostomy is the reimplantation of the ureter in the bladder.

PERCUTANEOUS NEPHROLITHOTOMY

Surgical Goal

In percutaneous nephrolithotomy (PCNL), large stones in the kidney or upper ureter are removed percutaneously through the nephroscope.

Pathology

Percutaneous nephrostomy, which involves the insertion of a tube into the renal pelvis for drainage, is indicated for selected patients with calculi lodged in the renal pelvis

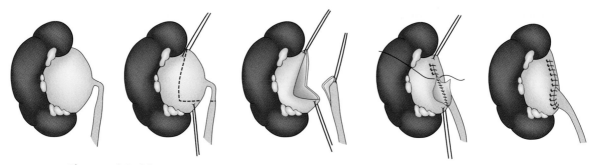

Figure 25-28 Pyeloplasty. *(From Garden O, Bradbury A, Forsythe J, Parks R: Principles and practice of surgery, ed 5, Edinburgh, 2007, Churchill Livingstone/Elsevier.)*

or upper ureter. It is performed under the following circumstances:

- The stone (or stones) are extremely large (larger than 2.5 cm), such as a **staghorn stone**.
- Conservative treatment, such as oral medication to dissolve the stones, has failed.
- The patient exceeds the weight limit (300 pounds [135 kg]) for extracorporeal shock wave therapy.
- The stone cannot be reached through the endoscopic ureteroscope.
- The stone is infected (the percutaneous method allows evacuation of infectious material at the time of the procedure).

Technique

1. The patient is placed in the prone position, and the flank and back are prepped and draped.
2. A hollow needle is inserted near the renal pelvis under ultrasound or fluoroscopy.
3. The first needle is replaced by a second needle with stylet, which is inserted into the renal pelvis.
4. A guide wire is passed into the renal pelvis.
5. A catheter is placed over the guide wire and inflated to expand the space.
6. A contrast medium is infused into the renal pelvis.
7. The nephroscope is inserted into the tunnel.
8. Stones are fragmented and removed through the nephroscope.
9. A ureteral catheter is positioned in the renal pelvis.
10. The scope is withdrawn.

Discussion

The procedure is performed under fluoroscopic guidance. Staff members must don lead aprons before the procedure. Intraoperative CT or ultrasound scanning also may be used.

A local anesthetic with monitored intravenous anesthesia is used. The patient is placed in the prone position, prepped, and draped for a midback procedure.

A rigid or flexible nephroscope may be used. The standard rigid scopes are available in sizes 19.5 to 26 Fr. Accessories include a working channel that accepts stone crushing and grasping instruments, a holmium:YAG laser fiber, and a ultrasonic lithotripter. A flexible nephroscope has a deflectable tip that is used to reach inside the calyx from its position in the renal pelvis. Warm isotonic irrigation fluid (0.9%

saline) is used to flush the operative site during nephroscopy. Precautions for preventing extravasation are same as those used in cystoscopic procedures. The surgical technologist and circulator must keep track of the amount of irrigation fluid used and the outflow to determine the amount absorbed.

To start the procedure, the surgeon uses a small-bore needle to puncture the skin near (but not into) the renal pelvis. The puncture site is located, under fluoroscopic or ultrasound guidance, between the twelfth rib and the ilium. The small needle then is replaced with a larger needle with a stylet. The stylet is removed, and a contrast medium is injected into the renal pelvis to identify the diseased calyx. The C-arm is rotated to provide optimal views. A guide wire is then passed through the needle sheath and positioned in the renal pelvis.

To pass the nephroscope, the surgeon must make a tract through the tissue. This is done by inserting balloon dilators over the guide wire, which is continually observed on the fluoroscope. When the tract is large enough to admit the nephroscope, the dilator is removed and the scope is inserted into the tract.

Stone-crushing forceps, stone baskets, and crushers are used to fragment the stone, which is flushed from the tract through the endoscope's working channels. Rigid and flexible endoscopes may be used during the same procedure. The surgical technologist should have accessories and equipment available for both sets. Large stones are fragmented and flushed through the working channel of the nephroscope. These must be retained as specimens. Staghorn stones are particularly sharp, and the fragments may require extraction with a grasping forceps.

When all stone fragments have been removed and the operative site has been irrigated, a nephrostomy tube is inserted into the tract. Foley or Malecot catheters are commonly used for this purpose. A Foley catheter provides continuous tamponade (pressure) within the operative site to control postoperative bleeding. A staged lithotomy may be required for several days after the surgery. In this case, a Malecot catheter is used. Occasionally a ureteral stent is implanted at the close of surgery.

Postoperative Considerations

Patients are monitored closely for postoperative bleeding and loss of kidney function. A chest radiograph may be taken in the PACU to make sure the lung was not punctured during insertion of the guide wire. Complications include recurrent stones, a urinary fistula, and ureteral obstruction.

SIMPLE NEPHRECTOMY (FLANK INCISION)

Surgical Goal
Simple nephrectomy is the surgical removal of one kidney.

Pathology
A nephrectomy is performed most often for severe hydronephrosis, obstruction, localized tumor, stones with infection, and trauma to the kidney. A kidney also may be removed from a live donor for transplantation.

Technique
1. A flank incision is made and carried through the oblique and transverse muscles.
2. A rib resection may be performed.
3. The ureter is cross-clamped, divided, and ligated.
4. The kidney pedicle is divided.
5. The kidney is removed.
6. The wound is closed.

Discussion
The patient is placed in the lateral position with the flank over the table break or kidney lift. The individual is then prepped for a subcostal flank incision. A Foley catheter is inserted before the start of surgery.

The surgeon makes the flank incision along the twelfth rib, extending to the border of the rectus muscle. If a rib must be resected, the eleventh or twelfth rib is first stripped of periosteum with a Doyen elevator or with osteotomes. This is necessary to allow the rib cutter to cut through the bone effectively. The surgeon grasps the rib with an Oschner or Kocher clamp and then uses a Bethune shears or rib cutter to cut the rib. The scrub should have bone wax available to be placed over the cut portions, which also may require some trimming to remove sharp edges.

The incision is carried through the subcutaneous and oblique muscles with the ESU. A self-retaining retractor is placed in the wound after the surgeon protects the edges of the wound with laparotomy sponges.

The Gerota capsule (perirenal fascia) is identified, and perirenal fat is removed. The scrub must preserve all perirenal fat in a small basin because it may be used to help control bleeding later in the surgery.

The ureter is identified, double-clamped with Mayo clamps, divided, and ligated with size 0 or 2-0 absorbable sutures. The surgeon mobilizes the kidney pedicle, including the renal vessels, by sharp and blunt dissection. To ensure that the renal artery is occluded securely, surgeon triple-clamps the vessels, and suture ligatures are placed through each vessel. An endovascular stapler can be used to ligate the vessels. This pedicle is then divided. The ligatures are not cut but are left long and tagged with a small hemostat.

The surgeon then removes the kidney from the wound. All bleeding is controlled with the ESU. The pedicle ligatures are cut, and the wound is irrigated with warm saline.

Before closure, the operating table is returned to a flat position to release tension on the flank tissues.

A Penrose drain is placed in the kidney fossa and brought out through a separate stab wound. If a rib was removed, the periosteum may be closed separately. The incision is then closed in layers. The fascia and muscle layers are closed with interrupted absorbable sutures. The skin is closed with staples.

LAPAROSCOPIC RADICAL NEPHRECTOMY

Surgical Goal
In a laparoscopic radical nephrectomy, the kidney and lymph nodes are removed to treat cancer.

Pathology
A primary tumor of the kidney arises from the renal cortex (the most common site) or the renal pelvis. The incidence is higher in men than in women. Risk factors include smoking, obesity, and exposure to industrial chemicals (e.g., petroleum products) and heavy metals.

Technique
1. Pneumoperitoneum is established, and trocar ports are placed.
2. The kidney and ureter are mobilized from the bowel, mesentery, muscle, and fascia attachments.
3. The renal artery and vein are isolated and divided.
4. The adrenal vessels are isolated, divided, and ligated with surgical clips.
5. The ureter is divided and ligated with surgical clips.
6. A specimen sac is introduced through a 12-mm cannula, and the kidney is placed inside.
7. The cannula is withdrawn, and the opening is exposed. (The kidney may be withdrawn through an extended incision in the abdomen.)
8. A morcellator is introduced inside the specimen sac, and the kidney is fragmented.
9. The specimen is removed with suction, and the sac is withdrawn.
10. The pneumoperitoneum is released, and the wounds are closed.

Discussion
General laparoscopic instruments, a vessel-sealing system, an ultrasonic scalpel, and vessel clips are needed for the procedure. The surgical technologist must also be ready to convert to an open procedure. A separate setup with laparotomy, kidney, and vascular instruments should be immediately available for conversion.

The patient is placed in the modified lateral position with the flank positioned over the table break. A soft, padded lift may be used to expand the flank, or the table may be flexed to achieve the same effect. Wide tape is placed over the ilium and secured to the table frame to maintain the patient in the lateral position. A combined flank and abdominal prep is performed, and a Foley catheter is inserted.

The initial trocar ports are inserted with the table rolled for access to the abdomen. After pneumoperitoneum has been established, the table is rolled back and the remaining ports are placed. A 10- or 12-mm port and one or two 5-mm ports are used.

With pneumoperitoneum established, the 10-mm trocar is inserted near the umbilicus. The table then is tilted, and the remaining ports are inserted. Sutures are used to secure the ports.

After examining the peritoneal cavity, the surgeon begins the dissection by using scissors, a Harmonic scalpel, and an ESU hook to separate the colorenal ligaments and mesentery from the kidney. This frees the bowel and provides access to the kidney and ureter.

The ureter is identified, and dissection continues along the lower pole of the kidney. The dissection may be completed using only the Harmonic scalpel, probe, and ESU hook, although dissecting scissors and forceps also may be used. The renal vein and artery are ligated with surgical staples before they are divided from the hilum. The adrenal vessels are ligated and smaller vessels are coagulated with the vessel-sealing system or clips.

To divide the ureter, the surgeon places two sets of surgical clips across the structure and incises the section between the clips. The kidney is moved to the abdomen by gentle manipulation.

The specimen can be removed by morcellization, or it can be brought out of the abdomen intact. Intact removal is performed through the 12-mm port using a specimen removal sac. The patient is rolled to expose the abdomen. The sac is inserted through the port and opened in the abdominal cavity. The specimen is pulled into the sac, which is pulled into the trocar. The trocar is withdrawn with the neck of the sac exposed. The incision is extended to accommodate the sac and specimen.

If the morcellization technique is used, the neck of the sack is brought out through the 12-mm trocar incision. The morcellator is inserted into the sac, and the specimen is fragmented. The fragments are removed from the sac with a suction tube, and the sac is withdrawn. The incision is closed.

The wound is then irrigated and checked for hemorrhage. All trocars are removed, and the incisions are closed with 2-0 and 3-0 absorbable sutures. The skin is approximated with interrupted monofilament sutures or skin staples.

KIDNEY TRANSPLANTATION

Surgical Goal
Kidney transplantation involves removing a kidney from a living donor or cadaver and implanting it into the patient.

Pathology
Kidney transplantation is performed for acute or chronic ESRD.

Discussion
Kidney transplantation is performed by a transplant team, and the routines are well established. In this procedure, surgeons operate on the living donor and recipient simultaneously. However, the kidney can be perfused to preserve the tissues. This discussion is limited to essential points in the procedure.

Before the transplantation process begins, the patient's name, date of birth, the side of the kidney, and the ABO blood compatibility should be confirmed with the team and transplant coordinator.

The operating rooms should connect to minimize contamination if the kidney is removed from a living donor.

The donor kidney is removed as described in the section Simple Nephrectomy (Flank Incision), with several major differences. The renal pedicle, which contains the vascular supply, is isolated and ligated before the kidney is removed. The Gerota fascia may be left intact on the donor kidney.

After removal, the donor kidney is preserved in cold solution and perfused with the surgeon's choice of electrolyte solution. When the recipient team is ready to receive the kidney, the surgeon transports it in a covered container, maintaining the correct temperature. The donor wound is closed as previously described.

The recipient patient is prepped and draped for a right iliac incision. An incision is made in the right lower quadrant and carried to the retroperitoneum. A self-retaining retractor is placed in the wound. The surgeon dissects through the rectus muscle and preserves the epigastric vessels for anastomosis later in the procedure. In a male, the spermatic cord is identified and retracted; in a female, the round ligament is identified and ligated. Vascular forceps and fine dissecting scissors are used to mobilize the hypogastric artery to the level of the bifurcation of the aorta.

The donor kidney then is brought to the field, and the vessels are trimmed as needed to accommodate the recipient structures. The kidney is returned to cold solution until the surgeon is ready for implantation.

The internal iliac artery is divided after it has been cross-clamped with a curved or an angled vascular clamp. The proximal side of the artery remains clamped. All the remaining venous tributaries must be ligated with 2-0 or 3-0 silk with the double-clamp and tie method. To prepare the iliac vein for the end-to-side renal anastomosis, the surgeon places Fogarty clamps proximal and distal. The iliac vein is flushed with heparinized saline, and six vascular sutures are put in place to secure the anastomosis later.

The kidney is secured in a slush "sling," and the anastomosis of the iliac vein and renal artery is sutured with 5-0 or 6-0 vascular sutures. The renal artery then is anastomosed to the proximal arm of the iliac artery. The iliac artery clamps are removed, and the anastomosis is observed.

To begin ureteral implantation, the surgeon incises the anterior bladder. The donor ureter is then placed through the bladder wall, and the edges are anastomosed to the inner bladder lining with fine absorbable sutures. A catheter stent is placed into the ureter through the anastomosis. It is advanced into the renal pelvis superiorly and brought out through the urethra. The surgeon then closes the bladder incision in two layers, using 4-0 or 5-0 absorbable sutures for the bladder lining and 2-0 sutures for the muscle layer. The bladder is irrigated to check for leakage.

The fascia is closed with size 0 running absorbable suture. The subcutaneous tissue is closed with a 2-0 or 3-0 interrupted stitch, and the skin is closed with fine nylon. One or two suction drains may be placed in the wound during closure. The wound is dressed with gauze fluffs and tape.

Postoperative Considerations

Patients are monitored closely for acute organ rejection, hemorrhage, and infection in the immediate postoperative period. Immunosuppression therapy leaves patients who have undergone transplantation at increased risk of infection and cancer.

ADRENALECTOMY

Adrenalectomy is the removal of one or both adrenal glands. Adrenalectomy usually is performed by conventional (open) surgery, or minimally invasive approach may be used in selected patients.

Adrenalectomy is indicated for pheochromocytoma, Cushing syndrome, adrenocortical carcinoma, renal carcinoma, and hyperaldosteronism. Hypersecretion of adrenocorticotropic hormone (ACTH) may cause neuroblastoma and affect the growth of other tumors that depends on adrenal secretions. Adrenal diseases are often life-threatening, and the procedure has many potential postoperative metabolic complications.

A number of techniques may be used for adrenalectomy, including open surgery through an abdominal, or thoracoabdominal, back (posterior), retroperitoneal incision or laparoscopic surgery. However, the choice of approach depends on many factors, such as the size and location of the tumor, associated structures, the length of the procedure, and the patient's condition.

CHAPTER SUMMARY

- Kidney stones are formed by crystalline mineral and salts precipitated from filtrate produced in the kidney. Stones are removed to prevent infection and obstruction.
- Renal cysts originate in the nephron as a result of obstruction. Fluid-filled cysts impinge on vascular structures, causing loss of kidney function. Cystic disease may be acquired or congenital. Polycystic disease is hereditary and has no treatment.
- End-stage renal disease is renal failure that cannot be reversed. The condition has many causes, including diabetes, hypertension, systemic lupus erythematosus, nephrotic syndrome, and infection (*E. coli* ingestion is a common cause of renal failure).
- Hydronephrosis is distension and loss of function of the ureter or renal pelvis as a result of urinary reflux (backward movement of the urine) caused by an obstruction such as a stricture, stone, or tumor.
- A UTI is an infection of the lower urinary tract and is commonly caused by *E. coli* contamination of the distal urethra or by a sexually transmitted disease. Chronic UTIs may result in scarring of the urethra that requires surgery.
- Benign prostatic hyperplasia is age-related enlargement of the prostate gland. It causes urethral constriction, which leads to reflux and incontinence.
- Hypospadias is a common congenital defect in which the urethra fails to develop fully. This results in urethral shortening and displacement of the urethral meatus on the back side of the penis.
- Testicular torsion is rotation of the testicle, usually related to a congenital anomaly. It is a medical emergency, because blood flow to the testicle may be obstructed, leading to ischemia and necrosis of the testicle.

- Varicocele is a condition of enlarged, dilated veins in the scrotum that develops as a result of venous valve failure.
- Dialysis is a procedure in which waste products are removed from the blood in patients with chronic kidney disease or end-stage renal disease.
- During hemodialysis, the blood is shunted into the heparinized hemodialysis machine, where it passes through a series of membranes and dialyzing solution, which filter waste and return the blood to the body.
- During peritoneal dialysis, dialyzing solution is instilled into the abdominal cavity through a suprapubic catheter and the peritoneum acts as a filter to remove metabolic wastes. The solution is then removed.
- Many laboratory tests for GU disease focus on the presence or absence of substances found in the blood and urine. Imaging tests are performed to outline the structures of the GU system, to observe its function, and to detect tumors.
- The serum creatinine or glomerular filtration rate measures the rate of creatinine clearance from the blood.
- A number of patient positions are used in GU surgery, depending on the type of surgery and the techniques used.
- Open GU procedures require specialty general surgery instruments. The ureters are extremely delicate and require atraumatic clamps (e.g., Babcock clamps).
- Minimally invasive surgical instruments are used in percutaneous nephroscopy, laparoscopy, and transurethral (cystoscopic) surgery.
- A rigid cystoscope is passed through the urethral meatus to perform diagnostic or operative procedures.
- The sheath is a hollow tube that serves as a passageway for the instruments used during cystoscopy and

- resection. The telescope is inserted into the sheath before it is passed into the urethra.
- Before the sheath is placed inside the urethra, a blunt, round-tip obturator is placed inside the sheath. The obturator tip advances ahead of the sheath and protects the wall of the urethra from abrasion during insertion.
- A resectoscope is a transurethral instrument used to remove small fragments of tissue. It consists of an endoscope, sheath, obturator, and electrosurgical loop, which cuts and coagulates target tissue inside the bladder.
- A variety of ureteral and urethral catheters may be used during GU procedures. The lumen or bore of the catheter is measured in French (Fr) sizes, ranging from 7 to 26 Fr.
- Transurethral procedures take place in a specialized cystoscopy ("cysto") room. This dedicated surgical suite has all the equipment needed to perform diagnostic or therapeutic procedures.
- Most facilities have a cystoscopy (cysto) assistant. This is a trained technologist or nurse whose main duty is to work in this specialty.
- Skin prep for cystoscopic procedures includes the entire perineum, external genitalia, and pubis. Digital imaging of the operative site during endoscopy is performed through the camera head of the flexible endoscope. Imaging systems used in endoscopic GU surgery are similar to those used in other specialties.
- During cystoscopic procedures, the bladder is distended with fluid to enhance visualization of the internal structures.
- Whenever electrosurgical instruments are used, the irrigation fluid must be nonelectrolytic. This means that the fluid cannot transmit or disperse electricity.
- The most commonly used solutions with electrosurgery are sorbitol and glycine.
- Water is not used during endoscopic resection procedures, because water causes hemolysis (rupture of red blood cells). During resection of the prostate, significant contact occurs between the irrigation solution and open veins of the prostate.
- Absorption of irrigation fluid (extravasation) may result in vascular overload. The assistant must accurately monitor the amount of fluid used and collected as runoff during a procedure to assess the amount absorbed.
- Cystoscopy is surgery of the distal GU system performed with an operative cystourethroscope.
- A lithotrite is a specialized instrument that grasps and crushes renal calculi (stones).
- During transurethral resection of the prostate, the prostate is removed with a resectoscope inserted through the urethra.
- Complications after prostatectomy include incontinence, impotence, and retrograde ejaculation. Nerve-sparing procedures have been developed to prevent these complications.

- Transurethral ureteroscopy is performed with a flexible or rigid ureteroscope. The flexible ureteroscope is inserted with the aid of a guide wire made of Teflon-coated stainless steel.
- During endoscopy, laser energy is delivered through a small quartz fiber (filament) to fragment a stone. An accessory, such as a wire prong grasper or basket, then can be used to extract the fragments.
- Circumcision is the removal of the prepuce (foreskin) to improve hygiene and for cultural and religious reasons.
- Chordee is a congenital downward curvature of the penis caused by a band of connective tissue between the urethral opening and the glans.
- Hypospadias is a common congenital anomaly involving incomplete development of the distal urethra.
- A hydrocele is a painless accumulation of fluid or blood around the testicle. The condition may arise from trauma, infection, tumor, or as a result of peritoneal dialysis.
- Orchiectomy (orchidectomy) is surgical removal of one or both testicles, usually for the treatment of cancer.
- Vasovasostomy is the surgical anastomosis of the vas deferens to restore continuity after vasectomy.
- Cystostomy is the insertion of a suprapubic catheter into the bladder for drainage. The catheter is inserted through a percutaneous or open approach.
- Total cystectomy is indicated for small invasive tumors that penetrate the bladder wall. A more conservative partial cystectomy may be performed when cancer staging reveals no lymph node metastasis.
- In an ileal conduit procedure, a functional bladder is constructed with a loop of bowel that is brought out of the abdominal wall. A stoma is created for drainage of urine.
- Vesicourethral suspension (Marshall-Marchetti-Krantz procedure) is a suspension of the bladder neck and urethra from the cartilage of the pubic symphysis to treat urinary stress incontinence in the female.
- A perineal approach to prostatectomy may include laparoscopic lymph node removal during a combined or separate procedure. Lymph node analysis is performed for cancer staging.
- Ureteral diversion surgery is performed to restore continuity between the kidney and bladder after damage to the ureter.
- Large stones in the kidney or upper ureter are removed percutaneously through the nephroscope.
- A simple nephrectomy is surgical removal of one kidney. A radical nephrectomy is removal of the kidney and regional lymph nodes.
- Kidney transplantation involves removing a kidney from a living donor or cadaver and implanting into the patient.
- Minimally invasive surgery is preferred for removal of an adrenal gland.

REVIEW QUESTIONS

1. Explain the purpose of continuous irrigation during transurethral surgery.
2. What safety considerations are necessary for using continuous irrigation during electrosurgery? Consider the type of irrigation fluid, the placement of the inactive electrode, and the condition of the patient (age, nutritional status).
3. Explain how a urethral catheter is used as a tamponade.
4. What is a French (Fr) size? What is the most common catheter size for an adult?
5. Explain why testicular torsion is an emergency.
6. The lateral position is used for many procedures of the genitourinary tract. List at least five critical safety considerations for this position. Include specific anatomical locations and risk factors.
7. What surgical approaches are used to enter the retroperitoneal cavity?
8. What specific psychological considerations are important for the male patient undergoing surgery of the external genitalia?
9. Many patients undergoing transurethral surgery are elderly. List four methods you would use to communicate with these patients.
10. Testicular cancer is the most common cancer among young men. How would you approach a 25-year-old patient undergoing surgery for testicular cancer? Be specific. Define the patient's emotional needs at the time of surgery as part of your response.

BIBLIOGRAPHY

Arthur D: *Smith's textbook of endourology*, ed 2, London, 2007, BC Decker.

Graham SD: *Glenn's urologic surgery*, ed 6, Philadelphia, 2004, Lippincott Williams & Wilkins.

Pietrow P, Karellas M: Medical management of common urinary calculi, *American Family Physician*, July 1, 2006. Retrieved August 15, 2008, at http://www.aafp.org.

Tanagho EA: *Smith's general urology*, ed 17, New York, 2008, McGraw Hill.

Walters MD: *Urogynecology and reconstructive pelvic surgery*, ed 3, Philadelphia, 2007, Elsevier.

Ophthalmic Surgery

LEARNING OBJECTIVES

After studying this chapter the reader will be able to:

- Discuss the specific psychological needs of the patient having eye surgery
- Describe the anatomy of the eye
- Describe ocular diseases and disorders
- Describe the diagnostic tests used in ophthalmology

- Define safe practice and techniques as they apply to eye surgery
- Explain how to prepare the microscope for use and how to care for it
- Recognize and name commonly used eye instruments
- Differentiate the types of ophthalmic drugs and their uses

TERMINOLOGY

Accommodation: A process in which the lens continually changes shape to maintain the focus of an image on the retina.

Bridle suture: In ophthalmic surgery, a temporary traction suture placed through the sclera and used to pull the globe laterally for exposure of the posterolateral surface. It is called a *bridle suture* because of its resemblance to the reins of a horse's bridle.

Cataract: Clouding of the eye, caused by a disease in which the crystalline lens of the eye, its capsule, or both become opaque. This prevents light from focusing on the retina, resulting in visual distortion. Cataracts may develop as a result of disease or injury.

Conformer: A device placed in the socket after enucleation or evisceration to fill the orbital space.

Cryotherapy: A technique in which a cold probe is used to freeze tissue, such as the sclera, ciliary body (for glaucoma), or retinal layers, after detachment.

Diathermy: Low-power cautery used to mark the sclera over an area of retinal detachment.

Enucleation: Surgical removal of the globe and accessory attachments.

Evisceration: Surgical removal of the contents of the eyeball, with the sclera left intact.

Exenteration: Removal of the entire contents of the orbit.

Focal point: The point where light rays converge after passing through a lens.

Glaucoma: A group of diseases characterized by elevation of the intraocular pressure. Sustained pressure on the optic nerve and other structures may result in ischemia and blindness.

Keratoplasty: Surgery of the cornea. The term *penetrating keratoplasty* refers to corneal transplantation.

Muscle recession: Surgery in which the eye muscle is moved back to release the globe.

Muscle resection: Surgical shortening of an eye muscle to pull the globe into correct position.

Phacoemulsification: A process whereby high-frequency sound waves are used to emulsify tissue, such as a cataract.

Pterygium: A triangular membrane that arises from the medial canthus; the tissue may extend over the cornea, causing blindness.

Refraction: A phenomenon of physics in which light rays are bent as they pass through a transparent medium that is denser than air. In the eye, refraction occurs as light enters the front of the eye and passes through the cornea, lens, aqueous humor, and vitreous.

Spatula needle: A flat-tip suture needle commonly used in ophthalmic surgery.

Strabismus: Inability to coordinate the extraocular muscles, which prevents binocular vision.

Trabeculectomy: Surgical removal of a portion of the trabecula to improve the outflow of aqueous humor for the treatment of glaucoma.

INTRODUCTION

The goal of ophthalmic surgery is to restore vision lost as a result of disease, injury, or congenital defect. Procedures include those performed on the external and internal structures of the eye.

Eye procedures are particularly delicate and precise. Teamwork and attention to detail are critical in ophthalmic surgery, because the surgeon's attention is focused on the focal area of the microscope, and it cannot be diverted from the operative site. Ophthalmic surgery is purposefully slow paced because of the precise, delicate nature of the procedures.

Ophthalmic surgery is performed in a variety of health care settings, including the hospital, and outpatient center. Regardless of the setting, preparations and procedures for the patient's safety are fully implemented in the perioperative period. Of particular concern are verifying that the operative site and the implants are correct, positioning precautions, and drug and environmental safety.

SURGICAL ANATOMY

ORBITAL CAVITY

The basic structure of the eyeball, the globe, is contained within the orbital cavity (also called the *bony orbit*). Seven separate bones come together to form the orbit: the frontal, lacrimal, sphenoid, ethmoid, maxillary, zygomatic, and palatine bones. The cavity is lined with connective tissue to cushion the eye. Although most of the orbit is composed of thin bone, the rim is particularly thick and therefore more protective. The optic nerve enters the posterior orbital cavity through the optic foramen (Figure 26-1).

EYELIDS

The eyelids are composed of fibrous connective tissue (referred to as the *tarsal plate*) covered with skin. The lids protect the eye from injury and light. The term *palpebral* refers to the eyelids. The space or interval between the upper and lower lids is called the *palpebral fissure*. Each juncture of the eyelids is called a *canthus*. Sebaceous glands located along the lid margin and in the lacrimal caruncle secrete a waxy oil that seals the eyelids when they are closed. The eyelashes, which extend along the tarsus, protect the eye from airborne particles (Figure 26-2).

GLOBE

The globe has separate cavities, each of which contains functional structures. The posterior cavity lies at the back of the eyeball. The anterior cavity is divided into two spaces, the anterior chamber and the posterior chamber.

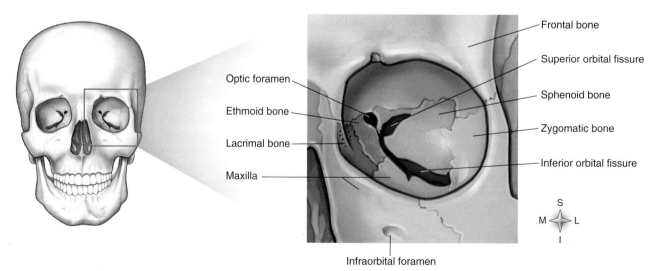

Figure 26-1 The orbital cavity (bony orbit) showing the composite bones. *(From Thibodeau G, Patton K: Anatomy and physiology, ed 6, St Louis, 2007, Mosby.)*

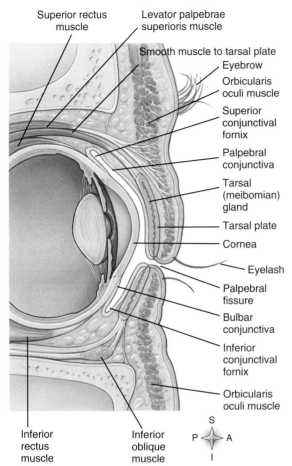

Superior rectus muscle

Levator palpebrae superioris muscle

Smooth muscle to tarsal plate

Eyebrow

Orbicularis oculi muscle

Superior conjunctival fornix

Palpebral conjunctiva

Tarsal (meibomian) gland

Tarsal plate

Cornea

Eyelash

Palpebral fissure

Bulbar conjunctiva

Inferior conjunctival fornix

Orbicularis oculi muscle

Inferior rectus muscle

Inferior oblique muscle

Figure 26-2 The external structures of the eye. *(From Thibodeau G, Patton K:* Anatomy and physiology, *ed 6, St Louis, 2007, Mosby.)*

The globe is enclosed by separate tissue layers, each very distinctive in structure and function (Figure 26-3).

EYE MUSCLES

Six muscles attach the sclera to the bony orbit and move the eyeball around various axes. This allows both eyes to focus on a single point. Each eye has four rectus muscles: the superior, inferior, lateral, and medial rectus muscles. Each eye also has two oblique muscles, the superior and inferior oblique muscles. The visual field is the area we see when the eyes are focused on a single point. Vision normally is binocular; that is, each eye has a nearly separate visual field, and the two are brought together as one image in the brain. The visible area consists of central and peripheral vision (Figure 26-4).

CONJUNCTIVA

The conjunctiva is a thin, transparent mucous membrane that lines each eyelid and covers the sclera. It is divided into the palpebral and bulbar regions. The palpebral conjunctiva is highly vascular and therefore pink. It lines the eyelids and extends over the cornea. The bulbar conjunctiva covers the anterior portion of the eyeball up to the junction of the sclera.

The bulbar conjunctiva appears white, because the sclera lies directly beneath it.

CORNEA

The cornea is a clear tissue layer overlying the front of the eyeball. Light enters the eye through the cornea and is refracted (bent); this allows images to be focused on the retina. The cornea has no blood vessels. It is composed of three tissue layers: the epithelium (superficial layer), the stroma, and the endothelium. The circular boundary of the cornea extends to the sclera. The two tissues come together at the limbus. During cataract surgery, the initial incision is made in the limbus.

SCLERA

The sclera is a thick, white, fibrous tissue that encloses about three fourths of the eyeball. It is the external supporting layer of the eyeball. The sclera is contiguous with the cornea at the front of the eye. The sclera communicates with the optic nerve sheath.

CHOROID AND CILIARY BODY

The highly vascular, pigmented choroid layer lies directly beneath the sclera. The primary function of the choroid is to prevent the reflection of light within the eyeball. An extension of the choroid layer, the ciliary body, is located at the periphery of the anterior choroid. It is composed of smooth muscle tissue to which suspensory ligaments are attached.

IRIS

The iris is a pigmented membrane composed mainly of muscle tissue that surrounds the pupil. The actions of the muscle fibers cause the pupil to close or open, to exclude light, or to admit light into the inner eye. The pupil may appear dilated or constricted, depending on the action of the iris.

RETINA

The innermost layer of the posterior globe is called the *retina.* The retina is the photoreceptive layer of the eye; it receives and transmits images to the brain via the optic nerve. Light energy projected onto the retina from the front of the eye is converted into nerve impulses that are transmitted to the brain, creating sight. The two types of photoreceptive cells are those that transmit black and white and those that enable color perception. The macula is a distinct area of acute vision that lies near the optic nerve. The center of this structure is called the *fovea centralis.* The optic nerve exits the globe in an area of dense neurons called the *optic disc.* The optic disc has no photoreceptors.

LENS

The lens lies directly behind the iris in the anterior chamber. It is a clear, biconcave disk contained in a transparent capsule.

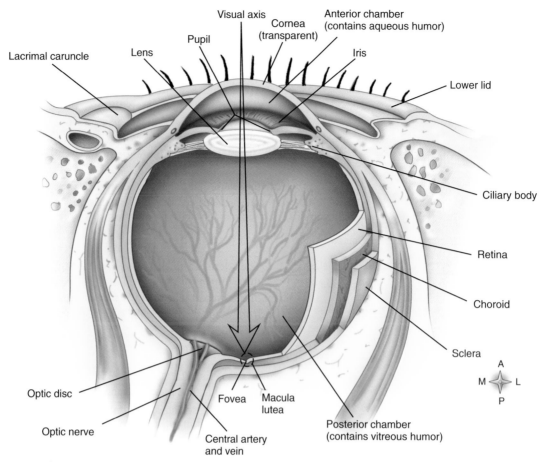

Figure 26-3 The interior of the globe showing the layers of the inner eye, chambers, lens, retina, and optic nerve. (From Thibodeau G, Patton K: Anatomy and physiology, ed 6, St Louis, 2007, Mosby.)

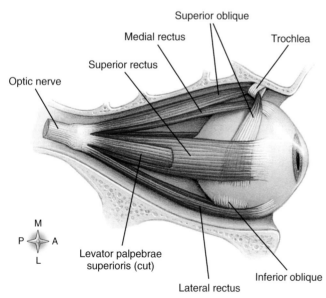

Figure 26-4 The extrinsic muscles of the eye. (From Thibodeau G, Patton K: Anatomy and physiology, ed 6, St Louis, 2007, Mosby.)

The lens is held in place by suspensory ligaments called *zonules*, which are attached to the capsule and ciliary body. The suspensory ligaments change the shape of the lens to bend light that passes through the lens. This focuses the images that are projected onto the retina.

ANTERIOR AND POSTERIOR CHAMBERS

The anterior space of the eye is divided into two separate chambers by the lens and the iris. The anterior space in front of the lens and iris is called the *anterior chamber*. Immediately behind the lens and iris is another space called the *posterior chamber*. A clear fluid produced by the ciliary epithelium, called *aqueous humor*, fills the anterior chamber. The pupil allows aqueous humor to pass between the two chambers through a space between the lens and the iris. From there it passes into the canal of Schlemm and is shunted directly into the venous system.

The posterior chamber lies between the posterior lens and the retina. It is filled with vitreous humor. Vitreous humor is a gel-like substance that fills the posterior chamber and nourishes the inner tissue layers. It also gives shape to the posterior globe and acts as a refractive medium for light.

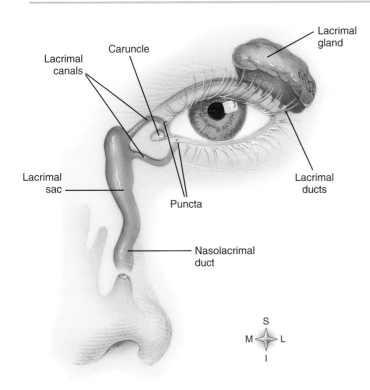

Figure 26-5 The lacrimal apparatus, including the lacrimal gland and ducts, lacrimal canals and sac, and the nasolacrimal duct. *(From Abrahams P, Marks S, and Hutchings R: McKinn's color atlas of human anatomy, ed 5, 2003, Mosby Ltd.)*

LACRIMAL APPARATUS

The lacrimal apparatus produces tears. This group of structures includes the lacrimal gland, caruncle, tear ducts, lacrimal sac, and nasolacrimal duct (Figure 26-5). Tears are produced by the lacrimal gland located laterally in the orbit. Each gland has numerous ducts that drain into the conjunctiva. The lacrimal ducts extend from the inner canthus to the lacrimal sac. The opening of each duct is called the *lacrimal punctum.* The lacrimal sac is an enlarged portion of the nasolacrimal duct, which is a passageway that connects the punctum and the nasal sinus.

Tears are composed of many chemicals, including proteins, mucus, sodium chloride, glucose, and enzymes capable of breaking down the cell membrane of bacteria. Tears continually bathe the eye and protect it from dehydration and infection. Tearing is stimulated by chemical and physical irritants and strong emotion. Tears produced as a result of emotion have a different composition than those arising from irritation and pain.

REFRACTION

Refraction is the bending of light rays through a transparent medium. Refraction occurs as light enters the front of the eye and passes through the lens. The light rays are refracted as they pass through the cornea, aqueous humor, lens, and vitreous, and the rays converge at the **focal point.** The image produced by the light rays is brought into focus by **accommodation.**

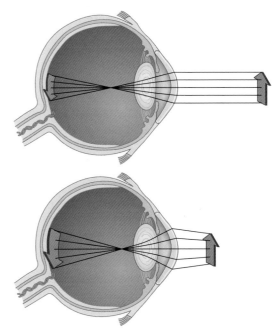

Figure 26-6 Light rays are refracted as they enter the eye and are bent through the lens. Images are focused on the retina and transmitted as nerve signals to the brain. *(From Thibodeau G, Patton K:* Anatomy and physiology, *ed 6, St Louis, 2007, Mosby.)*

This is a complex process in which the lens continually changes shape to keep the image focused on the fovea. This enables us to view objects at various distances and keep them in focus (Figure 26-6).

PATHOLOGY OF THE EYE

Table 26-1 presents common diseases of the eye.

DIAGNOSTIC TESTING

Refraction is a test for visual acuity, and the test is performed with a *photo-opter.* This device has a range of corrective lenses that allow the patient to compare different combinations while viewing an eye chart.

A *slit lamp* is used to examine the anterior chamber of the eye. Details of the lid margins, conjunctiva, tear film, cornea, and iris can be studied. The pupil can be dilated and the lens and anterior vitreous examined. Fluorescein is used to stain the cornea and highlight irregularities of the epithelial surface. A tonometer is used to measure the intraocular pressure (IOP).

Direct examination of the eyes is performed with an *ophthalmoscope.* This is a handheld instrument that magnifies the focal point, allowing the examiner to evaluate the fundus and other internal eye structures. An indirect binocular ophthalmoscope is used to examine the retina and other structures within a wider focal point.

Fluorescein angiography is used extensively in the diagnosis and evaluation of retinal and choroid diseases. It delineates areas of abnormality and is essential for planning laser treatment of retinal vascular disease. In this test, fluorescein dye is injected intravenously. When the dye reaches the retina and

<u>**Table 26-1**</u>

Pathology of the Eye

Condition	Description	Considerations
Cataract	A cataract is an opaque lens. Aging is the most common cause of a cataract. Other factors can be involved, including genetics, trauma, toxins, systemic disease (e.g., diabetes), and certain medications (e.g., corticosteroids).	Surgical treatment is necessary for treatment of advanced cataracts. (See Extracapsular Cataract Extraction.)
Corneal trauma	Penetrating wounds, a foreign body, and burns are the most common causes of corneal trauma. Minor abrasions heal quickly. Trauma to the stromal layer results in permanent scarring and opacification.	Eye trauma is a medical emergency. Severe corneal trauma may result in infection or blindness.
Corneal ulcer	A corneal ulcer, or ulcerative keratitis, may be caused by infection or irritation of the epithelial and stromal layers.	The condition is treated medically. Advanced disease may require corneal transplantation. (See Penetrating Keratoplasty [Corneal Transplantation].)
Dacryocystitis	Dacryocystitis is an inflammation or infection of the lacrimal sac. It usually arises from obstruction of the lacrimal canal.	Mild cases are treated medically. Advanced disease may require dacryocystorhinostomy.
Entropion/ectropion	An *entropion* is inversion of the eyelid, which occurs in the lower lid. This causes the eyelashes to rub on the cornea. An *ectropion* is drooping or eversion of the lid.	Surgical treatment is required for advanced disease. (See Repair of an Ectropion and Repair of an Entropion.)
Glaucoma	Glaucoma is a disease characterized by optic nerve and visual field damage, usually caused by inadequate drainage of aqueous humor. Unrelieved pressure damages the optic nerve and may result in progressive blindness.	Conservative treatment is medical. Surgery may be performed for more advanced disease. (See Filtering Procedures and Trabeculectomy.)
Intraocular foreign body	An accident, trauma, or an occupational injury may result in penetration of the eye by a foreign body.	A foreign body can be removed surgically. Objects in the posterior cavity may be treated by a pars plana vitrectomy.
Macular degeneration	A condition of degeneration of the rod and cone photoreceptor cells of the retina, macular degeneration results in central vision blindness. Age-related macular degeneration (ARMD) is the most common cause of blindness in people over age 65. The cause is unknown.	Photocoagulation has been used in the past to slow the disease; however, current treatment focuses on medical therapy with a number of drugs. Currently, no definitive cure is available.
Ocular and orbital trauma	Trauma to the eye is commonly caused by motor vehicle and sports accidents. Explosions, industrial accidents, and intentional violence are other common causes.	Rupture of the globe and bony fracture are characteristic of trauma. Surgical treatment is necessary. Severe trauma may require enucleation. (See Chapter 28 for a discussion of surgery of the bony orbit.)
Retinal detachment	A separation or tear in the retina allows vitreous to seep between the layers and delaminate them. Tears occur as a result of trauma or shrinking of the vitreous, which normally occurs with age.	Retinal detachment is a medical emergency that requires surgery to prevent further separation and blindness. (See Scleral Buckling Procedure for a Detached Retina.)
Strabismus (squint)	**Strabismus** is the inability to coordinate the extraocular muscles, which prevents binocular vision. The cause is weakness or paralysis of the muscles. The condition may be congenital or acquired.	The condition is corrected surgically. (See Muscle Resection and Recession.)
Uveitis/iritis	Uveitis/iritis is inflammation of the iris, ciliary, body, choroid, and commonly the retina.	Corticosteroids and cycloplegic/mydriatic agents are used to control the inflammation. If complications occur, surgical intervention for progressive glaucoma and cataract extraction may be necessary.

choroid, the vessels and epithelium are clearly delineated and images are recorded.

Ophthalmic ultrasonography is used to measure the density of eye tissues and detect abnormalities. Two types of ultrasound can be used, A-scan ultrasound or B-scan ultrasound. B-scan ultrasound produces an image of the target tissue that shows a series of spots, the brightness of which corresponds to tissue density. As tissue density increases, the image appears darker. For example, vitreous appears very dark or black on ultrasound. The A-scan ultrasound depicts tissue density as amplitude on two axes. The output is represented in waveform, resembling an electrocardiogram (ECG). High-density tissue produces an amplified wave.

Magnetic resonance imaging (MRI) and computed tomography (CT) are used in the evaluation of the orbital and intracranial structures. CT may have some disadvantages in ophthalmology, because it is unable to differentiate between structures of similar density and those that are very small.

PERIOPERATIVE CONSIDERATIONS

PSYCHOLOGICAL CONSIDERATIONS IN EYE SURGERY

Ophthalmic surgery can be frightening to patients. Although many look forward to correcting medical problems to improve or restore their eyesight, they often have unspoken fears that a poor outcome will result in blindness. In most ophthalmic surgeries, the patient receives a regional anesthetic, and monitored sedation is used. The patient therefore is awake and able hear sounds in the surgical environment. In addition, the patient can see the objects and instruments that are placed in the eye. This increases preoperative anxiety.

A reassuring environment is always important to the patient's psychological and physical well-being; however, it is particularly important in ophthalmic surgery, because anxiety can result in increased hemorrhage and intraocular pressure. The surgical technologist can help the patient by maintaining a calm, supportive atmosphere. Patients find it reassuring to be given simple explanations of what they will feel or sense as the procedure starts. During the procedure, the surgeon always warns the patient of any steps that involve pressure or pain, such as the initial sting of an anesthetic or loss of sensation.

VERIFICATION OF THE OPERATIVE SITE

The entire surgical team is responsible for verifying that surgery is performed on the correct patient at the correct site. The Joint Commission recommends that the surgeon write on or mark the skin near the operative site to identify the correct side. Timeout (see Chapter 16) to perform the universal protocol is implemented before every procedure to verify the correct patient, site, and side. In ophthalmic surgery, particular concerns arise because marks around the eye may be covered by drapes before the verification process is started.

Verification of implants also is a problem in ophthalmic surgery.

❖ *The protocol for preventing wrong site, wrong procedure, wrong person surgery can be found at http://www. jointcommission.org/PatientSafety/UniversalProtocol/.*

The surgical technologist shares in the responsibility for preventing wrong site surgery and also for errors in lens implants. All facilities have a protocol for timeout. However, mistakes occur because of human error, often related to a busy surgery schedule.

Intraocular implants (IO implants) *must be verified before insertion.* Lens implants are treated in much the same way as a drug distributed to the field (see Chapter 12). To prevent insertion of the wrong implant, the American Association of Ophthalmologists (AAO) has developed a sample protocol. The surgical technologist participates in this protocol:

1. Before surgery, the surgeon selects the intraocular lens (IOL) based on the patient's records available *in the operating room.*
2. The circulating nurse shows the surgeon the box and verbally verifies the IOL model number and lens power. The surgeon acknowledges this communication.
3. The circulating nurse *repeats this procedure with the surgical technologist.*
4. The scrubbed surgical technologist *verbally states the model number and lens power* as the IOL is passed to the surgeon.

Documentation of implants is discussed later in the chapter.

POSITIONING THE PATIENT FOR OPHTHALMIC SURGERY

Ophthalmic surgery is performed with the patient in the supine position with the head stabilized on a circular headrest (sometimes called a *doughnut*). The top of the head may be level with the end of the table, or the patient may be positioned several inches lower (toward the feet), depending on the surgeon's operating needs. A wrist rest is attached to the head of the table to aid the surgeon in steadying the hands during the procedure (Figure 26-7).

Many health facilities use a combination stretcher–operating table for transporting the patient and performing surgery. Shifting the patient immediately after surgery may result in increased IOP and eye injury.

If a standard stretcher is used, the patient must be transferred cautiously and slowly. Many eye surgery patients are elderly and may have difficulty moving across the stretcher onto the operating table. The patient should be warned of the narrow table, and the safety strap should be secured as soon as possible. The circulator then can stabilize the patient into a comfortable position with gel or foam supports as needed. The patient should be covered with warm blankets to prevent hypothermia and for comfort.

As mentioned, most eye procedures involve a regional block and monitored sedation. The position of the patient for eye surgery must be safe and comfortable. An uncomfortable patient may become restless during surgery, and this can result in injury to the eye. It is critical that patients remain still. Some patients may benefit from lumbar support and a

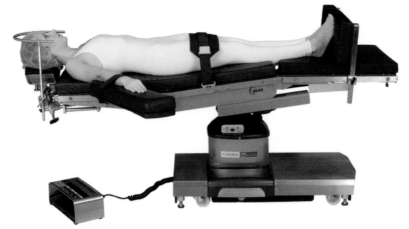

Figure 26-7 Positioning of the patient, showing a wrist rest at the head of the bed. (© 2008 by STERIS corporation. All rights reserved.)

cushion for the popliteal region. The arms may be tucked at the sides, but without contacting with any part of the metal frame or attachments.

PREPPING AND DRAPING

The skin prep commonly is performed after the patient has been anesthetized. Because regional anesthesia often is used, the circulator should have all prepping supplies ready before anesthesia is induced to prevent delay. Antiseptics used for eye prep include dilute povidone-iodine (5% or as directed by the surgeon) and hexachlorophene. Supplies needed for the sterile prep setup include the following:

- Small basins for the solutions
- Surgical towels
- Plastic towel drapes
- Lint-free gauze sponges
- Cotton balls
- Cellulose eye sponges
- Balanced salt solution (BSS)

Skin prep of the eye may include instillation of drugs to prepare the eye for surgery. The prep area includes the eyelid and margins, inner and outer canthus, brows, and face, ending usually at the chin. Before starting the prep, the circulator secures an adhesive towel drape at the hairline. Surgical towels are placed to absorb any solution runoff. However, runoff is prevented by squeezing excess solution from each sponge. A small piece of cotton may be placed in the operative side ear and the head turned toward the operative side. Irrigation of the eye may be required before the skin prep. BSS or a mild antiseptic of the surgeon's choice is used. The prep is performed starting at the eyelid and extending outward. The eyelid margins are cleansed using cotton-tip applicators. The canthus is considered a contaminated area, and any sponge that touches this area is discarded.

A number of techniques are used to drape the eye. It is important to isolate the hairline and nonoperative side of the face. Some surgeons use a head drape (see Chapter 11). This usually is followed by a fenestrated drape to expose the operative eye. A body sheet is used to maintain a wide sterile field,

or the procedure drape may be large enough to extend over the sides of the operating table.

ANESTHESIA

Most ophthalmic surgery is performed using a regional anesthetic with monitored sedation. A topical anesthetic, local infiltration, or a peribulbar nerve block, or a combination of these, is most often used. A retrobulbar block may be used in selected patients. However, this approach is associated with a number of serious risks and has more limited uses. Pediatric patients receive a general anesthetic.

For local anesthesia, a dedicated setup is prepared according to the surgeon's preferences. Anesthetic, syringes, infiltration needles (size 25 to 27 gauge), transfer needles, and sponges are needed. Lidocaine with epinephrine may be used to maintain vasoconstriction at the operative site. A topical anesthetic is applied over the cornea before injection. Patients generally tolerate the local anesthetic procedure well. The circulator is present at the patient's side to assist and to reassure the patient.

OPHTHALMIC DRUGS

Ophthalmic surgery requires the use of many types of drugs, which are administered preoperatively, during surgery, and in the postoperative period. Many of these drugs have potent effects, and a medication error could irreparably damage the eye. Chapter 12 discusses the appropriate protocol for receiving drugs on the sterile field. Important highlights are:

- *All drugs on the sterile field must be labeled as soon as they are received; this is critical.*
- Every drug passed to the surgeon must be identified and acknowledged by the surgeon—no exceptions.
- Preoperative topical drugs may be administered by the surgeon or the circulating registered nurse.
- The amounts of all drugs used must be recorded on the intraoperative report.

Table 26-2 presents a list of ophthalmic drugs and their uses.

Table 26-2

Medications Used During Ophthalmic Surgery

Drug/Brand Name	Description/Uses

Mydriatics (Drugs that dilate the pupil but permit focusing)

Phenylephrine (Neo-Synephrine, Mydfrin), 2.5%, 10%	Objective examination of the retina, testing of refraction, and easier removal of lenses; mydriatics may be used alone or with a cycloplegic drug.

Cycloplegics (Drugs that paralyze accommodation and inhibit focusing)

Tropicamide (Mydriacyl), 1%	Anticholinergic, dilation of the pupil, examination of the fundus, and refraction.
Atropine, 1%	Dilates the pupil, inhibits focusing; anticholinergic, potent, and has a long duration of action (7 to 14 days).
Cyclopentolate (Cyclogyl), 1%, 2%	Anticholinergic; dilates the pupil, inhibits focusing
Scopolamine hydrobromide (Isopto Hyoscine), 0.25%	Anticholinergic; dilates the pupil, inhibits focusing
Homatropine hydrobromide (Isopto Homatropine), 2%, 5%	Anticholinergic; dilates the pupil, inhibits focusing
Epinephrine (1:1000) preservative free (PF)	Dilates the pupil; added to bottles of balanced salt solution (BSS) for irrigation to maintain pupil dilation during cataract surgery or vitrectomy.

Miotics

Carbachol (Miostat), 0.01%	Potent cholinergic; constricts the pupil, used intraocularly during anterior segment surgery.
Carbachol (Isopto Carbachol), 0.75%, 1.5%, 2.25%, 3%	Potent cholinergic; constricts the pupil, used topically to reduce intraocular pressure (IOP) in glaucoma.
Acetylcholine chloride (Miochol-E), 1%	Cholinergic; rapidly constricts the pupil, used intraocularly during anterior segment surgery; reconstitute immediately before using.
Pilocarpine hydrochloride, 1%, 4%	Cholinergic; constricts the pupil, used topically to lower IOP in glaucoma.

Topical Anesthetics

Tetracaine hydrochloride (Pontocaine), 0.05%	*Onset:* 5–20 sec *Duration of action:* 10–20 min
Proparacaine hydrochloride (Ophthaine), 0.05%	*Onset:* 5–20 sec *Duration of action:* 10–20 min

Injectable Anesthetics

Lidocaine (Xylocaine), 1%, 2%, 4%	*Onset:* 4–6 minutes *Duration of action:* 40–60 minutes, 120 minutes with epinephrine
Methylparaben free (MPF)	Preservative free; adjunct to topical anesthetic.
Bupivacaine (Marcaine, Sensorcaine), 0.25%, 0.50%, 0.75%	*Onset:* 5–11 minutes *Duration of action:* 8–12 hr with epinephrine; often used in 0.75% strength in combination with lidocaine for blocks
Mepivacaine (Carbocaine), 1%, 2%	*Onset:* 3–5 minutes *Duration of action:* 2 hr (longer with epinephrine)
Etidocaine (Duranest), 1%	*Onset:* 3 minutes *Duration of action:* 5–10 hr

Additives to Local Anesthetics

Epinephrine, 1:50,000 to 1:200,000	Combined with injectable local anesthetics to prolong anesthesia and reduce bleeding.
Hyaluronidase	Enzyme mixed with anesthetics (75 units per 10 mL) to increase diffusion of anesthetic through tissue, improving the effectiveness of the block; contraindicated if skin inflammation or malignancy is present.

Viscoelastics

Sodium hyaluronate (Healon, Amvisc, Provisc, Vitrax) in a sterile syringe assembly with blunt-tip cannula	Lubricant and support; maintains separation between tissues to protect the endothelium and maintain the anterior chamber intraocularly; removed from anterior chamber to prevent postoperative increase in pressure; should be refrigerated (except Vitrax); allow 30 min to warm to room temperature.

Continued

Table 26-2

Table 26-2
Medications Used During Ophthalmic Surgery—cont'd

Drug/Brand Name	Description/Uses
Sodium chondroitin–sodium hyaluronate (Viscoat) in a sterile syringe assembly with blunt-tip cannula	Maintains deep chamber for anterior segment procedures, protects epithelium of cornea, and improves visualization; may be used to coat intraocular lens before implantation; should be refrigerated.
Duovisc	Packages of separate syringes of Provisc and Viscoat in the same box.

Viscoadherents

Drug/Brand Name	Description/Uses
Hydroxypropyl methylcellulose 2% (Occucoat) in a sterile syringe assembly with blunt-tip cannula	Maintains a deep chamber for anterior segment procedures, protects epithelium of cornea, and may be used to coat intraocular lens before implantation; removed from anterior chamber at end of procedure; stored at room temperature.
Hydroxyethylcellulose (Gonioscopic Prism Solution)	Bonds gonioscopic prisms to the eye; stored at room temperature.
Hydroxypropyl methylcellulose 2.5% (Goniosol)	Bonds gonioscopic prisms to the eye; stored at room temperature.

Irrigants

Drug/Brand Name	Description/Uses
Balanced salt solution (BSS, Endosol)	Used to keep the cornea moist during surgery; also used as an internal irrigant in the anterior or posterior segment.
BSS enriched with bicarbonate, dextrose, and glutathione (BSS Plus, Endosol Extra)	Used as an internal irrigant in the anterior or posterior segment; must be reconstituted immediately before use by adding part I to part II with the transfer device.

Hyperosmotic Agents

Drug/Brand Name	Description/Uses
Mannitol (Osmitrol)	Intravenous (IV) osmotic diuretic; increases the osmolarity of the plasma, causing the osmotic pressure gradient to pull free fluid from the eye into the plasma, thereby reducing the IOP.
Glycerin (Osmoglyn, Glyrol)	Oral osmotic diuretic given in chilled juice or cola; increases the osmolarity of the plasma, causing the osmotic pressure gradient to pull free fluid from the eye into the plasma, thereby reducing the IOP.

Antiinflammatory Agents

Drug/Brand Name	Description/Uses
Betamethasone sodium phosphate and betamethasone acetate suspension (Celestone)	Glucocorticoid; injected subconjunctivally after surgery for prophylaxis; also used to treat severe allergic and inflammatory conditions.
Dexamethasone (Decadron)	Adrenocorticosteroid; injected subconjunctivally after surgery for prophylaxis; also used to treat severe allergic and inflammatory conditions and intraocularly for endophthalmitis.
Methylprednisolone acetate suspension (Depo-Medrol)	Glucocorticoid; injected subconjunctivally after surgery for prophylaxis; also used to treat severe allergic and inflammatory conditions.

Antiinfective Drugs

Drug/Brand Name	Description/Uses
Polymyxin B/bacitracin (Polysporin ointment)	Topical treatment of superficial ocular infections of the conjunctiva or cornea; also used prophylactically after surgery.
Polymyxin B/neomycin/bacitracin (Neosporin ointment)	Topical treatment of superficial infections of the external eye; used prophylactically after surgery; hypersensitivity to neomycin is possible.
Neomycin and polymyxin B sulfates and dexamethasone (Maxitrol ointment or suspension)	Topical treatment of steroid-responsive inflammatory ocular conditions or bacterial infections of the external eye; hypersensitivity to neomycin is possible.
Tobramycin/dexamethasone (TobraDex)	Topical treatment or prevention of superficial infections of the external part of the eye; also has antiinflammatory properties.
Cefazolin (Ancef, Kefzol)	Injected subconjunctivally for prophylaxis after eye procedures; also used topically, intraocularly, and systematically for endophthalmitis.
Gentamicin sulfate (Garamycin)	Injected subconjunctivally for prophylaxis after eye procedures; also used topically, subconjunctivally, and intraocularly for endophthalmitis.
Ceftazidime (Fortaz, Tazicef, Tazidime)	Injected subconjunctivally and intraocularly for the treatment of endophthalmitis.

Other Drugs

Drug/Brand Name	Description/Uses
Cocaine, 1% to 4%	Used topically only, never injected; used on cornea to loosen epithelium before debridement and on nasal packing to reduce congestion of mucosa.

Continued

<u>Table 26-2</u>

Medications Used During Ophthalmic Surgery—cont'd

Drug/Brand Name	Description/Uses
5-Fluorouracil (5-FU)	Antimetabolite used topically to inhibit scar formation in glaucoma-filtering procedures; handle and discard in compliance with the regulations of the Occupational Safety and Health Administration (OSHA) and health facility's policies for safe use of antineoplastics.
Mitomycin (Mutamycin)	Antimetabolite used topically to inhibit scar formation in glaucoma-filtering procedures and pterygium excision; handle and discard in compliance with OSHA's and health facility's policies for safe use of antineoplastics.
Tissue plasminogen activator (TPA) (Activase)	Thrombolytic agent; used for the treatment of fibrin formation in patients who have had vitrectomy and for the lysis of clots on the retina.
Fluorescein	*IV diagnostic aid:* Used in fluorescein angiography to diagnose retinal disorders. *Topical stain:* Fluorescein strip temporarily stains the cornea yellow-green in areas of denuded corneal epithelium.
Timolol maleate (Timoptic)	Beta-adrenergic receptor blocking agent; used in the treatment of elevated IOP in ocular hypertension or open angle glaucoma.
Acetazolamide sodium (Diamox)	Carbonic anhydrase inhibitor; given IV to reduce the secretion of aqueous humor, resulting in a drop in IOP; also has a diuretic effect.
Dextrose, 50%	Added to BSS, Endosol, BSS Plus, or Endosol Extra for diabetic patients during intraocular procedures.

From Rothrock JC: *Alexander's care of the patient in surgery,* ed 13, St Louis, 2007, Mosby.

Adverse reactions to medications used during eye surgery are a serious consideration. Many different drugs are used in combination, and the circulator must be vigilant in observing for signs and symptoms that might indicate allergy or sensitivity. The scrub should notify the circulator and surgeon of any symptoms reported by the patient. The technologist does not assess the patient medically but should immediately report any observed changes in the patient's appearance or behavior.

INSTRUMENTS

Ophthalmic instruments (Figures 26-8 to 26-11) are delicate and expensive. All surgical personnel must take special care to ensure that the edges and tips of microsurgical eye instruments are not dulled or damaged by careless handling. Before the procedure begins, the scrub should check all instruments. Sharp items must be smooth, and scissor blades must align properly. Needle holders are particularly susceptible to injury. The scrub should make sure that catches and spring mechanisms are working properly. Suction tips should be checked for patency. All instruments must be kept in order on the Mayo stand. Surgery often is performed with the overhead lights dimmed. A neat instrument table is essential.

EQUIPMENT AND SUPPLIES

Electrosurgical Unit

Two types of electrosurgical systems are commonly used in eye surgery: the single-use, battery-powered cautery and the bipolar unit. The handheld battery unit has a very small filament tip that becomes hot when the unit is activated. Unlike monopolar or bipolar electrosurgical units (ESUs), this unit is a true cautery instrument. The filament is used to coagulate very small vessels of the eye; however, it does not have cutting capability. The bipolar or radio-frequency ESU is used for procedures in which fine cutting and coagulation are required. The bipolar unit is used in conjunction with bipolar instruments, which are connected to the unit by a thin cable. (A complete discussion of these technologies and safety precautions can be found in Chapter 21.)

Eye Sponges

Eye sponges are made of lint-free cellulose or similar material. These are supplied commercially attached to a short plastic rod (Figure 26-12). Sponges must be separated from supplies that might discharge lint particles. During surgery, the scrubbed surgical technologist may be required to blot blood or fluid from the surgical site. The sponge is never used on the cornea. The sponge absorbs fluid by wicking. This is done by holding the tip of the sponge in contact with the fluid and allowing the sponge to absorb it. Fresh sponges must always be available to maintain a clean operative site.

Sutures

Eye sutures are supplied in a wide range of materials in sizes 4-0 to 12-0. These must be handled gently and carefully. Sutures should be handled as little as possible, and the points

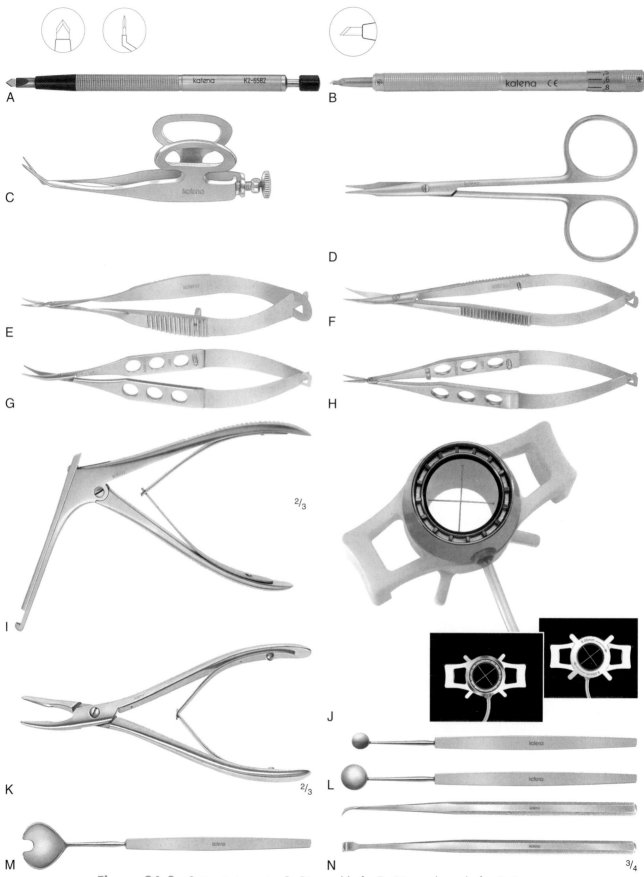

Figure 26-8   Cutting instruments. **A,** Diamond knife. **B,** Diamond step knife. **C,** Barraquer iris scissors. **D,** Stevens scissors. **E,** Vannas scissors. **F,** Westcott stitch scissors. **G,** Westcott tenotomy scissors. **H,** Katena-Vannas scissors. **I,** Kerrison rongeur. **J,** Barron vacuum trephine. **K,** Beyer rongeur. **L,** Enucleation spoon. **M,** Wells enucleation spoon. **N,** Freer lacrimal chisel. (Courtesy Katena Eye Instruments, Denville, New Jersey.)

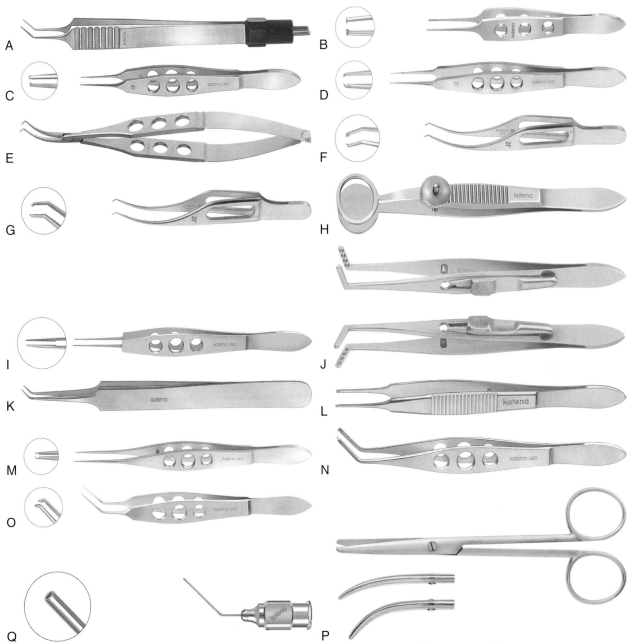

Figure 26-9 Forceps, calipers, and needle holders. **A,** Bipolar forceps. **B,** Bishop-Harmon forceps. **C,** Bonn forceps. **D,** Castroviejo needle holder. **E,** Clayman lens holding forceps. **F,** Colibri forceps. **G,** Harms-Colibri forceps. **H,** Hunt chalazion forceps. **I,** Jaffe tying forceps. **J,** Jameson muscle forceps. **K,** Jeweler forceps. **L,** Lester fixation forceps. **M,** Pierce corneal forceps. **N,** Troutman rectus forceps. **O,** Utrata capsulorrhexis forceps. **P,** Enucleation forceps. **Q,** Castroviejo caliper. *(Courtesy Katena Eye Instruments, Denville, New Jersey.)*

of the needles should be protected from damage. Double-arm sutures frequently are used in eye surgery to close circumferential incisions. Ophthalmic needles may be as small as 4 mm at the widest part. A magnetic needle pad is necessary for tracking needles during surgery. Sutures should not be allowed to contact cloth towels, which can transfer lint to the needle and suture material.

Ophthalmic Dressings

A soft dressing or hard shield may be used to protect the eye after surgery. Soft, lint-free gauze eye patches are supplied for

a simple dressing that absorbs fluid and prevents debris from entering the eye. A rigid eye shield is taped over the eye to provide protection from bumping or abrasion, which may cause dehiscence of an incision.

SURGICAL TECHNIQUES IN EYE SURGERY

MICROSURGERY

Microsurgery presents challenges to the scrub for several reasons:

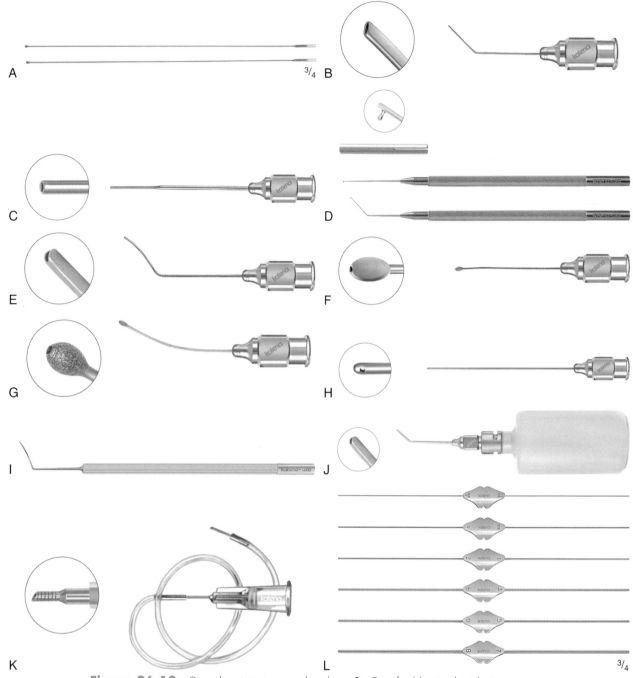

Figure 26-10 Cannulas, irrigators, and probes. **A,** Crawford lacrimal intubation. **B,** Hydrodissection cannula. **C,** Lacrimal cannula (23 gu). **D,** Lester interocular lens (IOL) manipulator. **E,** Randolph cyclodialysis cannula. **F,** Welsh olive-tip cannula. **G,** Jensen polisher. **H,** Air injection cannula. **I,** Barraquer iris spatula. **J,** Bishop-Harmon A/C irrigator. **K,** Chamber maintainer. **L,** Bowman lacrimal probe set. *(Courtesy Katena Eye Instruments, Denville, New Jersey.)*

- The surgeon's field of vision is magnified, but the scope (i.e., the area of vision) is very limited. Special technique is required for passing instruments, because the surgeon must not look away from the field to receive them.
- When required to look away from the field, the surgeon loses concentration and the rhythm of the surgery. To prevent such interruptions, the scrub should prepare for each step of the procedure. Using the proper method to pass instruments reduces the risk of patient injury.
- The patient and surgical field must be completely still. The scrub must prevent even slight movement of the microscope. When passing instruments or preparing items near the field, the scrub must have a steady hand and create as little movement as possible. Remember that if the patient raises the head or if any instruments are jarred while touching the eye, the patient can be injured.

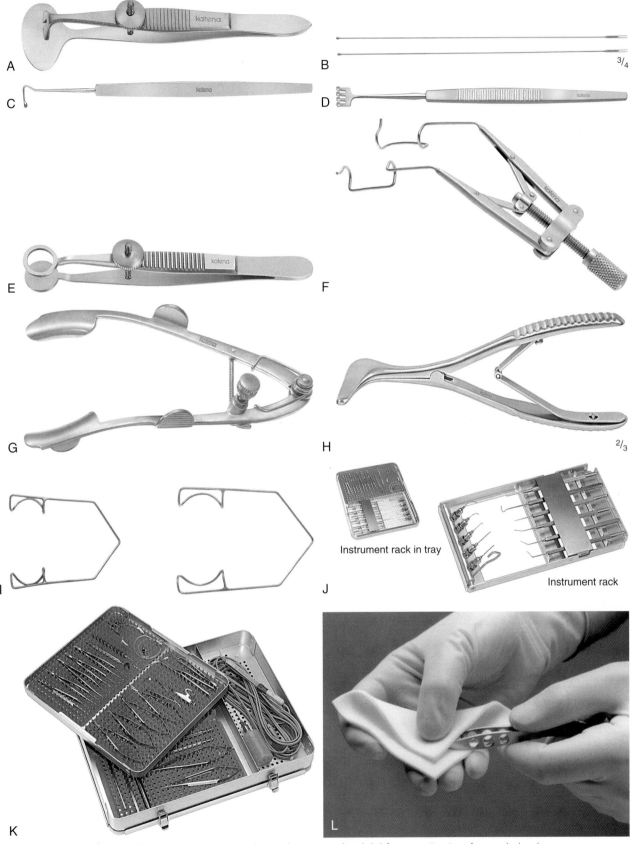

Figure 26-11 Retractors and speculums. **A,** Erhardt lid forceps. **B,** Graefe muscle hook. **C,** Jameson muscle hook. **D,** Knapp retractor. **E,** Lambert chalazion forceps. **F,** Lieberman speculum. **G,** Lester-Burch eye speculum. **H,** Nasal speculum, adult. **I,** Barraquer wire speculum. *Instrument Care:* **J,** Instrument rack. Eye instruments must be maintained in racks to prevent damage. **K,** Sterilization case for eye instruments. **L,** Lint-free instrument wipe. *(Courtesy Katena Eye Instruments, Denville, New Jersey.)*

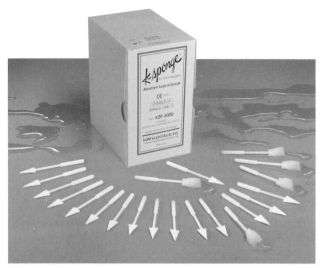

Figure 26-12 Eye sponges and K-sponge spears. *(Courtesy Katena Eye Instruments, Denville, New Jersey.)*

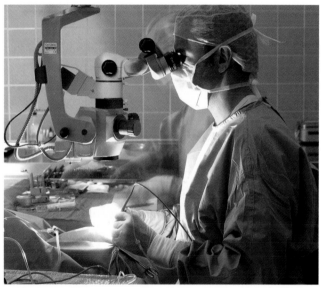

Figure 26-13 The surgeon at the microscope. *(Courtesy Carl Zeiss, Dublin, California.)*

OPERATING MICROSCOPE

The operating microscope is a heavy piece of equipment, but it also has delicate components (Figure 26-13). The technologist should become familiar with all components to prevent injury to the patient and to protect the microscope from damage. Box 26-1 lists common microscope terminology.

Handling the Microscope

The following guidelines should be observed when the microscope is handled:

1. Before moving the microscope, secure the arms. This prevents them from swinging out and striking the wall or other equipment.
2. The microscope must be balanced before use. This is necessary to ensure that the head of the microscope

---

Box 26-1

Microscope Terminology

Assistant binoculars: A separate optical body with a nonmotorized, hand-controlled zoom.
Beam splitter: A device that transmits an image from the primary ocular to an observer tube, producing an identical picture.
Broad-field viewing lens: A low-power magnifying glass attached to the front of the oculars that produces an overview of the field.
Coaxial illuminator: A light source (usually fiberoptic) transmitted through the lens or body of the microscope. It illuminates the area in the field of view of the objective lens.
Compound microscope: A microscope that uses two or more lenses in a single unit.
Illumination system: The lighting system of the microscope.
Magnifying power: The ability to enlarge an image.
Objective lens: The lens that establishes the working distance and produces the greatest magnification.
Ocular or eyepiece: The component of the microscope that magnifies the field of view.
Paraxial illuminators: One or more light tubes that contain incandescent bulbs and focusing lenses. Light is focused to coincide with the working distance of the scope.
X-Y attachment: A mechanism that allows the scope to move precisely along a horizontal plane.
Zoom lens: A lens that increases or decreases magnification and is operated by the foot pedal.

---

does not drift up or down. Always consult the manufacturer's instructions for balancing.
3. The microscope must be adjusted to accommodate the surgeon's and assistant's eyesight. Always test the microscope before moving it to the surgical field.
4. Check the brake and other controls to ensure that they are tight before using the microscope.
5. Take special care to ensure that the microscope head control knob is secure before surgery.
6. Check all cords for fraying or loose wires. Light bulbs also should be tested before surgery, and an extra bulb should be kept in the surgical suite.
7. Some microscopes are equipped with an X-Y axis carrier; this must be centered before the microscope is positioned at the field.
8. When moving the microscope, handle it with *both hands* on the vertical column. Moving the microscope by the head can cause it to tip over.
9. Make all adjustments to the vertical oculars before surgery.

Care of the Microscope

1. The microscope should be damp dusted before use. Follow the manufacturer's recommendations for use of a disinfectant. Never use detergent or disinfectant on the lenses. They should be cleaned with a lens cleaner or water and wiped with lens paper. Do not use cloth, which leaves lint on the lens.

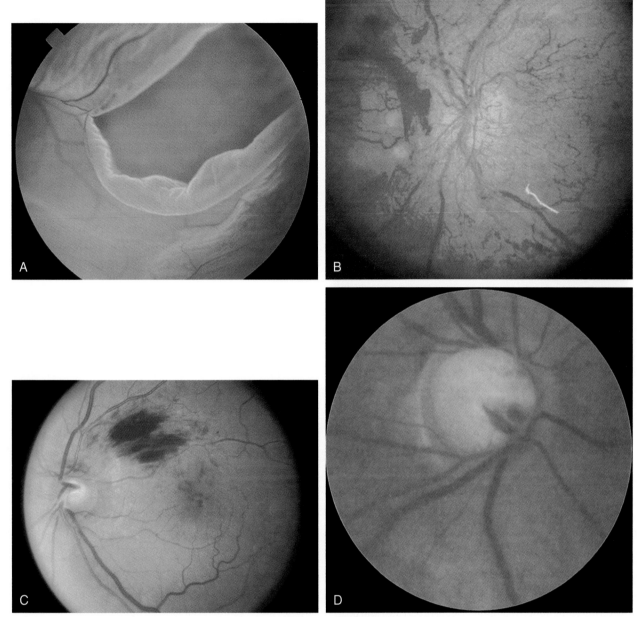

Figure 26-22 Pathological conditions of the retina. **A,** Retinal tear and detachment. **B,** Diabetic retinopathy, showing hemorrhages. **C,** Hypertensive retinopathy, showing the "flame hemorrhages" characteristic of the condition. **D,** Glaucoma (note the cupping of the optic disc caused by intraocular pressure). *(From Thibodeau G, Patton K:* Anatomy and physiology, *ed 6, St Louis, 2007, Mosby.)*

Technique

1. The Tenon capsule is separated from the sclera with blunt dissection.
2. Diathermy is applied to the area of detachment or tear.
3. Sutures are placed in the sclera.
4. The buckling components are implanted.
5. The site is examined under the indirect headlight for the position of the retinal detachment and break.
6. Intravitreous gas may be injected.
7. The Tenon capsule and the conjunctiva are closed.

Discussion

Retinal detachment requires immediate repair. Several techniques are used to repair detached tissue. A common technique is to produce adhesions between the layers using **cryotherapy** (freezing of the tissue) or **diathermy** (mild heat created by a diathermy unit or laser). Neither treatment damages the eye, and both create points of scar tissue. This is followed by immediate scleral buckling, in which a Silastic or foam band is attached to the sclera. Several synthetic "buckles" are placed over the band, causing it to indent. This technique puts the tissue in close contact with the retina during healing.

Another common technique is to perform a vitrectomy in conjunction with scleral buckling. In this procedure, the vitreous gel is replaced with Healon or gas through a small puncture wound. This method is used to eliminate traction and tearing on the retina. Two puncture sites are made in the sclera to accommodate microinstruments used to perform cryotherapy or diathermy. The eye remains pressurized throughout the microsurgical procedure. The procedure described here is for scleral buckling and cryotherapy.

The patient is placed in the supine position, prepped, and draped for an eye procedure. Conscious sedation is used for the surgery unless the procedure is expected to last longer than 2 hours. A retrobulbar block also may be used.

An open-ended retractor is placed in the eye. Toothed forceps and Wescott scissors are used to make two incisions in the Tenon capsule one under each rectus muscle. Some surgeons place two 4-0 bridle sutures under the rectus muscles for traction. The bridle suture is left long and used to retract the globe for access to the posterolateral surface.

Using the diathermy unit, the surgeon makes many small burn marks or "spot welds" over the area of detachment. The diathermy electrode produces a high-frequency electrical current that causes mild burning. If the cryosurgical probe is used, the detached area is treated in the same manner.

The assistant steadies the eye by holding the bridle sutures while the surgeon compresses the globe with cotton-tip applicators. The sclera then is approximated with fine suture of 4-0 Prolene. A double-arm suture of Dacron or other synthetic material is placed in the sclera and secured over Silastic sponges. This compresses the eye inward at the area of detachment. A Silastic band may be placed 360 degrees around the eye and a scleral buckle sutured into place under the muscles. Sutures are secured to the buckle so that it remains in place.

Intravitreous Gas Injection

Intravitreous gas injection is the injection of intraocular gas through a handheld syringe. The gas infusion exerts pressure on the retina while subretinal fluid is reabsorbed and scarification takes place. The gases include sulfur hexafluoride (SF6) and perfluoropropane (C3F8).

The scleral buckling procedure is illustrated in Figure 26-23.

FILTERING PROCEDURES AND TRABECULECTOMY

Surgical Goal

A **trabeculectomy** is performed to create a channel from which the aqueous humor may drain from the anterior chamber. This procedure is performed for the treatment of glaucoma.

Pathology

Glaucoma is a group of diseases characterized by optic nerve damage and visual field loss. In the past, glaucoma was defined by intraocular pressure above normal range in association with nerve damage. However, more recent definitions include

cases in which IOP is normal. In most types, IOP is elevated, and the unrelieved pressure can result in ischemia of the optic nerve, which leads to progressive blindness. The IOP is normally maintained by the aqueous humor, which is secreted by the ciliary epithelium (posterior chamber) and drained between the lens and iris, through the pupil into the anterior chamber. Fluid exits through the trabecular network and the canal of Schlemm. The balance in pressure is maintained by the rate of secretion and drainage. A number of pathological conditions can disturb this balance. In nearly all cases of glaucoma, the problem is with drainage rather than overproduction of aqueous humor (Figure 26-24).

There are many different types of glaucoma. The most common are described below[1]:

- *Primary angle closure glaucoma*: This type of glaucoma accounts for 30% of all cases. The incidence is higher in women. A sudden rise in IOP is caused by total blockage or obstruction of the aqueous humor at the root of the iris (the limbal drainage system). This is considered a medical emergency, because blindness may result if the blockage is not relieved.
- *Primary open angle glaucoma*: POAG is a chronic disease occurring in both eyes. It develops in the middle years or later. In this condition, the outflow of aqueous humor is obstructed in the trabecular meshwork which can be caused by different factors.
- *Normal tension glaucoma:* This is a subtype of open angle glaucoma in which intraocular pressure is normal. There is retinal damage and visual field loss with migraine and optic disc hemorrhage.
- *Congenital glaucoma*: In congenital glaucoma, the fluid drainage system is abnormal at birth. The infant's eye distends, and corneal haziness occurs. Symptoms include light sensitivity and excessive tearing. Surgery is indicated to prevent blindness.

Technique

1. The limbus is incised.
2. A scleral flap is created.
3. A small portion of the trabecular meshwork is excised and removed.
4. An iridectomy may be performed.
5. The conjunctiva is closed.
6. The anterior chamber is reinflated as needed.

Discussion

The patient is prepped and draped in routine manner. To begin the procedure, the surgeon inserts a lid speculum. Size 4-0 bridle sutures may be placed in the superior rectus muscle. The conjunctiva is incised at the limbus with toothed forceps and the knife. The Tenon capsule is separated from the sclera with Westcott scissors in the direction of the limbus. This creates a conjunctival flap.

The limbal area is gently scraped with a Beaver blade to remove any blood clots. This technique prevents accidental puncture of the conjunctiva. The sclera then is cauterized in the shape of the flap. The surgeon uses the Beaver blade to make an incision in the sclera, following the outlines of the

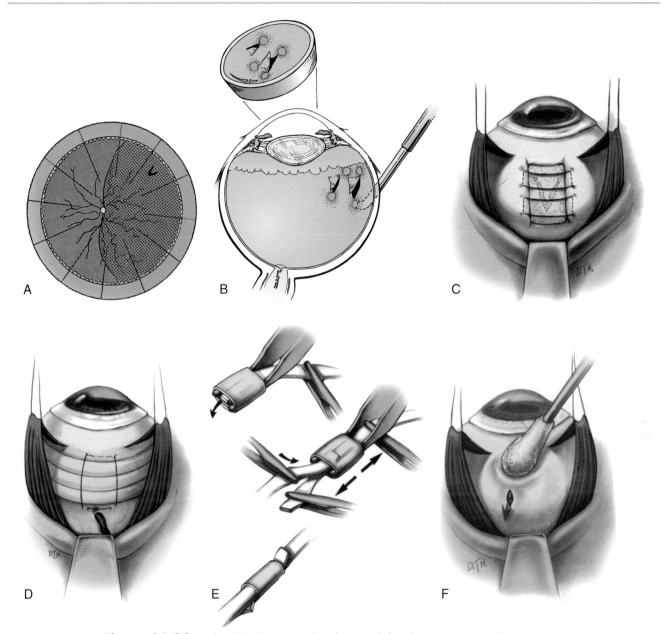

Figure 26-23 Scleral buckling procedure for retinal detachment. **A,** A retinal tear at equator of glove at 1:30 o'clock position. **B,** The surgeon visualizes the field and places the electrode beneath the retinal tear; a burn mark is made on sclera at the site of the retinal tear with the diathermy electrode. **C,** A sponge is sutured in place over the treated site of the retinal tear. **D,** A band and tire are used to encircle the eye. **E,** A Watzke silicone sleeve is placed to secure the encircling band. **F,** An incision is made in the sclera, and a fine incision is made in the choroids to allow subretinal fluid to drain. *(From Ryan S et al: Retina, ed 2, St Louis, 1994, Mosby.)*

cautery. Dissection of the scleral flap starts at the apex and extends upward toward the iris.

A stab wound is made through the cornea to drain the aqueous humor. This incision is self-sealing and can be used later to reinflate the anterior chamber. If necessary, the scleral flap is retracted, and Vannas scissors are used to excise a portion of the trabecular meshwork.

A complication of the procedure may occur at this point; that is, the iris may spontaneously prolapse into the wound.

In such cases, an iridectomy is performed. The surgeon grasps the iris with forceps and removes a portion, taking care not to damage the ciliary body.

In an uncomplicated procedure, BSS is instilled into the anterior chamber to reinflate it. The scleral flap is closed with 10-0 nylon sutures. The conjunctiva and Tenon capsule are approximated with 8-0 absorbable suture. BSS then is instilled into the anterior chamber. An eye sponge is placed over the incision site to check for leakage. Subconjunctival antibiotics

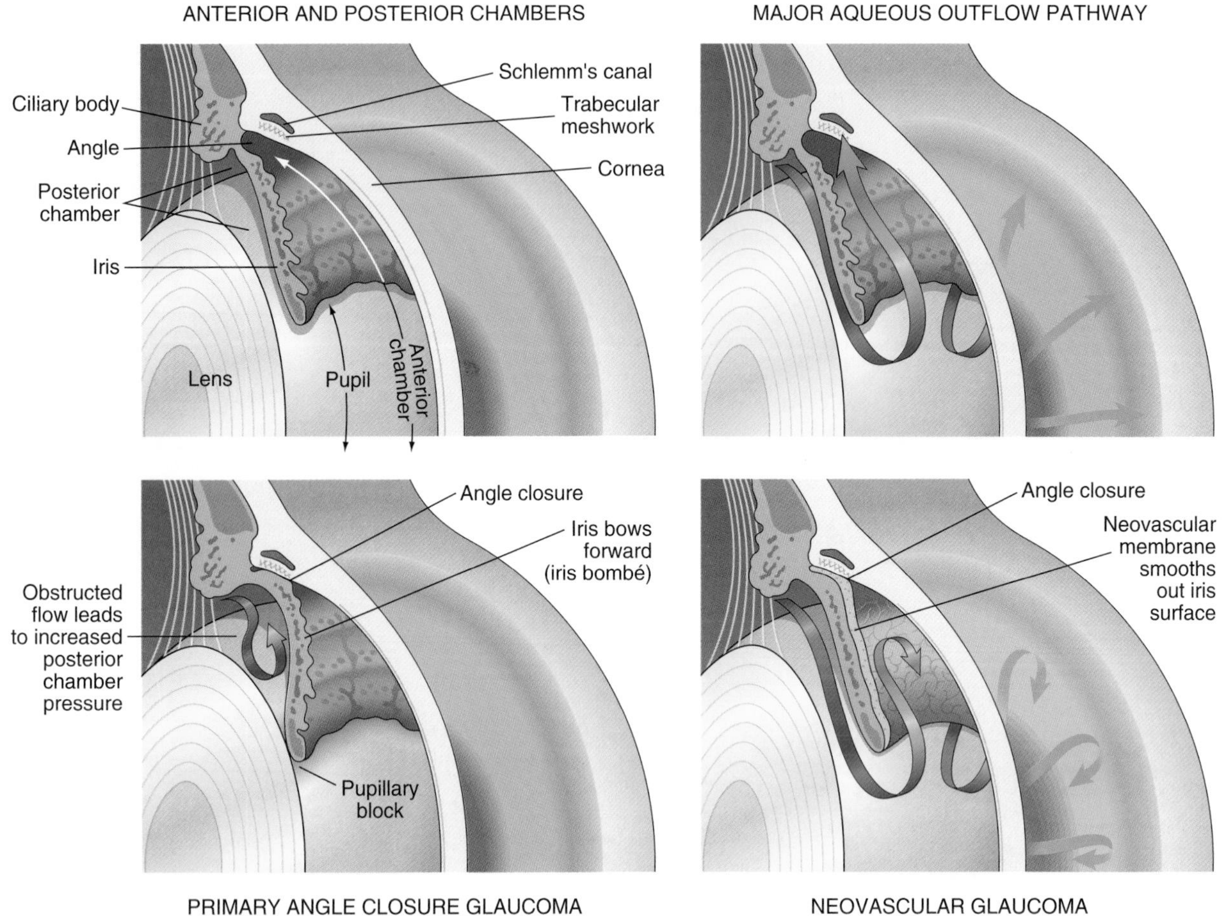

ANTERIOR AND POSTERIOR CHAMBERS

Schlemm's canal
Ciliary body
Trabecular meshwork
Angle
Cornea
Posterior chamber
Iris
Lens
Pupil
Anterior chamber

MAJOR AQUEOUS OUTFLOW PATHWAY

Angle closure
Iris bows forward (iris bombé)
Obstructed flow leads to increased posterior chamber pressure
Pupillary block

Angle closure
Neovascular membrane smooths out iris surface

PRIMARY ANGLE CLOSURE GLAUCOMA

NEOVASCULAR GLAUCOMA

Figure 26-24   Pathology of glaucoma. *Upper left,* A normal eye, showing the drainage pathway of the aqueous humor. *Lower left,* Primary closure glaucoma, in which the iris is in close contact with the lens. Increased pressure obstructs the trabecular meshwork. *Lower right,* Contraction of the myofibroblasts in the vascular membrane causes the iris to obstruct drainage. *(From Kumar V, Abbas A, Fausto N: Robbins and Cotran pathologic basis of disease, ed 7, Philadelphia, 2004, WB Saunders.)*

and steroids are injected, and antibacterial ointments are instilled into the eye.

Adjunctive Chemotherapy

If the filtering procedure is at risk of failure or if a low IOP is indicated, the surgeon may use a chemotherapeutic agent, such as 5-fluorouracil (5-FU), and mitomycin. If this is the case, a sponge soaked with the agent is placed at the surgical site for approximately 1 minute. After removal of the sponge, the entire field is irrigated with BSS, and the instruments that were exposed to mitomycin are removed from the field. Because of the potential toxicity of the drugs, protocols for their disposal and for instrument decontamination are required in most health care facilities.

Postoperative Considerations

The trabeculectomy will fail if a flat bleb does not form in the first postoperative days. If a bleb leak develops, a bandage contact lens may be inserted, and repair may be necessary. Cataract formation may occur as a result of the trabeculectomy, and additional surgery may be required.

The trabeculectomy procedure is illustrated in Figure 26-25.

ARGON LASER TRABECULOPLASTY

Surgical Goal

In argon laser trabeculoplasty, the argon laser is used to shrink collagen and stretch the canal of Schlemm, thereby expanding the canal, increasing drainage, and reducing IOP.

Pathology

Glaucoma is classified as open angle or closed angle and then further categorized as primary or secondary. Argon laser trabeculoplasty is indicated for primary and secondary open angle glaucoma. Primary open angle glaucoma has a genetic component and is more common in individuals with diabetes and African Americans. Secondary open angle glaucoma is differentiated by the obstruction of the outflow of aqueous humor, which causes an increase in IOP (see Filtering Procedures and Trabeculectomy).

Evert: To turn outward or inside out.

Goiter: Benign enlargement of the thyroid gland.

Hypertrophy (Hypertrophic): Enlargement of an organ or tissue.

Innervation: The supplying of a body part or organ with nerves or nervous stimuli.

Keratin: A substance created by the squamous epithelium.

Nasolaryngoscope: A flexible endoscope that is passed through the nose to visualize the larynx.

Neoplasm: An abnormal growth of cells.

Nystagmus: Rapid oscillation of the eye, a symptom of certain nervous system diseases.

Ossicles: The bones of the middle ear that conduct sound (i.e., the malleus, incus, and stapes).

Otitis media: Middle ear infection.

Ototoxic: A substance that can injure the ear.

Packing: A method of applying a dressing to a body cavity. In nasal procedures, ¼- or ½-inch (0.63 or 1.25 cm) gauze strips are inserted into the nasal cavity to absorb drainage, control bleeding, or expose the mucosa to topical medication. "Packing" a wound may refer to any dressing that is introduced into an anatomical space or cavity.

Papilloma: A benign epithelial tumor characterized by a branching or lobular tumor. Also called a *papillary tumor.*

Paranasal sinuses: Air cells surrounding or on the periphery of the nasal cavities. These are the maxillary, ethmoid, sphenoid, and frontal sinuses.

Paresis: Paralysis of a structure (e.g., vocal cord paresis).

Perforation: A defect in the tympanic membrane caused by trauma or infection.

Perichondrium: Tissue overlying the cartilage that provides its vascular and nervous supply.

Periosteum: Tissue overlying the bone that provides its vascular and nervous supply.

Phonation: Vibration of the vocal cords during speaking or vocalization.

Polyp: Excessive proliferation of the mucosal epithelium.

Sensorineural hearing loss: Hearing impairment arising from the cochlea, auditory nerve, or central nervous system.

Sublingual: A term for the region under the tongue, which is highly vascular. Specific medications may be administered sublingually, because they are rapidly absorbed through the mucous membrane.

TM: The tympanic membrane.

Transsphenoidal: Literally, "across or through the sphenoid bone." Surgery of the pituitary gland may be performed by approaching it through the sphenoid bone.

Tympanostomy tube: A tube that is placed in a myringotomy to produce aeration of the middle ear.

Uvulopalatopharyngoplasty (UPP): A procedure in which the tonsils, uvula, and a portion of the soft palate are removed to reduce and stiffen excess oropharyngeal and oral cavity tissue in patients with obstructive sleep apnea.

Vertigo: A symptom rather than a disease, *vertigo* is a general term referring to sensory disturbances in which the patient is unable to maintain balance or has the perception of spinning, falling, or the environment turning.

SECTION I: THE EAR

INTRODUCTION

Otorhinolaryngology is the medical specialty concerned with the ear, nose, and throat. Surgery of the ear includes procedures of the outer, middle, and inner ear. Procedures are performed under microscopy.

Many patients undergoing ear surgery have a hearing deficit. The perioperative team should adjust their communication methods to accommodate the patient's needs. The patient may state which method is best for communication and which ear has the deficit, and whether written communication is needed.

Many patients with a hearing deficit develop a sense of isolation. The hearing world often is impatient when individuals are unable to communicate quickly and easily. Equality in patient care sometimes requires extra effort for patients with sensorial loss. One of the primary goals of the perioperative protocol is to provide comfort and healing whenever possible. This begins with compassionate patient communication.

SURGICAL ANATOMY

The anatomy of the ear is divided into three regions: the *external ear,* the *middle ear,* and the *inner ear.*

EXTERNAL EAR

The structures of the external ear include the outer surface of the *tympanic membrane* (**TM**) and all structures lateral to it (Figure 27-1). This includes the *auricle* or *pinna,* the *external auditory meatus,* and the *external auditory canal.* The auricle is a cartilaginous structure covered by skin. Its function is to gather sound waves. The center of the auricle contains the external auditory meatus, which leads to the external auditory canal. The lateral one third of the external auditory canal is surrounded with cartilage and is lined with glands that secret a waxy substance called **cerumen.** The external auditory canal measures approximately 1 inch (2.5 cm) and terminates at the tympanic membrane. The TM also serves as a barrier between the external and middle ears.

MIDDLE EAR

The middle ear extends from the TM to the medial wall of the middle ear cleft. It includes the TM, the *ossicles* (i.e., the *malleus, stapes,* and *incus*), the opening to the eustachian tube, the opening of the mastoid cavity, and the intratympanic portion of the facial nerve.

The TM, which is elliptical and conical in shape, aids in the process of hearing by transmitting sound waves to the ossicles,

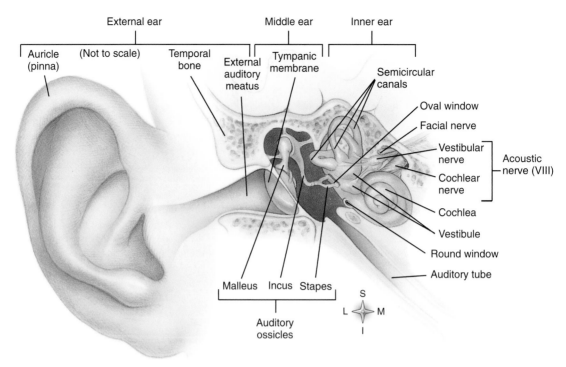

Figure 27-1 Structures of the ear. *(From Thibodeau G, Patton K:* Anatomy and physiology, *ed 6, St Louis, 2007, Mosby.)*

which are just posterior to it. The three ossicles together can fit on a dime. The malleus (hammer bone), the most lateral of the ossicles, is partly embedded in the TM. The incus (anvil) connects the stapes to the malleus. The stapes (stirrup) transmits the vibrations of the TM and the other ossicles to the inner ear via the oval window.

The proximal *eustachian* tube is composed of connective tissue and lined with mucous membrane. It extends into the nasopharynx at its distal end and assists in equalizing pressure between the external environment and the middle ear. It also is a pathway for bacteria to spread from the nasopharynx to the inner ear, causing **otitis media** (middle ear infection).

INNER EAR

The inner ear contains receptors for hearing and balance and is composed of a series of hollow tunnels called *labyrinths.* The inner ear has two separate labyrinth systems. The *bony labyrinth* is formed by the temporal bone and is filled with *perilymph fluid.* Within the bony labyrinth is the *membranous labyrinth.* This structure has three parts: the cochlea, the semicircular canals, and the vestibule.

The spiral-shaped *cochlea* contains the cochlear duct and the organ of hearing, the *organ of Corti.* This organ extends along the length of the membranous labyrinth in the cochlea. The organ of Corti is lined with cilia, which project into the endolymph and receive the sound waves transmitted by the middle ear.

The *semicircular canals* communicate with the middle ear via the oval and round windows. These are located within the temporal bone and contain endolymph. Each of the semicircular canals contains an enlarged space called the *ampulla.* The *crista ampullaris,* located within the ampulla, is responsible for equilibrium of the body in motion (called *dynamic equilibrium*). Figure 27-2 illustrates the structures of the inner ear.

SOUND TRANSMISSION IN THE EAR

Hearing is the neural interpretation of sound transmission. Sound waves in the air enter the ear and are transmitted to the tympanic membrane. The membrane vibrates against the malleus, which is attached on the posterior side. This causes vibration in the incus and in the stapes, which is connected to the oval window. From there, sound is transmitted into the perilymph of the cochlea, through the vestibular membrane, to the basil membrane of the organ of Corti. Nerve transmission occurs from the basil membrane to the cochlear nerve. This pathway is illustrated in Figure 27-3.

PATHOLOGY OF THE EAR

Table 27-1 presents conditions of the ear.
Figure 27-4 shows some pathological conditions of the ear.

DIAGNOSTIC PROCEDURES

CLINICAL EXAMINATION OF THE EAR

- The external auditory canal, auricle, mastoid, and surrounding tissues are examined for signs of infection, inflammation, neoplasm, scars, and lesions.

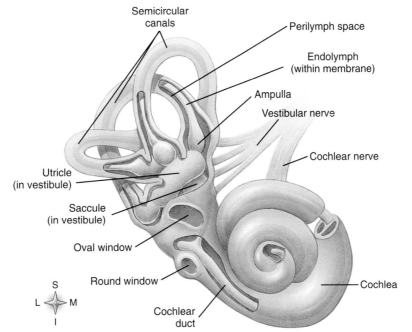

Figure 27-2   Structures of the inner ear. *(From Thibodeau G, Patton K: Anatomy and physiology, ed 6, St Louis, 2007, Mosby.)*

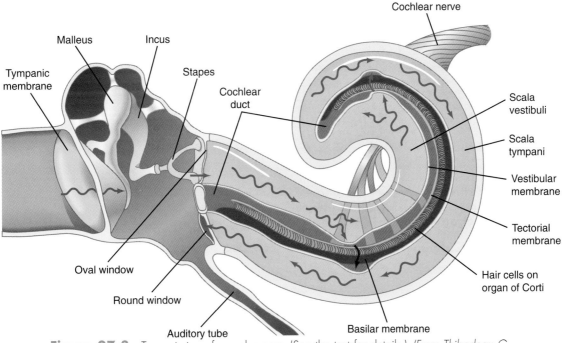

Figure 27-3   Transmission of sound waves. (See the text for details.) *(From Thibodeau G, Patton K: Anatomy and physiology, ed 6, St Louis, 2007, Mosby.)*

- An *otoscope* is used for the initial examination of the TM. If necessary, any cerumen is removed to allow complete visualization of the tympanic membrane.
- If further examination of the TM is warranted, microscopic examination may be performed with a 250-mm lens and an ear speculum.
- Nasal and oropharyngeal examinations are performed with a tongue blade and a penlight (or the light from an oto-scope) to detect any blockage of the eustachian tube by infection, inflammation, or tumor.
- Computed tomography (CT) or magnetic resonance imaging (MRI) scans may be ordered if any abnormalities are noted, such as asymmetrical hearing loss on the audiological examination or masses in the nasopharynx, oropharynx, or ear; or if cholesteatoma or infection are suspected.

Table 27-1

Pathology of the Ear

Condition	Description	Considerations
External Ear		
Trauma	Injury to the external ear can result in avulsion of the ear or hematoma.	Avulsion of the ear must be repaired through surgical reattachment of the ear, if possible; a hematoma must be drained to prevent necrosis of surrounding tissues.
Infection	The most common infections are otitis externa (swimmer's ear) and atopic dermatitis. Other causes can be viruses (e.g., herpes simplex) and bacteria (e.g., *Pseudomonas*).	These conditions usually are managed in the physician's office with antibiotics.
Tumors/cancers	Primary cancers of the external ear and external ear canal are basal cell carcinoma and squamous cell carcinoma.	Treatment is excisional biopsy for diagnosis and, if necessary, excision and closure to guarantee complete removal of the cancerous lesion.
Middle Ear		
Trauma	Laceration or perforation of the tympanic membrane may be caused by sudden high pressure or by a foreign body.	Small perforations heal spontaneously; larger defects require surgical repair. (See Tympanoplasty.)
Otitis media	Infection of the middle ear may be acute or chronic. It is more common in childhood, especially when children are exposed to cigarette smoke and other air pollutants.	Acute otitis media is treated with antibacterial drugs. Chronic infection may require drainage through a myringotomy and tube implant. Left untreated, chronic otitis media can spread to the mastoid cells and inner ear. (See Myringotomy and Mastoidectomy/Tympanomastoidectomy.)
Cholesteatoma	Cholesteatoma is a common complication of chronic otitis media. It is caused by shedding of **keratin** from the tympanic membrane. The tumor can extend into the middle ear and erode the mastoid bone.	Surgical treatment is necessary for advanced cholesteatoma. (See Tympanoplasty.)
Otosclerosis	Otosclerosis is abnormal thickening of the bone.in the middle and inner ear. This restricts the footplate of the stapes, the most common cause of conductive hearing loss.	Surgical treatment is necessary, with or without ossicular chain reconstruction. (See Stapedectomy/Ossicular Reconstruction.)
Inner Ear		
Meniere disease	The cause of Meniere disease is unknown. It is characterized by recurrent **vertigo** (dizziness) that lasts several hours, **sensorineural hearing loss** at low frequency, and ringing in the ears (tinnitus).	Treatment is nonsurgical; it includes management of symptoms and a low-sodium diet.

DIAGNOSTIC TESTS OF THE EAR

Table 27-2 presents diagnostic tests of the ear.

PERIOPERATIVE CONSIDERATIONS

As mentioned previously, many patients undergoing ear surgery have a hearing deficit. Sensitivity to the patient's needs is extremely important, because the environment can be frightening, and communication can be difficult. A dry erase board, hand signals, and other alternative methods of communication should used.

POSITIONING

Surgical procedures of the ear generally are performed with the patient in the supine position with the head turned. A doughnut headrest is used to stabilize the head and prevent pressure on the opposite ear. It is important that the patient remain perfectly still during surgery. The slightest movement while under the microscope can cause injury. Special positioning accommodations may be required for a patient with a previous neck injury or other skeletal problems that might cause discomfort during surgery.

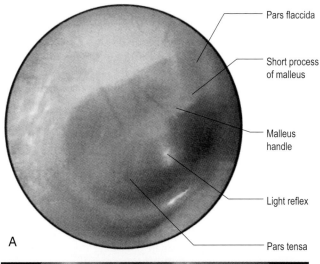

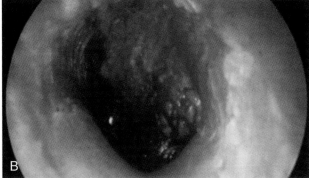

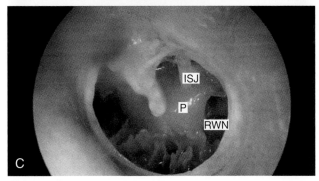

Figure 27-4 Pathology of the ear. **A,** Normal tympanic membrane. **B,** Otitis media. **C,** Subtotal perforation of the tympanic membrane. Round window *(RWN),* incostapedial joint *(ISJ),* promontory *(P). (From Dhillon RS, East CA: Ear, nose, and throat and head and neck surgery, ed 3, Edinburgh, 2006, Churchill Livingstone.)*

PREPPING AND DRAPING

Prepping and draping for ear procedures focuses on the ear and postauricular area. A secondary site is prepped for a skin graft. Selected procedures require the removal of a small amount of hair in the preauricular region.

Before prepping begins, the circulator verifies that the correct prepping solution is being used, because some prepping solutions are **ototoxic** and may damage the ear if allowed to drain into the middle ear through the incision or a puncture in the TM. A sterile cotton ball is placed in the ear canal

Table 27-2
Diagnostic Tests of the Ear

Test	Description
Tuning fork test (Rhine and Weber tests)	Test bone conduction and sensorineural hearing function of cochlea.
Audiological testing (hearing test)	Usually conducted by an audiologist; can include air conduction, bone conduction, and speech recognition tests.
Electronystagmography (ENG) testing	Tests for **nystagmus.**
Head positioning tests	Test for benign paroxysmal positional vertigo (BPPV).
Balance testing	Tests stance, gait, and balance for signs of vertigo.
Caloric testing	Tests for vertigo and nystagmus; warm or cool water is instilled into the external ear canal to determine whether those conditions are elicited.
Auditory brainstem response (ABR)	Usually conducted by an audiologist or neurologist; measures the response of the brainstem to electrical stimulus as it relates to the ear.

to prevent prep solution from entering the canal. The circulator then preps the surgical site, extending to the cheek medially, the occiput laterally, the temporal bone superiorly, and the upper neck inferiorly.

The ear is draped with four towels, which are covered with a fenestrated, transparent drape. The drape may be stapled in place. Next, a split sheet is draped over the patient and around the ear.

IRRIGATION

Irrigation is used frequently during surgery to remove blood and tissue debris from the operative field. Because the site is extremely small, even small particles of tissue or blood can obscure the entire field. A suction irrigator provides a fine stream of saline or lactated Ringer solution and removes fluid from the field. The suction irrigator also is used to remove bone fragments and to irrigate the drill tip during bone drilling. The suction irrigator is a combination Frazier suction tip and a smaller irrigator.

INSTRUMENTS

The primary instruments used in ear surgery include a small number of plastic surgery instruments: hook retractors, mosquito forceps, #15 knife, and delicate skin forceps. Ear instruments are designed with a short fulcrum and long shanks, which are extremely delicate and easily damaged. The working tips are short (2 to 5 mm). These include grasping forceps,

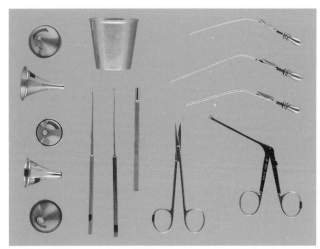

Figure 27-5 Instruments used in ear surgery. *(From Tighe SM: Instrumentation for the operating room, ed 7, St Louis, 2007, Mosby.)*

cup forceps, scissors, picks, elevators, and knives with different-shaped cutting surfaces. Several types of small spring retractors are also used. Various sizes of ear speculums are included in the set. These are designed to fit into the outer ear canal without external support. Ear instruments are maintained in a rack on the instrument table or Mayo stand. They must be arranged so that the tips are easily visible.

Microinstruments are considerably smaller than regular ear instruments. A dedicated light source should be directed over the Mayo stand so that the instruments can be identified. Like all microinstruments, ear instruments must be handled gently and protected from damage. Ear instruments are shown in Figure 27-5.

Speculum Holder

The speculum holder provides external structural support to the ear speculum; this allows the surgeon to use both hands to operate in the external auditory canal. Several styles of speculum holders are available. They include a bed (table) bracket, a blade that connects to the bed bracket, a flexible arm, and the speculum holder itself, which attaches to the flexible arm.

Otology Endoscope

The otology endoscope is used occasionally during surgery. Endoscopes are available in 2.7 and 4 mm and are 4.4 inches (11 cm) long. The endoscope is used with a standard fiberoptic light source and digital imaging equipment (see Chapter 21).

EQUIPMENT AND SUPPLIES

Power Drill

A power drill is needed in all ear surgery that involves bone. For example, a drill is used to open the mastoid bone, enlarge the bony portion of the ear canal, and to drill through the small stapes footplate.

All drills are used with small cutting or diamond burrs, which vary in size from 0.5 to 7 mm. The scrub must irrigate the tip of the drill during operation to prevent tissue heating. A suction irrigator or a mL3- to 5 mL syringe fitted with an 18-gauge angiography catheter is used for irrigation. If an angiography catheter is used, it is important that only the tip of the Angiocath be visible in the operating field so that the surgeon's vision under the microscope is not obscured.

Operating Microscope

The operating microscope is used in all procedures of the middle or inner ear. The standard operating lens for ear surgery has a focal length of 250 mm. However, some surgeons prefer a 200- or 300-mm lens. For simple procedures, such as a myringotomy, a small operating microscope on a floor stand may be used. Complex procedures, such as a tympanoplasty or mastoidectomy, require a larger, more mobile operating microscope on a floor stand or ceiling mount. Gross adjustments are made before surgery, and the microscope is draped within an hour of use. (Chapter 26 presents a complete discussion of the use and care of the operating microscope.)

Sponges

Cotton pledgets, such as those used during neurosurgery, are commonly used in ear procedures. Square 4 × 4 sponges should also be available. Even though the operative site may be small, sponge and sharps counts are routinely performed for all ear surgeries.

Dressings

Two types of dressings are used in ear procedures: the mastoid dressing and the Glasscock dressing. The mastoid dressing is applied after complex procedures of the ear, especially those that require drilling of the mastoid. The dressing consists of several fluffed gauze sponges to cover ear and incision, as well as rolled gauze (Kling or Kerlix), which is wrapped around the patient's head to hold the dressing in place. The Glasscock dressing is used after minor procedures of the ear, such as a stapedectomy or tympanoplasty. This dressing, which comes prepackaged, is composed of gauze sponges with Velcro straps to secure the dressing in place.

MEDICATIONS

Medications used during ear surgery include anesthetics, hemostatic agents, antibiotic solutions, and irrigation solutions. Lidocaine with epinephrine is used in most ear surgeries to control bleeding by vasoconstriction.

Hemostatic agents are used to control active bleeding. The primary hemostatic agents are Gelfoam and Helistat. Pledgets of Gelfoam may be soaked in epinephrine and applied directly to bleeding tissue.

Antibiotic solution often is instilled into the ear. Gelfoam soaked in a solution composed of an antibiotic and a corticosteroid may be used at the end of a procedure to control postoperative inflammation.

SURGICAL PROCEDURES

MYRINGOTOMY

Surgical Goal

A myringotomy is a surgical opening made in the tympanic membrane to release fluid from the middle ear.

Pathology

Fluid in the middle ear is referred to as an **effusion.** This can be caused by inflammation of the mucosa. It also can be caused by eustachian tube dysfunction, in which airflow between the nasopharynx and the middle ear is inadequate; the result is negative pressure in the middle ear and retraction of the TM. Eustachian tube dysfunction can be caused by a congenital anomaly, inflammation of the nasal mucosa, or enlarged adenoids. If left untreated, the effusion may lead to infection, mastoiditis, hearing loss, or perforation.

Technique

1. A speculum is placed in the ear canal, and the microscope is used to visualize the tympanic membrane (TM).
2. Excess cerumen is removed from the ear canal.
3. A small incision is made in the TM.
4. Fluid is suctioned.
5. A tympanostomy tube is placed if necessary.

Discussion

A middle ear effusion can be treated by making a small incision in the tympanic membrane (myringotomy). This allows trapped fluid to drain. To maintain open drainage, a **tympanostomy tube** often is placed in the incision. A myringotomy allows equalization of the pressure between the middle ear and the outside barometric pressure. Tubes usually are not removed, but are left in place until they fall out (Figure 27-6). The procedure most often is performed on children.

The patient is placed in the supine position with the head supported on a doughnut headrest. Skin prep and draping

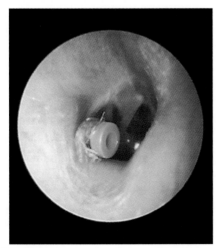

Figure 27-6 Myringotomy tube in place. *(From Thibodeau G, Patton K: Anatomy and physiology, ed 6, St Louis, 2007, Mosby.)*

usually are omitted. General anesthesia is administered by mask, because the procedure is brief. The surgeon sits while operating and uses a microscope with a 250-mm lens. The microscope is brought into position as soon as the surgeon is seated.

To begin the procedure, the surgeon inserts a Farrior speculum into the external ear canal. The speculum size is determined by the diameter and depth of the ear canal. With the speculum in place, the surgeon removes any wax or debris from the external auditory canal with a cerumen curette. Then, a 2- to 3-mm incision is made in the TM with a myringotomy knife. Fluid behind the TM is suctioned with a small Frasier microsuction (#3 or #5). If a tympanostomy tube is to be implanted, the scrub uses alligator forceps to grasp the tube. The surgeon inserts the tube into the myringotomy incision. Next, a Rosen needle is used to seat the tube in the incision. A combination of antibiotic and steroid drops or antibiotic drops alone are then instilled into the external canal, and the speculum is removed. The external canal is packed with cotton.

MYRINGOPLASTY

Surgical Goal

A myringoplasty is performed to close a small, nonhealing hole in the tympanic membrane. The procedure is performed without entering the middle ear.

Pathology

Causes of **perforation** of the TM may include a persistent opening after removal of a tympanostomy tube, a blast injury, or a penetrating foreign body in the ear.

Technique

1. A speculum is placed in the external canal for microscopic examination.
2. Debris is removed from the ear canal.
3. The edges of the tympanic membrane are everted and roughened.
4. A fat graft is removed if necessary.
5. A small patch (or fat graft) is placed over the perforation.

Discussion

The patient is placed in the supine position with the head positioned on a doughnut headrest. General anesthesia is administered by mask. Endotracheal intubation seldom is required, because the anesthesia time is short. The patient is prepped and draped for an ear procedure. Because the tympanic membrane is open during the prep, special care is taken to prevent any prep solution from entering the ear canal.

The operating microscope is fitted with a 250-mm lens. The microscope usually is not draped for the procedure. To begin the procedure, the surgeon places a Farrior speculum into the external auditory canal. The external canal is cleaned with a cerumen curette and Frasier suction. The surgeon then can **evert** (turn back) the edges of the perforated TM and score them with either a fine Rosen needle or a fine right-angle pick. Several types of patches can be used to close the defect (e.g., Gelfoam, Gelfilm, Steri-Strip, or a fat graft).

Fat Graft

The surgeon makes a small incision (approximately 5 to 8 mm) on the posterior side of the ear lobe with a #15 blade. Single skin hooks are used to expose the subcutaneous tissue. A small piece of the tissue is excised with a #15 blade and a hemostat or toothed Adson forceps. The graft is placed in a small amount of saline to keep it moist until the surgeon is ready to implant it. The graft site is closed with 4-0 Vicryl suture.

The graft is positioned over the defect in the TM. The external auditory canal is packed with gelatin sponges soaked in a steroid-antibiotic solution, and a Glasscock-style dressing is applied.

TYMPANOPLASTY

Surgical Goal

A tympanoplasty is the surgical removal of a **cholesteatoma** and mastoid bone, with or without reconstruction.

Pathology

A tympanoplasty is performed to treat a number of disorders affecting the TM. These conditions include a nonhealing perforation of the TM, a dysfunction of the eustachian tube that causes retraction of the TM, and a cholesteatoma. As mentioned previously, in dysfunction of the eustachian tube, inadequate airflow between the nasopharynx and the middle ear causes negative pressure in the middle ear and retraction of the TM. This causes the TM to vibrate improperly and can lead to a perforation or cholesteatoma. A cholesteatoma may cause infection, otorrhea, bone destruction, hearing loss, and paralysis of the facial nerve.

Technique

1. An incision is made posterior to the ear.
2. A fascia graft is removed.
3. The native tympanic membrane (TM) is removed or prepared for grafting.
4. The ear canal is enlarged with a drill (canalplasty).
5. The TM is reconstructed.
6. The incision is closed, and the ear canal is packed.

Discussion

Two methods are commonly used to perform a tympanoplasty. The approach depends on the condition of the TM, the size and position of the perforation, and the surgeon's preference.

In the underlay technique, the TM is lifted away and the middle ear is filled with Gelfoam to support a graft on the under surface of the TM perforation. This is used for a small, visible perforation with minimal signs of infection.

The overlay technique is used for a large perforation, a severely damaged TM, or for extensive infection. In this procedure, the TM remnants and bony canal skin are removed. The bony canal is enlarged with a drill, and the TM is recre-

ated with a fascia and skin graft (usually from the abdomen, upper arm, or pinna).

The patient is placed in the supine position with the head supported on a doughnut headrest. The arm on the operative side is tucked at the patient's side. General anesthesia is used.

If a skin graft from the arm or abdomen is planned, it may be removed before the skin prep and draping. The arm is prepped and draped with towels. The surgeon removes the graft with a sharp double-edged razor blade (e.g., a Gillette or a Watson) or a Weck skin graft knife. The graft is placed in a small basin and protected from damage or contamination. A small amount of saline is used to keep the graft moist. The graft site is covered or may be dressed. The patient is prepped and draped for the ear procedure.

The surgeon makes a postauricular (behind the ear) incision and carries it through the temporalis fascia to the mastoid tip. A temporalis fascia graft is harvested with Brown Adson forceps and a #15 blade. A *fascia press* is used to flatten and shape the graft. A separate sterile table may be set up for this, or the surgeon may use an area of the back table to prepare the graft. The fascia press with the graft on it should be left in the open position unless the surgeon requests otherwise. This allows the graft to dry so that it can be trimmed and placed in the ear later in the procedure.

The microscope is fitted with a 250-mm lens and moved into position. The TM is exposed with a gimmick or House knife and removed with Bellucci scissors or knife. If a **canalplasty** (reconstruction of the canal) is to be performed, the ear canal is enlarged with a small cutting drill and a small 4 × 5 suction irrigator. This permits better visualization of the middle ear and a larger space in which to work.

The middle ear is then prepared to receive the graft. The surgeon trims the fascia to the appropriate size using the fascia press and a #15 blade. The graft is grasped with a smooth alligator forceps and removed from the fascia press. The surgeon reconstructs the middle ear by placing the fascia graft in position with the alligator forceps and a fine Rosen needle. The skin grafts, if taken, are then laid over the fascia graft with alligator forceps and Rosen needle. The ear is packed with small pledgets of Gelfoam or Helistat to hold the graft in position. The wound is closed in layers with 3-0 absorbable sutures, and the skin is closed with 4-0 absorbable sutures. The ear is dressed with a mastoid dressing.

MASTOIDECTOMY/ TYMPANOMASTOIDECTOMY

Surgical Goal

A mastoidectomy or tympanomastoidectomy is the removal of diseased bone, the mastoid air cells, and the soft tissue lining the air cells of the matoid.

Pathology

The mastoid is composed of many air cells similar to the nasal sinuses. Inadequate flow of air through the sinuses can lead to infection and erosion of the surrounding bone. Cholesteatoma, eustachian tube dysfunction, **neoplasm,** or congenital malformation of the middle ear may block airflow to the mastoid and cause chronic mastoiditis. An advanced cholesteatoma may spread into the mastoid. In this case, mastoidectomy with tympanoplasty is performed.

Technique

1. A postauricular incision is made.
2. The skin flaps are elevated.
3. Temporalis fascia is harvested.
4. Diseased mastoid is removed with a drill.
5. The ossicles are removed if diseased.
6. The cholesteatoma is removed.
7. The mastoid cavity and middle ear are packed.
8. The incisions are closed, and dressings are applied.

Discussion

The patient is placed in the supine position, and the arm on the operative side is tucked at the patient's side. General anesthesia is used. A skin graft is taken before the ear prep, as described previously. A 27-gauge needle is used to inject the ear incision site with lidocaine with epinephrine. The patient is then prepped and draped for an ear procedure.

The surgeon makes a postauricular incision. The temporalis fascia graft is removed, smoothed onto the fascia press, and allowed to dry. The incision is carried to the bone, and the diseased mastoid tissue is excised with a power drill with a large cutting burr. The surgeon may use a variety of burrs to remove the bone. A Rosen needle, gimmick, or picks are used to assess the patency of the mastoid and determine the need for continued drilling. The surgeon removes the cholesteatoma with a gimmick or Rosen needle.

With the cholesteatoma removed, the surgeon places the fascia graft over the remaining ossicles; this is done as described for a tympanoplasty. The skin graft is placed in position over the fascia. The surgeon then uses a serrated alligator forceps and a gimmick to pack the mastoid cavity and middle ear with Gelfoam sponges that have been soaked in saline solution or a combination steroid-antibiotic. The incisions are closed in layers with 3-0 absorbable sutures. The skin is closed with 4-0 absorbable sutures. The external auditory canal is also packed with Gelfoam, as for the mastoid cavity. A mastoid dressing is applied.

STAPEDECTOMY/OSSICULAR RECONSTRUCTION

Surgical Goal

A stapedectomy is the reconstruction of the ossicles to restore conduction to the oval window.

Pathology

A stapedectomy, or ossicular reconstruction, is performed to treat profound hearing loss related to sclerosis of the stapes. Sound normally is received at the TM, which transmits vibrations through the ossicles and the oval window, which amplifies the sound. If the bony chain is immobile or discontinuous, not only is amplification lost, but sound

perception can be severely dampened. The most common cause of ossicle immobility is *otosclerosis* of the stapes. This is abnormal bone growth that locks the stapes into place and prevents it from vibrating and carrying the stimulus (Figure 27-7). Otosclerosis generally begins at age 30 and progresses with age. After surgery, 90% of patients have a permanent hearing gain, and 1% have a permanent hearing loss.

The most common cause of a break in the ossicle chain is a cholesteatoma, which erodes the ossicles. The shape and articulation of the ossicles provides minimal sound amplification (1.7 : 1). The size ratio between the TM and the oval window provides most of the amplification (17 : 1). This is important, because a mobile connection between the TM and the oval window can improve hearing.

Technique

1. The auditory canal is injected with lidocaine and epinephrine.
2. A speculum is placed in the external auditory canal.
3. The tympanic membrane (TM) is elevated.
4. The affected ossicles are freed or removed.
5. A hole is drilled in the stapes footplate.
6. The prosthesis is implanted and secured.
7. The TM is replaced.
8. The external canal is packed, and a dressing is applied.

Discussion

The patient is placed in the supine position, and the arm on the operative side is tucked at the patient's side. General anesthesia is used. The external ear canal is injected with a local anesthetic before prepping. The patient is prepped and draped for an ear procedure.

The operative microscope with a 250-mm lens is used to examine the middle ear. The external ear canal is irrigated and cleaned with a 7 Fr Frazier suction tip. In this procedure, a speculum holder is used. The surgeon places the speculum in the external canal and attaches it to a universal speculum holder for stabilization. This allows the surgeon to operate with both hands while the speculum is held in the external canal. The surgeon then changes to a 5 Fr Frazier suction tip to clear any fluid from the ear.

The TM is elevated, and the posterior bony ledge is removed with a House knife. With the TM elevated, the surgeon can visualize the ossicular chain. The incostapedial joint is cut with a joint knife, and the stapedial tendon is severed with Bellucci scissors. The stapes superstructure is then fractured with a fine Rosen needle and microcup forceps.

The surgeon then drills a hole in the stapes footplate with a Skeeter drill or similar microdrill using a 1-mm cutting burr. The prosthesis, which has been previously loaded onto a serrated alligator forceps or hook, is implanted in the hole in the footplate. The surgeon secures the prosthesis in place by **packing** the ear with gelatin sponges soaked in normal saline or steroidantibiotic ointment. A gimmick and a fine Rosen needle are used to replace the TM. The external auditory canal is packed with gelatin sponges soaked in saline or an

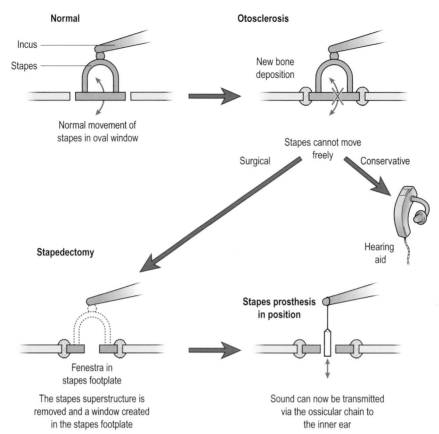

Figure 27-7   Stapedectomy for the treatment of otosclerosis. *(From Dhillon RS, East CA: Ear, nose, and throat and head and neck surgery, ed 3, Edinburgh, 2006, Churchill Livingstone.)*

antibiotic-steroid solution. A Glasscock or mastoid dressing is applied.

COCHLEAR IMPLANT

Surgical Goal

A cochlear implant is used to transmit external sound directly to the eighth cranial nerve. It is used in the treatment of sensorineural deafness (Figure 27-8).

Pathology

Sensorineural deafness can be congenital or acquired. It has many different causes including:

- Viral or bacterial infection causing damage to the cilia
- Acoustic trauma (caused by loud noise) which result in permanent injury to the cilia
- Tumor of the ocular nerve
- Drugs such as certain antibiotics that cause permanent hearing loss
- Autoimmune disease, stroke, brain tumor

A cochlear implant provides the perception of sound. However, significant postoperative rehabilitation is required for the patient to turn this into cognitive information. Congenital deafness in the child can be treated with a cochlear implant, but surgery is delayed until age 2.

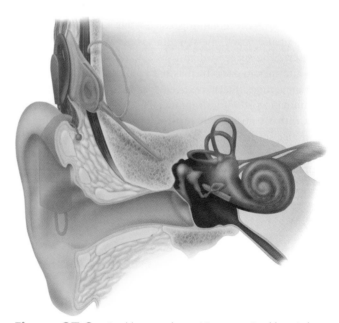

Figure 27-8   Cochlear implant. *(Courtesy Cochlear Ltd, 2009.)*

Technique

1. A postauricular incision is made and extended superiorly.
2. The cranium is exposed.
3. A recessed space for the internal receiver is created in the bone.
4. The facial nerve is identified.
5. The medial wall of the middle ear is identified.
6. The internal electrodes of the implant are placed into the cochlea via the round window.
7. The internal receiver is implanted and secured.
8. The incision is closed.

Discussion

Patients with sensorineural hearing loss have functional outer and middle ear structures. However, the cilia, which receive and transmit sound to the ocular nerve and brain, are damaged or absent. The cochlear implant is a device which receives sound and transmits them as electrical impulses to the brain.

The cochlear implant has two primary components: an electronic processor, which is implanted outside the ear over the temporal bone captures sound and sends it in digital form to an internal transmitter. The transmitter conveys signals to electrodes, which are implanted in the cochlea. The transmitter takes over the functions of the cochlear cilia. Instead of moving the cilia to transmit sound, the signals are interpreted directly by the acoustic nerve. The patient must learn to interpret the sounds and make sense of their meaning. This requires extensive postoperative rehabilitation and psychological support.

A facial nerve monitor is used to protect the nerve during surgical dissection and implantation of the implants. The monitoring electrodes are placed before the prep and draping.

The patient is placed in the supine position. The surgeon shaves the hair in the temporal region and outlines the incision with a skin scribe. The site is injected with 1% lidocaine with epinephrine 1:100,000. The surgeon implants the electrodes for facial nerve monitoring and connects them to the monitor. The patient then is prepped and draped for an ear procedure.

The surgeon makes a postauricular incision and extends it superiorly using a #15 blade. A skin flap is elevated with a needle-tip electrosurgical unit (ESU) and retracted with double-prong skin hooks or wire rakes. The flap is extended deeper to include the muscle. With the flaps elevated, the surgeon places a Beckman-Adson retractor or similar self-retaining retractor under the flaps to expose the cranium. The receiver template is placed in position and outlined with a skin scribe or the ESU. The surgeon then drills out the circumscribed area of the temporal bone using a medium cutting burr with irrigation. The template periodically is positioned in the drilled space to ensure a correct fit. A medium diamond burr is used to finish the edges of the temporal bone. Suture tunnel holes are placed, two on each side of the recess. These are used to secure the processor.

Next, a mastoidectomy is performed. The surgeon drills the mastoid with a large cutting burr and suction irrigator, preserving the bony ear canal and the opening of the facial recess. The medial wall of the middle ear is identified.

The implant is opened onto the sterile field. Implants are packaged individually and must be opened in a manner that limits or prevents the discharge of static electricity created during opening, because a static charge can interfere with the function of the implant electrodes. The circulator opens the outer package slowly onto the instrument table. The inner (sterile) package may then be submerged in a basin of normal saline and opened below the surface.

The surgeon places the internal processor into the drilled recess of the temporal bone. The active electrode is passed through the facial recess and round window into the cochlea. This is done using the electrode positioner provided in the implant kit. The active electrode is secured in the round window with a gimmick or Rosen needle.

The surgeon secures the internal processor by placing a 2-0 or larger Prolene suture through the suture holes and tying the knots diagonally across the holes. Bleeding is controlled with the bipolar ESU (monopolar ESU is not used, because it could cause current to be passed through the receiver). With the implant secured, the fascia overlying the cranium is closed with 2-0 absorbable suture. A 3-0 absorbable suture is used to close the subcutaneous tissue. The skin then is closed with a nonabsorbable suture. A mastoid dressing is placed over the wound.

Postoperative Considerations

To allow wound healing, the implant is activated several weeks after surgery. It is activated slowly so that the patient can adjust to the hearing world.

SECTION II: SURGERY OF THE NASAL CAVITY, OROPHARYNX, AND LARYNX

INTRODUCTION

Surgery of the nose, oropharynx, and larynx is performed by an otorhinolaryngologist. Most of the structures in these anatomical regions are related to respiration and vocalization, although some share functions with the digestive system. Surgery of lymph and secretory glands in the oropharynx are included in this specialty.

Procedures for pharyngeal and laryngeal tumors may extend into the neck, which contains large blood vessels and nerves that must be protected. Head and neck surgery requires meticulous dissection to avoid injury to these vital structures. (Procedures involving the skeletal structures of the face and oral cavity are described in the Chapter 28; p. 729.)

SURGICAL ANATOMY

EXTERNAL NOSE

The external nose is formed by two U-shaped, cartilaginous structures called the *lower lateral cartilages,* two rectangular structures called the *upper lateral cartilages,* and two nasal bones. The nares are the flared portions of the lower nose (nostrils). These are lined with skin. Fine hairs in this area filter the air as it enters the nasal cavity. The right and left nostrils are divided by the nasal septum, which is composed of cartilage.

NASAL CAVITY

The nasal cavity is located over the palatine bone, which is the "floor" of the nose; the "roof" of the nose is formed from the cribriform plate in the ethmoid bone. This is a significant structure, because it separates the nasal cavity from the cranial cavity. Infection or disease arising from the nose may enter the cranial cavity and spread to brain tissue. The nasal cavity has **paranasal sinuses,** or spaces. These are formed by extensions of the ethmoid bone and the frontal, maxillary, and sphenoid bones. The extensions are referred to as the *turbinates* or *nasal conchae.* The sinuses are lined with a highly vascular mucosa. As air passes through the sinuses, it is warmed, humidified, and filtered.

The nasal cavities drain into the superior, inferior, and middle meatus. The nasolacrimal duct drains into the inferior meatus. The posterior aspect of the nasal cavities is the choana, which separates them from the nasopharynx. This is an important structure because of the congenital anomaly choanal atresia. In this condition, infants are born with one or both choanae obstructed, requiring emergency surgery to restore airflow (see Chapter 34).

PARANASAL SINUSES

The paired *maxillary sinuses* are the large sinuses below the ocular orbits. The apices of the tooth roots are found in the floor of these sinuses. The paired frontal sinuses lie behind the lower forehead. The ethmoid sinuses consist of many small air cells in the lateral wall of the nasal cavity between the lateral nasal wall and the turbinates. The sphenoids lie at the posterosuperior extent of the nasal cavity. The optic nerves and carotid arteries are within the lateral wall of these sinuses, and the pituitary gland lies behind and above them. Surgery of the pituitary gland may be performed through a **transsphenoidal** approach. The anatomy of the sinuses is shown in Figure 27-9.

NASOPHARYNX

The *nasopharynx* is situated behind the nasal cavity and above the oral cavity. It communicates with the nasal sinuses and the oropharynx below it.

ORAL CAVITY

The oral cavity is divided into two sections, the vestibule and the oral cavity proper. The *vestibule* lies between the inner surface of the lips, buccal mucosa (cheeks), and the lateral aspects of the mandible and maxilla. The oral cavity proper lies within the medial surface of the maxillary and mandibular teeth. The roof of the oral cavity proper consists of the hard and soft palates, which separate it from the nasal cavity (Figure 27-10). The soft palate meets in the middle to form the uvula.

The floor of the mouth contains the ducts for the paired submandibular and lingual salivary glands. The tongue is attached in the midline to the floor of the mouth by a membranous structure called the *frenulum.* The tongue is a muscular structure covered by mucous membrane. The surface of the tongue is covered by papillae, or projections that contain taste buds. These are divided by type and regions of the tongue. Various types of papillae and taste buds are capable of separate sensations of taste. The undersurface of the tongue is highly vascular and has large blood vessels. The **sublingual** salivary gland ducts open into each side of the sublingual area.

PHARYNX

The *pharynx* is a tubular structure extending from the nose to the esophagus. It is separated into three areas: the *nasopharynx, oropharynx,* and *hypopharynx* (Figure 27-11). The nasopharynx extends from the posterior *choanae* of the nose to the palate. The adenoids lie in the posterosuperior aspect of the nasopharynx, and the eustachian tubes open on each side of the adenoids. The oropharynx extends from the palate to the hyoid bone. The soft palate, tonsils, and posterior third of the tongue (the base of the tongue) lie in the anterior portion of the oropharynx. The **hypopharynx** extends from the hyoid bone to the esophagus.

LARYNX

The larynx is composed of nine segments of cartilage, three paired sets and three unpaired segments. The unpaired cartilages are the cricoid, thyroid, and epiglottis segments; the paired sets are the arytenoids, corniculate, and cuneiform segments.

The larynx is separated into three spaces (Figure 27-12). The *supraglottis* lies above the true vocal cords and contains the vestibule, false vocal cords, and *epiglottis,* which is composed of cartilage. The *glottis* extends from the true vocal cords to about ½ inch (1 cm) below the free edge of the true vocal cords. The subglottis extends below this position to the inferior edge of the cricoid cartilage. The arytenoid cartilages lie in the posterior larynx and have processes that extend anteriorly (the vocal processes) and that lie within the true vocal cords. The area between the arytenoids is called the *posterior commissure.*

The true vocal cords meet anteriorly at the anterior commissure and connect to the thyroid cartilage. The free edge of the true vocal cords has a loosely covered membrane that vibrates to produce the voice.

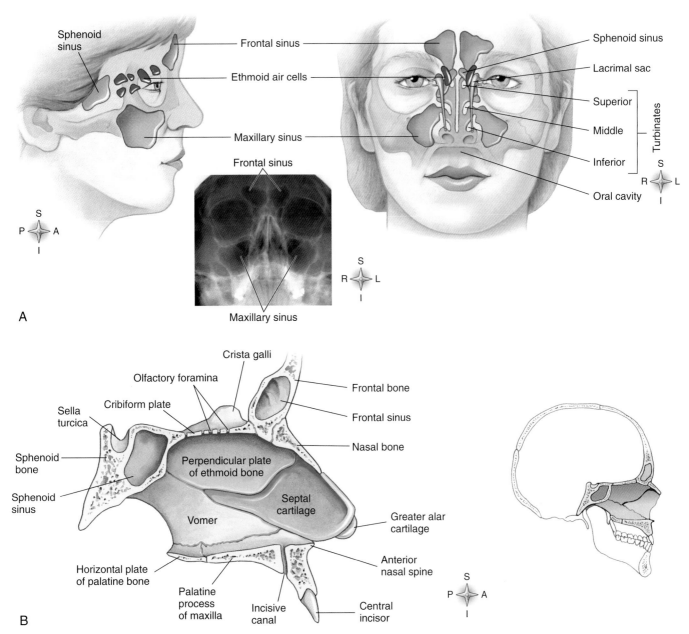

Figure 27-9   A, Paranasal sinuses. **B,** Bones of the nasal cavity. (**A** *from Abrahams PH, Marks SC, Hutchings RT: McKinn's color atlas of human anatomy, ed 5, St Louis, 2002, Mosby;* **B** *from Thibodeau G, Patton K: Anatomy and physiology, ed 6, St Louis, 2007, Mosby.)*

The trachea extends from the cricoid to the carina. It is composed of approximately 20 incomplete cartilaginous rings. The cricoid is the only closed ring of the upper airway. The posterior aspect of the trachea is membranous and has no cartilaginous structure.

PATHOLOGY OF THE NASAL CAVITY, PHARYNX, AND LARYNX

Table 27-3 presents pathological conditions of the nasal cavity, pharynx, and larynx.

DIAGNOSTIC TESTS

Diagnostic endoscopy procedures of the upper respiratory tract (larynx and pharynx) are commonly performed to direct visualization of the anatomy. Procedures include sinusoscopy, laryngoscopy, and bronchoscopy. Selected operative procedures such as biopsy and removal of small lesions may also be performed using endoscopic techniques. Pathology specimens are obtained by removing tissue or by cell washing, in which the mucosa is irrigated with saline and cells are collected with a biopsy brush. Fine needle aspiration and biopsy are also used before surgical excision.

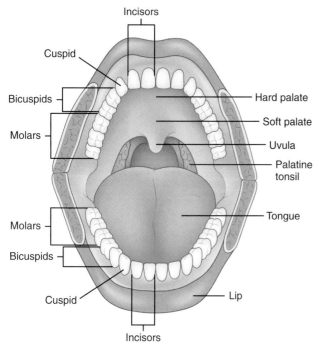

Figure 27-10 Anatomy of the oral cavity. *(From Herlihy B, Maebius NK: The human body in health and illness, ed 2 Philadelphia, 2003, WB Saunders.)*

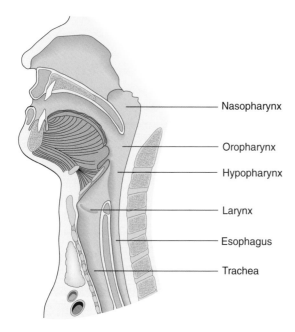

Figure 27-11 The pharynx. *(From Garden O, Bradbury A, Forsythe J, Parks R: Principles and practice of surgery, ed 5 Edinburgh, 2007, Churchill Livingstone.)*

Imaging studies such as MRI, CT, and ultrasonography are commonly used to confirm or rule out of disease or structural abnormalities.

PREPPING AND DRAPING

Patients undergoing nasal procedures generally are prepped from the forehead to the upper neck, including the entire face.

Patients having intranasal and endoscopic procedures may not be prepped, because these are considered clean rather than sterile cases. For nasal procedures, the patient is draped with a head drape. A three-quarter sheet is placed under the patient's head. The face then is draped with four towels secured with towel clips, and a split sheet is placed over the patient's body and around the face.

Procedures of the pharynx and larynx are approached transorally, and little or no prep is necessary because these are clean procedures. Often these patients are draped with a three-quarter sheet over the chest. A head drape may be applied and the eyes protected.

EQUIPMENT AND SUPPLIES

Microscope

The operating microscope is used frequently in surgery of the upper airway. The microscope is not draped for procedures of the mouth and throat. While the microscope is in use, the scrub must insert and guide the microinstruments into the laryngoscope, because the surgeon does not turn away from microscope to receive instruments. (Chapter 26 presents a complete discussion of the use and care of the operating microscope.)

Sponges

Flat cottonoid sponges (patties), cotton pledgets, and round gauze sponges are commonly used in procedures of the nasal cavities, mouth, and throat. All sponges have strings sewn into them for identification and retrieval to prevent loss and aspiration, which can result in injury or death. All sponges are counted according to routine policy.

Dressings

No dressings are applied to the mouth and throat after the procedure. A variety of nasal dressings may be used, depending on the procedure. The interior nasal passages may be "splinted" or packed with a continuous ¼- or ½-inch gauze strip (Figure 27-13). **Packing** material may be impregnated with a bacteriostatic agent before insertion. Packing is the process of placing long strips of fine gauze material inside the nose to provide support and absorb fluid.

Nasal packing also helps control bleeding or drainage after septoplasty or rhinoplasty. Exterior nasal splints are used to maintain the shape of the nose in the immediate postoperative period. Several types of external splints are available, including metal, foam, and fiberglass types.

Medications

Medications used for procedures of the nose, mouth, and throat include regional anesthetics, vasoconstrictive agents, and decongestants. A local anesthetic with epinephrine is injected into the nasal mucosa and turbinates for most nasal procedures. Cocaine in solution may be used as a vasoconstrictive agent in the nose or larynx. Solutions are administered by infiltration (injection) or may be applied topically with flat cottonoid sponges.

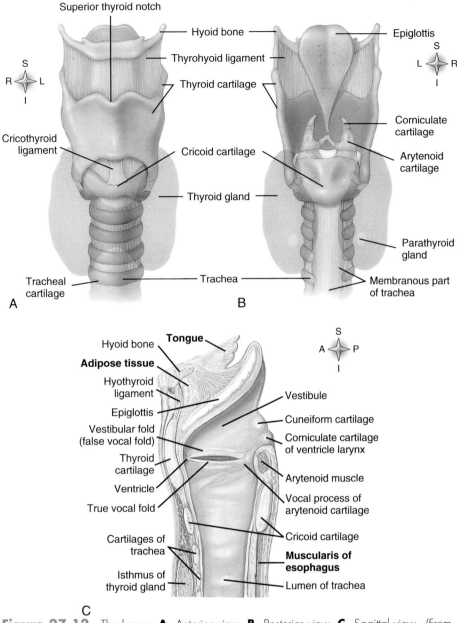

Figure 27-12   The larynx. **A,** Anterior view. **B,** Posterior view. **C,** Sagittal view. *(From Thibodeau G, Patton K: Anatomy and physiology, ed 6, St Louis, 2007, Mosby.)*

NASAL INSTRUMENTS

Specialty nasal instruments are designed for use on soft tissue and bone. Soft tissue instruments are needed for skin, submucosa, and soft connective tissue; bone and cartilage require heavier instruments. In many cases, the complex structure of the nasal cavity requires the surgeon to alternate frequently between these two types of instruments during a surgical procedure. All nasal instruments must be designed to reach deep into the nasal cavities from the outside. Instruments are balanced so that the hinge or fulcrum is much farther from the finger rings than in general surgery instruments. Instrument tips are available in an angled configuration for optimum access. Figure 27-14 shows commonly used nasal instruments.

Retractors

A nasal speculum is used for viewing tissue just inside the nares. Fine skin hooks or rakes are used to retract skin tissue in this area. Common retractors include the following:

- Alar retractor
- Fomon retractor
- Aufricht retractor
- Cottle retractor

Knives

Knives must have a delicate tip so that they can be manipulated in the small space of the nasal cavity. A #15 scalpel blade (knife) mounted on a #7 knife handle often is used for skin and submucosal incisions in the naris. The following are used for deeper dissection:

Table 27-3

Pathology of the Nasal Cavity, Pharynx, and Larynx

Condition	Description	Considerations
Nasal Cavity		
Choanal atresia	Congenital stricture of the choana.	Requires emergency surgery of the neonate to restore respiratory function. (See Chapter 24.)
Trauma	May be caused by a motor vehicle accident, fall, personal violence, or some other forceful injury.	Laceration or fracture may require surgical repair.
Infection/inflammation	Infections of the nose may be caused by bacteria or fungi. The most common causes of inflammation of the nose are allergies and nasal polyps.	Allergic rhinitis is treated with antihistamines. Nasal polyps and sinusitis may be treated with endoscopic sinus surgery. Cellulitis may require only antibiotics, or incision and drainage of the affected area may be needed.
Nonmalignant tumor	Nonmalignant tumors include juvenile nasal angiofibroma (JNA) and inverting papilloma. Although these are not cancerous, they can cause nasal obstruction.	If the patient is symptomatic, surgical removal of the tumor may be indicated.
Cancer	The most common types of cancer are squamous cell carcinoma and basal cell carcinoma. Squamous cell carcinoma can occur both internally and externally. Other common internal nasal cancers are salivary neoplasm, lymphoma, and malignant melanoma.	Surgical excision of the tumor and reconstruction are indicated. (See Endoscopic Sinus Surgery.)
Pharynx and Larynx		
Adenoiditis	Infection of the adenoid bed.	If the condition is chronic or causes significant obstruction, adenoidectomy may be performed.
Cancer	Squamous cell carcinoma, lymphoma, and malignant melanoma are the most common cancers found in the nasopharynx. All head and neck cancers have a high association with smoking or tobacco use and alcohol intake.	Surgical excision is indicated to remove the cancerous lesion. Radiation and chemotherapy are commonly used in treatment of cancers. Radical neck surgery may be indicated in selected cases.
Tonsillitis	Infection of the tonsils may be acute or chronic. Acute infection is treated with antibiotics.	Chronic infection or chronic streptococcal pharyngitis generally are treated with tonsillectomy.
Peritonsillar abscess (PTA)	A PTA is a collection of purulent fluid that arises from a blockage of a tonsil crypt.	The diagnosis is made with a computed tomography (CT) scan. The PTA may be drained surgically or in the clinic or emergency department.

- Joseph knife
- Ballenger swivel knife
- Button knife

Elevator or Dissector

Elevators are used to lift the periosteum or submucosa from the surface of bone or cartilage. They are available in a wide variety of designs to conform to the complex structure of the nasal cavity. The edge of the elevator is beveled but not sharp. Commonly used elevators include the following:

- Cottle knife or elevator
- Lempert elevator
- Freer elevator
- Penfield dissector

Forceps

Forceps are used for grasping and modeling tissue. The tips of the forceps may be cupped or beveled for cutting, or flat and serrated. An example of the cutting type of forceps is the Takahashi ethmoid forceps, which has small, cupped tips. The term *alligator forceps* refers both to a design and to an instrument. Alligator forceps have a long shank, short "working" tips, and two hinges, one at the base of the movable tips and one at the fulcrum that opens the tips. The distinction is made clear by the individual surgeon during the procedure. Dressing forceps are bayonet shaped and used to handle nasal packing.

Commonly used tissue forceps include the following:

- Takahashi ethmoid forceps
- Noyes alligator forceps
- Blakesley Wilde forceps
- Walsham septum straightening forceps
- Knight septum forceps

Rongeur

The rongeur is used specifically to cut bone. To provide enough leverage to cut through bone, many rongeurs have

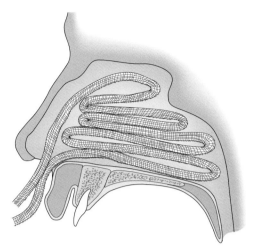

Figure 27-13 Nasal packing is placed in the nasal cavity for tamponade. Packing material is available in ¼- and ½-inch (0.63- and 1.25-cm) long gauze and often is identified by its brand name, Adaptic. *(From Garden O, Bradbury A, Forsythe J, Parks R: Principles and practice of surgery, ed 5, Edinburgh, 2007, Churchill Livingstone.)*

two hinges; these are identified as *double-action* rongeurs. A common double-action rongeur is the Jansen-Middleton rongeur.

Rongeurs with long shanks are used to reach deep into small spaces, such as the nasal sinus. Some of the rongeurs used in nasal surgery also are used in other specialties, such as neurosurgery. An example is the Kerrison rongeur. Commonly used rongeurs include the following:

- Kerrison rongeur
- Hartman rongeur
- Wilde rongeur
- Jansen-Middleton septum-cutting forceps

Gouge, Chisel, and Osteotome

The gouge, chisel, and osteotome are used with a small mallet to model nasal bone. Those used in nasal surgery are smaller and finer than those used in orthopedics. The sharp end of the instrument is angled against the bone and lightly struck with the mallet. This cuts the tissue by increments, producing bone shavings, which are removed with a forceps. The gouge is V-shaped, although the chisel and osteotome are straight. The chisel tip is beveled on both sides, but the osteotome has only one bevel.

Rasp and Saw

A nasal rasp is used to shave bone tissue. The handheld rasp usually is bayonet shaped. Note that the endoscopic shaver or microdebrider is used for the same purpose (discussed later). The bayonet saw is angled (right and left) and used to reduce small defects in bone.

TONSIL AND ADENOID INSTRUMENTS

Tonsil and adenoid instruments include the Crowe-Davis mouth gag, tonsil snares, adenoid curettes, elevators, clamps,

and scissors. The Crowe-Davis mouth gag is placed in the patient's mouth and attached to the edge of the Mayo stand during surgery. Tonsil snares are loaded with short strands of stainless steel wire. The snare is looped around the tonsil and retracted to transect the tonsillar fossa and release the tissue. Basic tonsil and adenoid instruments are shown in Figure 27-15.

Shaver and Drills

The microdebrider is used to excise tissue during nasal and laryngeal surgery. It is a small, powered handpiece with rotating blades (Figure 27-16). The microdebrider removes small segments of tissue and suctions them, removing blood and debris from the surgical field. Blades are available in a variety of lengths and as straight blades or blades with a 15- or 30-degree bend. A high-speed drill is used to drill bone in the ear and in nasal surgery.

Sinus Scope

The sinus endoscope (sinus scope) is used to visualize the sinus passages of the nose and face. The endoscope is available in focal angles of 0, 30, and 70 degrees. The 0-degree scope is used for sinus exploration and evaluation in all procedures. The 30-degree scope is used for maxillary, sphenoid, and ethmoid sinus procedures. The 70-degree scope is used for procedures of the frontal sinus.

NASAL PROCEDURES

ENDOSCOPIC SINUS SURGERY

Surgical Goal

Endoscopic sinus surgery is performed to treat disease of the paranasal sinuses, nasal cavity, and skull base and to improve nasal airflow. Endoscopic techniques are used in the following procedures:

- Polypectomy
- Maxillary antrostomy
- Ethmoidectomy
- Turbinectomy
- Sphenoidectomy

Pathology

Most endoscopic procedures of the nose are done to treat inflammatory or infectious diseases. A **polyp** is redundant mucosal tissue that prevents airflow and drainage of the paranasal sinus. In rare cases, intranasal neoplasms, **epistaxis** (nasal bleeding), and cerebrospinal fluid (CSF) leakage may be treated endoscopically.

Technique

1. The nasal mucosa is injected with a local anesthetic.
2. The nasal cavities are treated with decongestant compresses.
3. The endoscope is inserted into the nasal cavity.
4. Diseased tissue is removed.
5. Bleeding is controlled.
6. Nasal packing is inserted if needed.

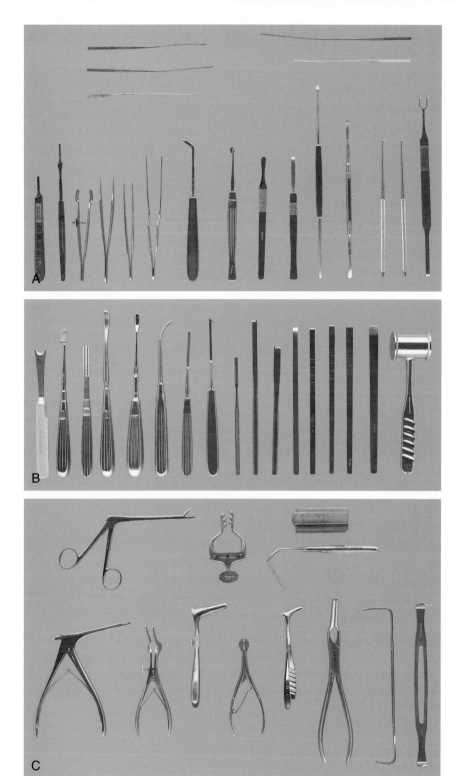

Figure 27-14 Basic nasal instruments. **A,** *Top,* 5 Ludwig wire applicators. *Bottom, left to right,* 1 Bard-Parker knife handle, #3; 1 Bard Parker knife handle, #7; 1 Cottle columella forceps; 1 Brown-Adson tissue forceps with teeth (7 × 7); 1 Beasley-Babcock tissue forceps; one Jansen thumb forceps, bayonet shaft, serrated tips; 1 Joseph button-end knife, curved; 1 Freer septum knife; 1 Cottle nasal knife; 1 McKenty elevator; 1 Cottle septum elevator; 1 Freer elevator; 2 Joseph skin hooks; 1 Cottle knife guide and retractor. **B,** *Left to right,* 1 Bauer rocking chisel; 1 Lewis rasp; 1 Maltz rasp; 1 Aufricht rasp, large; 1 Aufricht rasp, small; 1 Wiener antrum rasp; 2 Ballenger swivel knives; 1 Ballenger chisel, 4 mm; 2 Converse guarded osteotomes; 1 Cottle osteotome, round corners, curved, 6 mm; 4 Cottle osteotomes, straight (4, 7, 9, and 12 mm); 1 mallet, lead-filled head. **C,** *Top, left to right,* 1 Ferris-Smith fragment forceps; 1 mastoid articulated retractor; 1 Cottle bone crusher, closed; 1 Aufricht retractor. *Bottom, left to right,* 1 Kerrison rongeur, upbite; 1 Killian nasal speculum, 2 inch (5 cm), front view; 1 Killian nasal speculum, 3 inch (7.5 cm), side view; 1 Vienna nasal speculum, 1⅜ inch, front view; 1 Vienna nasal speculum, 1⅛ inch, side view; 1 Asch septum forceps; 2 Army-Navy retractors, side view and front view. *(From Tighe SM: Instrumentation for the operating room, ed 6, St Louis, 2003, Mosby.)*

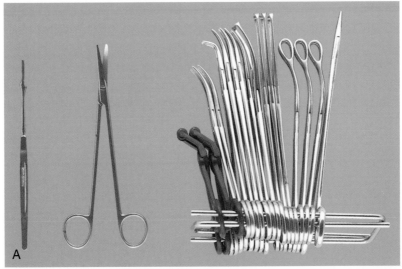

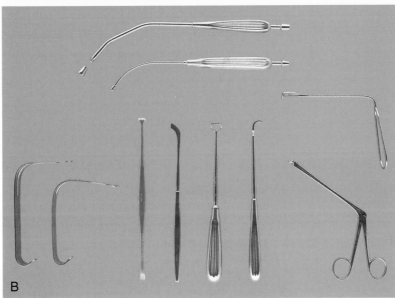

Figure 27-15 Basic tonsil and adenoid instruments. **A,** *Left to right,* 1 Bard-Parker knife handle, #7; 1 Metzenbaum scissors, 7 inch (17.5 cm); 2 drape clips; 3 Crile hemostatic forceps, 6½ inch; 1 Westphal hemostatic forceps; 4 tonsil hemostatic forceps; 1 Allis tissue forceps, long, curved; 1 Allis tissue forceps, long; 3 Ballenger sponge forceps, curved; 1 Crile-Wood needle holder, 8 inch (20 cm). **B,** *Top to bottom,* 1 Andrews-Pynchon suction tube with tip; 1 adenoid suction tube, tip connected. *Bottom, left to right,* 2 Weider tongue depressors; 1 Hurd tonsil dissector and pillar retractor; 1 Fisher tonsil knife and dissector; 1 LaForce adenotome, small, front view; 1 LaForce adenotome, large, side view. *Right, top to bottom,* 1 Lothrop uvula retractor; 1 Meltzer adenoid punch, round, with basket.

Discussion

The patient is placed in the supine position with the head stabilized on a doughnut headrest and the arms tucked at the sides. General anesthesia is used. A local anesthetic (usually 1% lidocaine with epinephrine 1:100,000) is injected into the nasal mucosa to provide hemostasis. The surgeon uses a nasal speculum and bayonet forceps to pack the nose with small cottonoids soaked in topical anesthetic or a vasoconstrictor (e.g., cocaine solution, topical adrenaline 1:1000, or Afrin). The patient is prepped and draped for a nasal procedure. The 0-degree sinus endoscope is inserted.

Polypectomy

Under direct visualization with the nasal endoscopes, the surgeon uses either a Wilde forceps or microdebrider to remove the nasal polyps. A #12 Frazier suction device is used to remove the morcellized tissue.

Maxillary Antrostomy

Under direct visualization with the 0-degree endoscope, the surgeon displaces the middle turbinate with a Freer elevator. The uncinate process is then removed with the sickle knife and Cottle elevator. An alternative technique is to displace the

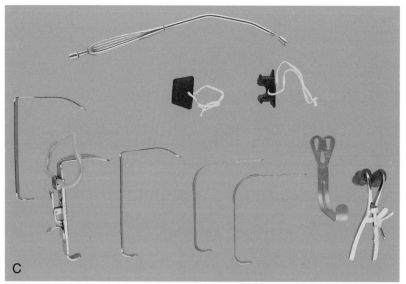

Figure 27-15, cont'd **C,** *Top to bottom,* 1 Andrews-Pynchon suction tube with tip; 2 bite blocks: child and adult. *Left to right,* 1 McIvor mouth gag frame with blade and two additional blades; 3 Weider tongue depressors, two side views and one front view; 1 side mouth gag. *(From Tighe SM: Instrumentation for the operating room, ed 6, St Louis, 2003, Mosby.)*

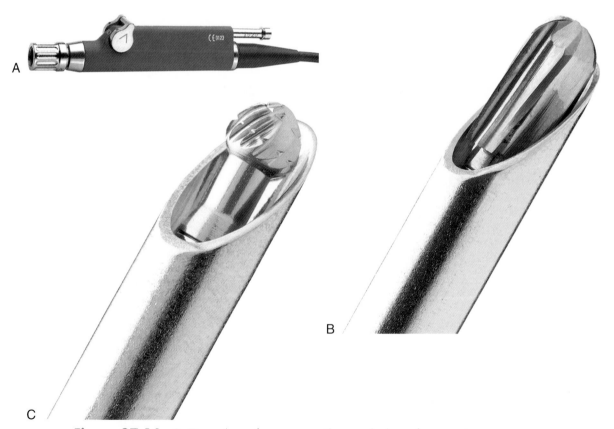

Figure 27-16 **A,** Tissue shaver for use on cartilage and other soft connective tissue. **B,** Shielded shaver blade. **C,** Shielded spherical blade. *(Courtesy Conmed Corp., Inc, Utica, NY.)*

mucosa with a Lusk osteum-seeking probe and then use the microdebrider.

A ball-tip suction probe is used to identify the maxillary antrum. The surgeon may change to a 30-degree endoscope at this point to view the maxillary sinus. The antrum is enlarged with a microdebrider or a reverse biting forceps. Redundant mucosa and polyps are removed from the maxillary sinus with a microdebrider, Wilde forceps, or Takahashi forceps.

Ethmoidectomy

Under direct visualization with a 0-degree endoscope, the surgeon removes (medializes) the middle turbinate up to the midline and removes the uncinate, as in the maxillary antrostomy. This allows visualization of the middle meatus. The ethmoids are removed with either a microdebrider or a Wilde forceps.

Turbinectomy

Under direct visualization with a 0-degree endoscope, the middle turbinate is displaced and the uncinate is removed, as in the maxillary antrostomy. This allows visualization of the middle meatus. The surgeon changes to a 30- or 70-degree endoscope. Any bony obstruction at the frontal sinus osteum is excised with a Wilde forceps or with a microdebrider with a curved blade.

Sphenoidectomy

The posterior ethmoids are removed with a microdebrider or Wilde forceps. A 30-degree endoscope is used to view the sphenoid sinus. The osteum is opened with the microdebrider or Wilde forceps. Diseased tissue is removed with the Wilde forceps or Takahashi forceps.

Bleeding is controlled with nasal packing saturated with a vasoconstrictive agent. The packing is removed after several minutes, and if necessary, fresh packing saturated with antibiotic ointment is inserted.

CALDWELL-LUC PROCEDURE

Surgical Goal

A Caldwell-Luc procedure is a technique used to enter the maxillary sinus in which an incision is made in the gingival-buccal sulcus (the junction of the gum and upper lip). The procedure is commonly performed for drainage of abscess in the maxillary sinus and surgical removal of granulation tissue that has accumulated as a result of chronic sinus infection.

Pathology

Access to the maxillary sinus and orbital floor is required for treatment of neoplasms and infectious diseases of the orbital cavity.

Technique

1. An incision is made in the gingival-buccal sulcus.
2. The periosteum over the canine fossa is elevated.
3. The infraorbital nerve is identified.
4. The anterior wall of the antrum is opened.
5. Cysts and tumors are removed.
6. The gingival-buccal incision is closed.

Discussion

The patient is placed in the supine position with the head on a doughnut headrest and the arms tucked at the sides. General anesthesia is used. Skin prep is omitted for procedures in which an oral approach is used. The patient is draped as for a nasal procedure.

The lip is retracted upward with a gauze sponge, and the gingival-buccal sulcus (gum line) is incised with the ESU. The incision is extended from the lateral incisor to the second molar and carried to the periosteum. The mucous membrane is retracted superiorly to expose the periosteum overlying the canine fossa. The periosteum is elevated with a periosteal elevator to the level of the infraorbital nerve. The nerve is identified and preserved.

Once the periosteum has been removed, the surgeon uses a drill and small cutting burr to enter the maxillary sinus. The opening is enlarged with Kerrison bone-cutting forceps; this exposes the diseased tissue. Cysts and tumors are removed with small cutting instruments, such as a Wilde or Takahashi forceps. Small bone curettes may also be used. The sinus is irrigated, and small fragments are removed with suction. The gingival-buccal incision is closed with 3-0 absorbable sutures. The Caldwell-Luc procedure is illustrated in Figure 27-17.

TURBINECTOMY/TURBINATE REDUCTION

Surgical Goal

Turbinectomy is removal of the bony turbinate to increase airflow through the nose.

Pathology

Nasal airflow may be impaired by chronic engorgement of the inferior turbinate or congenital malformation of the middle turbinate, called *concha bullosa*. Turbinectomy generally is performed at the same time as septoplasty.

Technique

1. A local anesthetic is injected, and a vasoconstrictive agent is applied to the nasal mucosa.
2. A nasal speculum is inserted into the nose to expose the affected turbinate.
3. The affected turbinate is removed or reduced.
4. The nasal cavity is packed if necessary.

Discussion

The patient is placed in the supine position with the head on a doughnut headrest and the arms tucked at the sides. General or local anesthesia may be used. The patient is prepped and draped for a nasal procedure. The surgeon begins by infiltrating the turbinate with a local anesthetic with epinephrine. The nose may be temporarily packed with gauze packing (gauze strips) impregnated with a vasoconstrictive agent such as lidocaine with epinephrine. The surgeon then places a nasal speculum in the nose to retract the nostril and expose the turbinates.

If a turbinectomy is to be performed, a #15 blade is used to make an incision into the mucosa at the anterior border of the inferior turbinate. The mucosa is elevated from the underlying bone with a Freer or Cottle elevator. A portion of the

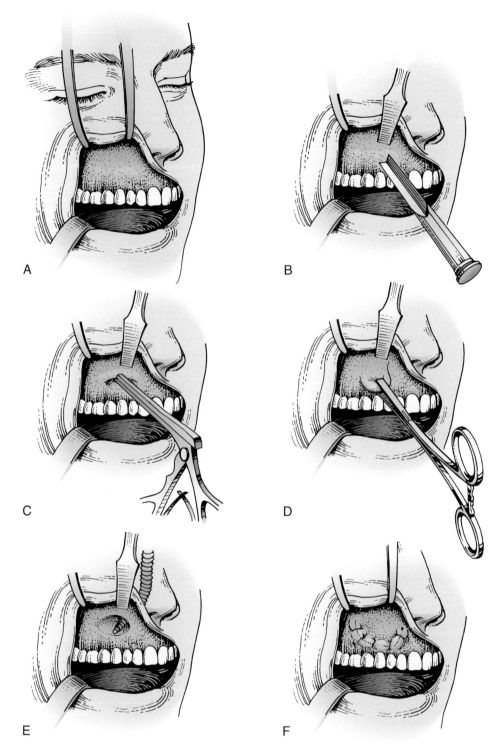

Figure 27-17 Caldwell-Luc procedure. **A,** An incision is made under the upper lip, creating a flap. **B,** The flap is retracted, and a perforation is made in the canine fossa. **C,** The perforation is enlarged with a Kerrison rongeur. **D,** The diseased antral membrane is removed. **E,** An antral window is created with a rasp. **F,** The incision is closed. *(Modified from Rothrock JC: Alexander's care of the patient in surgery, ed 12, St Louis, 2003, Mosby.)*

bone is removed with a Wilde forceps. The mucosa may be closed with 3-0 chromic suture.

If a turbinate reduction is planned, a sharp, two-prong bipolar electrode (ESU), sometimes called a *turbinate bipolar*, is inserted into the turbinate and activated for several seconds, causing desiccation of the tissue. The surgeon also may use coblation or somnus cauterization, which uses radiofrequency energy to desiccate the turbinate. This will result in physical shrinkage of the turbinates, allowing greater flow of air. The nasal cavity is packed as necessary to absorb draining.

SEPTOPLASTY

Surgical Goal

A septoplasty is surgical manipulation of the septum to return it to the correct anatomical position or to gain access to the sphenoid sinus for removal of a pituitary tumor.

Pathology

Septal deformity may be caused by trauma, infection, neoplasm, or birth trauma, and it may contribute to nasal obstruction, disrupted sleep patterns, headaches, and cosmetic deformities. Septoplasty may be performed with other procedures, such as rhinoplasty or sinus surgery.

Technique

1. Local anesthetic is injected into the nasal mucosa.
2. An incision is made ahead of the obstruction on one side.
3. The nasal septum is freed.
4. The deviated bone is removed.
5. The incision is closed.
6. Internal nasal splints are placed.

Discussion

The patient is placed in the supine position with the head on a doughnut headrest and the arms tucked at the sides. General anesthesia often is used, but local anesthesia with monitored intravenous (IV) sedation also may be employed. Before prepping and draping, the surgeon instills the nose and turbinates with a local anesthetic (1% lidocaine with epinephrine 1:100,000) and then packs the nose with ½- × 6-inch (0.63 × 15 cm) cotton strips soaked in a vasoconstrictive agent (e.g., adrenaline 1:1000, cocaine, Afrin, or a local anesthetic with epinephrine). The patient is then prepped and draped for a nasal procedure.

The surgeon removes the nasal packs and inserts a nasal speculum. An incision is made in the nasal septum below the obstruction with a #15 blade. Small tenotomy scissors are used to gently dissect the membranous nasal septum and expose the cartilaginous portion of the septum. The septum is raised from the underlying tissue with a Freer or Cottle elevator. With the nasal septum free, the surgeon removes the deviated bone with a 4-mm chisel and a small mallet. The fractured portions of the septum are grasped with a Takahashi forceps and removed. The incision is closed with 4-0 chromic suture, and internal nasal splints are positioned bilaterally to stabilize the septum. These are sutured to the membranous septum with 3-0 nonabsorbable suture.

RHINOPLASTY

Surgical Goal

Rhinoplasty is performed to reshape the external nose for aesthetic or functional purposes.

Pathology

Deformity of the external nose is caused by injury, congenital defect, or disease. These conditions may lead to functional obstruction, including narrowing and collapse of the cartilage on inspiration. Aesthetic surgery is performed to provide a smooth slope to the nose or to change the width. Rhinoplasty often is performed in conjunction with septoplasty, especially if cartilage is needed for support of external nasal structures.

Technique

1. Local anesthetic is injected into the nasal mucosa.
2. An incision is made in the nasal skin and carried to the periosteum.
3. The periosteum and perichondrium are elevated.
4. The nasal bone is remodeled.
5. Septoplasty is performed if necessary.
6. Soft tissue correction and grafting are performed if necessary.
7. The incisions are closed.
8. Internal splints are placed.
9. An external nasal splint is applied.

Discussion

Each rhinoplasty is approached differently, depending on the specific pathological condition. This section provides an overview of the techniques.

The patient is placed in the supine position with the head on a doughnut headrest and the arms tucked at the sides. General anesthesia is used. Before prepping and draping, the surgeon instills a local anesthetic (1% lidocaine with epinephrine 1:100,000) into the nose and turbinates and then packs the nose with ½- × 6-inch (0.63 × 15 cm) cotton strips soaked in a vasoconstrictive solution (e.g., adrenaline 1:1000, cocaine, Afrin, or local anesthetic with epinephrine). The patient then is prepped and draped for a nasal procedure, including a head drape.

After removing the nasal packs, the surgeon makes an incision in the nasolabial angle with a #11 or #15 blade, and double-prong hooks are inserted to retract the edges of the incision. Frazier suction is used on the incision margins. The **perichondrium** and the **periosteum** are elevated with a Freer elevator and tenotomy scissors. Bony overgrowth is removed with either a rasp or chisel and a small mallet.

Next, the surgeon performs a septoplasty, if necessary. Any cartilage or bone removed from the septum should be placed in normal saline and protected on the back table, because it may be used for grafting later in the procedure. The surgeon then reconstructs the nasal tip, if necessary, by inserting cartilage or bone grafts to provide support or shape.

Finally, lateral osteotomies (bone removal) may be performed with a 3- or 4-mm chisel and small mallet. This is done to straighten a curved nose or to make it narrower. The mucosa then is closed with 3-0 and 4-0 chromic sutures. After the wounds have been closed, internal and external nasal splints are placed. These splints may be made of metal, fiberglass, or tape.

TONSILLECTOMY

Surgical Goal

Tonsillectomy is performed to eradicate infection, improve the airway, or remove a cancer.

Pathology

Tonsillectomy is indicated for a number of different diseases. Among the most common are chronic infection, **hypertrophy** (enlargement), and suspected cancer. Recurrent tonsillitis, chronic tonsillitis, or peritonsillar abscess can lead to hypertrophy, causing disturbed sleep. Hypertrophy also may interfere with swallowing. The tonsil is a common site of cancer in adults, especially smokers.

Technique

1. The Crow-Davis mouth gag, including tongue blade, is inserted into the mouth and attached to the Mayo stand.
2. The tonsil is retracted medially with an Allis clamp.
3. The tonsil is separated from the underlying musculature.
4. Bleeding is controlled.

Discussion

The patient is placed in the supine position with a doughnut headrest and a shoulder roll, and the arms are tucked at the side. General anesthesia is administered so that the airway can be supported by endotracheal intubation. The patient is rotated 90 degrees to give the surgeon full access to the head. Draping is done with a head drape and a body sheet (usually a three-quarter sheet). Prepping is not necessary, because this procedure takes place in the mouth, which cannot be prepped to reduce bacteria. The surgeon uses a headlight to illuminate the surgical site.

A Crow-Davis retractor is inserted into the oral cavity and secured to the edge of the Mayo stand. This is mechanical retraction, not under direct control of the assistant, surgeon, or scrub. After the retractor has been positioned in the mouth and attached to the Mayo stand, the stand is slowly elevated. This holds the jaw open and provides access to the throat. When the retractor has been secured, the Mayo stand cannot be moved or jarred, because this can cause injury. During a tonsillectomy, suction must be available at all times. It is important to protect the lip from burns when a suction-ESU is used.

The surgeon grasps the tonsil with a straight or curved Allis clamp and retracts it toward the midline. A peritonsillar incision is made with the ESU or a #12 blade. The initial incision exposes the tonsillar capsule. The tonsil is separated from the underlying muscle and tonsillar fossa (tonsil bed) with Metzenbaum scissors, a Fisher knife, or a Hurd dissector. Schnidt clamps are used to clamp large bleeding vessels. A tonsil snare may be used to sever the pillar from the tonsil bed. The snare is prepared by inserting fine, precut lengths of stainless steel

through the tip. This forms a loop, which is used to encircle the tonsil and sever it. Throughout the procedure, the assistant uses suction to remove smoke from the oral cavity and to remove blood and oral secretions. The tonsils are kept as separate specimens and identified right and left.

Bleeding from the fossa usually is brisk after tonsillectomy. Large vessels are clamped with Schnidt clamps and ligated with 3-0 absorbable suture, or suture ligatures may be used. Tonsil sponges are placed in the tonsil fossa to control bleeding. The oral cavity is irrigated with warm saline, and a final assessment of the operative site is made. The tension of the retractor is then released.

Postoperative Consideration

Bleeding is a primary concern after a tonsillectomy. Instruments must remain available for immediate use until the patient has been extubated and transported to the post-anesthesia care unit (PACU), where immediate surgical care is available in case of postoperative bleeding after extubation.

ADENOIDECTOMY

Surgical Goal

An adenoidectomy is the surgical removal of the adenoids.

Pathology

The primary reasons for an adenoidectomy are chronic infection and obstruction caused by hypertrophy of the tissue. This often leads to obstruction of the eustachian tube and chronic otitis media. Enlarged adenoids may also contribute to upper airway obstruction, resulting in snoring and sleep apnea. Children are affected more often than adults, because the tissue naturally atrophies during adolescence. Adenoidectomy often is performed during tympanostomy and insertion of myringotomy tubes or tonsillectomy.

Technique

1. The Crow-Davis mouth gag is inserted.
2. Retraction is applied to the soft palate.
3. The adenoid tissue is removed, and bleeding is controlled.

Discussion

The patient is placed in the supine position, and a doughnut headrest and shoulder roll are used. The arms are tucked at the sides. General anesthesia is administered so that the airway can be supported by endotracheal intubation. The patient is prepped and draped as for a tonsillectomy.

The surgeon stands at the head of the bed and uses a headlight to light the field. A Crow-Davis retractor is inserted into the oral cavity and secured on the edge of the Mayo stand, as described previously. All precautions regarding the Crow-Davis retractor are observed.

The surgeon retracts the palate using a straight (Robinson) catheter (12 or 14 Fr) inserted through the nose and brought out of the mouth. The ends of the catheter are secured with a clamp. Next, the surgeon uses a dental mirror to inspect the

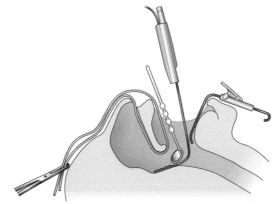

Figure 27-18 Adenoidectomy using suction ESU. *(From Dhillon RS, East CA: Ear, nose, and throat and head and neck surgery, ed 3, Edinburgh, 2006, Churchill Livingstone.)*

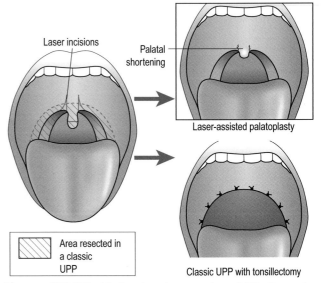

Figure 27-19 Uvulopalatopharyngoplasty (UPP). Surgical options for shortening the palate in the treatment of upper airway obstruction. *(From Dhillon RS, East CA: Ear, nose, and throat and head and neck surgery, ed 3, Edinburgh, 2006, Churchill Livingstone.)*

adenoids. Dipping the mirror in antifog or Hibiclens solution helps prevent fogging.

If the adenoid tissue is substantial, the surgeon uses an adenoid curette to remove it. The size of the curette depends on the size of the nasopharynx. Adenoid tissue may also be treated with suction ESU (Figure 27-18). After the tissue has been removed, the oral cavity and nasopharynx are irrigated with an Asepto syringe. The surgeon again uses the mirror to ensure that bleeding has stopped and that all of the adenoid tissue has been removed. Tension is carefully released from the Crow-Davis mouth gag, and the catheter and mouth gag are removed.

UVULOPALATOPHARYNGOPLASTY

Surgical Goal

Reconstruction of the uvula and oropharynx, or **uvulopalatopharyngoplasty (UPP),** is performed to reduce and tighten oropharyngeal tissue.

Pathology

Enlarged or redundant oropharyngeal mucosa may collapse on inspiration during the deep stages of sleep as muscles lose tone (Figure 27-19). This leads to high intrathoracic pressure as air is pulled through the obstruction, causing sleep apnea or interruption of deep sleep. Obstructive sleep apnea can cause a variety of sleep disorders, ranging from sleep deprivation to dangerous pulmonary and cardiovascular complications, including hypertension, cardiac arrhythmias, and neurological dysfunction.

Technique

1. The Crow-Davis mouth gag with tongue blade is inserted.
2. A tonsillectomy is performed.
3. The uvula and soft palate are retracted posteriorly with an Allis clamp.
4. The uvula and a portion of the soft palate are excised.
5. Bleeding is controlled.
6. The soft palate is closed.

Discussion

The patient is positioned as for a tonsillectomy. General anesthesia is used to protect the airway. A tracheotomy setup should be available in case of difficult intubation. The patient then is draped as for a tonsillectomy. Prepping is unnecessary.

A Crow-Davis retractor is inserted and secured to the Mayo stand. The tonsils are removed as necessary, as described previously. After the tonsillectomy, the uvula is grasped with an Allis clamp and retracted posteriorly. The surgeon excises the redundant soft palate and uvula with the ESU. The incision is approximated with 2-0 absorbable sutures. The oropharynx is irrigated, and any residual bleeding is controlled with the ESU. The tension on the retractor then is released. The tonsils and uvula are preserved as separate specimens and labeled appropriately.

Postoperative Considerations

Instruments are kept for immediate use until the patient has been transported to the PACU because of the risk of bleeding after extubation. Selected patients remain in the hospital overnight to ensure that no airway complications arise.

LARYNGOSCOPY

Surgical Goal

Laryngoscopy is endoscopic assessment of the larynx. Tissue specimens may be removed for pathological examination. Instruments for direct laryngoscopy are shown in Figure 27-20.

Pathology

Laryngeal lesions include neoplasms, foreign bodies, papillomas, laryngeal polyps, leukoplakia, and laryngeal web

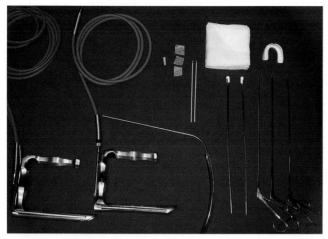

Figure 27-20 Direct laryngoscopy instruments. *Left to right,* Rigid laryngoscopes, suction tips, sponge carriers, and forceps for biopsy. *(From Shah JP, Patel SG: Head and neck surgery and oncology, ed 3, London, 2003, Mosby.)*

(Figure 27-21). A **papilloma** is a benign proliferative overgrowth of epithelium. Leukoplakia is a benign lesion of the laryngeal epithelium.

Technique

Indirect Laryngoscopy
1. A mirror is inserted into the oral cavity.
2. The tongue is retracted manually.
3. The patient is asked to phonate.
4. The vocal cords are visualized.

Discussion: Indirect Laryngoscopy

The patient is placed either in the sitting position or supine with a doughnut headrest. If the patient can cooperate throughout the procedure, no anesthetic is necessary. However, sedation or general anesthesia may be needed. After examining the mouth, the surgeon retracts the patient's tongue manually with a gauze sponge. The surgeon then positions an examination mirror against the uvula to inspect the larynx, base of the tongue, and pharyngeal wall. The patient may be asked to speak (**phonation**) if possible, so that the surgeon can observe the larynx in motion. The mirror then is removed.

Technique

Direct Laryngoscopy
1. A tooth guard is positioned in the mouth.
2. The laryngoscope is introduced into the mouth.
3. The laryngoscope is advanced through the vocal cords.
4. Biopsies are performed.
5. The laryngoscope is removed.

Discussion: Direct Laryngoscopy

The patient is positioned supine with the neck hyperextended using a shoulder roll as described in Chapter 10. The head is

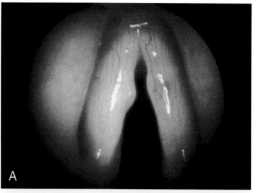

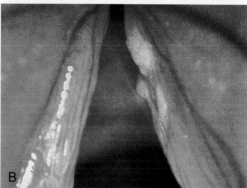

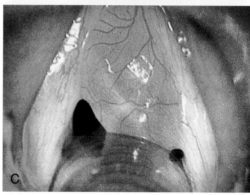

Figure 27-21 Lesions of the vocal cords. **A,** Vocal cord nodules. **B,** Hyperplastic leukoplasia. **C,** Polyp of the right vocal cord. *(From Dhillon RS, East CA: Ear, nose, and throat and head and neck surgery, ed 3, Edinburgh, 2006, Churchill Livingstone.)*

stabilized on a doughnut headrest. General anesthesia is used. The operating table is tilted into reverse Trendelenberg to allow full access to the operative area.

The surgeon introduces a tooth guard to protect the teeth from injury during the procedure. The rigid laryngoscope is introduced on the right side of the mouth and advanced into the upper airway.

Oral secretions are suctioned with an open-tip or a velvet-tip laryngeal suction device. The scrub assists by guiding the instruments into the working channel of the laryngoscope and advancing them a short distance into the scope. The surgeon then continues to advance the scope to the level of the larynx and vocal cords. The surgeon also examines the subglottic region and the upper portion of the trachea.

Any suspicious tissue is biopsied with a long cupped biopsy forceps. The scrub receives biopsy tissue and ensures that all specimens are kept separate and identified by the exact location and side. *It is extremely important that all tissue is collected from the tips of the biopsy instrument and carefully labeled.*

Bleeding is controlled by applying flat pledgets soaked in a vasoconstrictive agent (adrenaline, Afrin, or cocaine). The scope is gently withdrawn after all specimens have been removed and bleeding has been controlled.

TRACHEOTOMY/TRACHEOSTOMY

Surgical Goal

Tracheotomy or tracheostomy is performed to provide a patent airway.

Pathology

Tracheostomy is indicated for patients who require emergency or elective airway management for prolonged ventilator dependence or acute or chronic upper airway obstruction. Upper airway obstruction may be the result of mechanical obstruction, redundant pharyngeal mucosa (causing sleep apnea), a tumor, foreign body, infection, or secretions. Obstruction also may be caused by congenital, neurological, or traumatic conditions. Such obstructions can include a foreign body in the larynx or hypopharynx, acute laryngotracheal bronchitis in children, laryngeal edema, or some other condition that obstructs the airway.

Technique

1. An incision is made over the anterior tracheal wall.
2. The tracheal wall is visualized.
3. A tracheal incision is made, usually between the third and fourth tracheal rings.
4. The endotracheal (ET) tube is partly removed, to the point superior to the tracheal incision.
5. The tracheotomy tube is inserted.
6. Bleeding is controlled.
7. The tracheotomy tube is secured.
8. Dressings are applied.
9. The obturator from the ET tube is sent with the patient.

Discussion

The patient is placed in the supine position with the head on a doughnut headrest and the arms tucked at the sides with the neck hyperextended. General anesthesia is used. The patient is prepped and draped for a neck procedure.

Using a #15 blade, the surgeon makes an incision to the midline of the neck; the incision may be vertical or horizontal. The skin flaps are elevated with double-prong skin hooks and a #15 blade. With the flaps elevated, the strap muscles are separated in the vertical midline, at the median raphe, with a hemostat or the ESU. The isthmus of the thyroid also may be divided to allow visualization of the anterior tracheal wall. A tracheal hook then is placed into the cricoid cartilage to elevate the trachea.

An incision is made into the trachea between the second and third or third and fourth tracheal rings with a #15 blade. In adults, the tracheal incision is vertical and may include removal of an anterior square of tracheal cartilage. In infants, the tracheal incision is made vertically, and no tracheal cartilage is removed.

After the tracheal incision is made, the anesthesia provider withdraws the endotracheal (ET) tube to the level just above the tracheal incision. A tracheotomy tube then is placed into the tracheal incision with the obturator in place.

When patient ventilation through the tracheotomy tube has been established, the ET tube is completely removed. Bleeding is controlled with the ESU. The tracheotomy tube may be sutured to the skin with 2-0 nonabsorbable suture (e.g., Prolene or silk). Drain sponges and tracheotomy ties are then applied. The obturator must be sent along with the patient after surgery. Figure 27-22 shows an assortment of tracheotomy tubes, and a tracheostomy is illustrated in Figure 27-23.

Postoperative Consideration

The obturator of the tracheotomy tube is kept with the patient as long as the tracheal tube is in place. If the tube becomes dislodged or is traumatically removed, the obturator is needed to replace the tube.

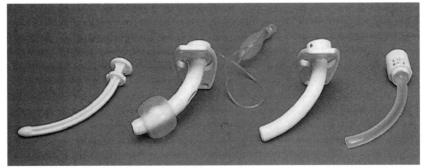

Figure 27-22 Tracheostomy tubes. *Left to right,* Introducer, cuffed fenestrated outer tube, uncuffed nonfenestrated outer tube, inner tube. *(From Dhillon RS, East CA: Ear, nose, and throat and head and neck surgery, ed 3, Edinburgh, 2006, Churchill Livingstone.)*

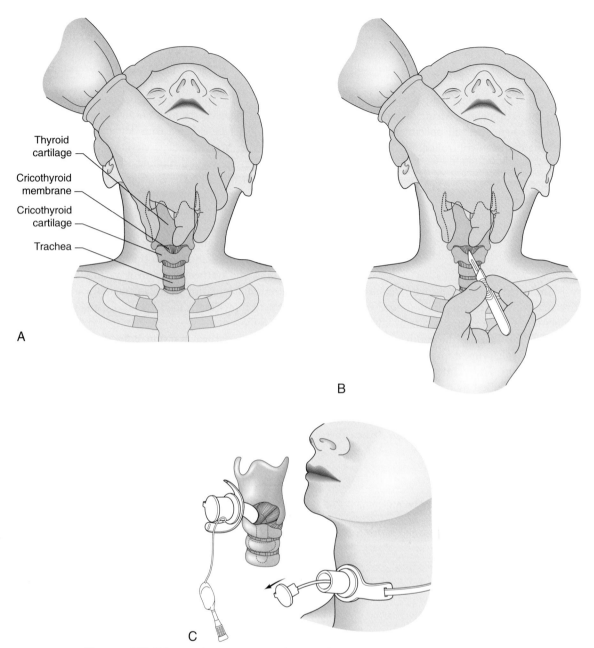

Figure 27-23 Tracheostomy. **A,** Palpation of the thyroid cartilage. **B,** An incision is made through the cricoid cartilage. **C,** Insertion of the tracheostomy tube. *(From Garden O, Bradbury A, Forsythe J, Parks R: Principles and practice of surgery, ed 5, Edinburgh, 2007, Churchill Livingstone.)*

SECTION III: THE NECK

INTRODUCTION

Surgery of the neck most often is performed to remove or debulk tumors arising from the mouth or upper respiratory system and for surgery of the salivary and thyroid glands.

SURGICAL ANATOMY

NERVES, VASCULAR SUPPLY, AND MUSCLES OF THE NECK

The neck is anatomically organized into triangles for identification. These triangles are called anterior and posterior triangles. Each side of the neck is divided into two large triangles separated by the sternocleidomastoid muscle, which attaches at the superior end to the mastoid process below the ear and inferiorly to the sternum and clavicle. Below the sternocleidomastoid muscle is the carotid sheath, which contains the carotid artery and its bifurcation, the internal jugular vein, and the vagus nerve (Figure 27-24).

The spinal accessory nerve (cranial nerve XI) crosses the posterior triangle of the neck behind the sternocleidomastoid muscle. The anterior cervical triangle is located anterior to the sternocleidomastoid. The digastric muscle crosses

this triangle. Finally, the submandibular triangle occurs above the digastric muscle. This section contains the submandibular gland and the hypoglossal nerve (cranial nerve XII).

The space below the digastric muscle contains an important structure, the carotid sheath. The larynx, pharynx, thyroid gland, and parathyroid glands lie on the medial side of the carotid sheath.

Cervical lymph nodes are located throughout the anterior neck. The thoracic duct, which connects the body's entire lymphatic system to the vascular system, is located in the left lower neck behind the carotid sheath, where it inserts at the junction of the left internal jugular vein and subclavian vein.

SALIVARY GLANDS

The body has three pairs of salivary glands: the parotid, submandibular, and sublingual salivary glands. Many minor salivary glands are found throughout the oral cavity and pharynx. The largest of the glands, the parotid gland, is situated over the mandible, anterior to the ear. It extends anteriorly to the masseter muscle. The tail of the parotid gland extends below the mandible into the upper neck. The parotid duct drains into the mouth and the cheek opposite the upper second molar. The facial nerve passes through the gland where it branches and then exits from the anterior aspect (Figure 27-25, A).

The submandibular gland is the second largest salivary gland. It is C-shaped and wraps around the lower (inferior) border of the mandible (Figure 27-25, B). The subman-

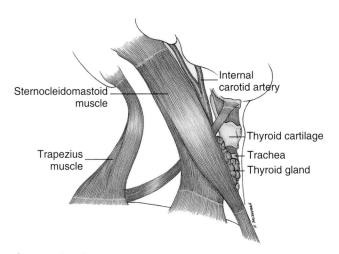

Figure 27-24 Anatomy of the neck. (From Potter PA, Perry AG: Fundamentals of nursing, ed 5, St Louis, 2001, Mosby.)

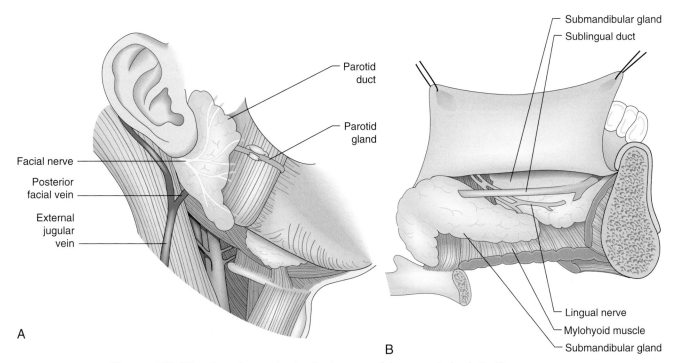

Figure 27-25 The salivary glands. **A,** Anatomy of the parotid gland. **B,** The submandibular gland. (From Garden O, Bradbury A, Forsythe J, Parks R: Principles and practice of surgery, ed 5, Edinburgh, 2007, Churchill Livingstone.)

dibular duct, or Wharton duct, emerges from the deep anterior portion of the gland and drains into the anterior floor of the mouth. A branch of the facial nerve lies within the superficial fascia of the gland. The hypoglossal nerve (cranial nerve XII) and the lingual nerve lie beneath the gland.

The smallest of the salivary glands, the sublingual glands, lie in the floor of the mouth just beneath the mucosa and empties into the oral cavity via multiple small ducts (ducts of Rivinus).

The salivary glands produce saliva, which irrigates the oral cavity and contains enzymes for breaking down simple carbohydrates. Buffers in saliva reduce acidity in the mouth and protect against pathogenic bacteria and demineralization of the teeth.

THYROID GLAND

The thyroid gland is located in the midneck and overlies the trachea below the larynx. It has two lobes, which are connected by a central band of thyroid tissue called the *isthmus*. A thin strip of thyroid tissue also projects from the superior edge of the isthmus (Figure 27-26). The thyroid secretes the hormones thyroxine (T_4) and triiodothyronine (T_3). These thyroid hormones (THs) are necessary for regulating cell metabolism and growth. Calcitonin, which also is secreted by the thyroid, is necessary for calcium regulation. The

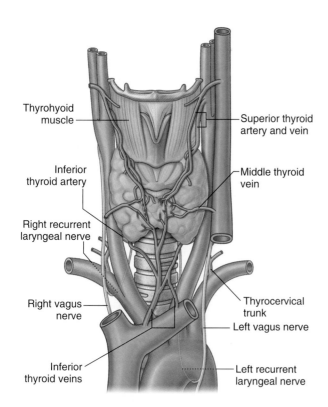

Figure 27-26 Relationship of the thyroid to the trachea and larynx. *(From Drake R, Vogl W, Mitchell A: Gray's anatomy for students, Edinburgh, 2004, Churchill Livingstone.)*

Labels in figure:
Thyrohyoid muscle
Inferior thyroid artery
Right recurrent laryngeal nerve
Right vagus nerve
Inferior thyroid veins
Superior thyroid artery and vein
Middle thyroid vein
Thyrocervical trunk
Left vagus nerve
Left recurrent laryngeal nerve

parathyroid glands are situated within the lobes of the thyroid. These small glands produce parathyroid hormone (PTH), which influences calcium and phosphate levels in the blood.

The thyroid gland is highly vascular and is composed of follicles that synthesize the thyroid hormones.

PATHOLOGY OF THE SALIVARY AND THYROID GLANDS

Table 27-4 lists pathological conditions of the salivary and thyroid glands.

PERIOPERATIVE CONSIDERATIONS

POSITIONING THE PATIENT FOR NECK SURGERY

Procedures of the neck are performed with the patient in the supine position with the head stabilized on a doughnut headrest. The arms are secured on arm boards at an angle of less than 90 degrees for venous access during general anesthesia. The neck may be hyperextended for better access; this is achieved by placing a padded roll at the shoulders. The roll must be carefully positioned to prevent compression of the cervical nerve.

DRAPING

Patients undergoing procedures of the neck are draped to exclude the face and to maintain a sterile field. The surgical site is draped with towels, which are secured with towel clips or skin staples. A clear incise drape commonly is used to cover the towels and operative site. The patient then is draped with a split sheet that surrounds the head. It may be helpful to cover the patient's chest with a towel and place a magnetic drape on top of the towel to prevent instruments from dropping to the floor during surgery.

INSTRUMENTS

General surgical instruments are required for procedures of the head and neck. Additional special instruments are included in tracheal and thyroid sets. These include neck retractors and thyroid grasping clamps. Vascular clamps may be added for radical neck procedures. Numerous vital nerves and large blood vessels in the neck require soft retraction with a Penrose drain or surgical vessel loops made of Silastic or cotton. Numerous right-angle clamps are needed during extensive neck dissection.

Neck dissection involves a significant risk of injury to peripheral nerves. A peripheral nerve stimulator or nerve monitoring device often is used to prevent this injury.

DRESSINGS

Neck dressings vary according to the procedure. Tracheotomy incisions generally are dressed with drain sponges (4 × 4 gauze

Table 27-4

Pathology of the Salivary and Thyroid Glands

Condition	Description	Considerations
Salivary Glands		
Sialith	A salivary gland stone (sialith) may block the salivary duct, resulting in swelling, pain, and infection.	The stone may be removed surgically or with ultrasonic lithotripsy.
Mucocele	A mucocele is an extravasation (movement of fluid into tissue) of saliva into adjacent tissue, causing a cyst. This usually is the result of trauma to the salivary gland or duct.	Treatment is surgical excision of the mucocele.
Neoplasm	Primary cancer of the salivary gland cancer is rare and usually is related to tobacco use.	Treatment involves chemotherapy, radiation therapy, or surgical excision.
Thyroid Gland		
Hypothyroidism	Hypothyroidism may be congenital or acquired. Thyroid hormone (TH) is essential for brain development in the fetus. In adults, hypothyroidism is caused by thyroidectomy or radiation of the thyroid for cancer treatment.	The disease is controlled by oral administration of thyroid hormone.
Hyperthyroidism	Overproduction of thyroid hormone may develop into a life-threatening condition characterized by hypermetabolism. Graves' disease is an autoimmune condition characterized by hyperthyroidism and goiter (enlargement of the thyroid gland).	Treatment is medical or surgical. (See Thyroidectomy.)
Neoplasm	Primary cancer of the thyroid is more common in women than in men. Excessive exposure to radiation increases the risk. The prognosis is good.	Thyroid cancer is commonly treated by thyroidectomy.

that has been slit to include the tracheotomy tube) and tracheal ties. Other procedures of the neck may be dressed with Telfa and Tegaderm or 4 × 4 sponges and tape. After radical neck procedures, a sump-type drain may be placed in the wound before closure.

MEDICATIONS

The medications most often used in head and neck surgery are local anesthetics and hemostatic agents. Hemostatic agents such as Gelfoam and thrombin should be available for extensive neck dissection.

SURGICAL PROCEDURES

EXCISION OF THE SUBMANDIBULAR GLAND

Surgical Goal

The submandibular gland is removed.

Pathology

The submandibular gland may be removed because of chronic infection (bacterial or viral), stone formation, or neoplasm (benign or malignant). These conditions are much more common in adults than in children. In children, however, about 60% of salivary gland masses are malignant.

Technique

1. A skin incision is made 0.8 inch (2 cm) below the mandible.
2. The submandibular gland is exposed.
3. The facial artery and vein are ligated.
4. The gland is separated from the mandible.
5. The submandibular duct and nerve are ligated.
6. The gland is removed.
7. Bleeding is controlled.
8. The incision is closed.

Discussion

The patient is positioned for neck surgery. General anesthesia is used. The patient is prepped and draped for a neck procedure, which includes inferior mandibular access.

The surgeon makes an incision with a #10 or #15 blade just below the inferior border of the mandible within a naturally occurring tissue fold. The incision is carried through the platysma muscle with the knife or Metzenbaum scissors. The skin-muscle flaps are retracted with double-prong skin hooks or small rake retractors. The surgeon does this carefully to avoid injuring the marginal mandibular branch of the facial nerve.

The knife or Metzenbaum scissors are used to make an incision in the inferior border of the gland. The facial artery and vein are identified, clamped, and ligated with 2-0 or 3-0 silk ties.

The tissue and vessels overlying the gland are retracted superiorly with a dull Senn retractor or three-prong dull rake.

The gland then is retracted with an Allis clamp or manually with a surgical sponge. Metzenbaum scissors and bipolar ESU are used to separate the gland from the inferior border of the mandible. The submandibular branch of the lingual nerve is identified, clamped, and ligated with 2-0 or 3-0 silk ties.

Next, an Army-Navy retractor is inserted to retract the myohyoid muscle anteriorly. This exposes the hypoglossal nerve. The submandibular duct is identified and ligated. The remaining soft tissue attachments are excised with a monopolar ESU. Bleeding is controlled with the ESU. The wound is irrigated, and a drain is put in place as necessary. The incision is closed in layers with 3-0 absorbable sutures. The skin may be closed with absorbable or nonabsorbable sutures.

PAROTIDECTOMY

Surgical Goal
A parotidectomy is the surgical removal of the parotid gland.

Pathology
A parotidectomy most often is performed for the treatment of a neoplasm. The facial nerve splits the parotid gland into superficial and deep lobes. Disease most often occurs in the superficial lobe and rarely involves the deep lobe. Involvement of the deep lobe usually indicates malignancy. However, most neoplasms of the parotid are benign.

Technique
1. A skin incision is made anterior to the ear.
2. The parotid gland is exposed.
3. The gland is mobilized, and the sternocleidomastoid muscle is retracted.
4. The gland is separated from the cartilaginous portion of the external auditory canal.
5. The facial nerve is identified.
6. The superficial portion of the parotid gland is removed.
7. The deep portion of the parotid gland is excised if necessary.
8. Bleeding is controlled.
9. The wound is closed.

Discussion
The patient is positioned and draped for a neck procedure. General anesthesia is required. However, neuromuscular blocking agents are not used to allow stimulation of the facial nerve for identification.

The skin incision begins just anterior to the helix of the ear and extends downward to the tragis. If necessary, the incision can be extended for greater access.

The surgeon creates skin flaps by dissecting the subcutaneous layer with Metzenbaum scissors. The skin flaps are retracted with skin hooks or dull rakes. The gland is separated from the sternocleidomastoid muscle and the cartilaginous portion of the external auditory canal with Metzenbaum scissors. The facial nerve trunk then is identified. A nerve stimulator or monitoring device may be required to identify the nerve.

Dissection is continued along the facial nerve branches, either superiorly or inferiorly, with a mosquito clamp and bipolar ESU until the superficial portion of the gland is removed. If the deep lobe of the parotid must be excised, the facial nerve is elevated and retracted with vessel loops. With the facial nerve retracted, the facial nerve branches are elevated off the underlying deep lobe of the parotid gland with a hemostat and bipolar ESU.

Dissection continues using the same technique to separate the gland from the underlying masseter muscle. Allis clamps are used to grasp the gland and provide countertraction as it is elevated. After the gland is removed, the wound is irrigated and a drain is placed. The wound then is closed in layers with absorbable sutures. The skin may be closed with either absorbable or nonabsorbable sutures. A parotidectomy is illustrated in Figure 27-27.

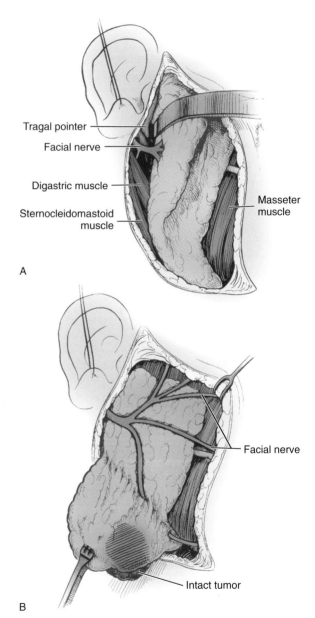

A

B

Figure 27-27 Parotidectomy. **A,** Blunt dissection of the parotid gland, exposing the facial nerve. **B,** Removal of tissue with the facial nerve intact. *(From Cummings CW, Haughey BH, Thomas JR et al: Otolaryngology: head and neck surgery, ed 3, St Louis, 1998, Mosby.)*

THYROIDECTOMY

Surgical Goal

A thyroidectomy is the surgical removal of one or more lobes of the thyroid gland.

Pathology

A thyroidectomy is performed to treat known or suspected malignancy or for the treatment of hyperthyroidism in selected cases. Benign enlargement of the thyroid (**goiter**) may compress the airway or esophagus. Removal of all or one lobe of the thyroid relieves the obstruction. In hyperthyroid disorders, such as Graves' disease, the patient may select partial removal of the hyperfunctioning gland or treatment with radioactive iodine.

Technique

1. The neck is incised.
2. The platysma muscle is divided.
3. The thyroid is mobilized.
4. The recurrent laryngeal nerve is identified and preserved.
5. The parathyroids are identified and preserved.
6. The thyroid is removed.
7. Bleeding is controlled.
8. The wound is closed.

Discussion

The patient is positioned for a neck procedure with the neck hyperextended. General anesthesia is administered. Before beginning the procedure, the surgeon may mark the proposed incision in a naturally occurring tissue fold over the thyroid.

The neck is incised with a #10 or #15 blade. The subcutaneous tissue is incised with the ESU, exposing the platysma muscle. The assistant retracts the tissue layers with rake retractors. The surgeon then divides the muscle layer with the deep knife or ESU. The incision is carried deeper with the ESU and Metzenbaum scissors. Numerous bleeders are encountered in the deep tissue, and these are controlled with the ESU.

As the dissection continues, deeper retractors are used, such as a Green retractor designed for thyroid surgery. When the thyroid gland finally is exposed, two Lahey spring retractors, or a Mayhorn thyroid retractor, are placed in the wound. The surgeon then grasps the gland with one or two Lahey tenacula. As the surgeon dissects the gland from the surrounding tissues, the parathyroid glands, the superior laryngeal nerves, and the recurrent laryngeal nerve are identified and preserved.

The thyroid gland is an extremely vascular structure. Therefore, to mobilize it, the surgeon successively double-clamps small sections of tissue, divides the tissue between the clamps, and ligates each section. Most surgeons use Kelly or mosquito clamps for mobilization. The scrub should have at least 12 to 15 clamps available for dissection of the thyroid. Large arteries of the thyroid are ligated with suture ligatures of 2-0 or 3-0 silk mounted on a fine needle. When mobilization and excision are complete, the gland is passed to the scrub. A frozen section may be required for determination of malignancy.

The wound is irrigated, and a Penrose drain is placed in the wound if necessary. The tissue layers of the neck are closed individually. The skin is closed with staples or fine nonabsorbable suture. The incision is dressed with flat gauze. Fluff gauze may be used if a drain has been inserted.

Technique

1. The skin is incised, and the skin flaps are elevated using sharp dissection.
2. The platysma muscle is divided.
3. The thyroid sheath is dissected.
4. Bleeders are serially clamped and ligated.
5. The upper and lower poles of the thyroid are explored bilaterally for parathyroid glands.
6. Affected glands are dissected and removed.
7. The wound is closed.

Postoperative Considerations

Injury of the recurrent laryngeal nerve can alter airway function. The surgeon may want a flexible laryngoscope available to examine the vocal cords in the recovery room when the patient is sufficiently awake to follow commands. A tracheotomy set should be available in the event of a bilateral cord paralysis. A thyroidectomy is illustrated in Figure 27-28.

THYROPLASTY

Surgical Goal

A thyroplasty involves moving the vocal cord to one side and stabilizing it with a Silastic or Gore-Tex implant.

Pathology

Unilateral vocal cord paralysis, or **paresis,** is the primary reason for performing a thyroplasty. Paralysis may be caused by a variety of conditions, including surgical trauma to the laryngeal nerves or prolonged intubation. Cord paralysis may prevent the vocal cords from meeting at the midline during speaking. Open, closed, or unilateral paralysis can cause difficulty with speech, such as hoarseness and aspiration. The most common type of thyroplasty is medialization, in which the paralyzed cord is fixed in the midline so that the moving cord may push against the fixed cord in to close the glottis. This improves speech volume and stamina and reduces aspiration. A paralyzed cord may also obstruct the airway and require lateral fixation.

Technique

1. An incision is made over the larynx.
2. The incision is carried to the thyroid cartilage.
3. A "window" is cut into the thyroid cartilage to expose the paraglottic space.
4. A nasolaryngoscope is inserted to view the vocal cords.
5. The true vocal cord is medialized.
6. The patient is asked to speak to assess the position of the vocal cord.
7. An implant is positioned in the paraglottic space.
8. The incision is closed.

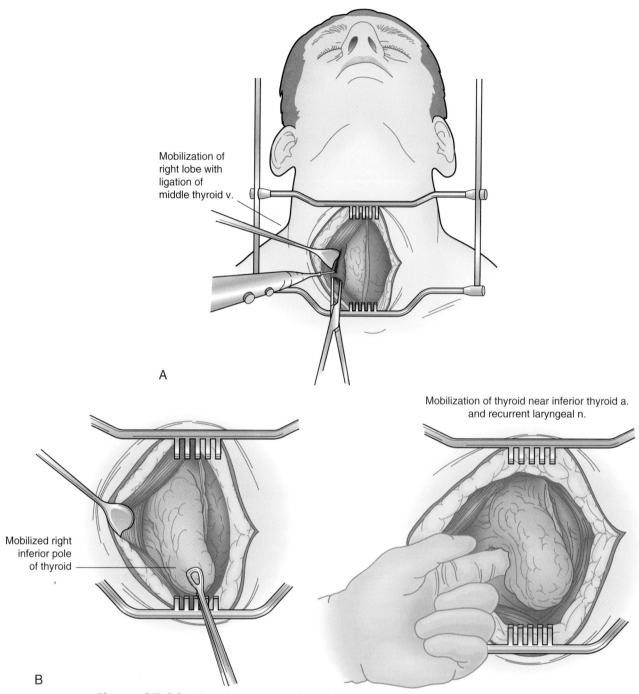

Mobilization of
right lobe with
ligation of
middle thyroid v.

Mobilization of thyroid near inferior thyroid a.
and recurrent laryngeal n.

A

Mobilized right
inferior pole
of thyroid

B

Figure 27-28   Thyroidectomy. **A,** A lateral incision is made in the neck, and the strap muscles are retracted with a Green retractor. The thyroid vein is exposed and ligated. **B,** Traction is placed on the thyroid for continued mobilization.

Discussion

The patient is positioned for a neck procedure as described previously. The patient is awake for most of the procedure, therefore it is important that the person be comfortable. IV sedation is given, and a local anesthetic (1% lidocaine with epinephrine 1:100,000) is infiltrated into the surgical site.

The surgeon makes a 0.8- to 1.2-inch (2 to 3 cm) incision in the neck at the midline with a #15 blade. The skin edges are retracted with double-prong skin hooks. The skin and subcutaneous tissue are dissected from the underlying tissue and

elevated. This exposes the platysma, which is divided with a #15 blade and toothed Adson forceps. A small Weitlaner retractor is placed to expose the strap muscles, which are retracted laterally to expose the thyroid muscle.

A Freer elevator is used to release the thyroid muscle from the thyroid cartilage. With the thyroid cartilage exposed, the surgeon marks the cartilage for the window (Figure 27-29, *A* to *E*). This can be done with a caliper or free-hand.

When the window has been marked, a small sagittal saw is used to cut a window measuring 5 × 10 mm. The assistant

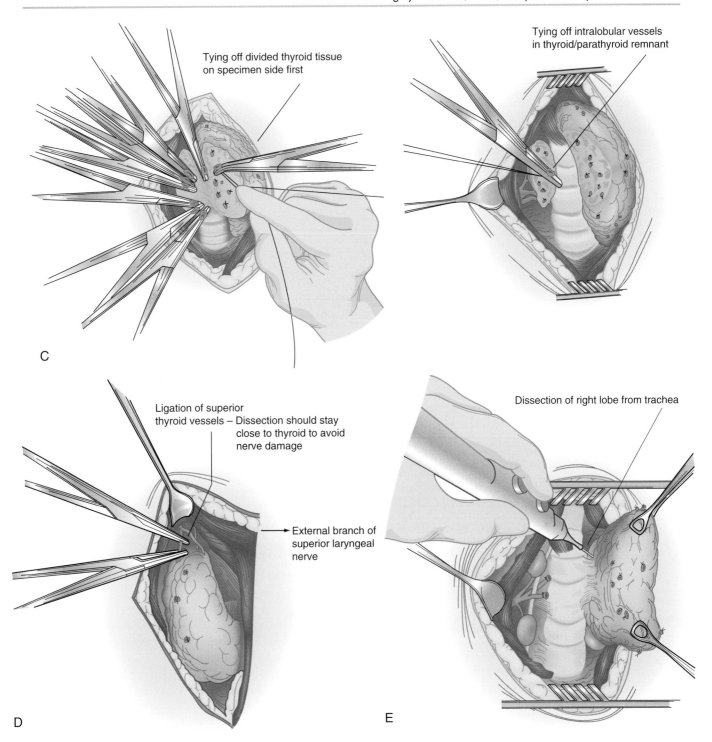

Tying off divided thyroid tissue on specimen side first

Tying off intralobular vessels in thyroid/parathyroid remnant

C

Ligation of superior thyroid vessels – Dissection should stay close to thyroid to avoid nerve damage

→ External branch of superior laryngeal nerve

D

Dissection of right lobe from trachea

E

Figure 27-28, cont'd   C, Bleeders are serially clamped and ligated with 3–0 and 4–0 suture ties. **D,** The thyroid vessels are carefully dissected free and ligated. **E,** The lobe is dissected from the trachea with the ESU. *(From Sabiston DC Jr, Gordon RG, editors: Atlas of general surgery, Philadelphia, 1994, WB Saunders.)*

keeps the cartilage moist with sterile saline to prevent the cartilage from being burned during dissection with the sagittal saw. The surgeon then dissects the incised tissue with a single-prong skin hook and a Freer elevator (Figure 27-29, *F* and *G*).

Medialization of the cord is performed by pushing the thyroarytenoid cartilage to the midline. The anesthesiolo-

gist passes a flexible **nasolaryngoscope** to visualize the medialization.

The surgeon asks the patient to speak while the nasolaryngoscope is in place. This step is taken to confirm that the paralyzed cord has been medialized. Upon confirmation of medialization, the surgeon places an implant. Medialization

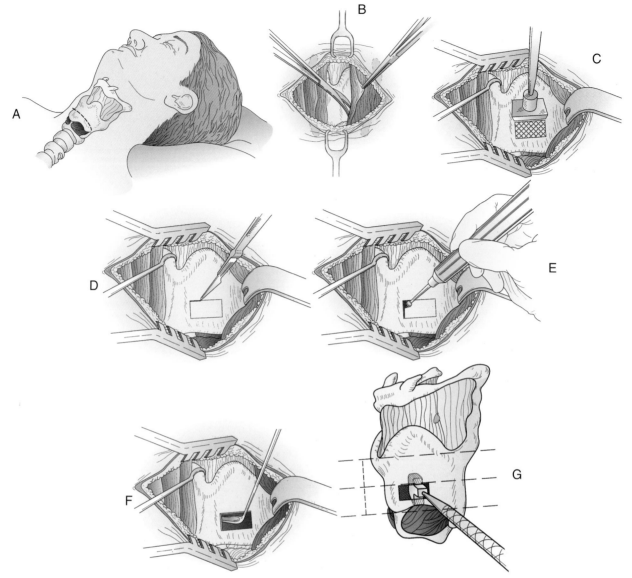

Figure 27-29   Thyroplasty (vocal cord medialization). **A,** An incision is made in the midline in the neck. **B,** Skin flaps are created to expose the platysma. **C,** The template for the window is positioned. **D,** The cartilage is marked. **E,** The window is removed. **F,** The window is elevated. **G,** The vocal cord is shifted medially, and the implant is positioned. (*Modified from Cummings CW, Haughey BH, Thomas JR et al: Otolaryngology: head and neck surgery, ed 3, St Louis, 1998, Mosby.*)

can be achieved with a portion of a Silastic block that has been carved by the surgeon; a Gore-Tex patch, mesh, or implant; or a prefabricated implant.

The surgeon reapproximates the strap muscles with 3-0 or 4-0 absorbable suture. A small drain may be placed below the platysmal layer. The platysma is closed with absorbable suture. The skin then is closed and dressed.

NECK DISSECTION

Surgical Goal
Neck dissection is performed to remove a tumor and affected lymph nodes.

Pathology
Many head and neck cancers, including malignant tumors of the oral and pharyngeal cavities, cutaneous malignant melanoma, and skin cancer, metastasize to the cervical lymph nodes.

Three types of neck dissections may be performed, depending on tumor staging. *Radical neck dissection* is the removal of all cervical lymph nodes and surrounding structures, including the spinal accessory nerve, the internal jugular vein, and the sternocleidomastoid muscle. *Modified radical neck dissection* is the excision of all lymph nodes with the preservation of one or more of the nonlymphatic structures (i.e., spinal accessory nerve, internal jugular vein, or sternocleidomastoid muscle). *Selective neck dissection* is the removal of the upper two thirds of the cervical lymph nodes and structures with preservation of the neurovascular and musculoskeletal structures.

Technique

1. A skin incision is made.
2. The structures of the neck are exposed.
3. The affected structures are removed.
4. Bleeding is controlled.
5. A tracheotomy is performed if necessary.
6. A drain is placed, and the wound is closed.

Discussion

The patient is placed in the supine position on a doughnut or Mayfield headrest with the affected side of the neck upward. The arms are tucked at the patient's sides, and a shoulder roll is placed to hyperextend the neck slightly. General anesthesia is used. The patient is prepped, including the face, neck, and chest, and draped for a head and neck procedure.

The surgeon begins the procedure by outlining the incisions with a skin scribe. The skin incision is made with a #15 blade. The incision is extended through the platysma, and the ESU and double-prong skin hooks are used for retraction. Bleeding vessels may be ligated with 2-0 or 3-0 silk ties.

The surgeon mobilizes the sternocleidomastoid muscle (SCM) using blunt dissection and then retracts it laterally with an Army-Navy retractor. If the SCM is to be sacrificed, it is cut with the ESU. This allows the surgeon to visualize the neurovascular sheath. Dissection continues along the neurovascular sheath to expose the anterior portion of the specimen. This dissection is performed bluntly with hemostats.

With the neurovascular sheath exposed, the surgeon identifies the carotid artery, internal jugular vein, and vagus nerve. The neurovascular sheath is retracted with a Cushing vein retractor. If the internal jugular vein is to be sacrificed, it is double-clamped, transected, and ligated with multiple 2-0 silk ties and 2-0 stick ties. The surgeon then retracts the SCM anteriorly, exposing the lateral cervical triangle. The subcutaneous tissue is removed with blunt dissection or Metzenbaum scissors. Bleeders are clamped with hemostats and 2-0 silk ties or the ESU. A tracheotomy is performed if necessary. The wound is then irrigated with normal saline. A drain is placed in the wound, and the wound is closed in layers with absorbable suture. A radical neck dissection is illustrated in Figure 27-30.

GLOSSECTOMY

Surgical Goal

A glossectomy is the removal of the tongue for the treatment of cancer. A partial glossectomy is removal of less than half of the tongue (*hemiglossectomy*). Simple excision includes primary closure or application of a split-thickness skin graft (STSG) to the anterior tongue. A secondary goal is to ensure that closure of the floor of the mouth prevents a fistula or leakage of saliva from the oral cavity into the neck tissues.

Pathology

The entire neurovascular supply of one side of the tongue passes through the base of the tongue; therefore, if one side of the base of the tongue requires excision, that entire side needs to be removed. A total glossectomy is the excision of tissue in the anterior two thirds of the tongue. A pectoralis myocutaneous (PMC) flap or free flap is constructed to produce a watertight seal. A total glossectomy is almost always combined with a total laryngectomy to treat laryngeal metastasis or problems with aspiration. A PMC or free flap is required to provide a water tight seal.

Technique

Partial Glossectomy

1. The tongue is grasped with a towel clip, or heavy silk sutures are placed through the tongue.
2. The affected portion of the tongue is excised with the electrosurgical unit (ESU).
3. The defect is closed, or a split-thickness skin graft (STSG) is placed.

Discussion: Partial Glossectomy—Primary Closure or STSG Closure

Radical procedures of the neck require instruments used in general surgery and vascular surgery, as well as fine orthopedic instruments, including a drill.

The patient is placed in the supine position on a doughnut or Mayfield headrest with the arms tucked at the sides. General anesthesia is used. The patient is prepped and draped for a head and neck procedure.

The surgeon grasps the tongue either by using large towel clips at the midline or by suturing the midline with a size 0 silk suture and grasping the ends of the suture with a hemostat. The tongue is pulled anteriorly to expose the affected tissue. The surgeon excises the tumor and a wide margin with the ESU blade or needle tip. The tongue is then closed. If primary closure is possible, the tongue is closed with 3-0 absorbable sutures. If primary closure is not possible, the defect is closed with a split-thickness skin graft. The graft is sutured into place with 3-0 absorbable suture.

Technique

Hemiglossectomy

1. An incision is made at the midline of the lip and extended to the submental region.
2. The soft tissue is retracted to expose the anterior surface of the mandible.
3. A titanium plate is placed over the proposed site of division and then removed.
4. The mandible is divided at the midline.
5. The tongue is divided at the midline for hemiglossectomy.
6. An incision is made in the floor of mouth between the tongue and the mandible.
7. The tumor is excised.
8. The mandible is reapproximated and internally fixated.
9. The incision is closed.

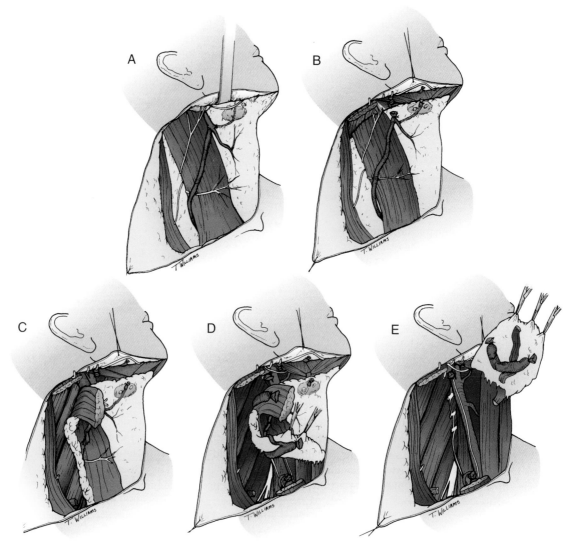

Figure 27-30 Radical neck dissection. **A,** Elevation of the skin flaps. **B,** Dissection and ligation of the facial vessels and dissection of the submandibular fascia. **C,** Sacrifice of the sternocleidomastoid muscle (SCM) superiorly. **D,** Sacrifice of the SCM inferiorly and ligation of the internal jugular. **E,** Removal of the specimen. *(Modified from Cummings CW, Haughey BH, Thomas JR et al: Otolaryngology: head and neck surgery, ed 3, St Louis, 1998, Mosby.)*

Discussion: Glossectomy with Mandibulotomy and PMC Flap

The patient is placed in the supine position on a doughnut or Mayfield headrest with the arms tucked at the sides. General anesthesia is used. Often a tracheotomy has been performed or will be performed before the glossectomy. The patient is prepped and draped for a head and neck procedure, including the chest in case a PMC flap is needed.

A #15 blade is used to make an incision through the midline lip; the incision is extended to the submental border. Skin flaps are elevated with the ESU. Senn rakes are used for retraction.

When the mandibular surface is exposed, a titanium plate is positioned in the region of the planned division. The screw holes are drilled with a small power drill. The plate is secured to the mandible with screws. The surgeon removes the plate after placement and splits the mandible at the midline, using a small power saw with a medium saw blade.

The surgeon then grasps the mandible with atraumatic rake retractors or a self-retaining retractor (e.g., a Weitlaner retractor). In a hemiglossectomy, the anterior part of the oral floor and the body of the tongue are divided at the midline with the ESU. The incision is extended to the tongue base. The affected side of the tongue is then excised with the ESU.

The incision is closed primarily or with a skin graft. The mandible is reapproximated and internally fixed with the plate. The incision is closed in layers with absorbable suture. For a total glossectomy, the incision is made between the floor of the mouth and the mandible and extended to the base of tongue with the ESU. The tongue is excised from the epiglottis with the ESU. A neck dissection is performed on one or both sides of the neck (see neck dissection).

If the incision cannot be closed primarily or with a split-thickness skin graft, a PMC flap is harvested (see the section Pectoralis Myocutaneous and Deltopectoral Flaps later in the chapter). The flap is sutured into the defect with the skin taking the place of the tongue. The skin is sutured to the remaining mucosa of the floor of the mouth (and to the epiglottic or pharyngeal mucosa if a total laryngectomy was performed concomitantly). Closure is done with 3-0 absorbable suture. The mandible is reapproximated and internally fixed with the titanium plate.

The lip incision, oral mucosa, and deep portions of the skin incisions are closed with 3-0 absorbable sutures. The skin is closed with fine nonabsorbable suture. A nasal feeding tube is placed and secured with 2-0 silk suture through the nasal septum. The skin incisions are then coated in antibiotic ointment.

Postoperative Considerations

The patient is transferred to the intensive care unit (ICU) for airway monitoring. A gastrostomy tube may be inserted to provide nutrition.

LARYNGECTOMY

Surgical Goal

A laryngectomy is the removal of the larynx, usually with wide excision and tissue grafting.

Pathology

A laryngectomy may be performed for four reasons:
- Cancer of the larynx
- Diversion for total separation of the respiratory and digestive tracts
- Chondroradionecrosis
- Major trauma that precludes open reduction and internal fixation

Technique

1. A skin incision is made.
2. The larynx and neck contents are exposed.
3. A neck dissection is performed if necessary.
4. A tracheotomy is performed.
5. The larynx is removed.
6. The pharynx is closed
7. Bleeding is controlled.
8. Drains are placed.
9. The wound is closed.

Discussion

The patient is placed in the supine position on a doughnut or Mayfield headrest with the arms tucked at the sides. A shoulder roll may be placed to hyperextend the neck. General anesthesia is used. The patient is prepped from the level of the nose to the level of the umbilicus and draped for a head and neck procedure, including the face, neck, and chest.

Using a #15 blade, the surgeon begins by making an apron incision, either from mastoid to mastoid (for laryngectomy with neck dissection) or from midsternocleidomastoid muscle

to midsternocleidomastoid muscle (for laryngectomy alone). The flaps are elevated about ½ to 1 inch (1 to 2 cm) above the sternal notch from below and ½ to 1 inch (1 to 2 cm) below the hyoid bone. The flaps generally are secured back with fishhook retractors or suture.

The surgeon detaches the strap muscles from the sternum using the ESU or Mayo scissors and retracts them laterally with Army-Navy retractors. This exposes the carotid sheath, thyroid, and a portion of the trachea. The carotid sheath is dissected laterally and retracted with a Cushing vein retractor. The thyroid veins may be ligated with hemostat clamps and 2-0 silk ties. The surgeon removes the thyroid lobe on the affected side by dividing the isthmus of the thyroid down the middle with the ESU or scissors.

The thyroid lobe then is dissected free. Scissors are used to remove the fat and lymph tissue from the gland. The inferior thyroid artery is ligated and transected, and the recurrent laryngeal nerve is transected. The dissection of the thyroid continues with blunt dissection to the level of the trachea. The remaining portion of the gland is grasped with a Kocher clamp and divided from the trachea with the ESU.

A cricoid hook is placed in the right-side larynx to allow rotation of the larynx and exposure of the constrictor muscles on the thyroid cartilage. These muscles are detached from the cartilage with the ESU.

A periosteal elevator then is used to remove the soft tissue from the underside of the thyroid cartilage. The larynx is rotated to the left with a cricoid hook to free the larynx from the remaining muscle and soft tissue of the thyroid. The surgeon then uses Metzenbaum scissors or a hemostat clamp to dissect the thyroid cartilage from the hyoid bone. Any vessels and nerves that are exposed at this point in the dissection are ligated. All muscular attachments between the tongue base and hyoid bone are separated with the ESU.

With the hyoid bone exposed and free, the surgeon uses heavy Mayo scissors to sever the attachments of the hyoid bone. The tracheotomy is performed at this point because the surgeon is ready to enter the airway. The surgeon sews the anterior tracheal wall to the posterior skin flap to secure it in place. The ET tube then is removed, and the anesthesia circuit is switched to the tracheotomy tube.

The surgeon then uses scissors or the ESU to make an incision into the hypopharynx in the midline over the hyoid bone. The hypopharynx is opened with a hemostat, and the epiglottis is grasped with an Allis clamp and rotated out of the larynx. The lateral pharyngeal walls are incised with heavy Mayo scissors, with as much mucosa as possible spared. The larynx then is opened out. The tracheal tube is removed, and the posterior membranous trachea is incised with a #15 blade. The trachea is dissected from the anterior esophageal wall with Metzenbaum scissors. The surgeon also transects any fibrous attachments to the larynx at this point. The larynx is removed, and the tracheal tube is replaced.

With the larynx removed, the pharyngeal mucosa is closed with or without a PMC flap (discussed later) in two layers. The first layer is closed with a long 3-0 absorbable suture on a tapered needle, and the second layer is closed with 3-0 absorbable horizontal mattress sutures. With the pharynx closed, the surgeon creates a stoma by closing the anterior tracheal wall to the inferior skin flap and the posterior tracheal wall to the superior skin flap, using either absorbable or non-absorbable sutures, depending on the surgeon's preference. The wound is irrigated with normal saline. Drains are placed, and the skin is closed in layers with absorbable suture.

Postoperative Considerations

The patient is transferred to the ICU. Chemotherapy and radiation are initiated as soon the wound is sufficiently healed to tolerate them. Laryngectomy is illustrated in Figure 27-31.

Related Procedure

Partial cricoidectomy is subtotal and submucosal resection of the cricoid performed in the treatment or control of chronic aspiration after radical pharyngeal surgery, including removal of the tongue. In this procedure the pharyngeal inlet is enlarged, and the laryngeal inlet reduced so that the voice is preserved and aspiration is controlled.

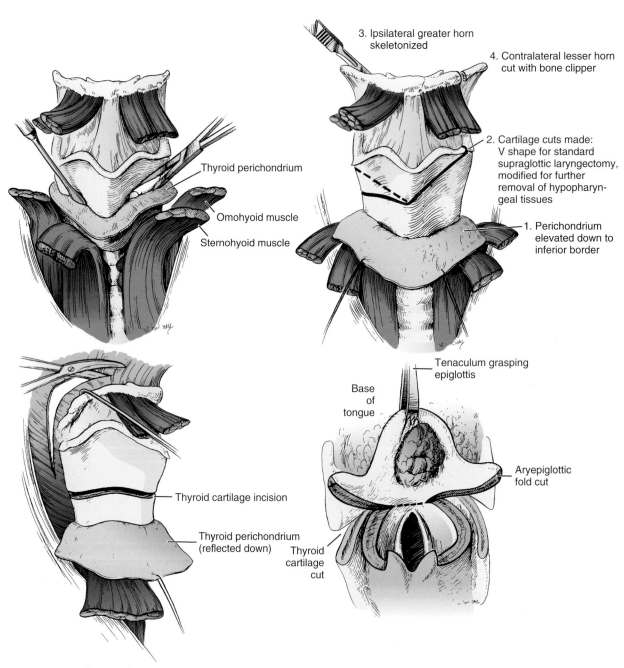

Figure 27-31 Laryngectomy. *(Modified from Cummings CW, Haughey BH, Thomas JR et al: Otolaryngology: head and neck surgery, ed 3, St Louis, 1998, Mosby.)*

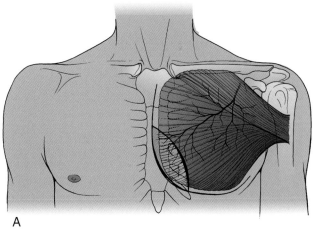
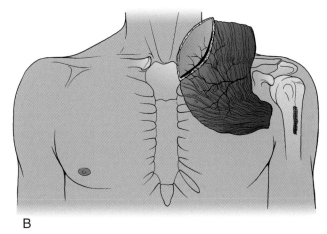

A   B

Figure 27-32 Pectoralis myocutaneous (PMC) flap. **A,** Location of skin flap outlined and incised down to the underlying fascia. **B,** The skin flap is elevated, and the lower border of the pectoralis is identified. *(Modified from Silver CE, Rubin JS: Atlas of head and neck surgery, ed 2, Philadelphia, 1999, Churchill Livingstone.)*

PECTORALIS MYOCUTANEOUS AND DELTOPECTORAL FLAPS

Surgical Goal

PMC and deltopectoral (DP) tissue flaps are created to provide coverage for a soft tissue defect.

Pathology

PMC and DP flaps replace soft tissue, usually after surgical excision of cancer in the head and neck region. A DP flap usually is used to close postirradiation fistulas and to resurface large cutaneous defects in the neck. A PMC flap may be used in the reconstruction of the pharynx, tongue, face, or neck. It is especially useful for covering the carotid artery when it may be at risk because of previous irradiation.

Technique

Deltopectoral (DP) Flap
1. The DP flap incision is made.
2. The flap is elevated.
3. The flap is rotated.
4. The flap is inset.
5. The donor site is closed with a skin graft.

Discussion: Deltopectoral Flap

The patient is positioned, prepped, and draped as for a neck dissection or laryngectomy, because the DP flap often is performed in conjunction with either of these procedures. The surgeon begins by outlining the proposed incision with a skin scribe. The incision typically goes from the acromion process to the sternum, extending to the space between the third and fourth ribs.

The incision is made with a #10 blade, and the flap (skin, vascular supply, subcutaneous tissue, and fascia) is elevated from the underlying pectoralis major muscle in a lateral to medial fashion. This is done with the ESU or a scalpel. Bleeders are controlled with the ESU. The flap is left attached at the medial border (because this is where its vascular supply enters)

and is rotated to cover the defect of the neck (Figure 27-32). The flap then is sutured into place with 3-0 absorbable sutures. The donor site then is covered with a skin graft, which is secured with 3-0 absorbable sutures or skin staples.

Technique

Pectoralis Myocutaneous (PMC) Flap
1. An incision is made, and the tissue flap is elevated.
2. The flap is "tunneled."
3. The flap is inset into the defect.
4. The donor site is closed.

Discussion: Pectoralis Myocutaneous Flap

The patient is positioned, prepped, and draped as for a neck dissection or laryngectomy, because the PMC flap often is performed with one of these procedures. The surgeon begins by measuring from the inferior border of the defect to the midclavicle with a lap sponge. This distance marks the superior portion of the skin paddle, which is drawn as a rectangle with rounded edges between the nipple and the sternum inferiorly to the inferior border of the pectoralis major muscle. A line is then drawn from the superolateral portion of the rectangle to the axilla.

The incision is made with a #10 blade. The skin, subcutaneous tissue, and fascia superior to the incision are elevated off the underlying muscle over the clavicle, making a tunnel into the neck. The flap (skin, vascular supply, subcutaneous tissue, fascia, and pectoralis muscle) is elevated from the underlying chest wall in an inferior to superior fashion. This may be done with either a scalpel or the ESU. The ESU is used to separate the muscle from the sternum and humerus. The muscular portion of the flap should be slightly larger than the skin paddle.

When the flap has been elevated to the level of the clavicle, it is rotated 180 degrees and tunneled under the skin and over the clavicle to reach the defect. The flap then is sutured in place with 3-0 absorbable sutures. Two drains are placed in the donor site, which usually is closed with 3-0 absorbable suture.

CHAPTER SUMMARY

- The structures of the external ear include the outer surface of the tympanic membrane and all structures lateral to it. This includes the auricle or pinna, the external auditory meatus, and the external auditory canal.
- The middle ear extends from the tympanic membrane to the medial wall of the middle ear cleft. It includes the TM, the ossicles (malleus, stapes, and incus), the opening to the eustachian tube, the opening of the mastoid cavity, and the intratympanic portion of the facial nerve.
- The inner ear contains receptors for hearing and balance and is composed of a series of hollow tunnels called *labyrinths.*
- Within the bony labyrinth is the membranous labyrinth. This structure has three parts: the cochlea, the semicircular canals, and the vestibule.
- The spiral-shaped cochlea contains the cochlear duct and the organ of hearing, the organ of Corti.
- The semicircular canals communicate with the middle ear via the oval and round windows. The crista ampullaris is located within the ampulla of the semicircular canals and is responsible for equilibrium of the body in motion.
- Infection of the middle ear (otitis media) may be acute or chronic.
- Otosclerosis is an abnormal thickening of the bone in the middle and inner ear. This results in restriction of the stapes footplate and conductive hearing loss.
- Surgical procedures of the ear generally are performed with the patient in the supine position with the head turned. A doughnut headrest is used to stabilize the head and prevent pressure on the opposite ear.
- The primary instruments used in ear surgery include a small number of plastic surgery instruments: hook retractors, mosquito forceps, a #15 knife, and delicate skin forceps.
- The operating microscope is used in all procedures of the middle or inner ear. The standard operating lens for ear surgery has a 250-mm focal length.
- Medications used during ear surgery include anesthetics, hemostatic agents, antibiotic solutions, and irrigation solutions.
- A myringotomy is a surgical opening made in the tympanic membrane to release fluid from the middle ear.
- A mastoidectomy or tympanomastoidectomy is the removal of diseased bone, the mastoid air cells, and the soft tissue lining the air cells.
- In a stapedectomy, the ossicles are reconstructed to restore conduction to the oval window.
- Sound normally is received at the TM, which transmits vibrations through the ossicles and the oval window, which amplifies the sound. If the bony chain is immobile or discontinuous, not only is amplification lost, but sound perception can be severely dampened.
- The most common cause of ossicle immobility is otosclerosis of the stapes. This is abnormal bone growth that locks the stapes in place and prevents it from vibrating and carrying the sound stimulus.
- The most common cause of a break in the ossicle chain is a cholesteatoma, which erodes the ossicles.
- A cochlear implant transmits external sound directly to the eighth cranial nerve. This procedure is performed to treat sensorineural deafness.
- Sensorineural deafness can be congenital or acquired. It is characterized by the inability of the cochlear cilia to stimulate the cochlear nerve, usually as a result of destruction from sound exposure, autoimmune disease, or infection.
- Surgery of the nose, oropharynx, and larynx is performed by an otorhinolaryngologist. Most of the structures in these anatomical regions are related to respiration and vocalizing, although some share functions with the digestive system.
- The external nose is formed by two U-shaped cartilaginous structures called the *lower lateral cartilages,* two rectangular structures called the *upper lateral cartilages,* and two nasal bones. The nares are the flared portions of the lower nose (i.e., the nostrils).
- The nasal cavity is located over the palatine bone, which is the "floor" of the nose; the "roof" of the nose is formed from the cribriform plate in the ethmoid bone.
- The nasal cavity contains paranasal sinuses, or spaces. These are formed by extensions of the ethmoid bone and the frontal, maxillary, and sphenoid bones. The extensions are referred to as the *turbinates* or *nasal conchae.*
- The posterior aspect of the nasal cavities is the choana, which separates the nasal cavities from the nasopharynx.
- The paired maxillary sinuses are the large sinuses below the ocular orbits. The apices of the tooth roots are found in the floor of these sinuses. The paired frontal sinuses lie behind the lower forehead. The sphenoids lie at the posterosuperior extent of the nasal cavity.
- The nasopharynx is situated behind the nasal cavity and above the oral cavity. It communicates with the nasal sinuses and with the oropharynx below it.
- The oral cavity is divided into two sections: The vestibule lies between the inner surface of the lips, the buccal mucosa (cheeks), and the lateral aspects of the mandible and maxilla. The oral cavity proper lies within the medial surface of the maxillary and mandibular teeth.
- The floor of the mouth contains the ducts for the paired submandibular and lingual salivary glands. The tongue is attached in the midline to the floor of the mouth by a membranous structure called the *frenulum.*
- The pharynx is a tubular structure extending from the nose to the esophagus. It is separated into three areas: the nasopharynx, oropharynx, and hypopharynx.

- The larynx is composed of nine segments of cartilage, three paired sets and three unpaired segments. The unpaired cartilages are the cricoid, thyroid, and epiglottis segments; the paired cartilages are the arytenoids and the corniculate and cuneiform segments.
- The arytenoid cartilages lie in the posterior larynx and have processes that extend anteriorly (the vocal processes) and that lie within the true vocal cords.
- The trachea extends from the cricoid to the carina. It is composed of approximately 20 incomplete cartilaginous rings. The cricoid is the only closed ring of the upper airway.
- Choanal atresia is congenital stricture of the choana, which may require emergency surgery at birth to restore respiration.
- Specialty nasal instruments are designed for use on soft tissue and bone. Soft tissue instruments are needed for skin, submucosa, and soft connective tissue; bone and cartilage require heavier instruments.
- Tonsil and adenoid instruments include the Crowe-Davis mouth gag, tonsil snares, adenoid curettes, elevators, clamps, and scissors.
- Endoscopic sinus surgery is performed to treat disease of the paranasal sinuses, nasal cavity, and skull base and to improve nasal airflow.
- In the Caldwell-Luc procedure, a technique used to enter the maxillary sinus, an incision is made in the gingival-buccal sulcus (the junction of the gum and upper lip).
- A turbinectomy is the removal of the bony turbinate to increase airflow through the nose.
- Septoplasty is the surgical manipulation of the septum to return it to its anatomical position or to gain access to the sinuses for removal of pituitary tumors.
- Rhinoplasty is performed to reshape the external nose for aesthetic or functional purposes. Each rhinoplasty procedure is approached differently, depending on the specific pathology.
- Reconstruction of the uvula and oropharynx (uvulopalatopharyngoplasty) is performed to reduce and tighten oropharyngeal tissue. Enlarged or redundant oropharyngeal mucosa may collapse on inspiration during the deep stages of sleep as muscles lose tone.
- Laryngoscopy is endoscopic assessment of the larynx. Tissue specimens are removed for pathological examination.
- Tracheostomy is indicated for patients who require emergency or elective airway management for prolonged ventilator dependence or acute or chronic upper airway obstruction. The obturator of the tracheostomy is kept with the patient as long as the tracheal tube is in place. If the tube becomes dislodged or is traumatically removed, the obturator is needed to replace the tube.

- Surgery of the neck most often is performed to remove or debulk tumors arising from the mouth or upper respiratory system and for surgery of the salivary and thyroid glands.
- The three pairs of salivary glands are the parotid, submandibular, and sublingual salivary glands. Many minor salivary glands are found throughout the oral cavity and pharynx.
- The thyroid gland is located in the midneck, overlying the trachea below the larynx. It has two lobes, which are connected by a central band of thyroid tissue called the *isthmus.*
- The thyroid secretes the hormones thyroxine (T_4) and triiodothyronine (T_3). These thyroid hormones are necessary for regulating cell metabolism and growth. Calcitonin, which also is secreted by the thyroid, is necessary for calcium regulation.
- A sialith is a salivary gland stone. Such stones may block the duct, resulting in swelling, pain, and infection.
- Hypothyroidism (inadequate levels of thyroid hormone) may be congenital or acquired. Thyroid hormone is essential for brain development in the fetus. In adults, hypothyroidism is caused by thyroidectomy or radiation of the thyroid for cancer treatment.
- Overproduction of thyroid hormone may develop into a life-threatening condition characterized by hypermetabolism. Graves' disease is an autoimmune condition characterized by hyperthyroidism and goiter (benign enlargement of the thyroid gland).
- The submandibular gland may be removed for chronic infection (bacterial or viral), stone formation, or neoplasm (benign or malignant). Thyroidectomy is performed to treat known or suspected malignancy or for the treatment of hyperthyroidism.
- The parathyroids produce parathyroid hormone, which controls (elevates) calcium. Disease of the parathyroid gland commonly causes hyperparathyroidism.
- During thyroplasty, the vocal cord is moved to one side and stabilized with a Silastic or Gore-Tex implant.
- Radical neck dissection is the removal of all cervical lymph nodes and surrounding structures, including the spinal accessory nerve, the internal jugular vein, and the sternocleidomastoid muscle.
- Modified radical neck dissection is the excision of all lymph nodes with preservation of one or more of the nonlymphatic structures (i.e., spinal accessory nerve, internal jugular vein, or sternocleidomastoid muscle).
- In selective neck dissection, the upper two thirds of the cervical lymph nodes and structures are removed and the neurovascular and musculoskeletal structures are preserved.
- A glossectomy is the removal of the tongue for the treatment of cancer. A partial glossectomy is removal of less than half of the tongue (hemiglossectomy). Simple excision includes primary closure or a split-thickness skin graft to the anterior tongue.

REVIEW QUESTIONS

1. Name the three regions of the ear.
2. Why is a myringotomy performed?
3. Describe the two methods of performing tympanoplasty.
4. What is otosclerosis? How is this treated?
5. When is a cochlear implant procedure performed on a child?
6. Why is it important to submerge the cochlear implant in normal saline after it is opened onto the sterile field?
7. Why is septoplasty not performed in children?
8. What are the three indications for a tonsillectomy?
9. Why are children more likely to be affected by adenoiditis than adults?
10. Explain the difference between indirect laryngoscopy and direct laryngoscopy.
11. What three procedures are included in a panendoscopy?
12. List three causes of upper airway obstruction that result in the need for placement of a tracheostomy.
13. What is the most common site of pathology of the parotid gland?
14. Which nerve is identified and preserved in thyroidectomy?
15. Why is a thyroplasty performed?
16. List the different types of incisions that can be used for neck dissection.
17. Describe the uses of a DP flap.
18. Describe the uses of a PMC flap.

BIBLIOGRAPHY

Bailey BJ (Editor): *Head and neck surgery: otolaryngology*, ed 2, vol 1 and 2, Philadelphia, 1998, Lippincott–Raven.

Boston Medical Products: *Montgomery thyroplasty system: surgeon's implant guide*, Westborough, Mass, 1998, Boston Medical Products.

Brackmann D, Shelton C, Arriaga MA: *Otologic surgery*, ed 2, Philadelphia, 2001, Saunders.

Coker NJ, Jenkins HA: *Atlas of otologic surgery*, Philadelphia, 2001, Saunders.

Cummings CW, Haughey BH, Thomas JR: *Otolaryngology: head and neck surgery*, ed 3, St Louis, 1998, Mosby.

Dhillon RS, East CA: *Ear, nose, and throat and head and neck surgery*, ed 3, Edinburgh, 2006, Churchill Livingstone.

Herman C: *Medialization thyroplasty for unilateral vocal cord paralysis*, AORN J Mar, 75(3): 511–522, 2002.

Marks SC: *Nasal and sinus surgery*, Philadelphia, 2000, Saunders.

Montgomery WW: *Surgery of the upper respiratory system*, ed 3, Baltimore, 1996, Williams & Wilkins.

Seiden AM, Tami AM, Pensak ML, Gluckman JL, Cotton RT (Editors): *Otolaryngology: the essentials*, New York, 2002, Thieme.

Silver CE, Rubin JS: *Atlas of head and neck surgery*, ed 2, Philadelphia, 1999, Churchill Livingstone.

Weerda H: *Reconstructive facial plastic surgery: a problem-solving manual*, New York, 2001, Thieme.

CHAPTER 28

Oral and Maxillofacial Surgery

CHAPTER OUTLINE

LEARNING OBJECTIVES

After studying this chapter the reader will be able to:
- Identify the bony structures of the face
- Describe common fractures and congenital anomalies of the face
- Describe common incisions used in maxillofacial surgery
- Identify instrumentation used in facial reconstruction surgery

TERMINOLOGY

Arch bars: Metal plates wired to the teeth to occlude the jaw during maxillofacial surgery or during healing. Arch bars maintain the patient's normal bite (occlusion).

Bicoronal incision: An incision made between the frontal and the parietal bones bilaterally.

Bicortical screws: Screws that penetrate both cortical layers and the intervening spongy layer of the bone.

Blowout fracture: A severe fracture of the orbital cavity in which a portion of the globe may extrude outside the cavity.

Dentition: The number, type, and pattern of the teeth.

Le Fort I fracture: A horizontal fracture of the maxilla that causes the hard palate and alveolar process to become separated from the rest of the maxilla. The fracture extends into the lower nasal septum, lateral maxillary sinus, and palatine bones.

Le Fort II fracture: A fracture which extends from the nasal bone to the frontal processes of the maxilla, lacrimal bones, and inferior orbital floor, and it may extend into the orbital foramen. Inferiorly, it extends into the anterior maxillary sinus and the pterygoid plates.

Le Fort III fracture: This fracture involves separation of all the facial bones from their cranial base. It includes fracture of the zygoma, maxilla, and nasal bones.

Mastication: Chewing.

Maxillomandibular fixation (MMF): See arch bars.

Occlusion: Normally to "close." In maxillofacial surgery this refers to the patient's bite pattern when the jaw is closed.

Odontectomy: Tooth extraction.

Oromaxillofacial surgery: Surgery involving the bones of the face, primarily for repair of fractures and reconstruction for congenital anomalies.

Subciliary incision: Skin incision made approximately 2 mm inferior to the lower eyelashes.

Transconjuntival incision: Incision made through the conjunctiva.

Transosteal implant: A bone plate with retaining posts used in the procedure for dental implants.

INTRODUCTION

Surgery for facial trauma may involve the many bones of the face and frontal sinus. The face is vulnerable to injury in motor vehicle and industrial accidents, high-speed sports, and intentional violence. Maxillofacial injuries can be quite complex, involving skin, muscle, nerves, and blood vessels. The long-term physiological effects of injury or congenital anomalies can affect speech, **mastication** (chewing), and development of the teeth. The psychological effects are equally important, because disfigurement often results in social and emotional isolation. Maxillofacial procedures are performed primarily by surgeons specializing in oromaxillofacial, plastic, or otorhinolaryngology surgery.

SURGICAL ANATOMY

BONES OF THE FACE

The bones of the face are divided into three regions: the upper face, the midface, and the lower face.

Upper Face

The upper face is composed of:
* The frontal bone

The frontal bone is part of the cranium. It forms the forehead and contains portions of the nasal sinuses (see Chapter 27 for more detail on ear, nose, and throat surgery). The superior margin of the bony orbit is formed by the frontal bone. This area generally is injured in a blow to the forehead, and trauma may involve the nasal duct as well. Injury to the dura (one of the protective layers of the brain) also may be sustained in trauma to this area.

Midface

The midface is composed of:
* The ethmoid
* The nasal bone
* The zygoma
* The maxillary bones

The ethmoid bone is a complex structure that contributes to the floor of the cranium and also contains a number of sinus cavities.

The nasal bone forms the bridge of the nose and articulates with the ethmoid and the maxilla. Fractures of the nasal ethmoid area may injure the lacrimal apparatus, including the ducts and lacrimal gland. The dura also is vulnerable and may require neurological surgery.

The zygoma forms the lateral walls and floor of the bony orbit, which houses the eyeball. The zygomatic arch is the cheekbone. Fractures in this area are important because of their association with injury to the eye, especially in displaced fractures. The most common causes of injury are assault, motor vehicle accidents, and sports injuries. The bony orbit is formed by the frontal bone, but it also contains portions of other bones of the face, including the zygoma, maxilla, lacrimal, ethmoid, sphenoid, and palatine bones. The orbital floor is formed by the maxillary sinus.

The bilateral maxillae come together to form the upper jaw, anterior hard palate, and a portion of the orbital cavities.

Lower Face

The lower face is composed of:
* The mandible

The mandible is the only movable bone of the face. It is a U-shaped bone suspended from the temporal bone. The condyles insert into the glenoid fossa of the temporal bones to form the temporomandibular joints. The ramus extends inferiorly from the condyle to the angle, where it joins the body of the mandible and extends anteriorly and medially to join the other half of the mandible. The teeth are embedded in the alveoli of the body of the mandible. Fractures of the alveoli frequently require dental surgery. Figure 28-1 shows the bones of the face and cranium. Figure 28-2 illustrates the skull as viewed from below, and Figure 28-3 illustrates the mandible.

PATHOLOGY OF THE MIDFACE AND MANDIBLE

Table 28-1 presents common pathological conditions of the midface and mandible.

DIAGNOSTIC PROCEDURES

Facial fractures and structural deformities are most commonly assessed by imaging studies. Plain radiographs are taken for a baseline assessment or for simple fractures. However, extensive tissue swelling may obscure complex anatomical features and injuries. Computed tomography (CT) scanning therefore is used for complex facial fractures and reconstruction procedures.

EQUIPMENT AND INSTRUMENTS

Oromaxillofacial surgery focuses on reconstruction and repair of the facial bones and may include structures of the oral cavity. The instrumentation used for these procedures, therefore, includes fine orthopedic instruments, implants, and grafting materials. (Chapter 30 presents a complete discussion of the biomechanical and surgical techniques used in bone trauma and reconstruction, including power drills and techniques for their use.) Nasal instruments may be required for surgery of the midface (see Chapter 27). Facial facture instruments are shown in Figure 28-4.

POWER DRILL

For procedures involving facial fractures, a small power drill is required to prepare bone for plates and screws and to remodel bone. The drill bits for the screws are included as components of the plate system used. (Chapter 30 presents a complete discussion of drills and techniques.)

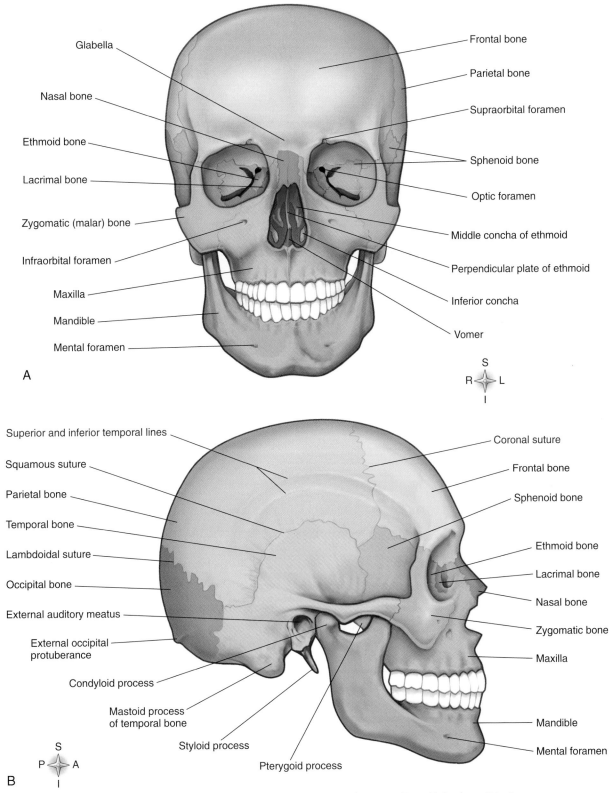

Figure 28-1 The cranium. **A,** Anterior view. **B,** Side view. *(From Thibodeau GA, Patt KT: Anthony's textbook of anatomy and physiology, ed 17, St Louis, 2003, Mosby.)*

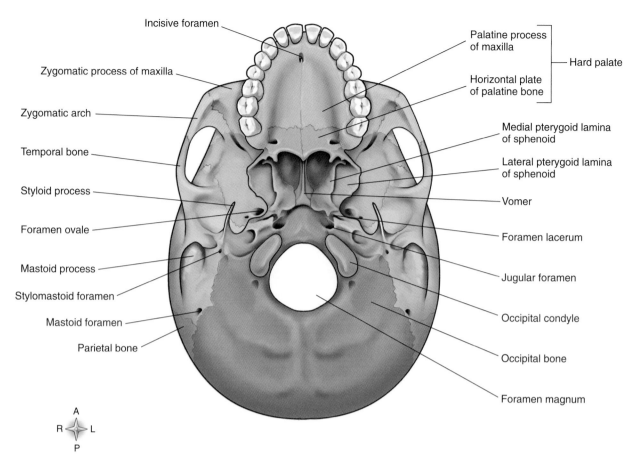

Figure 28-2 The skull (viewed from below). *(From Thibodeau GA, Patt KT: Anthony's textbook of anatomy and physiology, ed 17, St Louis, 2003, Mosby.)*

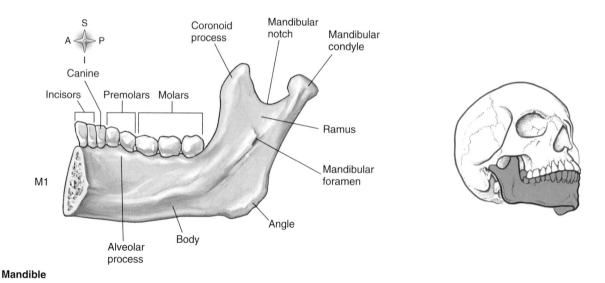

Mandible

Figure 28-3 The mandible. *(From Thibodeau GA, Patt KT: Anthony's textbook of anatomy and physiology, ed 17, St Louis, 2003, Mosby.)*

Table 28-1

Pathology of the Midface and Mandible

Condition	Description	Considerations
Torous palatinus/torus mandibularis	Bony outgrowth of the palatine bones or mandible; may develop into adulthood and continue to grow slowly throughout the individual's lifetime.	No treatment is necessary unless the growth becomes so large that it interferes with denture placement (in later life) or causes repeated injury while eating.
Facial trauma	Trauma to the face is most commonly caused by assault (intentional trauma) and motor vehicle accidents.	A facial fracture usually requires surgical intervention (i.e., reduction and fixation).
Dental caries	Bacterial infection and structural damage to the teeth are most commonly associated with poor oral hygiene and diet.	Dental extraction may be necessary.
Malocclusion	Malposition of the upper and lower jaw can result in misalignment of the teeth; the condition can affect oral health and may be associated with structural oromaxillofacial defects.	Conservative treatment includes orthodontics (braces, retainers). Surgery may be required for severe malocclusion.
Mandibular hyperplasia/maxillary hyperplasia	These are conditions of overdevelopment of bone; they may be acquired or congenital. The growth is nonneoplastic and may occur unilaterally or bilaterally.	Treatment, if necessary, is surgical.
Mandibular micrognathia	A congenital defect that results in an abnormally small lower jaw. This can affect feeding in the infant and alignment of the teeth as the infant grows.	The condition usually resolves without treatment during childhood development. If further correction is needed, surgery is performed after puberty.
Maxillary hypoplasia	Undergrowth of the maxilla, usually associated with bilateral cleft lip and palate.	Surgical correction is performed during adolescence when jaw growth is complete.

PLATES AND SCREWS

Plates and screws are the primary means of repairing facial fractures. Miniplate systems are small, malleable mesh plates that can be molded to fit over the contours of facial bone. Small cortical screws or **bicortical screws** are used to implant the titanium or stainless steel mesh plates, which provide stability during healing. Many systems are available, including Synthes, Leibinger, W Lorenz, Osteomed, and KLS. Each of these systems includes implants and the instrumentation required for the repair, including the following:

- Plates with screws
- Plate benders
- Plate cutters
- Holding forceps
- Screwdriver handles and blades
- Depth gauge

For mandibular fractures, the plates and screws most often are at least 2 mm in size. For midface, orbital, and frontal sinus fractures, the plates and screws are 1 to 2 mm. The scrub must keep track of all plates and screws used during surgery for documentation in the patient's record.

PREPPING AND DRAPING

Facial fractures are prepped with dilute Betadine scrub and paint because it has been shown to be the safest and most effective antiseptic for use on the face. Note that hexachlorophine and chorhexadine are not used on the face because they are ototoxic. The entire face is prepped, from the hairline to the sternal notch as described in Chapter 11. An endotracheal (ET) tube usually is part of the surgical field and therefore must be included in the prep. If a bicoronal incision (behind the hairline) is planned, the patient's head may be shaved, and the prep may be carried from the posterior head to the sternal notch. After the patient has been draped, the mouth may be irrigated with diluted Betadine paint and the teeth gently cleaned as a part of the presurgical medical assessment to assist the surgeon in identifying bone fragments and foreign bodies.

The patient is draped with four towels secured with towel clips to expose the surgical site. A split sheet then is draped over the patient and around the face, with the mouth, nose, and eyes included in the surgical field.

SPONGES AND DRESSINGS

SPONGES

Both 4 × 4 sponges and cottonoids may be used. As with all surgical procedures, all sponges and sharps are counted before, during, and at the end of the procedure.

DRESSINGS

Dressings are used to protect the wound from becoming infected and to absorb exudate. Antibiotic ointment may be applied to the incision, and Telfa or some other nonadherent dressing may be placed directly over the site. Flat gauze or gauze fluffs may be placed on top of the dressing. Kerlix

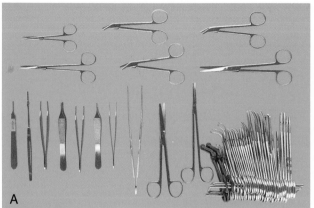
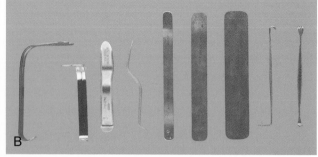
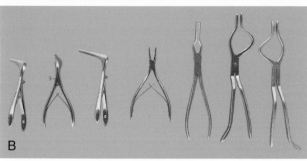
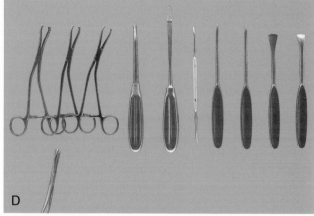
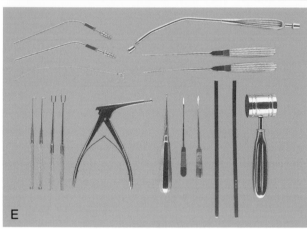
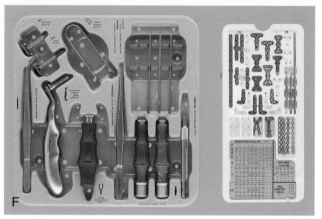

Figure 28-4 Instruments used in the repair of facial fractures. **A,** *Top, left to right,* 1 Stevens tenotomy scissors, curved; 1 plastic scissors, straight, sharp; 3 wire-cutting scissors; 1 Mayo dissecting scissors, straight. *Bottom, left to right,* 1 Bard-Parker knife handle, #3; 1 Bard-Parker knife handle, #7; 2 Adson tissue forceps with teeth (1 × 2), front view and side view; 2 Adson tissue forceps without teeth, front view and side view; 1 Brown-Adson tissue forceps with teeth (9 × 9), front view; 1 bayonet dressing forceps, 7½ inches (18.75 cm); 1 Mayo dissecting scissors, curved; 1 Metzenbaum scissors; 2 paper drape clips; 2 Backhaus towel forceps, small; 2 Backhaus towel forceps; 6 Halsted mosquito hemostatic forceps, curved; 2 Halsted mosquito hemostatic forceps, straight; 2 Providence hemostatic forceps, curved; 2 Halsted hemostatic forceps, straight; 4 Crile hemostatic forceps, curved; 2 Allis tissue forceps; 2 Webster needle holders, 4 inch; 2 Crile-Wood needle holders, 6 inch; 2 Johnson needle holders, 6 inch. **B,** *Left to right,* 1 Weider tongue retractor, large, side view; 1 Weider tongue retractor, small, front view; 2 University of Minnesota cheek retractors, front view and side view; 3 ribbon retractors, assorted sizes; 2 Senn-Kanavel retractors, side view and front view. **C,** *Left to right,* 1 Cottle nasal speculum, #1, side view; 1 Cottle nasal speculum, #2, front view; 1 Cottle nasal speculum, #3, side view; 1 Friedman rongeur, single action; 1 Asch forceps; 2 Rowe disimpaction forceps, left and right. **D,** *Top, left to right,* 3 Dingman bone-holding forceps; 1 Dingman zygoma elevator; 1 Gilles malar elevator; 1 Freer elevator; 2 Langenbeck elevators; 1 Langenbeck periosteal elevator, straight; 1 Langenbeck periosteal elevator, angled. *Bottom left,* Tip of Dingman bone-holding forceps. **E,** *Top, left to right,* 2 Frazier suction tubes with stylets; 1 Yankauer suction tube with tip; 2 zygomatic arch awls. *Bottom, left to right,* 2 Joseph skin hooks, single; 2 Joseph skin hooks, double; 1 Kerrison rongeur, 90-degree upbite; 1 Lucas curette, #0, short; 2 mandibular awls; 1 Cottle osteotome, curved; 1 Cottle osteotome, straight; 1 metal mallet. **F,** Titanium 2-mm microfixation system instrumentation, trays 1 and 2 of 3 (labeled). Facial fracture set.

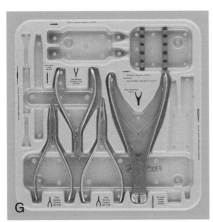

Figure 28-4, cont'd G, Titanium 2-mm microfixation system instrumentation, tray 3 of 3 (labeled). *(From Tighe SM: Instrumentation of the operating room, ed 6, St Louis, 2003, Mosby.)*

(rolled) wrap can be used to secure dressings on the head or face. Kerlix is soft and expandable and conforms to the contours of the skull and facial bones.

SURGICAL PROCEDURES OF THE FACE

MAXILLOMANDIBULAR FIXATION (APPLICATION OF ARCH BARS)

Surgical Goal

Arch bars are applied to realign the teeth or to maintain the patient's normal bite position. A fundamental goal of any maxillomandibular procedure is to preserve the patient's unique bite pattern or normal occlusion between the mandible (lower jaw), the maxilla (upper jaw), and the midface bones. Therefore, in many maxillofacial procedures, the teeth are aligned and fixated in a closed (occluded) position. This is called **maxillomandibular fixation (MMF).** In this procedure, a thin metal strap, called an **arch bar** is wired to each row of teeth. The bars are then wired together with stainless steel suture to occlude the jaw. MMF preserves the patient's normal bite position during repair and healing. MMF may be removed at the end of surgery if the fractures are stable and do not need the support of the arch bars during the healing process. If the fracture is still unstable, the bars may be left in place for several weeks.

❖ *If the arch bars remains in place postoperatively, wire cutters must be sent with the patient to the postanesthesia care unit so that the mouth can be opened in the event of an airway emergency.*

Technique

1. Arch bars are wired to the teeth with 24- or 26-gauge wire sutures.
2. The arch bars are wired together.

Discussion

Application of arch bars requires a basic facial fracture instrument setup, which includes wire and plate cutters, stainless steel suture, and arch bar material. Stainless steel suture ends are counted as sharps and isolated to prevent glove puncture or loss in the surgical wound. Wires are always cut with wire cutters rather than suture scissors.

Steel wire is passed to the field mounted on a needle holder. The ends of the suture must be controlled to prevent contamination or injury. A designated clamp may be fixed to the end of the suture for this purpose.

The surgeon shapes an arch bar fit over the patient's upper teeth and gums. With the cheek and tongue retracted by a cheek retractor, intraoral sweetheart or cloverleaf retractor, the bar is wired into place with 24- or 26-gauge stainless steel suture wires, which are cut into thirds. A wire is clamped with a Rubio needle holder, threaded between the teeth, wrapped around the bar, and twisted to tighten. The suture ends are cut with a wire cutter. Three wires are placed on each side of the mouth, if room is sufficient. The procedure is repeated for the lower teeth.

When the arch bars have been applied to both the upper and lower teeth, the jaw is closed in normal position, and the top and bottom arch bars are approximated with pre-cut lengths of steel suture. Size 24- or 26-gauge stainless steel suture is twisted into a clockwise loop and wrapped around the upper and lower bars with the needle holder. The wire is twisted clockwise until tight against the arch bars and then is cut with a wire cutter. To prevent the suture ends from injuring the soft tissues, a "rosebud" is made in the suture ends by grasping the wire with a hemostat and crimping it inward. The end may be buried in the patient's gingiva.

❖ *Standard protocol dictates that wires be tightened in a clockwise fashion so that any other surgeon knows to remove them in a counterclockwise direction.*

Postoperative Considerations

Wire cutters are kept with the patient at all times to allow access to the mouth in the event of an airway emergency. Figure 28-5 shows the application of arch bars.

OPEN REDUCTION/INTERNAL FIXATION: MIDFACE FRACTURE

Surgical Goal

In open reduction and internal fixation (ORIF) of midface fractures, fractures of the midface are reduced and fixated. The buttressing structures (those under force during dental occlusion) are reinforced.

Pathology

Fractures of the midface historically have been classified for treatment and identification. These classifications do not reflect the realities of high-impact facial fractures, which often exceed the boundaries defined. However, they are still used by some.

- **Le Fort I fracture:** This is a horizontal fracture of the maxilla that causes the hard palate and alveolar process to become separated from the rest of the maxilla. The fracture extends into the lower nasal septum, lateral maxillary sinus, and palatine bones.
- **Le Fort II fracture:** This type of fracture is pyramidal in shape. It extends from the nasal bone to the frontal processes of the maxilla, lacrimal bones, and inferior orbital floor, and it may extend into the orbital foramen. Inferiorly, it extends into the anterior maxillary sinus and the pterygoid plates. This type of fracture also is associated with leakage of cerebrospinal fluid (CSF) into the nasal sinuses.
- **Le Fort III fracture:** This fracture involves separation of all the facial bones from their cranial base. It includes fracture of the zygoma, maxilla, and nasal bones. The fracture line extends through the ethmoid bone and bony orbit, with severe facial flattening and swelling. Figures 28-6 and 28-7 show Le Fort fractures.

Technique

1. Arch bars are applied as required.
2. An incision is made transorally or externally.
3. The fracture is exposed and reduced.
4. The fracture is fixated internally with miniplates and screws.
5. The incisions are closed.
6. The arch bars may be removed.

Discussion

The patient is placed in the supine position on a doughnut or Mayfield headrest with the arms tucked at the sides. General anesthesia is administered through a nasotracheal tube. For extensive trauma, a tracheotomy may be performed first.

The patient is prepped and draped for a facial procedure. If other fractures are present, the patient may be placed in MMF. The surgeon makes the incision in the upper gingival mucosa on the affected side with a #15 blade. The incision is extended through the mucosa to the level of the maxilla. The surgeon then elevates the periosteum with a Freer or periosteal elevator. The zygoma is reduced with Hohmann retractors or a bone hook, or both.

The surgeon then chooses the size and type of plate to be used. The plates usually are 1.7 mm, or 2 mm. Cortical screws are used to secure the plate to the bone. The plate is secured in place with a plate-holding forceps or hemostat. The appropriate drill bit (according to the size of the screw) is loaded onto a small power drill, and the screw holes are drilled. The surgeon then chooses the screw length; a depth gauge may be used to determine the depth of the screw holes. The correct screw is loaded onto the screwdriver and is screwed into place. This process is repeated until all of the screws have been placed and the plate has been secured to the bone. The inci-

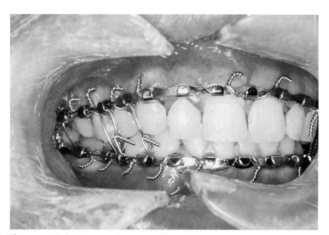

Figure 28-5 Application of arch bars. *(From Dingman RO, Natvig P: Surgery of facial fractures, Philadelphia, 1964, WB Saunders.)*

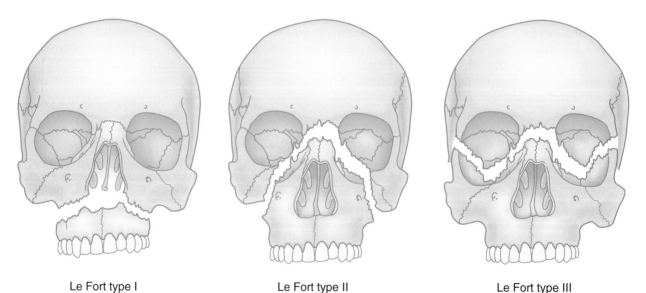

Le Fort type I   Le Fort type II   Le Fort type III

Figure 28-6 Overview of Le Fort fractures. *(From Townsend CM, Beauchamp DR, Ever MB, Mattox KL: Sabiston textbook of surgery, ed 18, Philadelphia, 2008, WB Saunders.)*

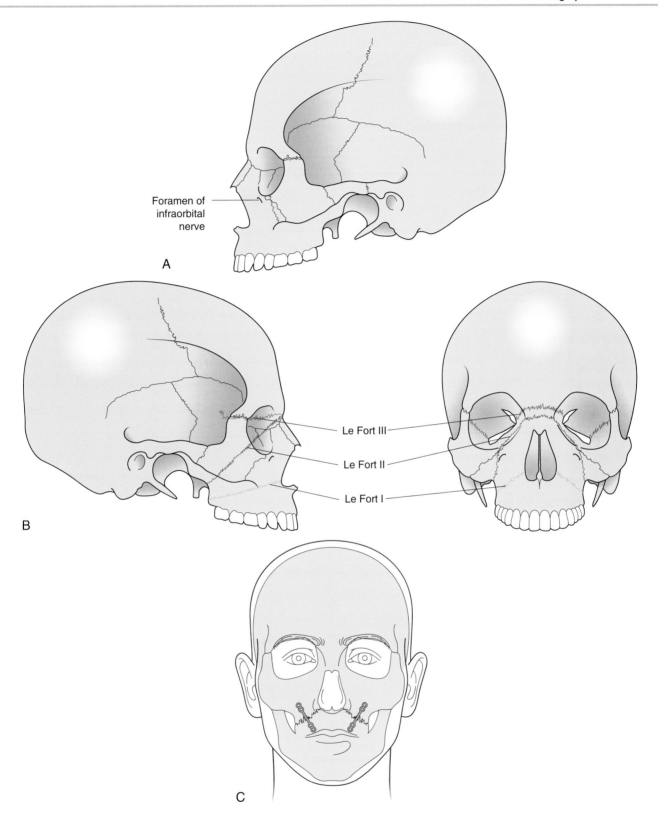

Foramen of
infraorbital
nerve

A

Le Fort III

Le Fort II

Le Fort I

B

C

Figure 28-7 Detail of Le Fort fractures. **A,** Malar fracture. **B,** Side and front views of Le Fort factures. **C,** Maxillary fracture with manipulation used for fixation. *(From Dhillon RS, East CA: Ear, nose, and throat and head and neck surgery, ed 3, Edinburgh, 2006, Churchill Livingstone.)*

sion then is closed with 3-0 absorbable suture. The wound is dressed with flat and fluffed gauze. A Kerlix wrap is used to secure the dressing. If the patient is to remain in MMF, a wire cutter must accompany the patient to the recovery room.

Postoperative Considerations

Patients are closely observed for hemorrhage, CSF leakage, and a patent airway. Healing usually requires 4 to 8 weeks. Complications include dehiscence of oral lesions, especially when oral hygiene is suboptimal. Nerve injury may occur as a result of tissue retraction during the surgery or from the injury itself.

OPEN REDUCTION/INTERNAL FIXATION: FRONTAL SINUS FRACTURE

Surgical Goal

ORIF of a frontal sinus fracture is performed to repair CSF leakage, prevent obstruction of the frontal sinus ducts, and restore an aesthetic contour to the forehead.

Pathology

Fractures of the frontal sinus are a result of direct trauma to the frontal bone, which may result in bone impaction and combination. As with other facial fractures, the most common causes are intentional violence and motor vehicle accidents. Fractures of the posterior wall of the frontal sinus may result in CSF leakage or herniation of brain tissue. These fractures present a real risk of life-threatening complications, including brain abscess and meningitis. Other complications include damage to the ducts that interferes with normal drainage. This can lead to chronic infection or a mucocele (a cyst arising from a mucous gland).

Technique

1. A bicoronal incision is made.
2. The periosteum is separated from the skull.
3. The fractures are exposed.
4. A fat graft is implanted in the sinus, and the fractures are repaired.
5. The incision is closed.

Discussion

Before frontal sinus fractures are repaired, the sinus mucosa must be removed and the duct occluded. The sinus then is often filled with a fat graft. In rare cases, a small leak can be patched and the anterior walled plated. Severe fracture of the posterior sinus wall may require *cranialization* of the sinus. In this procedure, the posterior wall of the sinus is removed, the sinus ducts are plugged, and the frontal sinus mucosa is removed. The brain is allowed to move into the previous frontal sinus space, and the fractures are repaired. A neurosurgeon usually is present to participate in the surgery.

The patient is placed in the supine position with the head on a Mayfield or simila headrest and the arms tucked at the sides. General anesthesia is administered. The incisions are made based on accessibility through the existing wounds or the need for entry through an alternative site. If the existing wounds are not used, a **bicoronal incision** may be made (i.e., following a line starting at the junction of the coronal and frontal sutures on one side of the head and extending to the other side, behind the hairline).

Using a #10 blade or the ESU with a Colorado needle tip, the surgeon makes the incision from the root of the helix of one ear to the root of the helix of the other ear. If a knife is used, Raney clips are applied to the scalp with a Raney clip applier to aid hemostasis (see illustrations in Chapter 35). The incision is carried deep to the periosteum. The periosteum is elevated to the level of the superior orbital rims and anterior wall of the frontal sinus with a periosteal elevator.

The surgeon examines the anterior and posterior walls of the frontal sinus. If the posterior wall of the frontal sinus is fractured, the frontal sinus will be obliterated. The surgeon does this by removing the posterior wall of the sinus and then removing the mucosal lining of the frontal sinus. The fractured portions of the posterior wall of the sinus are removed with hemostats. The mucosa is obliterated with a medium cutting or diamond burr loaded onto a small power drill. The mucosa of the frontal osteum is removed with a small acorn burr. The frontal osteum is packed with muscle or fascia. This separates the frontal sinus cavity from the rest of the sinuses. The cavity then is packed with a fat graft taken from the abdomen.

Fat Graft

The surgeon makes a small incision (approximately 2 to 3 mm) in the abdomen with a #15 blade. A small portion of fat tissue is excised using a #15 blade, and hemostat, or a toothed Adson forceps for teasing out and grasping the tissue. Double-prong skin hooks are used to retract the wound edges. Bleeders are controlled with the ESU. The graft is placed in normal saline to keep it moist until the surgeon is ready to place it in the frontal sinus. The graft site is closed with 4-0 Vicryl suture.

Repair

The anterior wall of the frontal wall is repaired with micromesh plates. Commonly used sizes are 1 or 1.3 mm. The free portions of the bone are secured to the mesh before it is secured to the stable portions of the bone. The appropriate drill bit is loaded onto a small power drill, and holes are drilled for the mesh plate. Screws are inserted as described in the previous procedure. These steps are repeated until the mesh is secured in place and the fracture has been reduced.

The incision is closed in layers. The periosteum is replaced over the cranium, and the subcutaneous tissue is closed with 3-0 absorbable suture. The skin is closed with skin staples or a locking silk stitch. The wound is covered with antibiotic ointment or with a Telfa and gauze dressing.

Postoperative Considerations

Patients are monitored carefully for symptoms of infection and CSF leakage. Bone fragments remaining in the sinuses can cause injury in the postoperative period. Patients are followed with CT scans for at least 1 year after surgery.

OPEN REDUCTION/INTERNAL FIXATION: ORBITAL FLOOR FRACTURE

Surgical Goal

ORIF of an orbital floor fracture is performed to reduce a fracture of the orbital floor, to prevent entrapment of the extraocular muscles, and to support the orbital contents.

Pathology

Orbital floor fractures, or "**blowout**" fractures, are caused by high-speed blunt force to the globe (Figure 28-8). Fractures of the orbital floor usually result from the increased orbital pressure caused by the impact on the globe. A portion of the globe may extrude into the nasal sinus (enophthalmus), or the globe can be displaced posteriorly. Entrapment of the eye muscles can result in diplopia, (double vision). The most common causes of the injury are assault and being struck by a high-velocity object.

Technique

1. A subciliary or a transconjunctival incision is made.
2. The orbit is exposed.
3. The fractures are reduced and repaired.
4. The incision is closed.

Discussion

The patient is positioned and prepped as for a facial fracture. General anesthesia is administered. Ophthalmic ointment may be placed in the eyes before the skin prep. The prep is performed carefully to prevent prep solution from draining into the eyes and ears.

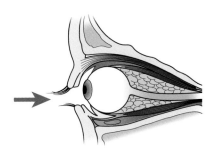

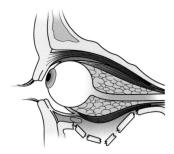

Figure 28-8   Orbital blowout fracture. *(From Dhillon RS, East CA: Ear, nose, and throat and head and neck surgery, ed 3, Edinburgh, 2006, Churchill Livingstone.)*

The surgeon begins by placing corneal protectors in the operative eye. Balanced salt solution (BSS) is instilled into the eye to provide moisture at this stage and as needed throughout the case.

With the cornea protected, the surgeon makes the incision. Either of two incisions can be used: a subciliary incision or a transconjunctival incision. A **subciliary incision** is made 2 mm under the eyelashes with a #15 blade. A **transconjunctival incision** is made in the conjunctiva of the inferior eyelid. The surgeon exposes the orbit by placing small, malleable retractors or brain spatula retractors into the wound and retracting superiorly and inferiorly. The wound is exposed to the level of the orbital rim, and the periosteum is elevated with a Freer elevator. The surgeon then elevates and retracts the orbital contents superiorly with a small, malleable retractor.

After assessment the surgeon may reconstruct the floor of the orbit using nylon sheeting, mesh, Gelfilm, Silastic sheeting, or an orbital floor plate. Typically, a 1-, 1.3-, or 1.5-mm plate or mesh is selected for orbital fractures. The surgeon cuts the selected material to size with plate cutters or scissors (depending on the material) and positions it between the orbital floor and the orbital contents. An orbital floor plate is secured in place with screws in the infraorbital rim. This technique is performed as previously described (see Prepping and Draping above).

With the orbital contents supported, the retractors are removed and the wound is closed. Subciliary incisions are closed with 5-0 absorbable suture. Transconjunctival incisions are not closed. The surgeon removes the corneal protector after the incisions have been closed. Antibiotic ophthalmic ointment may be placed in the eye and on the incision. A small dressing may be applied.

Postoperative Considerations

Patients frequently experience blurred vision immediately after surgery because of the use of the corneal shield and the antibiotic ointment. Patients are monitored for double vision, which can indicate muscle entrapment.

OPEN REDUCTION/INTERNAL FIXATION: MANDIBULAR FRACTURE

Surgical Goal

In ORIF of a mandibular fracture, the mandibular fracture is repaired and occlusion is restored.

Pathology

ORIF of the mandible is performed to treat facial trauma involving the mandible. Assault is the most common cause of a mandibular fracture.

Technique

1. Arch bars are applied.
2. A transoral or external incision is made.
3. The fracture is exposed and reduced.
4. Miniplates and screws are used to fix the fracture.
5. The incisions are closed.
6. The arch bars may be removed.

Discussion

The patient is placed in the supine position with the head stabilized on a doughnut headrest and the arms tucked at the sides. General anesthesia is administered through a nasotracheal tube. Extensive trauma of the face results in massive swelling and risks airway occlusion. Therefore, a tracheotomy may be performed before the ORIF. The patient is prepped and draped for a facial procedure.

After administration of anesthesia, the surgeon assesses the fractures. If necessary, arch bars may be applied before fracture reduction and fixation. An incision is made in the gingival-buccal mucosa with the ESU or in the skin over the fracture site with a #10 or #15 blade. The skin incision depends on the location and extent of the fracture. After the skin incision is made, Senn retractors are used to retract the skin and subcutaneous tissue. This exposes the mandible and periosteum, which can be elevated with a Freer or other type of periosteal elevator. The surgeon then reduces the fracture with a small bone clamp. Radiographs or fluoroscopy may be used to evaluate the reduction.

The surgeon then selects the plates needed for fixation. The 2-, 2.4-, and 2.7-mm plates are commonly used. Most mandibular fractures require two plates per fracture: a large plate is used on the inferior side, and a miniplate or tension band device is used on the superior aspect. A small drill bit is fitted to a high-speed drill. The plate is stabilized against the mandible with a plate-holding forceps, and the screw holes are drilled. A drill guide may be used to stabilize the drill bit. If a drill guide is used, a depth gauge is used to measure the required screw length. The appropriate screw is loaded into a screwdriver and inserted. When all of the fractures have been reduced and fixed, the incisions are closed. Transbuccal incisions are closed with 3-0 absorbable suture; external incisions are closed in layers with 3-0 absorbable suture; and the skin is closed with 4-0 absorbable suture. The arch bars may be removed or left in placed as needed.

ORAL SURGERY

Procedures involving the teeth are performed primarily by an oromaxillofacial surgeon.

DENTAL IMPLANTS

Surgical Goal
Dental implants are used to replace lost teeth.

Pathology
An implant may replace a single tooth or multiple teeth. Three types of dental implants are commonly used: endosteal implants, subperiosteal implants, and transosteal implants.

Discussion
An endosteal implant is a threaded screw, cylinder, or flat blade that is implanted in the alveolus of the maxilla or mandible and then covered with soft tissue. After several months (3 months for the mandible and 6 months for the maxilla,) a post is connected to the implanted fixture. This post extends slightly above the gingiva, allowing the artificial tooth to be attached.

Subperiosteal implants are placed beneath the periosteum directly on the alveolar bone. This type of implant is used primarily when bone is insufficient to support an endosteal implant.

Transosteal implants are bone plates with retaining posts; they resemble a staple. This type of implant is used only when the patient has severe loss of bone in the mandibular alveolar ridge.

TOOTH EXTRACTION

Surgical Goal
Extraction is the surgical removal of one or more teeth.

Pathology
Odontectomy, or tooth extraction, may be performed for a variety of reasons, including damaged or decayed teeth or impaction, which often affects the third molars (wisdom teeth).

Technique
1. An incision is made in the gingiva of the affected tooth.
2. The tissue surrounding the tooth is elevated to the level of the bone.
3. The tooth is elevated out of the alveolus, making it mobile.
4. The tooth is extracted with a dental extractor of the appropriate size.
5. The incision is closed if necessary.

Discussion
The patient is placed in the supine position with the arms tucked at the sides. A prep is unnecessary, because the procedure is performed inside the mouth. Betadine may be available on the field for irrigation. The patient is draped to allow adequate access to the mouth. The surgeon reviews radiographs to ensure that the correct teeth are extracted. A #15 blade is used to make a gingival incision to the level of the bone. A Molt elevator is used to elevate the tissue, including the periosteum, surrounding the tooth.

The surgeon then elevates the tooth out of the alveolus with an elevator; this breaks the attachment of the ligament holding the tooth in place, allowing the tooth to become mobile. The tooth is extracted with the appropriate-size dental extractor. The size of the extractor varies, depending on the tooth being extracted and the patient's age. If necessary, the incision is closed with absorbable 3-0 suture (this is usually required with impactions). Dental packs may be placed to prevent postoperative bleeding.

ORTHOGNATHIC PROCEDURES

MANDIBULAR ADVANCEMENT

Surgical Goal
Mandibular advancement is performed to correct a bony deformity of the mandible.

Pathology

Mandibular defects may be acquired or congenital and usually are represented by a recessed mandible. Surgical correction of the defects may help the patient for medical and psychological reasons. Surgery generally is delayed until the patient has developed sufficiently and has most of the permanent teeth.

Technique

1. Arch bars are applied.
2. Intraoral incisions are made.
3. The maxilla is cut at a predetermined location.
4. The bone is advanced.
5. Grafts are placed if necessary, and the bones are wired in place.
6. The intraoral incisions are closed.

Discussion

The patient is placed in the supine position with the arms tucked at the sides. A general anesthetic is used. The patient is prepped and draped to allow full exposure of the lower third of the face. Preoperative radiographs must be available in the room for the surgeon.

The surgeon begins by placing arch bars. This aligns the teeth and provides postoperative immobilization. Then, intraoral incisions are made to expose the mandible. This may be done with the scalpel or ESU. The incisions are carried to the periosteum. The periosteum is elevated with a periosteal elevator to expose the bony surface of the mandible. An oscillating saw is used to make cuts through the mandible at predetermined locations. After the mandible has been split, it can be advanced to the proper position. Bone grafts or biosynthetic material may be used to fill any space between the advanced mandible and the fixed mandible.

The grafts and mandible are fixed in place with wire or a mandibular plating system. The incisions are closed with 3-0 absorbable suture. The patient remains in MMF for several weeks.

Postoperative Considerations

Wire cutters are kept with the patient at all times in the postoperative period in case of an airway emergency.

MIDFACE (MAXILLARY) ADVANCEMENT

Surgical Goal

Midface advancement is performed to correct a bony deformity of the maxilla.

Pathology

Maxillary defects may be acquired or congenital. The most common presentation is a recessed mandible. This can result in misalignment of the teeth and social isolation. Surgery generally is delayed until the permanent teeth have developed.

Technique

1. Arch bars are applied.
2. Intraoral incisions are made.
3. The mandible is incised.
4. The bone is advanced.
5. Grafts are placed if necessary, and the bones are wired in place.
6. The intraoral incisions are closed.

Discussion

The patient is placed in the supine position with the arms tucked at the sides. The patient is prepped and draped to allow full exposure of the lower third of the face. Preoperative radiographs must be available in the room for the surgeon.

Arch bars are placed at the start of surgery. This allows alignment and stabilization of the dentition and provides postoperative immobilization.

The surgeon makes intraoral incisions to expose the maxilla. This may be done with the scalpel or ESU. The incisions are carried to the periosteum. A small area of the periosteum is removed with a periosteal elevator. The surgeon then uses an oscillating saw to make cuts through the maxilla at predetermined locations. After the maxilla has been split, it can be advanced to the proper position. Bone graft or biosynthetic material is used to fill any space between the advanced maxilla and the fixed maxilla.

The grafts and maxilla are fixed in place with wire or a mandibular plating system. The incisions are closed with 3-0 absorbable suture. The patient remains in arch bars for several weeks. Postoperative considerations are the same as for previously described procedures in which arch bars were placed.

TEMPOROMANDIBULAR JOINT ARTHROPLASTY

Surgical Goal

Temporomandibular joint (TMJ) arthroplasty is performed to reduce pain and increase mobility of the joint.

Pathology

TMJ disease is characterized by persistent pain and dysfunction of the temporomandibular joint. It usually is associated with stress-related muscle tension and grinding of the teeth (bruxism), malocclusion, trauma, or arthritis.

Technique

1. A preauricular or postauricular incision is made.
2. The temporalis fascia is exposed.
3. The joint capsule is incised and opened.
4. The disk is replaced or repositioned.
5. Drains are placed.
6. The wound is closed.

Discussion

The patient is placed in the supine position with the arms tucked at the sides. General anesthesia is administered. The patient then is prepped and draped to expose the temporomandibular joint, including a head drape.

The surgeon begins by making a preauricular or postauricular incision with a #15 blade. The skin flaps are elevated with either the ESU or scissors to expose the temporalis fascia. Retractors are placed to allow visualization of the wound. A #9 Molt elevator is used to dissect the underlying periosteum to the level of the arch. Next, blunt dissection is performed with a hemostat.

A horizontal incision is made into the joint capsule, and a flap is created to expose the condyle. The condyle is distracted inferiorly. Any adhesions are lysed with the ESU or mobilized with a scalpel. If any perforations are noted in the disk of the joint, the joint usually is removed and an artificial joint is placed. If the disk has rotated, it is repositioned and sutured in place with 2-0 nonabsorbable suture. A drain then is placed if necessary, and the wound is closed.

NOTE: endoscopic surgery for this procedure is now available in some dental and oromaxillofacial institutions.

CHAPTER SUMMARY

- The face is divided into three regions: the upper face, the midface, and the lower face.
- The upper face is composed of the frontal bone and the frontal sinus. The midface is composed of the ethmoid, zygoma, maxillary bones, and nasal bone. The lower face is composed of the mandible.
- Oromaxillofacial surgery focuses on reconstruction and repair of the facial bones and may include structures of the oral cavity. Therefore, the instrumentation for these procedures includes fine orthopedic instruments, implants, and grafting materials.
- The most common causes of facial fracture are intentional violence (assault), motor vehicle accidents, and sports.
- Plates and screws are the primary means of repairing facial fractures. Miniplate systems are small, malleable mesh plates that can be molded to fit over the contours of facial bone.
- Mandibular micrognathia is a congenital defect that results in a small lower jaw. This can affect feeding in the infant and alignment of the teeth as the infant grows.
- Facial fractures are prepped with Betadine scrub and paint. The entire face is prepped, from the hairline to the sternal notch.
- Arch bars are implanted to realign the dentition of the mandible and midface.
- A fundamental goal of any maxillomandibular procedure is to preserve the patient's unique bite pattern or normal occlusion between the mandible (lower jaw), the maxilla (upper jaw), and the midface bones. If the arch bars remain in place postoperatively, wire cutters must be sent with the patient to the PACU so that the mouth can be opened in the event of an airway emergency.
- ORIF of the mandible is performed to treat facial trauma involving the mandible. Assault is the most common cause of a mandibular fracture.
- Extensive trauma of the face results in massive swelling and risks airway occlusion. Therefore, tracheotomy may be performed before surgery.
- A Le Fort I fracture is a horizontal fracture of the maxilla that causes the hard palate and alveolar process to become separated from the rest of the maxilla. The fracture extends into the lower nasal septum, lateral maxillary sinus, and palatine bones.
- A Le Fort II fracture is pyramid shaped. It extends from the nasal bone to the frontal processes of the maxilla, lacrimal bones, and inferior orbital floor, and it may extend into the orbital foramen. Inferiorly, it extends into the anterior maxillary sinus and the pterygoid plates. This type of fracture also is associated with leakage of CSF into the nasal sinuses.
- A Le Fort III fracture involves a separation of all the facial bones from their cranial base. It includes fracture of the zygoma, maxilla, and nasal bones. The fracture line extends through the ethmoid bone and bony orbit, with severe facial flattening and swelling.
- Fractures of the frontal sinus are a result of direct trauma to the frontal bone, which may result in bone impaction and combination.
- ORIF of frontal sinus fractures is performed to repair CSF leakage, prevent obstruction of the frontal sinus ducts, and restore aesthetic contour to the forehead.
- Orbital floor fractures, or "blowout" fractures, occur as a result of high-speed blunt force to the globe. The increased orbital pressure produced by the impact on the globe usually is the cause of the orbital floor fracture.
- Complications of orbital floor fractures include extrusion of the globe into the nasal sinus and entrapment of the eye muscles.
- Endosteal implants are a threaded screw, cylinder, or flat blade that is implanted in the alveolus of the maxilla or mandible and then covered with soft tissue.
- Odontectomy, or tooth extraction, may be performed for a variety of reasons, including damage or decay in teeth, or impaction, which often affects the third molars (wisdom teeth).
- Mandibular advancement is performed to correct a bony deformity of the mandible.
- Mandibular defects may be acquired or congenital and usually are represented by a recessed mandible.
- Maxillary defects may be acquired or congenital. The most common presentation is a recessed mandible. This can result in misalignment of the teeth and social

isolation. Surgery generally is delayed until the permanent teeth have developed.
- TMJ disease is characterized by persistent pain and dysfunction of the temporomandibular joint. It usually is associated with stress-related muscle tension and grinding of the teeth (bruxism), malocclusion, trauma, or arthritis.
- TMJ arthroplasty is performed to reduce pain and increase mobility.

REVIEW QUESTIONS

1. Why are wire cutters sent with the patient after maxillomandibular fixation?
2. Why are arch bars used during open reduction and internal fixation of facial fractures?
3. How should stainless steel sutures be handled? (Review Chapter 17 if necessary.) Expand your answer to include care of sharp ends, threading, and preparation.
4. What are the three types of Le Fort fractures? What are the differences between them?
5. What type of facial fracture might result in leakage of cerebrospinal fluid?
6. Give two reasons for performing tooth extraction.

BIBLIOGRAPHY

Bailey BJ et al: *Head and neck surgery: otolaryngology,* ed 2, vol 1 and 2, Philadelphia, 1998, Lippincott-Raven.

Fortunato N, McCullough SM: *Plastic and reconstructive surgery: perioperative nursing series,* St Louis, 1998, Mosby.

Marks SC: *Nasal and sinus surgery,* Philadelphia, 2000, WB Saunders.

Moody FG: *Atlas of ambulatory surgery,* St Louis, 1999, Mosby.

Phillips N: *Berry and Kohn's operating room technique,* ed 10, St Louis, 2004, Mosby.

Porth C: *Pathophysiology: concepts of altered health states,* ed 6, Philadelphia, 2002, Lippincott Williams & Wilkins.

Rothrock JC: *Alexander's care of the patient in surgery,* ed 12, St Louis, 2003, Mosby.

Silver CE, Rubin JS: *Atlas of head and neck surgery,* ed 2, Philadelphia, 1999, Churchill Livingstone.

Thibodeau GA, Patt KT: *Anthony's textbook of anatomy and physiology,* ed 17, St Louis, 2003, Mosby.

Thumfart WF et al: *Surgical approaches in otorhinolaryngology,* New York, 1999, Thieme.

Weerda H: *Reconstructive facial plastic surgery: a problem-solving manual,* New York, 2001, Thieme.

CHAPTER 29

Plastic and Reconstructive Surgery

CHAPTER OUTLINE

LEARNING OBJECTIVES

After studying this chapter the reader will be able to:
- Describe the anatomical structures of the skin
- Identify the psychological and social pressures for a "normal" appearance

- Differentiate the types of skin-grafting techniques
- Identify equipment and instruments used in plastic surgery
- Identify surgical techniques used in common plastic and reconstructive procedures

TERMINOLOGY

Aesthetic surgery: Surgery that is performed to improve appearance but not function; also called *cosmetic surgery.*

Allograft: A tissue graft in which the donor and recipient are of the same species.

Augment: To enlarge a structure.

Autograft: The surgical transplantation of tissue from one part of the body to another in the same individual.

Biological graft: A graft derived from live tissue, whether human or animal.

Biosynthetic: A type of graft or implant material made of synthetic absorbable material.

Burn intensive care unit (ICU): A critical care unit for severely burned patients.

Composite graft: A biological graft composed of different types of tissues such as skin and muscle.

Debridement: The surgical removal of dead skin, debris, and infectious material from a wound.

Dermatome: A medical device used for removing single thickness skin grafts.

Desiccation: Drying or dehydration of tissue.

Eschar: Tissue that has been burned (second- and third-degree burns) but remains adherent to the wound. Eschar is nonelastic

and may constrict underlying structures, impairing vital functions.

Escharotomy: Excision of eschar to release stricture in surrounding tissues.

Fasciotomy: Multiple longitudinal incisions made in the fascia to release severe swelling or stricture which can result in necrosis.

Full-thickness skin graft (FTSG): A skin graft composed of the epidermis and dermis.

Hydrodressing: A dressing impregnated with a water-based gel. This type of dressing prevents the wound from drying and encourages healing.

Hypertrophic scar: A scar which contains excess tissue and may be inflamed. This type of scar usually reduces within 6 months.

Implant: A synthetic, natural, or biosynthetic substance used to fill in or replace an anatomical structure.

Keloid: A hypertrophic scar occuring in dark-skinned individuals. The scar may become bulbous and usually does not reduce over time.

Mohs surgery: A procedure in which a malignant tissue mass is removed and cut into quadrants before frozen section. These quadrants are used to map the tumor and determine the exact location of malignant margins. Further excision is performed until the specimen is clear of all malignancy.

Photodamage: Damage to the skin caused by ultraviolet light.

Plastic and reconstructive surgery: Surgery performed to restore form and function that have been lost because of trauma, radical surgery, or congenital anomaly.

Plicate: To fold tissue and secure it in place surgically.

Porcine: Derived from pig tissue.

Ptosis: Drooping or sagging of any anatomical structure.

Split-thickness (or partial-thickness) skin graft (PTSG): A skin graft that consists of the epidermis and a portion of the papillary dermis.

Stent: A surgical method of providing support to an anatomical structure; the term may also refer to the support device itself. In plastic surgery, a stent dressing is used to maintain contact between a skin graft and the graft site.

Synthetic graft: A graft derived from synthetic material compatible with body tissue. Synthetic grafts may be soft, semisolid, or liquid.

Undermine: A surgical technique in which a plane of tissue is created or an existing tissue plane is lifted, such as skin from the fascia.

Xenograft: A graft made up of tissue taken from one species and grafted into another species (e.g., porcine graft implanted in human tissue).

INTRODUCTION

Plastic and reconstructive surgery involves the treatment of congenital defects and anatomical abnormalities caused by disease and injury. Restoration of form and function is the primary goal of treatment. Plastic and reconstructive surgery crosses nearly all subspecialties and varies from simple procedures to extremely complex and technically demanding operations.

Aesthetic surgery, also called *cosmetic surgery,* is performed to improve the appearance but does not address function.

An individual's goals are deeply connected with social and cultural standards of acceptable appearance. In Western culture, body image is highly influenced by pressure to appear youthful (i.e., smooth, wrinkle-free skin; a slim body; and high definition of secondary sexual characteristics). Many plastic and reconstructive procedures are specifically intended to provide these changes. The basis of surgery is to fulfill a fundamental need for social acceptability. Individuals who have been disfigured by trauma, a congenital defect, or disease often experience a level of self-consciousness that prevents them from achieving a fulfilling life. For these patients, plastic surgery offers the hope of integration and acceptance into their social culture.

Whether the patient arrives in surgery for an elective or a nonelective procedure, special psychological needs must be met. Patients usually benefit from an honest, straightforward manner and should receive emotional support throughout the perioperative period.

SURGICAL ANATOMY

INTEGUMENTARY SYSTEM (SKIN)

The skin, or integumentary system (Figure 29-1), performs a number of vital functions:

1. It protects underlying tissues and organs.
2. It excretes organic waste and stores nutrients.
3. It excretes water and dissipates heat as a means of thermoregulation.
4. Its sensory organs transmit touch, pressure, pain, and temperature, which alert the body to possible injury.

Epidermis

The epidermis is the outer layer of the skin. The primary tissue cells of the epidermis are the keratinocytes. Five distinct epidermal layers represent various developmental stages of the keratinocyte:

- The *stratum corneum* is the most superficial layer. It is relatively transparent and composed of dead keratinocytes that are filled with a protein called *keratin*. The stratum corneum is thicker on areas of the body that are weight bearing or exposed to friction, such as the hands and feet.
- The *stratum lucidum* is composed of dead or dying cells that are flattened and densely packed. This layer is extremely thin (approximately five cells thick). It may not be found on regions of the body with thin skin.
- The *stratum granulosum* is several cells thick and produces keratin.
- The *stratum spinosum* contains undifferentiated cells that become specialized as they migrate to the skin surface.
- The *stratum germinativum,* also called the *stratum basale,* is the deepest layer of the epidermis attached to the dermis. The cells in this layer undergo mitosis, producing daughter keratinocytes that migrate through the layers of the epidermis. The melanocytes also are found in this layer; melanocytes are the cells responsible for the production of melanin, a substance that gives skin a particular color.

Dermis

The dermis lies between the epidermis and the subcutaneous fatty layer. The dermis provides nourishment and enervation to the epidermis. The blood vessels of the dermis are responsible for oxygenation of the tissue and thermoregulation. A large portion of the vascular plexus in the dermis bypasses the capillaries through an arteriovenous network in which small arteries flow directly into venules. This allows the vessels to dilate and constrict as the environmental temperature rises and falls. The dermis has numerous sensory receptors (i.e., for pain, touch, heat, cold, and pressure), which inform the brain about environmental change or danger.

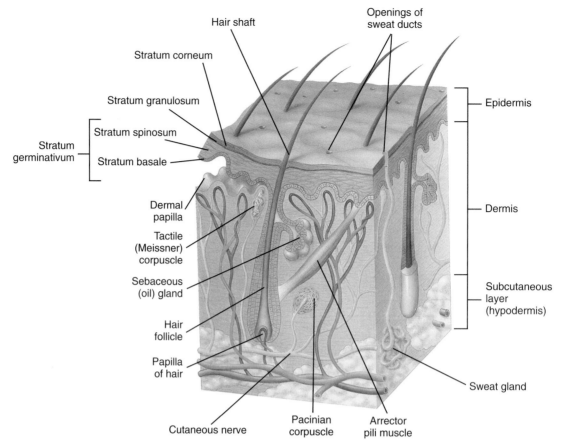

Figure 29-1   The skin, including the dermis and epidermis. *(From Thibodeau GA, Patton KT: Anthony's textbook of anatomy and physiology, ed 17, St Louis, 2003, Mosby.)*

Skin Appendages

Skin contains several specialized structures called *appendages*, such as hair, sweat, and oil glands, which have protective functions.

Hair is a protective structure that covers most areas of the body, except the palms and the soles of the feet. Each hair is surrounded by a follicle located in the dermis. The follicle consists of the hair itself, a sebaceous gland, muscle, and sometimes an apocrine (sweat) gland. The hair shaft, the visible portion of the hair, varies in size, shape, and color. The *sebaceous glands* discharge a waxy, oily secretion called *sebum* into the hair follicles. Sebum acts as a lubricant. The hair muscle (erector pili muscle) aids thermoregulation of the body by producing "goose bumps" in a cold environment; goose bumps reduce the surface area of the skin and prevent heat loss.

Two types of *sweat glands* are found in the human body. The *apocrine sweat glands* arise from the dermis and are located mainly in the axilla and groin. They open out into the hair follicle. The oily secretion has no odor unless it comes in contact with bacteria. The *eccrine glands* secrete sweat over the surface of the body through small tubules. Sweat helps regulate the body temperature by cooling it through evaporation.

As mentioned, sebaceous glands produce sebum, a combination of wax, lipids, cholesterol, and triglycerides. These glands are distributed over the entire body except on the palms and the soles of the feet. Their functions are to lubricate the skin and hair and to prevent evaporation in a cold environment. The sebaceous glands are responsive to hormonal influence, and their size is proportional to the amount of sebum produced.

ANATOMY OF THE FACE

The soft tissues of the face include skin, fat, muscle, fascia, and ligaments (Figure 29-2). The subcutaneous fatty tissue is separated into deep and superficial layers by a tissue plane called the *superficial musculoaponeurotic system* (commonly called the SMAS). The fat of the superficial layer is composed of lobes, which are deposited unevenly over the surface of the face and integrated within the fibrous tissue of the SMAS. The fat is densest in the cheek and neck region. The deep fat layer, under the SMAS, is thinner and divided by fibrous bands. The ligaments of the face support the soft tissue and attach it to the bone.

PATHOLOGY OF THE SKIN AND FACE

Table 29-1 presents common pathological conditions of the skin and face.

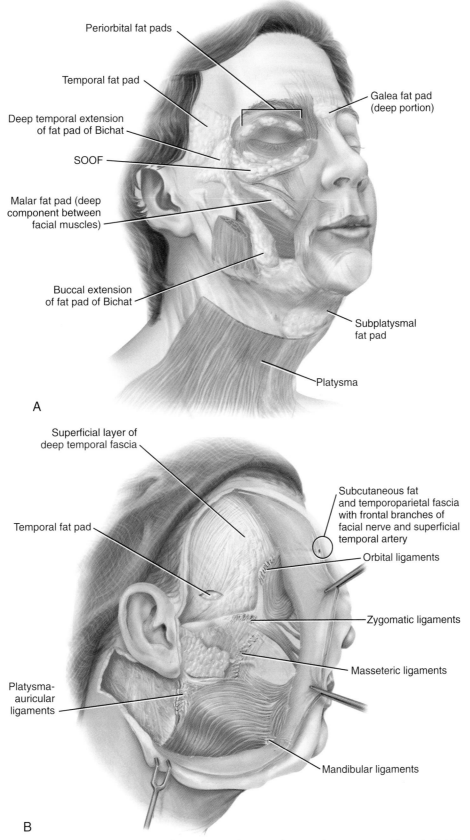

Figure 29-2 Anatomy of the face. **A,** Fat deposits deep to the SMAS. **B,** The sub-SMAS anatomy, showing muscles and ligaments. (**A** from Fortunato N, McCullough SM: Plastic and reconstructive surgery, St Louis, 1998, Mosby; **B** from LaTrenta G: Atlas of aesthetic face and neck surgery, Philadelphia, 2004, WB Saunders.)

Table 29-1

Pathology of the Skin and Face

Condition	Description	Considerations
Cleft palate	Defect of the palate resulting in separation. It is a congenital defect that occurs during development of the midface.	The cleft defect is repaired surgically. (See Cleft Palate Repair Chapter 34.)
Cleft lip	Defect of the lip resulting in a split that may be partial or complete, unilateral or bilateral.	Surgical treatment is necessary and usually is performed at 10 to 12 weeks for initial repair. (See Cleft Lip Repair Chapter 34.)
Basal cell carcinoma	The most common type of skin cancer. It is slow growing and arises from the basal layer of the epidermis.	Easily treated if detected early. Diagnosis is by biopsy, and treatment is by excision. Large lesions require excision and grafting. (See Excision of Superficial Lesions.)
Squamous cell carcinoma	The second most common type of skin cancer. It arises from the squamous cells of the epidermis.	If detected early, it is relatively easy to treat with biopsy and excision. However, if detected late, it may have metastasized to other areas of the body, making treatment much more difficult. (See Excision of Superficial Lesions.)
Melanoma	Rarest of the skin cancers but accounts for the most fatalities from skin cancer. It arises in the melanocytes.	Early detection leads to almost 100% cure. The metastasis rate is high. Treatment is surgical excision with possible chemotherapy. (See Excision of Superficial Lesions.)
First-degree burn	A burn involving the epidermis only (e.g., sunburn); referred to as a *partial-thickness burn*.	Heals within a few days without treatment.
Second-degree burn	Damage occurs to both the epidermis and dermis; referred to as a *partial-thickness burn*.	Heals within a few weeks with topical treatment. (See Debridement of Burns.)
Third-degree burn	May be electrical, chemical, or thermal; results in permanent damage to the skin and underlying tissues; referred to as a *full-thickness burn*.	These burns require debridement and skin grafting to maintain skin integrity. (See Debridement of Burns and Grafting.)
Keloid	A scar that continues to develop even after healing is complete.	Common in dark-skinned individuals. Surgical removal may be successful. (See Scar Revision.)
Hypertrophic scar	An overgrowth of scar tissue at the site of an injury or incision. Usually self-limiting, resolves to some degree over 18 to 24 months.	Surgical excision is the treatment if resolution does not occur. (See Scar Revision.)
Body dysmorphic disorder	An excessive preoccupation with a real or imagined defect in physical appearance.	A psychological disease that affects a very small percentage of the population; however, these individuals frequently seek cosmetic surgery to correct perceived defects in appearance.

PERIOPERATIVE CONSIDERATIONS

PREPPING AND DRAPING

Betadine is used to prep the skin for procedures other than the face. PHisoHex is commonly used for face prep. Graft sites are prepped with nonstaining solutions. Regardless of the prep solution used, care must be taken not to allow the prep solution to drain into the eyes or ears.

Draping routines in plastic and reconstructive surgery follow the general techniques described in Chapter 11. Extra draping towels, plain sheets, and adhesive drapes should be available for complex draping routines. For procedures involving the face, most surgeons use a head drape (see Figure 11-17). This prevents the hair from falling into the field and allows the surgeon to visualize the entire face during the procedure. If a head drape is used, the front edge of the drape may be placed behind the hairline. Fenestrated or split sheets are used for draping a limb. Whenever copious amounts of solution are required, such as during debridement, an impervious pocket drape should be used to collect and isolate runoff. Multiple draping sites are commonly required during plastic and reconstructive surgery.

INSTRUMENTS

Plastic surgery instruments (commonly called "plastic instruments") include a variety of devices for cutting, retracting, and grasping tissue. Most cosmetic surgery involves only the skin, therefore the instruments are short and have fine tips.

Sharp dissection is performed with tenotomy or fine Metzenbaum scissors and toothed tissue forceps. Many other delicate scissors are available, and most plastic surgeons have one or two favorites, which the scrub should have available.

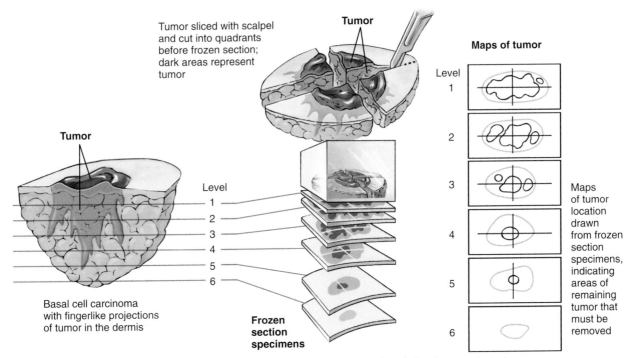

Figure 29-6 Mohs surgery. A frozen section is quartered and sliced into multiple layers to obtain a clear view of tumor margins. This technique preserves as much tissue as possible while excising any containing cancer cells. *(From Thibodeau G, Patton K: Anatomy and physiology, ed 6, St Louis, 2007, Mosby.)*

Discussion

The surgeon begins by marking the planned revision. The scar is incised with a #15 blade and Adson toothed forceps. The surgeon **undermines** the surrounding tissue with Metzenbaum scissors. The wound edges are closed with 4-0 or 5-0 absorbable synthetic suture.

DEBRIDEMENT OF BURNS

Surgical Goal

Debridement is the removal of nonviable tissue from a non-healing or traumatic wound. Burn wounds require repeated debridement to remove dying and dead tissue so that healing can continue.

Pathology

Burns are caused by flame, scalding (liquid), electrical current, radiation, or chemicals. The current system for classifying burns established by the American Burn Association, http://www.ameriburn.org/ describes the depth of tissue injury.

- *Superficial partial thickness first degree:* Only the outer layer of the epidermis is injured. The skin is red or pink, dry, and painful to touch.
- *Partial thickness second degree:* The epidermis and various degrees of the dermis are injured. The skin is blistered, red, and moist. The burn is very sensitive to environmental exposure and touch.
- *Full thickness second degree:* The epidermis and full dermis are injured. These burns are characterized by a white, smooth, shiny surface with dry blisters and edema.
- *Full thickness third degree:* The skin, subcutaneous tissue, muscle, and bone are burned. The third-degree burn is centered in an area of second-degree injury. The skin may be white, brown, or black and appears waxy. There is no pain because nerves have been destroyed.

Third-degree burns develop **eschar**, which is devitalized, nonelastic tissue that adheres to the wound site. Eschar is removed during debridement to allow healing and to reduce constriction.

Extensive second- and third-degree burns can result in fluid and electrolyte imbalance, infection, inadequate nutrition, respiratory deficit, and vascular damage. Circumferential eschar has a tourniquet effect on the affected body part and thus can extensively damage underlying muscle, bone, and vascular tissue. In this case, an **escharotomy** (eschar removal) or **fasciotomy** (multiple incisions through the fascia) is performed to release the stricture.

Technique

1. Nonviable tissue is removed.
2. Bleeding is controlled.
3. The debrided area may be covered with a graft.
4. Dressings are applied.

Discussion

Preparation of the burn patient requires extensive thermoregulation and physiological monitoring. The temperature in the operating room is raised to reduce the risk of hypothermia.

The patient is positioned to allow for adequate exposure of the burns. General anesthesia is used. The patient is prepped with Betadine spray and draped with towels and three-quarter sheets. A pneumatic tourniquet may be used on burns of the extremities.

The surgeon begins by removing all nonviable skin with a Braithwaite blade or USF debrider. The tissue is removed until only a viable layer remains. Lap sponges soaked in a solution of sterile saline and topical epinephrine (1:1,000) are applied to control bleeding. The concentration most often used is 1,000 mL of normal saline, with 4 mL of topical epinephrine (1:1,000) added according to the surgeon's orders.

When hemostasis has been achieved, an allograft may be applied. The graft is stapled over the debrided burns to create a layer of protection until autografting can be performed (usually several days after the initial debridement). Nonadherent dressings (e.g., Xeroform) and fluffs are applied. The extremities are wrapped with Ace bandages.

Postoperative Considerations

Patients may recover in the **burn intensive care unit (ICU)**. Multiple debridement surgeries and multiple skin grafts may be required before the rehabilitation process can begin. After the healing process, burn patients undergo extensive physical and occupational therapy to regain full use of the burned areas.

SPLIT-THICKNESS SKIN GRAFT

Surgical Goal

Skin grafting is performed to replace skin that has been lost as a result of trauma, disease, or infection.

Pathology

Skin is necessary for protection and nourishment of underlying tissues. Minor injuries or defects can regenerate sufficient skin to create a scar. Large defects require a skin graft to protect underlying tissues from infection, **desiccation** (drying), and injury.

Technique

1. The donor site is pulled taut.
2. The donor site is covered with lubricant.
3. The graft is removed with a dermatome.
4. The donor site is dressed.
5. The graft is applied to the prepared recipient site.
6. The recipient site is dressed.

Discussion

The patient is positioned to allow exposure of the donor site (i.e., supine position for the lower extremities and trunk; prone position for the buttocks and back). The donor and recipient sites are prepped and draped separately.

The surgeon removes the skin graft with either a free-hand skin graft knife (full-thickness graft) or a dermatome (split-thickness graft).

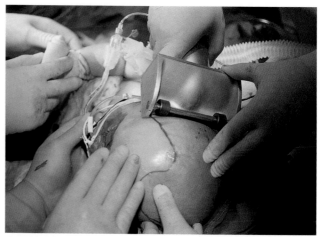

Figure 29-7   Removal of a split-thickness graft with a dermatome. *(From Barret JP, Herndon DN: Color atlas of burn care, Philadelphia, 2001, WB Saunders.)*

Dermatome

The scrub must prepare the dermatome, inserting the appropriate blade and guard. (In some facilities, the surgeon prepares the equipment.) The dermatome should always be handed to the field with the depth gauge set at 0. This allows the surgeon to select the depth setting for the blade, usually 0.012 to 0.015.

Mineral oil is applied to the graft site to reduce friction as the blade glides over the skin. To assist the surgeon in taking the graft, the assistant pulls the donor skin taut using either 4 × 4 gauze sponges or tongue blades. The surgeon positions the dermatome at the donor site and advances forward to remove the top layer of skin (Figure 29-7). The graft emerges from the back of the instrument as the dermatome is advanced across the skin. The assistant grasps and elevates the graft with forceps as it is produced (the surgical technologist may be asked to perform this task).

When sufficient skin has been removed, the dermatome is angled upward; this severs the graft. If it is not released, the graft can be separated from the donor bed with fine scissors. The scrub accepts the graft in a basin to protect it from contamination and injury. Alternatively, the surgeon may transfer the graft immediately to a carrier plate for meshing (see next section). The graft should be kept moist but not wet and covered with gauze, according to facility protocol.

The donor site is covered with a sponge soaked in saline or a solution of saline and topical epinephrine (1:1,000) to aid hemostasis. Xeroform gauze also is used to cover the wound.

Graft Preparation

Most split-thickness grafts require meshing before implantation. In this process, the graft is fed into a blade and roller mechanism that perforates the graft. The surgeon places the skin on a plastic carrier plate, spreading it evenly over the surface with the exterior side facing upward. The plate is inserted into the mesher, which is hand operated.

Placing the Graft

The recipient site may require debridement before grafting. When the site is ready, the carrier plate is held near the recipient site, and the skin is gently teased onto the prepared tissue bed. The surgeon spreads the graft over the defect and trims any excess with curved iris scissors. The graft is attached to the skin surrounding the defect with staples or absorbable suture. If the graft is implanted on an exposed area of the body, such as the hands or face, it is sutured in place. On areas that are not exposed, such as the abdomen or back, the graft may be stapled.

The donor site is dressed with an OpSite transparent dressing or a nonadherent dressing covered with Kerlix gauze roll.

A stent dressing may be placed over the graft (see Chapter 17).

Stent Dressing

A **stent** is a type of pressure dressing that is placed over the graft site to prevent the accumulation of serum or blood under the graft. To prepare a stent, four or more opposing sutures are placed at the periphery of the graft site. The ends are not cut but left long. Petroleum gauze is cut to fit over the entire graft. Saline-moistened gauze is molded to fit over the petrolatum. The gauze is tied in place with the long suture ends. The site is dressed with gauze fluffs. A soft splint made of cotton and gauze may be applied to prevent displacement of the graft in the immediate postoperative period.

PEDICLE GRAFT

Surgical Goal

Pedicle grafts provide coverage and vascularization to a soft tissue defect.

Pathology

A pedicle graft (also called a *flap graft*) is raised from the donor site but not immediately severed free. The donor site tissue is partly severed, and the flap is brought in contact with the recipient site. The graft is sutured in place to cover the defect. During the healing process, the graft tissue infiltrates and develops over the recipient wound. When healing is complete, the flap is released and the donor site defect is closed primarily with sutures. This type of graft is used when the recipient site requires skin and deep tissue to fill a large tissue defect resulting from radical surgery or trauma.

Types of Pedicle Graft

Pedicle grafts are classified as near or distant. A near graft is created in adjacent tissue (e.g., from the palm for use on the finger). Distant grafts are created from the trunk or other areas for use on a limb.

An advancement flap (see the following section) is raised from the tissues in the immediate area of the defect. Rotational flaps are semicircular and require some

degree of turning to reach and cover the recipient tissue defect.

Pedicle flaps have large blood vessels that infiltrate the recipient site during healing. A pedicle graft to the finger is shown in Figure 29-8. A rotational flap is shown in Figure 29-9.

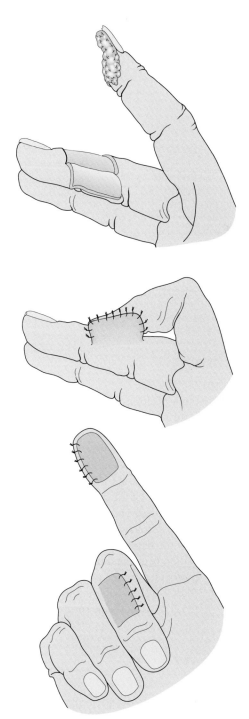

Figure 29-8   Pedicle graft of the finger. **A,** The flap is raised on the middle finger. **B,** The injured first digit is placed in contact with the flap and sutured in place. **C,** The flaps are closed after healing. *(From Garden O, Bradbury A, Forsythe J, Parks R: Principles and practice of surgery, ed 5, Edinburgh, 2007, Churchill Livingstone/Elsevier.)*

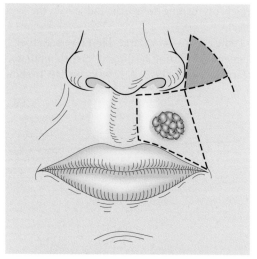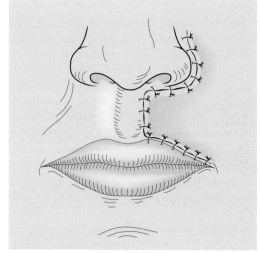

Figure 29-9 Rotational flap from the face. **A,** The lesion is removed, and a flap is raised from the perinalar area. **B,** The flap is rotated to fit over the defect, and the graft site skin is closed after healing. *(From Garden O, Bradbury A, Forsythe J, Parks R: Principles and practice of surgery, ed 5, Edinburgh, 2007, Churchill Livingstone/Elsevier.)*

Technique
1. The defect is measured.
2. The incision lines of the flap are measured and drawn on the skin.
3. The flap is elevated.
4. The flap is positioned over the defect.
5. The flap is sutured into place.
6. The donor site is closed.

Discussion
Advancement Flap
The patient is placed in a position that allows access to both the defect and the donor site. Depending on the size of the defect, general or local anesthesia may be used. The surgeon begins by measuring the defect and the proposed flap to ensure complete coverage. The incision lines are drawn with a skin scribe. Both surgical sites are prepped. The surgeon cleans any rough, uneven edges of the defect with a #15 blade.

Next, the donor site is incised. The flap is elevated with the knife or tenotomy scissors. Retraction is applied with double-prong skin hooks. When the flap has been raised sufficiently, it is advanced into position over the donor site. The surgeon does this by simply approximating the edges of the skin flap to cover the defect; 3-0 or 4-0 absorbable sutures are used for deep tissue, and 5-0 or 6-0 nonabsorbable sutures are used for the skin.

BLEPHAROPLASTY

Surgical Goal
Blepharoplasty resection of the eyelid is done to improve vision of the upper visual fields.

Pathology
With advancing age, the eyelids lose elasticity and tone and may obscure vision. The procedure also may be performed for cosmetic purposes.

Technique
1. The lids are injected with a local anesthetic.
2. The skin and subcutaneous tissue are incised.
3. The excess skin is removed from the eyelid.
4. The incision is closed.

Discussion
The patient is placed in the supine position with the head on a doughnut headrest and the arms tucked at the sides. General or local anesthesia may be used. A local anesthetic is instilled into the lid. The patient is prepped with pHisoHex and draped with a head drape and split sheet.

Upper Lid Blepharoplasty
The surgeon determines the exact location of the incisions and marks the sites with a skin scribe. The incision is made with a #15 blade. Dull rakes are used to retract the skin and expose the subcutaneous tissue. Depending on the amount, the fatty tissue may be excised with tenotomy scissors. A needle point bipolar ESU is used to control bleeding in the fatty tissue. If excess muscle also is present, it is removed with curved iris scissors. The incision is closed with nonabsorbable subcuticular suture and several interrupted sutures to reinforce the primary suture line. The ends of this suture are left long for easy removal. Upper lid blepharoplasty is illustrated in Figure 29-10.

Lower Lid Blepharoplasty: Subciliary Approach
Using a #15 blade, the surgeon makes the incision in the subciliary region, 2 to 3 mm below the lower lash line. The lower lid skin is elevated upward and outward to determine the amount to be removed. The skin is excised with a #15 blade. To gain access to the infraorbital fat pads, the surgeon makes an incision into the orbicularis muscle. Double-prong skin hooks are used to retract the skin. The excess fat is removed with iris scissors. The orbicularis oculi muscle is

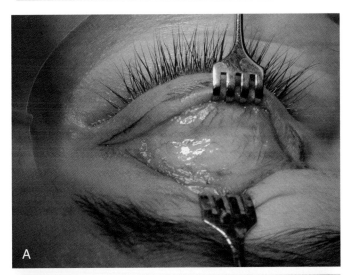

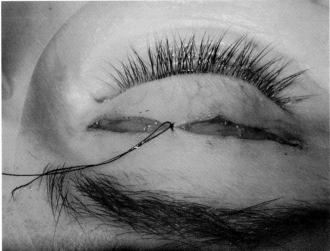

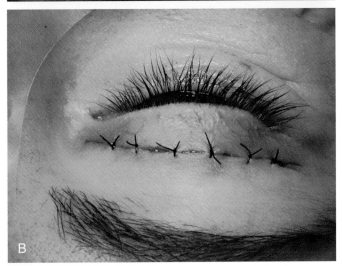

Figure 29-10 Upper lid blepharoplasty. **A,** The skin incision is retracted with dull rakes. Small bleeders have been coagulated with the bipolar ESU. The fat pad is exposed and may be removed with Westcott scissors. **B,** Closure with 6-0 Vicryl sutures. *(From Chen W, Khan J, McCord C: Color atlas of cosmetic oculofacial surgery, Edinburgh, 2004, Butterworth-Heinemann.)*

reattached to the periosteum at the lateral orbital rim with clear, nonabsorbable sutures. This prevents the lower lid from drooping after blepharoplasty. The incisions are closed as described previously. Lower lid blepharoplasty is illustrated in Figure 29-11.

BROW LIFT (OPEN AND ENDOSCOPIC TECHNIQUES)

Surgical Goal
Brow lift procedures are done to lift the supportive structures of the brow and alleviate drooping of skin, muscle, and fascia.

Pathology
The soft tissues of the brow may droop with age and deepen the furrows over the eyes. This may also lead to eyebrow **ptosis** and upper lid "hooding" of the eye.

Discussion
Open Technique
The patient is placed in the supine position with the head of the table raised. The arms are tucked at the sides. The surgeon pulls the hair back and secures it with rubber bands. The face is prepped with pHisoHex. Draping includes a head drape and split sheet.

A number of approaches can be used for a brow lift (Figure 29-12). These include the coronal approach (behind the hairline), the pretrichial approach (at the hair line), or the direct approach (at the level of the brow itself). The selected incisions are drawn carefully with a skin scribe. The incisions are made with a #15 blade. A periosteal elevator is used to lift the periosteum from the cranium to the level of the superior orbital rims. The periosteum is incised at the level of the orbital rim with the elevator. This allows for mobility of the brows. The muscles at the bridge of the nose are incised with scissors, electrocautery, or the elevator. The excess skin of the inferior flaps is excised with the #15 blade. The inferior flap is suspended from the superior periosteum with a nonabsorbable suture. The wound is closed in layers. Absorbable sutures are used for the deep layers. Absorbable or nonabsorbable sutures are used for the skin, or staples may be used in a coronal approach.

Endoscopic Technique
The patient is placed in the supine position with the head of the bed raised. The arms are tucked at the sides. The hair is pulled back and secured with rubber bands. The face is prepped and draped with a head drape and split sheet.

Using a #10 blade, the surgeon makes three central scalp incisions behind the hairline: one in the midline and two just medial to the superior temporal line. The incisions are extended, and a periosteal elevator is used to dissect the forehead flap from bone. The 30-degree 4- or 5-mm endoscope is passed through the rim of one of the incisions. Undermining is continued to a point approximately 0.8 inch (2 cm) above the supraorbital rim.

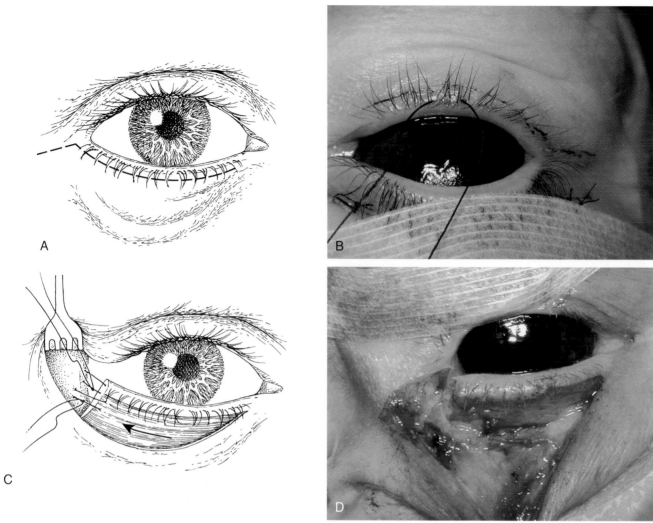

Figure 29-11   Lower lid blepharoplasty **A,** Infraciliary incision. **B,** Upside-down view of the lower lid margin. **C,** Canthotomy and resection. **D,** The lid after resection. *(From Chen W, Khan J, McCord C: Color atlas of cosmetic oculofacial surgery, Edinburgh, 2004, Butterworth-Heinemann.)*

Next, a straight periosteal elevator is used to elevate the temporal fascia with the endoscope in place. The two temporal dissections are connected with a straight periosteal elevator and the 30-degree endoscope. The surgeon elevates the frontal fascia to the level of the supraorbital rim.

When the periosteum has been mobilized, the surgeon elevates and fixes the lateral brow. (The medial brow usually is not fixed, because if it is elevated too much, the brow looks unnatural).

The tissue may be fixed by drilling into the bone and passing absorbable sutures through the holes and soft tissue. The incision is closed with staples. A head dressing consisting of Kerlix fluffs and rolled gauze is applied. An endoscopic brow lift is shown in Figure 29-13.

RHYTIDECTOMY

Surgical Goal

Redundant and sagging supportive tissue of the face is reduced or modified to provide a more aesthetic appearance.

Pathology

The aging process and gravity affect the skin and the structures that lie beneath it. This results in hollow infraorbital regions, nasolabial folds, jowls, and excess skin below the chin. Certain environmental factors contribute to laxity and wrinkling of the skin. Wrinkles are a normal product of aging. However, **photodamage** occurs with extended, excessive exposure to ultraviolet light. Smoking also causes extreme wrinkling of the skin.

Discussion

The patient is placed in the supine position with the head stabilized on a doughnut or Mayfield headrest and the head of the bed raised. The surgeon marks the skin with a skin scribe before the prep is performed. The patient is prepped and draped for a face procedure.

The excisional areas are injected with 1% lidocaine with epinephrine (1:100,000) to maintain hemostasis. A fine-gauge spinal needle and 10-mL syringe are used for the injection. This area includes the cheek to the submentum

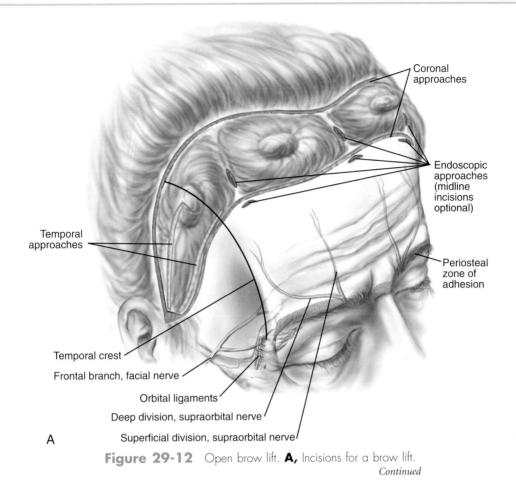

Coronal approaches

Endoscopic approaches (midline incisions optional)

Periosteal zone of adhesion

Temporal approaches

Temporal crest

Frontal branch, facial nerve

Orbital ligaments

Deep division, supraorbital nerve

Superficial division, supraorbital nerve

A

Figure 29-12 Open brow lift. **A,** Incisions for a brow lift.

Continued

(under the chin) and posteriorly over the mastoid and into the neck. Skin incisions are made with a #15 blade, and double-prong skin hooks are used for retraction. The surgeon may staple a sponge to the posterior aspect of the incision to reduce the amount of blood that collects in the hair.

The dissection continues with rhytidectomy scissors. The bipolar ESU is used to control small bleeders. The surgeon may use a fiberoptic retractor to aid exposure during dissection. At this point, the surgeon may overlap the underlying fascial attachment with 2-0 or 3-0 absorbable suture. A surgical option is to excise a strip of fascia in the preauricular area with Metzenbaum scissors. This tissue should be saved on the back table in saline in case it is needed for further augmentation procedures.

If the surgeon is performing a deep plane rhytidectomy, the fascia is elevated from the parotid gland and surrounding area in the neck. This dissection is performed with the rhytidectomy or Metzenbaum scissors. The two ends of the fascia are then folded over and secured with 2-0 or 3-0 absorbable suture.

Excess skin is excised with Metzenbaum scissors, and the subdermal layer is closed with 3-0, 4-0, and 5-0 absorbable sutures. A drain may be placed during closure. The skin is closed with a combination of staples and 5-0 absorbable or nonabsorbable sutures. A head dressing is placed to support the incisions. Gauze sponges with an Ace wrap or a fascio-

plasty splint are commonly used to dress the wound. Figure 29-14 shows rhytidectomy techniques.

LASER SKIN RESURFACING

Surgical Goal
Laser skin resurfacing removes the epidermis and a portion of the dermis to reduce facial lines and wrinkles.

Pathology
See Rhytidectomy.

Technique
1. The patient is anesthetized.
2. The operative area is draped with moist towels.
3. The skin is resurfaced with either the carbon dioxide or the erbium-YAG laser.
4. The wounds are dressed.

Discussion
All laser precautions must be followed before the start of surgery. This includes safety attire for the operating team (correct goggles for the type of laser), safety signs, and strict attention to sources of combustion on the operative field. (Chapter 19 presents a complete discussion of laser use.)

The patient is placed in the supine position with the arms tucked at the sides. The head of the operating table

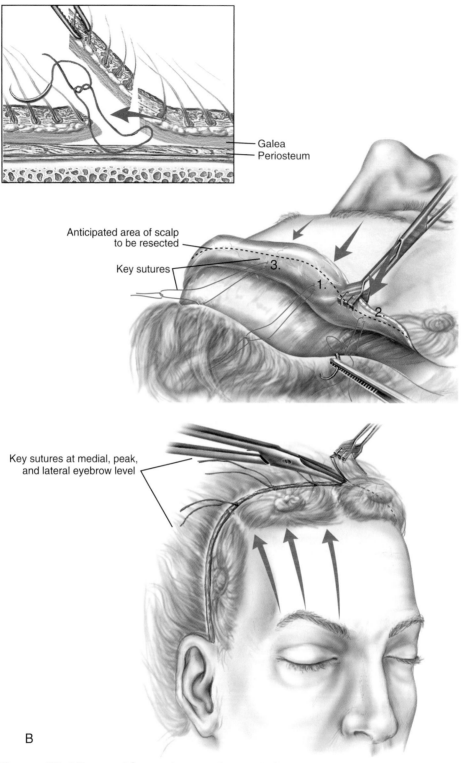

Galea
Periosteum

Anticipated area of scalp to be resected

Key sutures

Key sutures at medial, peak, and lateral eyebrow level

B

Figure 29-12, cont'd   B, Closure and removal of redundant scalp tissue. *(From LaTrenta G: Atlas of aesthetic face and neck surgery, Philadelphia, 2004, WB Saunders.)*

is elevated according to the technical requirements of the procedure. The type of anesthesia depends on the extent and length of the procedure. Short cases are done using local anesthesia, whereas more extensive surgery requires general anesthesia. If general anesthesia is used, a laser endotracheal tube must be used to prevent an airway fire.

The face is prepped with pHisoHex to remove debris and oil. Alcohol-based prep solutions must not be used when laser surgery is planned. The patient is draped with a head drape and split sheet. Moist towels are placed around the surgical site to reduce the risk of peripheral thermal damage and fire. The patient's eyes must be protected from injury with laser safety goggles.

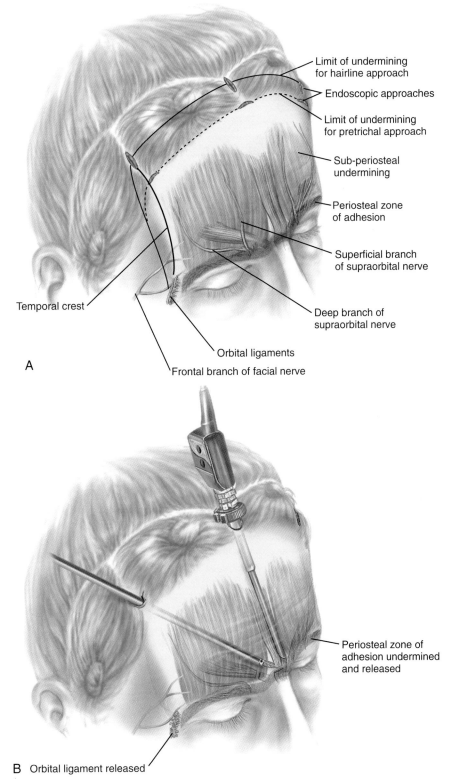

Limit of undermining
for hairline approach

Endoscopic approaches

Limit of undermining
for pretrichal approach

Sub-periosteal
undermining

Periosteal zone
of adhesion

Superficial branch
of supraorbital nerve

Deep branch of
supraorbital nerve

Temporal crest

Orbital ligaments

Frontal branch of facial nerve

A

Periosteal zone of
adhesion undermined
and released

B   Orbital ligament released

Figure 29-13   Endoscopic brow lift. **A,** Incisions for endoscopic lift. **B,** Subperiosteal dissection. *(From LaTrenta G: Atlas of aesthetic face and neck surgery, Philadelphia, 2004, WB Saunders.)*

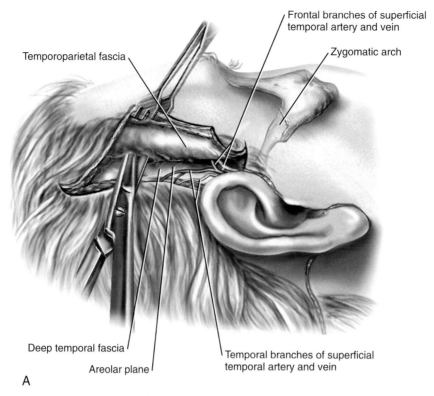

Temporoparietal fascia

Frontal branches of superficial temporal artery and vein

Zygomatic arch

Deep temporal fascia

Areolar plane

Temporal branches of superficial temporal artery and vein

A

SKIN TENSION VECTORS AND CLOSURE SEQUENCING
1 → 2 → 3

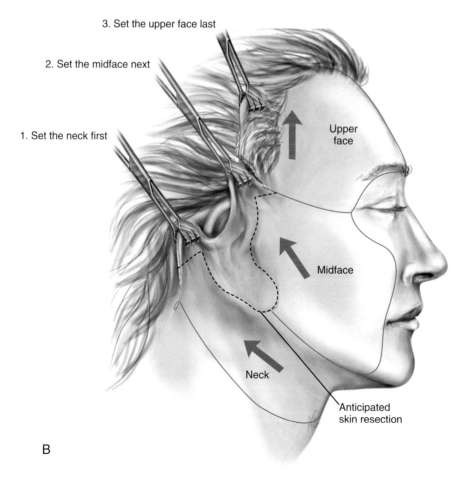

3. Set the upper face last

2. Set the midface next

1. Set the neck first

Upper face

Midface

Neck

Anticipated skin resection

B

Figure 29-14 Rhytidectomy techniques. **A,** Undermining in the temporal area. **B,** Closure of skin flaps and areas of resection. *(From LaTrenta G: Atlas of aesthetic face and neck surgery, Philadelphia, 2004, WB Saunders.)*

The surgeon adjusts the laser settings before resurfacing. The handpiece is passed over the skin using the computer guidance system of the unit. Each pass removes a layer of the epidermis, reducing the appearance of wrinkles. When the entire face has been resurfaced, a **hydrodressing** is applied.

FACIAL IMPLANT

Surgical Goal

Facial augmentation is performed to give normal contours to the chin or cheek. This is achieved by inserting a molded implant in the affected area. Many different materials are used as implants, including silicone, acrylic polymers, polyethylene, Gore-Tex, and mesh. Several types of subdermal and subcutaneous injectable filler materials can be used, such as Dermalogen, Alloderm, Restylane, collagen, and liquid silicone. An autograft (fat, bone, or cartilage) may also be used. The type of implant chosen depends on the surgeon's preference and the type of defect to be filled.

Pathology

Facial augmentation corrects malformation or loss of facial tissue caused by congenital anomaly, trauma, or radical surgery in which bone and other connective tissue was removed. Patients may also seek augmentation for aesthetic reasons in the absence of deformity.

Technique

1. The incision is planned, and the skin is marked.
2. The skin is incised.
3. The skin is undermined.
4. The superficial SMAS is imbricated, incised, and plicated.
5. The skin is closed.
6. Dressings are applied.

Description

Mentoplasty (Chin Augmentation)

The patient is placed on the operating table in the lounge chair position with the arms tucked at the sides. Before induction of anesthesia, the surgeon marks the anatomical landmarks by having the patient flex the neck. General anesthesia may be used. A local anesthetic is instilled into the region of the mental nerve, the incision line, and the surrounding soft tissue. The skin is prepped with Betadine scrub and paint or pHisoHex, including the entire face. The face is exposed during the procedure to allow the surgeon to assess the projection given by the implant. The patient is draped with a head drape and a split sheet.

A 10- to 15-mm incision is made vertically in the midline on the chin with a #15 blade. The incision extends through the subcutaneous fat and muscle to the layer of the periosteum. The assistant retracts the skin flaps with double-prong skin hooks. The periosteum is incised with a #15 blade.

Next, the surgeon elevates the periosteum with a periosteal elevator (e.g., Joseph elevator). The implant is eased into position; the periosteum is elevated with a Senn retractor during implantation. Absorbable sutures may be placed in the distal end of the implant and periosteum to prevent the implant from shifting.

The wound is closed in two layers. The periosteum is closed with interrupted 3-0 absorbable sutures, and the skin is closed with 6-0 nonabsorbable suture or a 5-0 fast-absorbing suture. Gauze dressings are applied.

Malar Augmentation (Cheek Augmentation)

The patient is prepped and draped as described previously. An intraoral incision is made below the parotid duct with a #15 blade and extended to the periosteum. The periosteum then is incised and elevated superiorly and laterally over the malar and zygoma. The implant is positioned, and the wound is closed in layers with 3-0 absorbable sutures. No dressing is applied, because the incision is intraoral.

Technique

1. The incision site is marked.
2. The surgical site is injected with a local anesthetic.
3. The incision is made.
4. The periosteum is elevated.
5. The implant is inserted.
6. The wound is closed.
7. The dressings are applied.

OTOPLASTY

Surgical Goal

Otoplasty is surgical creation of the external ear.

Pathology

Otoplasty is performed to correct a congenital malformation of the external ear or to create an ear destroyed by trauma.

Technique

1. Incisions are made in the periauricular skin.
2. Keith needles are inserted.
3. Sutures are placed.
4. The incisions are closed.

Discussion

Procedures for otoplasty often involve multiple surgeries. These procedures are somewhat complex, and many approaches can be used, depending on the pathological condition and the patient's needs.

The patient is placed in the supine position with the head of the table raised. A doughnut headrest is used to stabilize the head and allow access to the posterior ear. If the procedure is a bilateral one, the patient is prepped and draped to allow access to both ears.

An incision is made in the postauricular skin with a #15 blade to expose the cartilage. The soft tissue is dissected from the perichondrium. Keith needles are then used to recreate the antihelix on the anterior surface of the ear. The Keith needles are used as guides on the posterior surface to help the surgeon "break" the spring of the cartilage so that the antihelix can be recreated. This can be done by incising strips of skin with the #15 blade. Wedges of tissue are then released with a triangular

Farrior knife. A diamond-tip drill may be used to thin the strips. Once the spring has been broken, the cartilage is fixed in position with nonabsorbable sutures. If necessary, a strip of cartilage is removed from the lateral portion of the conchal bowl and the cartilage is reapproximated with nonabsorbable sutures. Techniques for pinning the ear usually involve suturing the posterior portion of the conchal bowl to the mastoid periosteum with nonabsorbable suture. The skin then is closed with absorbable suture.

The reconstructed ear is reinforced with ointment-impregnated cotton balls and a mastoid dressing.

AUGMENTATION MAMMOPLASTY

Surgical Goal

Augmentation mammoplasty is performed to increase the size and improve the shape of the breast.

Breast implants are constructed with a silicone outer layer and a saline or silicone inner space. Implants may be round or anatomical in shape. Round implants are used for an elective procedure on an intact breast, whereas anatomical implants are used after mastectomy or if the breast is very small.

Discussion

Postmastectomy Reconstruction

The patient is placed in the supine position, prepped, and draped for a breast procedure, including the sternal notch and xyphoid process. This allows the surgeon to use midline anatomical marks that have not been altered by previous surgeries.

The surgeon excises the mastectomy scar with Allis clamps and the skin knife. Hemostasis is maintained with the ESU. The scar is referred for pathological evaluation to ensure that no abnormal cells are present.

Technique

1. The mastectomy scar is excised.
2. A pocket is created under the pectoralis major muscle.
3. A tissue expander is implanted in the pocket with the saline port in the subcutaneous tissue of the midaxillary line (allowing easy access for expansion over the following weeks).
4. The saline reservoir is filled (the initial amount is 150 to 300 mL of saline solution).
5. The wound is closed.

The surgeon creates a pocket in the musculofascial tissue of the pectoralis major. This is done with a blunt hemostat or with gentle digital separation of the tissue. A tissue expander with a saline reservoir is inserted into the pocket. The reservoir is filled to 150 to 300 mL. The injection port is placed in the subcutaneous tissue at the midaxillary line of the affected side. The incision then is closed with 3-0 and 4-0 absorbable suture (e.g., Vicryl). The skin is closed with a running subcuticular suture of 4-0 synthetic absorbable material.

The surgeon uses the saline-filled tissue expander to slowly stretch the skin and underlying tissue by gradually filling the saline reservoir. When the tissue has stretched sufficiently, the tissue expander is removed and replaced with a permanent implant.

For insertion of the permanent implant, the patient is placed in the supine position, prepped, and draped as previously described.

A #15 blade is used to make an incision in the axillary region, around the lower half of the areola and nipple, or in the inframammary fold. Hemostasis is maintained with the ESU.

The surgeon creates a pocket under the pectoralis major. A tissue expander is inserted into the pocket and filled in 60-mL increments. The scrub must record the amount of fluid used in the expander, because the same amount will be used in the implant.

The surgeon may assess the symmetry and position of the breast by placing the patient in the sitting position. In this case, the patient's arms and head must be fully supported with the assistance of the anesthesia care provider. The permanent implant is inserted and filled with the appropriate amount of saline. The incision is closed with 3-0 and 4-0 absorbable suture. The skin is closed with a subcuticular suture.

Technique

Augmentation

1. The incision is made according to the selected approach.
2. A pocket is created under the pectoralis major muscle.
3. A temporary sizer is placed and filled with the appropriate amount of saline.
4. The sizer is removed, and the permanent implant is placed.
5. The wound is closed.

The procedure is repeated for the other breast. At the conclusion of the procedure, the scrub must document the amount of saline used in each implant.

REDUCTION MAMMOPLASTY

Surgical Goal

In a reduction mammoplasty, excess breast tissue is removed and the breast is reconstructed to provide an anesthetic appearance.

Pathology

Reduction mammoplasty may be performed for cosmetic or medical reasons. Macromastia (excessively large breasts) is related to the weight and size of the breast. The increased forward weight can cause cervical and thoracic pain. Patients also may suffer socially and psychologically. Macromastia in males is referred to as *gynecomastia*.

Technique

1. The incision lines are marked (this may be done before surgery admission).
2. An incision is made around the areola and extended in a wide triangle to the inframammary line.
3. The skin tissue is undermined.
4. The breast tissue is removed through the inframammary incision.
5. The inframammary and triangular incisions are closed.
6. A circular incision is made at the apex of the breast; the nipple is brought up and sutured in place.
7. The wound is closed and dressed with gauze fluff and a pressure dressing.

Discussion

Many different techniques are used to perform reduction mammoplasty. Preoperative preparation of the patient takes place in the surgeon's clinic. The procedure is planned using computer modeling and calibration. The incisions are clearly marked with an indelible skin scribe.

For the surgery, the patient is positioned in the supine or semi-Fowler position, prepped, and draped for a breast procedure as previously described.

The surgeon begins by making a circular incision around the areola with the breast held in extension. Next, the surgeon makes a triangular or anchor-shaped incision with the apex at the nipple margin and the base along the inframammary fold. The skin is undermined with a #15 blade, Adson toothed forceps, or Metzenbaum scissors. The breast then is manually retracted superiorly, and the glandular and fatty tissue is excised. This step is performed with sharp dissection. Any tissue removed is passed off the field to be weighed. This is done to ensure that approximately the same amount of tissue is removed from each breast.

The surgeon then approximates the breast tissue at the midline by bringing the sides of the triangle together and suturing them with absorbable 3-0 suture on a curved needle. Any excess skin at the inframammary incision is trimmed with Metzenbaum scissors or a #15 blade. The incision is closed with 3-0 absorbable suture. Both skin incisions then are closed with 4-0 subcuticular suture.

The surgeon uses a nipple marker to make a circular incision at the apex of the triangular incision. The tissue is excised with a #15 blade. This creates a new position for the areola and nipple, which are pulled through the incision line and sutured in place with nonabsorbable subcuticular suture. Gauze fluffs and supportive dressings are then applied.

TRANSVERSE RECTUS ABDOMINIS MYOCUTANEOUS (TRAM) FLAP

Surgical Goal

A TRAM flap is performed to reconstruct the breast without the use of implants.

Pathology

A TRAM flap can be used in a variety of plastic and reconstructive procedures, including breast reconstruction after mastectomy. In this procedure, a tissue flap containing skin, subcutaneous tissue, and muscle is raised from the lower abdomen and transferred to the mastectomy site. The flap continues to receive its blood supply from the pedicle (the portion of the flap that remains attached to the point of origin). This allows reconstruction of the breast without the use of implants.

Technique

1. The mastectomy scar is excised.
2. An elliptical incision is made in the transverse plane in the lower abdomen, at the level of the umbilicus, to include the umbilicus and the area above the symphysis pubis.
3. The incision is extended along the border, with attention paid to avoiding the large vessels of the rectus muscle.
4. The skin superior to the incision site is undermined at the level of the fascia.
5. The rectus sheath is incised.
6. The inferior epigastric artery and vein are ligated.
7. The flap is dissected up the costal margin, leaving the central edge of the rectus sheath attached to the rectus muscle.
8. The flap is delivered through the subcutaneous tunnel that has been created.
9. The transverse rectus abdominis myocutaneous (TRAM) flap is inserted into the area created by the elevated skin flaps of the mastectomy site.
10. The flap is trimmed to fit the defect, and a new breast is constructed.
11. Excess portions of the flap may be defatted and used to create a breast mound.
12. The flap is sutured in place.
13. The abdominal wound is closed, and a new umbilicus is created.

Discussion

The patient is placed in the supine position and prepped from the neck to the pubis. Draping exposes the abdomen and the breasts.

The surgeon grasps the mastectomy scar with Adson toothed forceps or Allis clamps and excises it with a #15 blade. The transverse abdominal incision extends from one iliac crest to the other. The upper margin includes the umbilicus. The surgeon then creates a subcutaneous tunnel that connects the mastectomy site with the abdominal incision, usually along the costal margin. This step is performed with large clamps and Metzenbaum scissors. The flap is elevated, and the upper border of the elliptical incision is carried into the abdominal wall. A small amount of subcutaneous tissue is left intact over the rectus sheath to preserve the vascular supply to the area.

The lower incision is carried to the level of the anterior fascia. The lateral margins, or "tails," of the incision are then mobilized. The rectus sheath and muscle are incised, and the inferior epigastric artery (found on the posterior surface of the rectus muscle) is ligated with a 2-0 silk tie. Sharp dissection is used to mobilize the rectus muscle, including the sheath, to the level of the costal margin.

The flap is brought through the subcutaneous tunnel in the direction of the mastectomy site. When the flap is in place over the mastectomy incision, it is trimmed. Excess skin is excised with scissors or a knife, and the flap edges are aligned with the skin flaps of the mastectomy incision.

The surgeon shapes the breast, trimming excess skin and subcutaneous tissue as needed with Metzenbaum scissors or the scalpel. The scrub must save all trimmed portions of the flap, because the subcutaneous tissue can be used to fill in the axillary region and to add more tissue to the breast mound itself.

A suction drain is placed in the wound before closure. Absorbable synthetic sutures (e.g., Vicryl) are used to secure the flap to the chest wall. Next, the skin flaps are closed with 4-0 nonabsorbable suture (e.g., Monocryl). Nipple reconstruction may be done at a later date if the patient desires. Additional surgeries also may be needed to contour the breast mound.

The surgeon closes the abdomen in layers. The rectus sheath is approximated with 2-0 absorbable synthetic suture. The skin is closed with staples or an absorbable subcuticular suture. Synthetic mesh may be used to reinforce the closure. (This process is described in Chapter 23.)

Nipple Reconstruction

After a TRAM flap reconstruction, some women may want the nipple and areola reconstructed to create a more natural appearance. The areola is constructed from a full-thickness graft taken from the medial thigh crease or postauricular region. The nipple is created with a full-thickness skin graft taken from the labia.

The nipple may be tattooed to provide color contrast at the time of reconstruction or at a later date. Figure 29-15 illustrates the process of TRAM flap breast reconstruction.

LIPOSUCTION

Surgical Goal

Liposuction is performed to remove excess deep fat.

Technique

1. The incisions are marked before surgery with a skin scribe.
2. Tissue to be removed is injected with a local anesthetic mixed with lactated Ringer solution.
3. The incisions are made.
4. The fat is aspirated.
5. The incisions are closed.
6. Dressings are applied if needed.

Pathology

No physical pathological condition requires the use of liposuction.

Discussion

Liposuction Instruments

Liposuction is performed with high-vacuum suction, a rigid cannula, and a large-bore suction tube (at least ⅜ inch [0.9 cm] in diameter). Large-bore tubing is required because adipose tissue is dense and would clog normal suction tubing. A high-vacuum apparatus is required to pull the tissue through the tubing.

The patient is placed in the supine position with the arms at a 90-degree angle to the body. Depending on the extent of the procedure, either general anesthesia or local anesthesia with IV sedation is used. The patient is prepped and draped with towels and three-quarter sheets to allow exposure of all the sites to be treated.

The surgeon begins by injecting an anesthetic into the soft tissue. A large volume of lidocaine and epinephrine diluted in lactated Ringer solution is injected into the targeted tissue until it is taut. The injection provides local anesthesia and hemostasis and expands the operative area, making it easier to insert the liposuction cannula.

Multiple incisions are made into each target area. This is done to allow easier access to the target tissue and to prevent depressions around the access sites. The liposuction cannula is connected to the large-bore suction tubing and high-vacuum suction. Superficial aspiration is performed with a 2- or 3-mm cannula. Deep aspiration requires a 4- or 5-mm cannula.

Aspiration is continued until the desired volume of fat has been removed or the desired shape has been achieved. The cannula is removed, and the incisions are closed with 3-0 absorbable suture. If the extremities have been treated, a compression stocking is applied to provide support and reduce postoperative swelling.

PANNICULECTOMY (ABDOMINOPLASTY)

Surgical Goal

Panniculectomy is performed to remove excess skin and adipose tissue from the abdominal wall.

Pathology

Abdominoplasty usually is performed as a cosmetic procedure, but it also can be performed for medical reasons. After significant weight loss, the skin of the abdomen hangs flaccid and can interfere with normal body movement. In some cases, the redundant skin can hang to the level of the knees. This "apron" makes movement and activities of daily living very difficult. In these cases, a panniculectomy is considered a medically necessary procedure.

Technique

1. With the patient in the standing position, the incision line is marked in the natural skin fold of the lower abdomen.
2. A low transverse incision is made, extending to both inguinal areas.
3. The skin or subcutaneous tissue flap is elevated away from the anterior abdominal wall.
4. **Plication** (folding) of the rectus abdominis may be performed from the level of the xyphoid process to the mons pubis.
5. The skin and subcutaneous tissue flaps are pulled inferiorly, and the excess tissue is excised.
6. A small midline incision is made through which the umbilicus may be delivered.
7. The umbilicus is sutured in place.
8. The abdominal incision is closed in two layers with drains in place.
9. Postoperatively the patient is placed in high Fowler position to reduce tension on the abdomen.

Discussion

Before the procedure, the surgeon marks the incisions while the patient is standing to assess the areas of excision.

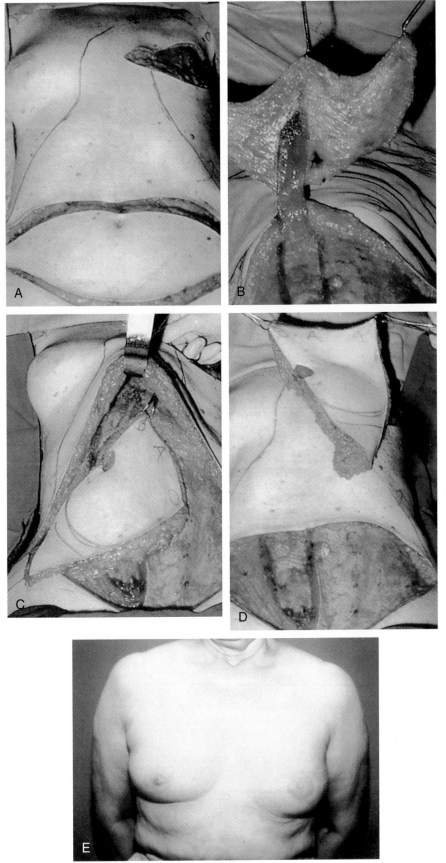

Figure 29-15 Transverse rectus abdominis myocutaneous (TRAM) flap for postmastectomy breast reconstruction. *(From Fortunato N, McCullough SM: Plastic and reconstructive surgery, St Louis, 1998, Mosby.)*

In the operating room, the patient is placed under general anesthesia. The individual is prepped from the nipples to the thighs and draped for an abdominal procedure. The patient is placed in semi-Fowler position to reduce tension on the abdominal tissue.

A transverse, U-shaped incision is made in the lower pelvis and extended to the fascia. Skin flaps are elevated with the ESU and Metzenbaum scissors. The umbilicus is excised and left in its natural position. The skin flap is further elevated to the level of the xyphoid process and the inferior sternal borders.

The abdominal wall may be folded (imbricated) from the xyphoid process to the mons pubis. This is done with 2-0 nonabsorbable suture (e.g., Prolene). The skin flap then is pulled inferiorly, and the excess skin is excised with the ESU. A small midline incision is made in the skin flap with a #15 blade to allow for delivery of the umbilicus into its natural position. The umbilicus is sutured into place with 3-0 absorbable suture. The abdominal wound is closed in two layers with absorbable suture. Dressings are applied, and the patient is maintained in semi-Fowler position to prevent tension on the suture line.

CHAPTER SUMMARY

- **Plastic and reconstructive surgery** involves the treatment of congenital defects and anatomical abnormalities caused by disease and injury. Restoration of form and function is the primary goal of treatment.
- **Aesthetic surgery,** also called *cosmetic surgery,* is performed to improve the appearance but does not address function.
- Most cosmetic surgery involves only the skin; therefore, the instruments are short and have fine tips.
- Reconstruction procedures may require fine orthopedic instruments, including small bone clamps, toothed tissue forceps, and small Kocher clamps. Rasps, small osteotomes, and fine curettes also should be available during procedures involving bone tissue.
- The dermatome is used to remove split thickness skin grafts. The Brown type dermatome is the most commonly used.
- Dressings in plastic and reconstructive surgery provide wound protection and physical support to remodeled structures. Complex reconstructive procedures require a variety of materials and techniques. Dressing routines in these procedures are exact and are considered a critical step of the procedure.
- Grafting is the surgical implantation of biological or manufactured material into an area of the body.
- Split-thickness skin graft (STSG) contains only the dermis while a full thickness skin graft (FTSG) contains both dermis and epidermis. A composite graft is one that contains two or more types of tissue.
- An implant is a synthetic, natural, or biosynthetic substance used to fill in or replace an anatomical structure.
- For diseased or traumatized tissue to heal, all devitalized or infected areas must be removed. The process of removing the disease, damaged, or infected tissue is called debridement.
- During **Mohs surgery**, a malignant skin lesion is removed and cut into quadrants before frozen section. These quadrants are used to map the tumor and determine the exact location of malignant margins

- (see Figure 29-6). Further excision is performed until the specimen is clear of all malignancy.
- Burns are classified according to the depth of tissue injury.
- In a superficial partial thickness, first-degree burn, only the outer layer of the epidermis is injured. The skin is red or pink, dry, and painful to touch.
- A partial thickness second-degree burn is one in which the epidermis and various degrees of the dermis are injured. The skin is blistered, red, and moist. The burn is very sensitive to environmental exposure and touch.
- In a full-thickness, second degree burn, the epidermis and full dermis are injured. These burns are characterized by a white, smooth, shiny surface with dry blisters and edema.
- Proper assembly of the dermatome blade and head is critical to prevent skin tissue from tearing during the procedure.
- The skin graft mesher is used to perforate a skin graft. This increases its surface area and prevents serum from accumulating under the graft once it is in place.
- In a full-thickness, third-degree burn, the subcutaneous tissue, muscle, and bone are burned. The third-degree burn is centered in an area of second-degree injury. The skin may be white, brown, or black and appears waxy. There is no pain because nerves have been destroyed.
- Third-degree burns develop **eschar,** which is devitalized, nonelastic tissue that adheres to the wound site.
- Mineral oil is applied to the donor skin graft site to reduce the friction between the skin and dermatome blade.
- A stent is a special dressing applied over a skin graft. The dressing provides continuous pressure on the site to keep the graft in contact with the wound during healing.
- A pedicle graft is a composite graft in which a flap of tissue is partially released from one area of the body and attached to the wound site. When healing is complete, the flap is released, and the donor site defect is closed primarily with sutures.

- Blepharoplasty resection of the eyelid is done to improve vision of the upper visual fields.
- Brow lift procedures are done to lift the supportive structures of the brow and alleviate drooping of skin, muscle, and fascia.
- The normal aging process and certain environmental factors such as smoking and exposure to excessive ultraviolet light contribute to sagging and wrinkling of the skin. Rhytidectomy is performed to remodle the skin and underlying tissue.
- Facial augmentation is performed to give normal contours to the chin or cheek. This is achieved by inserting a molded implant in the affected area.
- Otoplasty is performed to correct a congenital malformation of the external ear or to create an ear destroyed by trauma. Procedures for otoplasty often involve multiple surgeries. These procedures are somewhat complex, and many approaches can be used, depending on the pathological condition and the patient's needs.

- Augmentation mammoplasty is performed to increase the size and improve the shape of the breast. The procedure is performed in postmastectomy patients and those desiring larger breasts for aesthetic reasons.
- Reduction mammoplasty may be performed for cosmetic or medical reasons. Macromastia (excessively large breasts) is related to the weight and size of the breast. The increased forward weight can cause cervical and thoracic pain.
- A transverse rectus abdominus myocutaneous (TRAM) flap procedure is performed to augement the breast without the use of implants. In this procedure a flap is raised from the abdomen and transferred to the chest wall as a pedicle graft.
- Penniculectomy (abdominoplasty) is performed for cosmetic reduction of abdominal fat. An "apron" of tissue is removed in severe cases to improve the patient's quality of life.

REVIEW QUESTIONS

1. What are the three classifications of burns? Describe them.
2. When is debridement necessary for the treatment of burns?
3. What is compartment syndrome?
4. Differentiate full-thickness and split-thickness skin grafts.
5. Explain the purpose of a flap graft.
6. What is a biosynthetic material?

BIBLIOGRAPHY

Aston SJ, Beasely RW, Thorne CHM: *Grabb and Smith's plastic surgery,* ed 5, Philadelphia, 1997, Lippincott-Raven.

Cummings C, Flint P, Haughey B, Robbins K, Thomas J et al: *Cummings otolaryngology—head and neck surgery,* Philadelphia, 2005, Mosby.

Marks MW, Marks C: *Fundamentals of plastic surgery,* Philadelphia, 1997, WB Saunders.

Phillips N: *Berry and Kohn's operating room technique,* ed 11, St Louis, 2007, Mosby.

Rothrock JC: *Alexander's care of the patient in surgery,* ed 13, St Louis, 2007, Mosby.

Sandberg DJ, McGee WP, Denk MJ: Neonatal cleft lip and cleft palate repair, *AORN Journal* 75(3):490, 2002.

Tyers AG, Collin JRO: *Colour atlas of ophthalmic plastic surgery,* ed 2, Oxford, 2001, Butterworth-Heinemann.

Weerda H: *Reconstructive facial plastic surgery: a problem-solving manual,* New York, 2001, Thieme.

CHAPTER 30

Orthopedic Surgery

CHAPTER OUTLINE

LEARNING OBJECTIVES

After studying this chapter the reader will be able to:

- Identify major skeletal structures, including bones and joints
- Describe safety concerns when transporting and positioning an orthopedic patient
- Describe specific patient positions used in orthopedic surgery
- Identify common fracture types

- Identify common hardware used in fracture fixation
- Demonstrate the safe use of power equipment
- Discuss the principles of open and closed fixation
- Describe techniques used in arthroscopic surgery
- Identify the surgical goals of common orthopedic procedures

TERMINOLOGY

Abduction: Movement of a body part away from the midline.

Adduction: Movement of a body part toward the midline.

Alloys: Substances that are mixtures of pure metals.

Aponeurosis: A tendenous sheet which separates mucles or attaches a muscle to bone.

Arthrodesis: Surgical fusion of a joint.

Arthroscopy: Endoscopic assessment and surgery of a joint.

Bioactive implant: An orthopedic implant which releases calcium to enhance healing.

Biocompatibility: A term that describes a material that is compatible with tissue (i.e., causes no toxic or inflammatory effect).

Biomechanics: The relationship between movement and biological or anatomical structures.

Bone wax (Ostene): A waxy substance used to control capillary bleeding on the surface of bone.

Broach: A fin-shaped rasp used to enlarge the medullary canal for insertion of an implant. The broach is the same shape as the implant.

Cannulated: A device having a hollow core; for example, an instrument with a central channel that can be fitted over a guide wire or pin.

Casting: A method of immobilizing a limb by the application of rigid or semi-rigid material along the length of the limb. A cast can be fully or partially circumferential.

Closed reduction: Alignment of bone fragments into anatomical position by manipulation or traction.

Comminuted: A fracture in which there are multiple bone fragments.

Compression: Mechanical force in which a structures is compacted or pressed together. Compression is used to repair tissue. A compression injury (e.g., compression fracture) results when bone or other tissue is compacted.

Condyle: The rounded end of a long bone. A condyle plate is a contoured implant which fits over the condyle and also extends along the shaft of the bone, used to repair a fracture of the condyle.

Cruciate: Cross shaped.

Debridement: A process in which a contaminated, infected, avascular tissue or debris is cut away or removed from a wound.

Dislocation: Displacement of a joint from its normal position.

Distraction (distractor): A mechanical process in which a structure is elongated. Distraction can be used to suspend a limb (and thereby stretch the soft tissue) and bones during surgery. A distraction injury is caused by the pulling apart or stretching of tissue (the opposite of a compression injury).

Examination under anesthesia (EUA): Fracture and dislocation may be fully assessed when general anesthesia is used.

External fixation: A method of stabilizing bone fragments in anatomical position from outside the body. A cast is an example of an external fixation device.

Fasciotomy: A procedure in which fascia is incised to release pressure caused by swelling within a muscle bundle.

Inert: Nonreactive; causing little or no reaction in tissue. A desirable characteristic of tissue implants.

Internal fixation: A method of surgically repairing a fracture by inserting an implant a device that holds the bone fragments in place. Metal plates, rods, pins, and screws are examples of internal fixation devices.

Open reduction: Surgical access (through an incision) to bring bone fragments into anatomical alignment.

Orthopedic system: A specific (usually patented) set of instruments and implants used for an orthopedic technique. For example, arthroplasty implants are marketed as systems which include the joint components and instruments that are designed for use with that implant.

Osteophytes: Bony outgrowths found in an arthritic joint.

Osteotomy: A surgical cut into bone tissue.

Press-fit: To impact or press a joint implant into position. Press-fitted implants do not require bone cement.

Ream: To enlarge a pre-existing hole, depression, or channel, such as the medullary canal.

Replantation (reimplantation): Surgical attachment of the hand, thumb, or fingers after traumatic amputation.

Reduction: The process of manipulating a bone structure to restore anatomical position.

Revision arthroplasty: A repeat arthroplasty in which previously implanted joint components are replaced.

Skeletal traction: Traction device in which is connected by pins or rods which are surgically inserted into the bone.

Skin traction: Taping a traction system to the skin, used as a temporary measure only (e.g., Buck traction). Skin traction is seldom used in adults in modern medicine.

Slap hammer: A type of impactor used primarily in arthroplasty to seat a joint component into the bone.

Traction: A mechanical method of applying pulling force to fractured bone.

INTRODUCTION

Orthopedic surgery is a specialization of the body's connective tissues. These tissues are the framework of the body in a supporting and binding function. Surgery is performed to treat or to correct injuries, congenital anomalies, and disease of the bone, joints, ligaments, tendons, or muscle. Most orthopedic procedures focus on restoring bone and joint function, lost or diminished because of traumatic injury or disease. Alleviating pain is also a primary goal of surgical intervention.

Proficiency in orthopedic techniques relies heavily on a thorough understanding of the instrumentation and implants used for repair and reconstruction. Orthopedic techniques and **biomechanics** share many of the principles and language used in carpentry and engineering.

Many procedures rely on the use of an **orthopedic system**, which is a set of instruments and a technique specific for one surgical approach. For example, a fracture can be repaired with a plate, screws, wire, or a rod placed through the medullary canal for stability during healing. A typical system for any of these repairs might include the hardware (plate, screws, or rod) and specialty instruments designed for use with that particular company's hardware. Most manufacturers' system components are not interchangeable with those of another manufacturer, although some generic hardware does exist.

Although a daunting number of systems are available and in development, the biomechanical principles of orthopedics remain constant. The key to developing advanced skills is to learn basic principles and apply them to complex systems.

SURGICAL ANATOMY

SKELETON

The skeleton (Figure 30-1) provides structural support for the soft tissues of the body. For classification purposes the *skeleton* is divided into two parts: the *axial* skeleton, which includes the skull, face, ear bones, hyoid, sternum, and ribs; and the *appendicular skeleton*, which includes the bones of the legs, feet, hands, trunk, and spine. Individual bones usually articulate or join other bones at a joint.

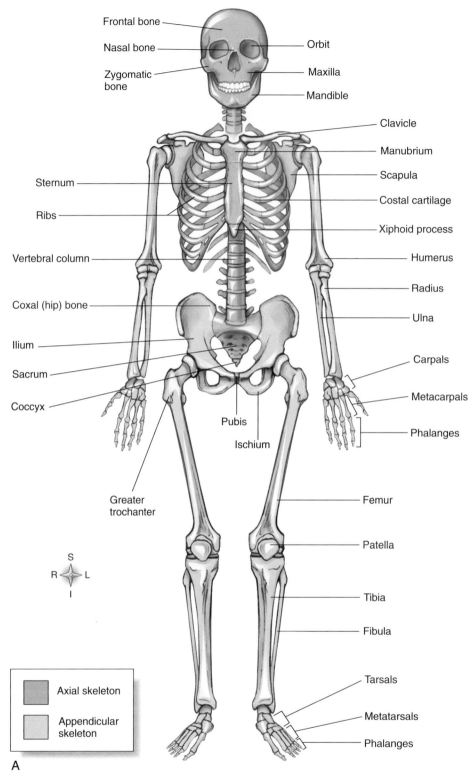

Frontal bone
Nasal bone
Zygomatic bone
Orbit
Maxilla
Mandible
Clavicle
Manubrium
Scapula
Costal cartilage
Xiphoid process
Humerus
Radius
Ulna
Carpals
Metacarpals
Phalanges
Femur
Patella
Tibia
Fibula
Tarsals
Metatarsals
Phalanges
Sternum
Ribs
Vertebral column
Coxal (hip) bone
Ilium
Sacrum
Coccyx
Greater trochanter
Pubis
Ischium

S
R — L
I

Axial skeleton

Appendicular skeleton

A

Figure 30-1 Axial and appendicular skeleton. *(From Thibodeau G, Patton K: Anatomy and physiology, ed 6, St Louis, 2007, Mosby.)*

Axial Skeleton

The axial skeleton is composed of the skull and facial bones, vertebral column, sternum, and ribs. The skull, or *cranium,* has eight main bones that are connected by tough connective tissue called *sutures.* The brain is encased within the cranium, which includes the floor of the skull, and the sphenoid bone. At birth, the cranial bones are loosely fused. In the prenatal period the sutures are wide and soft, which allows the head to mold as it passes through the mother's pelvis during birth. The *fontanels* are areas where the joint space is particularly wide. These occur in the posterior skull at the junction of the parietal and occipital bones and in the anterior skull between the parietal and frontal bones. The posterior fontanel usually closes by 8 weeks of age and the anterior fontanel at 3 to 18 months of age.

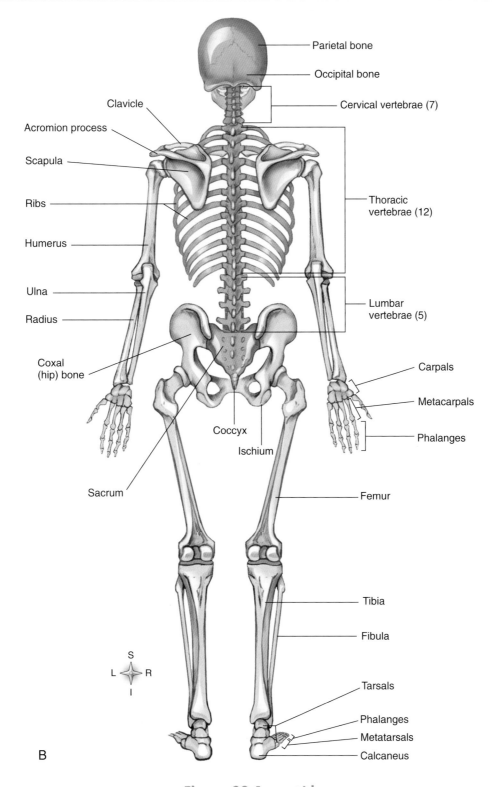

Figure 30-1, cont'd.

The fetal cranium is shaped to allow rapid growth of the brain, which occurs in the first several years of life. In infants, the head accounts for 25% of the total height of the body and is much wider from front to back than the adult skull.

The *facial bones* are more complex and form the structure of the nasal sinus, orbit of the eye, and jaw. Only the *mandible* (lower jaw) is freely moveable. The *zygoma* and *orbital rim* are common sites of fracture in sports and motor vehicle acci-

dents. These bones usually are repaired with small mesh plates. Reconstructive surgery of the face and cranium is a surgical specialty known as *oromaxillofacial surgery* (OMF). This type of surgery is performed to treat congenital malformations, as well as injuries or disease that result in disfigurement and loss of function (see Chapter 28).

The *vertebral column* consists of 24 individual vertebrae: 7 *cervical*, 12 *thoracic*, and 5 *lumbar*. In adults, the sacrum is composed of five vertebrae that are fused. The coccyx is formed by the fusion of four or five vertebrae.

The sternum forms the anterior chest wall and is composed of three sections: the *manubrium,* the *body,* and the *xiphoid process.*

Twelve pairs of ribs connect to their corresponding vertebrae. Ribs one through eight attach to the sternum and are connected by costal cartilage. The eleventh and twelfth ribs are "floating" ribs (i.e., they are not attached anteriorly.

Appendicular Skeleton

The appendicular skeleton is composed of the upper extremities, the lower extremities, and the pelvis.

Upper Extremities

The shoulder includes the *scapula* and *clavicle.* The long bone of the upper arm is the *humerus.* It articulates proximally with the *glenoid fossa.* The *ulna* and *radius* form the forearm, and the *carpel* and *metacarpal* bones form the hand and wrist.

Lower Extremities

The pelvis consists of the *ilium,* the *ischium,* and the *pubis.* The *femur,* or thigh bone, is the longest bone of the body. The *patella* is a sesamoid bone located between the femur and the lower leg. The lower leg bones are the *tibia* and the *fibula.* The foot is made up of the *calcaneus,* the *cuboid* and *navicular* bones, and the five *tarsals* and *metatarsals* (toes).

BONE TISSUE

The body has two types of bone tissue: *cortical* bone and *cancellous* bone. Cortical bone (also called *compact bone*) is found on the surface of bones and is organized in tubular units called *osteons.* Osteons resemble the rings of a tree. Each tubular unit has a central canal (the *haversian* canal), which provides nutrition and carries away cellular waste products. Blood vessels are located in the central canals. The concentric layers (lamina) of each osteon are composed of calcified tissue.

The ends of bones and the inner layer are composed of softer, less dense cancellous bone (also called *spongy bone*). Cancellous bone is less dense than cortical bone and has no geometric structure. Instead, the structure resembles a sponge, and the spaces are filled with red or yellow marrow, a soft connective tissue. Red marrow, which produces blood cells, is found in the center of certain long bones, in the vertebrae, and in pelvic bones. The structure of bone tissue is illustrated in Figure 30-2.

BONE MEMBRANES

Bones are covered with a tough, bilayered membrane called *periosteum.* The function of the periosteum is to protect the bone surface and provide attachment for tendons. It also contains osteoblasts. These are the bone's growth cells; they provide a source of development and repair in the same way that tree bark functions.

❖ *The periosteum is an important tissue in orthopedic surgery. It must be scraped away from the bone before cutting or remodeling. This is done with a periosteal elevator.*

The *endosteum* lines the inner channels of long bones. It also fills the *interstitial spaces* (i.e., the spaces between cells) of cancellous bone, as well as the haversian canals. The endosteum initiates bone growth and provides nutritional substances to bone.

BONE STRUCTURE AND SHAPE

The long bones are characterized by a middle shaft, called the *diaphysis,* and the two ends, called the *epiphyses* (sing., epiphysis). Bones with these features include the bones of the legs, arms, and digits (i.e., the fingers and toes). The shaft is composed mostly of compact bone and has a hollow center. The transition between the diaphysis and epiphysis is not readily apparent except during development, when the region is filled with cartilage. This developmental tissue is called the *epiphyseal plate* or *metaphysis.* It is significant in fracture pathology, because a break in this area may delay growth of the bone in a child. The hollow cavity inside a mature long bone is called the *medullary canal.* The epiphyses are wider and have bony outcroppings and protrusions where the ligaments are attached. The epiphyses, which are composed of cancellous bone, form the joints, which are covered with cartilage, a resilient connective tissue that increases the strength of the joint and reduces friction between the bones. Figure 30-3 illustrates the parts of a long bone and its membranes.

Bones can be classified by their shape. The *short* bones are those of the wrist and ankle. *Irregular* bones include the vertebrae, spine, and face. A few irregularly shaped bones occur singly; these are referred to as *sesamoid bones.* The patella is an example of a sesamoid bone.

Flat bones usually are thin compared to other types of bones. In adults, the inner cancellous layer of the flat bones contain red marrow. (In other types of bones, red marrow converts to yellow marrow during childhood and persists into adulthood). The ribs, cranial bones, scapula, and sternum are examples of flat bones.

LANDMARKS

Bones have many different irregularities, called *landmarks.* These function as areas of attachment for tendons and ligaments or provide a passageway for nerves and blood vessels. They appear as raised projections, bumps, ridges, channels, and tunnels. Some common types of landmarks are listed in Box 30-1. The body has many hundreds of bone landmarks. Differentiating the different types of landmarks is less important than recognizing them as identifiers of significant or common anatomical sites. Specific landmarks are referred to in surgical procedures to clarify the technique. For example, "an osteotomy was performed in the femoral neck." This means that the neck of the femur was incised, or cut. Another example of an important landmark is the iliac *crest,* which is a common site for harvesting a bone graft.

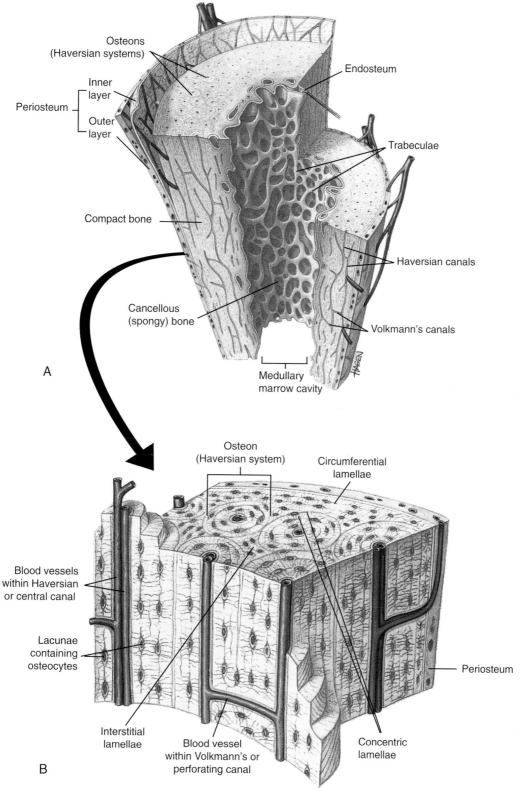

Figure 30-2 Structure of bone tissue. **A,** Longitudinal section of a long bone. **B,** Compact bone.

Continued

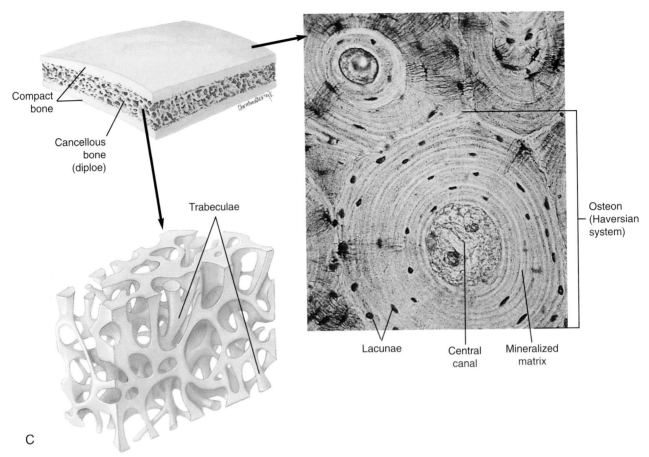

Compact bone

Cancellous bone (diploe)

Trabeculae

Osteon (Haversian system)

Lacunae

Central canal

Mineralized matrix

C

Figure 30-2, cont'd   C, Flat bone, showing compact and cancellous layers, haversian system, and trabeculae. *(From Thibodeau G, Patton K:* Anatomy and physiology, *ed 6, St Louis, 2007, Mosby.)*

BONE HEALING

Bone healing takes place through a complex process that resembles soft tissue repair. However, the process is slower. Return of full function may take 6 months or longer, especially in weight-bearing bones. The three phases of bone healing are the inflammatory phase, the reparative phase, and the remodeling phase.

Inflammatory Phase

When bone suffers a traumatic injury, blood arising from the bone itself and from the adjacent soft tissue accumulates at the fracture site. The body's clotting mechanism is triggered, and fibrin is released to form the basis of platelet aggregation and hematoma (congealed blood), which eventually is absorbed by the body. Fibroblasts in the region of the injury create a network of granulation tissue, which is a soft, spongy matrix of connective tissue and blood vessels.

Reparative Phase

During the reparative phase, growth cells originating from the periosteum develop into rudimentary bone cells and cartilage. These proliferate and form a callus, which fills in the space between the bone fragments. This normally occurs within a few days of injury. Ossification occurs as the soft callus is

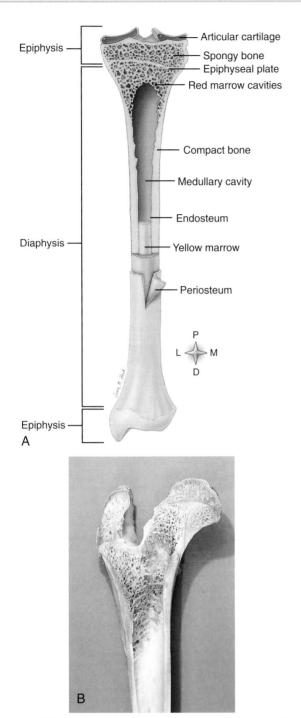

Figure 30-3   Parts of a long bone. *(From Thibodeau G, Patton K: Anatomy and physiology, ed 6, St Louis, 2007, Mosby.)*

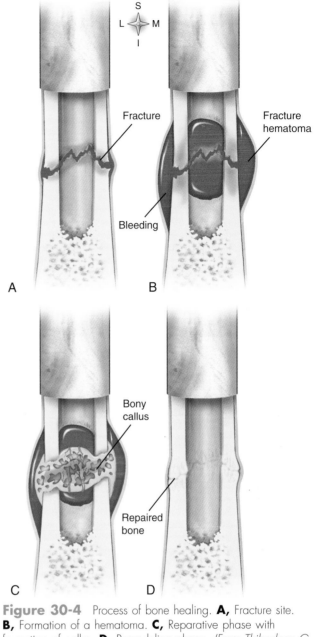

Figure 30-4   Process of bone healing. **A,** Fracture site. **B,** Formation of a hematoma. **C,** Reparative phase with formation of callus. **D,** Remodeling phase. *(From Thibodeau G, Patton K: Anatomy and physiology, ed 6, St Louis, 2007, Mosby.)*

replaced by bone minerals and bone cells. During this phase, a capillary vascular system develops within the matrix.

Remodeling
The remodeling stage is characterized by replacement of the initial bone matrix with compact bone cells and absorption of excess callus. This takes place over a period of weeks or months. The process of bone healing is illustrated in Figure 30-4.

The articular system (joints) includes the areas of the body where two bones meet and some degree of movement occurs. The movement may be small, as in the ossicles of the ear, or large, as in the hip joint.

CLASSIFICATION

Joints are classified according to the degree of movement they allow and also by the shape of the articulating surfaces (Figure 30-5). Joint classifications are as follows:

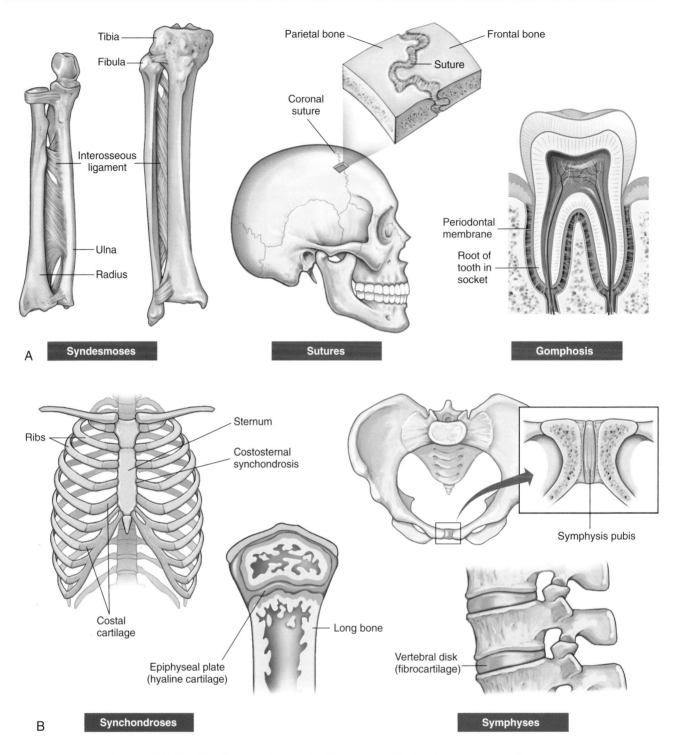

Figure 30-5 Classification of joints. **A,** Fibrous joints. **B,** Cartilaginous joints. *(From Thibodeau G, Patton K: Anatomy and physiology, ed 6, St Louis, 2007, Mosby.)*

- *Synarthrosis (suture joint)*: A joint with limited movement or fixed articular surfaces, such as between the skull bones.
- *Amphiarthrosis (cartilaginous joint)*: A joint in which the bones are connected by cartilage and only slightly moveable. The symphyses joints are included in this category (e.g., symphysis pubis).

- *Diarthrosis (synovial joint)*: A joint that is freely moveable, such as the hip or the shoulder. Most joints of the body are diarthroses. They are also called *synovial joints* because the joint capsule contains a fluid called *synovial fluid*. The synovial joint is the most important type for the study of surgical technology.

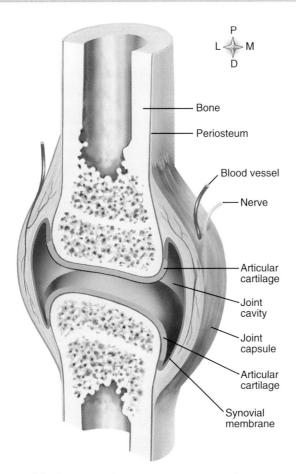

Figure 30-6 Synovial joint structure. *(From Vidic B, Suarez FR: Photographic atlas of the human body, St Louis, 1984, Mosby.)*

Synovial Joints

A synovial joint is composed of articulating bone ends and the connective tissues that surround them (Figure 30-6). The joint capsule surrounds the joint and contains nerves and blood vessels. The capsule is lined with a synovial membrane, which produces a viscous fluid that lubricates and nourishes the joint. The synovial fluid flows out of the joint capsule when it is injured or incised. The articular surfaces of the bones in the joint are covered with cartilage, which aids smooth gliding of one bone surface over the other. The space inside the joint capsule is called the *joint cavity*. During endoscopic joint surgery (**arthroscopy**), the telescope and instruments are inserted into the joint cavity through the capsule.

Nonsynovial Joints

Nonsynovial joints are separated by immoveable cartilaginous or fibrous tissue. These joints are said to have a *fixed* articulation and there is no joint cavity. Nonsynovial joints include the *sutures, synchondroses, symphyses,* and *syndesmoses.*

JOINT MOVEMENT

The flexibility of the joints is the basis of body movement. When a joint becomes diseased or is injured, movement becomes difficult or impossible because of mechanical restrictions or pain.

Joint movement is carefully described in medicine. In surgery, movement terminology often is used during assessment of a joint. Terms are also used to direct patient positioning. In both cases, the surgeon may ask other team members to move a limb in a certain direction or in a spatial orientation. For example, the surgeon may request "more internal rotation" or "increased abduction." Specific terminology is used because less precise terms may cause confusion, resulting in injury to the patient.

Anatomically, a joint moves within its normal range of motion. Each moveable joint of the body is classified according to specific anatomical movements (Figure 30-7). These are described in mechanical terms. The important point is that joints must be manipulated *only within their normal range of motion* to prevent injury. (Chapter 10 reviews terms and presents illustrations related to joint movement.) The types of moveable joints are as follows:

- *Hinge joint:* A joint that has rocker and cradle components, which allow extension and flexion only (e.g., the elbow).
- *Saddle joint:* A joint in which the two components have a complementary convex-concave shape, and the bones slide over each other. The body has only one saddle joint, which is in the thumb. This joint allows flexion, extension, **abduction**, and **adduction**.
- *Gliding joint:* A joint in which relatively flat surfaces of bone slide over each other (e.g., the vertebrae, movement of which allows the spine to flex).
- *Ball-and-socket joint:* A joint with a spherical component and a concave component. Movement occurs in several planes, making this joint the most freely moveable type (e.g., the hip and the humerus). Ball-and-socket joints allow flexion, extension, abduction, adduction, rotation, and circumduction.
- *Pivot joint:* A joint composed of a bony protuberance and an open collar component (e.g., the first and second vertebrae of the neck). This type of joint provides rotation.
- *Condyloid joint:* A joint in which a small protrusion (condyle) slides within a slightly elliptical component (e.g., the carpal bones of the wrist). Condyloid joints allow flexion, extension, abduction, and adduction.

SOFT CONNECTIVE TISSUES

TENDONS AND LIGAMENTS

Muscles and bones are attached by tendons and ligaments:

- Tendons attach muscle to bone.
- Ligaments attach bone to bone.

The fibers of tendons and ligaments can withstand very high levels of stress and tension along the fiber axis. Tendons move within a protective sheath filled with a type of synovial fluid. Their movement to move the muscles often resembles a pulley system. Tendons can take the form of a fibrous cord, or a sheet of connective tissue called an **aponeurosis**. Liga-

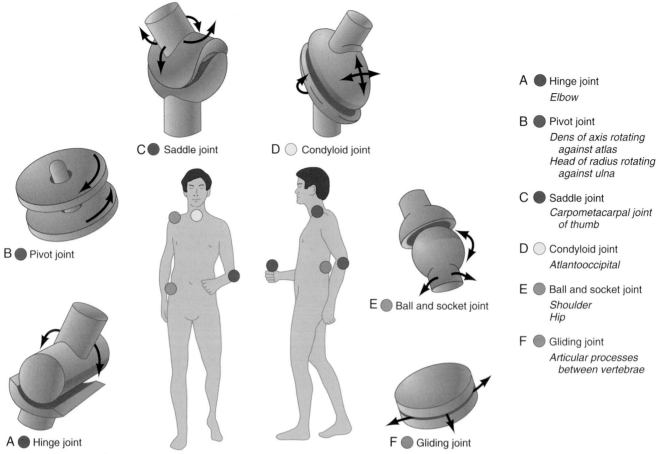

Figure 30-7 Types of moveable joints. *(From Thibodeau G, Patton K: Anatomy and physiology, ed 6, St Louis, 2007, Mosby.)*

ments attach bones to each other, providing flexibility and strength to the skeletal structure. When attached to the cartilage, they stabilize the joint and limit movements that might injure it. Neither tendons nor ligaments have a significant blood supply.

MUSCLE

The three major muscle types in the human body are striated muscle, smooth muscle, and cardiac muscle.

Striated Muscle

Striated muscle, also commonly called *skeletal muscle,* is composed of fibers that are bound together by sheaths of fascia. Each group of fibers and its associated sheath are bound together to form one muscle. Striated muscle is under voluntary control and makes up most of the body's muscle tissue (Figure 30-8).

Smooth Muscle

Smooth muscle is also called *involuntary muscle* because it is not under conscious control. These muscles are found principally in the internal organs, especially the digestive tract, respiratory passages, urinary and genital ducts, urinary bladder, and gallbladder and in the walls of blood vessels. In structures such as the bladder and intestine, smooth muscle

has two layers: an outer longitudinal layer and an inner circular layer. When the muscles such as those in the intestine contract and relax, the contents of the moved along the length of the intestine. This is referred to as *peristalsis.* Peristalsis occurs in many other tubular structures of the body such as the esophagus, ureters, and fallopian tubes that also contain smooth muscle.

Cardiac Muscle

As the name implies, cardiac muscle is the muscle of the heart. Like voluntary muscle, cardiac muscle is striated, but these muscles are involuntary. Cardiac muscle is responsible for the sustained contractions of the heart and for movement of blood into and out of the heart. This mechanism, as well as the rate of contraction, is driven by a complex series of impulses from the autonomic nervous system.

PATHOLOGY

Table 30-1 presents common pathological conditions of the bones and joints.

DIAGNOSTIC PROCEDURES

A variety of imaging procedures are used to diagnose orthopedic trauma and disease, including the following:

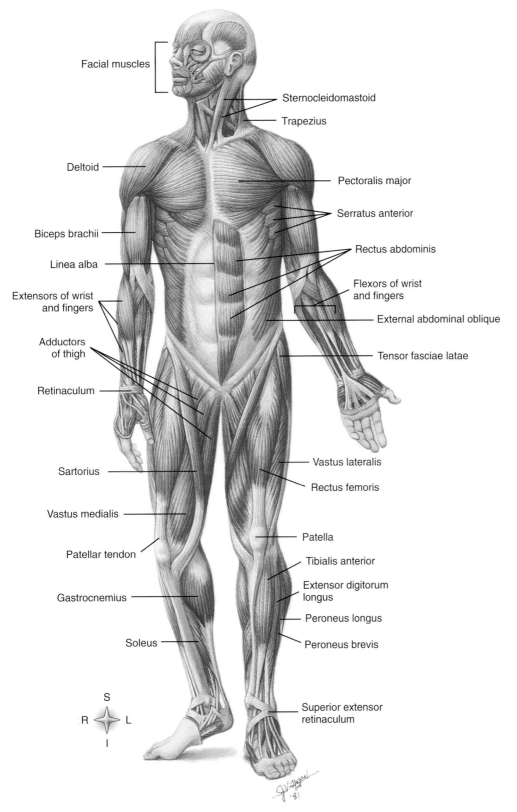

Figure 30-8 Striated muscles of the body. *(From Thibodeau G, Patton K:* Anthony's textbook of anatomy and physiology, *ed 17, St Louis, 2003, Mosby.)*

Continued

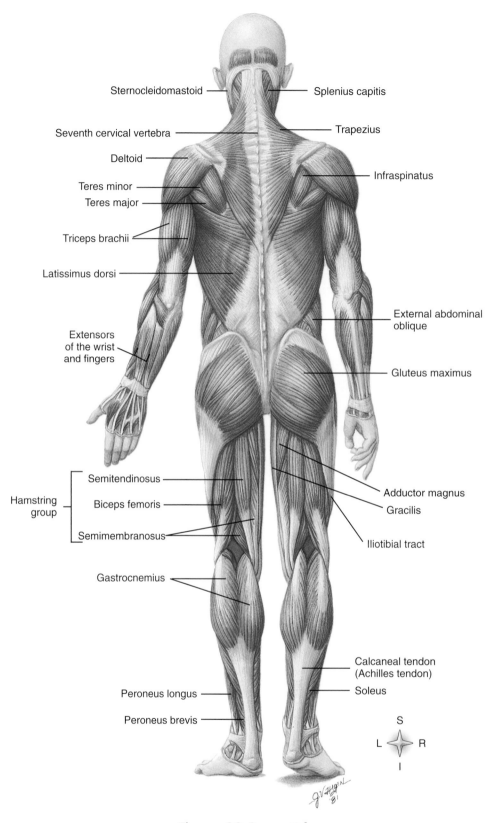

Figure 30-8, cont'd.

Table 30-1

Pathology of the Bones and Joints

Condition	Description	Considerations
Rheumatoid arthritis (RA)	RA is a systemic inflammatory disease that affects connective tissue. It is progressive and involves autoimmune factors that cause joint and soft tissue degeneration and deformity. It can be fatal.	The goals of medical treatment are to stop the progression of tissue damage and control pain. A number of drugs are used to treat various pathologies associated with the disease. Advanced joint degeneration may require joint replacement. (See the sections on arthroplasty procedures.)
Osteoarthritis	Joint disease characterized by swelling, pain, and loss of function. It most often is age related but can occur secondary to chronic overuse or injury of a joint with an intrinsic metabolic disorder of the cartilage. It does not cause deformity.	Conservative treatment is aimed at reducing inflammation and pain, especially when activities of daily living are restricted. Joint arthroplasty is performed in advanced disease.
Malignant bone tumor	Primary bone tumors are relatively uncommon; most are metastatic tumors of another tissue. About 1% of tumors are primary to bone. The most important are malignant osteosarcoma and Ewing sarcoma, which are quickly metastatic.	Treatment is surgical to debulk or remove the tumor, followed by radiation and chemotherapy.
Metastatic bone disease	Bone is a frequent site of tumor metastasis, which occurs commonly in breast, lung, prostate, kidney, and thyroid cancer. The primary symptom is pain and pathological fracture. The diagnosis is made with imaging studies and selected blood tests.	Treatment is palliative using radiation and chemotherapy. Medical goals include restoring mobility and flexibility and pain control.
Osteoporosis	Osteoporosis is a metabolic disease of bone involving increased porosity, which leads to decreased bone mass and pathological fracture. It is most commonly associated with advancing age in females but is also related to malignancy or an endocrine disorder.	Lowering risk factors is the most important means of preventing osteoporosis. For more information on prevention, refer to the National Osteoporosis Foundation Web site at http://www.nof.org.
Scoliosis	Scoliosis is a disease that affects the spinal column, resulting in rotation and curvature. Postural scoliosis can be corrected with physiotherapy and exercise. Structural disease is a congenital defect arising during fetal life or as a result of neurological or muscle disease.	Early screening in childhood is required in most states. Structural scoliosis is treated with bracing or surgically with rod or plate implants. (See Chapter 35.)
Avascular necrosis	Necrosis of bone tissue occurs when the blood supply is interrupted. The resulting ischemia can affect all areas of the bone, including the medullary canal. The cause of the disease often is trauma; it may be a complication of a complex fracture in which soft tissues, including blood vessels, are crushed. Other causes are thrombosis, embolism, and prolonged use of corticosteroids.	Treatment includes resting the area, and administration of nonsteroidal antiinflammatory agents. Osteonecrosis of a joint may be treated with joint arthroplasty.
Osteomyelitis	Osteomyelitis is infection of the bone and medullary canal. It usually is associated with an open fracture or communication to the bone through a traumatic wound, including those made during surgery. The disease is characterized by pain, inflammation, purulence, and destruction of bone.	Rigorous antibacterial therapy is initiated as soon as possible after diagnosis. Continuous irrigation and debridement of the wound help remove dead and infected tissue. Recovery usually is long.
Compartment syndrome	Compartment syndrome is tissue damage and necrosis resulting from increased pressure in any anatomical space; the term usually refers to the muscle compartment of a limb. The syndrome results in permanent loss of function because of nerve and vascular injury.	An emergency response is needed to relieve the pressure. A **fasciotomy** is performed, in which multiple longitudinal incisions are made through the fascia of the affected limb.
Pathological fracture	A pathological fracture is a fracture caused by disease (e.g., osteoporosis, cancer) rather than injury.	Treatment depends on the type and severity of the fracture.
Benign neoplasm	Benign neoplasms are noncancerous tumors that arise from connective tissue. Examples are osteoma (arising from bone), chondroma (arising from cartilage), and osteochondroma (arising from the growth plate).	Surgical excision is necessary when benign tumors interfere with function or impinge on other vital structures.
Systemic lupus erythematosus (SLE)	SLE is a chronic, often lift-threatening inflammatory disease that may affect any organ; it commonly causes nondegenerative arthritis.	Treatment is medical and varies widely, depending on the target tissue and systemic effects of the disease.

- *Radiography:* Radiographs are the first-level assessment in most cases of orthopedic trauma.
- *Magnetic resonance imaging (MRI):* MRI scans generally are not used for routine diagnosis of fractures, but they commonly are done for spinal cord injuries and for tumors of the musculoskeletal system.
- *Computed tomography (CT):* CT scans are used for complex fractures, joint disease, and trauma. The scans produce cross-sectional images that are valuable in the diagnosis of tumors and internal injury caused by trauma.
- *CT-angiography:* In orthopedics, angiograms are used to diagnose vascular injury caused by trauma.
- *Ultrasonography:* Ultrasound scans routinely are done in cases involving complex traumatic injuries.

SPECIAL STUDIES

Selected trauma cases require assessment for soft tissue damage associated with injury and disease.

PATIENT TRANSPORT AND TRANSFER

Patients undergoing an orthopedic procedure arrive for surgery either shortly after a traumatic injury or as "well" patients who are having reconstructive or joint replacement surgery. Trauma patients and those with a chronic skeletal injury require special handling during transport and transferal to the operating table.

Trauma patients may arrive in traction (explained later), an external splinting device, or an antishock garment. The transfer may be completed after administration of an anesthetic to reduce the patient's discomfort. It is important to maintain anatomical alignment of the body at all times during the transfer. This may require extra personnel to complete the transfer safely. Traction equipment must be monitored carefully to ensure that weights and pulleys are not dislodged. Teamwork is essential in transferring a trauma patient.

POSITIONING

Patients are positioned for orthopedic surgery on the standard operating table or on a specialty table. (Chapter 10 presents a complete description of important safety precautions for preventing patient injury during positioning.)

The modern orthopedic table (also called a *fracture table*) is used mainly for surgery of the femur and lower leg. This table supports the operative leg while providing open access to the femur. The open design of the table also allows safe and rapid positioning of the C-arm fluoroscope. Features of the orthopedic table include:

- Jointed (articulated) components to hold the leg in traction
- Open design of the lower portion to allow positioning of the C-arm
- Translucent support surfaces

Many standard operating tables can be converted to allow femoral or lower extremity surgery by removing the foot section and replacing it with adjustable leg suspension devices.

The Fowler position can be created for shoulder surgery by adjusting the articulated sections of the table, and replacing the normal headboard with an open-design head stabilizer. It is important to allow adequate time to make these modifications before the patient arrives in surgery. Table accessories can be quite heavy, therefore adequate personnel should be available for assembly.

Positions associated with a specific surgical exposure are described in Table 30-2 and shown in Figures 30-9 through 30-13.

HEMOSTASIS

Bone tissue bleeds profusely when cut. However, the bleeding arises from capillaries that cannot be ligated. Hip arthroplasty and open reduction of a hip fracture have been associated with a high risk of significant blood loss. However, refined instrumentation and improved surgical techniques have reduced this risk. Total blood loss is determined by weighing surgical sponges and measuring the volume of blood in the suction canister. Trauma patients are evaluated before surgery, and blood products are administered as needed.

PNEUMATIC TOURNIQUET

The pneumatic tourniquet (discussed in Chapter 17) is used in all extremity surgery. The components of the tourniquet are the cuff, the regulator, and the tubing. An appropriate-size cuff must be selected according to the patient's size. The tourniquet cuff is placed proximal to the surgical site before the patient is prepped. Webril bandaging material is wrapped over the tourniquet site carefully to reduce any folds or pinching in the skin. The cuff then is secured over the bandaging. The regulator is adjusted for the patient's blood pressure but not activated. After the surgical prep and draping, a rubber bandage (Esmarch bandage) is used to exsanguinate the limb. The bandage is applied in a proximal direction, causing blood to flow out of the limb. The tourniquet then is inflated, providing a nearly bloodless surgical field.

Pneumatic tourniquets have been associated with skin, nerve, and vessel damage and embolus when used improperly. Numerous safety protocols guide their application and use. Before and after application, the skin must be assessed for injury or potential damage. Tourniquet times depend on the patient's overall medical condition and tissue status. (Chapter 17 presents illustrations and a more detailed discussion of the pneumatic tourniquet.)

A Web site covering all clinical aspects of tourniquet use, including current guidelines from the Association of periOperative Registered Nurses (AORN), can be found at http://www.tourniquets.org/aorn.html.

HEMOSTATIC AGENTS

During surgery, a waxy preparation called **bone wax (Ostene)** is pressed into bleeding areas to control oozing. Beeswax combinations traditionally have been used for this purpose. Other hemostatic agents, such as topical thrombin, are used in peripheral tissues during microsurgery of the hand.

Table 30-2

Positions for Surgical Exposure in Orthopedic Surgery

Anatomical Area	Position	Special Features*
Shoulder and humerus	Beach chair (modified Fowler position)	• Head is stabilized with a Mayfield headrest or similar attachment. • Upper body is flexed 45 to 60 degrees. • Operative shoulder is slightly over the table edge. • Nonoperative shoulder is padded at the scapula. • Vertical foot board may be required.
Forearm and elbow	Supine with hand table extension	• Operative arm is extended on a hand table at no greater than 90 degree of abduction.
	Supine or semilateral using "over chest" extension	• Operative arm is abducted and elevated over the thorax with the elbow flexed. • Stabilizers are used to maintain the semilateral position (table supports, foam wedges).
Wrist and hand	Supine with hand table extension	• Operative arm is extended on a hand table at no greater than 90 degrees of abduction. • Pad or "bump" is placed under the wrist for stabilization.
	Supine with hand suspended in sterile distracter	• Separate sterile accessories are required for the distracter.
Pelvis	Supine	• Precautions are taken to protect nerves and blood vessels.
	Prone	• Lower extremities may be held in traction. • Precautions are taken for respiratory clearance. • Lower table section may be removed.
Hip and femur	Supine using standard operating table	• No special accessories are required.
	Supine using fracture table	• Operative leg is in traction or distraction. • Nonoperative leg rests on a perpendicular crutch or is extended in a boot accessory. • Perineal stop (post) requires substantial padding. • Allows complete clearance above and below lower extremities.
	Lateral	• Stabilizers are used to maintain the lateral position (table supports or padded wedges).
Knee and lower leg	Supine	• Operative knee is supported in variable flexed position with foot or knee-crutch support. • Operative leg may be suspended over the table edge for intraoperative manipulation.
Ankle and foot	Supine	• Supine or prone position is used with the operative leg in free position or elevated on padding.

*Normal precautions to protect nerves, vessels, and respiratory clearance are observed for all positions.

INFECTION CONTROL

Orthopedic surgery is performed with particular attention to the risk of airborne contaminants and droplet contamination. Postoperative infection after joint replacement (arthroplasty) can result in destruction of the joint, with no recourse for further treatment. Osteomyelitis after any orthopedic surgery can result in long-term disability.

Orthopedic procedures are commonly performed in operating suites with laminar airflow, or "super clean" air capability. In laminar airflow, air moves in linear patterns, entering at one wall and exiting at another. Super clean air is created with fresh air exchanges that occur at a rate of more than 300 changes per minute. Laminar airflow and systems used to create super clean air significantly reduce the number of airborne organisms.

Other methods of reducing airborne contaminants include ultraviolet light and the use of vented operating attire, or "space suits," which consist of a vented head bubble and body suit.

FRACTURES

Fractures occur as a result of trauma or disease. Traumatic bone injury may be complicated by soft tissue injury, with critical damage to nerves and blood vessels.

CLASSIFICATION OF FRACTURES

Fractures are medically classified for reporting and treatment purposes. Several classification systems are used. Classification is important to the surgical technologist, because it provides information needed for preparation of the appropriate instrumentation, for positioning, and for the surgical approach. Systems of classification vary by the type of criteria they use:

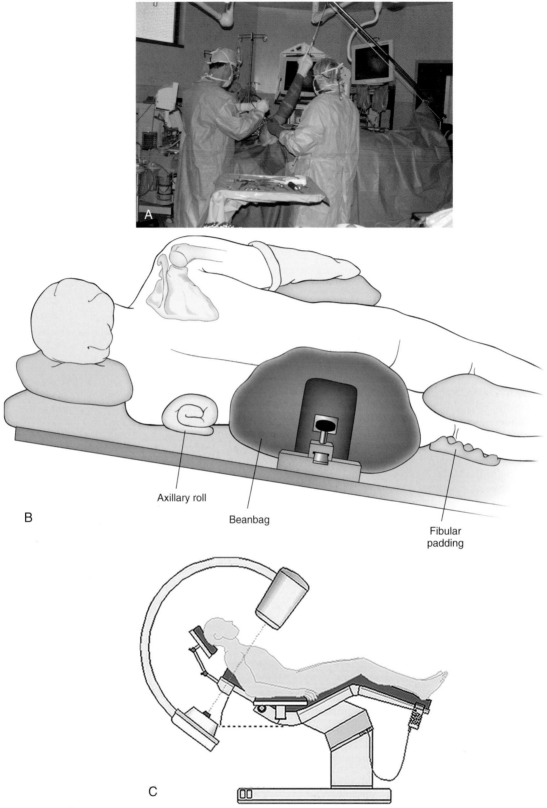

Figure 30-9 Positioning for shoulder surgery. **A,** Supine position with the arm suspended in an overhead distractor to allow manipulation. **B,** Lateral position using an arm board for a posterior approach to the shoulder. **C,** Semi-Fowler (beach chair) position with the C-arm in place. (**A** from Canale S, Beaty J: Campbell's operative orthopaedics, ed 11, St Louis, 2007, Mosby; **B** from Miller MD, Chhabra AB, Hurwitz SK, Mihalko WM: Orthopaedic surgical approaches, St Louis, 2008, WB Saunders.)

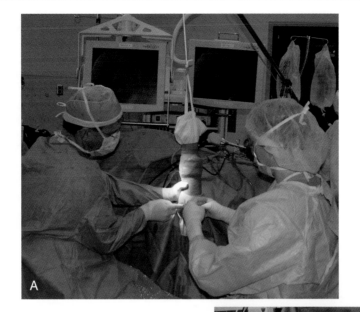

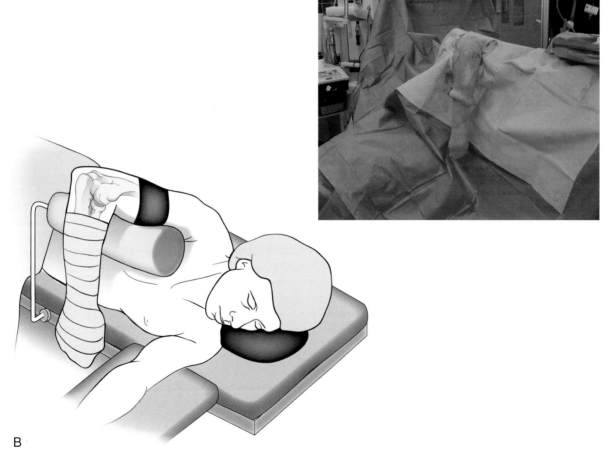

Figure 30-10   A, Positioning for elbow surgery using an overhead distractor. The arm can also be left in a free position. **B,** Lateral position using an arm holder for arthroscopy. (**A** from Canale S, Beaty J: Campbell's operative orthopaedics, ed 11, St Louis, 2007, Mosby; from Miller MD, Chhabra AB, Hurwitz SK, Mihalko WM: Orthopaedic surgical approaches, St Louis, 2008, WB Saunders.)

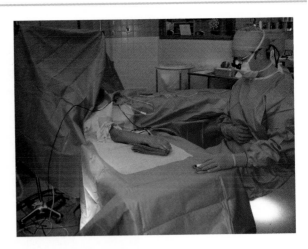

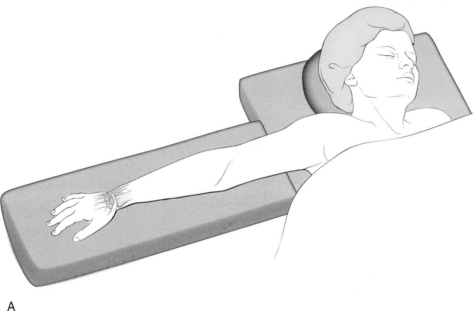

A

Figure 30-11   Positioning for hand surgery. **A,** The patient is in the supine position with the hand in the prone or supine position.

- *Name of the bone and location:* The distinguishing features are the name of the bone (e.g., tibia, femur, third phalanx) and the anatomical area (distal or proximal). For example, a fracture might be located in the distal tibia or the proximal humerus.
- *Pattern of fracture:* Fractures may be described by the pattern of the break (explained later). This helps identify the forces involved and the methods required for repair.
- *Level of comminution:* This is the extent of fragmentation. For example, a severely **comminuted** fracture is one that has many fragments. Mild comminution describes a fracture with few fragments. A highly comminuted fracture requires a longer surgical time and complex instrumentation.
- *Displacement:* This factor describes whether the bone fragments are in anatomical alignment. A nondisplaced fracture is one in which the bone fragments are in alignment.

- *Pathological origin:* A pathological fracture can occur with normal load. It is caused by any disease that weakens the structure and composition of bone.

FRACTURE PATTERNS

Fracture patterns can be associated with the impact and environment that caused them (Figure 30-14). Common fracture patterns include the following:

- *Transverse:* The fracture occurs perpendicular to the long axis of the bone.
- *Oblique:* A type of transverse fracture that occurs at an angle.
- *Spiral:* A fracture of the long bone that occurs in a spiral pattern as the result of twisting or torsion on the bone.
- *Impacted:* A fracture in which bone fragments are driven into each other or into another bone.
- *Comminuted:* A fracture with two or more pieces.

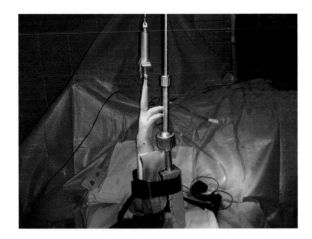

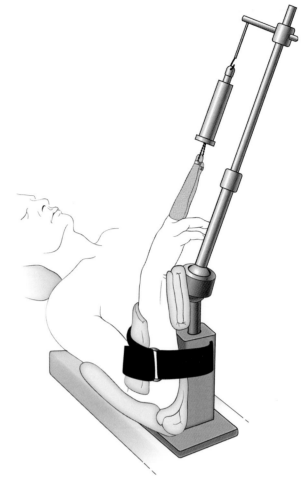

B

Figure 30-11, cont'd **B,** The hand is stabilized with a sterile distractor. *(From Miller MD, Chhabra AB, Hurwitz SK, Mihalko WM: Orthopaedic surgical approaches, St Louis, 2008, WB Saunders.)*

* *Open:* A fracture in which the fractured end penetrates the skin.
* *Greenstick:* A fracture of immature bone that is soft and less brittle than mature bone. The fracture is incomplete, or the impact results in severe bending and bruising.

BIOMECHANICAL FORCES ON BONE

Different types of stress or impact and the type of bone determine the pattern of a fracture (Figure 30-15). The following terms are used in biomechanics. They are relevant to fractures and also to methods of repairing bone.

* *Torque or torsion (twisting force):* Torque is the type of force applied to a screwdriver to implant a screw. Torsion injury results when tissue is twisted on itself.
* *Shear force (bending):* The force of an object acting perpendicular or at an angle to another surface. Shear force can apply to any surface or structure acting on tissues, such as skin. For example, shear injuries occur when a patient is dragged across a bed sheet (rather than rolled or lifted). The friction of the sheet can cause tissue injury that may not be immediately visible as the injury can occur in the deeper tissues.

* *Axial or* **compression** *force:* This force or load occurs parallel to the long bone. For example, the weight of the upper body exerts axial force on the long bones of the legs.

FRACTURE REPAIR

Common surgical goals for all types of fractures are:
1. Alignment of the bones (reduction)
2. Stabilization of the bone until healing is complete (fixation)

Reduction

Reduction is the process of bringing the bone fragments into anatomical alignment. Mechanical or manual reduction of the bone fragments is performed with the patient under anesthesia. Reduction is a physical (kinetic) process and may require the mechanical advantage of a traction device that pulls the injured bones into alignment. If the fracture is minor, manual reduction may be adequate. The two types of reduction are open and closed:

* **Open reduction** takes place through an incision as part of the surgery.

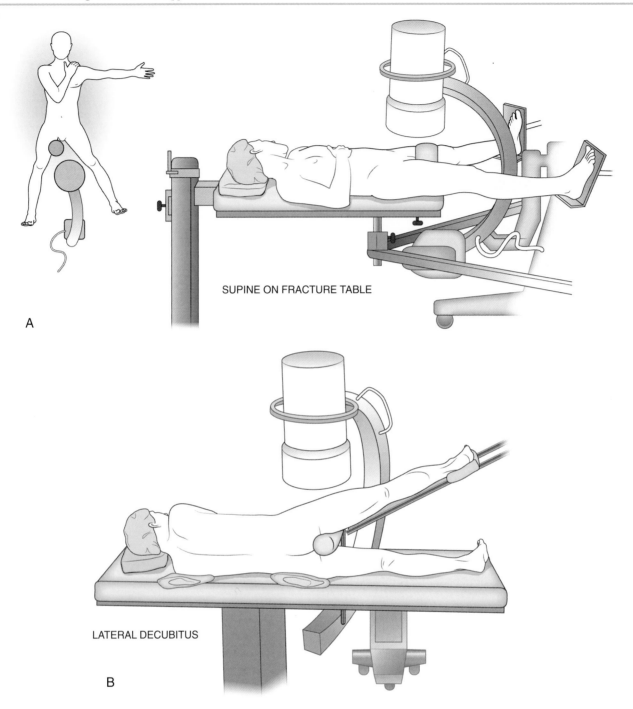

SUPINE ON FRACTURE TABLE

A

LATERAL DECUBITUS

B

Figure 30-12 A, Orthopedic table used for procedures of the hip and femur. The open configuration use allows positioning of the C-arm fluoroscope. The hips may be distracted by adjusting the leg extensions. **B,** Patient in the lateral position. *(From Miller MD, Chhabra AB, Hurwitz SK, Mihalko WM: Orthopaedic surgical approaches, St Louis, 2008, WB Saunders.)*

• **Closed reduction** is performed by manipulation of the bone or with an external traction device which pulls the bone fragments into position. No incision is made in the skin.

The patient may arrive in surgery with a traction device in place, or reduction may be performed internally as part of the surgery. **Distraction** and traction are not quite the same. A **distractor** is used to elongate a limb or structure during

surgery. This is done to aid positioning or to increase the "compartment" space that the bones occupy in the tissue.

Fixation

Fixation is the mechanical or structural method used to hold bone fragments in anatomical position during healing. Much of orthopedic surgery focuses on various methods of fixation. The two main types of fixation are:

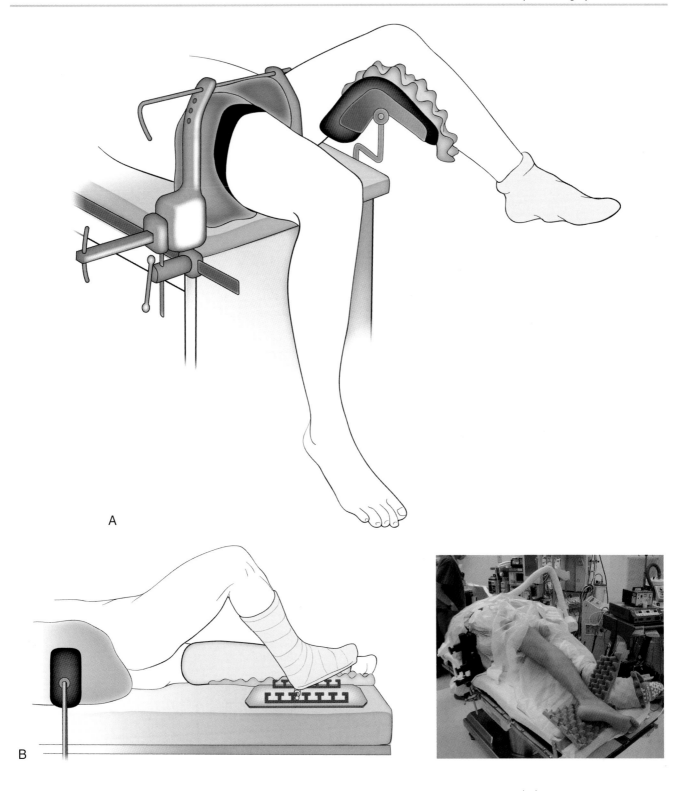

Figure 30-13 Positions for knee and lower leg surgery. **A,** Supine position with the leg in a holder, suitable for arthroscopy. The knee also can be left in the free position. **B,** Posterolateral position with foot support. *(From Miller MD, Chhabra AB, Hurwitz SK, Mihalko WM: Orthopaedic surgical approaches, St Louis, 2008, WB Saunders.)*

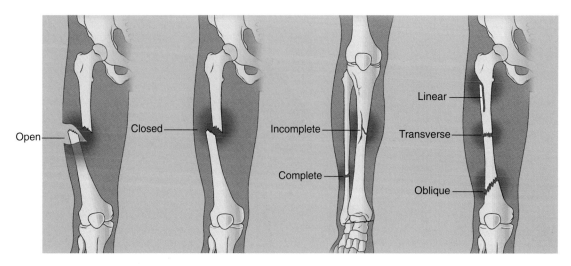

Figure 30-14 Common fracture patterns. *(From Thibodeau G, Patton K: Anthony's textbook of anatomy and physiology, ed 17, St Louis, 2003, Mosby.)*

LOADING MODE

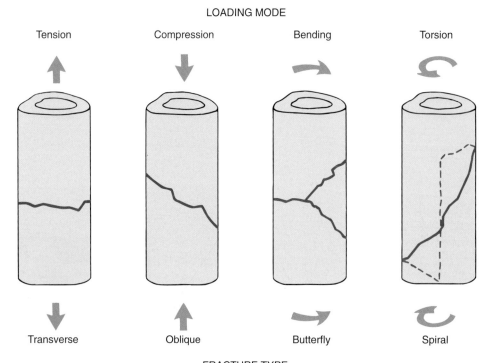

FRACTURE TYPE

Figure 30-15 Fracture loading. *(From Browner B, Jupiter J, Levine A, Trafton P: Skeletal trauma: basic science, management, and reconstruction, ed 3, Philadelphia, 2003, WB Saunders.)*

- **Internal fixation**, which requires surgery to insert or implant a device that holds the bone fragments in place. Metal plates, rods, pins, and screws are examples of internal fixation devices.
- **External fixation**, which is a means of stabilizing bone fragments in anatomical position from outside the body. A cast is an example of an external fixation device. Other devices, including external frames and cages, are also used. Pins or wires may be inserted through the skin and into the bone to support the external fixation device.

Orthopedic procedures are specifically described according to the type of reduction and repair. The surgical options are:

- *Open reduction and internal fixation:* This procedure involves open surgery to expose the bone and reduce the fracture (i.e., replace the bones in anatomical position). Internal orthopedic implants are used to achieve fixation.
- *Open reduction and external fixation:* In this procedure, reduction requires an incision to align the bones. However, an external device (e.g., a frame or cast) is

used to stabilize and hold the bone fragments during healing.

- *Closed reduction and external fixation:* The fracture is reduced manually or with a traction device. Except for casting, and other types of noninvasive splinting, an external fixation device requires the insertion of wires, pins, or other devices to support the external structure. Some devices can be inserted transcutaneously. A very small incision is made in the skin, and the pin or wire is drilled into the deeper tissue and bone.

ORTHOPEDIC TECHNOLOGY

POWER EQUIPMENT

Power equipment is used in orthopedic surgery to cut, drill, and remodel bone. The surgical technologist should be familiar with the safety and mechanical features of power equipment. The most important points are:

- Safety features of the equipment and power source
- How to connect the power equipment to the power source
- Types of accessories and their function
- How to attach accessories
- Assisting the surgeon during use of the equipment
- Cleaning and reprocessing the equipment

Safety

Most power equipment used in surgery uses compressed nitrogen (pneumatic energy). The force exerted through the hose and instrument is very powerful and can cause serious injury. A complete discussion of gas cylinder and regulator safety can be found in Chapter 15. The following are general safety precautions for use of pneumatic instruments:

1. Inspect the instrument and hose before use. Make sure the instrument is properly assembled.
2. Place the instrument in the safe position before attaching accessories or the power hose.
3. Make sure that accessories are attached correctly, using guards where applicable. A drill or saw attachment that is incorrectly seated can be propelled from the handpiece with extreme force and may cause serious injury.
4. Inspect accessories before attaching them. Never attach a bent drill tip or other accessory, because it can wobble and become disengaged from the handpiece. Never use a cracked or chipped cutting accessory.
5. Put the instrument in the safe position before passing it to the surgeon.
6. Test the pressure before using the instrument. Make sure the pressure does not exceed the approved level.
7. Always bleed the air hose before detaching the handpiece. With the nitrogen tank valve turned off, activate the instrument to remove any remaining gas from the hose.
8. Follow the manufacturer's guidelines for decontamination and sterilization.

9. Power instruments generate heat as a result of friction between the tissue and tip. The temperature can be high enough to destroy tissue in the vicinity of the tip. To prevent tissue injury, make sure to irrigate the tip while the instrument is in use. Irrigation solution is always used with power drills and saws.

Drill

An orthopedic drill is similar to a carpenter's drill. The drill has two main components, the head and the handle. Attachments for the drill are inserted at the drill head. Many different kinds of attachments are available. The surgical technologist must be familiar with the specific functions and handling of surgical drills (Figure 30-16). Drills are used whenever torque is required (torque is energy applied to an object that rotates).

Drill Attachments and Accessory Tools

The following are the most commonly used drill attachments and accessories:

- *Burr*—A round, conical, or tapered tip used for making narrow holes or for smoothing very small areas. Burrs are composed of stainless steel, titanium, or diamond.
- *Chuck*—The chuck is attached to the drill head. A drill bit, reamer, burr, or other rotational cutting tip is inserted into the chuck. A chuck key is used to open and close the chuck's jaws, which are shaped like a clover leaf. Some types of chucks are tightened and loosened manually.
- *Depth gauge*—A small, calibrated rod used to measure the depth of a drilled or reamed hole in bone.
- *Drill bit*—A pin with wide cutting threads that is used to make a smooth-sided hole in the bone. Flutes (phalanges) in the drill bit allow cut bone to escape from the thread channels. Drill bits are supplied singly or in standard sizes in a metal rack.
- *Drill guide (drill sleeve)*—An instrument inserted near or at the screw hole to correctly aim the angle of a screw, pin, nail, or wire as it enters the bone. The drill guide may be a single instrument or part of an assembly. Although many designs are available, the function is the same for all types.
- *Reamer*—A rod-shaped or chisel-pointed cutter used to **ream**, or clear, the medullary canal. A rounded or cup-shaped reamer is used for dishing surfaces such as the acetabulum. Reaming may be done to prepare the bone for an implant. A reamer may be attached to a power drill or used manually.
- *Shaver*—A type of burr used mainly on cartilage for shaping and removing tissue such as the meniscus.
- *Tap*—An instrument similar to a screw that is used to cut threads in the bone. The tap corresponds to the diameter of the screw, its shape, and the pitch. Pretapping prevents bone from becoming embedded in threads of the screw as it is inserted.

Saws

Power saws are used to cut bone in a precise direction and angle. The saw blades generally are fine toothed and vibrate

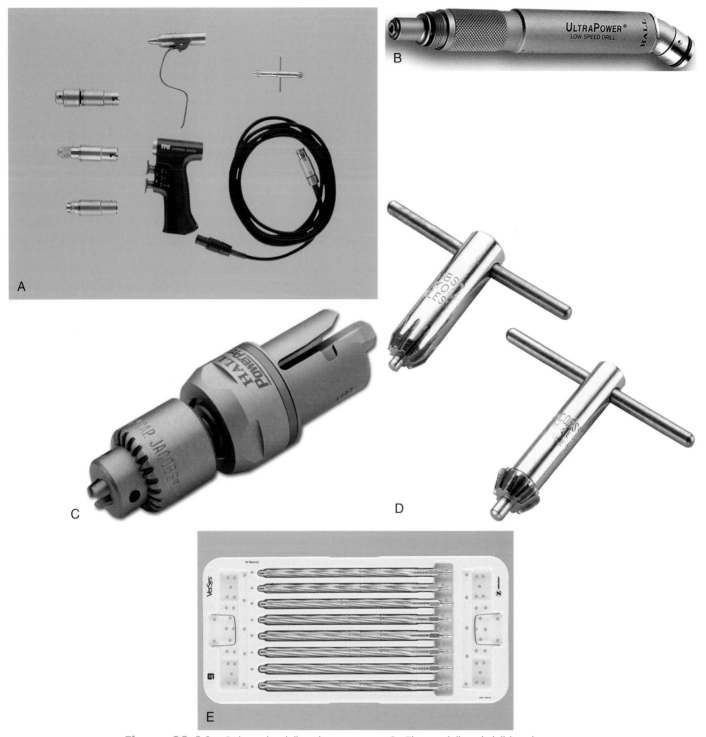

Figure 30-16 Orthopedic drill and accessories. **A,** Electric drill and drill heads. **B,** Pneumatic low-speed drill. **C,** Jacob chuck. **D,** Jacob chuck keys. **E,** Reamers used for canalization of the long bones.

or oscillate rapidly. This produces a smooth cut with little bone loss. Orthopedic saws are identified mainly by the movement of the blade. The name of the saw is also the category of blade the device uses:

- *Reciprocating saw*—The blade moves "in and out" of the handpiece.

- *Sagittal saw:* The blade is fixed at a right angle (90 degrees) to the handpiece and moves along a perpendicular axis.
- *Oscillating saw:* The blade is mounted along the same axis as the handle and moves "back and forth."

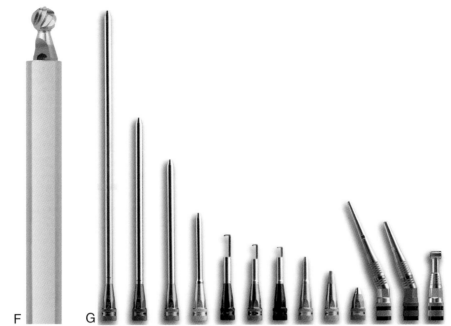

Figure 30-16, cont'd *F,* Diamond burr. **G,** Drill tips. (**A** *and* **E** *from Tighe SM: Instrumentation for the operating room, ed 6, St Louis, 2003, Mosby;* **D, F,** *and* **G** *courtesy Zimmer, Warsaw, Ind.)*

Each type of blade is available in many shapes, which are identified by the length of the blade shaft, the type, and the width of the blade edge.

HAND INSTRUMENTS

Many orthopedic instruments have been designed for use with a specific system. These specialized instruments are classified by type (e.g., impactor) and system (e.g., Syrus tibial nail). Generic instruments, which are not associated with a specific system, are classified by type and sometimes more specifically by anatomical region, (e.g., hip, knee). Surgical technologists should be familiar with the standard instruments used in their facility.

Retractors and Bone-Holding Clamps

Because bone does not yield to retraction the way soft tissue does, the surgeon most often retracts the surrounding tissue away from the bone or uses a bone-holding clamp or hook to grasp a bone for manipulation. Certain types of bone retractors (e.g., Blount and Bennet retractors) are designed to be used as levers against the bone, to shift its position. Soft tissue retractors are designed for a specific anatomical location, such as the shoulder, and some general surgery retractors (e.g., Army-Navy and Weitlaner retractors) are also used in orthopedic surgery. Figures 30-17 and 30-18 illustrate common bone-holding clamps and retractors.

Rongeurs and Bone Cutters

Rongeurs and bone cutters are used for trimming and modeling bone and cartilage. Double-action instruments have two hinges for increased force at the tips (from increased lever-age). Cutting edges may be cupped, anvil tip, or double bladed. Figure 30-19 shows common rongeurs and cutters. Specialty cutting instruments used in ear, nose, and throat (ENT); plastic surgery; and neurosurgery are shown in Chapters 27, 29, and 35.

Chisels, Osteotomes, Gouges, and Curettes

Chisels, gouges, and osteotomes are used with a mallet to model bone or to remove bone for a graft. Each has a specific type of cutting tip. Instruments in this group usually are supplied in graduated sizes and secured in a metal rack.

- *Chisel:* Beveled on one side only
- *Osteotome:* Beveled on both sides
- *Gouge:* V-shaped chisel

A curette is used without a mallet. It has a cup-shaped cutting edge and is used for scooping out bone and other dense tissue. Figure 30-20 shows instruments in this category.

Elevators and Rasps

A periosteal elevator (or simply, elevator) is used in nearly every open orthopedic procedure. Although it has many uses, its main function is to remove or scrape away the periosteum (the tough outer membrane of the bone) from the bone surface. This is necessary to cut or saw through bone tissue, because the periosteum tends to shred or tear on contact with a rongeurs or cutting instrument, preventing a clean cut. Many sizes and types of elevators are available. The most common are the smooth-tip joker elevator and the larger, square-tip Key elevator. Figure 30-21 shows common elevators.

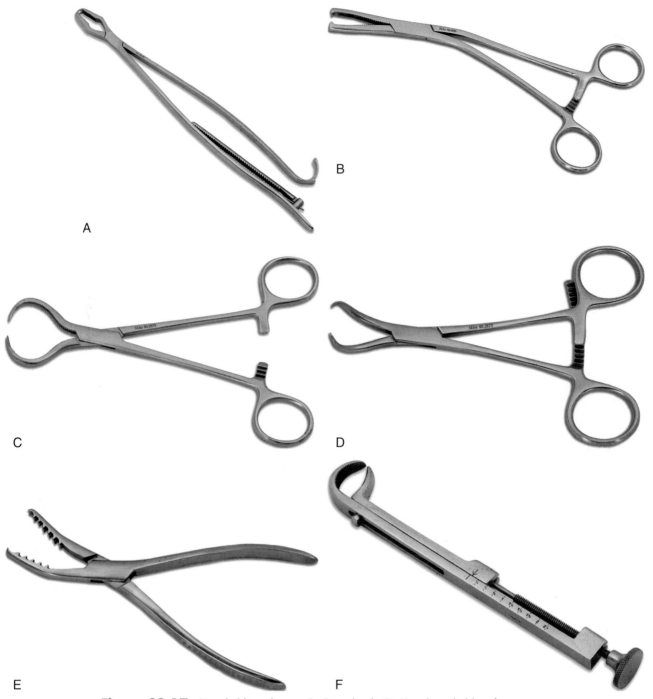

Figure 30-17 Bone-holding clamps. **A,** Bone hook. **B,** Kern bone-holding forceps. **C,** Bone and cartilage clamp. **D,** Lane clamp. **E,** Dingman clamp. **F,** Lewin clamp. *(Courtesy of Sklar Instruments, West Chester, Pa.)*

A bone rasp is used to model and shape bone or to roughen the bone surface.

Measuring Devices

Measuring devices commonly used in orthopedic procedures include the protractor, caliper, screw depth gauge, and ordinary ruler (Figure 30-22). Computerized mapping has replaced some but not all of the measuring techniques previously used in joint replacement surgery.

ORTHOPEDIC IMPLANTS

Orthopedic implants or hardware are the devices used to attach or fix bone and other connective tissue (joint replacement implants are discussed separately). Many hundreds of different implants are available for orthopedic repair. However, a relatively simple classification system (i.e., implant type and use) is used for them. The manufacture and use of orthopedic hardware are regulated to protect the public. The

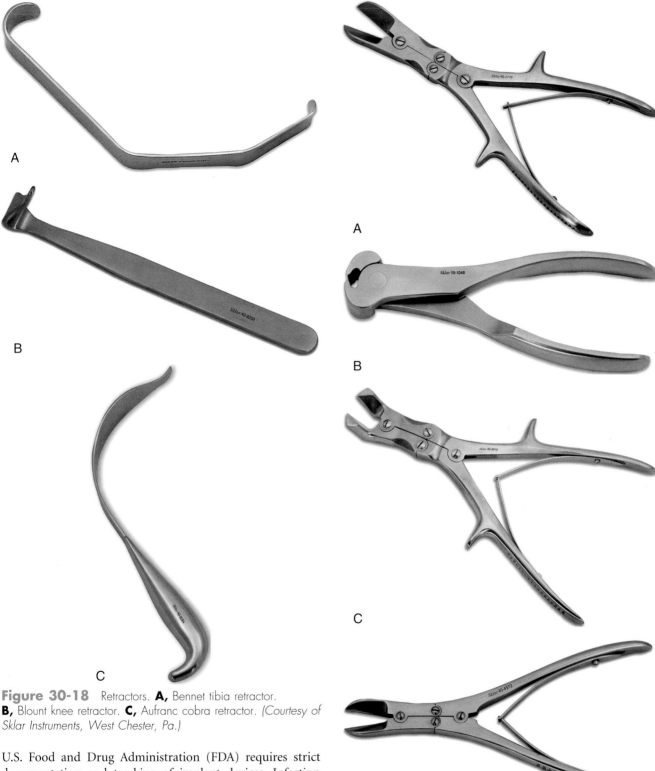

Figure 30-18   Retractors. **A,** Bennet tibia retractor.
B, Blount knee retractor. **C,** Aufranc cobra retractor. *(Courtesy of Sklar Instruments, West Chester, Pa.)*

Figure 30-19   Rongeurs and bone cutters. **A,** Stille-Liston rongeur. **B,** Liston cutting forceps. **C,** Stille-Horsley rongeur. **D,** Ruskin forceps. *Courtesy of Sklar Instruments, West Chester, Pa.)*

U.S. Food and Drug Administration (FDA) requires strict documentation and tracking of implant devices. Infection related to implants is prevented by strict protocols for sterilization.

Hospitals and other health care facilities maintain an inventory or supply of sterile implants for surgical cases routinely performed in that facility. The inventory is organized in a way that protects the implants from contamination and damage while making it easy for staff members to select the correct implant for surgery. A database of all implants is maintained for regulatory purposes and restocking. A surgical tech-

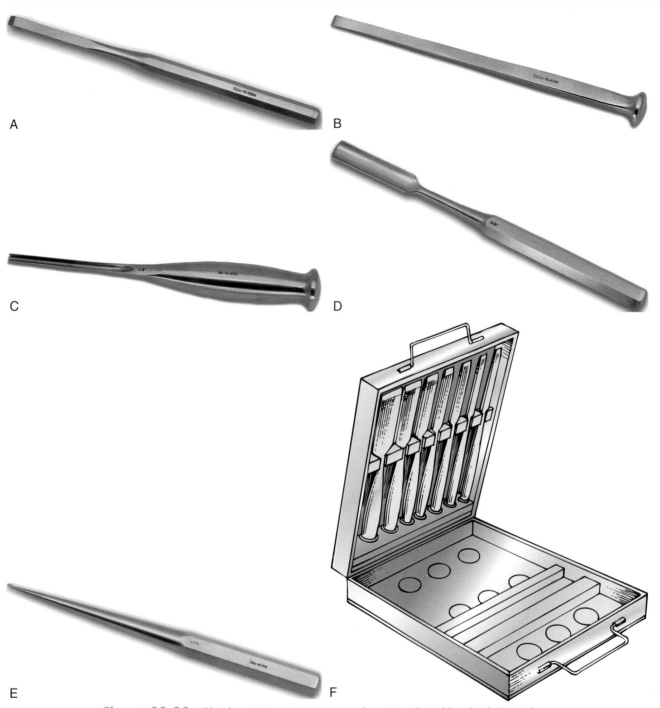

Figure 30-20 Chisels, osteotomes, gouges, and curettes. **A,** Hibbs chisel. **B,** Hoke chisel. **C,** Army pattern osteotome. **D,** Lambotte osteotome (often called simply a "Lambotte"). **E,** Smith Peterson gouge. **F,** Instrument rack. *(A-E Courtesy of Sklar Instruments, West Chester, Pa. F from Phillips N: Berry and Kohn's operating room technique, ed 11, St Louis, 2007, Mosby.)*

nologist (team leader or orthopedic specialist) may be designated to maintain implant inventories and implement the documentation and supply system.

Materials

Metals are commonly used in the manufacture of implants, because metal can withstand the load required of bone. Current research is aimed at creating new metal **alloys** (made from a mixture of different metals) that are highly biocompatible and inert. Stainless steel remains the alloy most commonly used for implants.

Bioactive implants (e.g., absorbable fixation screws that release calcium) are absorbed by the body and stimulate or enhance bone repair. **Biocompatibility** means that the implant is compatible with tissue and does not cause injury. This includes a possible allergic reaction or other immune response.

A material that is **inert** does not react with other nonorganic or biological substances. This quality is also critical because metals, in particular, can interact at the molecular level, creating ions that are harmful to the body. Reactions also can lead to corrosion or oxidation of the implant, leading to weakness or breakdown. For these reasons, it is important to make sure that devices composed of different metals are not implanted near each other in the body.

Documentation

All implants stored in the operating room must be documented on a database for tracking, retrieving, and stock

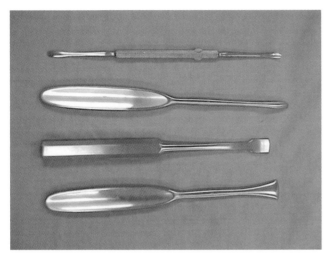

Figure 30-21 Elevators. *Top to bottom,* Freer elevator, used mainly in ear, nose, and throat (ENT) and plastic surgery; Joker elevator; Key elevator; and Langenbeck elevator. *(Courtesy the College of Southern Idaho, Twin Falls, Idaho.)*

replacement. When an implant is used, specific information about the implant is recorded in the patient's record. This includes but is not limited to:

- Date and name of the facility
- Type of implant and size (where applicable)
- Location of implant in the body
- Name of the surgeon
- Manufacturer's identification number, including the batch, lot, and serial numbers

Implant Log

The facility keeps information about each implant in a permanent log. This can be an electronic database or a written log. The FDA requires the following information:

- Name and address of the surgical facility
- Manufacturer's identification information
- Implant serial number, lot number, batch number, and any other identifying information (e.g., size, type)
- Patient's identification details
- Surgeon's identification details
- Implant expiration date (if applicable)

Implant Sterilization

Many implants, including joint components, are supplied by the manufacturer individually in sterile packages. Plates, screws, pins, and rods are not wrapped individually but supplied in sterile sets, from which the appropriate size is selected during surgery. Joint and other specialty implants that are sterilized and packaged by the manufacturer are opened onto the sterile field only after the exact size and type have been determined. This reduces environmental exposure during surgery, as well as the need for an excessive implant inventory.

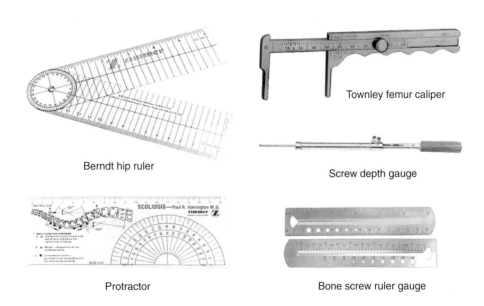

Figure 30-22 Measuring devices. *(From Phillips N:* Berry and Kohn's operating room technique, *ed 11, St. Louis, 2007, Mosby.)*

Implants must not be flash sterilized except in extreme emergency. The Association for the Advancement of Medical Instrumentation (AAMI), which institutes international protocols for patient safety, states that "careful planning, appropriate packaging, and inventory management in cooperation with suppliers can minimize the need to flash sterilize implants."[1] AORN recommends that if an emergency situation makes flash sterilization unavoidable, a biological monitoring device must be used, along with a chemical indicator. The implant must not be used until the biological indicator provides a negative result.[2]

The patient's permanent operative record must reflect the details of the sterilization process and the outcome of the biological and chemical indicators. The sterilizer log (computer printout), which includes all sterilization parameters achieved when the implant was flashed, must be included in the patient's chart. The Association for the Advancement of Medical Instrumentation provides yearly updates of accepted sterilization practices through its *Standards Registry*. Standard *ST79* provides current practices regarding steam sterilization for implants and should be consulted yearly for updated information.

Screws

An orthopedic screw is the most commonly used type of orthopedic implant (Figure 30-23). Screws are supplied in different types, sizes, shapes, and designs. They are made of titanium, stainless steel, or bioabsorbable material. To maintain order and allow quick identification of the size needed during surgery, screws are held in screw racks that are color coded or imprinted with the sizes. The surgical technologist should be able to recognize different types of

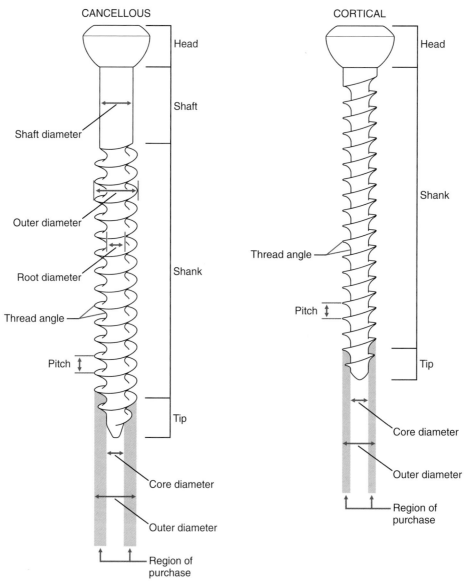

Figure 30-23 Components of the cancellous and cortical screw. *(From Browner B, Jupiter J, Levine A, Trafton P: Skeletal trauma: basic science, management, and reconstruction, ed 3, Philadelphia, 2003, WB Saunders.)*

screws and understand their application. Screws are commonly used to:

- Attach a metal implant to bone
- Attach bone to bone or bone to soft tissue

Parts of a Screw

The parts of a screw are as follows:

- *Head*—The flat or conical part of the screw. The recess of the screw may be hexagonal, a straight slot, or cruciform (cross shaped).
- *Shaft*—The long section of the screw. The outside of the threads (thread diameter) determines the screw's numerical diameter. The main shaft, or root diameter, determines the strength of the screw. The root diameter is measured where there are no threads.
- *Threads*—The spiral-shaped ridges along the screw shaft. The threads on most screws are asymmetrical (i.e., flat on the top and rounded underneath). This provides a wide surface for pulling the screw into the bone. The depth of the thread determines contact with the bone and its "pullout" strength. The number of threads in relation to the length of the shaft determines the pitch. As the pitch increases, so does contact with the bone, giving the screw greater gripping strength. Some screws have no threads near the head. These partly threaded screws have a specific biomechanical function (discussed later).
- *Tip*—The pointed end of the screw may be blunt, corkscrew, or trocar shaped. The shape determines whether the screw is self-tapping or requires a predrilled hole.

Types of Screws

Screws can be classified according to type:

- *Cancellous*—Used mainly in dense (cancellous) bone; large diameter and greater pitch to increase contact with the bone.
- *Cortical*—Small diameter and decreased pitch; used in cortical bone. The bicortical screw is inserted into the cortical bone on one surface and passes through the cancellous portion into the cortical surface on the opposite face of the bone.
- *Lag*—All screws that exert compression on bone fragments, either directly or with a plate.
- *Herbert*—Used for fixation of small bones; a cannulated screw with variable pitch and threads at both ends.
- *Locking*—Used with a special plate that has threaded holes to secure the screw head to the plate.
- **Cannulated**—A screw with a hollow core that is used to join bone fragments. The hollow center allows the screw to be fitted over a prepositioned guide wire to ensure precise placement.
- *Self-tapping*—Has flutes at the tip that cut a passage for the threads as the screw is inserted. Tapping is the process of making a hole in the material to accommodate the screw. A drill bit is used for tapping a hole (Figure 30-24).

The function of a screw is to hold two or more objects together. It can be used to attach a plate that bridges a fracture,

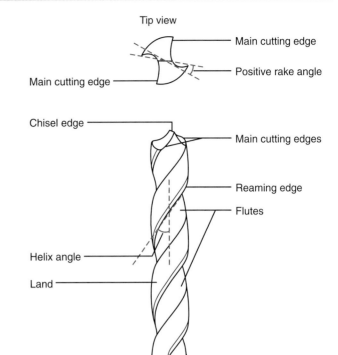

Figure 30-24 Drill bit. A bit is fitted to the head of a power drill for tapping (i.e., making a hole to accommodate the screw). *(From Browner B, Jupiter J, Levine A, Trafton P: Skeletal trauma: basic science, management, and reconstruction, ed 3, Philadelphia, 2003, WB Saunders.)*

and it can be used by itself to join two or more bone fragments or bone and soft tissue. When a screw is implanted across two objects, it compresses the materials together by cutting a spiral path in the material. This prevents the screw from backing out. The strength of a screw depends on several factors:

- The depth of the threads
- The pitch of the threads
- The shape of the threads

It is important that surgical technologists understand the lag screw principle. The screw thread applies compression only on the object farthest from the screw head. For example, in the case of two bone fragments, the fragment farthest from the screw head is drawn into the first. This is an important concept for the scrub assisting in orthopedics cases. When tapping is done for this type of screw, the size of the drill tap is slightly larger than the screw diameter. The near side of the hole is drilled out to produce a space for countersinking the screw head. This allows the smooth part of the screw to glide easily through the hole (sometimes called the *glide hole*). When the screw engages in the second fragment, it grabs it and pulls it into position. Figure 30-25 illustrates the application of a lag screw through two bone fragments.

Plates

Plates span bone and provide stability and support during healing. They are used in simple or comminuted fractures.

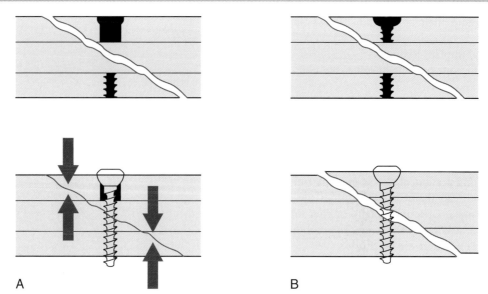

Figure 30-25 Application of a lag screw. The black sections indicate drilling areas. **A,** The cortex is drilled on the near side to produce a glide (countersink hole). **B,** Lack of a countersink results in a gap in the bone. *(From Browner B, Jupiter J, Levine A, Trafton P: Skeletal trauma: basic science, management, and reconstruction, ed 3, Philadelphia, 2003, WB Saunders.)*

Plates are made of titanium or stainless steel and are available in a matte or a polished finish. All have screw holes, because screws are used to fix them in place and to aid compression. Plates can be straight, contoured, or beveled to fit smoothly over bone and joint surfaces. The screw holes can be smooth sided, threaded, oblique, or straight.

Different forces are exerted on the fracture, the plate, and the soft tissue, depending on the type of plate used. To be effective at stabilizing, the implant must provide a means of preventing normal movement of the fracture area. This means that twisting, bending, and shearing (force at a right angle to the long axis) must be prevented. Functions of various plating systems are to:

- Protect and neutralize the fracture
- Span the fracture
- Provide compression
- Reduce the fracture (bring the bone fragments together)
- Buttress structures or fragments

Static (Neutralization) Plate

A static, or neutralization, plate spans a two-fragment fracture and is fixed in place with lag screws. This is a simple means of stabilizing (i.e., neutralizing) force acting on the bone fragments with no mechanical action on the fracture line. This type of plate is used when the fragments can be compressed manually and the fracture is stable (Figure 30-26). The plate also is used to reduce a fracture (Figure 30-27).

Reconstruction Plate

A reconstruction plate may be bent to fit the contours of the bone surface. First, an aluminum template is fitted over the bone to duplicate its contour. The template then is taken to the back table, and the implant plate is shaped with pliers, a plate press, and other instruments. More delicate reconstruction plates may be shaped and cut to size by hand. This type of plate is used commonly in facial, cranial, and pelvic fractures (Figure 30-28).

Locking Plate

A locking plate has threaded screw holes that lock the screws into the plate. This prevents toggling of the screws, which tends to loosen them or cause them to back out.

Dynamic Compression Plate

A dynamic compression plate (DCP) has screw holes that are inclined (sloped) and offset. This design feature provides reduction and compression of the fragments. Anchor screws are inserted into one fragment. As the screws are tightened, the plate slides along the bone, drawing the two bone fragments together (Figure 30-29). The term *dynamic* refers to the compression of bone fragments produced by the natural load exerted on the bones by the body itself.

A low-contact dynamic compression (LCDC) plate is designed to reduce contact between the plate and the bone. The plate sits just above the surface of the bone, secured by screws. This prevents direct pressure on the periosteal vascular supply and may enhance healing. Another type of plate used to reduce contact with the periosteum is the wave plate, which is contoured to intermittently curve away from the bone. This type of plate is used in fractures that have failed to heal by other methods (Figure 30-30).

Tension Band Plate

A tension band plate provides a mechanical advantage in fixation of the long bones. Asymmetrical loading occurs in all long bones; that is, more weight is carried on the concave

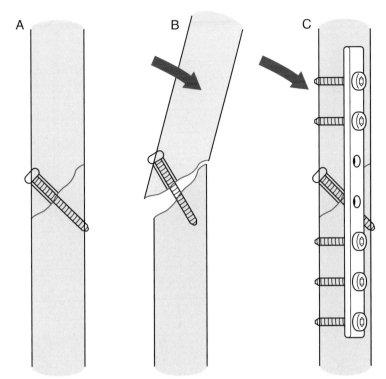

Figure 30-26 Neutralization plate. **A,** Screw fixation without a neutralization plate. **B,** The bone is loaded transversely, showing failure. **C,** The plate is effective at resisting the load as force is distributed across the length of the bone. *(From Browner B, Jupiter J, Levine A, Trafton P: Skeletal trauma: basic science, management, and reconstruction, ed 3, Philadelphia, 2003, WB Saunders.)*

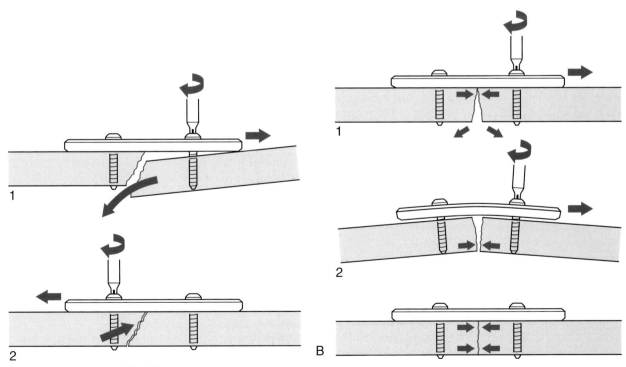

Figure 30-27 The plate as a means of reducing a fracture. **A,** the screws are tightened to produce inward loading and alignment. **B,** the rigid plate draws the displaced fragments into horizontal alignment with the plate. *(From Browner B, Jupiter J, Levine A, Trafton P: Skeletal trauma: basic science, management, and reconstruction, ed 3, Philadelphia, 2003, WB Saunders.)*

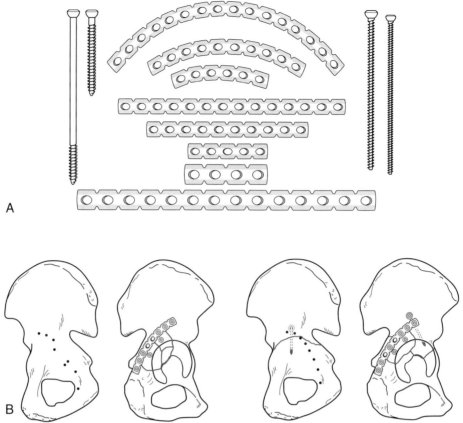

Figure 30-28 A, Examples of reconstruction plates. Plates are notched along the sides so that they can be easily bent in all directions to fit the contours of the bone. **B,** Use of plates for fixation of the posterior acetabular wall. *(From Browner B, Jupiter J, Levine A, Trafton P: Skeletal trauma: basic science, management, and reconstruction, ed 3, Philadelphia, 2003, WB Saunders.)*

side of the long axis of the bone. A partial fracture on the convex side tends to widen under load. The tension band plate is placed on the convex or gap side of the fracture to counteract the load and prevent the gap from widening. The principle of tension banding is also used without plates (Figure 30-31).

Buttress Plate

A buttress is a supporting structure that prevents an adjoining object or structure from collapsing. An example of common buttressing is a lean-to shed. The structure supporting the roof at its highest point is a buttress. The supporting structure is "pushing" on the roof to support it at an angle. In orthopedics, a buttress plate is used to give added strength or to "prop" one structure against another. This technique is commonly applied in fractures of the tibia (Figure 30-32).

Condylar Plate

A condylar plate often is used in conjunction with a compression screw for fixation of fractures of the **condyle** (the rounded end of a long bone). The end of the plate is contoured to fit over the surface of a condyle, and compression lag screws are inserted through the fracture fragments (Figure 30-33).

Intertrochanteric Nail and Plate Combination

Fractures that occur across the trochanter of the hip often require stabilization from a side plate, which is implanted at the proximal end of the femur. An older prototype of this device is the Jewett nail. Although the Jewett nail is still occasionally used, it has been largely replaced by more efficient systems, such as the dynamic hip screw (DHS) and the dynamic compression-sliding hip screw. This implant has two primary pieces: a lag screw, which is inserted into the trochanter, and a locking plate, which is inserted over the screw and extends along the proximal femur. During healing, the plate-nail combination shifts the load from the trochanter (normal loading) to the long axis of the femur, removing excess pressure from the trochanter (Figure 30-34).

Intramedullary Nail or Rod

An intramedullary (IM) nail is a thick rod inserted into the medullary canal of long bones to provide structural support from inside the bone. This device is used for fractures of long bones, such as the femur, tibia, and humerus. IM nails are made of titanium and stainless steel. They are supplied as slotted, cannulated (hollow), or solid. Nails are inserted by reaming the intramedullary canal or by impacting the nail

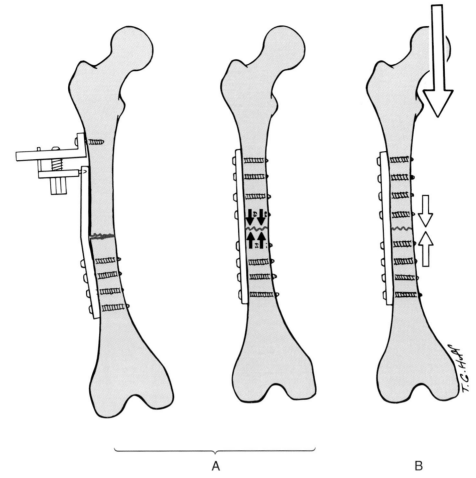

Figure 30-29 Compression plate technique. Both static and dynamic compression are shown. **A,** The plate is applied to the femur to produce static compression. **B,** Normal weight (loading) on the femur further compresses the fragments at the fracture site. *(From Browner B, Jupiter J, Levine A, Trafton P: Skeletal trauma: basic science, management, and reconstruction, ed 3, Philadelphia, 2003, WB Saunders.)*

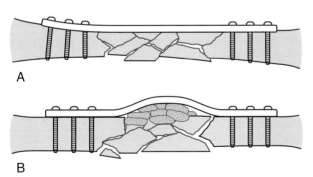

Figure 30-30 Wave or bridge plate. This type of plate is contoured away from an area of severe comminution to preserve blood supply and encourage the growth of new bone cells without external pressure. **A,** Conventional plating. **B,** Wave plate. *(From Browner B, Jupiter J, Levine A, Trafton P: Skeletal trauma: basic science, management, and reconstruction, ed 3, Philadelphia, 2003, WB Saunders.)*

through the marrow tissue to seat it. The Ender nail and Rush rod are older style nails that are used in multiples and impacted with a mallet. Modern IM systems include the nail itself plus two or more transverse locking bolts, which increase contact with the bone and provide structural support. Locking bolts are placed at the proximal and distal ends of the nail and prevent it from drifting or backing out of the medullary canal. They also provide rotational support. Figure 30-35 shows a femoral nail with locking bolts.

Wires and Cables

Flexible wire and cable are used in a variety of techniques to approximate bone and soft tissue and for stabilization. Wire most often is used to reduce small bone fragments. This is done by drilling holes in the fragments, inserting a wire through the holes, and drawing the fragments together. The wires are then twisted, and the resulting knot is buried in adjacent soft tissue or flattened against the bone. Wire or cable also is used in cerclage (encircling) reduction to provide added strength to another type of implant, such as an IM nail. Cables are closed at their ends with a cable clamp.

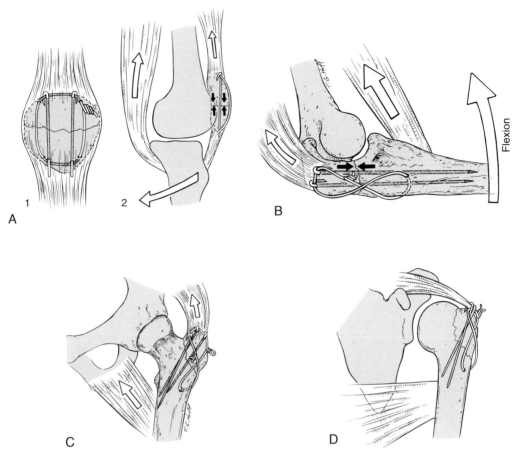

Figure 30-31 Tension band technique. *(From Browner B, Jupiter J, Levine A, Trafton P: Skeletal trauma: basic science, management, and reconstruction, ed 3, Philadelphia, 2003, WB Saunders.)*

Kirschner Wires and Steinmann Pins

Kirschner wires (K-wires) and Steinmann pins are thick wires that are inserted with a drill. The wires have a sharp, diamond-shaped point that penetrates bone and soft tissue. They are inserted directly into tissue with a drill. They are extremely sharp and can easily puncture gloves and drapes with little impact. They should be handled with caution. After insertion, the surgeon often cuts the excess wire with cutters. All pieces must be retrieved from the surgical field and placed in a magnetic container to prevent injury.

The main advantages of K-wires and Steinmann pins are their size and ease of insertion. They cause little trauma to bone and can be easily withdrawn. They commonly are used:

- As a guide wire for cannulated screws and instruments
- To provide temporary or final stabilization for a fracture
- As an intramedullary device to span a fracture in a small bone (e.g., the digits)
- To position multiple fragments of a comminuted fracture
- As a template for cannulated nails
- As an aid in traction devices

JOINT REPLACEMENT IMPLANTS

Joint implants are metal or synthetic components used to replace the diseased or injured tissue. The load placed on a joint requires that the implant meet certain criteria. When implant surfaces (called the *bearing surfaces*) rub on each other, minute particles of the implant materials are released into the joint cavity. These particles cause a cellular reaction that leads to the destruction of bone tissue. Different types of implant materials are designed to help overcome this problem through greater resistance to wear. No implant material or design is suitable for all patients. The selection is based on the patient's bone type, age, activity level, and general health.

Materials

Metals

Metal alloys are used in the manufacture of joint implants. The metals and alloys most commonly used are:

- Cobalt-chromium-molybdenum
- Titanium-aluminum-vanadium
- Pure titanium
- Tantalum

Metal-on-metal components were the first type to be used in joint replacement. Some researchers have returned to this

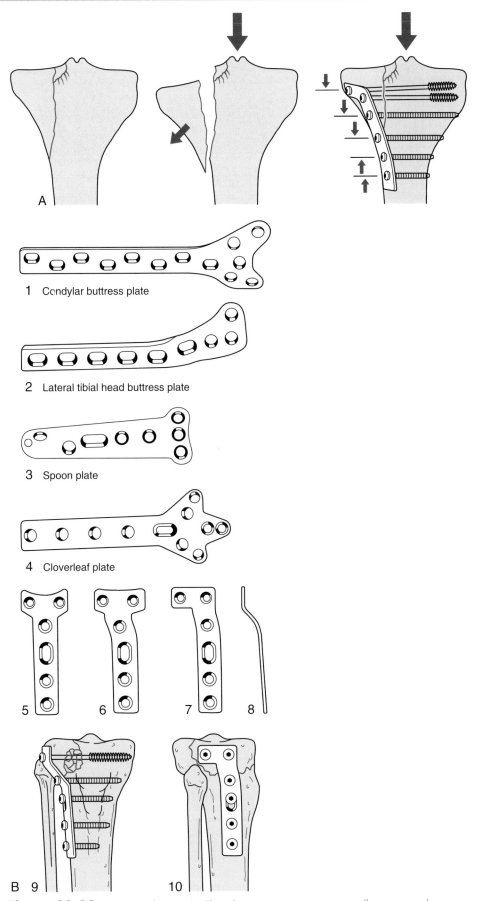

Figure 30-32 Buttress plating. **A,** The plate acts as a retaining wall to support the fractured component. **B,** Types of buttress plates. Views *9* and *10,* Lateral plate used with a cancellous bone graft to buttress a tibial plateau fracture. *(From Browner B, Jupiter J, Levine A, Trafton P: Skeletal trauma: basic science, management, and reconstruction, ed 3, Philadelphia, 2003, WB Saunders.)*

1 Condylar buttress plate

2 Lateral tibial head buttress plate

3 Spoon plate

4 Cloverleaf plate

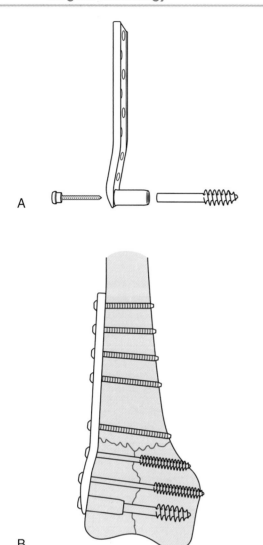

Figure 30-33 Condylar plate and screw. *(From Browner B, Jupiter J, Levine A, Trafton P: Skeletal trauma: basic science, management, and reconstruction, ed 3, Philadelphia, 2003, WB Saunders.)*

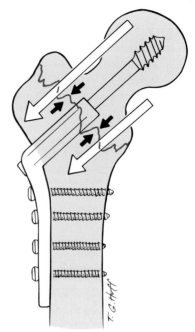

Figure 30-34 Dynamic compression plate with sliding hip screw for fracture of the trochanter. *(From Browner B, Jupiter J, Levine A, Trafton P: Skeletal trauma: basic science, management, and reconstruction, ed 3, Philadelphia, 2003, WB Saunders.)*

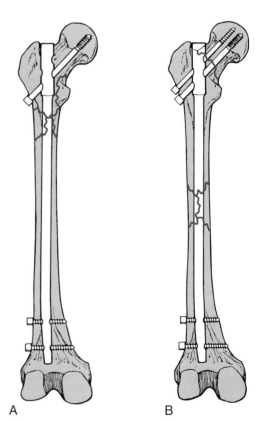

Figure 30-35 Femoral intramedullary nail. This is the second-generation intramedullary nail, which adds locking bolts at each end for added strength and to prevent the nail from backing out or rotating. This type of nail is used for femoral and tibial fractures. *(From Browner B, Jupiter J, Levine A, Trafton P: Skeletal trauma: basic science, management, and reconstruction, ed 3, Philadelphia, 2003, WB Saunders.)*

design, using more advanced metallurgy. However, metal can release ions into the body, causing toxicity. This type of system is not used in patients with kidney disease or in women of childbearing age.

Polyethylene

Polyethylene is a highly durable, low friction plastic in the form of ultra high molecular weight, highly cross-linked polyethylene (UHMWPE). This is a modified form of polyethylene made through a process of irradiation. Although very strong, highly-cross linked polyethylene breaks down through wear and delamination (separation of layers). UHMWPE components are commonly used in hybrid joint systems, which use both metal and polyethylene.

Ceramic

Ceramic materials were developed to increase resistance to wear. This type of component is mainly limited to hip replacement. Three types of ceramic materials currently are used: alumina, zirconium, and oxidized zirconium. Ceramic materials have been used for the manufacture of femoral heads for several decades. Ceramic-on-polyethylene, ceramic-on-ceramic, and ceramic-on-metal implants currently are available.

The advantages of ceramic are that it is very hard, it can be highly polished, and it remains resistant to scratching. The greatest disadvantage is that the material is brittle and can fracture or shatter.

Surface Materials

Some implants are roughened and coated to enhance healing and resist wear. Metal fibers or "beads" may be applied to the surface of the implant to create microscopic pores that accept bone cement during implantation. In **press-fit** implants, bone tissue infiltrates the pores during healing. Metal coatings are used, or the original surface material may be altered by infusing it with gas or exposing it to nitrogen ions.

Design Structure

The structure and surface of a joint implant are extremely important to the safety and function of the joint postoperatively. Joint stability is achieved by the basic design and surface coating.

Modular and Nonmodular Design

Modular components are now used in many joint replacement systems. These are joint systems that contains several parts. Modular components can be manufactured from different materials or the same material and assembled inside the patient. An inventory of modular components allows surgical facilities to maintain a variety of sizes of components within a single system. Nonmodular systems may provide greater longevity because they have fewer components.

Joint implants may be cemented in place with bone cement, or they may be press-fit by impaction. The choice of cemented or press-fit design depends on the bone quality and the patient's age, health, and desired level of activity.

GRAFTS, BONE CEMENT, AND BIOACTIVE MATERIALS

Grafts

Bone transplantation usually is performed using a segment of the patient's own bone (autograft) or cadaver bone (allograft). Cadaver bone is reprocessed to remove minerals and protein and then is freeze dried. Bone is stored in the hospital bone bank and supplied in sterile form.

Bone Graft Substitutes

Bone graft substitutes are commonly used to repair and reconstruct bone. A shortage of graft materials and interest in bioactive materials have led to the development of new graft substitutes:

- Ceramic—Composites of calcium phosphate, calcium sulfate, and bioactive glass (paste, chips, granules)
- Polymer—Cross-linked collagen based or hydroxyapatite coated, resin based

Bone graft substitutes are supplied in the following forms:

- Injectable paste
- Block form
- Granules
- Putty
- Chips

Materials are mixed with intravenous (IV) fluids or solutions using a graft preparation device.

BONE CEMENT

Implants used in arthroplasty (joint replacement) may be cemented in place with polymethylmethacrylate (PMMA). Bone cement is an interface or a grout (rather than a glue) between the joint implant and tissue. It is formed by mixing two components, PMMA powder and a liquid monomer of methylmethacrylate. When dry, the cement forms a strong radiopaque filler. Bone cement is supplied plain or with an antibiotic additive that is released into the bone.

Bone cement is prepared during surgery to a doughy consistency. It is instilled into the joint manually or with a cement gun. After mixing, it hardens within 15 minutes. During mixing, the two components create an exothermic (heat releasing) reaction.

PMMA is a hazardous chemical and must be handled according to regulations established by the National Institute for Occupational and Safety Health (NIOSH) and the hospital's policies and protocols. Exposure to PMMA vapor is an occupational risk, and use of the cement is associated with toxic and cardiovascular events in the patient.

Occupational Risk

Vapors released when the dry and liquid components of PMMA are mixed are known to cause serious eye damage and respiratory tract and skin irritation. An allergic reaction may also occur. The effects of vapor inhalation are cumulative and are associated with kidney and liver damage. Inhalation also may cause neurological symptoms and pregnancy complications. NOTE: More information on occupational risk is available on the NIOSH Web site at http://www.cdc.gov/niosh/database.html.

Patient Risks

Patient risks associated with PMMA include toxicity and vascular events. Acute toxicity causes sudden cardiovascular complications and possible cardiac arrest. Increased intramedullary pressure may force marrow tissue into the circulation, resulting in embolism. Bone cement implantation syndrome (BCIS) includes life-threatening hypotension, pulmonary edema, and cardiogenic shock. These hazards can be reduced by the use of good surgical technique, such as using pulse lavage (Figure 30-36) to clear the medullary canal before the cement and implant are inserted.

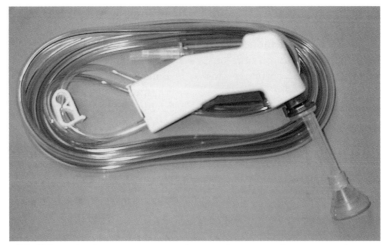

Figure 30-36 Pulse lavage system. Antibiotic solution or saline commonly is used to apply a pulsed stream of pressurized solution to the wound for debridement and irrigation. *(From Townsend CM: Sabiston textbook of surgery, ed 17, Philadelphia, 2001, Saunders.)*

Safety Precautions

The cement is supplied to the sterile field in its two components, as a dry powder and a liquid solvent. These are combined and mixed in a closed container specially designed for use with PMMA. The bone cement mixer is fitted with a vacuum tube that shunts vapors away from the surgical field. They then are dissipated through a charcoal filter. The vacuum system also removes air pockets, which destabilize the cement. Surgical technologists must become familiar with the operation and assembly of bone cement mixers used in their facility.

Preparing Bone Cement

The manufacturer's instructions for mixing bone cement should always be consulted before the process is started. Cement is injected into a prepared joint with cement gun. Some mixers have a cartridge that is transferred directly to the cement gun after mixing. General preparation includes the following steps:

1. Assemble the mixing apparatus according to manufacturer's specifications. Attach one end of the vacuum tubing to the mixer. The circulator receives the other end and attaches it to a vacuum pump, which is operated with compressed nitrogen.
2. Pour the powered and liquid cement components into the mixer.
3. Secure the lid of the mixer. Rotate the lid handle to mix the components.
4. Continue to mix the cement until it reaches a doughy consistency. At this stage, it is removed from the mixer and molded to shape. When it is no longer sticky, it is ready for use.
5. If a cartridge mixer is used, remove the cartridge from the mixer and transfer it immediately to the cement gun.
6. Change sterile gloves when the cement no longer requires handling.
7. Discard any unused cement according to hospital policy. Do not handle unused cement.

CASTING

Casting is a method of external fixation in which a limb is immobilized by applying plaster or synthetic resin. Acute or open fractures are not treated with a cast because of the high risk of complications, such as compartment syndrome and infection.

Casts differ by location and medical objectives. A cylinder cast is a simple wrap along the length of the limb to immobilize a fracture. A spica cast is used in pediatrics to immobilize hip fractures or deformities. The spica cast covers the trunk and one or both limbs. Casting splints sometimes are applied longitudinally over the arm or wrist to provide rigid support after surgery. The splints do not occlude the surgical incision or encase the limb.

Casting materials include plaster and polyurethane resin. Plaster is used less commonly than resins, which are stronger and resistant to breakdown by moisture. Resin casts also are more manageable for the patient because of their light weight. Casting materials are available in 2- to 6-inch (5 to 15 cm) widths.

Before a cast is applied, the limb is wrapped with padding. Two types of padding are commonly used. A stockinet is first applied to the limb. This is followed with felted (batted) cotton Webril. Rolled Webril is applied from distal to proximal. At least two layers of Webril are needed. Extra padding is needed for bony prominences.

Rolls of cast material are immersed in water before use. During application, the limb is lightly supported by the assistant. Plaster hardens within 30 minutes but requires 24 to 48 hours to set completely. Resin casts dry in 15 to 30 minutes.

TRACTION

Traction is a mechanical method of applying pulling force or elongation to fractured bone. Traction is used to:

- Prevent injury to soft tissues, especially blood vessels and nerves near the fracture site

- Align bone after a fracture or **dislocation**
- Prevent movement of a fractured limb
- Reduce pain in acute orthopedic trauma before surgical repair
- Reduce muscle spasm in orthopedic injuries

Traction is used much less often in modern orthopedics than it was in the past. Advances in orthopedic implant surgery and techniques have replaced long-term traction as a primary method of treatment except in certain circumstances. The two types of traction are:

- **Skin traction**, which involves taping a traction system to the skin. It generally is used only as a temporary measure (e.g., Buck traction). Skin traction is seldom used in adults. Modern external traction frames provide temporary traction for emergency use (Figure 30-37, *A*).

- **Skeletal traction**, which requires surgical insertion of metal pins or rods through the bone distal to the fracture. The pins are attached to a traction device that applies force or is drawn by a weighted pulley (Figure 30-37, *B*).

MODULAR ROD AND PIN FIXATION

Modular rod and pin fixation is used mainly for temporary external stabilization of a fracture. The system is very flexible and can be used for fractures of the long bones and pelvis and also for joint lengthening procedures involving bone loss. This type of system also is used to distract bone in which loss has occurred as a result of trauma or disease. The external framework maintains alignment with expansion of the limb to create space for new bone growth.

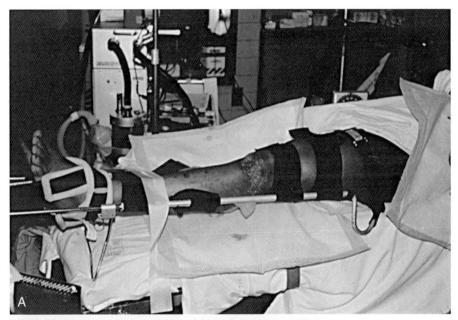

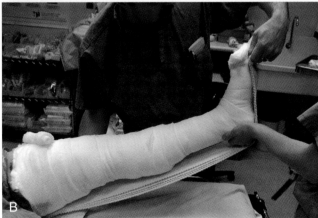

Figure 30-37   Traction. **A,** Emergency traction using soft straps and rods. **B,** Skeletal traction of the femur after surgery to insert traction pins. (**A** *from Wolinsky PR, Johnson KD: Femoral shaft fractures. In Browner BD, Jupiter TB, Levine AM, Trafteon PG, editors: Skeletal trauma, ed 2, Philadelphia, 1998, WB Saunders;* **B** *from Townsend CM: Sabiston textbook of surgery, ed 17, Philadelphia, 2001, WB Saunders.)*

The basic design is based on external metal rods, which act as a superstructure to the bone. The rods are held in place with bolts and pins, which are inserted through the bone to support the outer framework. The modular system can be used as a unilateral frame (a single rod attached by internally placed pins) or a modular frame constructed with multiple rods and pins, which are inserted into the bone fragments and connected with clamps (Figure 30-38). The pins do not require predrilling and are inserted with a power drill.

ARTHROSCOPIC SURGERY

Arthroscopic surgery is minimally invasive surgery (MIS) of the joints. This technique is used mainly for diagnostic procedures and for repair and reconstruction of soft tissue. Most open soft tissue procedures of the joints can be performed arthroscopically.

Before studying the minimally invasive techniques presented in the chapter, the reader should review Chapter 21. The principles are the same; only the instrumentation, patient preparation, and specific operative techniques are different.

Instruments

Many orthopedic MIS instruments resemble those used in open procedures. However, where retraction normally would require an instrument with strong leverage, a hook or probe is used. Because the endoscope penetrates the joint area, mechanical retraction usually is not necessary. Dissection is performed with heavy endoscopic scissors, an electrosurgical unit (ESU) probe, and shears. Power shavers, drills, burrs, and cutters are supplied in endoscopic sets. Graspers contain biting tips for use on cartilage and other fibrous tissues.

A number of sophisticated devices are available for passing sutures through bone and cartilage. The basic principle in all the designs is similar. An eyed, awl-type instrument is used to run the suture through the tissues, or a hole is placed first and the eyed tool with suture mounted is passed through it. Anchoring devices, which contain a biosynthetic screw with suture attached at the distal end, are easily passed through a large trocar for attachment of the joint capsule to ligaments and muscle. Some common arthroscopic instruments are shown in Figure 30-39.

Joint Distension

Joint distension with saline or lactated Ringer solution is necessary for arthroscopy of the shoulder and knee. Fluid is instilled into the joint through one port and exits through another. Inflow tubing and outflow tubing are required to maintain continuous flushing of the joint.

As with other forms of MIS, expansion of the operative field from within allows greater visibility of the structures. Free-flowing solution keeps the operative field free of tissue debris and blood, which can obscure the endoscopic image transmitted to the monitor.

Fluid distension also acts as a tamponade (pressure to control bleeding). This is particularly important in rotator cuff surgery, in which bleeding can be brisk. In knee surgery, the synovial capsule may be inflamed, which can contribute to capillary bleeding. When tamponade is required, the inflow of fluid must be adjusted to keep up with the outflow. The circulator is responsible for making adjustments in the pump system (or gravity system) as necessary. An arthroscopic fluid system is shown in Figure 30-40.

SHOULDER AND ARM

The shoulder is composed of three main bones: the scapula, the clavicle, and the humerus. The head of the humerus fits into the glenoid socket of the scapula; this forms the glenohumeral joint. The socket is surrounded by a rim of cartilage called the *labrum,* which helps stabilize the head of the humerus. The labrum also attaches to several ligaments, which further support the joint.

The clavicle moves in coordination with the humerus and is a primary site of sports injury. Clavicular joints include:

- Acromioclavicular (AC) joint—Clavicle to acromion
- Sternoclavicular (SC) joint—Clavicle to sternum

The shoulder is a mechanically unstable structure. It is suspended from the skeleton by soft tissue and is mobile in all directions. The head of the humerus technically is a ball-and-socket joint, but the glenoid socket, which holds the head of the humerus, is shallow. As mentioned earlier, the labrum encircles the rim of the glenoid. The labrum is a cartilaginous structure similar to the meniscus in the knee. It increases the amount of contact between the humeral head and the glenoid, but joint stability relies on the ligaments, muscles, and tendons. The muscles that attach the humerus to the glenoid socket are jointly called the *rotator cuff.* These muscles also add to the stability of the joint; however, they can be torn as a result of sports injury or other traumatic stress (Figure 30-41).

The shoulder joint is shown in Figure 30-42. Inside the joint capsule is a layer of connective tissue that is thickened at three points; these are referred to as the *glenohumeral ligaments.* When these soft tissues fail because of injury or repetitive stress, shoulder dislocation and subluxation can occur. Recurrent dislocation and subluxation requires surgical treatment in most cases. In the past, techniques were used to bind and restrict soft tissues in the shoulder to prevent recurrence of the injury. In modern surgery, the goal is to restore function and range of motion, especially in active patients who want to return to their usual activities. This goal is not always possible; the surgeon discusses surgical alternatives with the patient to determine the best approach to meet the individual's needs.

The *Bankart* and *Putti Platt* procedures, which involve soft tissue repair and replantation to secure the shoulder, are commonly used for recurrent shoulder dislocation. In the Bankart procedure, the glenoid rim is reattached to the joint capsule; in the Putti Platt procedure, the subscapularis tendon is severed and attached to the glenoid. Sutures or anchoring devices are used to attach the cartilaginous structures. The Bankart procedure is described in the following section as a representative procedure for recurrent shoulder dislocation. Many variations on the two procedures have been developed, but the principles are similar.

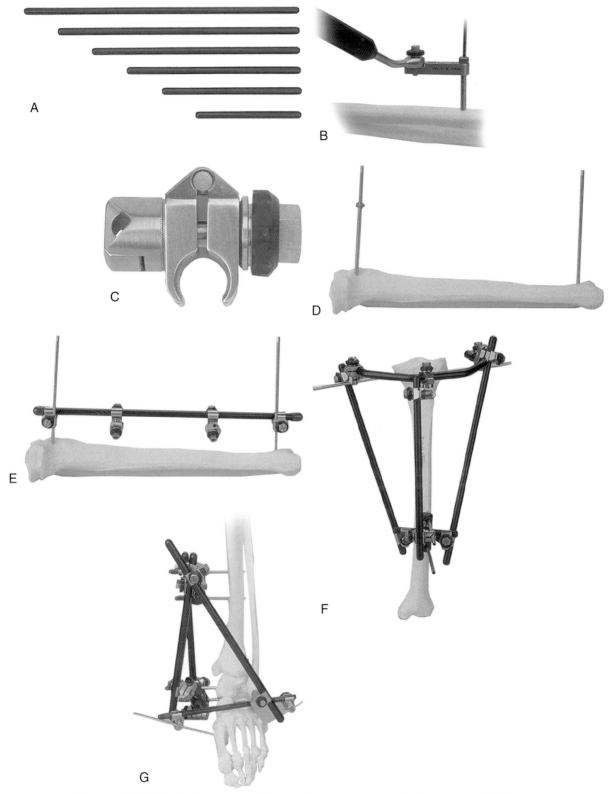

Figure 30-38   Modular external fixation/distraction device. **A,** Modular pins. **B,** Setting the pins. **C,** Clamp. **D,** Building the frame. **E, F,** Building the frame. **G,** Ankle frame in place. *(Courtesy Zimmer, Warsaw, Ind.)*

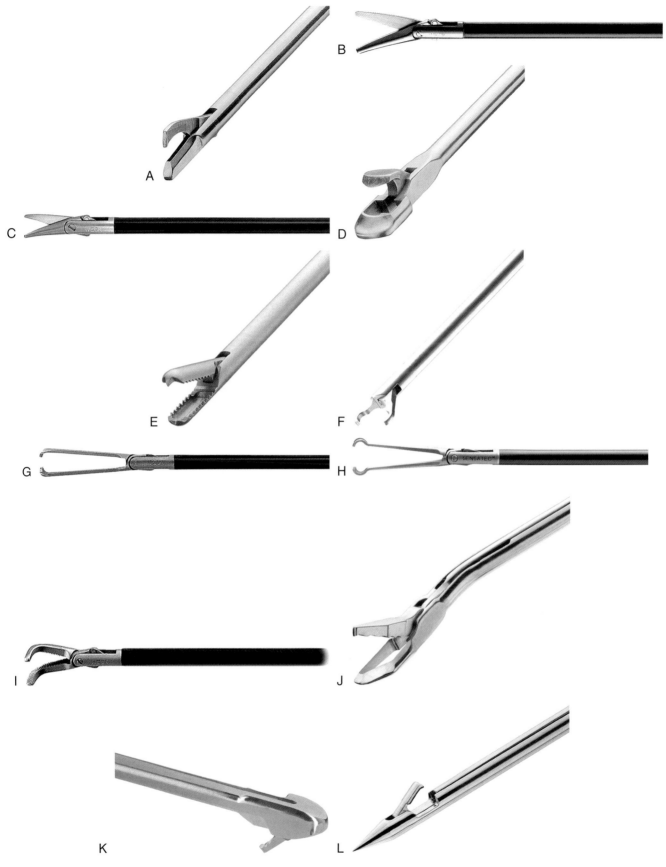

Figure 30-39 Arthroscopy instruments. **A,** Microscissors. **B,** Mayo scissors.
C, Metzenbaum scissors. **D,** Shovel-nose forceps. **E,** Alligator grasper. **F,** Retrieval forceps.
G, Allis grasper. **H,** Babcock grasper. **I,** Mixter forceps. **J,** Linear grasper. **K,** Retro punch.
L, Suture carrier. *(Courtesy Zimmer, Warsaw, Ind.)*

NOTE: The *Bristow* procedure, used in the past, has been replaced by safer techniques. In this procedure the coracoid process is severed and transferred as a sling. This technique has largely been abandoned because of intraoperative risk and postoperative complications, including recurrent subluxation.[3]

SURGICAL APPROACHES TO THE SHOULDER

During open surgery, an anterior approach is used for many types of shoulder procedures (Figure 30-43, *A*). Another common approach is directly over the deltoid at the acromion (Figure 30-43, *B*). The posterior approach also is used is some cases.

BANKART PROCEDURE

Surgical Goal

In the Bankart procedure, the glenoid rim is reattached to the joint capsule with a biosynthetic or other anchoring device or with heavy sutures.

Pathology

An important cause of recurrent glenohumeral dislocation is separation of the labrum (the rim of the glenoid capsule) from the joint capsule. This usually is caused by sports trauma in which the humeral head is forced out of the glenoid anteriorly. The condition may affect young, healthy individuals.

Technique

1. An anterolateral or anterior incision is made and extended to the joint.
2. The conjoined tendon is mobilized and retracted.
3. The joint capsule is incised.
4. The glenoid rim is elevated and trimmed.
5. The capsule is attached to the glenoid with biosynthetic bone anchors, staples, or heavy sutures.
6. The capsule is closed.
7. The wound is closed.

Discussion

The Bankart procedure has been modified since it was developed in the 1920s. It has become less traumatic with the

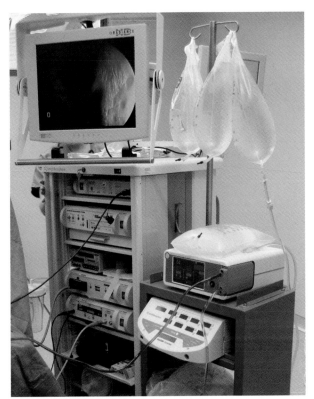

Figure 30-40 Continuous irrigation system used in arthroscopy. Flow pressure is monitored by the control unit. *(From Canale S, Beaty J: Campbell's operative orthopaedics, ed 11, St Louis, 2007, Mosby.)*

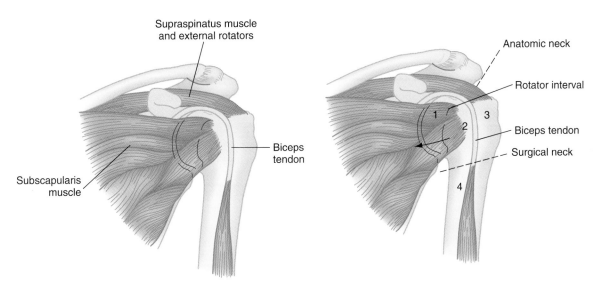

Figure 30-41 Structures of the rotator cuff. *(From Marx J, editor: Rosen's emergency medicine: concepts and clinical practice, ed, 6, Philadelphia, 2006, Mosby.)*

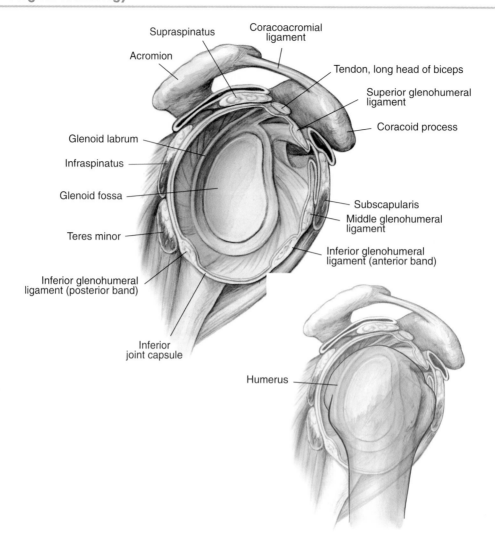

Figure 30-42 Anatomy of the shoulder joint. *(From Miller MD, Chhabra AB, Hurwitz SR, Mihalko WM: Orthopaedic surgical approaches, Philadelphia, 2008, WB Saunders.)*

development of absorbable anchoring devices attached to heavy sutures. The device is placed through the joint capsule, and the sutures are placed through the glenoid rim to repair the lesion. Heavy sutures may also be used to reattach the glenoid.

The patient is placed in the beach chair position. A pad is placed under the scapula to lift the shoulder and bring the scapula forward. The shoulder and arm are prepped and draped, and the arm is left free for intraoperative manipulation.

An anterior or anterolateral incision is made near the axillary crease. The incision is carried into deep tissue using sharp dissection with Metzenbaum scissors and the ESU. Rake retractors are used superficially to expose the muscles. As the incision is extended, deep handheld or a self-retaining retractor are used to expose the joint (Figure 30-44).

When the muscles have been exposed, the conjoined tendon is dissected free and retracted. The capsule is divided, and the glenoid rim is elevated with a retractor such as a ring retractor. The glenoid is prepared for the anchoring devices.

In some cases the tear may require slight remodeling with small rongeurs. An osteotome or rasp is used to score the glenoid rim and produce a raw surface on the bone to which the capsule will be attached.

The capsule is attached with biosynthetic bone anchors, staples, or heavy sutures (Figure 30-45). If anchors are used, the scrub should have several anchors available. For thick bone, a pilot hole may be required. Size 0 or 2-0 Mersilene sutures are the traditional method of repair.

After inspecting the repair, the surgeon uses the long suture ends to close the joint capsule. The shoulder then is manipulated into all ranges of motion to test the repair. The wound is irrigated and closed with continuous or running sutures. A simple dressing is applied, and the shoulder is placed in a soft immobilizer.

Postoperative Considerations

After an open procedure for shoulder instability, dislocation can recur in 30% to 60% of cases. The patient may return to some activity within several months. Physical therapy is

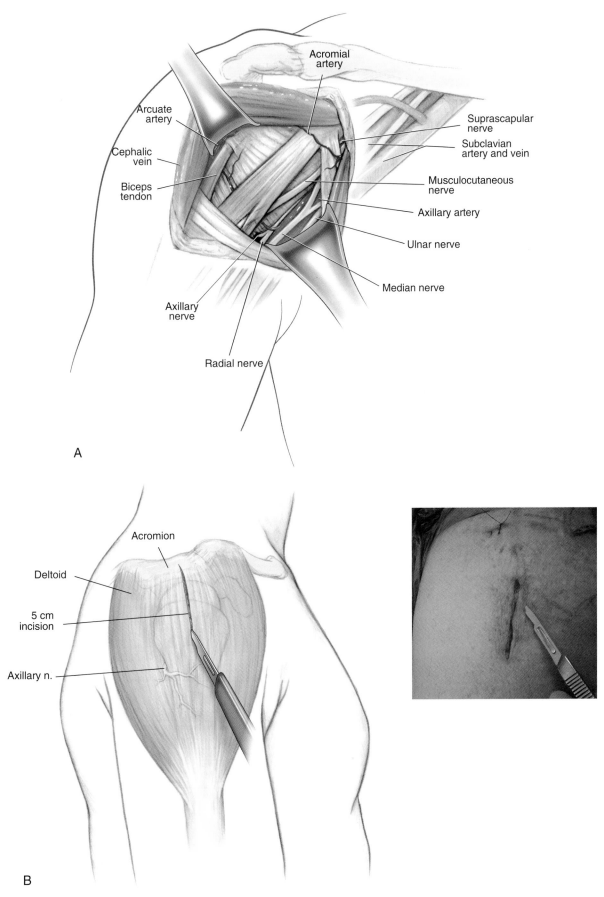

Acromial
artery

Arcuate
artery

Suprascapular
nerve

Cephalic
vein

Subclavian
artery and vein

Biceps
tendon

Musculocutaneous
nerve

Axillary artery

Ulnar nerve

Median nerve

Axillary
nerve

Radial nerve

A

Acromion

Deltoid

5 cm
incision

Axillary n.

B

Figure 30-43 Surgical approach to the shoulder. **A,** Deltopectoral approach. **B,** Deltoid splitting incision. *(From Miller MD, Chhabra AB, Hurwitz SR, Mihalko WM: Orthopaedic surgical approaches, Philadelphia, 2008, WB Saunders.)*

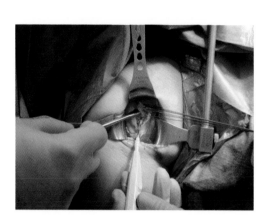

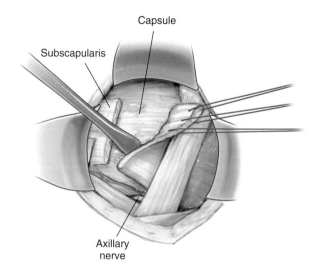

Figure 30-44 Exposure of the shoulder. The subscapularis has been divided, and traction sutures have been placed. Note the conjoined tendon at right. *(From Miller MD, Chhabra AB, Hurwitz SR, Mihalko WM: Orthopaedic surgical approaches, Philadelphia, 2008, WB Saunders.)*

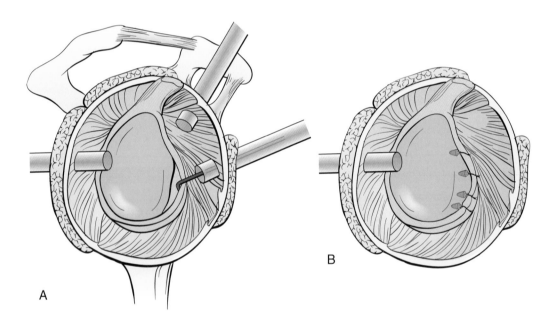

Figure 30-45 Surgical repair for recurrent shoulder dislocation. Multiple sutures are placed in the glenoid rim. *(From Rakel R: Textbook of family medicine, ed 7, Philadelphia, 2007, WB Saunders.)*

required to strengthen the rotator cuff muscles. Healing usually is complete within 6 months.

OPEN ROTATOR CUFF REPAIR

Surgical Goal

The goal of rotator cuff repair is to reattach torn muscles of the rotator cuff to the humerus with sutures or anchor-suturing devices. An open or arthroscopic approach can be used.

Pathology

The rotator cuff is composed of four tendons that attach to the humerus. Each tendon is continuous with a muscle that originates at the scapula. The muscles are the supraspinatus, the subscapularis, the infraspinatus, and the teres minor. One or more tendons may be damaged by traumatic injury or as a result of recurrent shoulder dislocation. A rotator cuff tear usually occurs where the supraspinatus tendon inserts into the humerus. The injury can be superficial or can involve the entire tendon. Degenerative conditions, in which the tissue is weakened because of past injury or previous surgery, can also result in tearing.

Technique

1. An anterior or deltopectoral incision is made in the shoulder and carried to the coracoacromial ligament.
2. The ligament is incised, and traction sutures are placed through the edge.
3. For suture repair, several suture holes are made in the humerus with a drill or an awl.
4. Sutures are passed through the bone and tendon.
5. Biosynthetic screws or a collagen patch may be used in the repair.
6. The deltoid is attached with heavy synthetic sutures.
7. The wound is closed.

Discussion

The patient is positioned, prepped, and draped for a shoulder procedure with the arm free. In addition to general surgery instruments, the technologist should have a shoulder set, drill, and small drill bits available. The incision is carried to the joint capsule with the ESU and Metzenbaum scissors. A self-retaining retractor (e.g., Gelpi or Beckman retractor) is used to expose the rotator cuff tendons and muscles.

The deltoid muscle may be split with a needle-tip ESU, or it may be dissected from the acromion, depending on the exposure needed and the type of repair. The coracoacromial ligament is incised with the ESU. A heavy polyester suture is inserted through the ligament, and the long suture ends are tagged with a hemostat. The supraspinatus tendon and bursa are then exposed, and the injury is evaluated.

If sutures are used to repair the tear, the acromion must be prepared. Several small holes are made in the surface of the humerus with an awl. Braided polyester sutures are passed through the bone and the tendon; two lines of sutures may be placed. The suture ends are left long and tagged with hemostats. This step is repeated until all sutures are in place. The arm then is raised and the shoulder is adducted to reduce tension on the suture line. The sutures are then tied.

Newer techniques for rotator cuff repair involve the use of biosynthetic or collagen material, which is secured over the repair site to strengthen the tissue. If anchor screws are used for the repair, pilot holes are drilled before insertion of three or more anchors, depending on the size of the tear. The anchor is implanted, and the sutures are drawn through the edge of the tendon and then tied. If the deltoid muscle was severed, it is reattached to the acromion with several heavy sutures passed through drill holes. The wound is irrigated with antibiotic solution, and bleeding is controlled with the ESU.

The incision is closed with 2-0 and 3-0 absorbable suture. The subcutaneous tissue is closed with staples or 4-0 absorbable suture and Steri-Strips. The incision is covered with 4 × 4 gauze and a bulky dressing and is immobilized with a sling or shoulder immobilizer. A repair using collagen patch material is illustrated in Figure 30-46.

PLATING OF THE PROXIMAL HUMERUS

Surgical Goal

A fracture of the proximal humerus is repaired using open reduction and internal fixation. A metal plate is secured across the fracture with locking screws.

Pathology

A direct blow to the proximal humerus may result from a fall. This type of injury is common among the elderly. Other accidents, such as a fall from a horse or during construction work, are also common causes. Only about 20% of proximal humeral fractures require open reduction or pinning. Most heal with immobilization.

Technique

1. The patient is placed in beach chair position and prepped for a shoulder procedure.
2. An anterior deltopectoral approach is used.
3. The fracture is reduced and stabilized with K-wires.
4. K-wires are placed in the proximal and distal screw holes with a drill guide.
5. Screw holes are drilled and measured. Screws are inserted and hand-tightened.
6. The K-wires are removed, and locking caps are placed on each screw.
7. The wound is irrigated and closed in layers.

Discussion

Humeral plating is a method of restoring continuity after a displaced fracture of the proximal humerus. A number of systems are available. Cannulated screws or a screw-plate combination are commonly used. Plates may be fixed to the lateral side of the humerus, with additional smaller plates on the anterior side.

The instruments required are a basic orthopedic set, power drill, Kirschner wires, the implant plates and screws, plus any specialty instruments packaged with the plate set (i.e., a drill guide, screwdriver, and bone spacers). C-arm fluoroscopy is needed, and the equipment should be adjusted and draped before the start of the case.

The patient is placed in supine or semi-Fowler's position, and a general anesthetic is administered. An anterior (deltopectoral) approach is used to expose the humerus (see the description of the Bankart procedure). Rake and right-angle retractors are placed in the wound.

The fracture is reduced by manipulation and then stabilized with 2-mm K-wires or heavy synthetic sutures. At least two or three wires are used. These are inserted with the power drill. The plate then is fitted over the curve of the proximal humerus and temporarily attached with a K-wire.

A bone spacer may be used, depending on the surgeon's preference. Spacers elevate the plate slightly to prevent direct contact with the periosteum, which can compromise the blood supply to the fracture during healing. Spacers are available in thicknesses of 1 to 3 mm. The position of the plate is assessed fluoroscopically. If the reduction is satisfactory, screws may be inserted.

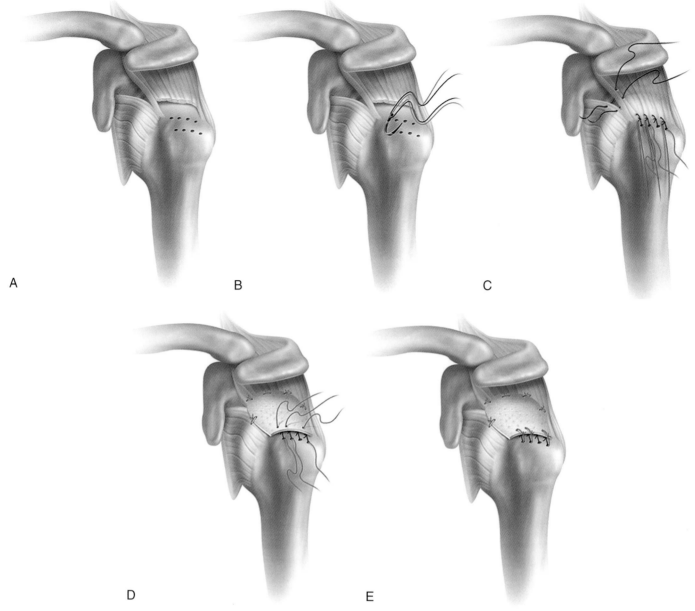

Figure 30-46 Rotator cuff repair. **A,** Preparation of the humerus. Holes are made with a drill or an awl. **B,** Insertion of Mersilene or braided nylon sutures through the bone holes. **C,** The rotator cuff tendon is attached. Additional sutures are placed through the rotator cuff gap *(top)*. **D,** A collagen patch is trimmed and fitted over the repair site. Additional sutures are placed. **E,** Completed repair. *(Courtesy Zimmer, Warsaw, Ind.)*

In preparation for setting the screw holes and fixing the plate, the scrub should have drill bits, a screw rack, drill guide, screwdriver, and depth gauge available. The drill guide and drill bit are needed to drill the screw holes. The drill guide fits over the plate and guides the angle of insertion. The screw holes are drilled under fluoroscopy. A depth gauge is used to measure the depth of the hole and the screw length. The screws are selected and implanted, and a torque screwdriver is used to hand-tighten the screws. The same technique is used for proximal and distal screws. The K-wires are removed.

The last step in the procedure is to set the locking caps on the screws. This is done with the torque screwdriver. The bone spacers then can be removed and replaced with additional screws. Surgical options include use of a small bendable side plate that is attached to the main plate with wire and to the bone with small screws. The technique is illustrated in Figure 30-47.

The wound is dressed with Telfa and flat and fluffed gauze for protection. The arm may be put in a sling or an immobilizer.

Postoperative Considerations

Physical therapy is required to regain flexibility and strength in the shoulder. Adhesions (scarring) and limited range of

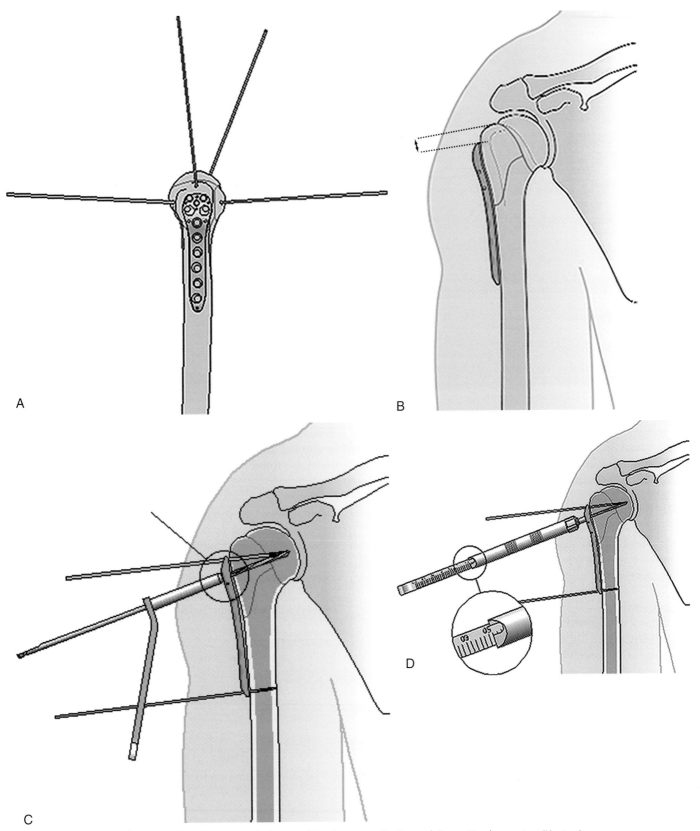

Figure 30-47 Proximal plating of the humerus. **A,** Several 2-mm Kirschner wires (K-wires) are inserted through the humerus to hold the fragments in place. **B,** The plate is positioned with one or two K-wires inserted through the screw holes. **C,** With the K-wires still in place, a drill guide is positioned to align drill holes for screws. **D,** Drill holes are made with a 3-mm drill bit. The length of the hole is measured with a calibrated depth gauge.

Continued

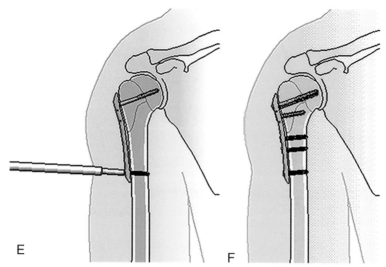

Figure 30-47, cont'd   E, Bicortical screws are inserted into the proximal and distal ends of the plate. **F,** Completed repair. *(Courtesy Zimmer, Warsaw, Ind.)*

motion may result in a stiff arm. Healing normally occurs within about 12 weeks.

SHOULDER ARTHROSCOPY

Surgical Goal

The surgical goals are the same as for open procedures and depend on the nature of the injury.

Pathology

An arthroscopic approach can be used for most types of shoulder injury and disease, except for total joint arthroplasty procedures and when the injury is extensive and wider exposure is needed.

Discussion

The patient is placed in the semi-Fowler or lateral position. The shoulder and arm are prepped and draped free or suspended with a shoulder distracter. A marking pen is used to identify the bony landmarks. The surgeon uses an 18-gauge spinal needle and 60 mL of saline with or without epinephrine to infiltrate and expand the joint space. A small puncture is then made with a #11 blade, and the inflow cannula is inserted.

Irrigation is connected, and the tubing is unclamped. While the joint is being infiltrated, a third incision is made. The scope sleeve and the 30-degree scope are inserted, and the biceps tendon is identified. Figure 30-48 illustrates the placement of the operative scopes and instruments during a routine shoulder arthroscopy.

The patient's arm is rotated and moved as needed to allow the surgeon to visualize the various structures in and around the joint. The shoulder is irrigated, incisions are closed with 4-0 nylon, 4 × 4 dressings are applied, and either a shoulder immobilizer or an arm sling is applied.

SHOULDER ARTHROPLASTY

Surgical Goal

During total shoulder arthroplasty, the humeral head and glenoid capsule are replaced with artificial components to restore function and relieve pain. In hemiarthroplasty, only the humeral component is replaced.

Pathology

The indications for shoulder arthroplasty are persistent pain that is not relieved by more conservative surgery and an inability on the part of the patient to perform activities of daily living because of loss of function. Osteoarthritis is the primary cause of these symptoms. Rheumatoid arthritis, traumatic arthritis, and shoulder instability related to rotator cuff disease are less commonly indicated for joint replacement.

Technique

1. An anterolateral incision is made in the shoulder and carried to the glenohumeral joint.
2. The shoulder is dislocated.
3. The humeral head is resected.
4. The humeral shaft is reamed and shaped to receive the implant.
5. The humeral implant is inserted with or without cement.
6. The glenoid fossa is assessed, and osteophytes are removed. The rim is lowered as necessary.
7. Holes or a trough is drilled into the fossa as required to receive the glenoid component.
8. The glenoid component is cemented in place.
9. The joint is reduced.
10. The wound is closed.

Discussion

Many shoulder replacement systems are available. The appropriate system for any patient depends on the pathology, the

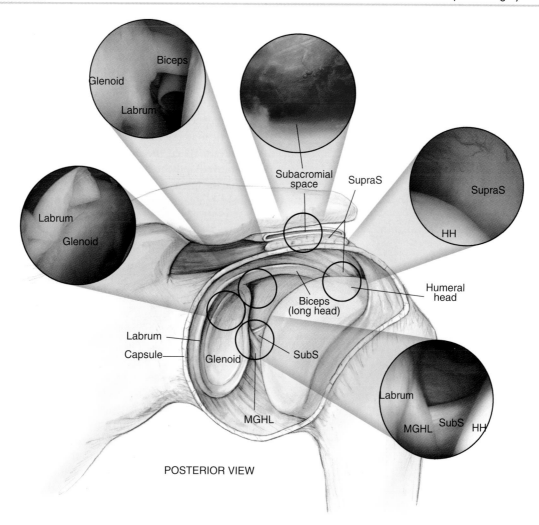

Figure 30-48 Arthroscopy of the shoulder. Posterior view for procedures of the glenohumeral joint and subacromial space. *HH,* Humeral head; *MGHL,* medial glenohumeral ligament; *SubS,* subscapularis; *SupraS,* suprascapularis. *(From Miller MD, Chhabra AB, Hurwitz SR, Mihalko WM: Orthopaedic surgical approaches, Philadelphia, 2008, WB Saunders.)*

condition of the tissues at the time of surgery, and the patient's age and level of activity. A total joint system includes a humeral component, which is similar to the femoral component used in hip arthroplasty. The stem portion may be press-fit or cemented. The glenoid component is replaced with a pegged cup, usually constructed of polyethylene. Figure 30-49 shows a total shoulder system (i.e., the Zimmer Anatomical Shoulder).

In preparation for shoulder arthroplasty, the surgical technologist should have all the components and sizers needed for the selected system. A major orthopedic set and shoulder instruments are added, and ample table room should be provided to accommodate the instrument trays. A pneumatic oscillating saw is needed to perform the osteotomy. Reamers are required for medullary canalization of the humerus. **Broaches** (fin-shaped rasps that closely match the contour of the medullary implant) that fit the specific system implant are also needed for canalization. If a cemented prosthesis is planned, provisions should be made for these components

(e.g., mixer, tubing). A magnetic instrument pad should be used to prevent instruments placed on the surgical field from falling. ESU and suction are used continuously during the procedure, and holsters should be provided for these on the field.

A total arthroplasty procedure has three parts: the approach to the joint, replacement of the humerus, and replacement of the glenoid. The patient is placed in semi-Fowler position with the affected side near the edge of the operating table. The shoulder and upper body are prepped as previously described. An anterior (deltopectoral) approach is most commonly used for the procedure. The incision extends to the joint capsule, which is incised to allow the humerus to be lifted from the glenoid fossa. Slotted retractors and a bone hook may be used to release the humerus.

Humeral Component

With the humerus removed from the glenoid fossa, the humeral neck may be severed. A template measuring device

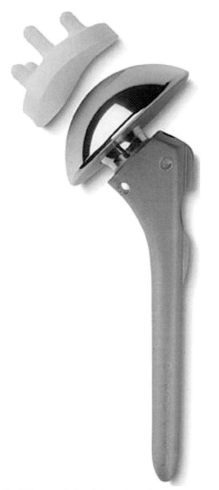

Figure 30-49 Total shoulder arthroplasty components. *(Courtesy Zimmer, Warsaw, Ind.)*

is placed either directly over the humerus or the x-ray to determine the angle of osteotomy. The surgeon may mark the cutting line with the ESU. The technologist should have a sagittal saw and irrigation prepared at this point. A retractor may be placed under the humerus to protect the soft tissues during the osteotomy. The sagittal saw then is used to the divide humerus. The removed portion is passed to the scrub as a specimen and may be used during bone grafting.

The medullary canal is prepared for reaming by delivering the humerus out of the incision. A pilot hole is made in the cancellous bone with a small reamer, and increasingly larger reamers (8- to 12-mm) are used to enter the medullary canal. An osteotome is used to remove a "fin" of bone to fit the shape of the prosthesis. When the cancellous bone has been penetrated, modular broaches are used to form a space for the humeral stem. When the last modular rasp has been used, it is left in place. Test heads are fitted onto the modular rasp with the attachments specific to the system used. The modular broach then is removed, and the actual head component is assembled.

The humeral component now can be inserted. Before insertion, pulse lavage is used to irrigate the medullary canal and clean it of all debris. Antibiotic solution may be used for irrigation. NOTE: Sutures used to repair the subscapularis may be placed just before the prosthesis is fitted into the canal. Several drill holes are made in the neck of the humerus, and Mersilene or other braided suture is passed through the holes. The sutures are tied during closure.

The stem is fitted to the system impactor (driver), and the prosthesis is inserted into the canal with or without bone cement, depending on the type of implant used. Bone or biosynthetic material may be used to fill in any gaps in a press-fit prosthesis. When the prosthesis is fully seated, the impactor is removed and the ball prosthesis is fitted on the stem. If a hemiarthroplasty is planned, the humerus can be replaced in the glenoid cavity by manipulation.

Glenoid Component

When complete arthroplasty is planned, the disarticulated joint is examined before the glenoid side is prepared. The glenoid rim often needs to be trimmed, and osteophytes and other bony growths must be removed. The fossa can be lowered (the rim taken down) with rongeurs or by reaming the fossa with a high-speed burr or cup-shaped reamers.

Two types of glenoid prostheses are commonly used, a pegged design or a keeled design. Holes may be drilled to accommodate a pegged component. Pegged systems provide a drill guide for exact placement of the holes. For a keeled component, a trough is drilled with a high-speed drill and round burr. After creation of the holes or trough, the surface is cleaned with pulse lavage. If a cemented prosthesis is used, the cement may be impacted into the peg holes with a sponge and hemostat. The prosthesis is fitted into the holes and held in place manually or with a system tool until the cement has set. Before the humerus is replaced in the glenoid, the joint is irrigated and all bits of cement are removed from the field. The scrub assists by making sure all debris has been removed from the drapes and that fresh sponges are supplied. The joint then is reduced and assessed for mobility and function.

The incision is closed in layers. The subscapularis sutures are secured, and the rotator cuff is closed with synthetic nonabsorbable sutures. The superficial layers are closed with absorbable synthetic sutures. A sump drain may be placed before closure. The wound is dressed with Kerlix fluffs and an abdominal pad. A shoulder brace is applied for stability. Shoulder arthroplasty is illustrated in Figure 30-50.

Postoperative Considerations

Patients begin passive range of motion exercises within 24 hours of surgery. A rigorous physiotherapy routine is begun within the first week and continues for 3 to 6 months.

ELBOW ARTHROPLASTY

Surgical Goal

Elbow arthroplasty is performed to relieve pain and restore function to the elbow. The elbow joint system is illustrated in Figure 30-51.

Pathology

Arthroplasty of the elbow most often is performed to treat rheumatoid arthritis or a severe traumatic injury.

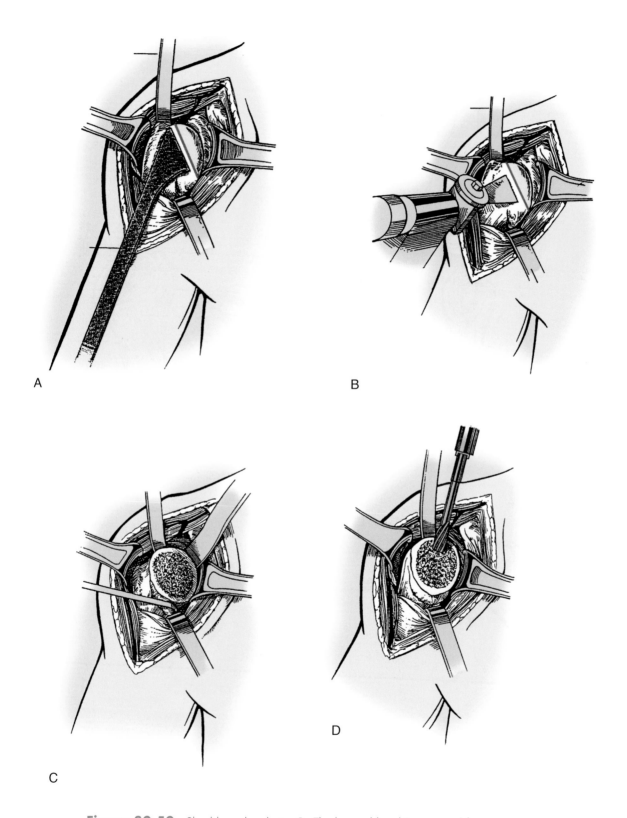

A

B

C

D

Figure 30-50 Shoulder arthroplasty. **A,** The humeral head is measured for an osteotomy with a template. **B,** A sagittal saw is used to perform the osteotomy. **C,** The cut surface of the humerus. **D,** Reamers are used to penetrate the cancellous bone.

Continued

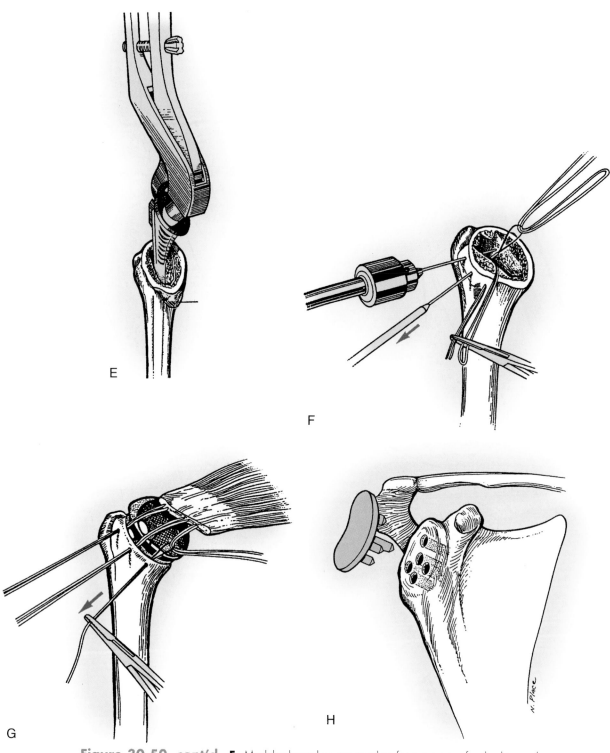

Figure 30-50, cont'd **E,** Modular broaches are used to form a space for the humeral stem. **F,** Holes are drilled in the humeral neck, and sutures are threaded through them. **G,** After the humeral implant is inserted, the sutures are used to secure the subscapular tendon. **H,** Placement of the glenoid component. *(From Matsen FA III, Rockwood CA Jr, Wirth MA et al: Glenohumeral arthritis and its management. In Rockwood CA Jr, Matsen FA III, Wirth MA et al, editors: The shoulder, ed 3, Philadelphia, 2004, WB Saunders.)*

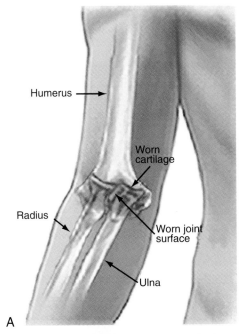

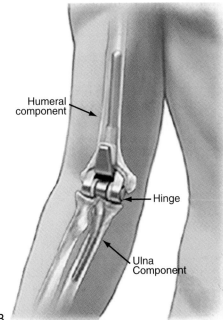

Figure 30-51 Elbow arthroplasty. **A,** Areas of worn cartilage. **B,** Implant design. *(Courtesy Zimmer, Warsaw, Ind.)*

Discussion

Elbow arthroplasty is a procedure that currently is in development, and it is performed much less often than shoulder or knee reconstruction.

The instruments required for elbow arthroplasty include an orthopedic set, power drill, K-wires, Steinmann pins, pulse lavage, and the selected joint replacement system. A general anesthetic is used.

A pneumatic tourniquet is applied to the upper arm. The patient is placed in the supine position, and the operative arm, and hand, are prepped and draped. The hand is usually wrapped with an occlusive drape to exclude it from the surgical site.

The surgeon makes a posteromedial incision at the elbow. The ulnar nerve is identified and protected. The medial half of the triceps is elevated, and the tip of the olecranon is removed. The medial collateral ligament (MCL) is released to improve exposure. The forearm then is rotated in the lateral position to produce exposure of the distal humerus. An oscillating saw is used to remove a portion of the trochlea. Access to the medullary canal of the humerus is complete. An IM canal finder is inserted and exchanged for an alignment stem with an attached cutting block. An oscillating saw is used to remove the distal humerus.

The surgeon enters the medullary canal of the ulna using a high-speed drill or burr. Additional bone is removed from the tip of the olecranon to make room for the reamers. After reaming, a rasp is impacted down the ulna, with care taken to prevent a proximal ulnar fracture or other complication.

After the humerus and ulna have been prepared, the surgeon inserts the trials. When the trials are in place, range of motion, including flexion and extension, is tested. The trials are removed, and the surgical site is irrigated.

Bone cement is mixed and placed in a cement gun for injection into the humeral and ulnar canals. Bone graft is placed in any open spaces and behind the humeral implant. The bone graft helps the humerus resist posterior and rotational displacement. The humeral implant is impacted, and the ulnar implant is inserted.

When the bone cement has cured, the tourniquet is deflated and hemostasis is obtained with the ESU. The surgical site then is irrigated with an antibiotic irrigant. The incision is closed, a dressing is applied, and the elbow is placed in neutral position with a posterior splint and an arm sling.

WRIST AND HAND

Wrist and hand surgery is a specialty that combines orthopedics, vascular surgery, and neurosurgery. Technological advances in instrumentation within the past 15 years have greatly improved recovery after complex hand trauma and soft tissue diseases such as fascial contraction and nerve entrapment. Innovative joint replacement procedures are now common for the treatment of joint diseases, such as degenerative arthritis.

The arm and hand are prepped using standard techniques. The hand may require scrubbing to remove embedded dirt, especially from under the fingernails. Trauma cases involving shards of glass, metal, wood, or other foreign objects that are embedded in soft tissue require more complex **debridement** and lavage. This usually is performed outside the operating room, often in the emergency department. Industrial accidents may result in tissue injection of oil and other chemicals, which also require extensive debridement.

A regional or local anesthetic is used for most hand surgery. A combination of lidocaine and a long-acting local anesthetic (e.g., bupivacaine) is commonly used. Vasoconstrictive agents (e.g., epinephrine) are not used, because they can cause damage to delicate vessels and nerves. A pneumatic tourniquet is used for all hand cases.

Short plastic surgery instruments are used for all hand procedures. Delicate orthopedic instruments are required for joint and trauma surgery involving bone. A small drill and fine Steinmann pins or K-wires are commonly used for internal fixation. Reconstruction procedures require small vascular clamps and short right-angle clamps. The bipolar ESU with a fine-needle point and bipolar forceps is used to prevent lateral heating. Silastic vessel loops are used to retract tendons and ligaments. The surgeon may use magnifying loupes or the operating microscope during surgery. Instruments commonly used in hand surgery are shown in Figure 30-52.

Delicate tendons, ligaments, nerves, and blood vessels are critical for precise movement of the hand. These tissues must be kept moist during surgery. The surgical technologist assisting in hand procedures irrigates the surgical wound with saline. A small bulb syringe or standard syringe fitted with an irrigation tip may be used. Low-pressure suction with fine angled suction tips is used to prevent injury to the tissue. Neurosurgical patties and small gauze sponges dipped in saline are also required.

In reconstructive hand surgery, sutures are required for tendon, nerve, and ligament repair. These tissues must heal with as little scar formation as possible to preserve function. Inert suture materials, such as 6-0 and 7-0 polypropylene (Prolene), stainless steel, and polyester (Ti-Cron), are commonly used. A fine ⅜ cutting curve is commonly used. Vascular sutures are required for trauma, reconstruction, and **replantation**, also called **reimplantation** (reattachment of a digit or a portion of the hand). Sutures of 5-0 and 7-0 polyester and polypropylene are commonly used. Double-arm sutures are used for anastomosis of vessels, tendons, and nerves. Figure 30-53 presents an anterior view of the hand.

OPEN REDUCTION AND INTERNAL FIXATION OF THE WRIST

Surgical Goal
Screws or pins are used to repair a fracture of the wrist to stabilize the bone fragments so that healing can occur in their correct anatomical position.

Pathology
The scaphoid is the most common site of a wrist fracture because of its vulnerable location. A common cause of fracture is a fall when the wrists are flexed to break the impact. Simple, nondisplaced fractures are treated with casting. Open reduction and internal fixation are required for a displaced fracture.

Discussion
One or more cannulated screws are used for fixation of the scaphoid. The Herbert screw, the Synthes 3.0 cannulated screw, or Steinmann pins are surgical options. C-arm fluoroscopy should be available for the procedure.

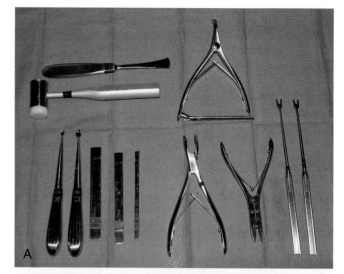

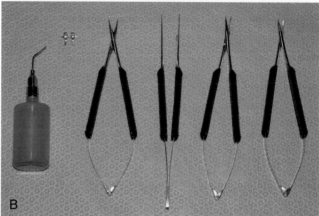

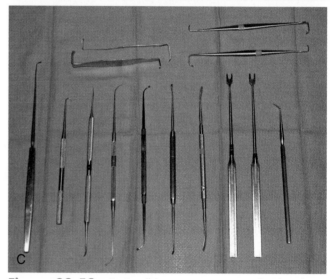

Figure 30-52   A, Small bone instruments used in hand surgery. **B,** Selected microinstruments. **C,** Dental and ear, nose, and throat (ENT) instruments useful in hand surgery. *(From Canale S, Beaty J: Campbell's operative orthopaedics, ed 11, St Louis, 2007, Mosby.)*

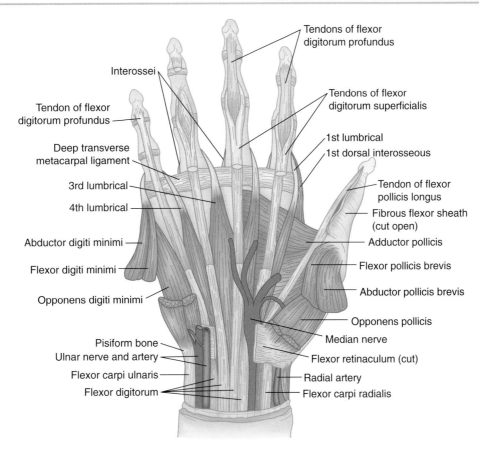

Interossei

Tendon of flexor
digitorum profundus

Deep transverse
metacarpal ligament

3rd lumbrical

4th lumbrical

Abductor digiti minimi

Flexor digiti minimi

Opponens digiti minimi

Pisiform bone

Ulnar nerve and artery

Flexor carpi ulnaris

Flexor digitorum

Tendons of flexor
digitorum profundus

Tendons of flexor
digitorum superficialis

1st lumbrical
1st dorsal interosseous

Tendon of flexor
pollicis longus

Fibrous flexor sheath
(cut open)

Adductor pollicis

Flexor pollicis brevis

Abductor pollicis brevis

Opponens pollicis

Median nerve

Flexor retinaculum (cut)

Radial artery

Flexor carpi radialis

Figure 30-53 Anatomy of the anterior hand. *(From Snell RS, Smith MS: Clinical anatomy for emergency medicine, St Louis, 1993, Mosby.)*

The patient is placed in the supine position with the operative arm on a hand table. A tourniquet is applied, and the hand and arm are prepped and draped in routine manner. The instruments required for insertion of a cannulated or Herbert screw include a minor orthopedic set, a small drill, K-wires, and a screw system. A compression fracture may require bone grafting.

Exposure

A rolled towel may be placed under the wrist to stabilize it, or the hand may be placed in a distracter. A common approach for repair is the volar approach (Figure 30-54). The surgeon makes a small incision over the scaphoid bone and inserts two rake retractors to expose the flexor carpi muscle. This is divided with a curved hemostat and scissors. The tendon sheath is incised. The flexor tendon is isolated and retracted. Depending on the approach, a branch of the radial artery may be encountered. This is divided and ligated with 3-0 or 4-0 nonabsorbable suture. The joint capsule then is incised to expose the scaphoid bone. A small Weitlaner retractor is placed in the wound.

Cannulated Screw and Threaded Washer

The cannulated screw and washer set includes instruments required for the procedure described here. For placement of

a cannulated screw, a threaded guide wire is inserted over the fracture site. A drill sleeve may be used to direct the wire at the correct angle. The screw hole may be predrilled with a small power drill. A cannulated drill bit is used. A space for the threaded washer also is created.

The washer is inserted with the cannulated driver. A measuring device similar to a drill tap is inserted over the guide wire to measure the depth of the predrilled hole and washer. The screw is threaded over the guide wire and tightened with a screwdriver. The guide wire is removed by using the power drill in reverse mode.

The wound is irrigated with saline and closed in layers. The capsule is closed with 4-0 synthetic absorbable suture. Skin and subcutaneous tissue are closed with 4-0 nonabsorbable sutures. The wound is dressed with flat gauze. A plaster cast usually is applied over the wrist and arm.

CARPAL TUNNEL RELEASE

Surgical Goal

The goal of surgical carpal tunnel release (CTR) is to free an entrapped median volar nerve and restore function of the wrist. An open or a minimally invasive technique may be used.

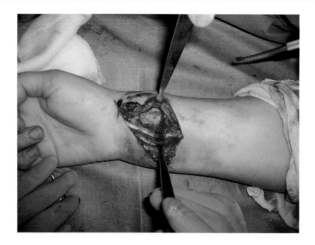

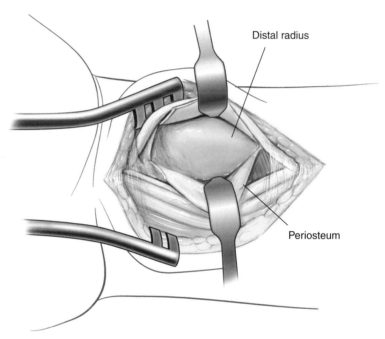

Distal radius

Periosteum

Figure 30-54   Volar approach to the hand. *(From Miller MD, Chhabra AB, Hurwitz SR, Mihalko WM: Orthopaedic surgical approaches, Philadelphia, 2008, WB Saunders.)*

Arthroscopic instruments used in carpal tunnel release are shown in Figure 30-55.

Pathology

Carpal tunnel syndrome occurs when the median nerve in the carpal tunnel of the wrist is compressed. A variety of factors may contribute to nerve compression. These include an anatomical decrease in the size of the carpal tunnel, wrist fracture, post-traumatic arthritis, and inflammatory disease, such as rheumatoid arthritis. External conditions, such as vibration, prolonged direct pressure, and repetitive movement, may contribute to or trigger the condition. Carpal tunnel syndrome occurs most often in adults 30 to 60 years of age and is more common in women than in men. Patients experience numbness and tingling in the fingers and pain in the hand that often radiates up the forearm.

Technique

1. A curvilinear or longitudinal incision is made in the palm and extended to the wrist.
2. The carpal ligament is retracted and divided.
3. The tourniquet is deflated, and the wound is inspected for bleeding.
4. Hemostasis is maintained.
5. The wound is closed.
6. A compression bandage and splint are applied.

Discussion

The patient is positioned supine on the operating room bed with the affected arm resting on a hand table. The procedure is performed using local infiltration, a regional nerve block (Bier block), or general anesthesia. A pneumatic tourniquet is used to create a bloodless field. The open technique is described here.

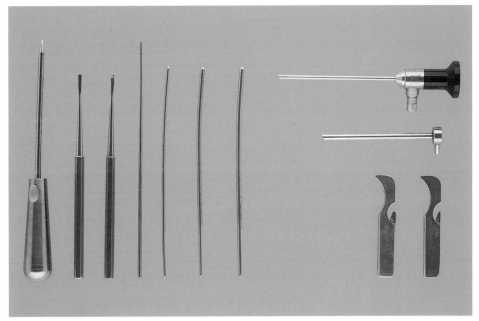

Figure 30-55 Arthroscopic carpal tunnel instruments. *Left to right,* 1 obturator; 2 dissectors; 1 probe; 3 Hegar dilators; small arthroscope and handles for carpal tunnel blades. *(From Tighe SM: Instrumentation for the operating room, ed 6, St Louis, 2003, Mosby.)*

The surgeon uses a #15 blade to create a longitudinal or curvilinear incision in the skin (Figure 30-56.) Blunt dissection with small Metzenbaum scissors exposes the fascia, which is retracted with small Weitlaner retractors, skin hooks, or sharp Senn retractors. The flexor tendon is exposed and retracted. The surgeon identifies both the flexor tendon and the neurovascular bundle that lies close to the tendon.

The carpal ligament then is well visualized, and the midsection is cut either with scissors or with a knife blade to release the carpal ligament and median nerve. The incision is irrigated with sterile saline.

The tourniquet pressure is released, and the wound is checked for bleeders, which are controlled with the bipolar ESU. The surgeon may inject the incision with bupivacaine to control postoperative pain. The skin is closed with an absorbable subcuticular suture. A bulky compression dressing using gauze fluffs and a splint is applied.

Arthroscopic Technique

Carpal tunnel release may also be performed as minimally invasive surgery using Endowrist instruments. The anesthesia considerations, prepping, draping, and tourniquet use are as described for open carpal tunnel release. An advantage of the endoscopic approach is that it uses one or two small incisions over the palm of the hand instead of the extensive incision described for the open approach. The carpal ligament is directly below the incisions, in the distal area of the palm just below the wrist. The carpal ligament is cut longitudinally. This releases the pressure on the nerve as it passes through the ligament. Wound closure and dressing application are as described for the open technique.

Postoperative Considerations

Carpal tunnel release most often is performed in the outpatient setting, and the patient is discharged within hours of the procedure. Immediate and long-term postoperative complications are rare.

METACARPOPHALANGEAL JOINT ARTHROPLASTY

Surgical Goal

The surgical goal of metacarpophalangeal (MCP) joint arthroplasty is to eliminate pain and align the joints, producing joint stability.

Pathology

The primary cause of MCP joint disease in adults is advanced rheumatoid arthritis.

Discussion

The patient is placed in the supine position with the affected arm extended on an arm table. A tourniquet is applied. The arm is prepped from the fingertips to the elbow. The arm then is draped with an extremity drape. A small bone set, the implant instruments, and a microburr are needed.

A transverse incision is made over the dorsum of the metacarpals, exposing the tendon. Note that a volar (palm side) approach may be used. Tenotomy scissors and a #15 blade are used to release the extensor tendon. The joint capsule and collateral ligaments are elevated on both sides of the metacarpal and on the proximal phalanx. A microsaw is used to resect the metacarpal head. Two small (Hohmann) retractors should be placed under the bone to protect the underlying tissue

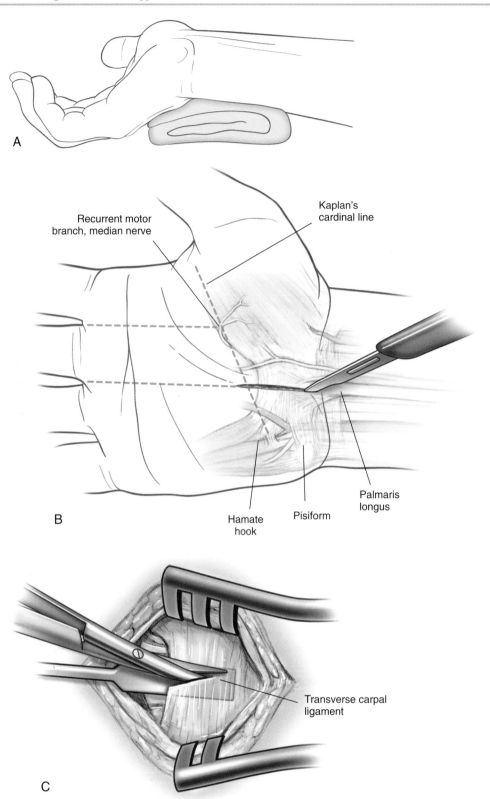

Figure 30-56 Open carpal tunnel release. **A,** Position on the hand. **B,** Skin incision and anatomy. **C,** Exposure of the median nerve with fine dissecting scissors. *(From Miller MD, Chhabra AB, Hurwitz SR, Mihalko WM: Orthopaedic surgical approaches, Philadelphia, 2008, WB Saunders.)*

when the saw is used. A small diamond rasp is used to smooth the ends of the bones.

The surgeon uses a microburr to enter the medullary canal. This burr also widens the canal for the implant. When the intramedullary canal is open, trials are used to measure the implant size, and the site is irrigated. The implants are inserted, the joint is again irrigated, and the wound is closed. Dressings are applied, and the hand is placed in a posterior splint with the finger or fingers held in extension. This procedure is illustrated in Figure 30-57.

DUPUYTREN CONTRACTURE

Surgical Goal

Constricted palmar fascia is incised and released to restore mobility to the hand and fingers.

Pathology

A Dupuytren contracture is a common condition in which the fascia of the palm or fingers contracts. The disorder has a strong familial component, particularly when the onset is in younger men. The deformity progresses rapidly.

Discussion

The patient is placed in the supine position with the operative arm on an arm board. A Bier block or general anesthetic may be used. The hand and lower arm are prepped and draped.

The surgeon uses a #15 blade to make the incision on the ulnar side of the palmar fascia, as well as the apex of the fascia. Tenotomy scissors and fine forceps are used to dissect the tissue and expose the tendons. After the tendons have been freed, and the fingers can be moved without impingement, the tourniquet is released and the wound is checked for

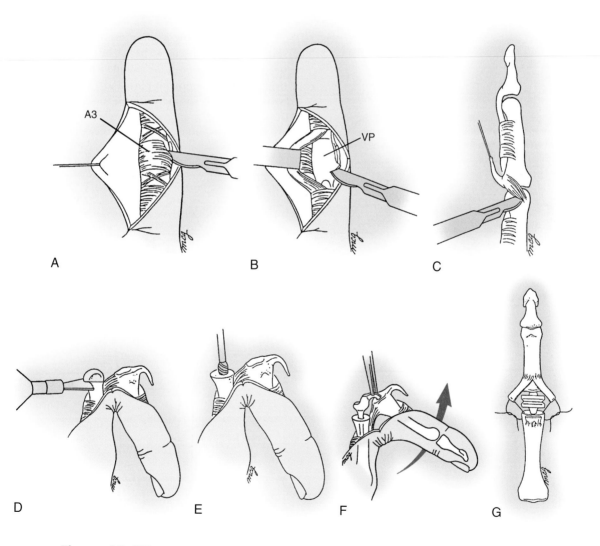

Figure 30-57 Metacarpophalangeal (MCP) joint arthroplasty. **A,** A V-shaped incision is made. **B,** The flexor tendon is retracted. **C,** The collateral ligaments are released. **D,** The articular surface exposed. **E,** The medullary canal is prepared. **F,** Trial implants and the permanent implant are inserted. **G,** The ligaments are reconstructed. *(From Canale S, Beaty J: Campbell's operative orthopaedics, ed 11, St Louis, 2007, Mosby.)*

hemostasis and then irrigated. The skin is closed with interrupted nonabsorbable sutures. A bulky compression dressing using gauze fluffs is applied.

HIP AND PELVIS

FEMORAL NECK FRACTURES

Surgical Goal

A combination femoral plate and compression lag screw (intertrochanteric component) are inserted to stabilize a fracture of the femoral neck or proximal femur. Fractures that occur above the trochanter also may be repaired with a cannulated screw system using a similar technique.

Pathology

The femoral neck (trochanter) is a common site of injury in a fall. The fracture may occur alone or may be accompanied by a fracture of the femur itself. Figure 30-58 illustrates common femoral neck fractures.

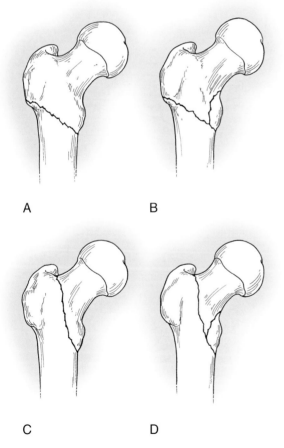

Figure 30-58 Femoral neck fractures. **A** does not involve the trochanter. **B** extends below the trochanter. **C** does not involve the lesser trochanter. **D** extends into lesser trochanter. *(From Canale S, Beaty J: Campbell's operative orthopaedics, ed 11, St Louis, 2007, Mosby.)*

Technique

1. A lateral or posterolateral incision is made over the hip.
2. A guide pin is inserted into the trochanter.
3. The pin is measured for length.
4. A cannulated reamer is fitted over the pin.
5. A lag (compression) screw is inserted through the trochanter.
6. The plate component is fitted over the screw and advanced.
7. The guide pin is removed.
8. Screw holes are drilled, and screws are inserted into the side plate.
9. The lag screw is removed.
10. The wound is closed.

Discussion

A number of options are available for surgical treatment of a fracture of the femoral neck (located across the trochanter or the neck itself). These include:

- Compression screw and plate system
- Dynamic compression screws alone
- Arthroplasty

A procedure using a compression screw and sliding plate (Figure 30-59) is discussed here. The instruments and supplies needed for the procedure include a major orthopedic set, a drill, K-wires, Steinmann pins, and a screw-plate system. The orthopedic table is used, with the lower extremities in abduc-

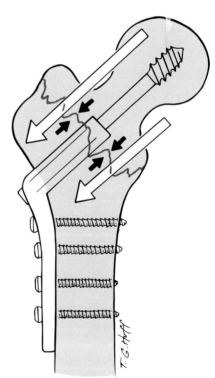

Figure 30-59 Compression screw-plate system. A plate-tube assembly is inserted through the trochanter, and a compression screw is inserted through the trochanter to pull the fragments together. The screw is then removed. *(From Browner B, Jupiter J, Levine A, Trafton P: Skeletal trauma: basic science, management, and reconstruction, ed 3, Philadelphia, 2003, WB Saunders.)*

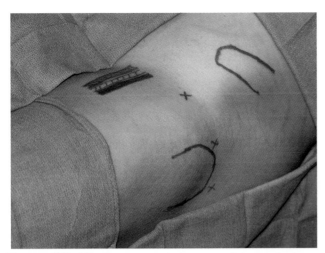

Figure 30-60 Exposure and alignment of the leg for hip surgery using a fracture table. *(From Canale S, Beaty J: Campbell's operative orthopaedics, ed 11, St Louis, 2007, Mosby.)*

tion and the affected leg in traction (Figure 30-60). C-arm fluoroscopy and an image intensifier are used intermittently during the procedure.

A general anesthetic is administered, and the patient is placed in position for traction. The fracture is reduced using table traction, and the position is verified on fluoroscopy. The operative leg is prepped from the lower leg to the chest. The leg is draped with wide exposure.

A lateral or posterolateral incision is used for surgical treatment of a hip fracture (Figure 30-61). Rake retractors are placed in the wound, and the ESU is used to divide the subcutaneous tissue and fascia. The muscle then is divided and retracted. Richardson, Army-Navy, Hibbs, or Deaver retractors may be used for deep retraction.

A guide pin is inserted to establish the correct angle for the trochanter compression screw and plate. A Steinmann (guide) pin and drill are used for this purpose. The guide pin remains in place during most of the procedure, and cannulated instruments are inserted over it. For insertion of the guide pin, a 6.4-mm drill bit is used to make a pilot hole in line with the femoral neck. An angle guide is used to obtain the correct angle of the guide pin. The pin then is drilled following the angle of the guide, viewed under fluoroscopy. Next, the depth of the guide pin is determined with a cannulated depth gauge. An appropriate-size reamer is used to drill over the guide pin according to the depth gauge measurement. This is the starter channel, or tap. A long reamer designed for lag screw insertion is calibrated for the channel, which then is reamed to the appropriate depth. The reamer is cannulated and fits over the guide wire during this process. The angle of the pin may be checked with a trial plate. The scrub may receive the plate from the circulator at this time. The size should be verified with the surgeon before the sterile implant is opened.

The lag screw is inserted with or without pretapping. A calibrated tap drill (reamer) is used as necessary, and the

reading is taken from the back of the tap. The surgeon then determines the correct size for the lag screw. The plate component is fitted into the lag screw inserter, and the T-handle and lag screw are inserted into the assembly. The assembled unit is placed over the guide pin and into the prepared channel. The surgeon advances the lag screw and plate barrel. The guide pin is removed, and the traction is released.

The scrub should prepare a drill, drill guide, and drill bit for attaching the side plate to the femur. The surgeon then drills the holes and measures them with a depth gauge. The scrub selects the correct-size screw and passes it with the screwdriver. When the side screws have been placed, an impactor may be used to secure the plate barrel. A compression screw is inserted into the tube and tightened by hand. This brings the femoral neck fragments into contact. The compression screw then is removed.

The wound is irrigated and checked for bleeders. A sump or gravity drain or may be placed in the wound before closure. The muscle is closed with 2-0 or 3-0 interrupted absorbable synthetic sutures. The fascia is closed with a running suture of the same material. Subcutaneous tissue is closed with 3-0 absorbable sutures, and the skin is approximated with staples. A compression dressing consisting of flat gauze and an abdominal pad is placed over the incision. The steps of the procedure are illustrated in Figure 30-62. A related procedure is repair using a cannulated screw system (Figure 30-63).

Postoperative Considerations

The patient usually is able to begin weight bearing within 24 hours after surgery.

INTRAMEDULLARY FEMORAL NAILING

Surgical Goal

A femoral shaft fracture can be repaired with an intramedullary femoral nail. A femoral nail is a rigid rod that is seated in the medullary canal and held in position with locking screws placed at a 90-degree angle to the nail.

Pathology

The intramedullary technique for repairing a femoral fracture may be used for a comminuted fracture or a proximal and distal fracture.

Discussion

The instruments required for the procedure are an orthopedic set, including hip retractors, a drill, a Steinmann pin set, and a femoral nailing system.

The patient is placed in the supine position on an orthopedic or a standard operating table. A general anesthetic is administered. The operative leg may be placed in traction using the orthopedic table's boot attachment. The position then is assessed fluoroscopically. The prep includes the knee, hip, thigh, buttock, and trunk, including the axilla. Draping is standard, using a large U-drape that extends to the knee. The incision is drawn with a marking pen.

An incision is made over the trochanter and carried through the subcutaneous, fascial, and muscle layers. Richardson or

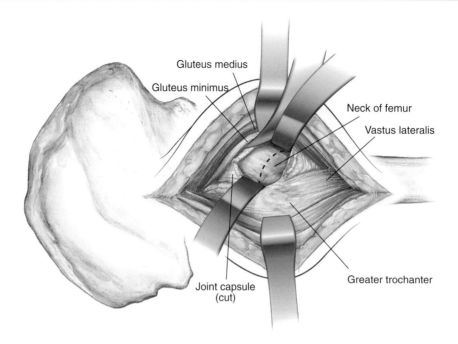

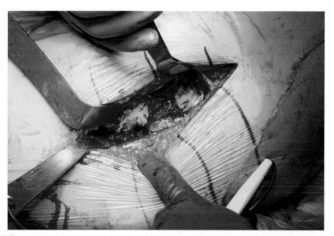

Figure 30-61   Lateral approach to the hip. Tissue layers usually are thin. After the skin incision has been made, the subcutaneous, fascial, and muscle layers are quickly incised with the ESU. Note the position of the Hibbs retractor *(top)*. Narrow Deaver or Richardson retractors also are used at this level. *(From Miller MD, Chhabra AB, Hurwitz SR, Mihalko WM: Orthopaedic surgical approaches, Philadelphia, 2008, WB Saunders.)*

large rake (Israel) retractors are used to expose the trochanter.

An awl is used to form the entry point into the medullary canal. As an alternative, a Steinmann pin can be inserted percutaneously. The awl is rotated to create the entry point. A ball-tip guide wire then is inserted into the canal.

To prepare for medullary reaming, a cannula (metal sleeve) and bushing are placed over the guide wire. The cannula is advanced over the guide wire until it is seated. A cannulated reamer is inserted over the pin to the trochanter. The guide wire then is replaced with a ball-tip wire, which is manipulated into the canal beyond the fracture site. A cannulated nail-length gauge is used to measure the depth

of the canal. Fluoroscopy is used to assess the position and depth.

Graduated intramedullary reamers are used to increase the space for nail insertion. The technologist should have several reamers of incremental sizes ready for this part of the procedure; sizes 5 to 7 mm commonly are used.

When the medullary canal has been prepared, the correct nail is selected and prepared on the back table. This describes use of an interlocking nail guide, which is used to align the cross-screw position in the nail. A driver and **slap hammer** attachment are used to drive the nail into the canal while the nail guide maintains correct position. The nail is driven into the medullary canal, and the driver is disengaged. Nail caps,

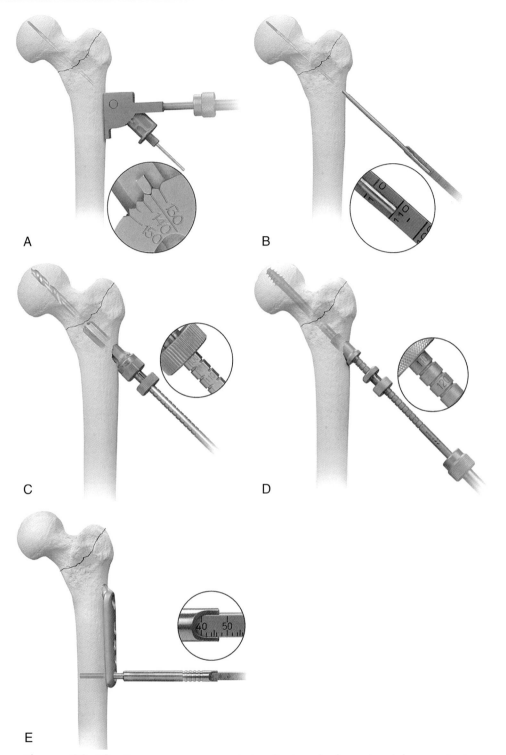

Figure 30-62 Compression screw and plate fixation of a femoral neck fracture. **A,** An angle guide is used to accurately place a Steinmann pin, which is inserted with a drill. **B,** A guide pin depth gauge is used to measure the length of the pin in place. This determines the length of the implant. **C,** A calibrated reamer is used to drill over the guide pin. **D,** Calibrations are shown on the bone tap. **E,** The tube/plate is inserted into the bone, and screw holes are drilled. A depth gauge is used to determine the tap hole depth. (Courtesy Zimmer, Warsaw, Ind.)

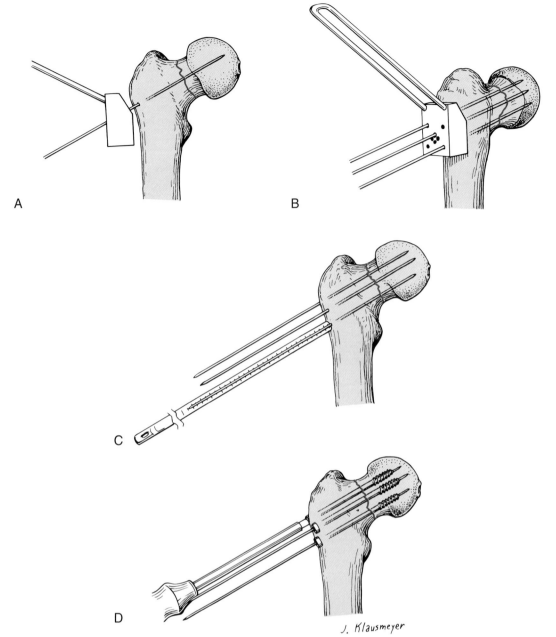

Figure 30-63 Cannulated screw system for a fracture of the trochanter. **A,** The fracture is reduced, and a guide wire (Steinmann pin) is inserted. **B,** Additional guide wires are placed as needed. **C,** A depth gauge is used to determine the length of the pins. **D,** Cannulated screws are placed over the guide wires, which are then removed. *(From Browner B, Jupiter J, Levine A, Trafton P: Skeletal trauma: basic science, management, and reconstruction, ed 3, Philadelphia, 2003, WB Saunders.)*

if used, are inserted by hand at this time with a nail cap inserter.

A screw guide with protective bushing is inserted into the targeting device, and the proximal screw holes are drilled. A depth gauge is used to measure the holes, and the appropriate-size screws are placed through the bone and nail by hand. A freehand targeting device is used to locate the distal screw hole with fluoroscopy. The targeting device is positioned over the distal nail hole, and a combination trocar-drill is used to penetrate the bone through the targeting device. The position is

confirmed with fluoroscopy. An incision is made over the trocar, and the nail hole is located with a hemostat. The trocar is centered in the nail hole, and the hole is completed. A depth gauge is used to measure the drill hole, and the appropriate-size screw is inserted and hand-tightened.

The scrub and circulator should note the size of the screws and nail used, because these must be documented appropriately. The position of the nail and screws is assessed, and the wound is irrigated. All tissue debris is removed from the wound, and any potential bleeders are checked with the ESU.

The wound is closed with interrupted absorbable synthetic sutures and skin staples. A flat dressing is placed over the incision.

NOTE: The techniques used in this procedure closely follow those used in tibial nailing, which is discussed later in this chapter.

Related Procedure: Repair of a Supracondylar Fracture

Distal femoral fractures may be repaired using a lag screw–plate combination. The techniques described previously are used for this procedure. The patient is placed in the supine position with the operative flank raised slightly for better exposure of the distal femur.

HIP ARTHROPLASTY

Surgical Goal

The goal of hip arthroplasty is to replace diseased components of the hip joint, including the acetabulum, trochanter, and ball of the femur, with one or more artificial implants.

Pathology

Hip arthroplasty is performed to treat a number of arthritic conditions:

- *Osteoarthritis:* Results in loss of cartilage and eventual erosion of bone. The disease usually is associated with the aging process.
- *Osteonecrosis:* Death of bone and marrow tissue, usually related to trauma or disease.
- *Acetabular fracture:* Hip trauma, commonly associated with falls and motor vehicle accidents.
- *Femoral neck fracture:* Commonly associated with falls.
- *Avascular necrosis:* Death of bone tissue related to interruption of the blood supply to the hip.

Technique

1. An anterior or posterolateral incision is made over the hip.
2. The hip is dislocated.
3. The femoral neck is incised, and the ball of the femur is removed.
4. The acetabulum is trimmed and reamed.
5. A trial shell is tested in the acetabulum, and the prosthesis is implanted with or without screws.
6. The femoral canal is created with reamers and broaches.
7. The cut end of the femur is trimmed.
8. The trial femoral head is inserted over the broach or femoral implant and tested by reducing the joint.
9. The joint is dislocated, and the femoral canal is cleaned.
10. The prosthesis is cemented or press-fit into place.
11. The wound is irrigated and closed.

Discussion

Many surgical approaches can be used for hip arthroplasty. Aside from variations in the implant design, the main technical differences important to the surgical technologist are:

- One or both components of the hip joint may be replaced.

- The implants may be cemented or press-fit.
- One incision or two may be used for the surgical approach.

The surgical options are chosen based on the patient's age and desired level of activity after surgery, the condition of the bone, and the surgeon's specific training.

Hip Components

Modular implant systems for hip arthroplasty include the following:

- *Femoral component:* Includes the stem, neck, and head. The neck usually is adjustable for angle (called the *offset*) and length. The femoral component may be press-fit or cemented.
- *Acetabular components:* Includes an acetabular liner, which is seated into the prepared acetabulum, and a shell, which fits into the liner. The outside of the shell may be spiked or smooth, or it may have drill holes for screws.

Figure 30-64 shows examples of hip arthroplasty components.

Instruments needed for hip arthroplasty include a standard orthopedic set and hip instruments, including large hip retractors, bone hooks, bone clamps, chisels, and osteotomes. The manufacturer commonly supplies any additional equipment intended for use with a specific type of implant. Special instruments include bone-cutting and measuring devices, an impactor, and screwdrivers. Broaches are used to create a space in the medullary canal for the femoral stem. A power saw and drill are also needed. If a cemented implant is used, components for mixing the cement and an exhaust system are required.

Implants are not opened until the surgeon requests them during surgery. Trial sizers are included in the system setup and are used to test an implant after measurements have been taken and the bone prepared.

The patient is placed in the lateral position, and a stabilizing device is used to maintain the position. The skin is prepped from the waist to the foot. Draping exposes the hip and thigh. The foot is not exposed but is wrapped in sterile towels so that the hip and leg can be manipulated during the procedure. The lower leg may be draped with impervious tube stockinet. An incise drape is used over the operative site.

The surgeon makes an anterior or posterolateral incision. An anterior approach is discussed here. After the skin incision has been made, the wound is opened with the ESU. Initially, medium Richardson retractors are placed in the wound edges. The fascia and muscle are then divided, and large rake retractors or right-angle retractors can be inserted in the wound. The technologist should have ample lap sponges and suction available during this part of the procedure.

Once the joint capsule has been exposed, the surgeon opens it with the deep knife and the ESU. Hohmann retractors are used to elevate and expose the proximal femur. The hip joint is dislocated using a large bone hook and manual traction. This exposes the acetabular surface. The surgeon trims diseased tissue, including a torn labrum (the rim of connective tissue around the acetabulum). This is done with the knife,

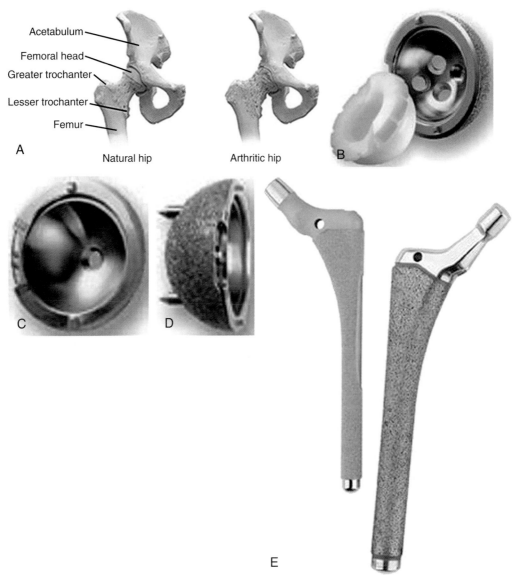

Figure 30-64 Components of a modular hip arthroplasty. **A,** Modular components include the femoral stem, ball, acetabular cup, and polyethylene liner. **B,** An acetabular cup and liner with screw holes for attachment. **C,** An acetabular cup with a single screw hole. **D,** An acetabular cup with pegs. Note the beaded coating. **E,** Femoral stems. *(Courtesy Zimmer, Warsaw, Ind.)*

ESU, and cup-tipped rongeurs. Pituitary-type rongeurs also may be used for this step of the procedure.

The next step is the osteotomy, in which the femoral head is removed. The technologist should prepare a narrow-width oscillating blade and power saw. A cutting guide or jig is placed over the proximal trochanter, and the femoral head is grasped with a sharp bone clamp. The saw then is used to divide the femoral neck. The assistant irrigates the bone during cutting to prevent heating. The scrub receives the femoral head, which is set aside on the back table and preserved with moist saline sponges. The surgeon may need to remove additional bone from the femoral neck after measurements are taken.

To prepare the acetabulum for the implant, the surgeon trims any loose tissue or **osteophytes** (bony spurs) from

the rim of the joint. A cup-shaped rongeur (e.g., pituitary rongeur), curette, ESU, and knife are used to remove the tissue. The surgeon then dishes out the surface of the acetabulum using power-operated reamers in graduated sizes.

The trial shell is fitted (but not impacted) into the acetabulum with a positioning instrument. The final component then is impacted by hand with a mallet or with the supplied positioner and slap hammer. If screws are to be inserted through the shell, these can be inserted by hand. The liner then is fitted into the shell.

To prepare the femoral side of the joint, the surgeon creates an intramedullary space in the femur to accept the femoral stem. The exact depth of the space is determined before surgery by comparing the radiograph with a transparent template. The surgeon may measure the femur again before reaming. A hand awl or chisel is used to start the opening for the femoral canal. This is followed by broaches. The technologist should have several sizes of intramedullary rasps (broaches). The broach is impacted into the canal with a mallet or slap hammer and guide, which is fitted over the broach. Broaches are used in successively larger sizes. Immersing the rasps in a basin of water is helpful for removing tissue debris from the instruments after each use. When broaching is nearly complete, the handle of the broach is removed and a planer is used to prepare the end surface (calcar) of the femur. This step is optional for some types of femoral implants. The broach may be tested for tightness. Final broaching then is completed, and the handle is removed.

In the next phase of the procedure, a trial femoral head is tested for fit. Two surgical options are available: the trial head can be fitted over the broach, or the broach can be removed and a trial stem inserted in its place. The hip is reduced and assessed. The hip is dislocated, and the femoral component and neck are implanted. If a broach is still in place, it is removed. A pulse lavage system is used to irrigate the femoral canal, which then is suctioned to remove debris.

Cement is prepared if required for the implant (see the earlier discussion of bone cement). The circulator then opens the appropriate-size implant and distributes it to the scrub. When the cement is ready, it is injected into the femoral space. The implant is impacted into the space by fitting it to a stem inserter. Press-fit components can be inserted by hand and then seated with the mallet and stem inserter. Figure 30-65 illustrates a technique for hip arthroplasty.

Postoperative Considerations

Patients are closely monitored for hemorrhage and embolism after arthroplasty. Deep vein thrombosis or fat embolism may occur in the immediate postoperative period or weeks after surgery. Patients are encouraged to begin walking within 24 hours of surgery.

FRACTURE OF THE PELVIS

Surgical Goal

The goal of surgical fixation of the pelvis is to reduce and stabilize a fractured pelvis.

Pathology

Fractures of the pelvis generally are the result of a high-impact injury and often are accompanied by soft tissue injury. An unstable pelvic fracture can be life-threatening as a result of damage to major blood vessels and pelvic organs.

Discussion

Open reduction is the preferred method of repair of an unstable fracture. A number of surgical options for fixation are available based on the location of the fracture:

- Fracture of the ilium is fixed internally with lag screws and fragment plates.
- Surgical options for fracture of the pubic rami are percutaneous pins or internally placed screws.
- Sacral fracture is treated with plates, screws, or rods (Figure 30-66).
- External fixation with a rod and pin system may also be used.

The patient is placed in the supine position for access to the pubic symphysis and also for a fracture of the acetabulum. A Pfannenstiel incision is used for access to the pubic rami.

The prone position is used for fractures of the iliac wings, ilium, sacroiliac joint, and some fractures of the acetabulum. When the prone position is used, a chest brace is placed under the thorax with the arms extended on arm boards. Soft

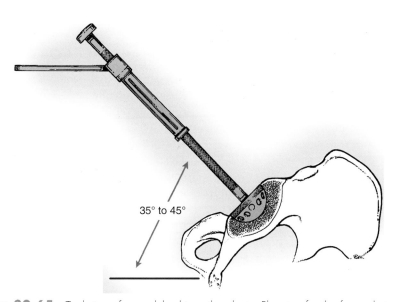

35° to 45°

Figure 30-65 Technique for modular hip arthroplasty. Planning for the femoral stem. A template is placed over the radiographic image to determine the depth of intermedullary reaming. *(From Canale S, Beaty J: Campbell's operative orthopaedics, ed 11, St Louis, 2007, Mosby.)*

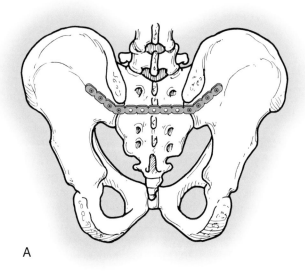
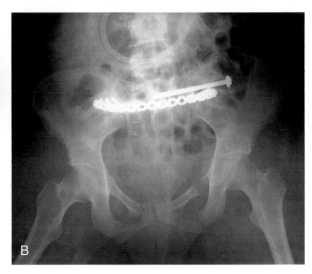

Figure 30-66 Tension band plate used for a sacral fracture. *(From Canale S, Beaty J: Campbell's operative orthopaedics, ed 11, St Louis, 2007, Mosby.)*

padding is placed under the thighs and feet. (Chapter 11 presents a discussion of precautions to use with the prone position and a chest brace.)

Patients with pelvic fractures often have other serious injuries, and the surgery is performed in conjunction with soft tissue repair or reconstruction. Bladder and urethral injury are common, and fluoroscopy is used during the procedure to maintain the safety of the pelvic organs. All assessment scans must be available during surgery. These may include CT, MRI, contrast angiogram, and cystogram. If the patient arrives in traction, weights are attached to the operating table until reduction is secured.

The surgical technologist and circulating nurse are informed about instrumentation for internal or external fixation. However, a decision may be changed during surgery. The scrub should have a major orthopedic set, general surgery instruments, a drill, and the designated implant system available. Extra drapes, towels, and laparotomy sponges are needed for trauma patients. A suprapubic catheter may be inserted during the procedure. Bone grafting instruments and materials should be readily available but not opened unless requested. Abdominal and pelvic injury may require bowel instruments.

Postoperative Considerations

Complications of a pelvic fracture include infection, pulmonary embolism, and urinary problems. Permanent nerve injury also may occur. Recovery from a pelvic fracture can be very long and difficult.

KNEE AND LOWER LEG

The knee is the most complicated joint of the body. It is vulnerable to a variety of injuries, which are caused mainly by sports and motor vehicle accidents. The knee is the largest joint, and it carries a great deal of body weight, especially

when in motion. It also has the longest mechanical levers of the body. Pathogenic conditions in the knee often are very disabling because of the weight-bearing function of the joint. Anterior and posterior views of the knee are shown in Figure 30-67. The joint is divided into separate compartments, which are created by the structures contained within it. However, no separate, fibrous capsule binds the joint together. The ligaments and tendons surround the two joints that make up the knee, the tibiofemoral joint and the patellofemoral joints. The patella forms part of the knee joint on the anterior side. The *menisci* separate the femoral and tibial condyles and provide shock absorption.

Many procedures of the knee are approached endoscopically. The open technique most often is used with a parapatellar, medial, lateral, or posterior approach.

KNEE ARTHROSCOPY

Surgical Goal

Knee arthroscopy is a common technique for assessing and correcting problems arising from injury and disease.

Discussion

The patient is placed in the supine position. Spinal or general anesthesia is used. The surgeon examines the knee under anesthesia (**examination under anesthesia [EUA]**), assessing flexion and extension. A tourniquet is applied to the operative leg. The nonoperative leg is placed in a padded leg holder, and the operative leg is placed in a stabilizing device that allows countertraction. The leg is prepped from midthigh to the ankle circumferentially and draped in routine manner.

An incision is made lateral to the patella and just above the joint line, allowing an inflow cannula to be inserted into the knee joint without damaging the cartilage.

When the knee has been infiltrated with fluid, a second incision is made medially, and a sharp trocar and sheath are

In extension: posterior view

In flexion: anterior view

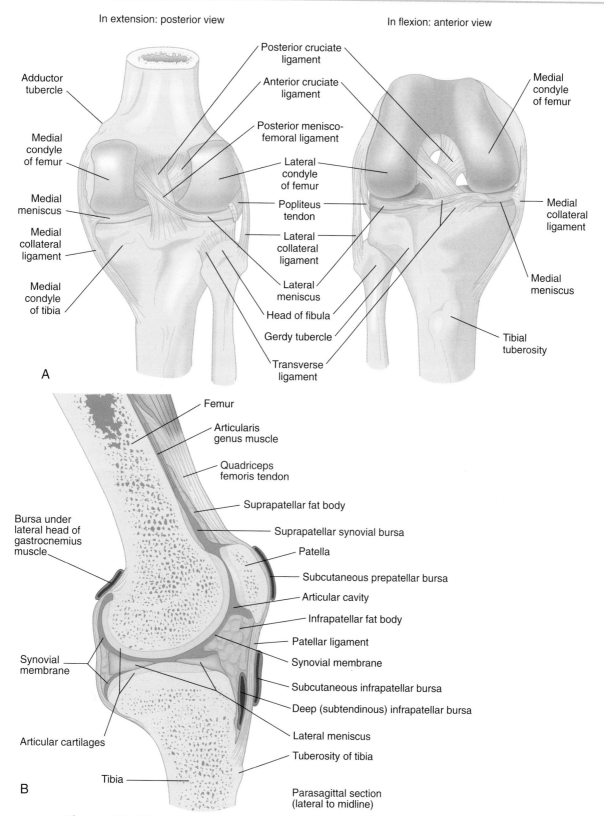

Posterior cruciate ligament
Anterior cruciate ligament
Posterior menisco-femoral ligament
Lateral condyle of femur
Popliteus tendon
Lateral collateral ligament
Lateral meniscus
Head of fibula
Gerdy tubercle
Transverse ligament

Adductor tubercle
Medial condyle of femur
Medial meniscus
Medial collateral ligament
Medial condyle of tibia

Medial condyle of femur
Medial collateral ligament
Medial meniscus
Tibial tuberosity

A

Femur
Articularis genus muscle
Quadriceps femoris tendon
Suprapatellar fat body
Suprapatellar synovial bursa
Patella
Subcutaneous prepatellar bursa
Articular cavity
Infrapatellar fat body
Patellar ligament
Synovial membrane
Subcutaneous infrapatellar bursa
Deep (subtendinous) infrapatellar bursa
Lateral meniscus
Tuberosity of tibia

Bursa under lateral head of gastrocnemius muscle
Synovial membrane
Articular cartilages
Tibia

Parasagittal section (lateral to midline)

B

Figure 30-67 Anatomy of the knee. **A,** Anterior and posterior views. **B,** Sagittal view. *(From Marx J, editor: Rosen's emergency medicine: concepts and clinical practice, ed, 6, Philadelphia, 2006, Mosby.)*

inserted into the knee joint. The trocar then is removed and replaced with a blunt trocar. The knee is irrigated, any fluid is removed, and a 30-degree scope is inserted.

An 18-gauge spinal needle is inserted into the knee joint under direct visualization to determine the placement of a third incision. This incision creates an opposite portal for the insertion of the probe and operative instruments. The location of this incision depends on the type of surgery to be performed. Figure 30-68 illustrates visualization of the knee through various ports.

ARTHROSCOPIC MENISCECTOMY

The meniscus is a horseshoe-shaped cartilage that distributes load across the joint and creates capsular stability. A tear in the meniscus is the most common knee injury. The medial meniscus is injured more often than the lateral meniscus.

Meniscectomy may be partial or complete. Complete meniscectomy leaves the medial rim of the structure to share load bearing and stabilize the knee.

When the meniscus is in view, the surgeon locates the tear with a probe. The attachment of the meniscus is divided with a hook knife. A motorized shaver is used to remove frayed edges from the cartilage. Complete removal, if required, is performed with meniscus knives and scissors. Figure 30-69 illustrates arthroscopic meniscal surgery.

ARTHROSCOPIC ANTERIOR CRUCIATE LIGAMENT REPAIR

Surgical Goal
The goal of surgery is to repair a torn anterior cruciate ligament and restore stability to the joint.

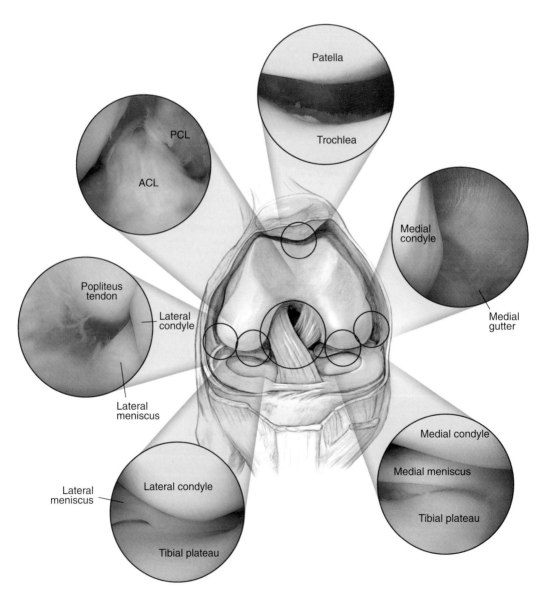

Figure 30-68 Arthroscopy of the knee. *(From Miller MD, Chhabra AB, Hurwitz SR, Mihalko WM: Orthopaedic surgical approaches, Philadelphia, 2008, WB Saunders.)*

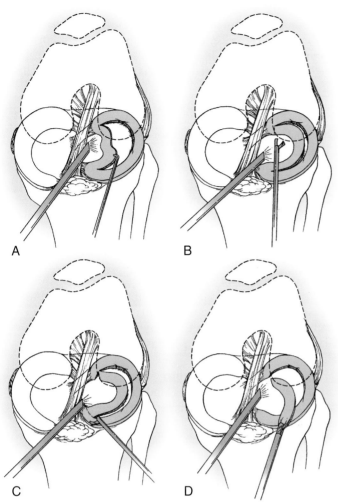

Figure 30-69 Arthroscopic meniscus repair. **A,** A bucket-handle tear is assessed with a probe. **B,** After reduction, the posterior attachment is divided with scissors. **C,** The anterior attachment is divided. **D,** A grasper is used to extract the fragment. *(From Canale S, Beaty J:* Campbell's operative orthopaedics, *ed 11, St Louis, 2007, Mosby.)*

Pathology

The ACL stabilizes the knee in the anterior-posterior position, preventing buckling of the knee. It crosses the center of the knee joint, attaching to the femur superiorly and the tibia inferiorly. ACL tears usually occur during a twisting motion of the leg, often during sports or other strenuous activity.

Technique

1. The knee is assessed arthroscopically.
2. A tendon graft is harvested from the patella tendon, including bone plugs at each end.
3. The graft is prepared at the back table.
4. The damaged anterior cruciate ligament (ACL) is removed from the knee joint.
5. Tunnels are drilled in the femur and tibia to receive the graft.
6. The graft is passed through the tunnels and secured with biosynthetic interference screws.
7. The repair is tested by manipulating the knee.
8. The wounds are closed and dressed.

Discussion

Repair of the anterior **cruciate** ligament (ACL) routinely is performed arthroscopically. A graft is taken from the central portion of the patellar tendon to replace the torn ACL. Surgical options include harvesting a graft from the hamstring or quadriceps tendon or using a cadaver graft. Many options can be used for arthroscopic repair of the ACL; however, the surgical principles are similar. A composite graft of bone and tendon is used to replace the ACL. The graft is secured by passing it through tunnels made in the tibia and femur. The graft is attached with sutures or biosynthetic interference screws, which prevent the graft from being pulled out of the tunnels.

The required instrumentation includes arthroscopy instruments, as well as ACL system instruments, including cannulated burrs, guide wires, and attachment devices. In this procedure, biosynthetic interference screws are used to attach the graft. Power equipment includes drills, a microsagittal saw, and a motorized arthroscopy shaver.

The patient is prepped and draped for a diagnostic arthroscopy. A pneumatic tourniquet is used. The foot of the operating table is lowered slightly. Before starting the procedure, the surgeon manipulates the knee with the patient under anesthesia to assess the injury. An arthroscopic examination is performed before the start of the repair.

Graft Harvesting (Open Surgery)

Although the ACL repair is performed arthroscopically, the graft is removed using open surgical technique. An anterior approach to the patellar tendon is used, which may involve either one or two incisions. After dividing the skin and subcutaneous tissue, the surgeon uses Metzenbaum scissors to separate the paratenon, which lies directly over the tendon. Senn retractors or small rakes are used for retraction. This exposes the patellar tendon. Army-Navy retractors should be available to expose the joint.

The graft is removed from the center patellar tendon. A disposable double-bladed knife or #15 knife blade is used to notch out a section of tendon, which remains attached to the patella at the upper pole and the tibia at the lower pole. An oscillating saw then is used to cut through the bone at each end of the graft. A ¼-inch (0.63 cm) osteotome is used to divide the bone plugs at both ends. This produces a strip of tendon with small bone plugs attached at each end. The scrub should have a small basin to receive the graft, which is removed to the back table for preparation.

The bone ends are trimmed with a small, single-action rongeur. The scrub must preserve any bone chips in a basin with a small amount of saline, because they may be replaced in the wound when the graft is placed. The surgeon passes the graft through a 10-mm metal tube to trial the graft to ensure that it fits. The bone plugs are trimmed as necessary. The surgeon then makes a small hole in each bone plug using a small drill and a fine drill bit. Size 0 nonabsorbable sutures are passed through each hole, and the ends are left long and tagged with hemostats. The surgeon then uses a surgical pen to mark the graft at the bone-tendon margin. These marks are used to align the graft in the joint during insertion. The graft is ready for insertion. It is preserved in a specimen basin until the surgeon needs it.

The surgeon irrigates the wound and closes the remaining patellar tendon with 2-0 absorbable suture. Skin closure is delayed until the end of the procedure.

Arthroscopic Insertion of the Graft

To start the arthroscopic portion of the procedure, the surgeon inserts two lateral trocars. The joint is distended with saline or lactated Ringer solution. The surgeon then examines the torn ligament and menisci. A probe is introduced into the joint for the examination.

The motorized shaver is used to remove the damaged ACL. The scrub should have a basin available for periodic outflow drainage. A torn meniscus may be removed at this stage. To prepare the joint for the graft, a drill guide is used to position the tunnel that will receive the graft. A guide wire is drilled into the tibia. A tunnel then is drilled over the guide wire with a cannulated reamer or burr. This step is repeated on the femoral side. A calibrated aiming device may be used to locate the exact angle of the tunnels before drilling.

An eyed pin is drilled through the bone tunnels and brought out through the skin. The scrub should bring the graft to the field. The preplaced sutures are threaded through the eye of the pin and pulled through the tunnel at both ends. Biosynthetic interference screws are placed in the tunnel against the bone plugs to provide a tighter fit. A small guide wire is placed first, and the screws are placed over the wire. The screws are seated with a screwdriver. The preplaced sutures are then removed.

The repair is inspected through the arthroscope, and the distension fluid is drained. The wounds are closed with synthetic absorbable suture. The wound is dressed with gauze, and a leg brace is applied. The technique for ACL repair is illustrated in Figure 30-70.

Postoperative Considerations

The patient remains on crutches for 2 to 3 weeks using a leg brace. Physical therapy is initiated within the first week of recovery. The total recovery period is 4 to 6 months. The patient usually is able to return to normal activities after a successful repair.

Related Procedure: Repair of a Torn Lateral Collateral Ligament

A torn lateral collateral ligament can be repaired using the techniques described for repair of the ACL. A patellar tendon graft is used to replace the damaged collateral ligament. With a less severe injury, the ligament may be reattached with biosynthetic screws, staples, or sutures of heavy Dacron.

KNEE ARTHROPLASTY

Surgical Goal

The goal of knee arthroplasty is to relieve pain and allow the patient to resume activity.

Pathology

Three common forms of arthritis affect the knee: osteoarthritis, rheumatoid arthritis, and post-traumatic arthritis. Inflammation and degeneration of the joint surfaces results in pain and loss of function. Osteoarthritis is the most common indication for arthroplasty.

Discussion

The knee has three cartilaginous surfaces: the patella, the tibia, and the femur. Any or all three surfaces may be involved in joint disease. In unicompartmental arthroplasty, the medial or lateral surfaces of the femur and tibia are replaced. In total knee replacement, all three components are replaced. Unicompartmental replacement often requires total knee replacement later in the patient's life and is suitable for patients with intact supporting structures.

Knee replacement is a complex procedure. Many systems are available and are continually being refined. In particular, the unicompartmental approach is under intense development. Electronic systems that aid precise alignment of the joint components are now used in some facilities.

As mentioned, during total knee replacement, three components are implanted. (Modular or partial arthroplasty also is performed.) Figure 30-71 shows the knee components:

- A metal femoral component inserted over the distal femur
- A tibial base plate, and metal tray which is placed in the proximal tibia. A polyethylene patellar component is inserted. The components may be implanted with bone cement, or they may be press-fit.

Summary of Total Knee Replacement

Technique

Femur
1. The knee is opened with an anterior or a midpatellar approach. The patella is retracted.
2. The intramedullary canal is located with a drill.
3. The distal femur cuts are planned with a computer-based system or an alignment system.
4. A distal femoral guide (block) is used to direct the cut.
5. The distal femur is cut with an oscillating saw.
6. Distal femoral holes are drilled to calibrate the femur.
7. The posterior femur is cut.
8. The anterior femur is cut.

Technique

Tibia
1. The proximal tibia is cut.
2. The proximal tibia is drilled and sized.
3. The tibia is reamed by hand if a stemmed component will be implanted.

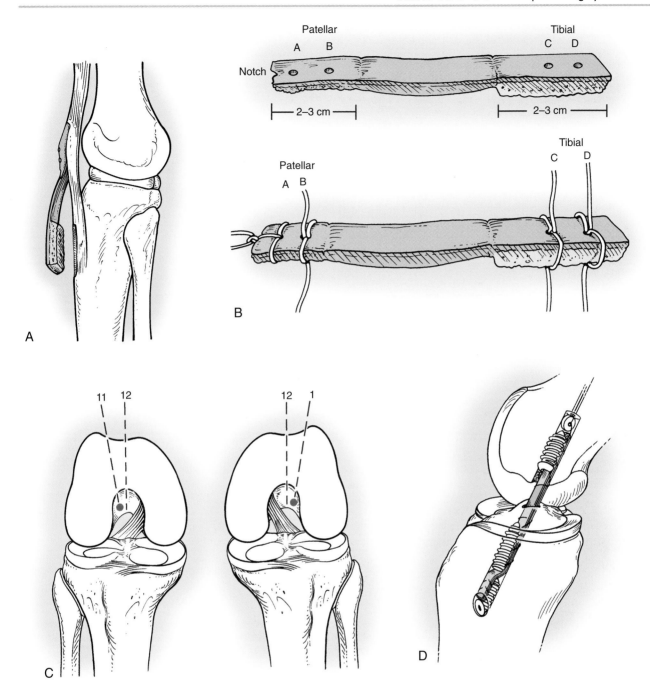

Figure 30-70 Anterior cruciate ligament repair with graft. **A,** Removal of the graft from the tibial tuberosity. **B,** Sutures may be placed at each end of the graft. **C,** The pilot holes are positioned to accommodate the graft. **D,** The graft is secured with biosynthetic screws. *(From Canale S, Beaty J: Campbell's operative orthopaedics, ed 11, St Louis, 2007, Mosby.)*

Technique

Implantation of Components

1. A press-fit tibial base plate is impacted over the tibial surface.
2. The base plate is stabilized with screws.
3. If a cemented base plate is used, a thin layer of cement is placed over the tibia.
4. The polyethylene insert is fitted over the base plate.
5. The femoral component is implanted with an impactor.

The wound is irrigated frequently during the procedure with pulse lavage to remove all debris, which might contribute to infection.

The incision is closed in layers with 2-0 and 3-0 absorbable synthetic sutures. The skin is closed with staples or 3-0 or 4-0 nonabsorbable sutures. An occlusive dressing is placed over the incision, followed by a support bandage or stocking. Knee arthroplasty is illustrated in Figures 30-72 and 30-73.

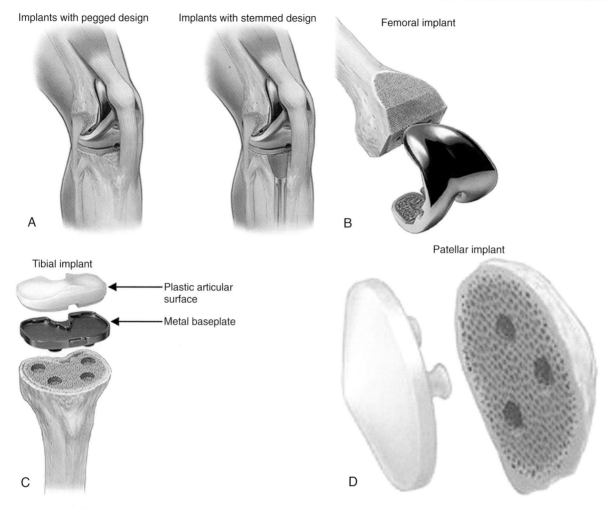

Implants with pegged design   Implants with stemmed design   Femoral implant

A   B

Tibial implant

— Plastic articular surface

— Metal baseplate

Patellar implant

C   D

Figure 30-71 Knee arthroplasty. **A,** Pegged and stemmed design. **B,** Femoral implant. **C,** Tibial implant. **D,** Patellar implant. *(Courtesy Zimmer, Warsaw, Ind.)*

Postoperative Considerations

The patient is encouraged to ambulate within 24 hours after surgery and is placed on anticoagulant therapy to prevent thrombosis. Continuous passive motion may be used immediately after surgery for a patient who is unable to ambulate. The patient generally is required to remain in the hospital for up to 3 days after surgery and may resume limited activity within 2 to 4 weeks.

INTRAMEDULLARY NAILING (TIBIA)

Surgical Goal

In intramedullary nailing of the tibia, an intramedullary rod (nail) is inserted into the tibia for fixation and stabilization of a fracture.

Pathology

Fractures of the tibia are commonly the result of a high-velocity impact caused by a motor vehicle accident or sports trauma.

Technique

1. The medullary canal is opened.
2. A guide wire is inserted into the canal.
3. The intermedullary canal is reamed.
4. The tibial nail is inserted using a targeting device.
5. The nail is impacted.
6. The guide wire is removed.
7. Locking screws are inserted using a targeting device.

Discussion

The selection of an IM nail for a fracture of the tibia is based on the type and severity of the fracture, the patient's age, and the surgeon's preference. Two types of IM nails are commonly used, the cannulated nail and the solid nail. Although called "nails," these devices are rod implants that are impacted into the intramedullary space along the parallel axis. Stabilizing screws may be placed at the proximal and distal ends to prevent the nail from slipping. The nail may be inserted without preparation of the medullary canal, or the canal may be reamed before insertion of the nail.

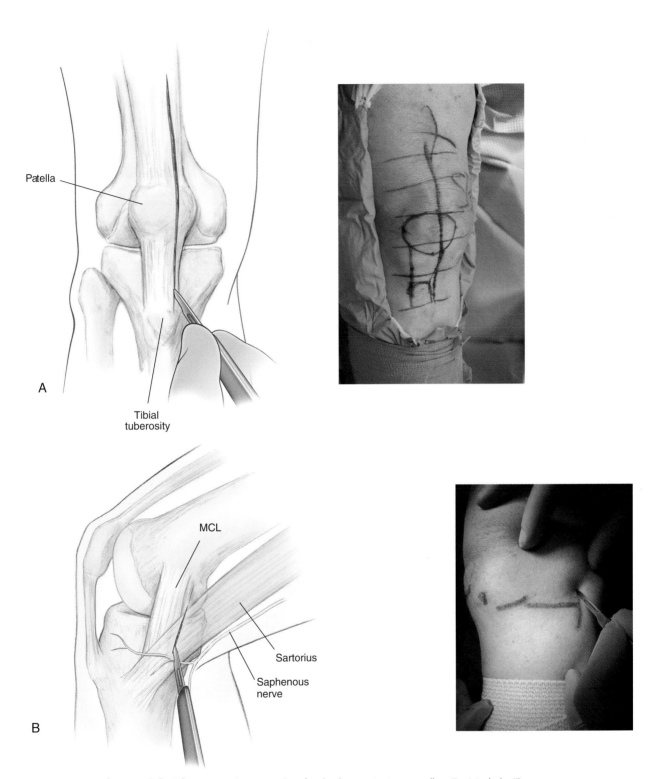

Figure 30-72 Surgical approaches for the knee. **A,** Parapatellar. **B,** Medial. *(From Miller MD, Chhabra AB, Hurwitz SR, Mihalko WM: Orthopaedic surgical approaches, Philadelphia, 2008, WB Saunders.)*

The patient is placed in the supine position on a translucent operating table or orthopedic table using distraction. C-arm fluoroscopy is used intraoperatively. The knee will be flexed to 90 degrees during the procedure, and appropriate padding and accessories are necessary to maintain safe positioning. A knee crutch or distraction device may be used to position the affected leg. The C-arm is adjusted before the skin prep to ensure full exposure of the operative site. A pneumatic tourniquet may be used to maintain hemostasis. The foot and leg are prepped up to and including the thigh, because the leg

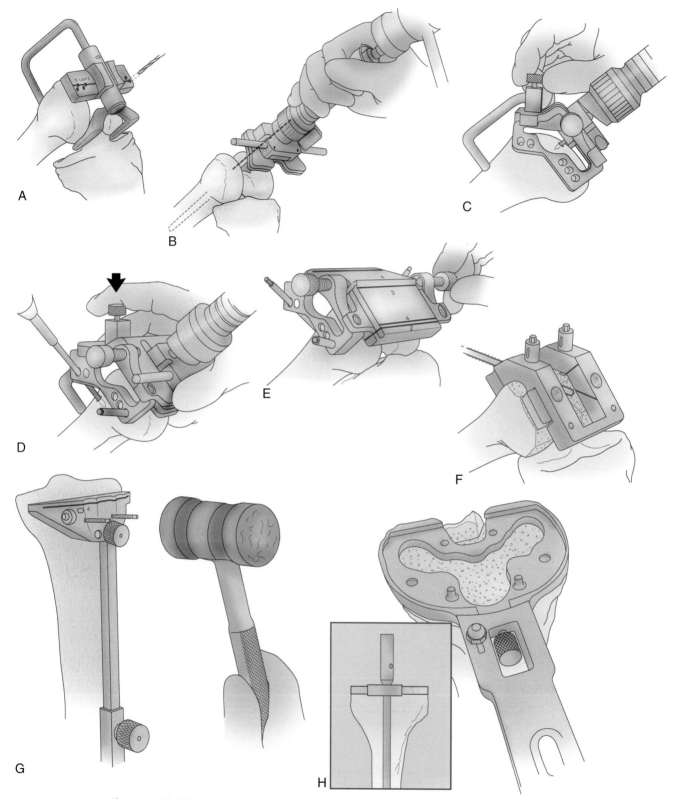

Figure 30-73 Knee arthroplasty. **A,** A femoral sizer is placed over the distal femur. **B,** The femoral canal is reamed, and an intramedullary alignment guide is inserted into the medullary canal. **C,** The femoral cutting guide is attached to the alignment guide. **D,** The femoral cutting guide is positioned. **E,** The femur is resected. **F,** The femoral cuts are completed. **G,** A tibial alignment guide is positioned, and the tibia incised. **H,** Tibial measurements are taken. *(Courtesy Zimmer, Warsaw, Ind.)*

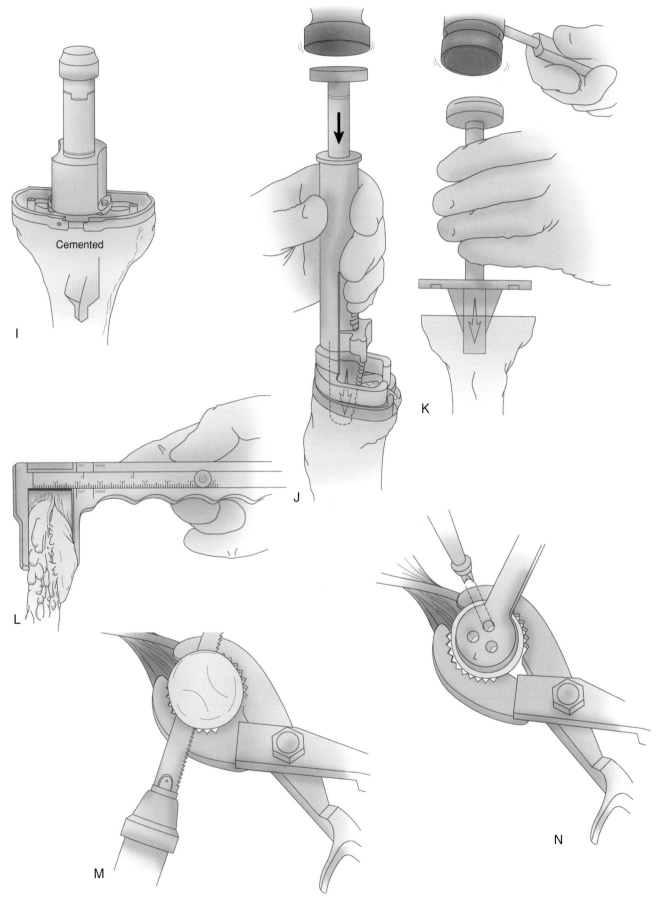

Figure 30-73, cont'd **I,** The tibia is reamed. **J,** The tibia is impacted. **K,** The tibial trial is inserted. **L** and **M,** The patella is measured and sized. **N,** The patella is drilled. *(From Rothrock J: Alexander's care of the patient in surgery, ed 17, Philadelphia, 2007, Mosby.)*

is manipulated during surgery. The foot may be wrapped in an occluding drape before the leg drapes are applied.

Before starting surgery, the surgeon measures the tibia using the image intensifier and a ruler, which is positioned along the long axis of the leg in two places. The skin is marked with a skin scribe. This determines the size of nail required. For complex, multiple fractures of the tibia, a distracter may be required to hold the leg in reduction.

The scrub should have a basic orthopedic set available, including knee retractors; general surgery instruments, including superficial retractors; and the instruments, implants, and accessories for the nailing set to be used. A pneumatic drill or hand drill also is required for setting the guide pins. Some types of IM nails are inserted with the drill. The nail may be inserted percutaneously (through the skin) or through an incision and preparation of the medullary canal.

After the prep, draping, and timeout, the knee is flexed and held in position by the assistant. The surgeon makes an incision over the proximal tibia along the midline of the bone. The scrub should have skin rakes and the ESU immediately available. The patellar tendon then is retracted with a dull rake or a shallow right-angle retractor (e.g., Senn retractor). In some procedures, the tendon is split.

To ensure correct positioning of the implant and precise removal of intramedullary tissue, a guide pin or rod and a tissue protection sleeve are positioned in the canal.

A guide wire (threaded Steinmann pin) is inserted into the medullary canal with a power drill or hand drill. A 2.5-mm wire is commonly used. The guide wire is advanced with a drill sleeve, which keeps the pin straight as it is drilled. The position of the pin then is verified fluoroscopically.

A cannulated reaming rod is used to ream the intramedullary canal. This step may be omitted if reaming is unnecessary. In the nonreamed method, a tissue protection sleeve may be inserted over the guide rod. If reaming is necessary, the cannulated reaming rod is placed over the guide wire and advanced with a hand drill. The turning motion of the reamer creates bits of tissue from the medullary canal. The scrub should be alert to clear these tissue fragments from the field and retain them as specimen. The scrub also must keep the reamer irrigated to reduce tissue heating.

After the canal has been reamed, the hand assembly is removed and the tissue or medullary tube is inserted over the reamer. The reamer then is removed and may be replaced with a guide rod, which is used to guide the IM nail into position.

The selected nail implant then is inserted. At each step, the position of the guide wires is verified, and the hollow medullary tubes are used to protect the tissue of the endosteum while drilling takes place. The medullary tube and guide wires are removed only when the IM nail is in place.

Depending on the system and the manufacturer, a number of methods can be used to insert the nail. A hollow nail can be grasped with a targeting device or guide, which keeps the nail strait and angled correctly as it is inserted over the guide wire. The nail is inserted manually with twisting or oscillating movement. A metal driver may be used to seat the nail.

The position of the implant is verified fluoroscopically, and the guide wire is removed. Locking pins are then inserted. These fit into the nail at a right angle through the proximal and distal ends of the nail. To line up the entry point of the locking bolts with the nail, a targeting guide or similar right-angle aiming device is used. The IM guide wire is removed, and the targeting device is attached. The skin is incised over the site for the locking bolts, and the tissue is dissected to bone. The drill holes then are made through the tissue protector. Screw length is determined with a depth gauge. The locking screws are inserted and tightened manually with the screwdriver. Tibial nailing is illustrated in Figure 30-74.

FOOT

REPAIR OF THE ACHILLES TENDON

Surgical Goal
The goal of repair of the Achilles tendon is to return strength and flexibility to the foot after a traumatic injury.

Pathology
The Achilles tendon may be torn or ruptured in active sports, especially those involving jumping, such as tennis, basketball, gymnastics, and volleyball. A low level injury may occur in other activities, such as cycling.

Discussion
Surgical treatment for Achilles tendon injuries varies widely. A graft may be used to replace a severely injured tendon. In some cases, the paratenon is stripped to provide a "fresh" wound for more rapid healing.

The patient is placed in the supine position with the affected leg supported by a soft support or sandbag. Spinal or general anesthesia is used, and a pneumatic tourniquet applied. The foot and lower leg are prepped and draped in routine manner.

A posterolateral approach is used. The incision is made parallel to the tendon on the lateral or median side with a #15 knife. The skin and subcutaneous tissue are retracted with skin rakes or a Weitlaner retractor. This exposes the fascia (paratenon), which is incised to expose the tendon. The tendon is irrigated and trimmed with Metzenbaum scissors. The ends of the torn tendon are approximated with size 0 heavy Mersilene or other synthetic suture. The paratenon is sutured with 2-0 absorbable synthetic sutures. The foot remains flexed while a short leg cast is applied.

Postoperative Considerations
The patient begins to regain mobility in 4 to 6 months.

TRIPLE ARTHRODESIS

Surgical Goal
Triple **arthrodesis** is the fusion of the talocalcaneal, talonavicular, and calcaneocuboid joints. This is performed by removing the cartilage from each joint and allowing them to heal in approximation. The surgical goal is to prevent move-

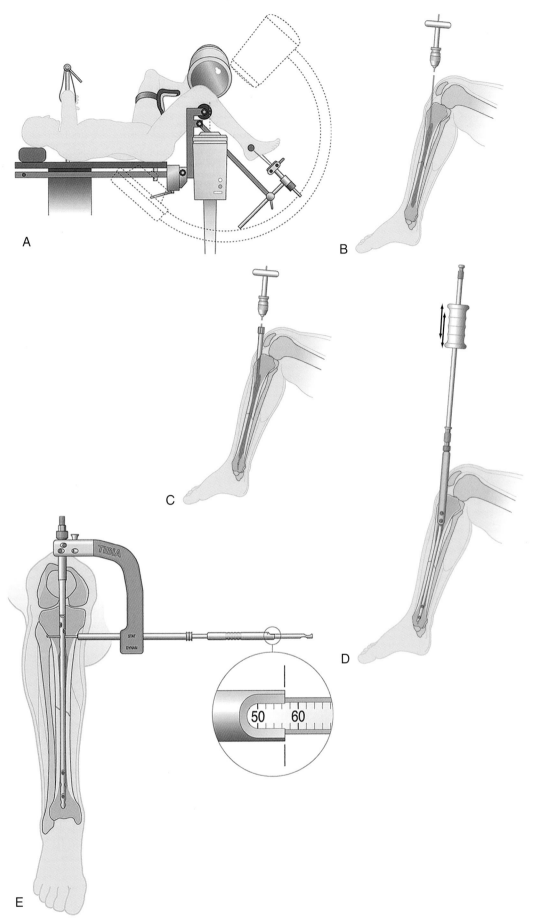

Figure 30-74 Intermedullary tibial nailing. **A,** Patient position using a fracture table. **B,** A guide rod is inserted into the medullary canal. **C,** A ball-tip is inserted under image intensification. **D,** The canal has been reamed and a nail has been inserted. A "slap hammer" is used to impact the nail. **E,** A targeting device is used to locate the screw holes. The screw length is measured (shown), and the locking screws are inserted. *(Courtesy Zimmer, Warsaw, Ind.)*

ment of these joints and thereby prevent pain and joint instability.

Pathology

Triple arthrodesis is performed to treat a number of painful, chronic joint diseases that are not helped by conservative therapy. These include rheumatoid arthritis, post-traumatic arthritis, and neuromuscular disease.

Discussion

The instruments required for triple arthrodesis include a foot and ankle orthopedic set, including a lamina spreader, bone saw, drill, K-wires, and burrs. Medium-size osteotomes and curettes also should be available, along with a cannulated screw system. A bone graft may be harvested from the iliac crest, or biosynthetic grafting material can be used.

The patient is placed in the supine position. General or spinal anesthesia is used. The foot and leg are prepped to the knee. The foot is draped in routine manner.

An anterior or anterolateral incision is made. This approach prevents injury to the superficial peroneal nerves. The cartilage and soft tissue are dissected and removed from the joints with single- and double-action rongeurs, a #15 blade, and tissue forceps. The capsules of the talonavicular, calcaneocuboid, and subtalar joints are incised circumferentially to obtain as much mobility as possible. The articular surfaces of the calcaneocuboid joint, the subtalar joint, and the talonavicular joint are removed with an osteotome, a power saw, or a rasp. Any bone removed is preserved on the back table for possible use in grafting.

When all articular surfaces have been cleaned, the foot is placed in correct anatomical position. Bone or biosynthetic grafting material may be used to fill gaps in the bone-to-bone surfaces. K-wires are inserted for temporary fixation. Cannulated screws then are used to bridge the three bones (Figure 30-75). Fluoroscopy is used to check the position of the K-wires and the cannulated screws inserted over them.

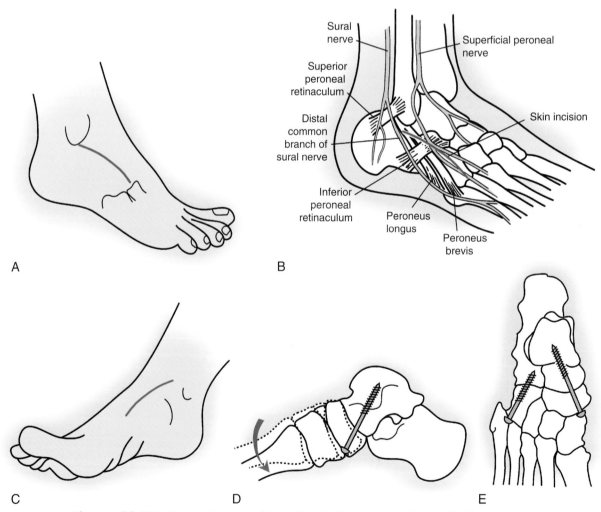

Figure 30-75 Triple arthrodesis of the ankle. **A,** Skin incision. **B,** Superficial anatomy. **C,** Medial incision. **D,** Talonavicular fixation. **E,** Calcaneocuboid and talonavicular screw fixation. *(From Canale S, Beaty J: Campbell's operative orthopaedics, ed 11, St Louis, 2007, Mosby.)*

Distal locking screws are placed over the cannulated screws. Surgical options include insertion of a cannulated arthrodesis nail, which is inserted from the calcaneus and locked in place with cannulated screws.

A closed drainage system (e.g., Hemovac drain) may be inserted, and the wound is closed in layers. A postoperative nerve block is used to reduce postoperative pain. The ankle is covered with a compression dressing, and a posterior splint is applied.

Postoperative Considerations

The patient is weight bearing after 2 weeks. Physical therapy is started as soon as possible to increase range of motion. Complications of triple or hindfoot arthrodesis include failed union, avascular necrosis of the talus, arthritis, and ankle deformity.

FRACTURE OF THE ANKLE

Surgical Goal

Open reduction and internal fixation of the foot is performed to stabilize fractures of the distal tibia, fibula, talus, and calcaneus.

Pathology

Fracture of the ankle is caused by overeversion or overinversion, usually as a result of a sports injury, missed step, or fall. Ankle injury also is common in motor vehicle, motorcycle, and bicycle accidents.

Discussion

Open reduction and internal fixation of the ankle is performed using cannulated screws, pins, wires, and plates. Preoperative assessment, including imaging studies, is performed to determine the best approach. Special instruments are selected based on the approach chosen. Basic instruments and supplies include a basic orthopedic set, soft tissue instruments, a drill, a K-wire set, drill bits, and shallow right-angle retractors. Trauma cases may require a pulse lavage irrigation system. C-arm fluoroscopy is used in most procedures.

The patient is placed in the supine position with the operative leg supported on a padded roll. A tourniquet is positioned around the upper leg. General or spinal anesthesia is used. The foot and leg are prepped to just above the knee.

Surgical options for internal fixation include the following:

- *Insertion of cannulated or lag screws:* K-wires (guide wires) are inserted across the fracture, and their position is verified fluoroscopically. Screw holes are made with a cannulated drill and measured with a depth gauge. The cannulated screws are inserted over the guide wires. The position is verified, and the K-wires are removed.
- *Bridge plates with screws:* Small plates (small fragment set) are cut and contoured to fit the fracture site.

BUNIONECTOMY

Surgical Goal

In a bunionectomy, an enlarged metatarsal head (hallux valgus) is reduced or removed. The goal of surgery is to alleviate pain and increase patient mobilty.

Pathology

Hallux valgus is a deformity of the first metatarsal head and is associated with various structural anomalies of the entire toe. Poorly fitting shoes contribute to the pathology. An enlarged metatarsal head is painful and often limits the patient's mobility.

Discussion

The patient is placed in the supine position with a sandbag or soft padding under the nonoperative hip. Regional anesthesia is administered, and a pneumatic tourniquet is applied. The foot is prepped and draped.

An incision is made in the anterior or medial side of the metatarsal shaft and extended through the fascia. Senn retractors are placed in the wound. The joint capsule is incised with the deep knife and tenotomy scissors. Repair is performed by removal of the proximal phalanx with an oscillating power saw. The bony outgrowth of the metatarsal head (bunion) is also removed. To maintain the toe in alignment, one or two fine K-wires are placed through the medullary canal of the phalanx and metatarsal head. Fluoroscopy is used to check the position of the K-wires. The wound is irrigated and closed with absorbable sutures. The foot is dressed with bulky padding and placed in a foot brace.

HAMMERTOE CORRECTION

A hammertoe is a condition in which a toe has contracted at the proximal interphalangeal (PIP) joint, the middle joint in the toe. Contracture of the ligaments and tendons causes the toes to curl downward. Pain arises from friction between the shoe and the top of the joint. Hammertoe may occur in any toe except the big toe.

To correct a hammertoe deformity, a flexor tenotomy is performed with a #15 knife. Surgical options include resection of the head of the proximal phalanx. A small K-wire is driven through the end of the toe and both joint edges to maintain alignment during healing (Figure 30-76).

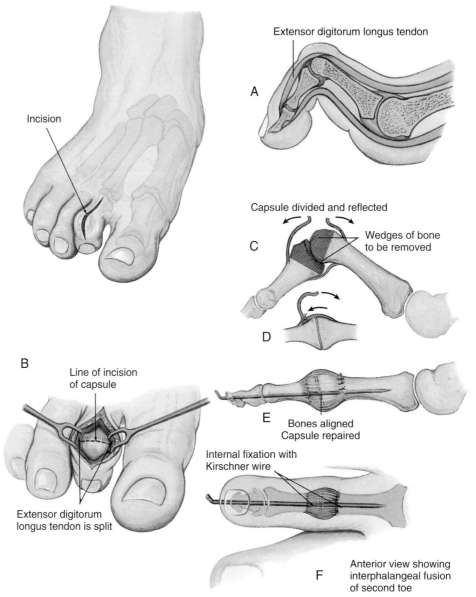

Figure 30-76 Hammertoe repair. *(From Herring JA: Tachdjian's pediatric orthopaedics from the Texas Scottish Rite Hospital for Children, ed 3, Philadelphia, 2002, WB Saunders.)*

CHAPTER SUMMARY

- Orthopedics is a surgical specialty of the connective tissues. Surgery is performed to treat or correct injuries, congenital anomalies, and disease of the bone, joints, ligaments, tendons, and muscle.
- The skeleton is divided into two parts for classification purposes. The axial skeleton includes the skull, face, ear bones, hyoid, sternum, and ribs. The appendicular skeleton includes the bones of the legs, feet, hands, trunk, and spine.
- Cortical bone (also called compact bone) is found on the surface of bones and is organized by tubular units called osteons.
- Cancellous bone is much more open than cortical bone and has no geometrical structure. The structure

resembles a sponge, and the spaces are filled with red or yellow marrow, a soft connective tissue.
- The hollow cavity inside a mature long bone is called the medullary canal.
- The outer membrane of bone is called periosteum; the medullary canal is lined with endosteum.
- The epiphyses are composed of cancellous bone and form the joints, which are covered with cartilage, a resilient connective tissue that increases the strength of the joint and reduces friction between the bones.
- Bones have many different irregularities, called landmarks. These function as areas of attachment for tendons and ligaments or provide a passageway for nerves and blood vessels.

- Bone healing takes place in three phases: the inflammatory, reparative, and remodeling phases. During these phases, specific physiological changes take place.
- The articular system (joints) includes the areas of the body where two bones meet and some degree of movement occurs.
- Anatomical movement of a joint refers to its normal range of motion. Each moveable joint of the body is classified according to its specific anatomical movements.
- Muscles and bones are attached by tendons and ligaments. Tendons attach muscle to bone; ligaments attach bone to bone.
- The three major muscle types in the human body are striated muscle, smooth muscle, and cardiac muscle.
- Trauma patients may arrive in traction, an external splinting device, or an antishock garment. The transfer may be completed after administration of an anesthetic to reduce the patient's discomfort.
- Many standard operating tables may also be converted for femoral or lower extremity surgery by removing the bottom section and replacing it with adjustable leg suspension devices.
- Fractures occur as a result of trauma or disease. Traumatic bone injury may be complicated by soft tissue injury with critical damage to nerves and blood vessels.
- Fracture classification systems vary according to the criteria used. Common criteria include the name and location of the fracture, the pattern of fracture, and the level of comminution.
- Common surgical goals for all types of fractures are alignment of the bones (reduction) and stabilization until healing is complete (fixation).
- Internal fixation requires surgery to insert or implant a device that holds the bone fragments in place. Metal plates, rods, pins, and screws are examples of internal fixation devices.
- External fixation is a means of stabilizing the bone from outside the body. A cast is an example of external fixation. Other devices, including external frames and cages, are also used in external fixation. Pins or wires may be inserted through the skin and into the bone to support the external fixation device.
- A modular rod and pin design is used mainly for temporary external stabilization of a fracture.
- Orthopedic implants or hardware includes the devices used to attach or fix bone and other connective tissue.
- Bioactive implants are absorbed by the body or stimulate or enhance bone repair (e.g., absorbable fixation screws that release calcium).
- All implants stored in the operating room must be documented on a database for tracking, retrieval, and stock replacement.

- Plates are designed to span bone and provide stability and support during healing. Plates are used in simple or comminuted fractures.
- The orthopedic screw is the most common type of orthopedic implant. Screws are supplied in different types, sizes, shapes, and design. They are made of titanium, stainless steel, or bioabsorbable material.
- An intramedullary nail is a thick rod inserted into the medullary canal of long bones to provide structural support from inside the bone.
- Flexible wire and cable are used in a variety of techniques to approximate bone and soft tissue and for stabilization.
- Kirschner wires (K-wires) and Steinmann pins are thick wires with a sharp, diamond-shaped point that penetrates bone and soft tissue. They are inserted directly into tissue with a drill.
- Joint implants are metal or synthetic components used to replace diseased or injured tissue.
- Bone graft substitutes are commonly used to repair and reconstruct bone. A shortage of graft materials and interest in bioactive materials have led to the development of new graft substitutes.
- Bone cement is an interface or grout (rather than a glue) that is used between the joint implant and tissue. It is formed by mixing polymethylmethacrylate powder with a liquid monomer of methylmethacrylate. The vapors released when the ingredients are mixed are known to cause serious eye injury, respiratory tract damage, and skin irritation.
- Casting is a method of immobilizing bone by applying a plaster or synthetic resin support to a limb.
- Traction is a mechanical method of applying pulling force to a fractured bone.
- Arthroscopic surgery is minimally invasive surgery of the joints. This technique is used mainly for diagnostic procedures and to repair and reconstruct soft tissue. Most open soft tissue procedures of the joints can be performed arthroscopically.
- In the Bankart procedure, the glenoid rim is reattached to the joint capsule with a biosynthetic or other anchoring device or with heavy sutures.
- The goal of rotator cuff repair is to reattach torn muscles of the rotator cuff to the humerus using sutures or anchor-suturing devices. An open or arthroscopic approach can be used.
- Open reduction and internal fixation may be used to repair a fracture of the proximal humerus. A metal plate is secured across the fracture with locking screws.
- An arthroscopic approach can be used for most shoulder repair procedures, except when injury is extensive. The surgical goals are the same as with open procedures and depend on the nature of the injury.
- Wrist and hand surgery is a specialty that combines orthopedic and vascular surgery and neurosurgery. The scaphoid is the most common site of wrist fracture

because of its vulnerable location. A common cause of fracture is a fall on the wrist when it is flexed to break the impact.

- Carpal tunnel syndrome occurs when the median nerve in the carpal tunnel of the wrist is compressed. The individual experiences numbness and tingling in the fingers, as well as pain in the hand that often radiates up the forearm.
- A Dupuytren contracture is a common condition in which the fascia of the palm or fingers contracts.
- A fracture of the femoral neck is a common injury caused by a fall. It may occur alone or with fracture of the femur itself.
- Intermedullary nails commonly are used to repair fractures of the tibia and femur. Locking screws are seated through the nail to prevent slipping in the medullary canal.
- Hip arthroplasty is performed using modular components, including the femoral stem and ball and the acetabular liner and shell.
- Fractures of the pelvis generally are the result of a high-impact injury and often are accompanied by soft tissue injury. An unstable pelvic fracture can be life-threatening because of damage to major blood vessels and pelvic organs.
- The knee is the most complicated joint in the body. It is vulnerable to a variety of injuries, mainly those caused by sports and motor vehicle accidents. Knee arthroscopy is a common approach for assessing and correcting problems that arise from injury and disease.
- The meniscus is a horseshoe-shaped cartilage that distributes load across the joint and ensures capsular stability. A tear in the meniscus is the most common knee injury.
- Damage to the anterior cruciate ligament routinely is repaired arthroscopically. A graft is taken from the central portion of the patellar tendon to replace the torn ACL.
- Repair of a torn lateral collateral ligament can be performed using techniques described for curiae ligament repair. A patellar tendon graft is used to replace the damaged collateral ligament.
- Triple arthrodesis is the fusion of the talocalcaneal, talonavicular, and calcaneocuboid joints. It is performed by removing the cartilage from each joint and allowing them to heal in approximation.
- In unicompartmental knee arthroplasty, a femoral and tibia component are implanted. In total knee arthroplasty all three components (femoral, tibial, and patellar) are replaced. A bunion is a medial mass on the metatarsal head (hallux valgus). The bunion is removed to reduce pain and allow return to routine activities.
- A hammertoe is a condition in which a toe has contracted at the proximal interphalangeal joint (the middle joint in the toe).

REFERENCES

1. Association for the Advancement of Medical Instrumentation. ANSI/AAMI ST79:2006 *Comprehensive guide to steam sterilization and sterility assurance in health care facilities.* Arlington, VA. Advancement of Medical Instrumentation. 2006.
2. Association of periOperative Registered Nurses (AORN): Recommended practices for sterilization in the perioperative practice setting. In *Standards, recommended practices and guidelines, 2007 edition,* Denver, AORN, 2007.
3. University of Washington Orthopedices and Sports Medicine: *Treatment of recurrent instability,* in Shoulder Dislocations, accessed January 24, 2007, at www.orthop.washington.edu/uw/tabID_3404Default.aspx.

BIBLIOGRAPHY

Browner B, Jupiter J, Levine A, Trafton P: *Skeletal trauma: basic science, management, and reconstruction,* ed 3, Philadelphia, 2003, WB Saunders.

Canale S, Beaty J: *Campbell's operative orthopaedics,* ed 11, St Louis, 2007, Mosby.

DeLee J, Drez D: *Delee Drez's orthopaedic sports medicine: principles and practice,* Philadelphia, 2003, WB Saunders.

Marx J, editor: *Rosen's emergency medicine: concepts and clinical practice,* ed 6, Philadelphia, 2006, Mosby.

Matsen FA III, Rockwood CA Jr, Wirth MA et al: Glenohumeral arthritis and its management. In Rockwood CA Jr, Matsen FA III, Wirth MA et al, editors: *The shoulder,* ed 3, Philadelphia, 2004, WB Saunders.

From Miller MD, Chhabra AB, Hurwitz SR, Mihalko WM: *Orthopaedic surgical approaches,* Philadelphia, 2008, WB Saunders.

Rothrock J: *Alexander's care of the patient in surgery,* ed 17, Philadelphia, 2007, Mosby.

Thibodeau G, Patton K: Anatomy and physiology, ed 6, Philadelphia, 2007, Mosby.

Townsend CM: *Sabiston textbook of surgery,* ed 17, Philadelphia, 2001, WB Saunders.

Peripheral Vascular Surgery

LEARNING OBJECTIVES

After studying this chapter the reader will be able to:
- Discuss the surgical treatment of atherosclerosis
- Describe drugs used for hemostasis and coagulation during surgery
- Discuss techniques used in peripheral vascular surgery
- Explain the principles of grafting in vascular surgery

TERMINOLOGY

Aneurysm: Ballooning of an artery as a result of weakening of the arterial wall. It may be caused by atherosclerosis, infection, or a hereditary defect in the vascular system.
Angioplasty: Dilation of an artery using endovascular techniques (i.e., an arterial catheter); may include insertion of a supportive stent inside the artery to maintain blood flow.
Arteriosclerosis: A disease characterized by thickening, hardening, and loss of elasticity of the arterial wall.
Arteriotomy: An incision made in an artery, usually to perform an anastomosis with a graft or another artery or to remove plaque or a thrombus.
Arteriovenous (AV) fistula: A naturally occurring or surgically created connection between an artery and a vein. In surgery, it is created to prepare a vessel for hemodialysis.
Atherosclerosis: The most common form of arteriosclerosis, which causes plaque to form on the inner surface of an artery.
Bifurcation: The Y-shape of an artery or graft.
Diastolic pressure: The lowest pressure exerted on the arterial wall during the resting phase of the cardiac cycle (**diastole**).

Doppler duplex ultrasonography: A type of ultrasonography that amplifies sounds that pass through tissue and produces a visual image of blood flow.
Electroencephalogram (EEG): A diagnostic tool that measures the electrical activity of the brain. During vascular surgery, an EEG may be used to determine the patient's neurophysiological response.
Embolus: A moving substance in the vascular system. An embolus may consist of air, a blood clot, atherosclerotic plaque, or fat.
Endarterectomy: The surgical removal of plaque from inside an artery.
Extracorporeal: A term meaning "outside the body." In extracorporeal hemodialysis, the blood is shunted outside the body for filtering and cleansing.
Hemodialysis: A process in which blood is shunted out of the body and passed through a complex set of filters for the treatment of end-stage renal disease (and in some cases, poisoning); also called *renal replacement therapy* (RRT).

Hemodynamic: A term referring to the pressure, flow, and resistance in the cardiovascular system.

Hypertension: An abnormal increase in blood pressure.

Hypotension: An abnormally low blood pressure.

Infarction: A blockage in an artery that leads to ischemia and tissue death.

In situ: A term meaning "in the natural position or normal place, without disturbing or invading surrounding tissues."

Intravascular ultrasound: A diagnostic tool in which a transducer is introduced into an artery and ultrasound is used to translate the physical characteristics of the lumen into a visible image.

Ischemia: The decrease in or absence of blood to a localized area, usually related to vascular obstruction.

Lumen: The inside of a hollow structure, such as a blood vessel.

Percutaneous: A term that literally means "through the skin." In a percutaneous approach in surgery, an incision is not made; rather, a catheter or other device is introduced through a puncture site.

Stasis (venous): Pooling of blood in the veins caused by inactivity or disease. Stasis can cause distension of the veins.

Stent: A tubular device placed inside an artery for dilation, support, and to prevent stricture.

Systolic pressure: The highest pressure exerted on the inside arterial wall during contraction of the heart (**systole**).

Thrombus: Any organic or nonorganic material blocking an artery; generally refers to a blood clot or atherosclerotic plaque but also includes fat or air.

Umbilical tape: A length of mesh tape used to loop around a blood vessel for retraction. See *vessel loop*.

Varicosity: Thinning and enlargement of veins as a result of stasis (pooling of blood in the vessel).

Vessel loop: A device used to retract a vessel during surgery. A length of thin Silastic tubing or cotton tape (umbilical tape) is passed around the vessel. The ends can be threaded through a bolster (a ⅛- to ¼-inch [0.3 to 0.6 cm] length of rubber or Silastic tubing) to secure the loop against the blood vessel.

INTRODUCTION

Peripheral vascular surgery includes procedures of the arteries and veins lying outside the immediate area of the heart or brain. Many vascular procedures are performed to treat arteriosclerosis, atherosclerosis, or thromboembolic disease. Surgical intervention for vascular disease includes open and minimally invasive procedures. Many conditions that required open surgery in the past may now be performed using an endovascular technique, with far less trauma and a more rapid recovery. Sophisticated diagnostic technology also has contributed to early diagnosis and a decrease in the number of open surgical procedures.

Reconstruction and grafting procedures often require temporary clamping of large vessels or those which contribute the main blood supply to vital organs. Timing is important to minimize the risk of **ischemia** (loss of blood supply) to tissue during selected grafting procedures. An example is clamping the carotid artery during carotid endarterectomy. Even if the blood flow to the brain is decreased because of the disease, complete occlusion presents a risk of ischemia to the brain, which must be managed. The surgical scrub must be attentive to the surgical site at all times, but especially when target vessels are clamped. A high level of knowledge going into surgery is required to anticipate steps in the procedure. Equipment and instruments must be well organized and ready for immediate use on the surgical field.

SURGICAL ANATOMY

The peripheral vascular system is a complex network of vessels, the function of which is to carry blood cell components and nutrients (including oxygen) to all parts of the body and to remove the waste products of metabolism. The organs of this system are the arteries, veins, and capillaries.

STRUCTURE OF BLOOD VESSELS

All blood vessels except the capillaries are composed of three layers or walls. From the outside to the inside, they are:

- The *tunica externa* (also called the *adventitia*), which is composed of connective tissue, which protects the vessel from injury and provides structural strength.
- The *tunica media,* which is composed of inner layers of smooth muscle bounded by connective tissue. Smooth muscle is under the control of the autonomic nervous system.
- The *tunica intima,* which secretes substances that cause vasodilation or constriction, as well as substances that prevent platelet aggregation in the vessel.

The structure of arteries and veins is shown in Figure 31-1.

Arteries

The *arteries* carry oxygenated blood from the heart to the rest of the body. The only exception is the *pulmonary arteries*, which carry deoxygenated blood to the lungs. Arteries and the smaller arterioles have distinct characteristics that enable them to transport a large volume of blood under pressure.

The arteries are thick walled, highly elastic, and contain mostly smooth muscle. The arteries branch into the arterioles, which transition to the capillaries, where oxygen is released into the tissues. The arterioles provide vascular resistance, regulating the flow of blood into organs and tissues.

The elastic nature of the arteries allows them to contract during **systole** (ventricular contraction) and relax during **diastole** (the resting phase of the heart) to maintain vascular pressure. The arteries dilate and contract to accommodate the metabolic needs of the body. For example, inflammation causes expansion of the arteries and the release of blood through the arterioles; this increases blood to the injured and infected tissue. Vascular dilation lowers the body tempera-

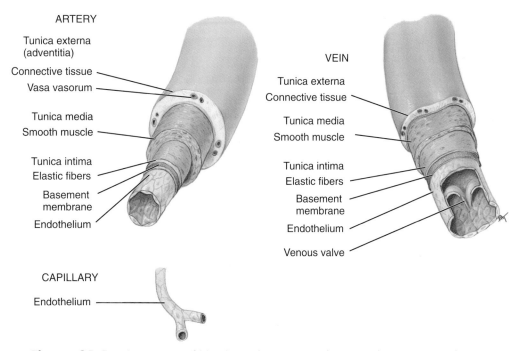

Figure 31-1 The structure of blood vessels. *(From Applegate E: The anatomy and physiology learning system, ed 2, St Louis, 2000, WB Saunders.)*

ture, because it exposes the blood to surface cooling provided by evaporation of sweat from the skin. Peripheral vasoconstriction occurs during shock and when the body's core temperature is subnormal; this concentrates the greatest volume of blood in the heart and brain and prevents further cooling at the surface of the body.

Capillaries

The *capillaries* are microscopic vessels that function as the transition and exchange mechanism for oxygen and other substances between the vessel walls and the tissue cells. Arterioles transition to the capillaries, which transition to venules and veins. Capillaries are composed of endothelial cells and have no muscle fibers. Precapillary sphincters control the flow of oxygenated blood into the capillary. The walls of the capillary are one cell thick and allow selected substances, including oxygen, to diffuse through the capillary membrane into the tissue. The microcirculation of the capillary system is illustrated in Figure 31-2.

Some tissues, such as the liver and spleen, have a rich supply of capillary networks. Because of this, these tissues bleed easily and profusely when injured. Capillary bleeding sometimes is difficult to control during surgery, and topical hemostatic agents are required to maintain hemostasis (see Chapter 17).

Veins

The venous system carries blood back to the heart from the peripheral tissues. After passing through the capillary network, blood enters venules, which transition to increasingly larger branches of veins that run roughly parallel to the arteries on their way to the heart.

Veins are thin walled, which allows them to expand. They function as vessels for transporting blood and also as storage units for blood. Like arteries, larger veins contain muscle fibers that allow them to constrict. However, unlike arteries, veins have valves that open only one way, preventing blood from backing up.

Blood is not pumped through the veins; rather, it is milked toward the heart by contractions in skeletal muscles in the peripheral system (Figure 31-3) and by intraabdominal and intrathoracic pressure in the trunk of the body. Malfunction of the veins' one-way valves results in venous **stasis** or pooling, which can cause the veins to dilate abnormally (called a **varicosity**). A number of physiological functions prevent blood from clotting in the vessels. Movement is among the most important. Stasis and pooling can cause thrombosis or blood clot in the peripheral or cardiac circulation.

Box 31-1 presents important differences between arteries and veins.

PULMONARY AND SYSTEMIC CIRCULATORY SYSTEMS

The circulatory system is divided into two pathways, the pulmonary system and the systemic system. The pulmonary system carries blood from the heart to the lungs for oxygenation (hemoglobin in the red blood cells picks up oxygen molecules). The oxygenated blood then returns to the heart and is pumped into the systemic circulation, which reaches all tissues of the body.

The systemic and pulmonary systems (Figure 31-4) function simultaneously. The ventricles provide the primary pumping action for the heart. As the ventricles contract, deox-

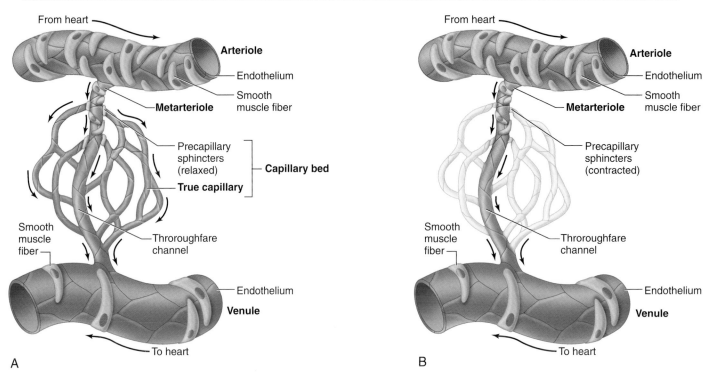

Figure 31-2 Microcirculation in the capillary system. *(From Thibodeau G, Patton K: Anatomy and physiology, ed 6, St Louis, 2007, Mosby.)*

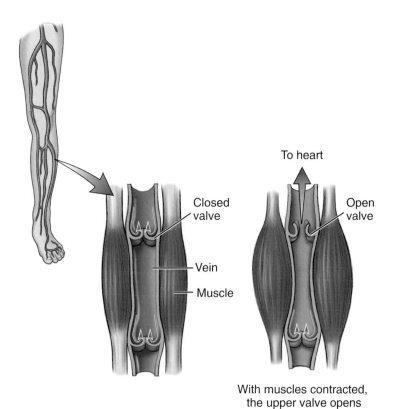

Figure 31-3 Skeletal muscle "pump." One-way valves in the veins prevent blood from backing up. Blood in the extremities is milked toward the heart by skeletal muscle contraction. *(From Herlihy B, Maebius NK: The human body in health and disease, ed 2, Philadelphia, 2003, WB Saunders.)*

<u>Box 31-1</u>

Comparison of Arteries and Veins

Arteries
- Thick walls
- Elastic
- Blood is moved through arteries by the pumping action of the heart.
- No internal valves
- Loss of function can lead to tissue injury or death
- When severed, spurt blood (because of pumping action of the heart)
- Blood loss can be rapid and severe
- Arterial pressure is higher than venous pressure

Veins
- Thin walls
- Less elastic than arteries
- Blood is moved through veins by contraction of skeletal muscles
- Internal valves prevent back flow
- Loss of function not as medically significant as with arteries
- When severed, tend to bleed slowly
- Tend to be closer to the skin surface than arteries

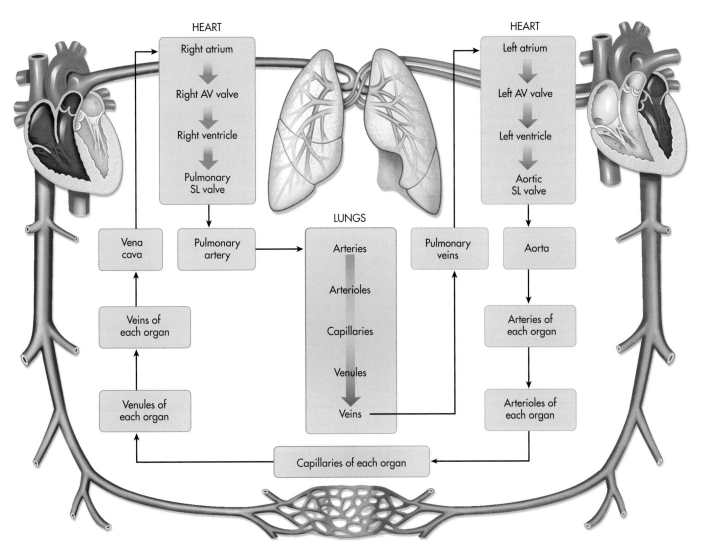

Figure 31-4   The systemic and pulmonary systems. In the pulmonary system, blood leaves the right heart, travels to the lungs and returns to the heart. In the systemic circulation, oxygenated blood leaves the left ventricle, travels through the ascending aorta, and is transported throughout the body. It passes through the capillary system and returns to the heart via the venous system. (See the text for further detail.) *(From Thibodeau G, Patton K:* Anatomy and physiology, *ed 6, St Louis, 2007, Mosby.)*

ygenated blood flows to the lungs through the pulmonary system while oxygenated blood is pumped into the systemic system. Both systems have arterial, venous, and capillary structures.

- *Systemic circulation:* Oxygenated blood in the left ventricle is pumped through the ascending aorta to the rest of the body. Blood returning from the body passes from the capillaries into the venous system and returns to the left atrium through the vena cavae.
- *Pulmonary circulation:* Deoxygenated blood in the right ventricle is pumped through the *pulmonary arteries* (the only arteries that carry deoxygenated blood) to the lungs. Blood is oxygenated in the capillaries of the alveoli (lungs) and returns to the left ventricle through the *pulmonary veins* (the only veins that carry oxygenated blood).

BLOOD PRESSURE

Blood pressure is the force exerted on the arterial wall by the pumping action of the heart. The **systolic pressure,** the higher pressure, occurs during contraction of the ventricles (systole). The lower pressure, the **diastolic pressure,** occurs during the relaxation phase of the cardiac cycle (diastole).

Regulation of blood pressure is influenced by many physiological conditions, including body position, temperature, pain, and emotion. The complex hormonal regulation of arterial pressure, which is called the *renin-angiotensin-aldosterone system,* is influenced by fluid volume and other factors.

Negative alterations in blood pressure (**hypotension**) can be caused by hypovolemia (a precipitous drop in blood or fluid volume), fluid shifts between the spaces in the body, shock, or infection.

Hypertension, or abnormally high blood pressure, often is caused by cardiovascular disease, such as arteriosclerosis, but it also occurs with chronic renal failure and hypermetabolic conditions (e.g., malignant hyperthermia and hyperaldosteronism).

Normal blood pressure is affected by the following factors:

- *Gender:* Adult females generally have higher blood pressure than males.
- *Age:* A gradual rise in blood pressure occurs from childhood to adulthood.
- *Weight:* Blood pressure is higher in individuals with a high body mass index, regardless of age.
- *Exercise:* Blood pressure rises with strenuous activity but returns to baseline level at rest.
- *Diurnal (daily) fluctuation:* Blood pressure tends to rise during the day and is lowest in the mornings.

Blood pressure also is influenced by specific physiological parameters:

- *Elasticity of the arterial walls:* The ability of the artery to expand and relax affects systemic pressure. Arteries stiffened by atherosclerosis result in hypertension.
- *Total blood volume:* The total amount of circulating blood has a direct effect on blood pressure. The body has mechanisms to constrict peripheral blood vessels when volume is low. However, this protective mechanism cannot overcome large blood loss or fluid shifts.
- *Peripheral vascular resistance:* Vascular resistance occurs when the muscular layer of the artery is unable to relax or arteries are stiff and their diameter is reduced.
- *Blood viscosity:* Viscosity is measured by the amount of fluid in the blood. Lower viscosity or "thicker" blood increases blood pressure.

BLOOD VESSELS OF THE BODY

In many cases, only the major arteries and veins and tributaries of the body are named. Names are often identical among arteries and veins, with a few exceptions.

Major Arteries

The largest artery of the body is the aorta. It emerges from the heart in an arch at the left ventricle and curves downward to descend through the thoracic cavity, passing in the heart but in front of the spinal column. As it enters the abdomen, it passes through the diaphragm behind the retroperitoneum space. The aorta terminates at the pelvic **bifurcation** (splitting into a Y), which forms iliac arteries.

Thoracic Cavity

The aorta arises from the left ventricle of the heart to form an arch (the *aortic arch*). Three major arteries arise from the top of the arch: the *brachiocephalic* artery, the left *common carotid* artery, and the *left subclavian* artery. Beyond these branches, the aortic arch curves downward and is called the thoracic *descending aorta.* It passes through the diaphragm and leaves the thoracic cavity. It is called the *abdominal aorta* at this level. There are many branches of the aorta at all levels.

Head

The *brachiocephalic artery* gives rise to the *right common carotid artery,* which branches to the *external carotid artery* and the arteries of the brain. The vertebral artery, which branches from the *brachiocephalic artery,* follows the cervical vertebra and branches distally to the arteries of the head.

Upper Extremities

The arteries of the upper body begin at the three vessels of the aortic arch discussed above. The brachiocephalic artery branches into the right common carotid and the right subclavian. These supply blood to the right side of the head, neck, right shoulder, and upper arm. The left common carotid artery supplies blood to the left side of the neck and head. The left subclavian artery provides blood to the left shoulder and right arm. The radial and ulnar arteries arise from the brachial artery. Figure 31-5 shows major arteries of the body.

Abdomen

The descending aorta continues through the abdomen and branches to the celiac trunk, a network that gives rise to the gastric, splenic, and hepatic arteries. Other significant arteries in the abdomen include the mesenteric arteries, which provide

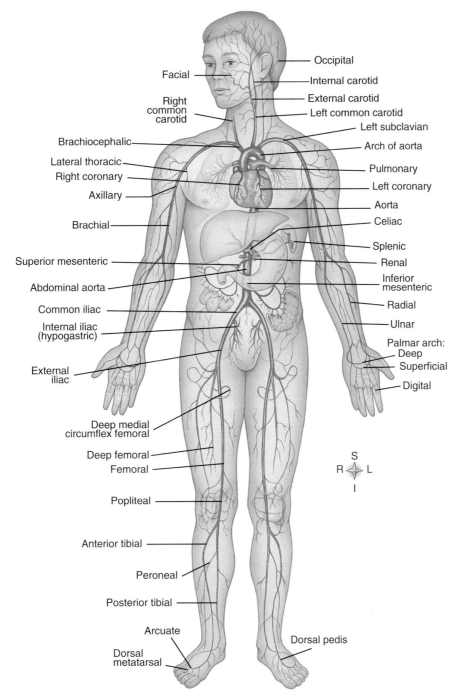

Facial — Occipital
Right common carotid — Internal carotid
External carotid
Left common carotid
Left subclavian
Brachiocephalic — Arch of aorta
Lateral thoracic — Pulmonary
Right coronary — Left coronary
Axillary — Aorta
Brachial — Celiac
Splenic
Superior mesenteric — Renal
Abdominal aorta — Inferior mesenteric
Common iliac — Radial
Internal iliac (hypogastric) — Ulnar
Palmar arch: Deep
External iliac — Superficial
Digital
Deep medial circumflex femoral
Deep femoral
Femoral
Popliteal
Anterior tibial
Peroneal
Posterior tibial
Arcuate — Dorsal pedis
Dorsal metatarsal

Figure 31-5   Major arteries of the body. *(From Thibodeau G, Patton K: Anatomy and physiology, ed 6, St Louis, 2007, Mosby.)*

the blood supply to the intestines, and the renal arteries, which branch directly from the aorta and supply blood to the kidneys.

Lower Limbs

The iliac arteries divide into the internal and external iliac arteries in the pelvis, and the external iliac artery converges into the femoral artery in the groin. Traveling distally, the femoral artery communicates with the popliteal artery in the knee area. The popliteal artery branches into the arterial tibial, peroneal, and posterior tibial arteries. The dorsal pedalis emerges from the anterior tibial artery and then further divides into smaller arteries of the foot and phalanges.

Major Veins

The largest vein of the body is the vena cava, which is divided into *inferior* and *superior* segments. The vena cavae communicate with the heart through the right atrium. The superior vena cava receives deoxygenated blood from the head, neck, and upper extremities, and the inferior vena cava receives blood from the lower body and extremities. The major veins are illustrated in Figure 31-6.

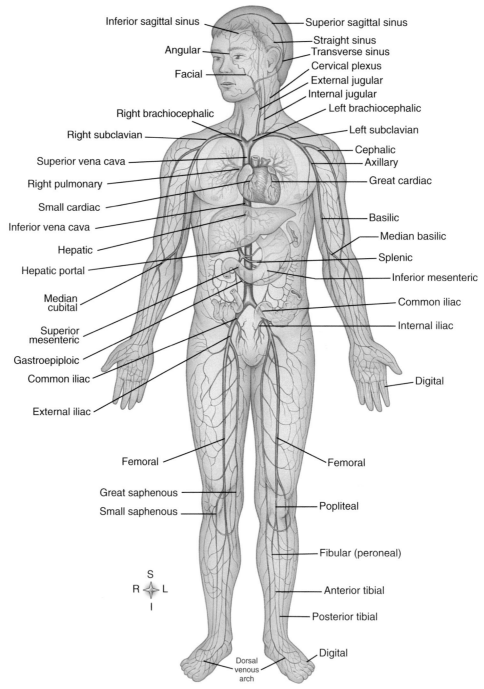

Inferior sagittal sinus
Superior sagittal sinus
Angular
Straight sinus
Transverse sinus
Facial
Cervical plexus
External jugular
Internal jugular
Right brachiocephalic
Left brachiocephalic
Right subclavian
Left subclavian
Superior vena cava
Cephalic
Right pulmonary
Axillary
Great cardiac
Small cardiac
Basilic
Inferior vena cava
Median basilic
Hepatic
Splenic
Hepatic portal
Inferior mesenteric
Median cubital
Common iliac
Superior mesenteric
Internal iliac
Gastroepiploic
Common iliac
Digital
External iliac
Femoral
Femoral
Great saphenous
Small saphenous
Popliteal
Fibular (peroneal)
Anterior tibial
Posterior tibial
Digital
Dorsal venous arch

S
R ✦ L
I

Figure 31-6 *Major veins of the body. (From Thibodeau G, Patton K: Anatomy and physiology, ed 6, St Louis, 2007, Mosby.)*

Portal Circulation

The hepatic portal circulation is unique in structure and function. The superior mesenteric and splenic veins converge to form the portal vein. This large vessel carries nutrients from the digestive system into the liver and also supplies about 60% of that organ's oxygen requirements. The hepatic veins carry blood out of the liver to the vena cava. However, a pressure difference between the hepatic and portal veins allows the liver to store approximately 450 mL of blood.

This can be released back into the systemic circulation as needed.

Microscopic sinuses (sinusoids) in the liver, which are lined with epithelium, filter and remove bacteria, toxins, and cell remnants from the blood. The blood then is shunted back into the hepatic veins and into the vena cava (Figure 31-7). Because of the structure of the liver and sinusoids, fibrotic diseases of the liver, such as cirrhosis, can prevent the flow of venous blood out of the sinusoids. Blood backs up into the

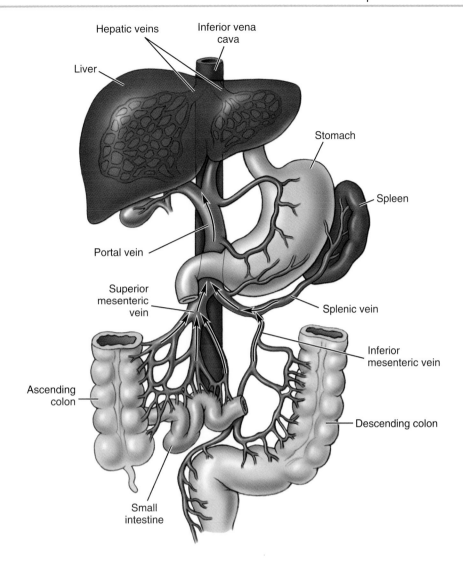

Figure 31-7 The portal circulation. *(From Herlihy B, Maebius NK: The human body in health and disease, ed 2, Philadelphia, 2003, WB Saunders.)*

veins of the digestive system, causing varicosities and rupture of the vessels.

LYMPHATIC SYSTEM

The lymphatic system is composed of ducts (vessels), regional lymph nodes, and lymph (fluid). Lymph contributes to the formation of plasma, the liquid portion of blood, which is derived from intercellular components. Lymph vessels follow the anatomical pattern of arteries and veins. Like veins, lymph vessels contain valves that prevent reverse flow. The complex lymph system drains into two primary collection ducts. The right lymphatic duct drains lymph from the head, neck, thorax, and right arm. Lymph from the right lymphatic duct enters the subclavian vein. The second collecting system is the thoracic duct, which receives lymph from other parts of the body and drains into the left subclavian vein. Occlusion of these ducts (e.g., during radical surgery) results in lymphedema or swelling of the lymph

vessels. Certain diseases and tumors also cause blockage of the lymph system.

Lymph nodes are located at intervals along the lymph ducts. Nodes are composed of lymphatic tissue that collects and filters fluid from the system. They also produce lymphocytes (white blood cells). Nodes occur in groups or chains in collection areas. For example, the axillary nodes drain lymph from the breasts. Lymph from the pelvic organs drains to nodes in the inguinal area. During lymph node dissection, specific nodes are removed and assessed according to the organ suspected of cancer to determine whether metastasis has occurred.

PATHOLOGY OF THE PERIPHERAL VASCULAR SYSTEM

Table 31-1 presents common pathological conditions of the peripheral vascular system.

<u>Table 31-1</u>

Pathology of the Peripheral Vascular System

Condition	Description	Considerations
Arteriosclerosis	A group of vascular diseases characterized by hardening and stiffening of the arteries caused by calcium deposits and fatty substances in the arterial wall. The disease is related to age, smoking, diabetes, and hypertension.	Treatment usually is medical and includes behavioral changes in lifestyle and medications that dilate the blood vessels. Surgical intervention includes artery stenting and angioplasty. Severe peripheral arteriosclerosis may require amputation. (See Above-the-Knee Amputation and Transluminal Angioplasty.)
Atherosclerosis	The most common form of arteriosclerosis; an obstructive disease of the arteries in which the vessels are infiltrated with calcium and fatty fibrous deposits, causing reduced elasticity as well as obstruction and ischemia. Risk factors include smoking, a high-fat diet, obesity, and inactivity.	Treatment includes behavioral changes in lifestyle and diet. Cholesterol-reducing drugs may help inhibit the disease. Surgery is required to remove fatty plaque from critical locations such as the carotid or coronary arteries. (See Carotid Endarterectomy.)
Peripheral vascular disease (PVD) (also called *peripheral arterial disease*)	An atherosclerotic disease characterized by arterial obstruction, pain, and ischemia. Most patients with PVD also have coronary artery disease.	Arterial obstruction is surgical treated by endarterectomy. See Arthrosclerosis above.
Embolus	A moving particle in the bloodstream, such as a blood clot, fat, or atherosclerotic plaque. An embolus may become lodged in a vessel, causing obstruction, local ischemia, and tissue death.	Treatment depends on the location and type of embolus. Emergency medical treatment is necessary in the event of stroke, pulmonary arrest, or sudden occlusion of a vital organ. Surgical treatment includes embolectomy.
Aneurysm	An area of thinning and ballooning of an arterial wall, usually near a bifurcation. Causes include atherosclerosis, infection, and congenital malformation. An aneurysm becomes life-threatening when the sac ruptures. In a dissecting aneurysm, blood seeps between the vessel layers, causing them to tear.	Surgery is necessary to remove the aneurysm and restore arterial circulation. (See Abdominal Aortic Aneurysm; also see Cerebral Aneurysm in Chapter 34.)
Varicose veins	A condition in which the veins becomes grossly distended. It is related to nonfunctional or incompetent valves, which result in poor venous circulation and stasis. Note: Varicosities may occur in other locations of the body, such as the esophagus.	Varicosities of the lower extremities are treated with sclerosing agents or laser therapy. Only severe conditions require surgery. (See Management of Varicose Veins.)
Deep venous thrombosis (DVT)	A thrombus that occurs in a deep peripheral vein of the leg (the condition is also called *thrombophlebitis*). A DVT may lead to pulmonary embolism, which can be fatal. Venous stasis related to immobility or lifestyle is a risk factor. Surgery that results in venous injury (e.g., transurethral resection of the prostate or repair of a hip fracture) increases the risk of DVT.	Prevention of DVT in surgery includes application of antiembolism stockings or a sequential compression device (SCD). Individuals who are at high risk for DVT may undergo implantation of a vena cava filter. (See Insertion of a Vena Cava Filter.)
Portal hypertension	A condition of the portal vein related to liver cirrhosis. It causes blood to reflux (back up) into the esophageal veins. Venous rupture and hemorrhage may be fatal.	Esophageal varices are treated with sclerosing agents or laser surgery. Portal bypass is treated by the radiological procedure, transjugular intrahepatic portosystemic shunt (TIPS).
Vascular trauma	Trauma of a large artery results in obvious blood loss and a threat to life. Injury can occur during motor vehicle or industrial accidents or as a result of intentional violence. Secondary injury can occur as a result of a fracture.	Emergency response to vascular trauma is undertaken by ambulance personnel and may include whole body or local compression until surgery can be performed.

DIAGNOSTIC PROCEDURES

Diagnosis of peripheral vascular disease is based first on the patient's history and the physical examination findings and on the results of routine blood tests. More specific studies may be performed based on the findings of these tests and the patient's signs and symptoms.

ARTERIAL PLETHYSMOGRAPHY

A pulse volume recorder is used to measure the arterial pulse waveform during systole. For this test, three blood pressure cuffs are placed on the leg and inflated to 65 mm Hg. Each cuff reading produces a waveform, which is compared with the waveforms from the other two cuffs. A reduced wave in one area may indicate reduced blood flow at that point.

DOPPLER SCANNING

Doppler scanning intensifies the sounds made by blood flowing through a vessel. The pitch, rhythm, and quality of the sound reflect pressure, volume, and flow rate. The tip of the Doppler probe is placed over a pulse point or other area that requires evaluation. The high-frequency sound waves generated by the probe are reflected back to a data recorder. Interpretative Doppler scanning is performed with a sterile probe. **Doppler duplex ultrasonography** combines Doppler scanning with ultrasound to produce visual images of the vessel. Blood flow, strictures, thrombi, turbulence (swirling motion of blood characteristic at a stricture, and other abnormalities are displayed on a monitor in real time and can be preserved for permanent documentation.

ARTERIOGRAPHY

Arteriography is radiographic imaging of the artery. This is done as an intraoperative, diagnostic, or interventional procedure to delineate the shape and interior surface of the arteries. A contrast medium is injected into the artery under fluoroscopy or computed tomography (CT). Complex studies that provide three-dimensional images and time-flow data are commonly used in diagnosis. Interventional arteriography is performed in conjunction with the insertion of stents and other devices.

INTRAVASCULAR ULTRASONOGRAPHY

Intravascular ultrasound is used in both peripheral and coronary surgery to map the **lumen** of a vessel. A rotating flexible catheter carrying a transducer is introduced into the vessel. Ultrasonic energy is generated and interpreted by the transducer. The lumen of the vessel can be mapped (including density, accumulation of atherosclerotic plaque, and wall thickness), and a visual image can be produced. Because the catheter is able to rotate, intravascular ultrasound produces a 360-degree image.

INSTRUMENTS

Vascular surgery is performed with general surgical instruments and vascular instruments. Other sets are added according to the regional anatomy. Nearly all vascular procedures require right-angle (Mixter type) clamps, tonsil (Schnidt) clamps, and Kelly, Crile, and mosquito forceps. General dissecting scissors and general surgery forceps also are used on nonvascular tissue.

VASCULAR CLAMPS

Vascular clamps are specifically designed to prevent trauma to blood vessels. The jaws contain finely serrated inserts that grip the tissue but do not crush or damage the surface of the vessel, even when fully closed. Clamps are available in a wide variety of shapes and sizes to fit around a vessel as it lies in normal anatomical position. Peripheral vascular clamps are much smaller than those used in cardiac surgery. Hundreds of types of vascular clamps are available, many with the same name (e.g., DeBakey clamps). The nature of vascular surgery is such that often little time is available for selection during surgery. It is common practice for the surgeon to specify which vascular clamps are needed before surgery so that the scrub can have them ready on the instrument table. In an emergency, such as sudden hemorrhage from a large vessel, the scrub should rely on common sense regarding the type of clamp needed, because the surgeon may not be able to turn away from the field to designate one.

SCISSORS

Vascular scissors are extremely sharp and fine. Many are angled so that the tips can be easily inserted into the vessel. The blades must be kept sharp to prevent tissue from buckling or folding between them. The most commonly used vessel dissection scissors are Potts (right angle) and De Martel scissors. Scissors are sharply pointed or have a probe tip. Fine Metzenbaum scissors are also used in vascular dissection. Vascular scissors must never be used to cut materials off the surgical field, because this damages them.

FORCEPS

Vascular forceps have very fine serrations at the tips to allow a secure grip without tearing or slipping. The most common vascular forceps are DeBakey forceps.

Surgeons generally do not ask for a specific type of vascular forceps during surgery. They assume that their personal preference is on record, and the scrub has placed these on the instrument table. Vascular forceps are always passed to the surgeon when it is apparent they will be used to grasp a blood vessel or other delicate tissue. Plain general surgical forceps are not suitable for use on vascular tissue, because they do not have the precision or gripping ability of vascular forceps. Toothed forceps are never used on blood vessels, because they can puncture the tissue.

RETRACTORS

There are few vascular-specific retractors except small vein retractors, which are also used in general surgery. Nonpenetrating, shallow retractors are commonly used during superficial vascular surgery. A dull Weitlaner (self-retracting) or spring retractor should be available for skin and subcutaneous retraction in the hand, arm, or superficial leg. Handheld retractors include the Senn retractor, vein retractor, and shallow Richardson retractor. Skin hooks occasionally may be needed.

For deeper surgery, general surgery retractors are used (e.g., Deaver, Richardson, and U.S. [Army-Navy] retractors). A standard Balfour self-retaining retractor is commonly used for procedures of the abdominal arteries.

SUCTION TIPS

Small suction tips, such as the Frazier tip, are commonly used in most vascular procedures. The suction pressure should be lowered for use on the actual vessels. Frazier suction tips are available in a wide variety of French (Fr) sizes, and the size used depends on the tissue. Suction tips must be kept clear of blood and tissue debris by suctioning a small amount of water through the tip. Larger suction tips are used according to the regional anatomy. General surgical tips, such as the Poole (vented) or Yankauer suction tip, are used in abdominal vascular surgery.

A dry surgical site is critical in vascular surgery, and suction must be available at all times. Because vascular suction tips (e.g., the smaller Frazier tip) clog easily, the scrub should keep one on the field and another in reserve. This allows the clogged tip to be flushed or cleared with a metal stylet while one remains in use.

Large vessels, such as the abdominal aorta, require larger suction tips. Two suctions may be necessary to maintain a dry field. In general, suction is used more often than sponges to maintain a dry operative field.

TUNNELER

A tunneler is used to burrow a channel through connective tissue to make space for a tubular vascular graft. Occasionally during surgery, the graft anastomosis sites are surgically exposed but located some distance apart. The tunneler is inserted into one site and pushed through the subcutaneous tissue to the other wound site. This creates a tunnel for the graft, which can then be pulled through before anastomosis.

Instruments used in vascular surgery are illustrated in Figures 31-8 to 31-10.

SUTURES

Vascular sutures range in size from 3-0 to 11-0. Cutting and taper needles used for anastomosis are $^{3}/_{8}$ curved needles. Synthetic monofilament or coated material is preferred over plain braided suture, because it is nonreactive and prevents endovascular clotting and emboli.

Vascular suture materials include polyester (Mersilene), polypropylene (Prolene), polyhexafluoroprophylene (Pronova), Gore-Tex, and silk. Suture-needle combinations are very delicate and require careful handling. Only fine-tip needle holders should be used. Cardiovascular (CV) sutures are available as single needles or double-arm needles.

The CV needle is grasped in the usual position behind the swage, and the suture is gently withdrawn from the

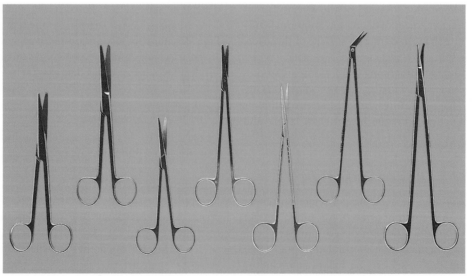

Figure 31-8   Vascular surgery scissors. *Left to right,* 1 straight Mayo scissors; 1 curved Mayo scissors; 1 Metzenbaum scissors; 1 Metzenbaum carbide insert scissors; 1 Lincoln scissors; 1 Potts-Smith scissors, 1 Strully scissors. *(From Tighe SM:* Instrumentation for the operating room, *ed 7, St Louis, 2007, Mosby.)*

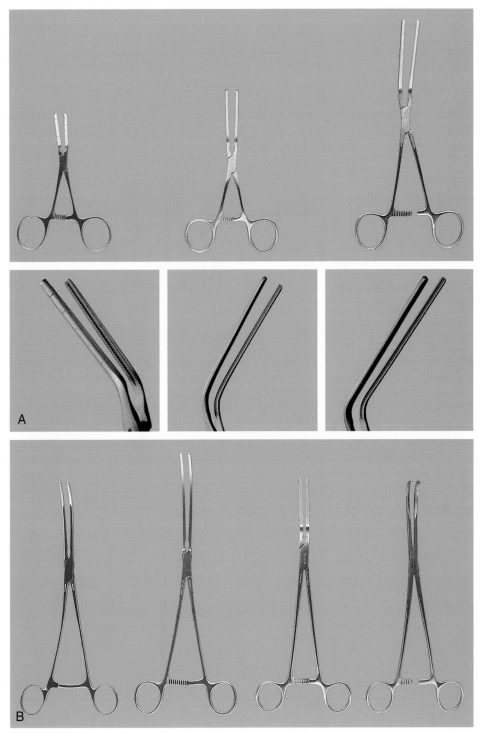

Figure 31-9   Cardiovascular clamps. **A,** *Left to right,* College clamp, angled; DeBakey clamp; DeBakey peripheral vascular clamp. **B,** *Left to right,* DeBakey aortic clamp, S-shaped; DeBakey aortic clamp, S-shaped, long; DeBakey multipurpose clamp; Semb ligature-carrying forceps. *(From Tighe SM: Instrumentation for the operating room, ed 7, St Louis, 2007, Mosby.)*

package. When vascular sutures are removed or passed, care must be taken to avoid snagging the needle on drapes or gloves. Passing of double-arm sutures may be problematic. As the loaded needle holder is passed, the other end may be easily snagged on drapes and instruments. Two needle holders may be used, or a small hemostat can be clamped

to one of the needles. The whole unit must be passed in a way that prevents tangling. An alternative method is to pass the nonoperative (mounted) needle on a folded towel while passing the mounted needle in the usual way. The towel is placed on the field in clear sight of the surgeon and assistant.

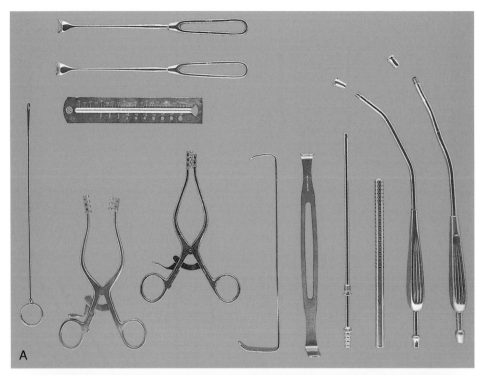

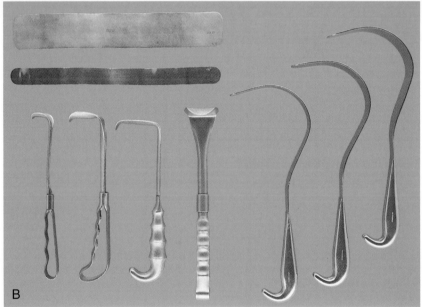

Figure 31-10 Instruments used in vascular surgery. **A,** *Top,* Vein retractors and metal ruler. *Left to right,* Obturator for Rummel tourniquet; 2 Weitlaner retractors; 2 Army-Navy retractors; Poole suction tip; Poole suction guard; 2 Yankauer suction tips **B,** *Top,* Ribbon retractors. *Left to right:* 4 Richardson retractors; 3 Deaver retractors.

❖ *During surgery, do not remove a loaded needle holder from the field unless you are certain it is free and clear of the anastomosis. Double-arm sutures are used in tandem, and removing one may drag the other out of the tissue.*

Vascular sutures are also supplied with felt pledgets (small squares of felted material) attached to the suture. The pledget prevents the stitch from tearing through the arterial wall.

VASCULAR GRAFTS

Vascular grafts are used to replace a blood vessel or to patch a vessel. Synthetic grafts are made of Dacron, polyester, or Gore-Tex. Sources of biological materials are banked human umbilical cord and autograft (usually from the saphenous vein). Grafts may be straight or bifurcated (Y-shaped). The length is measured in centimeters, and the diameter reflects the outside diameter (OD).

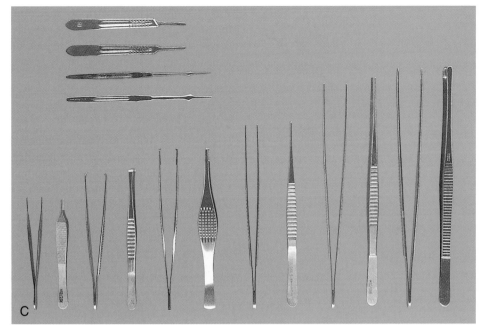

Figure 31-10, cont'd **C,** *Top,* Knife handles. *Left to right,* 2 Adson forceps; 2 Martin forceps; 2 Ferris Smith vascular forceps; 2 DeBakey vascular forceps, medium; 2 DeBakey forceps, long; 2 Russian forceps. *(From Tighe SM: Instrumentation for the operating room, ed 7, St Louis, 2007, Mosby.)*

Synthetic grafts require no preinsertion preparation except trimming. Patch grafts are cut into elliptical sections and sutured in place with a double-arm suture. Bovine grafts were commonly used in the past but are rarely used today. All prepared grafts are intended for use as directed by the manufacturer.

Vascular grafts are extremely expensive. They must not be opened until the surgeon is ready to insert them and has verbally requested the size required. All manufactured grafts are identified by size, lot, and identification number, which must be recorded on the patient's operative record.

CATHETERS

The most common method of removing thrombi is with a Fogarty-type embolectomy catheter. This is a narrow, flexible catheter with a firm tip and an inflatable balloon at the tip. The length of the catheter varies widely. Balloons are round or elliptical, and catheters are available in sizes ranging from 1 to 6 Fr. The balloon is filled with air or saline for testing purposes and saline, for actual use, according to the manufacturer's specification. A tuberculin syringe is used to fill the balloons, which have a volume of 1 mL or less. The balloon must be tested before use and must never be overinflated.

STENTS

An endovascular **stent** is a tubular mesh implant that fits against the wall of an artery. The stent thus provides a physical barrier between the atherosclerotic plaque and the vessel lumen. It also holds the vessel open so that blood can flow freely without platelet aggregation. Stents are made of stainless steel, titanium, or a metal alloy called Nitinol.

Stents are implanted permanently. Two common types of stents are the balloon stent and the self-expanding mesh stent. The balloon stent is a fine catheter with a balloon tip. The stent is fixed over the balloon, and when the balloon is expanded, the stent is pushed into position against the vessel wall. The self-expanding stent opens to provide a similar effect.

VESSEL RETRACTION

During vascular surgery, blood vessels are mobilized and positioned for incision and entry. Retraction is performed with a **vessel loop.** Several types of loops are available. The most common is a thin length of Silastic material, which is carried around the vessel with a right-angle clamp. The ends of the vessel loop are clamped together with a hemostat. An *umbilical tape* (18 inches [45 cm] by ⅛- or ¼-inch [0.3 or 0.6 cm] flat, mesh cotton) Umbilical tapes are available prepackaged for use as vessel loops. A vessel loop may also be used to occlude a blood vessel by acting as a tourniquet. In this case, the ends of the vessel loop are threaded through a 0.25 mm length of Silastic tubing (called a **bolster**). The ends of the loop are pulled taught through the bolster which tightens the loop around the blood vessel. When a bolster is used, the scrub threads the loop through the bolster and passes it on a right-angle clamp along with a hemostat to secure the ends. A Rummel tourniquet is a longer bolster (Figure 31-11).

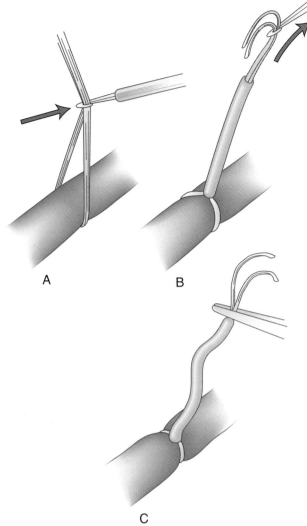

A

B

C

Figure 31-11 Application of a vessel loop (Rummel tourniquet). The two ends of the umbilical tape are grasped and threaded through the tubing. *(From Ouriel K, Rutherford R: Atlas of vascular surgery: operative procedures, Philadelphia, 1998, WB Saunders.)*

DRUGS

Vascular surgery requires a number of important and potentially harmful intraoperative drugs. Safety protocols for the distribution of drugs and proper labeling must be followed. (These protocols are discussed in detail in Chapter 14.) Specific drugs are used to prevent blood from clotting at the operative site (anticoagulation) or to encourage clotting (coagulation).

Anticoagulation

During vascular surgery, heparinized saline solution (usually 1:100) is used to prevent coagulation in the area of the operative vessels. This prevents thrombi from forming at the surgical site and reduces the risk of embolus. Systemic heparin may be administered just before arterectomy (incision into the operative artery) begins. Heparinized saline is prepared by the scrubbed surgical technologist. He or she receives both heparin

and injectable saline, which are mixed in ratio according to the surgeon's orders. For use on the field, the solution is drawn up with a 20- or 30-cc syringe fitted with a tapered irrigation tip. Systemic heparin is reversed with protamine sulfate, which is administered by the anesthesia care provider.

Coagulation

Hemostasis is maintained at anastomosis sites with collagen or fibrin products, such as microfibrillar collagen hemostat (Gelfoam, Avitene) or topical thrombin. Topical thrombin is a dry powder that is reconstituted with saline. Topical hemostatic collagen materials are used on anastomosis sites and capillary beds. Small squares (1 cm) of Gelfoam often are soaked in topical thrombin before use. Surgicel also may be placed on the site of the anastomosis.

> ❖ *Because both thrombin and heparin are distributed to the scrub, there is a risk that the wrong drug may be offered to the surgeon. It is critically important that all medications on the field be clearly marked as soon as they are received. Intravenous administration of thrombin can cause a fatal embolus.*

TECHNIQUES IN VASCULAR SURGERY

ENDARTERECTOMY

Many vascular procedures require removal of atherosclerotic plaque from the inside of the artery (**endarterectomy**). Plaque is a rubbery substance that adheres to the tunica intima, causing stenosis or occlusion. When the surgeon removes plaque, there is a risk it will break apart, causing an embolus when clamps are removed to test blood flow. Endarterectomy requires meticulous technique and fine instruments. Plaque can be removed in one piece (Figure 31-12). The surgeon may use a Penfield or Freer elevator to separate the plaque from the intima while applying gentle traction. An alternative technique is to open the artery at its bifurcation and remove the plaque circumferentially.

VESSEL ANASTOMOSIS

Longitudinal incisions in the blood vessel are closed with a double-arm suture. Traction sutures may be placed at one or both ends of the incision. Circumferential incisions (in an anastomosis) are closed with a double-arm suture (Figures 31-13 to 31-15).

Graft Tunneling

Vascular grafts often must be tunneled through subcutaneous tissue or other layers to connect one vessel to another. Two techniques are used. The surgeon may use the fingers to separate the tissue digitally, or a graft tunneler (discussed previously) can be used. The tunneler is a long metal shaft with bunt tips that is pushed manually through the tissue. As the tunneler is advanced, it leaves a tubular space through which the graft can be threaded. The surgeon usually performs this

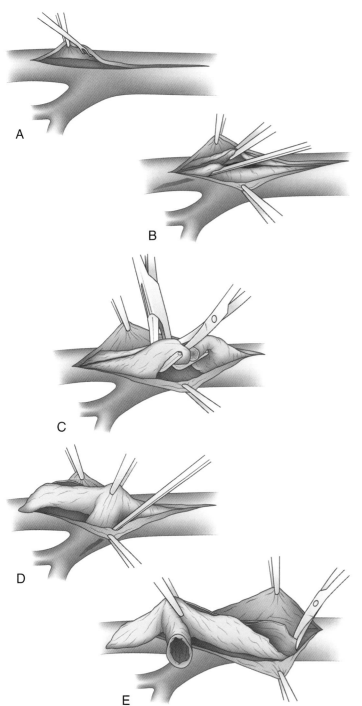

Figure 31-12   Endarterectomy technique. **A,** An arteriotomy is made. **B,** A plane is created between the vessel wall and plaque. **C,** The plaque is divided over a right-angle clamp. **D,** The plaque is mobilized distally. **E,** The proximal end of the plaque is trimmed. *(From Ouriel K, Rutherford R: Atlas of vascular surgery: operative procedures, Philadelphia, 1998, WB Saunders.)*

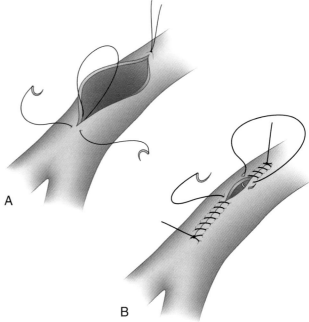

Figure 31-13   Suturing technique for closing a longitudinal arteriotomy. **A,** Double-arm suture is placed at each end. **B,** Continuous sutures are placed to provide a sealed closure. *(From Ouriel K, Rutherford R: Atlas of vascular surgery: basic techniques and exposures, Philadelphia, 1993, WB Saunders.)*

SURGICAL PROCEDURES

INTRAOPERATIVE ANGIOGRAPHY

Surgical Goal

Preoperative angiography (arteriography) is the injection of a contrast medium into a selected artery and its branches to determine the exact location of strictures, occlusion, or malformation. During surgery, intraoperative angiography is used in conjunction with angioplasty to allow the surgeon to see the position of the stricture and to place the catheter in the correct location.

Technique

1. All team members must wear a lead apron during a procedure involving radiography.
2. The circulator distributes the contrast medium to the scrub.
3. The scrub prepares the contrast medium and sterile saline.
4. The operative site is prepared for radiographs or C-arm fluoroscopy.
5. Metal instruments are removed from the field, and the operative site is covered with a sterile drape.
6. The surgeon injects the contrast medium into the artery, and images are recorded during injection.
7. The contrast medium is flushed from the artery with sterile saline.

Discussion

Intraoperative angiography is performed with intravascular ultrasound and other imaging techniques because it allows the

step by inserting a long clamp (e.g., a Péan clamp) into the tunnel and grasping the graft from the entry site. If the tunnel is short, the surgeon can pass it easily. Longer grafts may require an intermediate incision in the skin and subcutaneous tissue.

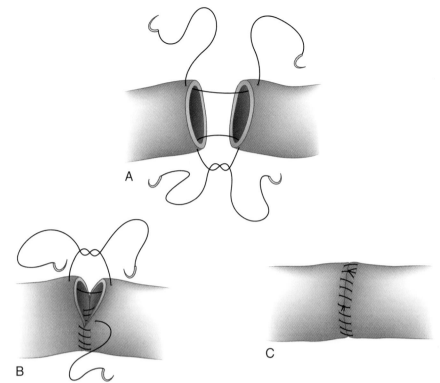

Figure 31-14   End-to-end anastomosis. **A,** Two double-arm sutures are placed in opposite locations. **B,** Continuous sutures are placed circumferentially. **C,** Completed closure. *(From Ouriel K, Rutherford R: Atlas of vascular surgery: basic techniques and exposures, Philadelphia, 1993, WB Saunders.)*

surgeon to see obstructions or emboli distal and proximal to the operative area.

In this procedure, the contrast medium is injected directly into the operative artery, and its branches and outline, as well as the interior configuration of the vessel, are observed on radiographs or fluoroscopy. The contrast medium is flushed through the vessel with sterile saline at the completion of the procedure. Repeat injections and data recording may be required to clarify an image.

Whenever angiography is planned, all personnel must wear a lead shield over their scrub attire. The equipment needed for intraoperative angiography includes:
- Two or more 30- or 50-cc syringes
- A contrast medium, as specified by the surgeon
- An arterial needle
- One or two vinyl catheters with a stopcock attached
- An intravenous (IV) catheter for injection of the contrast medium
- Sterile IV saline

The circulator distributes the contrast medium to the scrub, who draws it up into two syringes. A solution of 60% Renografin usually is used. A third syringe of IV saline is prepared to flush the contrast medium from the arteries when radiographs have been completed. The scrub attaches one end of the angiography needle to a short length of vinyl tubing and the other end to a syringe of dye. All air bubbles must be removed from the tubing to ensure that air is not introduced

into the artery. A Kelly or Mayo hemostat is placed across the tubing to prevent air from backing into it. If a stopcock is used, air bubbles are flushed out and the stopcock is secured in the closed position.

The surgeon may choose one of several techniques to inject the contrast medium:
- If the **arteriotomy** (incision in the artery) has already been sutured closed, an angiography needle is inserted between the sutures.
- A catheter can be inserted into the vessel and secured with a suture tie.

If standard radiographs are to be taken, the scrub uses sterile technique to receive the cassette in a cassette pouch. A deep fold is made in the edge of the cover, making a wide sterile cuff. After the cassette has been dropped inside, the edges of the pouch are turned up and secured. The cassette is placed under the limb, the radiography machine is positioned, and films are taken. The cassette and cover are removed from the field. If C-arm fluoroscopy is used, the C-arm is draped and images are observed during injection. The artery and branches are immediately flushed with saline.

TRANSLUMINAL ANGIOPLASTY

Transluminal angioplasty is the insertion of an arterial catheter or stent into an artery to establish patency and normal blood flow.

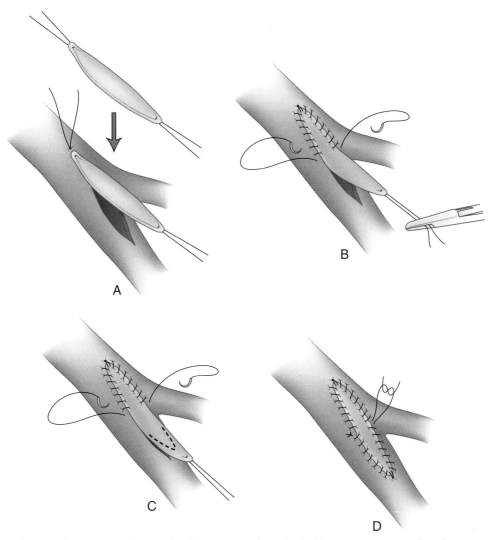

Figure 31-15 Technique for placing a patch graft. **A,** Traction sutures are placed at each end of the graft. **B,** Sutures are applied at both sides of the graft. **C,** The graft may be trimmed as needed *(dotted line)*. **D,** Completed graft. *(From Ouriel K, Rutherford R: Atlas of vascular surgery: basic techniques and exposures, Philadelphia, 1993, WB Saunders.)*

Pathology

Atherosclerosis is an obstructive arterial disease that causes stiffening and loss of elasticity of the artery wall. In peripheral atherosclerosis, fatty plaque and calcium are deposited on the tunica intima, causing stenosis and loss of circulation. Areas of plaque are most dense near arterial bifurcations. Circulatory obstruction in the lower limbs leads to intermittent **claudication** (severe pain related to obstructed arterial flow) and ischemia. Dry gangrene may develop in untreated severe obstruction.

Discussion

Angioplasty is performed during angiography with C-arm fluoroscopy. The contrast medium is injected to verify correct placement of the stent, embolectomy catheter, or intravascular shaving device. **Percutaneous angioplasty** is performed in interventional radiology.

Balloon Angioplasty

In balloon angioplasty, a stricture in the artery is expanded with a balloon catheter that has been inserted to the level of the plaque. The inflated balloon pushes the plaque against the vessel wall and releases the stricture. Angioplasty balloons are available in graduated lengths and widths.

Before the balloon angioplasty is performed, the contrast medium is injected into the artery, and the area of stricture is marked on films produced by the data recorder. The balloon catheter is inserted into the artery to the level of the stricture. The catheter is left in place at a specific pressure and for a specific length of time. The balloon catheter is filled with contrast medium, and both the vessel walls and catheter balloon are observed on fluoroscopy. The catheter is withdrawn, and final angiography films are taken.

Stent

For implantation of the balloon stent, the patient is placed in the supine position and a large-bore needle is inserted into the vessel distal to the stenting site. A flexible guide wire is passed over the needle, which is withdrawn, and the angioplasty balloon catheter is inserted and filled using a syringe. The stent is discharged, and the catheter is removed. A common type of balloon expandable stent is the Palmaz stent. The self-expanding stent is placed in the same manner except that the stent is preloaded into a delivery system that is passed over the guide wire. When the stent is discharged, it opens and adheres to the lumen wall. The Wallstent is a commonly used self-expanding stent. Figure 31-16 illustrates percutaneous transluminal angioplasty.

INSERTION OF A VENA CAVA FILTER

Surgical Goal

A vena cava filter is a metal, umbrella-shaped filter inserted into the inferior vena cava to prevent emboli from entering the pulmonary system. The filter can be temporary or permanent.

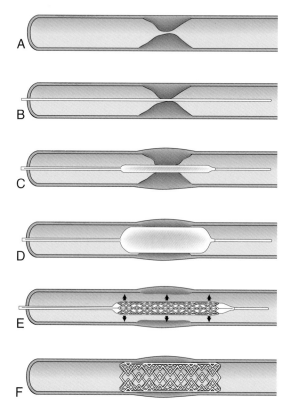

Figure 31-16   Percutaneous transluminal angioplasty (PTA). **A,** Stenosis of the artery. **B,** Insertion of a guidewire. **C,** A balloon catheter is inserted over the guide wire. **D,** The balloon is inflated. **E,** A mesh stent is inserted over the guidewire. **F,** The stent is inflated, and the guidewire is removed. *(From Garden O, Bradbury A, Forsythe J, Parks R: Principles and practice of surgery, ed 5, Edinburgh, 2007, Churchill Livingstone/Elsevier.)*

Pathology

Pulmonary emboli occur when one or more thrombi move from the venous system into the pulmonary vascular system. The vena cava filter is a method of capturing and preventing further movement of emboli. Candidates for the surgery include the following:

- Patients who have a venous thrombus but cannot tolerate anticoagulant therapy; these include patients who have had recent surgery or have a history of hemorrhagic stroke
- Patients who have had a massive pulmonary embolism and survived but for whom a subsequent embolism would be fatal.
- Patients with chronic or venous thromboemboli in spite of anticoagulant therapy.
- Patients at high risk for pulmonary embolism

Technique

1. An incision is made in the groin, and a guide wire is inserted.
2. The filter and introducer are inserted over the guide wire under fluoroscopy.
3. The filter is deployed from the introducer, and the introducer is withdrawn.
4. The position of the filter is verified.
5. A pressure dressing is applied to the insertion site.

Discussion

Insertion of a vena cava filter is commonly performed in the radiology department under fluoroscopy. New filter devices can be inserted at the patient's bedside in the intensive care unit (ICU).

The vena cava filter is inserted by percutaneous needle insertion. The procedure requires a guide wire and filter introducer. The guide wire is a fine, flexible wire coated with a chemical (e.g., polytetrafluorethylene [PTFE]), which prevents platelet aggregation and allows the wire to slide easily through the vessel. The filter itself, which resembles an umbrella without fabric, is made of titanium, stainless steel, or Nitinol. When the filter is deployed, it opens out to the edges of the vessel (Figure 31-17).

All personnel working in interventional radiology wear lead aprons over their scrub attire.

The patient is placed in the supine position on the fluoroscopy or radiology table. The groin is prepped with Betadine solution, and the area is draped in the usual manner. Local anesthesia with or without sedation is administered.

The surgeon or radiologist begins the procedure by inserting a large-bore needle into the femoral artery. A guide wire is inserted through the needle, and the needle is withdrawn. With the aid of fluoroscopy, the introducer is passed over the guide wire, and the filter is ejected from the tip. The introducer and guide wire are withdrawn, and pressure is applied to the puncture site for 10 to 15 minutes. A pressure dressing is placed over the site. The patient must remain in the flat supine position for at least 4 hours after the procedure to prevent postoperative hemorrhage.

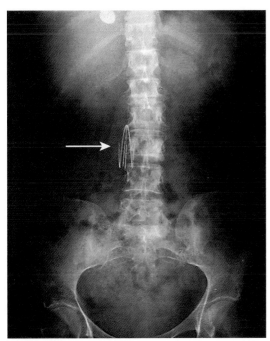

Figure 31-17   Radiograph showing the position of a vena cava filter inserted to prevent emboli. *(From Garden O, Bradbury A, Forsythe J, Parks R: Principles and practice of surgery, ed 5, Edinburgh, 2007, Churchill Livingstone/Elsevier.)*

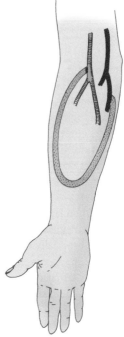

Figure 31-18   Arteriovenous shunt. A graft is implanted to form an anastomosis between the arterial and venous circulations. In this technique, the brachiocephalic vein and radial artery have been used. An alternative technique is direct anastomosis between the artery and vein. *(From Wilson SE: Vascular access: principles and practice, ed 3, St Louis, 1996, Mosby.)*

VASCULAR ACCESS FOR RENAL HEMODIALYSIS

Surgical Goal

Patients with severe or end-stage renal disease require frequent hemodialysis. This treatment requires long-term access to the patient's vascular system. An anastomosis between the arterial and venous systems is created surgically to produce this access. Two techniques usually are used to create vascular access: an arteriovenous shunt or an arteriovenous fistula.

Pathology

End-stage and severe renal disease results in severe electrolyte imbalance and uremia (nitrogenous wastes in the blood). When the kidneys' filtering ability drops below 5%, hemodialysis is necessary for survival. During **extracorporeal hemodialysis,** the patient's blood is shunted outside the body through an artery. The blood is pumped through a series of filters to remove the waste products and excess electrolytes that normally would be filtered by the kidneys. The blood then is returned to the body through a vein.

Discussion

Arteriovenous Shunt: Arm

The patient is placed in the supine position with the arm extended on a large arm board. The arm is prepped and draped free. A local anesthetic usually is administered.

A skin incision is made over the cephalic vein and carried through the fascial layer with a curved hemostat and tenotomy or other plastic surgery scissors. Two small vessel loops are placed around the vein, and the ends are clamped with

mosquito hemostats. A small bulldog or similar vascular clamp is placed over the proximal end of the vessel. The distal end is divided and ligated with silk or polypropylene suture. This technique is repeated on the artery. A graft tunneler may be used to bring the graft in close approximation to both vessels. The graft is sutured in place with 6-0 or 7-0 polypropylene suture. The incisions are closed in layers and dressed with dry gauze. The completed graft is shown in Figure 31-18.

Arteriovenous Fistula

An **arteriovenous (AV) fistula** is a direct anastomosis between an artery and a vein. The site is selected for patency and accessibility. After routine prep and draping of the area, an incision is made over the vessels. The vessels are mobilized with sharp dissection and anastomosed as for an arteriovenous shunt. The wound is closed in layers.

Postoperative Considerations

Several months may be required for complete recovery of the AV fistula before it can be used for dialysis. Postoperative complications include infection and thrombosis.

THROMBECTOMY (OPEN PROCEDURE)

Surgical Goal

The goal of thrombectomy is to remove a stationary clot in a blood vessel. This restores circulation and prevents emboli.

Thrombectomy is commonly performed with an embolectomy catheter.

Pathology

A **thrombus** is a stationary clot in the arterial or venous system. A thrombus that breaks away from the vessel wall is called an **embolus.** As an embolus travels through increasingly smaller vessels of the vascular system, it may lodge in the heart, brain, kidney, mesentery, or other vital organ. This causes vascular obstruction **(infarction),** leading to tissue death. Thrombectomy therefore can be a life-saving procedure. Common causes of thrombi are:

- Atherosclerosis
- Surgery, especially when large blood vessels are exposed to air and clots form at the surgical site
- Orthopedic trauma, especially of the hip or other large bone

Pulmonary emboli (those that lodge in the lung) usually originate from the venous system of the lower extremities.

Technique

1. The surgeon exposes and mobilizes the target vessel.
2. Vessel loops are placed around the artery.
3. The vessel is clamped.
4. An incision is made into the artery (arteriotomy).
5. The embolectomy catheter is threaded into the arteriotomy past the thrombus.
6. The balloon is inflated, and the catheter is retracted slowly, pulling the thrombus through the arteriotomy.
7. Intraoperative Doppler duplex ultrasonography may be performed.
8. The arteriotomy is closed.
9. The wound is closed.

Discussion

Patient preparation depends on the location of the thrombus as determined by angiograms, duplex Doppler ultrasonography, and magnetic resonance imaging (MRI). Thrombi from the lower extremities often are removed from the groin. Mesenteric thrombi require an abdominal approach (laparotomy). The following discussion presents the techniques of thrombectomy, beginning with isolation of the vessel and use of the embolectomy catheter. Surgical incisions and closures are found in chapters associated with a particular anatomical area.

The patient is placed in the supine position for abdominal, lower extremity, and upper extremity surgery. A general or regional anesthetic is used. The surgical site is prepped in normal fashion.

The scrub should have heparinized saline, vessel irrigation tips, vascular sutures, ties, and hemostatic agents available. A variety of vascular clamps matched to the size of the vessel (or the surgeon's preference) also should be available on the instrument table. Small-bore suction and larger atraumatic suction tips are needed. Vascular forceps are used throughout the procedure. Catheters should not be opened until the surgeon requests the size and type needed.

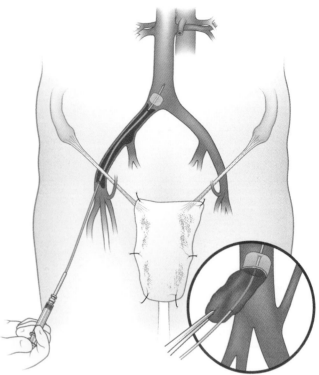

Figure 31-19 A thrombectomy catheter is inserted through a femoral venotomy and advanced past the thrombus. The balloon is inflated, and the catheter is carefully withdrawn, pulling the thrombus with it. *(From Ouriel K, Rutherford R: Atlas of vascular surgery: operative procedures, Philadelphia, 1998, WB Saunders.)*

After surgical exposure of the target vessel, the surgeon places several vessel loops around the vessel and its nearby tributaries. This allows manipulation of the vessel and traction as needed.

To perform the embolectomy, the surgeon clamps the vessel distal to the thrombus. A vascular clamp is selected to fit the configuration of the vessel and its position in the wound. An arteriotomy is made with a #11 scalpel blade. Suction is applied at the arteriotomy site.

The prepared embolectomy catheter is carefully threaded into the vessel past the site of the thrombus. The balloon is inflated, and the catheter is withdrawn (Figure 31-19). This pulls the thrombus back through the vessel. Angioscopy and angiography may be performed to ensure that the procedure was successful. The removed thrombus should be retained as a specimen.

The arteriotomy is closed with 6-0 or 7-0 nonabsorbable vascular suture. The wound is closed in layers according to the incision site.

CAROTID ENDARTERECTOMY

Surgical Goal

Carotid endarterectomy is the surgical removal of atherosclerotic plaque from the carotid artery. Plaque is removed through an open incision in the artery. This re-establishes the flow of oxygenated blood to the brain.

Pathology

Partial obstruction of the carotid artery forms at the bifurcation of the common carotid artery with the internal and external carotid branches. The obstruction causes restricted arterial blood flow to the brain, which may result in neurological symptoms resulting from transient ischemic stroke and high risk for major stroke. Patients with complete blockage of the carotid artery are generally not considered for carotic endarterectomy.

Technique

1. An incision is made along the anterior border of the sterno-cleidomastoid muscle and carried to deep tissue.
2. The common, external, and internal carotid arteries are mobilized and controlled with vessel loops.
3. The internal, common, and external carotid arteries are clamped.
4. The electroencephalogram is monitored.
5. An arteriotomy is made into the common carotid artery and extended upward.
6. An intraluminal shunt may be put in place to provide continuous cerebral blood flow.
7. Atherosclerotic plaque is dissected from the vessel wall.
8. A graft may be sutured over the arteriotomy, or the incision may be closed.
9. The graft is checked for leaks, and extra sutures are placed as needed.
10. All bleeders are controlled with the electrosurgical unit (ESU).
11. The wound is closed in layers.

Discussion

During carotid endarterectomy, the surgeon will temporarily occlude the carotid arteries while removing plaque. This is a critical phase in the procedure, because blood flow to the brain is severely compromised. The instruments and Mayo table must be kept neat and organized to ensure maximum efficiency during the procedure. All essential instruments, catheters, and vascular clamps must be prepared and in view. Attention to the surgical wound is important throughout the procedure.

Carotid endarterectomy may be performed using either a general or regional anesthesia. When a regional anesthetic is used, the patient will respond to simple neurological tests, such as hand strength tests or speaking. An **electroencephalogram (EEG)** commonly is used to measure the brain's electrical activity during the procedure. Electrical activity is affected by oxygen supply to the tissue, a critical component of carotid surgery.

The patient is placed in the supine position, and the head is turned away from the affected side. A small pad may be placed under the shoulders to hyperextend the neck. If EEG monitoring will be used, electrodes are placed. The skin prep extends from the face to the axillary line. Draping is similar to that for thyroidectomy.

The surgeon begins the procedure by incising the neck along the anterior border of the sternocleidomastoid muscle. The incision is carried deeper with the vascular forceps, elec-

trosurgical unit (ESU), Metzenbaum scissors, and sponge dissectors to the level of the common, internal, and external carotid arteries. The scrub should have a variety of retractors available, including two dull Weitlaners, dull rakes, and Army-Navy retractors. The rake retractors should have dull rather than sharp teeth to prevent trauma to the large vessels that lie nearby.

The common, external, and internal carotid arteries are mobilized with fine vascular tissue forceps and Metzenbaum scissors. The bifurcation itself is not mobilized fully. Vessel loops are placed around each of the three arteries. Small hemostats are used to clamps the ends of the loops. Small sections of tubing or Rumel tourniquets also may be placed around the loops for control.

Before the surgeon makes the arterial incision, the anesthesia care provider administers systemic heparin to the patient. This prevents clotting and reduces the risk of emboli. The carotid sinus may be injected with 1% lidocaine to prevent brachycardia and hypotension associated with manipulation with the carotid body.

Before the actual endarterectomy, the scrub should have a number of instruments ready: a #11 scalpel blade, Potts and DeMartel scissors, neurosurgical elevators (Penfield or similar), a Freer elevator, and straight hemostats. Wide-tip atraumatic suction also is needed. The surgeon indicates the preferred vascular clamps.

To begin the endarterectomy, the surgeon clamps the internal, common, and external carotid arteries. The surgeon then notifies the anesthesia care provider and circulator that the arteries have been clamped. The length of time the artery is occluded is timed. The EEG is closely monitored until the clamps are released.

The surgeon makes a small incision into the common carotid artery with the #11 scalpel blade. The incision is extended with Potts or DeMartel scissors. Arterial plaque is identified as a thick, yellow, rubbery material that adheres to the lumen (intimal layer) of the artery.

Internal Shunt Device

To provide continuous blood flow to the cerebrum while plaque is removed, the surgeon may insert a flexible internal shunt into the internal and common carotid arteries. Many types of shunts are available (e.g., *Javid shunt*). The scrub must flush the shunt with heparinized saline before passing it to the surgeon. Use of a shunt during the procedure is shown in Figure 31-20.

If a shunt is to be used, it is inserted at this point. A shunt ring clamp (called a *Javid clamp*) and vessel tourniquets are used to maneuver and hold the shunt in place. Cross clamps placed on the carotid before the arterectomy These may be released when the shunt is in place.

The surgeon grasps the edge of the plaque with vascular forceps or a straight hemostat and lifts it gently from the intima. Penfield or Freer elevators are used to create a dissection plane between the plaque and the inner lumen. The arterial plaque and lumen of the artery are flushed with heparinized saline during this part of the procedure.

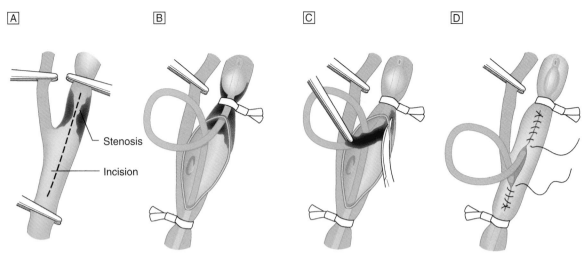

Ⓐ   Ⓑ   Ⓒ   Ⓓ

Stenosis

Incision

Figure 31-20   Use of the Javid shunt during endarterectomy. The arteriotomy is performed, and the shunt is inserted, allowing partial blood flow during the removal of plaque. *(From Garden O, Bradbury A, Forsythe J, Parks R: Principles and practice of surgery, ed 5, Edinburgh, 2007, Churchill Livingstone/Elsevier.)*

After dissection, the plaque is passed to the scrub as a specimen. The arterial lumen is flushed with heparinized saline solution.

The arterial incision is closed with 5-0 or 6-0 cardiovascular sutures, or a patch graft may be put in place at this time. The patch graft is cut to size from a sheet of PTFE or other grafting material.

Before the arteriotomy is closed, the external, internal, and common carotid artery clamps are opened and closed, in that order. This allows any debris to flow out and restores blood flow. At this point, the arteries are clamped.

NOTE: If a shunt has been placed, it is removed just before the arterial incision is completely closed. The ring clamp holding the shunt is released from the internal carotid artery, and the shunt is removed. The arterial clamps are removed sequentially (e.g., external, common, and internal).

When the arteriotomy has been closed, the surgeon removes the clamps from the external, common, and finally the internal carotid arteries.

The suture line is observed for leaks and blood flow tested with confirmed with Doppler. Any leaks are repaired with additional sutures and controlled with topical hemostatic agents. Protomine sulfate is administered to reverse the effects of systemic heparin.

Angiograms may be taken at this time to check the patency of the vessel superior to the surgical site. Doppler and intravascular ultrasound also may be used. All bleeders are controlled with the ESU, and the neck incision is irrigated with warm saline. The deep layers of the arterial incision are closed with 3-0 synthetic absorbable sutures. The skin is closed with 4-0 nylon or other synthetic, nonabsorbable material. The wound is covered with a gauze dressing. The procedure for carotid endarterectomy is shown in Figure 31-21.

Postoperative Considerations

Patients may be taken to the neurosurgical ICU after the procedure and observed closely for neurological deficit, hemorrhage, and respiratory complications. Damage to the carotid body, a structure between the external and internal carotid arteries, may result in disruption of the body's hypoxic drive to breathe. Alterations in cerebral perfusion may cause neurological deficit.

ABDOMINAL AORTIC ANEURYSM

Surgical Goal

An abdominal aortic **aneurysm** is a condition in which a section of the abdominal aorta becomes thin and bulges because of atherosclerotic plaque and progressive weakening of the aortic wall. The surgical goal is to implant a graft extending from the aorta to both iliac arteries. This restores circulation to the lower extremities and pelvis.

Pathology

Aortic aneurysms can occur at any location in the artery. However, they usually occur just below the renal arteries and extend to the bifurcation of the common iliac arteries or just above it. If the disease remains undiagnosed, the walls of the aorta become increasingly stretched and finally rupture. This usually results in death. A dissecting aneurysm is one in which blood seeps between the layers of the vessel, causing it to tear and split. Atherosclerosis and degeneration of the muscular layer of the vessel are the most common causes of aortic aneurysm. Although the aneurysm may not extend into the iliac arteries, a bifurcated graft often is used in the repair.

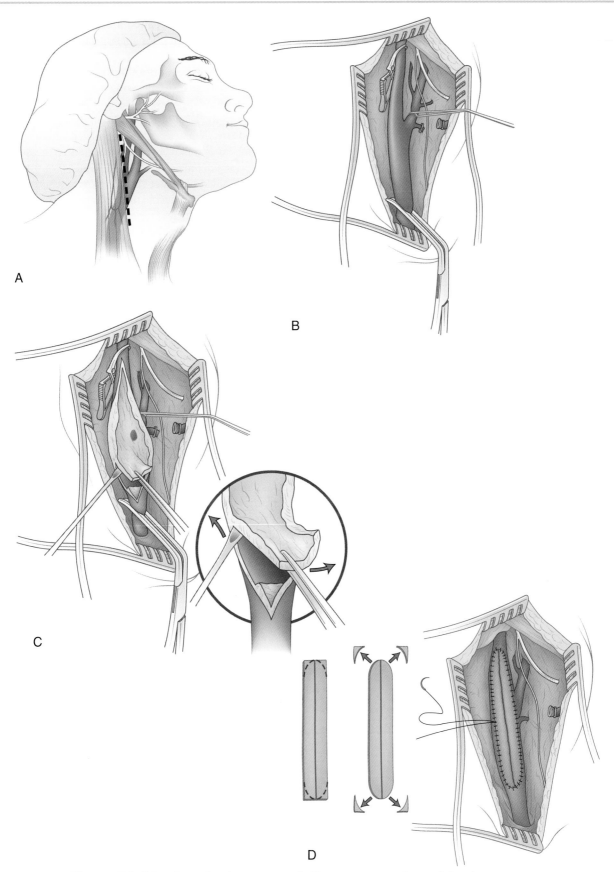

Figure 31-21 Carotid endarterectomy. **A,** The incision is made parallel to the sternocleidomastoid muscle. **B,** The internal jugular vein is mobilized, and the carotid vessels are exposed. **C,** An arteriotomy is performed, and plaque is extracted from the vessel. **D,** Closure with a patch graft. *(From Ouriel K, Rutherford R: Atlas of vascular surgery: operative procedures, Philadelphia, 1998, WB Saunders.)*

Technique

1. The surgeon performs a laparotomy through a midline incision extending from the xiphoid to the pubis.
2. The retroperitoneal space is entered.
3. The abdominal aorta is partly dissected.
4. The renal vein may be ligated for access to the perirenal aorta.
5. The aorta is cross-clamped.
6. The aneurysm is incised and opened.
7. Blood clots and plaque are removed from the aneurysm sac.
8. A graft is implanted in the aorta above the proximal end of the aneurysm, extending to the bifurcation of the iliac arteries.
9. Angiograms are taken.
10. The retroperitoneal space is closed.
11. The abdomen is closed as a single layer with polydioxanone surgical (PDS) suture or in multiple tissue layers.

Discussion

Repair of an aortic aneurysm may be scheduled (elective) or an emergency procedure. If the procedure is an emergency, recall that the most important stages of the surgery are exposure of or access to the target tissue, adequate visualization of the trauma site, immediate control of hemorrhage, and rapid repair or restoration of circulation.

The scrub should have long instruments immediately available because the target site is anterior to the posterior body wall or retroperitoneum. Right-angle clamps, the surgeon's choice of vascular clamps, abdominal suction tips, and an ESU are needed. A long Penrose drain and vascular loops also should be available for vessel retraction. Because of the depth of the wound, deep handheld retractors (e.g., a Deaver retractor) or a self-retaining retractor (e.g., a Thompson or Bookwalter retractor) with multiple attachments may be required. Grafts should be available but not opened until the surgeon has prepared the vessels. A blood-recovery system, such as the Cell Saver or Haemonetics system, usually is used in emergency surgery.

The patient is placed in the supine position, prepped, and draped for a midline incision extending from the xiphoid to the pubis. A Foley catheter is inserted before the skin prep.

The surgeon enters the abdomen through a long midline incision. Many moist laparotomy sponges are used to preserve tissue viability during the procedure. If the intestines must be brought out of the abdominal cavity, a plastic pouch may be used to keep them moist. Long vessel loops should be prepared at this time. Each should be tagged with a hemostat. Right-angle clamps are used to pass the loop under the vessels.

Retractors are placed, and the retroperitoneum is incised with a #10 blade mounted on a long scalpel handle. Using blunt and sharp dissection vascular forceps, the surgeon exposes the aorta and places a vessel loop around it.

Occasionally the left renal vein must be clamped and ligated to provide access to the perirenal aorta. (This does not usually have a long-term effect on the kidney, because collateral circulation is sufficient.) Using finger dissection and sponge dissectors, the surgeon frees the upper end of the aorta. There is a risk of damaging the vena cava at this stage.

If damage occurs, it is repaired immediately with 4-0 or 5-0 vascular suture. The inferior mesenteric artery are clamped, ligated, and divided.

Dissection continues until the aorta is freed from the vertebral column. If excessive bleeding occurs, pressure is applied with laparotomy sponges. Dissection of the distal aorta is performed to the level of the common iliac arteries for complete exposure. The arteries are mobilized carefully by blunt dissection. The lumbar arteries, which enter the aorta from the posterior side, may be occluded with 4-0 or 5-0 polypropylene or braided polyester sutures. When dissection is complete, the surgeon can decide the type and size of graft needed for the repair. If the iliac arteries are also disease (aneurysmal) the internal and external arteries are mobilized in order to provide space for cross clamping.

The aneurysm is prepared for opening. If a risk of excessive bleeding exists in spite cross-clamps on the aorta, a Foley catheter with a 30-mL balloon may be prepared for use as an intraluminal tamponade in the aorta. In any event, the scrub should be prepared for excessive bleeding when the aneurysm is opened. Extra aortic clamps, suction, and mounted sutures should be prepared. A basin is used to collect large clots and debris.

Before opening the aneurysm sac the patient is heparinized and the common iliac arteries are clamped using DeBakey or similar right-angle vascular clamps. The proximal aorta is then cross clamped using a Crafoord coarctation forceps, Satinsky clamp, Potts, or Cooley clamp is placed across the aorta to occlude. Some surgeons place the distal clamps first to prevent the flow of thrombi into the renal arteries. However, this is not a rigid practice and the proximal clamp may also be placed first.

The surgeon uses a #15 blade or the ESU to make a longitudinal incision into the aneurysm sac, leaving the anterior surface of the aorta and aneurysm intact. Any blood clots and debris are scooped out. The plaque is grasped with vascular forceps and gently separated from the wall of the aorta. The scrub should keep the basin on the field to collect the specimens. Any bleeding from the lumbar arteries can be repaired with polypropylene sutures. Bleeding from the IMA may require clamping or ligation with a vessel loop.

Each artery is opened, and the proximal ends are irrigated with heparinized saline. The bifurcated graft is trimmed and distal limbs anastomosed with 3-0 or 4-0 polypropylene suture. If only a straight graft is required (e.g., in the case of healthy iliac arteries). The aneurysm sac is approximated over the graft using size 3-0 polypropylene vascular suture. The surgeon checks the graft for leaks by slowly releasing the clamps. Additional sutures may be required. Hemostatic agents may be applied to the suture lines until all bleeding has been controlled. Angiograms and ultrasound are used to verify patency of the vessels.

The wound is irrigated with saline solution. The retroperitoneum is closed with a running suture of 2-0 or 3-0 absorbable suture. The abdominal contents are replaced, and the abdominal wound is irrigated before closure. A single-layer closure of polydioxanone surgical (PDS) suture may be used, or the abdomen can be closed in layers. Figure 31-22 presents the details of this procedure.

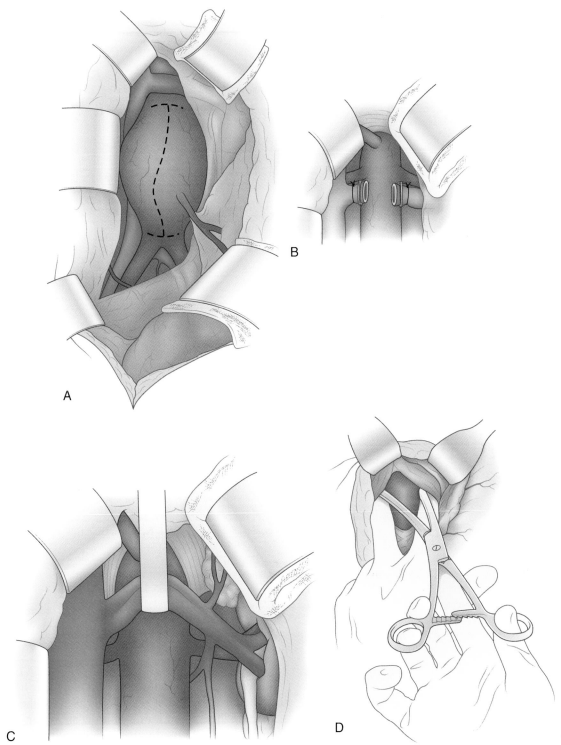

Figure 31-22 Abdominal aortic aneurysm with graft insertion. **A,** The retroperitoneum is incised over the aneurysm. **B,** The left renal vein can be safely divided to gain additional exposure. **C,** Alternatively, a narrow retractor can be used to provide exposure. **D,** The aorta is cross-clamped. *(From Ouriel K, Rutherford R: Atlas of vascular surgery: operative procedures, Philadelphia, 1998, WB Saunders.)*

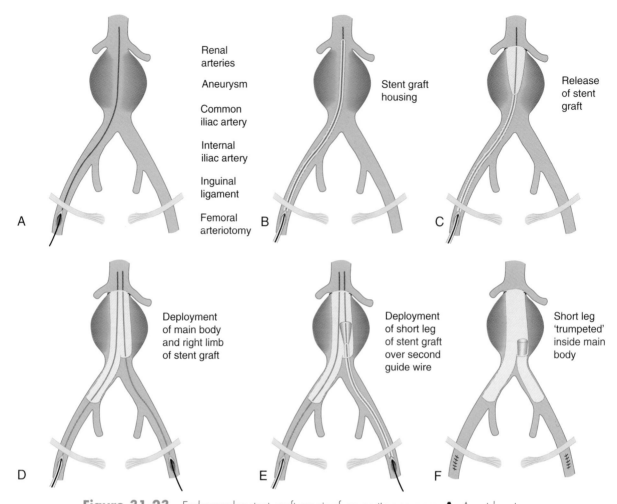

Renal arteries

Aneurysm

Common iliac artery

Internal iliac artery

Inguinal ligament

Femoral arteriotomy

Stent graft housing

Release of stent graft

Deployment of main body and right limb of stent graft

Deployment of short leg of stent graft over second guide wire

Short leg 'trumpeted' inside main body

A   B   C   D   E   F

Figure 31-23 Endovascular stent graft repair of an aortic aneurysm. **A,** A guide wire is passed through the aneurysm through the right common femoral artery. **B,** A catheter containing the stent graft is passed over the guide wire and into position in the aneurysm. **C,** The outer cover of the catheter is removed, allowing the proximal end to remain open. **D,** The rest of the graft is removed, allowing deployment of the main body and right limb of the sent graft in the common iliac artery. **E,** A second guide wire is passed through the short limb of the stent graft. **F,** Deployment is complete, and the aneurysm sac is excluded from the circulation. *(From Garden O, Bradbury A, Forsythe J, Parks R: Principles and practice of surgery, ed 5, Edinburgh, 2007, Churchill Livingstone/Elsevier.)*

Endovascular Approach (Endovascular Abdominal Aneurysm Repair)

In endovascular abdominal aneurysm repair (EVAR), the aortic aneurysm is approached through the femoral artery. A multi-sectional stent is introduced into the aorta through the femoral artery under fluoroscopy. Because the graft is expandable, once it is implanted, the vessel can be straightened to some degree, reducing the risk of rupture (Figure 31-23). The long-term effectiveness of the EVAR procedure is under statistical review. Short-term results have been favorable.

Discussion

During the procedure, correct placement of the stent graft is verified with a variety of catheters and guide wire systems. The devices used are based on the surgeon's experience and prefer-

ences. Each manufacturer of a stent system has a specific design and method of stent deployment. At the time of this writing there are at least four different systems in use. Sectional stents are used in order to accommodate anatomical variations of the aneurysm. Commonly used systems are based on multiple components and three main operative objectives. These are:

- Access to the ileofemoral region
- Placement (deployment) of the main body of the graft stent
- Deployment of the stent limbs. The components of the device are deployed separately, and connect by overlapping "barbs" in the neck of each stent. The devices are made of stainless steel, cobalt-chromium alloy, or nitinol while the grafts are usually polyester or ePTFE (expanded polytetrafluoroethylene). Components include:

1. The main body of the stent graft which is bifurcated (Y shaped).
2. A graft limb (iliac limb)
3. Extensions as needed
4. Cuffs

The patient is positioned on a radiolucent operating table with fluoroscopy available during the procedure. Skin prep and draping are the same as that used for bilateral femoral bypass (see above). Both groins are prepped because the stent is inserted into through one side while the opposite site is used for angiogram access during stent placement.

A femoral artery on the side of the stent insertion (operative side) introduces the stent guide wire through the femoral artery through direct puncture or mobilization and control of the artery in the standard fashion for arterial cutdown. The angiogram catheter is introduced into the opposite femoral artery. The operative guide wire is advanced under fluoroscopic guidance and advances the stent into the aorta. The stent is then positioned and the graft deployed. The graft barbs attach to the aortic wall and help to stabilize its position. The guide wire removed.

The angiogram catheter is now removed and the opposite side iliac limb stent and graft is inserted using a new guide wire under fluoroscopy.

Postoperative Considerations

One of the most common complications (and reasons for failure) of EVAR is endoleak in which blood flows outside the graft and into the aneurysm sac postoperatively. The components of the graft or device can separate at the site of attachment or the sac may enlarge. These complications can be repaired by re-entering the wound and placing additional stents or balloon dilation. In more severe cases, coil embolization or ligating the lumbar and IMA arteries may be necessary.

Abdominal aortic procedures commonly cause fluid shifts, which require continuous observation and treatment for **hemodynamic** abnormalities. The peripheral pulses are carefully monitored and chest radiographs and electrocardiograms are routinely obtained in the postoperative period. Complications include hemorrhage, infection, renal failure, and bowel obstruction.

AORTOFEMORAL BYPASS

Surgical Goal

An aortofemoral bypass is performed to treat aortoiliac occlusive disease. A graft is implanted between the aorta and the femoral arteries to bypasses the iliac arteries and restore circulation (Figure 31-24).

Pathology

The iliac artery is a common site of atherosclerosis. An aortofemoral bypass is performed instead of an endarterectomy or aortoiliac bypass because it produces increased patency and can be performed in patients with extensive calcification of the arteries.

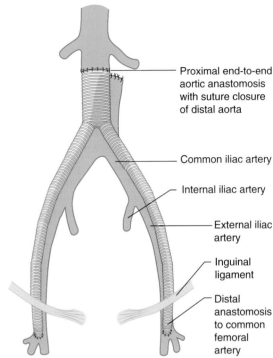

Figure 31-24 Aortofemoral bypass. A graft is implanted between the aorta and the femoral arteries to bypass the iliac arteries and restore circulation. *(From Garden O, Bradbury A, Forsythe J, Parks R: Principles and practice of surgery, ed 5, Edinburgh, 2007, Churchill Livingstone/Elsevier.)*

Labels in figure:
- Proximal end-to-end aortic anastomosis with suture closure of distal aorta
- Common iliac artery
- Internal iliac artery
- External iliac artery
- Inguinal ligament
- Distal anastomosis to common femoral artery

Technique

1. Bilateral groin incisions are made to expose the femoral arteries.
2. A laparotomy is performed through a long midline incision, and the aorta is exposed.
3. The patient is heparinized, and the aorta is clamped below or at the renal arteries.
4. The distal portion of the aorta is oversewn with heavy vascular sutures.
5. The proximal end of a bifurcated graft is anastomosed to the distal aorta.
6. Bilateral subcutaneous tunnels are made in the retroperitoneal tissue.
7. The graft is pulled through the tunnels.
8. Bilateral arteriotomies are made in the femoral arteries, and the graft limbs are anastomosed to each artery.
9. Angiography and ultrasound are used to verify patency.
10. The wound is checked for bleeders and closed in the routine manner.

Discussion

The patient is placed in the supine position. The prep area extends from the axillary line to the midthighs. Both legs are draped circumferentially, and the genitalia are covered with a towel and barrier drape. A Foley catheter is inserted before the skin prep.

The procedure begins with bilateral groin incisions, which are carried deeper to expose the femoral arteries. Dissection is performed with Metzenbaum scissors, sponge dissectors, and the ESU. Weitlaner or Gelpi self-retaining retractors are used superficially, and Richardson retractors are used for deeper hand retraction. After the femoral vessels have been exposed, the incisions may be covered with sterile towels during laparotomy.

A midline abdominal incision is made and carried to the aorta, as described in the previous procedure. The proximal portion of the aorta is dissected to the renal veins.

Heparin is administered to the patient, and the femoral arteries are clamped with right-angle vascular clamps. The inferior mesenteric artery is clamped to prevent an embolus from entering it when the aortic clamp is applied.

The surgeon mobilizes the aorta using blunt dissection and clamps it below the level of the renal arteries. The aorta is divided, and the distal end is oversewn with 2-0 or 3-0 polypropylene sutures. The proximal end of a bifurcated graft is trimmed to fit and anastomosed to the distal aorta with 3-0 polypropylene sutures.

Retroperitoneal tunnels are created in the loose connective tissue of the groin to accommodate the graft limbs. The finger is used to separate the tissue. The two limbs of the graft are pulled through the tunnels and into the femoral wounds. A vascular clamp may be placed across the graft limb to prevent it from twisting.

Suture scissors are used to trim the ends of the graft to a 45-degree angle, rounding the tips. Each limb of the graft is sutured into the femoral artery through an arteriotomy, commonly with 4-0 double-arm polypropylene sutures.

After completion of the anastomoses, the femoral clamps are slowly released. Angiograms and ultrasound scans are performed to verify the patency of the grafts. The wound is irrigated and closed as described in the previous procedure.

Postoperative Considerations

Patients recover in the ICU or the surgical unit. Doppler testing is performed throughout the first 48 hours of postoperative recovery to ensure that the peripheral circulation remains intact. Complications include infection, renal failure, hemorrhage, fluid shift, and respiratory complications.

AXILLOFEMORAL BYPASS

Surgical Goal

An axillofemoral bypass creates circulation between the femoral arteries and the axillary artery. This restores circulation to the lower extremity or, in an emergency procedure, bypasses an infected aortic graft or aneurysm.

Pathology

Circulation to the lower extremities derives from the descending aorta and the iliac and femoral arteries. Atherosclerotic disease of the aortoiliac region results in obstruction of the lower extremities.

Technique

1. A 45-degree incision is made in the subclavicular area on the affected side.
2. The pectoralis major muscle is bluntly divided, and the deep fascia is incised.
3. The pectoralis minor muscle tendon is divided.
4. The axillary artery is mobilized and clamped.
5. A synthetic graft is tunneled through the subcutaneous tissue from the axillary incision to the femorofemoral graft.
6. The axillary artery and tributaries are clamped.
7. The axillary artery is incised, and the proximal end of the graft is anastomosed to the artery.
8. The groin is entered, and the femoral graft is mobilized and controlled.
9. The distal graft is anastomosed to the femorofemoral graft.
10. The incisions are checked for leakage.
11. Angiograms are performed.
12. The wounds are closed in layers and dressed.

Discussion

An important indication for axillofemoral bypass is an infected aortic graft. Perfusion of the leg (i.e., blood flow and oxygen exchange in the leg tissues) can be restored after excision of the graft. Axillofemoral bypass offers an alternative. It avoids the risks of major aortic surgery, but long-term patency of the graft is possible only if outflow from the axillary artery is brisk.

The patient is placed in the supine position. The skin prep includes the affected arm, shoulder, clavicular and neck areas, abdomen, and groin. The arm is placed on a wide arm board and draped as for an upper arm procedure (excluding the hand). The groin is occluded with towels and an adhesive drape. Separate drapes are used to expose the operative area, and both legs may be draped with split sheets or U-drapes. A body sheet or procedure drape is placed on top of the drapes.

Two surgeons may work simultaneously, one at the subclavicular incision and the other at the groin. To begin the procedure, the surgeon makes a 45-degree incision in the subclavicular region. The subcutaneous layer is entered with the ESU, and a rake or retractors are placed at the incision edges. The pectoralis major muscle is divided manually, and the deep fascia is incised. However, the tendon attachment of the pectoralis minor must be severed with the ESU. A deep self-retaining retractor or small Richardson retractors replace the rakes.

The axillary artery is mobilized, and vessel loops are placed around it and nearby tributaries. Small branches are clamped with small bulldog or spring clamps, divided, and ligated.

A graft tunneler is used to make a tunnel in the subcutaneous incision between the upper incision and the groin. If the patient is very tall, an intermediary incision may be necessary.

The groin is entered as previously described, and the femoral artery graft and bifurcation are mobilized. Vessel loops are placed around the graft and controlled with Rummel tourniquets.

The patient is given heparin intravenously, and the axillary artery is clamped. The artery is incised with a #11 scalpel blade, and the anastomosis is performed with 5-0 or 6-0 polypropylene suture.

The distal end of the graft is brought in contact with the femoral graft. The distal tip of the graft is beveled with scissors and anastomosed with 6-0 Gore-Tex sutures. A double-arm suture is commonly used.

Suture lines are checked for leaks, and the heparin is reversed with protamine. An angiogram may be done to ensure patency of the graft. Both wounds are irrigated and closed in layers.

FEMOROFEMORAL BYPASS

Surgical Goal

A femorofemoral bypass involves implantation of a prosthetic graft that connects the femoral artery on the affected side to the opposite femoral artery. This is done to bypass unilateral atherosclerotic disease in the iliac artery.

Pathology

Refer to *Atherosclerosis* in Table 31-1. A femorofemoral bypass is used only when the iliac system on the donor side is free of disease. Iliac disease usually is bilateral, and in such cases, stenting or balloon angioplasty of the donor iliac system may be necessary.

Technique

1. Bilateral groin incisions are made, and the common femoral arteries are isolated.
2. A subcutaneous tunnel is created between the groin incisions.
3. A synthetic graft is pulled through the tunnel and anastomosed to each femoral artery.
4. The wounds are closed.

Discussion

The patient is prepped and draped for bilateral groin incisions. The genitalia are excluded from the prep with towels and an occlusive drape. A Foley catheter may be inserted. A general or regional anesthetic may be used.

The procedure begins with groin incisions, which are made with the scalpel and carried to the deeper layers with sponge dissectors, Metzenbaum scissors, and the ESU. Large bleeders may be clamped and ligated with 3-0 silk suture. The scrub should have right-angle clamps and two or more self-retaining retractors available for the dissection. Army-Navy retractors and small Richardson retractors also may be needed. The groin incision is carried to the level of the common femoral artery, which is isolated with Silastic loops. The iliac artery also may be looped for manipulation. The procedure is repeated on the opposite side.

The surgeon uses the fingers to create a subcutaneous tunnel in the skin between the two incisions. An aortic clamp is used to puncture the fascia attachments at the midline. The surgeon grasps one end of the graft with the curved aortic clamp and pulls it through the tunnel. The graft must be pulled through the tunnel without kinks or twists.

An end-to-side anastomosis is created between the graft and the profunda femoris on each side. Running sutures of 5-0 or 6-0 polypropylene are commonly used to perform the anastomosis. Air is pushed out of the graft, and the vascular clamps are removed. Hemostatic agents are applied to the suture lines. Protamine sulfate may be administered to reverse the effects of systemic heparin. However, this practice is under investigation and current research. When the wound is dry and the suture lines are secured, the wound is closed in layers. A femorofemoral bypass is illustrated in Figure 31-25.

IN SITU SAPHENOUS FEMOROPOPLITEAL BYPASS

Surgical Goal

In situ saphenous vein bypass is a surgical alternative to use of a synthetic graft to bypass a diseased femoral artery. The saphenous vein is not removed but is left in anatomical position. In the technique described here, a continuous incision is made along the entire saphenous vein. This is the safest method and allows complete ligation of tributaries. The distal or narrow end of the vein is anastomosed to the popliteal artery, and the proximal vein is anastomosed to the large end of the femoral artery. The goal is to produce vascular continuity with an autograft.

Technique

1. A single incision or multiple incisions are made on the medial thigh, following the path of the saphenous vein.
2. The branches of the vein are ligated and divided.
3. The proximal and distal ends of the vein are clamped and divided.
4. Internal valves are obliterated with microvascular valve scissors, a valvulotome and angioscope, or a valvulotome alone.
5. The saphenous vein is anastomosed to the femoral and popliteal arteries.

Discussion

The patient is prepped and draped with the operative leg and thigh exposed. The medial aspect of the thigh is incised from above the ankle to the groin, following the saphenous vein. The incision is carried deeper with dissecting scissors and the ESU. This exposes the saphenous vein, which is partly or completely mobilized. Vessel loops are placed along its length for manipulation.

The branches of the vein are clamped with mosquito hemostats or clipped. Each is divided from the vein. Fine silk sutures also may be used to ligate the tributaries. The distal and proximal ends of the saphenous vein are clamped and divided.

Before the anastomoses are performed between the saphenous vein and the femoral and popliteal arteries, the valves must be incised so that arterial blood can flow through the valves easily. Several techniques are used. The angioscope is passed through the lumen of the vein, and a system is used to both sever the valves and remove tributaries. This avoids extensive dissection of the vein. An alternative method is to

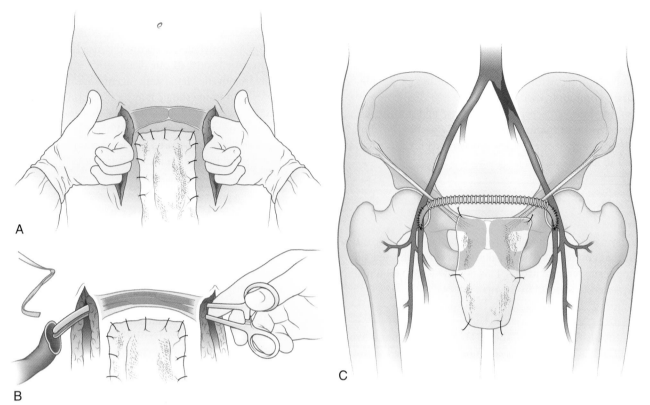

Figure 31-25 Femorofemoral bypass. **A,** A suprapubic tunnel is created digitally. **B,** The midline fascia is pierced with a long clamp, which grasps a Penrose drain or umbilical tape to facilitate delivery of the graft without kinks or twists. **C,** Bilateral end-to-side anastomoses are constructed; each anastomosis is run onto the profunda femoris artery if the superficial femoral arteries are occluded. *(From Ouriel K, Rutherford R: Atlas of vascular surgery: operative procedures, Philadelphia, 1998, WB Saunders.)*

incise the first two valves under direct vision with valve scissors and then to use a valvulotome, with or without the angioscope, to release the others.

Anastomoses are created between the saphenous vein and the femoral artery. The vein is trimmed to a bevel, and a small incision is made in the femoral artery with Potts scissors or a #11 scalpel blade. An end-to-side anastomosis is formed with 6-0 or 7-0 nonabsorbable sutures with a double- or single-arm needle. The profunda femoris also can be used for anastomosis. The distal anastomosis is made with the same technique.

Next, the small tributaries that branch from the saphenous vein must be occluded. These are located with Doppler ultrasound unless the vein is completely exposed. The surgeon applies digital pressure over the vein while observing the Doppler wave. Increased flow indicates an area of arteriovenous fistula (a vascular connection between the arterial circulation and the venous flow). These areas are exposed, and each individual tributary is clipped or ligated and incised.

Angiography is performed at this time to check for patency. The wounds are irrigated and closed in layers, with absorbable synthetic sutures used for subcutaneous and fascial tissue. The skin is closed with clips or nonabsorbable suture.

The wounds are dressed with a nonadherent dressing and then with gauze squares and roller gauze.

FEMOROPOPLITEAL BYPASS

Surgical Goal
In a femoropopliteal bypass, a synthetic graft or autograft is implanted between the femoral and popliteal arteries. As discussed previously, in situ grafting uses the greater saphenous vein as a shunt.

Pathology
Femoropopliteal bypass is indicated for atherosclerosis of the femoral artery (see *Atherosclerosis* in Table 31-1.)

Technique
1. An incision is made on the medial side of the thigh and carried to deep tissues with sharp and blunt dissection.
2. The femoral artery is mobilized, and vessel loops are placed around it.
3. The distal incision is made on the medial side of the knee, inferior to the patella.
4. The popliteal artery is located and mobilized.
5. Angiograms are taken.
6. A synthetic graft is tunneled through the subcutaneous tissue, connecting the two wound sites.

7. The femoral artery is clamped, and an arteriotomy is performed.
8. The proximal end of the graft is anastomosed to the femoral artery.
9. The popliteal anastomosis is performed.
10. Angiograms are taken, and pulses are verified.
11. The wounds are closed after all bleeding has been controlled.

Discussion

The patient is placed in the supine position, prepped, and draped with the affected leg and groin exposed. An incision is made on the medial side of the thigh, below the groin. Dissection is performed with the scalpel, Metzenbaum scissors, sponge dissectors, and the ESU. A Weitlaner or Gelpi retractor is used for superficial retraction. For deeper retraction, Army-Navy retractors or small Richardson retractors may be used.

The femoral artery is mobilized with careful dissection. One or more vessel loops are placed around the artery for retraction and manipulation.

A second vertical incision is made on the medial side of the knee below the patella. The subcutaneous, fascial, and muscle layers are dissected with both sharp and blunt dissection. A self-retaining retractor is used to expose the popliteal space. The popliteal artery is mobilized with sponge dissectors and scissors. A vessel loop is placed around the artery. Angiography may be done at this time to verify that the popliteal artery is patent.

The surgeon chooses the appropriate-size graft. The greater saphenous vein may be used instead of a synthetic graft (see the following section).

A tunnel is made in the subcutaneous tissue, and the graft is carried from the upper to the lower wound. The graft is then drawn back into the popliteal space. To perform the anastomosis, the surgeon first places a vascular clamp across the femoral artery. A small incision is made in the artery with a #11 scalpel blade or vascular scissors. Using running sutures of 5-0 or 6-0 polypropylene, the surgeon creates the anastomosis between the femoral artery and graft.

The popliteal anastomosis is created in the same manner as the femoral anastomosis. During both anastomoses, the scrub should have heparinized saline solution available for irrigation of the arterial sites. Hemostatic agents are used to check bleeding at the anastomosis, and additional sutures are placed if needed.

Angiograms are done at this time, and the patency of the arterial system is monitored with the Doppler or intravascular ultrasound. The wound is irrigated and closed in layers. The popliteal space is closed with 2-0 or 3-0 interrupted absorbable synthetic sutures. The skin commonly is closed with staples or nylon sutures. The groin incision is closed in layers and dressed with gauze squares.

A femoropopliteal bypass is illustrated in Figure 31-26.

Postoperative Considerations

During the immediate postoperative period, the patient's pedal pulses are monitored carefully. Possible complications include blockage of the graft and infection. Patients may experience some numbness of the lower leg. Swelling of the operative leg is common after surgery.

SAPHENOUS VEIN GRAFT

Surgical Goal

For a saphenous vein graft, the greater saphenous vein is removed to provide an autograft for peripheral or coronary artery bypass. The goal is to remove the vein yet retain its structural and physiological soundness.

Pathology

An autograft is an ideal graft for arterial bypass. The greater saphenous vein has been used more successfully than other materials for small-diameter arterial bypass. It is readily accessible, and its connective tissue layer thickens with increased pressure. This makes it strong and able to withstand high arterial pressure.

Technique

1. The groin and inner aspect of the leg are incised over the saphenous vein.
2. Branches of the vein are clamped, ligated, and divided.
3. The vein is injected with papaverine or lidocaine to prevent spasm.
4. The vein is mobilized and removed.
5. The vein is checked for leaks.
6. Tributaries are clamped and ligated.
7. The leg wound is closed.
8. The graft is preserved in saline.

Discussion

A general anesthetic usually is administered because the procedure is performed in conjunction with a peripheral or cardiac bypass surgery. The patient is placed in the supine position, and the selected leg is prepped from the groin to the foot. Drapes expose the leg and groin, with the foot occluded.

A common problem during vein harvesting arises from the practice of one surgeon harvesting the vein while the rest of the team prepares the implant site (e.g., during coronary artery bypass). In this case, the two overhead operating lights are dedicated to the top of the surgical field, leaving no direct light for the saphenous vein harvest. A third light or headlight should be available to provide lighting on the leg.

The knee is flexed to gain access to the medial aspect of the leg. To begin the surgery, the surgeon makes a long incision directly over the saphenous vein from the groin to the point of removal, usually below the knee.

The groin incision is made parallel to the upper thigh crease, directly over the saphenous vein. Bleeders are coagulated with the ESU or ligated with 3-0 silk suture. A dull Weitlaner retractor may be placed in the wound. Branches of the vein are clamped and ligated with silk or clipped and divided. The vein is ligated with heavy silk sutures and divided with scissors.

The surgeon performs the distal excision by first clamping tributaries and ligating them. The vein is carefully dissected

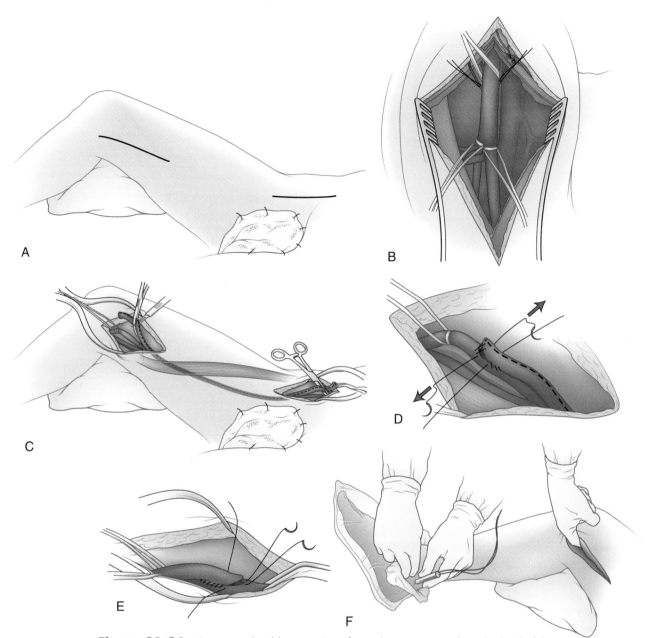

Figure 31-26 Femoropopliteal bypass. **A,** A femoral incision is made at the level of the inguinal ligament. A popliteal incision is made on the medial side of the distal thigh. **B,** The common femoral, superficial femoral, and profunda femoris arteries are exposed in the groin. **C,** A curved hemostat and the knife blade are used to bevel the graft for the anastomoses. **D,** Completion of the popliteal anastomosis. **E,** The proximal anastomosis is completed with a two-suture technique. **F,** Doppler ultrasound is used to assess the hemodynamic result intraoperatively. *(From Ouriel K, Rutherford R: Atlas of vascular surgery: operative procedures, Philadelphia, 1998, WB Saunders.)*

along its length to avoid creating wide tissue flaps on each side. The scrub or assistant must keep the vein and incision moist during the surgery. Frequent irrigation with saline solution is necessary. An Asepto syringe can be used for irrigation. Some surgeons inject papaverine or lidocaine into the subcutaneous tissue to prevent vein spasm.

The surgeon places Silastic vessel loops around the vein for retraction rather than using forceps, which can damage the

vessel. When all tributaries have been divided, the vein is removed and placed in a basin.

Preparation of the Vein

The scrub attaches a blunt-tip irrigation needle to a 30-cc syringe. The needle is inserted into the tip of the vein and secured with a heavy silk tie. Saline is used to irrigate the vein during the repair. If ordered, heparinized papaverine may be used. The surgeon injects solution into the vein and occludes the branches with silk ties. The vein must be kept moist at all times.

After preparation, the graft is maintained in a moist saline environment until needed. The vein also may be placed in a basin with heparinized papaverine and normal saline solution. This often is called a "vein bath." The vein must be carefully monitored and protected at all times.

The leg incision is closed with interrupted sutures. The skin is closed with staples or monofilament synthetic suture. Harvesting of a saphenous vein is illustrated in Figure 31-27.

MANAGEMENT OF VARICOSE VEINS

Surgical Goal
Surgical treatment of varicose veins involves the removal of dilated and tortuous (varicose) veins and their tributaries to prevent symptoms and to improve cosmetic appearance.

Pathology
Venous blood returns to heart from the extremities aided by the contraction of skeletal muscles. The intraluminal valves of the veins prevent blood from returning by gravity to the extremities. Valve incompetency or chronic inactivity may cause stasis of venous blood and distention in the veins. In primary varicose veins, the superficial saphenous veins are affected. Secondary varicose veins originate from the deep saphenous vein. Surgical treatment includes removal of the deep saphenous vein, superficial saphenous veins, or both. Tributaries of the veins visible through the skin are removed separately.

Technique
1. The greater saphenous vein is exposed at the medial malleolus.
2. The vein is ligated and divided.
3. A vein stripper is passed through the vein to the groin.
4. The groin is incised to expose the proximal end of the vein.
5. The proximal end is ligated, and all tributaries are divided and ligated.
6. The vein is removed by extracting the vein stripper.
7. Superficial veins are removed by excision.

Discussion
Before surgery, the paths of the superficial veins are marked with indelible ink. The patient is placed in the supine position, prepped, and draped with the affected leg and groin exposed. A general or regional anesthetic is administered.

The surgeon makes an incision anterior to the medial malleolus. The incision is carried deeper with a curved hemostat and Metzenbaum scissors. A small Weitlaner retractor or Senn retractors may be placed in the wound.

When the distal saphenous vein is located, it is dissected free. The severed distal end is ligated with 2-0 silk. The surgeon threads a disposable vein stripper through the lumen until resistance is felt. Small tributaries (perforators) that connect the deep saphenous vein to the superficial vein may impede passage of the stripper. A small incision is made over the

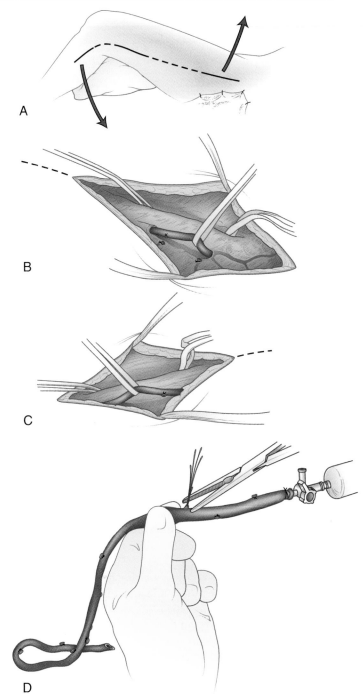

Figure 31-27 Harvesting the saphenous vein. The saphenous vein commonly is harvested to replace a diseased coronary artery and for other bypass procedures. **A,** External rotation of the hip exposes the line of incision. **B,** The saphenous vein and artery are exposed. Tributaries are clamped, tied, and divided. **C,** During surgery, the vein is preserved with saline solution (note the Asepto syringe). **D,** The vein has been removed and is tested for leaks, which are clamped and ligated. *(From Ouriel K, Rutherford R: Atlas of vascular surgery: operative procedures, Philadelphia, 1998, WB Saunders.)*

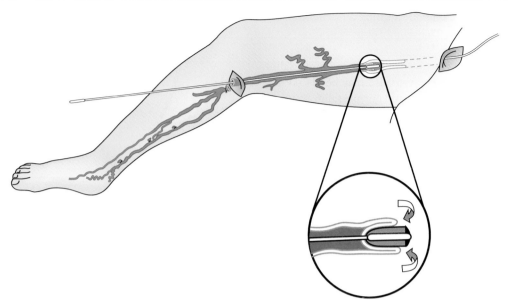

Figure 31-28   Stripping of the saphenous vein. (See the text for details.) *(From Townsend CM: Sabiston textbook of surgery, ed 17, Philadelphia, 2001, WB Saunders.)*

tributary, which is clamped, divided, and ligated. The stripper is advanced to the terminal end at the femoral junction.

The groin is incised with the scalpel, and bleeders are coagulated with the ESU. A rake, Army-Navy, or Weitlaner retractor is placed in the wound. The proximal end of the saphenous vein is isolated with a vessel loop. The branches are double-clamped, divided, and ligated with 3-0 silk suture.

When all branches have been secured, the vein stripper is pulled out at the groin incision while the assistant applies pressure over the calf and thigh using folded towels.

To remove small superficial tributaries, the surgeon makes an incision directly over them and mobilizes them with a curved hemostat and dissecting scissors. The vessels are double-clamped, divided, and ligated with silk ties.

The leg is dressed with nonadherent gauze strips and rolled gauze and then with an elastic compression bandage. Varicose vein stripping is illustrated in Figure 31-28.

Postoperative Considerations

Patients generally have pain, bruising, and swelling after surgery. Serious complications include arterial injury, deep vein thrombosis, and pulmonary embolism.

ABOVE-THE-KNEE AMPUTATION

Surgical Goal

Above-the-knee amputation involves the surgical removal of the leg.

Pathology

Although amputation may not be considered strictly a vascular procedure, it usually is performed when vascular insufficiency caused by arteriosclerotic or thromboembolic disease results in necrosis of the lower limb. Above-the-knee rather than below-the-knee amputation is chosen when the vascular supply in the lower limb is insufficient for proper healing at the amputation site. The procedures are very similar.

Technique

1. The skin and subcutaneous tissue are incised.
2. The incision is carried to the femur.
3. The femur is severed.
4. The popliteal vessels are ligated.
5. The sciatic nerve is ligated.
6. The wound is closed.

Discussion

The patient is placed in the supine position, and the affected leg is prepped. Many surgeons prefer to place the gangrenous foot in a plastic bag to protect the wound site from possible contamination. The foot is excluded from the scrub prep.

To begin the procedure, the surgeon incises the leg. The incision is carried through the subcutaneous, muscle, and fascial layers with the deep knife, heavy scissors, or electrocautery pencil. Large rake retractors (e.g., Israel rake retractors) often are useful for drawing the wound edges back to expose the femur. The surgeon may sever the femur with a Gigli saw or with an amputation saw (e.g., Satterlee saw).

When the femur has been severed, the surgeon completes the amputation by severing the soft tissues that lie on the posterior side of the femur. The scrub removes the limb from the field and may pass it directly to the circulator. The surgeon ligates the popliteal artery and vein and grasps the sciatic nerve with a Kocher or other heavy clamp. The end of the nerve is crushed with the clamp to prevent the formation of a neuroma (tumor at the end of a nerve). It is ligated with size 0 or 2-0 suture ligature. The end of the nerve is cut with the scalpel or scissors and allowed to retract into the femoral stump (Figure 31-29).

The stump is closed in layers with size 0 or 2-0 Dexon or other absorbable suture. The skin is sutured with the surgeon's choice of material and dressed with bulky gauze and an elastic wrap bandage.

Postoperative Considerations

Patients are monitored carefully for hemorrhage and pain in the immediate postoperative period. Complications of surgery include phantom limb pain (pain perceived in an area of the severed limb), limb edema, and damage to the incision area.

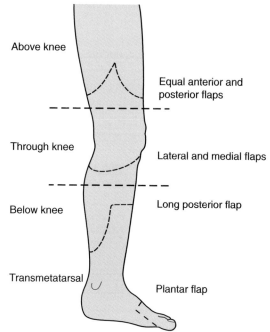

Figure 31-29   Amputation. **A,** Amputation levels with flap designs. **B,** Below knee amputation with an anterior flap. *(From Garden O, Bradbury A, Forsythe J, Parks R: Principles and practice of surgery, ed 5, Edinburgh, 2007, Churchill Livingstone/Elsevier.)*

CHAPTER SUMMARY

- The peripheral vascular system is a complex network of vessels, the function of which is to carry blood cell components and nutrients (including oxygen) to all parts of the body and to remove the waste products of metabolism.
- All blood vessels except the capillaries are composed of three layers or walls. From the outside to the inside, these are the tunica externa, tunica media, and tunica intima.
- The arteries carry oxygenated blood from the heart to the rest of the body. The only exception is the pulmonary arteries, which carry deoxygenated blood to the lungs.
- The elastic nature of the arteries allows them to contract during systole (ventricular contraction) and relax during diastole (the resting phase of the heart) to maintain vascular pressure.
- The capillaries are microscopic vessels that function as the transition and exchange mechanism for oxygen and other substances between the vessel walls and the tissue cells.
- The venous system carries blood back to the heart from the peripheral tissues. Veins have one-way valves, which prevent blood from backing up.
- The circulatory system is divided into two pathways, the pulmonary system and the systemic system. The

pulmonary system carries blood from the heart to the lungs for oxygenation (hemoglobin in the red blood cells picks up oxygen molecules). The oxygenated blood then returns to the heart and is pumped into the systemic circulation, which reaches all tissues of the body.
- Blood pressure is the force exerted on the arterial wall by the pumping action of the heart. The systolic pressure is the highest pressure, occurring during contraction of the ventricles (systole). The lowest pressure is the diastolic pressure, occurring during the relaxation phase of the cardiac cycle (diastole).
- The lymphatic system is composed of ducts (vessels), regional lymph nodes, and lymph (fluid). Lymph contributes to the formation of plasma, the liquid portion of blood, which is derived from intercellular components.
- Lymph nodes are located at intervals along the lymph ducts. Nodes are composed of lymphatic tissue, which collects and filters fluid from the system. They also produce lymphocytes (white blood cell).
- Arteriosclerosis is a group of vascular diseases characterized by hardening and stiffening of the arteries as a result of calcium deposits and fatty substances in the arterial wall.

- An embolus is a moving particle, such as a blood clot (thrombus), fat, or atherosclerotic plaque, in the bloodstream.
- An aneurysm is thinning and ballooning of an arterial wall, usually near a bifurcation. Causes include atherosclerosis, infection, and congenital malformation. An aneurysm becomes life-threatening when the sac ruptures.
- In a dissecting aneurysm, blood seeps between the vessel layers, causing them to tear.
- Deep vein thrombosis is a thrombus that occurs in a deep peripheral vein of the leg (also called *thrombophlebitis*). A DVT may lead to pulmonary embolism, which can be fatal.
- Arteriography is radiographic imaging of the artery. This is performed as an intraoperative, diagnostic, or interventional procedure to delineate the shape and interior surface of the arteries.
- Vascular clamps are specifically designed to prevent trauma to blood vessels. The jaws have finely serrated inserts that grip the tissue but do not crush or damage the surface of the vessel, even when fully closed.
- Vascular forceps have very fine serrations at the tips to allow a secure grip without tearing or slipping. The most common vascular forceps are DeBakey forceps.
- Vascular grafts are used to replace a blood vessel or to patch an area of tissue. Synthetic grafts are made of Dacron, polyester, or Gore-Tex. Sources of biological materials are banked human umbilical cord and autografts.
- Synthetic grafts require no preinsertion preparation except trimming. Patch grafts are cut into elliptical sections and sutured into place with a double-arm suture.
- All manufactured grafts are identified by size, lot, and identification number, which must be documented in the patient's operative record.
- The most common method of removing thrombi is with a Fogarty-type embolectomy catheter. This is a narrow, flexible catheter with a firm tip and an inflatable balloon at the tip.
- An endovascular stent is a tubular mesh implant that fits against the wall of an artery to maintain flow and prevent the release of atherosclerotic plaque.
- During vascular surgery, open vessels are irrigated with heparinized saline solution. This prevents thrombi from forming at the surgical site and reduces the risk of embolus.
- Because both thrombin and heparin are distributed to the scrub, the risk exists that the wrong drug may be offered to the surgeon. It is critical that all medications on the field be clearly marked as soon as they are received. Intravenous administration of thrombin can cause a fatal embolus.
- Many vascular procedures require removal of atherosclerotic plaque from the inside of the artery. Plaque is a rubbery substance that adheres to the tunica intima, causing occlusion.
- Angioplasty is performed during angiography, with C-arm fluoroscopy. A contrast medium is injected to verify correct placement of the stent, embolectomy catheter, or intravascular shaving device.
- The goal of thrombectomy is to remove a stationary clot. This restores circulation and prevents emboli. Thrombectomy commonly is performed with an embolectomy catheter.
- Patients with end-stage renal disease require frequent hemodialysis. This treatment requires long-term access to the patient's vascular system. An anastomosis between the arterial and venous systems is performed surgically to create this access.
- Carotid endarterectomy is the surgical removal of atherosclerotic plaque from the carotid artery. Plaque is removed through an open incision in the artery. This re-establishes the flow of oxygenated blood to the brain.
- The greater saphenous vein may be removed surgically to provide an autograft for peripheral or coronary artery bypass.
- An axillofemoral bypass creates circulation between the femoral arteries and the axillary artery to restore circulation to the lower extremity or, in an emergency procedure, to bypass an infected aortic graft or aneurysm.
- In a femoropopliteal bypass, a synthetic graft or autograft is implanted between the femoral and popliteal arteries. *In situ* grafting uses the greater saphenous vein as a shunt.
- Surgical management of severe varicose veins includes removal of the veins and their tributaries.
- An abdominal aortic aneurysm is a condition in which a section of the abdominal aorta becomes thin and bulges because of accumulation of atherosclerotic plaque and progressive weakening of the aortic wall.
- Surgical treatment of an aortic aneurysm involves implanting a graft to replace the diseased portion and restore continuity to the circulation.
- An aortofemoral bypass is performed to treat aortoiliac occlusive disease. A graft is implanted between the aorta and the femoral arteries to bypass the iliac arteries and restore circulation.
- Amputation of the leg for vascular insufficiency is performed in late-stage atherosclerosis in which significant necrosis of the lower limb has occurred.

REVIEW QUESTIONS

1. Define a stent.

2. The terms *arteriosclerosis* and *atherosclerosis* often are used interchangeably. What are the effects of these diseases on the arteries?

3. Why are double-arm needles used for arterial anastomosis?

4. What is the effect of venous stasis on the veins?

5. What are the three layers of the arterial wall?

6. What is the proper method of handling an amputated limb during surgery?

7. A Freer elevator or a Penfield elevator is used to remove atherosclerotic plaque from an artery. In what other surgical specialties are these instruments used?

BIBLIOGRAPHY

Eliason JL, Clouse DW: Current management of infrarenal abdominal aortic aneurysms, in *Surgical Clinics of North America*, 87:5, October 2007, WB Saunders.

Garden O, Bradbury A, Forsythe J, Parks R: *Principles and practice of surgery*, ed 5 Edinburgh, 2007, Churchill Livingstone/Elsevier.

Moody F: *Ambulatory surgery*, Philadelphia, 1999, WB Saunders.

Ouriel K, Rutherford R: *Atlas of vascular surgery: operative procedures*, Philadelphia, 1998, WB Saunders.

Porth CM: *Pathophysiology: concepts of altered health states*, ed 7, Philadelphia, 2004, Lippincott Williams & Wilkins.

Rutherford R: *Atlas of vascular surgery: basic techniques and exposures*, Philadelphia, 1997, WB Saunders.

Tinkmah MR: The endovascular approach to abdominal aortic aneurysm repair, *JAORN*, 89:2, pages 289–306, February 2009, Elsevier, St. Louis.

Thibodeau G, Patton K: *Anatomy and physiology*, ed 6, St Louis, 1997, Mosby.

Townsend CM: *Sabiston textbook of surgery*, ed 17, Philadelphia, 2001, WB Saunders.

CHAPTER 32

Thoracic and Pulmonary Surgery

CHAPTER OUTLINE

LEARNING OBJECTIVES

After studying this chapter the reader will be able to:
- Discuss the basic anatomy of the respiratory system
- Differentiate between ventilation, diffusion, and perfusion
- Describe the significance of negative pressure in the thoracic cavity and its role in ventilation

- Describe basic pulmonary pathology
- Discuss the purposes of and precautions in closed chest drainage
- Identify the instrument sets required for thoracic surgery
- Identify the techniques used in basic pulmonary procedures

TERMINOLOGY

Arterial blood gases (ABGs): A blood test that determines carbon dioxide and oxygen saturation, pH, and other important parameters of respiration and oxygen perfusion.

Blebs: Areas of overdistention in the lung tissue.

Closed chest drainage: A system of removing air from the thoracic cavity and restoring negative pressure so that the lungs can expand properly after thoracic surgery or trauma to the chest wall.

Diffusion: The molecular passage of oxygen across the alveoli and into the bloodstream.

Dyspnea: Difficulty breathing.

Empyema: A pus-filled area of the lung.

Expiration: The act of breathing out (exhalation).

Hemoptysis: Bloody sputum or bleeding arising from the respiratory tract.

Hemothorax: The presence of blood in the thoracic cavity or between the pleural sac and lungs, usually caused by trauma.

Hypoxia: Lower than normal oxygen perfusion.

Inspiration: The act of taking a breath (inhalation).

Perfusion (oxygen): The distribution of oxygen to tissues.

Pleur-Evac: The prototype of single-use, closed chest drainage systems, introduced in 1967.

Pleuritis: Inflammation of the pleural membrane, usually caused by an infection or a tumor.

Pneumothorax: Air in the chest cavity, which prevents the lungs from expanding and may displace the mediastinal structures.

Pulmonary function tests (PFTs): Tests performed to measure the function and strength of the pulmonary system.

Thoracoscopy: Minimally invasive surgery of the thoracic cavity; also referred to as video assisted thoracoscopic surgery or VATS.

Thoracotomy: Open chest surgery in which the thoracic cavity is entered; literally, an incision into the chest wall.

Valsalva maneuver: Voluntary closure of the epiglottis and contraction of the intraabdominal muscles, which results in increased thoracic pressure. Action used during "breath holding" and "bearing down."

Ventilation: The process of inflating and deflating the lungs during breathing.

INTRODUCTION

Thoracic and pulmonary surgery includes procedures of the respiratory system and thoracic cavity, excluding those that involve the heart and cardiac vessels. Most thoracic procedures within the specialty involve the lungs, bronchi, and peripheral bronchial system. Surgery involving other organs located within the thoracic cavity, such as the esophagus and thymus, may be performed by a thoracic surgeon or by a general surgeon with assistance of a thoracic specialist. This often depends on whether the surgery involves pulmonary structures.

Surgery of the lungs and other pulmonary structures in the thoracic cavity is frequently preceded by endoscopic assessment of the respiratory structures. Tissue biopsy is performed through the flexible or rigid bronchoscope. Open or video-assisted thoracoscopy may then be used to remove a mass or perform other procedures. Interventional procedures such as foreign body removal, biopsy, and removal of small tumors can be performed through the endoscope, especially the rigid bronchoscope, which has a larger diameter than the flexible scope.

Maintaining lung inflation is an important procedural consideration in thoracic surgery. The thoracic cavity is under *negative pressure*. Under normal circumstances, the lungs expand freely within a vacuum within the chest cavity. An incision, tear, or puncture of the chest wall allows atmospheric air to rush into the thorax. This results in immediate collapse of the lungs. During **thoracotomy** (open chest surgery), the lungs are inflated with the use of a mechanical respirator managed by the anesthesia care provider. In the immediate postsurgical phase and healing phase, the normally negative pressure within the thoracic cavity is maintained with a closed drainage system, which removes air and fluid to allow lung expansion (described later in the chapter).

SURGICAL ANATOMY

The diaphragm is a sealed barrier between the thoracic and abdominal cavities. The function of the respiratory system is to maintain a steady intake of oxygen from the air and eliminate carbon dioxide from the blood. Oxygen is necessary for life, and carbon dioxide is a waste product of normal metabolism.

Three processes are involved in respiratory function:
- **Ventilation:** The breathing process; it involves contraction of the diaphragm and accessory muscles and expansion of the ribs to pull air into the lungs.
- **Diffusion (oxygen):** The transfer of oxygen from the alveoli in the lungs to the bloodstream.
- **Perfusion:** The movement and absorption of oxygen molecules into body tissues; also called *oxygenation*.

UPPER RESPIRATORY TRACT

The nose is composed of cartilage and bone covered by skin. The external nose flares to form the nares. The internal nose is lined with mucous membrane and is highly vascular. It is divided by the nasal septum, which is composed of cartilage and bone. Nasal hairs in the anterior nasal cavity help filter the air as it enters the upper respiratory tract. Olfactory nerves, which are responsible for the sense of smell, are located in the superior nasal airway and septum.

The nasal sinuses are bilateral structures, each composed of three tiers of bony projections called the *conchae* or *turbinates*. These projections are the superior, medial, and inferior meati (sing., meatus). The projections form spaces called the *paranasal sinuses*. Each of these is named after the bone above it (i.e., the maxillary, ethmoid, frontal, and sphenoid bones). The nasal passages are lined with mucous membrane, which warms and humidifies air as it enters the body.

PHARYNX

The pharynx lies behind the oral cavity and communicates with the nasal cavities. It is subdivided into three sections: the oropharynx, nasopharynx, and laryngopharynx or larynx. The oropharynx lies immediately below the mouth. The nasopharynx communicates with the nasal cavities. Two important structures are located in the nasopharynx: the eustachian tube, which drains from the middle ear, and the pharyngeal tonsils (adenoids). The palatine tonsils, the structures commonly referred to as "the tonsils," are located in the oropharynx.

LARYNX

The larynx connects the trachea with the oropharynx. The anatomy of this region is complex and is best understood by studying illustrations of this anatomy. The larynx is a wide, circular cavity formed by cartilage. It contains the vocal cords and prevents food and other foreign bodies from entering the trachea.

The epiglottis is a cartilaginous structure that functions as a flap to close off the entrance to the trachea during swallowing. The epiglottis also is under voluntary control and is closed when a person holds the breath. During defecation, the glottis is voluntarily closed and the intraabdominal muscles are contracted. This is referred to as **Valsalva maneuver.** This action also causes a momentary decrease in intrathoracic pressure and an increased heart rate. The epiglottis often is confused with the uvula, which is the visible projection of epithelial tissue extending from the soft palate of the mouth.

The larynx is divided into bilateral sections by paired folds of tissue, which are extensions of the epithelial lining of the laryngeal cavity. The upper folds are called the *vestibular folds*. The lower folds form the vocal cords to produce speech. The space between the folds is the glottis, which is the entrance to the trachea.

Two other important cartilaginous structures in the larynx are the thyroid cartilage and the arytenoid cartilage. The thyroid cartilage is a large "shield" of tissue that forms the anterior wall and protects the larynx from injury. This structure is larger in men than in women. The horn-shaped arytenoids extend superiorly and support the vocal cords. Figure 32-1 illustrates the upper respiratory system.

TRACHEA

The trachea begins at the larynx and branches into two main airways, the right and left primary bronchi and bronchial tree. The trachea is a semirigid tube mainly composed of C-shaped rings. The cricoid cartilage is the only completely closed ring in the structure.

BRONCHI

The trachea branches into the right and left primary bronchi at the carina. Because the right bronchus is straighter than the left, inhaled foreign material is more likely to enter the right lung. As the bronchi enter the lung segments, they branch into smaller and smaller branches, or bronchioles, forming a treelike structure. Cartilaginous rings support the primary bronchi. However, as the branches become smaller, the walls are formed by cartilage plates until the level of the bronchioles,

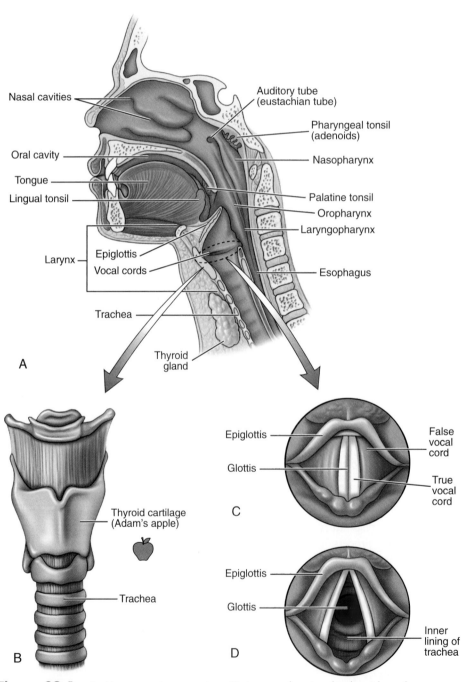

Figure 32-1 **A,** Upper respiratory system. **B,** Larynx, showing the thyroid cartilage. **C,** Vocal cords and closed glottis. **D,** Open glottis. *(From Herlihy B, Maebius NK: The human body in health and illness, ed 2, Philadelphia, 2003, WB Saunders.)*

where there is no cartilage. The bronchioles are composed of smooth muscle lined with epithelium.

LUNGS

The lung is divided into anatomical regions. The right lung has three lobes, and the left lung has two lobes. Each lung is composed of smaller segments, called *bronchopulmonary segments,* which contain branches of the main bronchi. The hilum (notch) of each lung is located on the medial side. Large blood vessels and primary bronchi enter the lung at the hilum. The apex of the lung is located at the upper portion and extends just above the clavicle.

The bronchioles terminate in small ducts, alveolar sacs, and individual alveoli. An alveolus exchanges incoming oxygen molecules with carbon dioxide molecules from the blood.

The lungs are separated in the thoracic cavity by the mediastinum. This space contains the heart, large vessels, bronchi, trachea, esophagus, and thymus gland. Each lung is enclosed in a pleural cavity and covered by a double membrane, the pleural sac. The outer membrane forms the parietal pleura, which lines the thoracic cavity and outer mediastinal walls. The inner, or visceral, pleura covers the lungs. A small amount of pleural fluid is secreted into the pleural space between the two membranes. **Pleuritis** is inflammation of the pleural membranes. An increase in fluid (e.g., serous fluid, pus, or blood) is called a *pleural effusion.* The pleural space is called a *potential space* because during respiration, the space increases or decreases as the lungs fill with air. In pleural effusion, the lungs cannot expand fully.

The pleural space normally maintains negative pressure in relation to atmospheric air and the alveoli. If the chest wall and pleural space are opened, such as during trauma or surgery, air rushes in and collapses the lungs in the same way vacuum-packed wrappers fill with air when punctured. Figure 32-2 illustrates the lungs and bronchial tree.

Mechanism of Breathing

Breathing is a complex physiological and mechanical process controlled by the autonomic nervous system but also under voluntary control. The thoracic cavity is a closed space. The diaphragm is continuous with the parietal pleural membrane. Recall that the pressure between the two pleural membranes is negative, whereas air pressure in the trachea, bronchi, bronchioles, and alveoli is equal to atmospheric pressure outside the body. When the diaphragm contracts during inhalation, the potential space between the two pleural membranes decreases, and air is pulled into the airways and lungs. When the diaphragm relaxes during exhalation, air flows passively out of the lungs (Figure 32-3).

A number of important factors affect breathing:

1. An intact pleural membrane is needed to maintain the negative pressure in the pleural space.
2. Penetrating trauma to the chest cavity causes air to rush in and collapses the lungs. Air (**pneumothorax**), blood (**hemothorax**) or exudate in the pleural space displaces and compresses the lungs. This prevents their expansion and may result in full collapse of the lung.
3. The alveoli must have sufficient elasticity to expand and fill with air. Diseases that constrict the alveola, such as emphysema results in loss of alveolar elasticity and therefore inability to exchange oxygen with carbon dioxide.
4. An intact central nervous system (CNS) is required to initiate transmission to the phrenic nerve, which controls the diaphragm. For example, barbiturate drugs can depress the CNS to the level that breathing stops.
5. The chest cavity must be able to expand freely. An example of pathological restriction is eschar from extensive third-degree burns.

PATHOLOGY OF THE THORACIC AND PULMONARY SYSTEMS

Table 32-1 presents common pathological conditions that affect the thoracic and pulmonary systems.

DIAGNOSTIC TESTS

Diagnostic tests for the respiratory system assess the function of the lungs, thoracic space, and bronchial system.

PULMONARY FUNCTION

Pulmonary function tests (PFTs) are a specific group of procedures that measure lung function. These noninvasive tests are performed with a complex breathing machine, which measures the parameters digitally. The following tests are included in this group:

- *Tidal volume:* The amount of air exhaled during normal respiration.
- *Minute volume:* The amount of air exhaled per minute.
- *Vital capacity:* The total volume of air exhaled after maximum **inspiration.**
- *Functional residual capacity:* The volume of air remaining in the lungs after exhalation.
- *Total lung capacity:* The total amount of air in the lungs when fully inflated.
- *Forced vital capacity:* The amount of air expelled in the first, second, and third seconds after exhalation.
- *Peak expiratory flow rate:* The maximum amount of air expelled in forced **expiration.**

LABORATORY TESTS

A complete blood count (CBC), including white blood cell differential, is performed as a basic screening tool for surgical patients. More specific laboratory tests, such as those for tumor markers, are performed according to the suspected pathological condition. Culture and sensitivity may be performed on exudate collected from the respiratory tract.

Among the most important blood tests for pulmonary function is determination of arterial blood gas values,

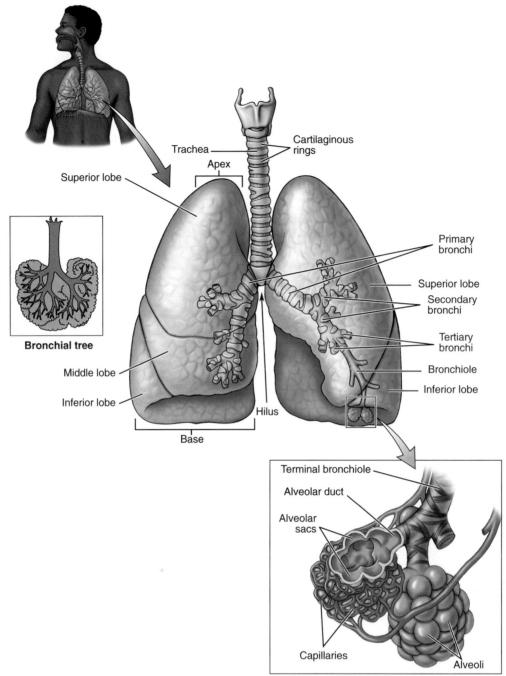

Figure 32-2 The lungs and bronchial tree. *(From Herlihy B, Maebius NK: The human body in health and illness, ed 2, Philadelphia, 2003, WB Saunders.)*

commonly called **arterial blood gases (ABGs).** In this test, the arterial blood is assessed for oxygen and carbon dioxide levels and pH (acid-base balance).

IMAGING STUDIES

Imaging studies of the pulmonary and thoracic structures include radiographs, magnetic resonance imaging (MRI), ultrasound scans, and computed tomography (CT) scans. Radiographs are used to screen patients for tuberculosis, acidosis, and other fibrotic diseases. Fluid and air in the pleural space, tumors, and anatomical deformities are also detected

on radiographs. MRI and CT scans are used for more definitive analysis of masses.

Pulmonary angiography is performed when CT scans are inconclusive for diagnosis of pulmonary embolism. During angiography, the blood vessels of the lungs are injected with a contrast medium, and fluoroscopy is used to detect any abnormalities (Figure 32-4).

Endoscopic procedures (discussed later in the chapter) are performed to obtain biopsy specimens of cells, fluid, and tissue. Visual examination of the respiratory tract by endoscopy, along with other diagnostic tools, assists in determination of the diagnosis.

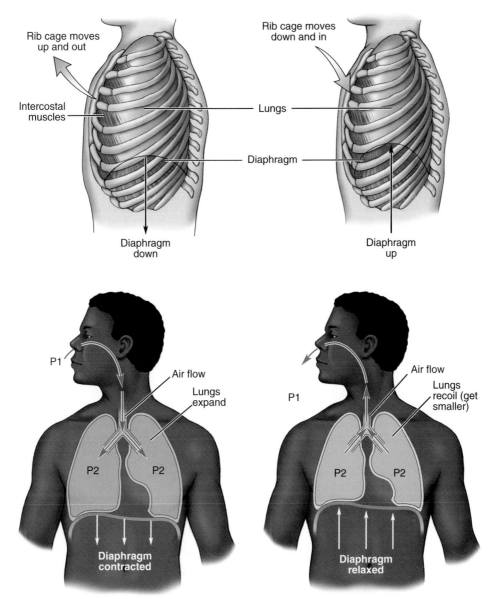

Figure 32-3 Mechanism of breathing. *(From Herlihy B, Maebius NK: The human body in health and illness, ed 2, Philadelphia, 2003, WB Saunders.)*

PERIOPERATIVE CONSIDERATIONS

PREPPING AND DRAPING

The incisions most commonly used in pulmonary surgery are the posterolateral and anterolateral thoracotomy, with the patient in the lateral position (see Chapter 10, especially Figure 10-22). The skin prep may extend from the neck to the iliac crest. Minimum draping includes a body sheet, towels for squaring the incision, an incise drape, and a fenestrated thoracotomy drape.

INSTRUMENTS

Open thoracic surgery of the respiratory structures requires the following instruments:

- General surgery instruments, including long instruments (shanks must be at least 9 inches [22.5 cm] for most adult patients).
- Chest wall instruments, including self-retaining chest, rib, and scapula retractors, and rib approximates. Orthopedic rongeurs, periosteal elevators, and rib-stripping instruments also are required for some procedures.
- Lung instruments, including atraumatic tissue-grasping clamps.
- Bronchus clamps, which are large, right-angle clamps used to occlude the primary bronchi. The jaws of the clamps are stippled for greater grip on the cartilaginous tissue.
- Surgical stapling instruments, which are commonly used in thoracic surgery (both open and endoscopic procedures). These are used in lung resection and for occlusion of the bronchial stem after resection.
- Vascular clamps are needed for some lung procedures.

Figures 32-5 and 32-6 show thoracic and tracheal instruments.

<u>Table 32-1</u>

Pathology of the Thoracic and Pulmonary Systems

Condition	Description	Considerations
Atelectasis	Atelectasis is inadequate or incomplete expansion of the lung. This may be caused by pneumothorax, hemothorax, or pleural effusion. The condition may also be present at birth.	Positive-pressure ventilation may re-expand compressed lung tissue, but if this fails to allow expansion, chest tubes are inserted to facilitate expansion. (See *Thoracostomy [Insertion of Chest Tubes.]*)
Bone malformations	Malformations of the sternal bone can include depression of the sternum (pectus excavatum) or projection of the xyphoid and lengthening of the costal cartilages.	Chest wall malformations are treated surgically when cardiac or respiratory function is impaired. (See Chapter 34.)
Bronchitis	Chronic bronchitis may be caused by infection, cigarette smoke, or other environmental pollutants that irritate the bronchi.	Treatment is medical, but a biopsy may be indicated to rule out the presence of cancer. (See *Bronchoscopy*.)
Cancer/neoplasms	Lung cancer is the leading cause of cancer death in the United States. It is associated with smoking and exposure to asbestos and other environmental toxins. Most lung cancers arise in the bronchus. The most common is adenocarcinoma.	The diagnosis usually is not established until metastasis has occurred. Treatment includes surgery, chemotherapy, and radiation therapy. (See *Lobectomy*.)
Emphysema	Emphysema is loss of elasticity and distention of the alveoli. This results in severely impaired gas exchange and reduced perfusion. The two primary causes are smoking and a genetic factor that results in antiprotease deficiency.	Surgical treatment includes excision of the emphysematous portions of the lung tissue. (See *Lung Volume Reduction Surgery*.)
Fibrosis	Fibrosis of the pleura may develop after infection, trauma, lung abscess, tumor, or other disease that causes chronic inflammation. Fibrosis impairs lung expansion and gas exchange.	Removal of the fibrous tissue is required to allow lung expansion. (See *Decortication of the Lung*.)
Hemothorax	Hemothorax is blood in the pleural cavity. In sufficient volume, it may compress the lungs and prevent adequate gas exchange. Hemothorax usually is caused by trauma.	A small amount of blood can be reabsorbed by the body. The cause of the hemothorax must be investigated and, if necessary, surgery must be performed to stop the hemorrhage and restore negative pressure. (See Thoracostomy [Insertion of Chest Tubes].)
Chronic obstructive pulmonary disease (COPD)	COPD is a progressive, irreversible condition characterized by reduced inspiratory and expiratory function of the lungs. COPD may result from asthma, cigarette smoking, chronic bronchitis, or pulmonary emphysema.	COPD is irreversible but may be treated medically. Surgical treatment may include lung transplantation. (See Lung Transplantation.)
Pleural effusion	Fluid or exudate in the pleural space most often is caused by infection and tumors. Control of effusion is critical to remove any impingement on the lungs.	Fluid is removed by thoracostomy. Chest tubes may be inserted, or fluid may be drawn off in a single or multiple treatments. Individual treatments are performed at the bedside using a local anesthetic.
Pneumothorax	Pneumothorax occurs when air enters the pleural cavity, which normally is at negative air pressure. This can occur because of trauma or surgery, or it may happen spontaneously.	Air must be removed to restore lung inflation. This is done by inserting chest tubes and using a closed drainage system. (See Thoracostomy [Insertion of Chest Tubes].)
Pulmonary embolism	Pulmonary embolism is an obstruction in the pulmonary vascular system that may result in ischemia to that portion of the lung. It may be caused by a blood clot, air, or fat that enters the bloodstream. Pulmonary embolism may be quickly fatal. The obstruction usually arises from deep vein thrombosis (DVT).	DVT is prevented by implementing protocols in the perioperative period (e.g., sequential compression stockings). Vulnerable patients are placed on anticoagulant therapy. Emergency measures to remove life-threatening embolism include venous ligation and plication. (See Chapter 31.)

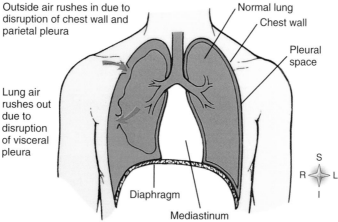

Figure 32-7 Pneumothorax. The pressure in the thoracic cavity normally is negative. Air rushes in through an opening in the pleural sac, causing the lung to collapse. *(From Thibodeau G, Patton K:* Anatomy and physiology, *ed 6, St Louis, 2007, Mosby.)*

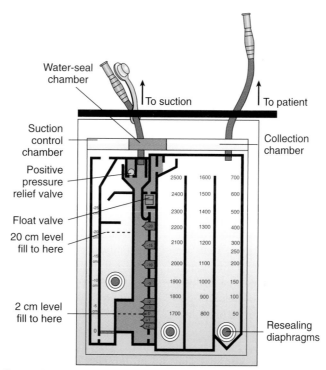

Figure 32-8 A closed chest drainage unit is used to maintain negative pressure in the thoracic cavity after surgery or trauma to the chest cavity. *(From Lewis SM, Heitkemper MM, Dirksen SR:* Medical surgical nursing, *ed 6, St Louis, 2004, Mosby.)*

Pathology

The effects of diseases of the bronchi often are visible with the aid of endoscopy. Pathological indications for bronchoscopy include:

- Bleeding arising from the respiratory tract (called **hemoptysis**).
- Suspected tumor
- Infection
- Evaluation of the extent of burn injury from toxic inhalation or smoke inhalation
- Aspirated foreign body (food or objects, usually in pediatric patients)
- Lesions seen during imaging studies

Technique

1. A bronchoscope is inserted into the trachea and slowly advanced.
2. The respiratory structures are examined.
3. Interventional procedures, such as removal of tissue or extraction of a foreign body, are performed.
4. Bronchial specimens are removed (washings, cytological biopsy, or sputum samples).
5. The bronchoscope is gently withdrawn.

Two types of bronchoscopy are discussed below—*rigid* and *flexible*. Each has particular advantages and used according to the patient's requirements:

- Flexible bronchoscopy utilizes a slender fiberoptic endoscope capable of entering the primary and peripheral bronchi. The modern flexible scope may also be used for interventional procedures such as cryosurgery and laser surgery.
- Rigid bronchoscopy is used for interventional procedures, which require a large bore endoscope and rigid instruments such as removal of a tissue mass or a foreign body. This is because the lumen of the rigid scope is larger than that of the flexible bronchoscope.

RIGID BRONCHOSCOPY

Surgical Goal
Refer to Bronchoscopy.

Pathology
Refer to Bronchoscopy.

Discussion
The patient is placed in the supine position with the neck slightly hyperextended. A body drape is applied. The patient's eyes may be protected with pads and a head drape. Before the procedure begins, the scrub should make sure all light cables and fittings are in good working order. An eyepiece adapter should be placed over the scope to protect the surgeon from contamination by the patient's body fluids. A tooth guard is placed in the patient's mouth to protect the teeth.

The surgeon inserts the rigid scope into the trachea. Side channels on the bronchoscope allow for insertion of irrigation and suction devices and other instruments. The scrub should assist by guiding the instruments into the side channels.

If sputum or fluid samples are to be taken, suction tubing adapted with a Lukens trap is attached to the tubing. Cells are washed free from the bronchus and retrieved with the suction cannula attached to a Lukens trap. This small vial collects solutions as they are suctioned. The trap must be held upright to avoid losing the specimen. The surgeon performs bronchial lavage by injecting saline into the side channel.

Biopsy tissue is removed with cup forceps. The scrub is responsible for removing the tissue from the forceps. The sample is placed on a moistened Telfa pad to prevent its loss. The tissue must be handled gently when removed from the forceps so that it is not crushed, because this may distort the pathology.

Foreign bodies are retrieved with a basket similar to that used to remove kidney stones. The basket instrument is threaded into the side channel. Grasping forceps also may be used to retrieve a foreign body.

At the close of the procedure, before the scope is withdrawn, the surgeon suctions the patient free of all secretions. The scope is then withdrawn.

Postoperative Considerations
An important complication of rigid bronchoscopy is injury to the tracheobronchial structures if the patient moves during the procedure. The autonomic gag reflex may cause the patient to arch and cough even during heavy sedation or light general anesthesia. This is called *bucking*. A local anesthetic is sprayed into the trachea before the endoscope is inserted to help prevent bucking during the procedure.

Complications include possible injury to the bronchial tree and lung tissue. Additional complications include laceration of blood vessels near the bronchial tissue and infection. Bronchoscopy is illustrated in Figure 32-9.

FLEXIBLE BRONCHOSCOPY

Surgical Goal
Refer to Bronchoscopy.

Pathology
Refer to Bronchoscopy.

Technique
1. A fiberoptic tube is inserted through the patient's mouth or nose.
2. The tracheobronchial tree is examined.
3. Cytology or biopsy specimens are taken.
4. The bronchial tree is suctioned.
5. Video data are recorded.
6. The scope is withdrawn.

Discussion
Flexible bronchoscopy is preferred over rigid bronchoscopy for patients in whom hyperextension of the neck or jaw manipulation is difficult or impossible. The flexible bronchoscope can provide a more extensive assessment. Rigid and flexible procedures may be performed sequentially during the same surgery.

Like all endoscopes, the fiberoptic bronchoscope has digital capability, and the images transmitted through the scope are projected onto a monitor. Instruments required include imaging equipment, various sizes and types of biopsy forceps, a cytology brush, a 10-cc syringe, and collection tubes for tissue washings. If cytology specimens are to be taken, microscope slides and fixative are needed. The patient is placed in semi-Fowler position. A local anesthetic is sprayed into the throat, and the patient usually is sedated. A bite block frequently is used to prevent the patient from biting on the endoscope and damaging it. The flexible fiberoptic tube is lubricated and passed through the patient's mouth or nose. Unlike rigid bronchoscopy, which allows the patient to be ventilated through the tube, the patient must breathe around the flexible endoscope.

The patient is placed in supine position. There is no prep, although a top drape is used to protect the patient and secure the instruments and leads. The eyes are protected with a towel or head drape. Monitored sedation is often use. The throat may be sprayed with local anesthetic before insertion of the scope, to prevent gagging.

The surgeon advances the endoscope through the trachea and bronchial tree. When cancer is suspected or known, the healthy lung is examined first to avoid seeding it with cancer cells.

The surgeon obtains cytology samples by inserting a small brush through the operating channel. The technologist must

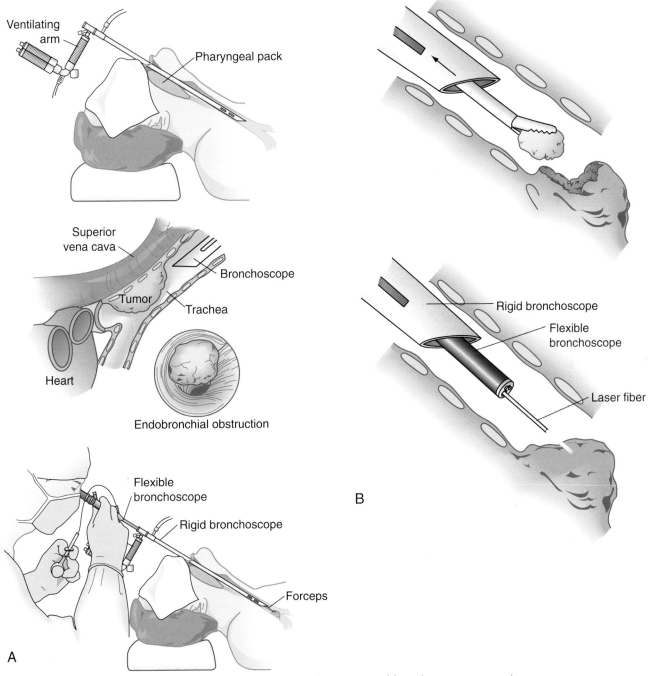

Figure 32-9 Bronchoscopy. **A,** *Top to bottom,* A rigid bronchoscope is inserted. Endobronchial obstruction. A flexible scope is placed inside the rigid scope for biopsy. **B,** The mass is removed with forceps. Laser removal. *(From Sugarbaker DJ, Strauss G, Fried MP: Laser resection of endobronchial lesions: Use of rigid and flexible bronchoscopes, Operative Techniques in Otolaryngology—Head and Neck Surgery 3:93, 1992.)*

make sure the instrument is long enough to extend outside the tip of the scope. After the brush is removed, the scrub dips it in a specimen container holding a small amount of saline. This process may be repeated several times. In some cases the tip of the cytology brush may be cut from the wire and placed in the fixative container.

Biopsy forceps may be used to obtain small tissue samples. These forceps must be handled carefully, because they are very small and easily lost. After the forceps is withdrawn from

the scope, the sample should be placed immediately in a specimen container or on a Telfa pad. A hypodermic needle is helpful for removing bits of tissue from the biopsy forceps.

A suction cannula is used to remove secretions. These are trapped in the Lukens specimen trap, just as in rigid bronchoscopy.

Recent innovations in tumor ablating devices have increased the use of flexible bronchoscopy for tissue debridement. The *microdebrider* used commonly in sinus surgery (see

Chapter 27) has been modified for use during flexible bronchoscopy. Cryotherapy and argon laser are also becoming more popular for interventional procedures. These techniques have been discussed in Chapters 19 and 27.

MEDIASTINOSCOPY

Surgical Goal
Mediastinoscopy is endoscopic examination of the mediastinum through an incision. Thymus and lymph node biopsy are performed to establish a diagnosis.

Pathology
Mediastinoscopy is performed for diagnostic or interventional surgery. The thymus gland, which is located in the mediastinal space in children, regresses in adulthood. Biopsy of the thymus gland and regional lymph nodes within the mediastinal space is performed to determine or rule out a cancer diagnosis.

Technique
1. An incision is made in the suprasternal notch.
2. The fascia is incised, and a tunnel is created into the mediastinum with digital pressure.
3. The mediastinoscope is inserted into the tissue space.
4. The trachea, bronchial tree, aortic arch, and lymph nodes are examined.
5. Lymph nodes may be removed.
6. The mediastinoscope is withdrawn.
7. The wound is closed.

Discussion
A rigid mediastinoscope is a stainless steel endoscope inserted through a small incision at the suprasternal notch. Video-assisted endoscopy allows the scope's field of vision to be projected on a monitor. Newer techniques, including natural orifice (transesophageal) mediastinoscopy, currently are being assessed and implemented in some facilities.

The patient is placed in the supine position with the neck hyperextended. The individual is prepped and draped for an upper thoracic incision. The procedure is performed using general anesthesia. The surgeon may stand at the patient's head or side.

A small incision is made over the suprasternal notch with a #10 knife blade. The incision is carried through the subcutaneous and muscle layers, commonly with Metzenbaum scissors and tissue forceps. The fascial layer on the anterior surface of the trachea is identified. The surgeon clamps small veins with mosquito hemostats and ligates them with fine silk ties. The electrosurgical unit (ESU) is used for smaller bleeders.

The surgeon uses blunt finger dissection to make a plane between the tissues into the superior mediastinum. The scope is then inserted into this tissue plane and carefully advanced.

Lymph node biopsy is performed routinely during the procedure. A specialized needle attached to a metal stylet is used to pierce the biopsy tissue and aspirate the contents. The technologist attaches a syringe to the stylet before handing it to the surgeon. This procedure is done to verify that the speci-

men is nodal tissue. When this is confirmed, the surgeon uses cup biopsy forceps to obtain a pathology specimen. The technologist removes the tissue from the forceps and places it in a specimen container or on a Telfa pad moistened with saline.

After specimens have been obtained, the surgeon dries the wound and checks for bleeding. The ESU and hemostatic agents (e.g., absorbable gelatin sponge) may be used to control bleeding. The surgeon then withdraws the scope and closes the incision with synthetic absorbable sutures and skin staples.

THORACOSCOPY (VIDEO-ASSISTED THORASCOPIC SURGERY)

Video-assisted thorascopic surgery (VATS) is a minimally invasive surgery of the thoracic cavity. This technique is similar to other types of minimally invasive procedures in which cannulae are inserted through the body wall and used to receive a rigid scope and telescope instruments. This technique is different from endoscopic (bronchoscopic) surgery in which a flexible or rigid scope is inserted through the airway via the trachea. The term *video-assisted thoracoscopy* or *VATS* was coined at a time when minimally invasive and endoscopic surgery was in its early development. At this time video display from the endoscope to a monitor was a relatively new technology. Thoracoscopy has now been developed to the extent that it has taken the place of most open procedures of the thorax.

Patient Preparation
The patient is placed in the lateral position with the operative side up, and a general anesthetic is administered through a double-lumen endotracheal tube. The double lumen allows the operative lung to collapse while the anesthetic and oxygen are administered to the opposite lung.

The patient is prepped from the neck to the iliac crest and from bedside to bedside. The exposed shoulder and arm also may be prepped and the arm placed on an overhead arm board.

Trocar and Cannulas
Endoscopic ports are placed according to the procedure. Three or four ports usually are required. A combination minithoracotomy (small thoracotomy incision) and thoracoscopy may be performed.

Instruments
Thoracoscopy in an adult requires 10-mm lenses in sizes 0 degrees and 30 degrees. The scope, camera, and light source are managed as with all minimally invasive endoscopic procedures (see Chapter 21). Thoracoscopy instruments are shown in Figure 32-10.

THORACOSCOPY: LUNG BIOPSY

Surgical Goal
In **thoracoscopic** lung biopsy, a small portion of lung tissue is removed for pathological assessment.

Pathology
Lung biopsy is performed to confirm a diagnosis.

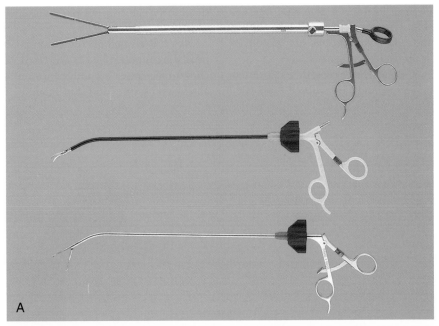

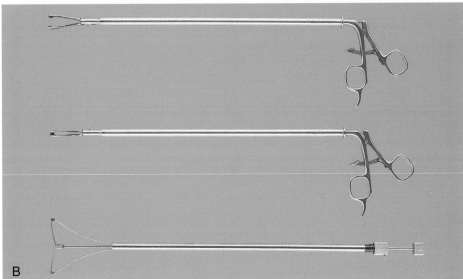

Figure 32-10 Thoracoscopy instruments. **A,** *Top to bottom,* 1 lung grasper;
1 roticulating scissors; 1 roticulating Babcock clamp. **B,** *Top to bottom,* 2 Duval lung clamps;
fan retractor. *(From Tighe SM: Instrumentation for the operating room, ed 6, St Louis, 2003, Mosby.)*

Technique

1. The cannulas and telescope are inserted.
2. One or more additional trocar sites are incised for instrumentation.
3. A small section of lung is removed.
4. The edges of the divided lung tissue are assessed for bleeding and air leakage.
5. A chest tube may be inserted through one puncture site.
6. The wounds are closed.

Discussion

The patient is placed in the lateral position and prepped and draped for a thoracostomy. A 2-mm skin incision is made to accommodate the first cannula. Size 10- or 12-mm trocars are used. A 10-mm thoracic telescope is introduced.

A wedge resection is a large tissue biopsy or the removal of a small peripheral lesion. These are commonly removed with the linear surgical stapler during thoracoscopy.

A small sponge forcep is inserted through one of the instrument ports, and a 30-mm endoscopic linear stapler is introduced through a separate port. The biopsy specimen is removed with the stapling device, which divides the lung and secures the opening. Additional specimens, including lymph node samples, may also be removed.

The surgeon carefully inspects the suture line for air leaks by filling the chest cavity with warm saline solution. The anesthesia care provider then inflates the lung and observes the suture line for bubbles. The surgeon or assistant applies pressure to the site, and additional sutures are placed as needed. Wedge biopsy is illustrated in Figure 32-11.

The instruments are withdrawn, and a chest tube is inserted into the lower incision. The wounds are sutured with syn-

thetic absorbable suture and skin staples. Steri-Strips may also be used to close the skin.

NOTE: If a small open incision is necessary for biopsy, the procedure is performed as described with the linear stapler. A chest tube is inserted, and the wound is closed with synthetic absorbable sutures and skin staples.

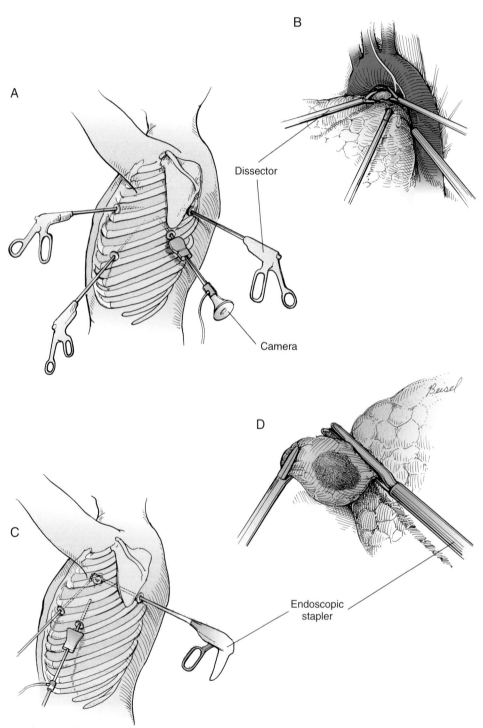

Figure 32-11   Video-assisted thorascopic surgery (VATS). **A,** The trocar is placed. **B,** The lung tissue is isolated. **C,** The endoscopic stapler is inserted. **D,** The wedge is resected. *(Modified from Waldhausen JA, Pierce WS, Campbell DB: Surgery of the chest, ed 6, St Louis, 1996, Mosby.)*

LUNG VOLUME REDUCTION SURGERY

Surgical Goal

In lung volume reduction surgery (LVRS), portions of the lung severely affected by chronic pulmonary emphysema are removed to improve pulmonary function. Segmental resection is performed by means of a VATS technique using surgical staples.

Pathology

Chronic pulmonary emphysema is marked by loss of elasticity and destruction of lung tissue, usually related to chronic cigarette smoking. The disease is characterized by stiffening of the tissue and inability to empty the alveoli, which results in abnormal enlargement of the lungs. Gas exchange is severely impaired, and the result is **dyspnea** (difficulty breathing) and **hypoxia.** Areas of overinflation, or **blebs,** develop in the most severely affected tissue. Segmental removal of diseased lung tissue improves pulmonary function, especially tidal volume.

Technique

1. Trocars and cannulas are placed for a video-assisted thoracoscopic surgery (VATS) procedure.
2. Adhesions are dissected.
3. The lungs are deflated to identify areas of trapped air.
4. Lung clamps are used to grasp the portion of the lung to be excised, and surgical stapling devices lined with bovine pericardium or polytetrafluorethylene (PTFE) are applied to each side of the lung tissue to be excised.
5. The lung is inspected to identify residual air leaks; these are closed.
6. Chest tubes are placed in each pleural space.
7. The incisions are closed.

Discussion

The patient is placed in the lateral or supine position and prepped and draped. General anesthesia is administered.

Trocars and cannulas are placed at strategic locations in the chest wall. To inspect the lung, the anesthesia care provider inflates and deflates areas of the pulmonary tissue. This reveals areas of trapped air, indicating severe damage caused by emphysema.

The surgeon uses Duval lung forceps or other atraumatic forceps to isolate areas to be resected. The edges of resected lung tissue must be sealed to prevent air from escaping after excision. A leakproof seal is achieved with a stapling device lined with bovine pericardium, or by placing a polytetrafluoroethylene (PTFE) graft on the edges of the resection. If the bovine implant is used, the scrub receives it from the circulator and rinses it in several baths of normal saline before insertion. PTFE strips do not require special preparation before use.

The selected blebs are transected and removed. The resected sections are examined for leaks. A chest drain is inserted, and the thoracoscopy cannulas are removed. Individual incisions are closed in two layers, and the chest drains are attached to a sealed chest drainage unit. The patient may be transferred to the postanesthesia care unit (PACU) or the intensive care unit (ICU).

Postoperative Considerations

Patients who undergo a VATS technique for resection of blebs may be placed on mechanical ventilation in the immediate postoperative period.

SCALENE NODE BIOPSY

Surgical Goal

Scalene node biopsy is performed on patients with palpable nodes in the area of the scalene fat pads. Biopsy is performed to establish cancer staging or to confirm a diagnosis.

Pathology

Lung cancer spreads through the intrathoracic and mediastinal lymphatics to the supraclavicular nodes. Excision and biopsy of the scalene fat pad is performed before thoracotomy. Scalene node biopsy is performed in conjunction with bronchoscopy and is used to identify patients most likely to benefit from thoracotomy for malignant disease.

Technique

1. An incision is made following the clavicle.
2. The incision continues through the platysma muscle.
3. The scalene fat pad is removed, exposing the phrenic nerve and the anterior scalene muscle.
4. The wound is closed.

Discussion

The patient is placed in the supine position with the head turned away from the surgical site. The individual is then prepped and draped for an upper thoracic incision. General anesthesia is used for the procedure. The surgeon makes a transverse incision 2 to 2.8 inches (5 to 7 cm) long approximately 0.8 inch (2 cm) above the clavicle. Small bleeders are coagulated using the ESU. The incision is carried through the subcutaneous tissue and loose connective tissue. The surgeon places a small, self-retaining retractor in the wound, or may use a shallow hand held retractor to exposed the lymph nodes.

An individual lymph node is dissected from the surrounding connective tissue using Metzenbaum scissors and fine tissue forceps. Fine silk ligatures or the ESU are used to control bleeders. The node is fully dissected free and passed off the field. A frozen section may be ordered.

The wound is closed using fine absorbable synthetic sutures size 3-0 or 4-0. Skin is closed with interrupted sutures of nylon or silk, or fine skin staples may be used. The wound is dressed with a flat gauze dressing.

THORACOTOMY

Surgical Goal

Thoracotomy is the general term for open surgery of the thoracic cavity. The procedure for opening and closing the chest generally is the same for any thoracotomy.

Pathology

Thoracotomy may be performed for any condition that requires opening of the chest.

Technique

1. The skin is incised.
2. The subcutaneous tissue and muscle layers are divided.
3. A rib may be removed.
4. The intercostal space is entered.
5. The thoracic cavity is entered.

Discussion

Thoracotomy requires a thoracotomy set and long general surgery instruments. Rib instruments usually are included in the thoracotomy set. Once the chest cavity is opened, lung-grasping forceps (Duval type), long tissue forceps, mounted sponges, and Metzenbaum scissors are required. Lung tissue is spongy and delicate and requires smooth rather than toothed instruments (e.g., forceps and other grasping instruments). Various sizes of right-angle (Mixter) clamps are needed to reach around vessels for hemostasis and dissection. Deep vascular clamps may be required for some resection procedures. Bronchial clamps (e.g., Sarot clamp) are required for resection. Many surgeons use long vascular forceps for handling tissue.

An extender or long spatula blade is needed for the ESU pencil to reach deeply into the wound. A Finochietto self-retaining retractor commonly is used. Handheld retractors include medium and wide Deaver and malleable ribbon retractors. A scapular retractor should also be available. Silastic vessel loops or a long Penrose drain is used for retraction of large vessels.

The patient is placed in the lateral position, prepped, and draped for a lateral thoracotomy. The incision is made following the curve of the rib. Subcutaneous and muscle layers then are divided with the knife or ESU. Bleeders are coagulated or clamped and ligated with silk ties.

The surgeon inserts a scapular retractor beneath the shoulder muscles and elevates the scapula. An intercostal incision is made with the knife or ESU. Occasionally a rib must be removed. If this is necessary, the surgeon incises the periosteum along its anterior surface. A periosteal elevator or rib raspatory is used to strip periosteum from the rib. The surgeon severs the rib from its attachment at the spine and sternum using Bethune rib shears. The entire rib is removed. The surgeon then trims the sharp edges of the remaining rib end using Sauerbruch rib shears.

The edges of the wound are covered with laparotomy sponges to protect them from bruising. A self-retaining retractor is placed in the wound and opened slowly. Surgery then continues as planned.

Closure

After chest tubes have been inserted and instruments have been removed, the surgeon places pericostal sutures (e.g., 1-0 or 2-0 absorbable suture) around the two ribs and tags the suture ends with a hemostat. Four to six sutures usually are required. A rib approximator (e.g., the Bailey approximator) is used to bring the ribs together. The pericostal sutures are tied securely while the approximator is in place.

A size 0 continuous absorbable suture may be used to approximate the periosteum between the two ribs. The surgeon then closes the muscles with a size 0 continuous or interrupted nonabsorbable suture. Subcutaneous tissue is closed with 3-0 nonabsorbable synthetic sutures. The skin is closed with staples or 4-0 nonabsorbable suture. Chest tubes are connected to the sealed drainage system, and the wound is dressed with absorbent pads and tape. A thoracotomy is illustrated in Figure 32-12.

LOBECTOMY

Surgical Goal

In a lobectomy, a lobe of the lung is removed to prevent the spread of cancer or to treat a benign tumor. Lobectomy may be performed as a VATS procedure or as an open procedure. The principles and anatomical divisions are the same for open and closed procedures. If thoracoscopy is planned, instruments for converting to an open procedure must be available.

Pathology

A lobectomy most often is performed to treat tumors, but it may indicated in other conditions, such as cysts, localized infection, or trauma to a portion of the lung.

Technique

1. A thoracotomy is performed.
2. The hilum of the lobe is identified, and individual arteries and veins are divided.
3. The bronchus is mobilized and separated from the hilum.
4. The lobe is removed.
5. The suture line is tested for leaks, and extra sutures are placed as needed.
6. The bronchial stump is covered with pleura.
7. Chest tubes are inserted and the incision or incisions are closed.

Discussion

The patient is placed in the lateral position, prepped, and draped for a thoracotomy incision.

A posterolateral thoracotomy is performed. The surgeon examines the entire lung and mediastinum closely to make certain no evidence of disease exists beyond that previously diagnosed. The lobe then is retracted with lung-grasping forceps, and the pleura is incised. The pulmonary artery and vein are dissected free at the hilum. Sponge dissectors are used to help separate the vessels from the connective tissue around the hilum.

Silastic vascular loops may be used to retract the bronchus and large vessels. Smaller vessels are mobilized with scissors and clamped with right-angle clamps. Ligation is done with 2-0 silk ties.

The bronchus is occluded with a bronchus clamp. Suction is very important while the bronchus is open to prevent blood

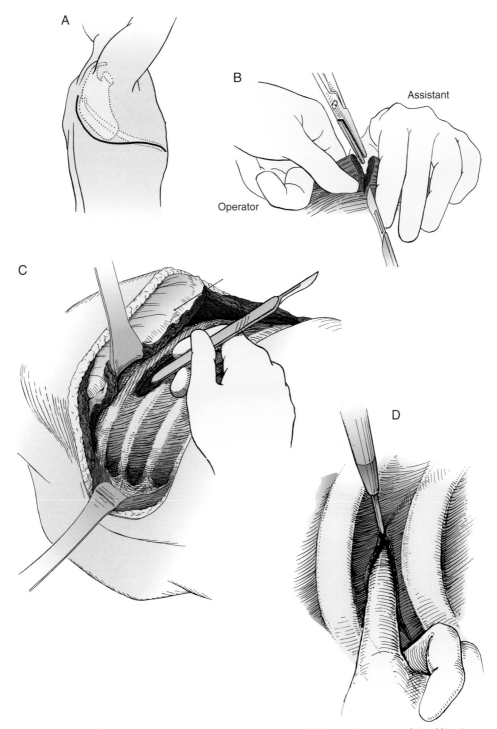

Figure 32-12 Thoracotomy. **A,** An incision is made following the curve of the fifth rib. **B,** The muscles are divided. **C,** A short incision is made in the intercostal muscles. **D,** The incision is extended with the ESU.

Continued

or fluid from draining into the opposite lung. The scrub may be needed to manage the suction while the surgeons transect and suture the bronchus. Interrupted sutures of 3-0 silk, 4-0 synthetic absorbable suture, or a linear stapler are used to occlude the proximal bronchus, which is divided with the knife.

When all vessels and the bronchus have been occluded, the lobe can be removed. The bronchial stump is covered with the pleura and sutured with interrupted 3-0 polyethylene sutures.

The wound is irrigated, and the lung is inflated to check for leaks. A chest tube is inserted, and the wound is closed in layers. A lobectomy is illustrated in Figure 32-13.

PNEUMONECTOMY

Surgical Goal

Pneumonectomy is the removal of the entire lung.

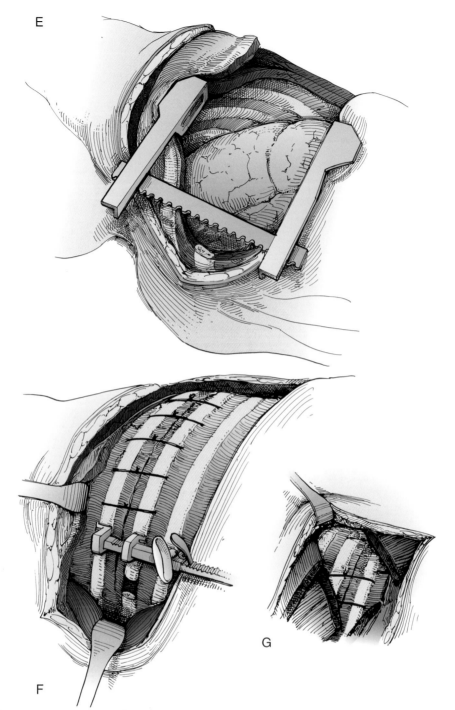

Figure 32-12, cont'd **E,** Rib retractor in place, exposing the lung. **F, G,** Closure. A Bailey rib approximator is used to close the ribs. *(Modified from Waldhausen JA, Pierce WS, Campbell DB: Surgery of the chest, ed 6, St Louis, 1996, Mosby.)*

Pathology

Removal of a lung reduces the size of a tumor that may be impinging on vital structures. Debulking is also a palliative measure to slow the progression of cancer. Other indications for lobectomy include extensive or chronic abscess or bronchiectasis, which is chronic dilation of the bronchi caused by infection, pulmonary obstruction, or tuberculosis.

Technique

1. A thoracotomy is performed.
2. The mediastinal pleura is incised.
3. The major vessels are divided (i.e., bronchus, pulmonary artery, and superior and inferior pulmonary veins).
4. The vagus, phrenic, and recurrent laryngeal nerves are identified.
5. Regional lymph nodes are dissected.
6. The bronchus is divided and closed.
7. The lung is removed, and the wound is closed; chest tubes may be inserted.

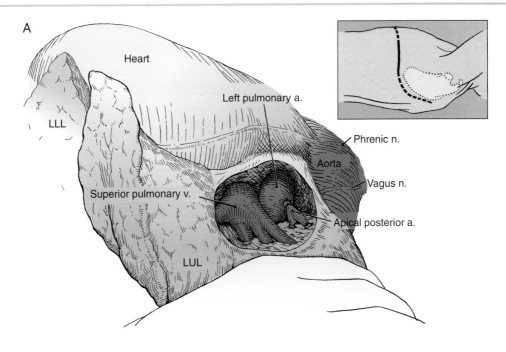

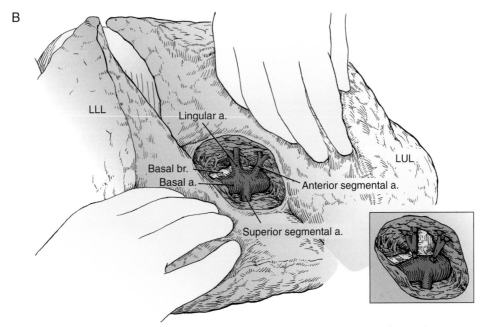

Figure 32-13   Open lobectomy. **A,** The left main pulmonary artery is identified and followed distally to the first upper lobe branch. **B,** The fissure is divided between the upper and lower lobes and opened to allow division of the arteries.

Continued

Discussion

The patient is placed in the lateral position, and a thoracotomy is performed. The entire lung and surrounding tissues are examined closely to evaluate the extent of the disease. The lung is retracted with nonmalleable or malleable retractors or Duval lung forceps to expose the mediastinal pleura. The pleura is incised with scissors and smooth tissue forceps. Blunt dissection along the edge of the parietal pleura is performed with sponge dissectors.

Dissection is carried to the hilum. The major structures connected to the lung are isolated, including the bronchus, pulmonary artery, and pulmonary vein. The pulmonary artery and vein are carefully separated, clamped with right-angle vascular clamps, and divided. Heavy silk sutures are used to ligate the vessels. The vagus, recurrent laryngeal (left side only), and phrenic nerves are retracted with vessel loops or moist umbilical tapes.

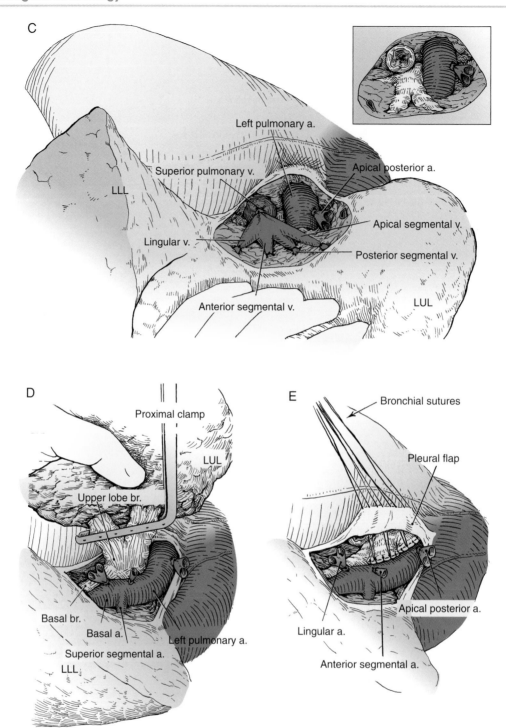

Figure 32-13, cont'd   C, Dissection of the superior pulmonary vein. **D,** Proximal clamp in place. **E,** Closure of the upper lobe bronchus. *(Modified from Waldhausen JA, Pierce WS, Campbell DB: Surgery of the chest, ed 6, St Louis, 1996, Mosby.)*

The pulmonary artery is clamped, divided, and ligated. The surgeon may oversew the cut edges of the artery with a fine suture, such as 4-0 or 5-0 silk or polypropylene. The superior and inferior veins are ligated and divided in similar fashion. Ligation clips may be used for smaller vessels.

The bronchus commonly is occluded with a Sarot clamp and divided with the knife. The lung then can be removed from the wound. The open end of the bronchus is closed with interrupted sutures (e.g., 3-0 polypropylene sutures) or the

stapler. The bronchus is divided, and the lung is removed from the wound.

The wound is irrigated with warm saline, and any leaks are identified and repaired with sutures. The pleura is sutured over the bronchus. Chest tubes may be inserted and brought out through stab wounds adjacent to the incision. These are secured with heavy silk sutures. The upper mediastinal pleura is closed with absorbable suture, and the wound is closed in layers.

RIB RESECTION FOR THORACIC OUTLET SYNDROME

Surgical Goal

Thoracic outlet syndrome (TOS) is a rare condition in which the subclavian vessels and the brachial plexus are compressed at the apex of the thorax. The surgical goal is to release the compression of the neurovascular tissue and restore function to the affected upper extremity, neck, or shoulder.

Pathology

The opening of the thoracic outlet is formed by the first ribs, the spine, and the sternum. TOS occurs when the brachial plexus and the subclavian vein or artery are compressed as they pass from the neck into the upper extremity (in the region between the thoracic outlet and the insertion of the pectoralis minor muscle). The obstructing structures may include the first rib, clavicle, or pectoralis tendon. The causes of TOS include trauma, structural anomaly, repetitive motion, and poor posture.

Complete rib resection may help to prevent recurrent symptoms. Soft tissue dissection instruments, as well as rib cutters, elevators, and rongeurs, are needed.

Technique

1. Technique
2. An axillary incision is made.
3. Dissection is carried to the cervical or first rib.
4. The rib is resected.
5. A drain is placed and the incision is closed.

Discussion

The patient is placed in the lateral position with the arm abducted up to 90 degrees and suspended by an assistant or mechanical device. The skin prep includes the arm, neck, and upper chest. An incision is made between the pectoralis muscle and the latissimus dorsi muscle on the affected side. The incision is carried to the level of the cervical rib (if present) or the first rib. The ESU is used for this step of the procedure.

A self-retaining retractor is placed in the wound with several lap tapes to protect the edges. The neurovascular bundle is identified, and the rib is exposed. The midportion of the rib is dissected using a periosteal elevator.

The midportion of the rib is removed, or the entire rib can be extracted using bone shears or double action rongeurs. A small Penrose drain may be placed in the wound, which is closed using interrupted sutures of absorbable synthetic material.

DECORTICATION OF THE LUNG

Surgical Goal

Decortication of the lung is the surgical removal of a portion of the parietal pleura.

Pathology

Chronic inflammation, infection (**empyema** or tuberculosis), or a lung tumor causes the formation of exudate in the pleural space. Because of the effusion or tumor, fibrin deposits form and the parietal pleura can adhere to the chest wall. Removal of the affected pleura aids the treatment of chronic infection and eases restriction of the pleura. Pleurectomy (removal of the pleura) is performed to treat pleural cancer, such as mesothelioma.

Technique

1. The patient usually is placed in a posterolateral thoracotomy position.
2. An incision is made in the fifth intercostal space.
3. Blood clots or exudate is removed.
4. Adhesions below the parietal and visceral pleura are sharply divided.
5. When the visceral pleura is reached, the dissection is continued alternately with a gauze pledget ("sponge stick") or the fingertip until the fibrotic covering is removed sufficiently to allow full expansion of the lung.
6. Drainage tubes are inserted.
7. The incision is closed.

Discussion

A thoracotomy set is required for the lung decortication. Curettes may also be needed for removal of tough fibrous deposits.

After the thoracic incision has been made, the skin, subcutaneous tissue, and muscle are dissected with scissors and electrocautery. A rib spreader is inserted to expose the affected portion of the lung. A portion of the fifth or sixth rib may be resected with rib shears. Empyema or other fluid is drained and cultured. The anesthesia care provider expands the lung intermittently to demonstrate areas requiring additional decortication. After sufficient dissection and removal of the fibrous membrane, drainage tubes are inserted, and the incision is closed.

LUNG TRANSPLANTATION

Surgical Goal

Transplantation of one or both lungs is performed to remove a diseased lung and replace it with a donor lung. Single lung transplantation increasingly is used as a way to maximize the allocation of donor lungs. If both lungs are diseased, bilateral transplantation is indicated.

Technique

Lung Donor
1. The donor is prepped from chin to knees. (The donor may be living or deceased.)
2. A median sternotomy is performed
3. A sternal (or rib) retractor is inserted.
4. The pleura is opened longitudinally, and the pericardium is divided.
5. Umbilical tapes are placed around the aorta and the superior and inferior venae cavae.
6. Pleural adhesions are divided, and the proximal pulmonary arteries are dissected.
7. The superior vena cava is ligated with heavy silk ties.

8. The aortic arch is dissected free, and the ligamentum arteriosum (the remnant ductus arteriosus) is divided.
9. The pulmonary artery is encircled with an umbilical tape and separated from the ascending aorta.
10. Cardioplegia solution is infused through the proximal aorta into the heart via the coronary arteries; pulmoplegia solution is infused into the pulmonary organs.
11. Cardiac veins and arteries are separated, and the heart is removed and placed in a cold preservative solution.
12. The pulmonary arteries are separated from the mediastinum.
13. The trachea is dissected free.
14. The lungs are inflated and then stapled and removed.
15. The lungs are placed in a cold preservative solution.

Pathology

Single and double lung transplantation are indicated for patients with restrictive lung disease, emphysema, pulmonary hypertension, and other noninfectious end-stage pulmonary diseases.

Discussion

The donor patient is placed in the supine position, which allows the best exposure of the various organs to be excised. Procurement of lung tissue (and other organs) is a very precise procedure that requires knowledge of protocols and procedures, and problem-solving abilities. Procurement teams are self-sufficient and usually do not require equipment or instruments from the host facility, such as basic thoracic and/or cardiac instruments and supplies (e.g., cold preservative solutions and sterile containers for the organs).

Speed usually is important, because many organs have a limited period of viability. Organ transplantation is a team effort, and all members of the staff play a role in a successful transplantation outcome.

Single Lung Transplantation (Recipient)

A patient undergoing single lung transplantation is placed in the lateral position with the affected side up. A double-lumen endotracheal tube is inserted to inflate either lung selectively. Generally, the groin is prepped and exposed in case a femoro-femoral bypass is required. Thoracotomy instruments are used in single lung transplantation; cardiopulmonary bypass instruments and supplies should be available in the operating room in case bypass is required. The choice of suture materials depends on the surgeon; the previous description may be different in other institutions.

Technique

Lung Recipient
1. The patient is placed in the lateral position with the operative side up. The individual is prepped from chin to knees.
2. A thoracotomy incision is made, and a retractor is inserted.
3. If the recipient's right lung is to be removed, the pulmonary vein, pulmonary artery, and azygous vein are isolated and divided.

4. If the recipient's left lung is to be removed, the ligamentum arteriosum is divided.
5. The lung to be removed is collapsed, and the proximal pulmonary artery is occluded. If hemodynamic instability is a factor, a femorofemoral bypass may be performed.
6. The lung is removed.
7. The pulmonary veins are divided, and branches of the pulmonary artery are separated.
8. The bronchus is divided, and the diseased lung is removed.
9. The bronchus-to-bronchus anastomosis is performed with 3-0 absorbable suture.
10. The pulmonary artery–to–pulmonary artery anastomosis is performed with a running 4-0 polypropylene suture.
11. The recipient pulmonary veins are attached to the donor atrial cuff with a running 4-0 polypropylene suture.
12. The new lung is inflated and inspected.
13. Chest tubes are inserted, and hemostasis is achieved.
14. The chest is closed.
15. Bronchoscopy may be performed to suction secretions and confirm an intact anastomosis.

Techniques used during the procedure include shortening the donor bronchial stump, wrapping the anastomosis with omentum or an intercostal muscle pedicle, or performing an intussuscepting (e.g., telescoping) bronchial anastomosis technique.

Bilateral Lung Transplantation (Recipient)

Bilateral lung procedures often require cardiopulmonary support. Bypass may be avoided with the bilateral sequential technique, in which the more diseased native lung is removed first if the other lung is capable of maintaining adequate oxygenation. Femoral cannulation supplies should be readily available.

Technique

1. The patient is placed in the supine position and prepped from chin to knees. The arms are placed above the head and supported with an ether screen or similar device.
2. A bilateral anterior thoracotomy ("clam shell") incision is made.
3. If bilateral sequential transplantation is to be performed, the most functional lung is inserted first and the process is repeated on the opposite side for the second lung. This often eliminates the need for cardiopulmonary bypass.
4. If a bilateral en bloc procedure is to be performed (both donor lungs are removed and implanted as one unit), cardiopulmonary bypass usually is required.
5. Bronchial pulmonary artery and atrial anastomoses are performed as described for single lung procedures.
6. The procedure is completed as described for single lung transplant.

Postoperative Considerations

Complications include rejection and infection. Transplant anastomoses may require repair if persistent bleeding develops. Lung biopsies are done in the postoperative period to detect possible rejection.

CHAPTER SUMMARY

- The respiratory system is divided into upper and lower tracts. The upper respiratory tract is composed of the nose, nasal sinuses, pharynx, and larynx. The lower respiratory tract is composed of the trachea, bronchial tree, and lungs.
- The nasal sinuses are bilateral structures, each composed of three tiers of bony projections called the *conchae* or *turbinates*.
- The pharynx lies behind the oral cavity and communicates with the nasal cavities. It is subdivided into sections: the oropharynx, nasopharynx, and laryngopharynx or larynx.
- The palatine tonsils (tonsils) are located in the oropharynx. The pharyngeal tonsils, or adenoids, are located in the nasopharynx.
- The larynx connects the trachea with the oropharynx. It contains the vocal cords and prevents food and other foreign bodies from entering the trachea.
- The epiglottis is a cartilaginous structure that functions as a flap to close the entrance to the trachea during swallowing.
- The epiglottis often is confused with the uvula, which is the visible projection of epithelial tissue extending from the soft palate of the mouth.
- The trachea begins at the larynx and branches into two main airways, the right and left primary bronchi and bronchial tree.
- The trachea branches into the right and left primary bronchi at the carina. Because the right bronchus is straighter than the left, inhaled foreign material is more likely to enter the right lung.
- Cartilaginous rings support the primary bronchi.
- The bronchioles are composed of smooth muscle lined with epithelium. Bronchioles terminate in small ducts, alveolar sacs, and individual alveoli. An alveolus exchanges incoming oxygen molecules with carbon dioxide molecules from the blood.
- The lung is divided into anatomical regions. The right lung has three lobes, and the left lung has two lobes.
- Each lung is enclosed in a pleural cavity and covered by a double membrane, the pleural sac. The outer membrane forms the parietal pleura, which lines the thoracic cavity and outer mediastinal walls. The inner or visceral pleura covers the lungs.
- The pleural space normally maintains negative pressure in relation to atmospheric air and the alveoli.
- When the diaphragm contracts (inhalation), the potential space between the two pleural membranes is decreased and air is pulled into the airways and lungs.
- Diagnostic tests for the respiratory system assess the function of the lungs, thoracic space, and bronchial system.
- Pulmonary function tests (PFTs) are a specific group of procedures that measure lung function.
- Among the most important blood tests for pulmonary function is determination of arterial blood gases (ABGs). In this test, arterial blood is assessed for oxygen and carbon dioxide levels and pH (acid-base balance).
- The incisions most commonly used in pulmonary surgery are posterolateral and anterolateral thoracotomy with the patient in the lateral position.
- Negative pressure in the thoracic cavity is lost when the chest wall and pleura are open or punctured. This occurs during trauma and thoracic surgery. For the lungs to expand, negative pressure must be restored. This is done by means of closed chest drainage, also called *closed underwater drainage*.
- A patient with chest drainage must be moved carefully so that the chest tubes are not disrupted. The closed drainage system must never be raised above the level of the patient's chest.
- Video-assisted thorascopic surgery is minimally invasive surgery of the thoracic cavity.
- During lung volume reduction surgery, portions of a damaged lung are removed to improve pulmonary function.
- Bronchoscopy is the insertion of a flexible fiberoptic or rigid telescope into the trachea and bronchi for assessment purposes or to perform a surgical procedure. Rigid bronchoscopy generally is used only for removal of a large amount of tissue or a foreign body.
- Lobectomy is the removal of a lobe of the lung; pneumonectomy is the removal of the entire lung.
- Thoracic outlet syndrome is a rare condition in which the subclavian vessels and the brachial plexus are compressed at the apex of the thorax. The condition is relieved by rib resection.
- Decortication of the lung is the surgical removal of a portion of the parietal pleura for the treatment of fibrosis.
- In lung transplantation, a diseased lung (or both lungs) is removed and replaced with a donor lung. Single lung transplantation increasingly is performed as a means of maximizing the allocation of donor lungs.

REVIEW QUESTIONS

1. Explain the process of breathing, including the influence of negative pressure in the thoracic cavity.
2. Why must a closed chest drainage unit be kept lower than the patient's body?
3. What is the difference between lobectomy, pneumonectomy, and segmental resection?
4. What is the difference between thoracotomy and thoracostomy?
5. Explain pneumothorax and why it occurs.
6. What is the purpose of debulking a tumor?
7. What instruments are needed to perform a rib resection?
8. What is the Valsalva maneuver? What is the affect of this maneuver on the heart rate?

Cardiac Surgery

CHAPTER OUTLINE

LEARNING OBJECTIVES

After studying this chapter the reader will be able to:

- Discuss the pathology associated with surgical procedures of the heart
- Identify common incisions used in cardiac surgery
- Identify the instrumentation and equipment used in cardiac surgery
- Explain the rationale for cardiopulmonary bypass
- Describe common cardiac procedures

TERMINOLOGY

Aneurysm: A bulge in an artery caused by weakening of the arterial wall. The weakening may be a congenital defect or the result of atherosclerosis, arteriosclerosis, infection, trauma, or degenerative disease.

Apex: The lower left tip of the left ventricle of the heart; also, the rounded upper portion of each lung.

Arrhythmia: An abnormal heartbeat (also called *dysrhythmia*).

Arteriosclerosis: Disease of the arteries characterized by loss of elasticity and hardening of the arterial walls.

Atherosclerosis: A disease characterized by the buildup of cholesterol deposits in the arterial lining.

Bradycardia: A slow heart rate (usually a heart rate under 60 beats per minute).

Cardiac cycle: The pumping action of the heart from one beat to the next.

Cardioplegia: Intentional stopping of the heart during cardiac surgery. This is achieved with a cardioplegic solution, which often contains a mixture of potassium chloride, lidocaine, dextrose, insulin, albumin, tromethamine, and Plasmanate.

Coarctation: A congenital narrowing or stricture in the descending thoracic aorta.

Congenital: A condition present at birth.

Cross-clamp: To place a clamp across a structure (usually a blood vessel) to occlude it.

Diastole: That phase of the cardiac cycle when the ventricles contract.

Endovascular repair: Endoscopic surgery of the vascular system.

Fibrillation: Uncoordinated muscular activity in the heart muscle, which results in "quivering" rather than pumping action. This results in pooling of blood.

Fusiform aneurysm: A type of aneurysm that involves the entire circumference of a blood vessel.

Heart lung machine: Medical device used during cardiac bypass. Systemic blood is shunted out of the body via cannulae, which are implanted in the heart. The device collects the blood, removes excess carbon dioxide, oxygenates it, and returns it to the body through separate cannulae.

Infarction: Necrosis and death of tissue related to obstruction of blood flow.

Ischemia: Reduced blood supply to tissue. Ischemia may be a result of obstruction within the blood vessels or external pressure, which acts as a tourniquet.

Mediastinum: An enclosed cavity in the chest that contains the heart, large vessels, trachea, esophagus, and lymph nodes.

Off-pump procedure: A procedure performed without a cardio-pulmonary bypass (i.e., "the pump").

Pacemaker: A device that stimulates the heart muscle to contract.

Preclotting: The process of soaking a graft or patch of synthetic graft material in the patient's blood or plasma before insertion. Most grafts no longer need preclotting.

Saccular aneurysm: A type of aneurysm in which a saclike formation with a narrow neck projects from the side of the artery.

Shunt: To bypass a structure or carry fluid from one anatomical location to another.

Stenosis: The narrowing of a hollow structure such as a blood vessel or duct.

Sternotomy: An incision made into the sternum.

Systole: The relaxation phase of the cardiac cycle when the ventricles are filling with blood.

Tachycardia: A fast heart rate (usually over 120 beats per minute).

Thoracotomy: An incision made into the thoracic cavity.

INTRODUCTION

Cardiac surgery includes procedures of the heart and associated great vessels performed to treat acquired or **congenital** disease. Open techniques and minimally invasive endoscopic procedures are used. The techniques used in cardiac surgery build on those used in thoracic, general, and vascular procedures. However, cardiac procedures generally are more complex and require equipment not used in other specialties (e.g., cardiac bypass). The surgical technologist may become a specialist in cardiac surgery after training in general, peripheral vascular, and thoracic surgery. This specialty requires a thorough understanding of cardiothoracic anatomy and cardiac function, as well as the ability to work in a complex surgical environment with multiple technologies.

SURGICAL ANATOMY

The thoracic cavity contains the heart and its great vessels, the lungs and their associated respiratory structures, the mediastinum, and a portion of the esophagus.

HEART

The heart is a muscular organ that consists of four hollow spaces, or chambers. The two upper chambers are the right atrium and the left atrium; the two lower chambers are the right ventricle and the left ventricle (Figure 33-1). The heart is contained within a closed cavity called the **mediastinum**, between the two lungs, posterior to the sternum, and anterior to the vertebrae and esophagus. Most of the heart lies to the left of the midline.

The heart is enclosed by a double-layered membrane called the *pericardium*. Pericardial fluid between the outer parietal and inner visceral pericardium lubricates the layers and prevents friction. The walls of the heart have three layers: the outer epicardium, the middle myocardium, and the inner endocardium. Myocardium is specialized muscle tissue (cardiac muscle) capable of generating electrical impulses, which cause the heart to contract.

The heart's four chambers are divided by a septum (Figure 33-2). The right ventricle receives deoxygenated blood from the right atrium. From the right ventricle, the blood is pumped through the pulmonary artery to the lungs, where it is oxygenated. The left ventricle receives oxygenated blood from the left atrium. From the left ventricle, the blood is pumped into the aorta and the systemic circulation. The valves of the heart maintain one-way flow through the cardiac chambers.

The heart's own blood supply is delivered by the coronary artery circulation (Figure 33-3).

HEART VALVES

The valves of the heart maintain unidirectional blood flow. The atria are separated from the ventricles by the atrioventricular (AV) valves. The tricuspid valve lies on the right side, and the bicuspid (mitral) valve lies on the left side. The leaflets of the valves open as blood is pumped and close when the pressure on the other side of the valve exceeds the entry pressure. The AV valve leaflets are attached to the papillary muscle of the ventricles by connective tissue called *chordae tendineae*. The large vessels of the heart also have valves. The semilunar valves connect the ventricles to the large vessels. The pulmonary valve connects the right ventricle with the pulmonary artery. The left aortic valve connects the left ventricle to the aorta.

CARDIAC CYCLE

The pumping action of the heart from one beat to the next is called the cardiac cycle. The cycle occurs in two phases, systole and diastole. During systole, the ventricles contract; in diastole, they relax and fill with blood. The cycle is fully defined by the electrical impulses that occur in specific areas of the heart, the muscular activity, and the flow of blood through the chambers and vessels. The electrical activity of each cycle is demonstrated on an electrocardiogram (ECG). The complete cycle is shown in Figure 33-4.

CONDUCTION SYSTEM

The electrical conduction system contains a network of specialized cells, which generate electrical activity along conduction pathways. These cells, which are found in several areas of the heart, transmit nerve signals that cause the heart muscle to contract in a coordinated way.

The sinoatrial (SA) node initiates the cardiac cycle and is sometimes called the heart's pacemaker. Impulses travel from the SA node to the AV node in the interatrial septum. From the AV node, they travel to the bundle of His at the AV junction. Conduction continues through the right and left bundle

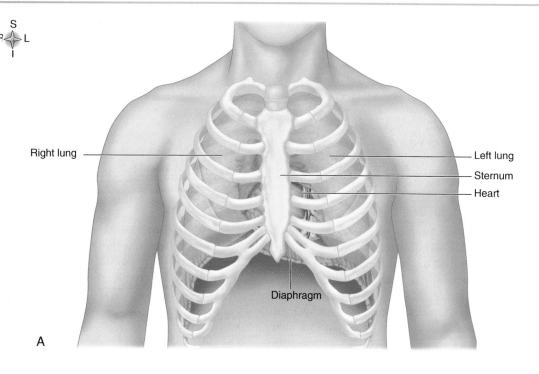

Right lung

Left lung

Sternum

Heart

Diaphragm

A

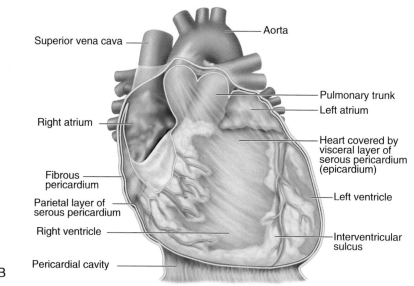

Superior vena cava

Aorta

Right atrium

Pulmonary trunk

Left atrium

Heart covered by visceral layer of serous pericardium (epicardium)

Fibrous pericardium

Parietal layer of serous pericardium

Right ventricle

Left ventricle

Interventricular sulcus

Pericardial cavity

B

Figure 33-1 **A,** Location of the heart in the thoracic cavity. **B,** Anterior view showing the heart in relation to the lungs. **C,** Detail of the heart with the pericardial sac open. *(From Thibodeau G, Patton K: Anatomy and physiology, ed 6, St Louis, 2007, Mosby.)*

branches, ventricular walls, and Purkinje fibers. Disease or interference in the conduction system results in uncoordinated electrical activity in the cardiac muscle and may cause ineffective contractions. The conduction system is illustrated in Figure 33-5.

PATHOLOGY OF THE HEART

Table 33-1 presents common pathological conditions of the heart.

DIAGNOSTIC PROCEDURES

Before surgery, the patient undergoes diagnostic studies to identify pathological conditions or anomalies. Many of these studies are performed in the interventional radiology department, and the surgical technologist occasionally may be involved in the procedures. Cardiac function tests may require sophisticated imaging techniques, injection of radionuclide, and physical stress tests.

Routine laboratory tests are performed to identify abnormalities of the blood, urine, cardiac enzymes, and waste

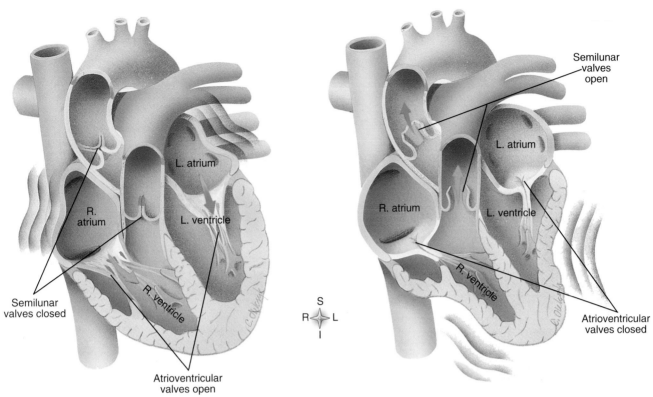

Figure 33-2 Chambers and valves of the heart. *(From Thibodeau G, Patton K: Anatomy and physiology, ed 6, St Louis, 2007, Mosby.)*

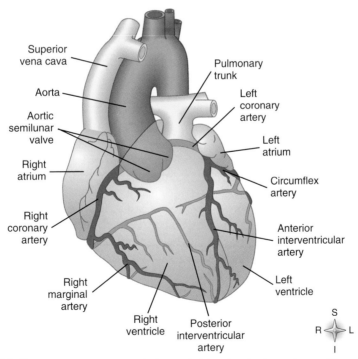

Figure 33-3 Coronary arteries, which supply blood to the heart tissue. *(From Thibodeau G, Patton K: Anatomy and physiology, ed 6, St Louis, 2007, Mosby.)*

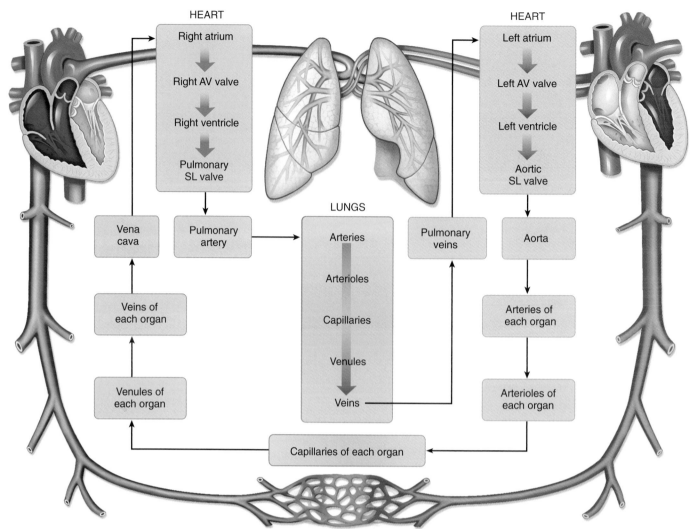

Figure 33-4   Cardiac cycle. *(From Thibodeau G, Patton K: Anatomy and physiology, ed 6, St Louis, 2007, Mosby.)*

products, which may indicate myocardial damage. Common tests are listed in Box 33-1.

CARDIAC CATHETERIZATION

Cardiac catheterization is an interventional radiology procedure that involves insertion of a cardiac catheter into the heart chambers and large vessels via a peripheral artery or vein. Specific tests are then performed inside the heart and vessels, such as intravascular ultrasonography, angiography (including coronary artery imaging), and endocardial biopsy.

Left heart catheterization most often is performed to assess the coronary arteries, systemic vascular resistance, aortic and mitral valve function, and left ventricular pressure. These tests are performed through a percutaneous puncture of the femoral, radial, or brachial artery, with catheterization through these vessels.

Right heart catheterization is performed to assess the right atrium and ventricle and the pulmonary artery. Pulmonary artery occlusion pressure (PAOP) is a significant test that determines cardiac volume and output. Valve function may also be tested through right heart catheterization. In this pro-

cedure, a catheter is inserted percutaneously through the femoral, subclavian, or internal jugular vein, advanced into the right atrium, and then advanced farther, into the pulmonary artery, via the tricuspid valve, right ventricle, and pulmonary valve.

Cardiac imaging has become increasingly complex in the past 10 years. In addition to standard angiography, in which a contrast medium is injected to obtain real-time images of the cardiac system, digital subtraction angiography also is used. In this process only the vessels and chambers in which contrast medium is injected are shown on the fluoroscopic image. All other tissues are masked or subtracted. Aortic imaging is performed for the assessment of **coarctation** of the aorta, valve regurgitation, congenital anomalies, and **aneurysm**. Ventricular angiography demonstrates the movement of blood through the valves and can be used to measure the ejection fraction (the amount of blood pumped from the ventricles) and end systolic and end diastolic volumes. Cardiac imaging data are shown in Table 33-2.

Intravascular ultrasound is performed with an end-catheter transducer, which can be advanced into the lumen of the blood vessel to determine the rate of blood flow.

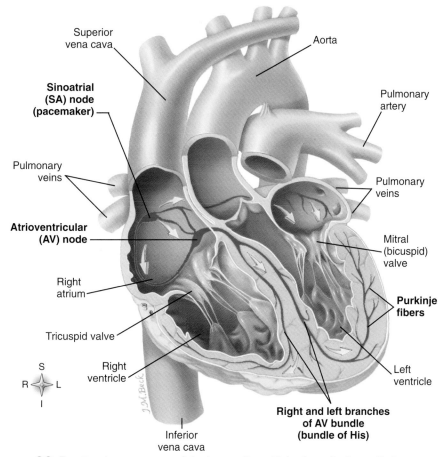

Figure 33-5 Conduction system of the heart. *(From Thibodeau G, Patton K:* Anatomy and physiology, *ed 6, St Louis, 2007, Mosby.)*

Table 33-1

Pathology of the Heart

Condition	Description	Considerations
Aneurysm	A weakening in the wall of an artery or heart chamber, leading to thinning and ballooning. This can lead to separation of the vessel or chamber walls or complete rupture. Aneurysm is associated with atherosclerosis, arteriosclerosis, infection, and congenital defects in the tissue.	Medical treatment to reduce hypertension usually is the initial treatment unless rupture is impending. (See Resection of a Left Ventricular Aneurysm.)
Atherosclerosis	A type of arteriosclerosis (hardening of the arteries) that results in stiffness and loss of function; characterized by the formation of fibrous fatty deposits in the intimal layer of medium and large blood vessels. Risk factors include hypercholesterolemia, age, and a family history of the disease.	Atherosclerosis affects the blood vessels and heart tissue, causing vascular obstruction, tissue ischemia, and weakened vessel walls. Any organ can be affected by the disease. Cardiac involvement is seen in coronary artery disease. (See Coronary Artery Bypass Grafting.)
Atrial fibrillation (AF)	Cells in the atrium quiver (rather than contract in an effective manner). The atria do not contribute to efficient filling of the ventricles. Stasis of blood also occurs, which can create a thrombus that can embolize.	Medical management is first attempted; a patient with prolonged AF may undergo surgery to redirect the impulses. (See Surgery for Atrial Fibrillation [Cardiac Ablation].)
Bradycardia	Portions of the conduction system may not function because of aging, infection, toxicity, or trauma, causing the heart rate to become too slow (under 60 beats per minute) to provide adequate blood flow to the tissues.	Treatment includes insertion of a pacemaker to provide a heart rate that is high enough to provide adequate blood flow to the tissues. (See Insertion of an Artificial Cardiac Pacemaker.)

Continued

Table 33-1

Pathology of the Heart—cont'd

Condition	Description	Considerations
Congenital anomalies of the heart	Some congenital anomalies involve defects (i.e., missing tissue) between the atrial and ventricular septa. If the defect is large, blood flow to the lungs is increased (which can develop into pulmonary hypertension), or mixing of oxygenated and unoxygenated blood occurs, which can reduce the amount of oxygen delivered to the cells.	Some small defects close spontaneously. If the child fails to thrive, surgery may be required to correct the defect. (Refer to Chapter 34.)
Congestive heart failure (CHF)	A condition in which the heart is unable to eject a sufficient amount of blood to perfuse the body's tissues.	Severe CHF requires surgery. (See Insertion and Removal of an Intraaortic Balloon Catheter and Heart Transplantation.)
Coronary artery disease (CAD)	In CAD, scarring of the arterial wall, calcification, thrombosis, and uptake of cholesterol results in decreased blood flow to the heart muscle. This can cause myocardial infarction, angina, conduction defects, and death. The cause in most cases is atherosclerosis.	Conservative treatment includes lifestyle modifications and drug therapy. Surgery is required to restore function to the heart and blood vessels. (See Coronary Artery Bypass Grafting.)
Infection	Infection of the lining of the heart and valves usually is caused by streptococcal and staphylococcal bacteria. Infections can lead to significant tissue destruction, requiring valve replacement, and may be fatal.	Early diagnosis and antibacterial treatment may prevent permanent cardiac damage. Valve replacement may be necessary.
Myocardial infarction (MI)	Blockage in one or more coronary arteries can produce myocardial infarction. This is vascular blockage of an area of the heart, resulting in tissue death and cessation of effective heart contraction.	Treatment includes excising ischemic or infracted portions of the myocardium. (See Resection of a Left Ventricular Aneurysm.)
Neoplasm	Primary tumors of the heart are rare. Sarcomas (malignant) and myxomas (nonmalignant) are the most common types.	Operable tumors are removed surgically to restore function.
Pericardial effusion	Excess fluid in the pericardium compresses the heart and restricts ventricular filling.	Fluid may be surgically removed to restore cardiac function. (See Creation of a Pericardial Window.)
Pericarditis	Chronic inflammation of the pericardium may result in fibrosis or calcification of the pericardium. This restricts the heart's ability to fill.	Removal of the fibrotic covering over the heart improves cardiac function. (See Pericardiectomy.)
Rheumatic heart disease	An immune-mediated disease occurring after group A beta-hemolytic streptococcal throat infection. The disease is a significant factor in the cause of chronic heart valve disease and endocarditis. It mostly affects school-aged children.	Valve injury related to rheumatic fever may require valve replacement. (See discussions of valve replacement surgeries.)
Trauma	Trauma by intentional injury or accident is an important source of cardiac pathology.	Emergency surgery is required for life-threatening injury.
Valve regurgitation	The aortic and mitral valves produce back flow into the preceding chamber when the leaflets (or other portions of the valve) are stretched, torn, or ruptured. In some valves, changes in the valvular tissue produce a weakening of the valve components.	Mitral and tricuspid valves may be repaired; they may require replacement if they are severely diseased. Aortic valves commonly require replacement with a prosthetic valve. (See Mitral Commissurotomy.)
Valve stenosis	The aortic and mitral valves may become narrowed (stenosis) as a result of increased calcification, fibrosis, rheumatic fever, or hypertension.	Mitral and tricuspid valves may require replacement if repair is not feasible. Aortic valves commonly require replacement with a prosthetic valve. (See discussions of valve replacement surgeries.)
Ventricular tachycardia/ ventricular fibrillation	Cardiac muscle that has been damaged by disease may be easily triggered to beat abnormally fast (tachycardia), or to quiver rather than beat (fibrillation).	Medical treatment often is attempted; if it is unsuccessful, an internal defibrillator is inserted. (See Insertion of an Implantable Cardioverter-Defibrillator.)

Box 33-1

Cardiac Diagnostic Tests

Resting electrocardiogram (ECG)
Exercise ECG (stress test)
Chest radiography
Echocardiogram
Radionucleotide scanning
Computed tomography (CT) scan
Positron emission tomography (PET) scan with or without stress test
Magnetic resonance imaging (MRI) and magnetic resonance angiography (MRA)
Pulmonary function tests
Aortography
Electrophysiology
Cardiac catheterization
Endomyocardial biopsy
Mediastinoscopy

Table 33-2

Angiographic Data

Angiographic Data	Findings
Coronary arteries	Anatomy/function of the coronary vascular bed, distal coronary flow, atrioventricular (AV) fistula, atherosclerosis, anomalous origin of coronary arteries
Ventriculography	Anatomy/function of ventricles and associated structures, left ventricular (LV) aneurysm, congenital abnormalities, valvular stenosis/regurgitation, shunts
Valvular angiography	Intact mitral/tricuspid complex, valvular incompetence/stenosis/regurgitation
Pulmonary angiography	Pulmonary embolism, congenital abnormalities
Aortography	Patency of aortic branches; normal mobility, competence, and anatomy of aortic valve; aneurysms (saccular, fusiform); origin of aortic dissection; shunts or anomalous connections; congenital defects or obstructions

Modified from Pagana KD, Pagana TJ: *Mosby's diagnostic and laboratory test reference*, ed 7, St Louis, 2005, Elsevier/Mosby.

Oxygen saturation can be measured at various points in the heart and large vessels during catheterization. This information determines whether blood is being shunted (taking an abnormal route).

Cardiac output is measured by calculating the amount of blood ejected through the heart per minute.

Cardiac muscle biopsy is performed to detect tissue rejection after heart transplantation.

PERIOPERATIVE CONSIDERATIONS

POSITIONING

Procedures of the heart and associated structures are performed with the patient in the supine or lateral position with the affected side up. The following are the incisions most commonly used in open cardiac surgery:

- Median **sternotomy** (supine): A partial or full midline incision is made through the sternum.
- Paramedian (supine): The incision is made to the right or left of the sternum. This position is used for minimally invasive procedures and lymph node biopsy.
- Anterolateral, posterolateral: This is a modification of the lateral position in which the patient is supine with soft padding under the hip and shoulder of the affected side. This rolls the thorax slightly upward. The shoulder of the affected side then is abducted, and the arm is suspended safely on an overhead table brace.
- Minithoracotomy (supine): The 2-inch (5 cm) right or left minithoracotomy is made between the ribs for access during minimally invasive and robotic procedures.

Common thoracic incisions are described in Table 33-3.

INSTRUMENTS

Cardiac surgery requires a general surgery set augmented with cardiac instruments, general thoracic instruments (including stapling devices), and lung instruments, depending on the procedure. Specific instruments for coronary artery, valve, aneurysm, chest wall, and lung surgery may be added (Figure 33-6). Instrumentation can be quite complex, requiring experience and advanced organizational skills to anticipate the steps of a procedure.

The Rumel tourniquet, commonly used in cardiovascular surgery, is a short length of rubber tubing either commercially prepared or cut from a straight (Robinson) urinary catheter. The tourniquet is threaded over cannulation sutures to help hold them in place. The Rumel tourniquet also is used when large vessels are occluded or isolated with a vessel loop or umbilical tape (a length of cotton passed under a vessel for retraction). A stylet, such as that from a Rumel tourniquet, is used to snare the strands of suture or tape and bring them through the lumen of the tubing. The tubing is tightened against the cannula or vessel by pulling on the strands, which are held using a hemostat placed at the upper end.

Coronary Artery Instruments

Coronary artery instruments are extremely delicate. They include scissors, forceps, and needle holders, which are similar to routine vascular instruments. Many are angled at the tips.

Minimally invasive coronary procedures require longer instruments with the same precision tips. In off-pump coronary anastomosis, a flexible, suction-tip coronary stabilizing device can be positioned on either side of the coronary artery to minimize cardiac movement. Figure 33-7 shows the stabilizer attached to a sternal retractor and an apical suction device to expose the posterolateral heart.

Table 33-3

Thoracic Incisions

Incision	Position	Indications	Special Patient Needs
Median sternotomy: Incision down the center of the sternum	Supine	Most adult cardiac procedures except those on branch pulmonary arteries, distal transverse aortic arch, and descending thoracic aorta; OPCAB	Padding for the hands, elbows, feet, back of head, and dependent bony prominences
Ministernotomy: Partial upper or lower sternal incision starting either from the sternal notch or the xiphoid process and extending to the midportion of the sternum; lower end sternal splitting (LESS)	Supine	MAS, on-CPB or off-CPB procedures	Same as for a median sternotomy
Parasternotomy: Resection of the right or left costal cartilages (from the second to the fifth cartilage, depending on the surgical target)	Supine; a small roll may be placed under the affected side	Left: MAS CABG Right: MAS CABG, valve procedures	Same as for a median sternotomy; risk of postoperative chest wall instability
Anterolateral thoracotomy: Curvilinear incision along the subpectoral groove to the axillary line	Supine with a pad or pillow under the operative site; arm on the affected side is supported in a sling or overarm board; the arm on the unaffected side may be tucked along the side	MAS, MIDCAB, trauma to the anterior pericardium and left ventricle; repeat sternotomy	Padding for extremities; pillow or other device to elevate the affected side; armboard or sling for the arm on the affected side
Left anterior small thoracotomy (LAST), right anterior minithoracotomy: Curvilinear incision along the subpectoral groove, right or left side	Supine with a small roll under the affected side	Left: MAS, MIDCAB Right: MAS valve procedures or CABG	Same as anterolateral thoracotomy
Lateral thoracotomy: Curvilinear incision along the costochondral junction anteriorly to the posterior border of the scapula	Placed on the side with the arms extended and the axilla and head supported; the knees and legs are protected	Lung biopsies; first rib resection; lobectomy	Armboard, overarm board, axillary roll, padding for extremities, pillow between the legs; sandbags, straps, wide tape, or other devices to support the torso
Posterolateral thoracotomy: Curvilinear incision from the subpectoral crease below the nipple, extended laterally and posteriorly along the ribs almost to the posterior midline below the scapula (the location of the intercostal incision depends on the surgical site); used less often with the availability of VATS techniques	Lateral with the arms extended and the axilla and head supported; the knees and legs are protected	First rib resection; lobectomy	Similar to needs for a lateral thoracotomy
Transsternal bilateral anterior thoracotomy (clamshell): Submammary incision extending from one anterior axillary line to the other across the sternum at the fourth interspace	Supine	Lung transplantation; emergency access to the heart when a sternal saw is not available	Same as median sternotomy; requires transection of left and right IMA

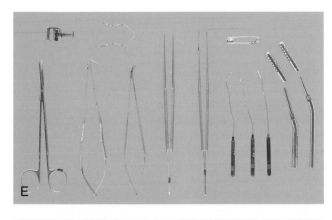

E

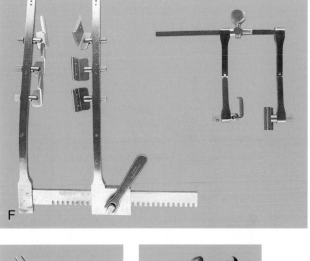

F

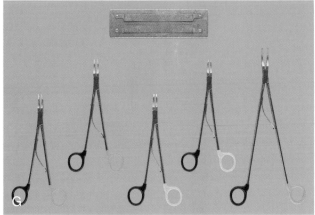

G

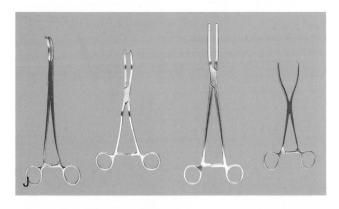

J

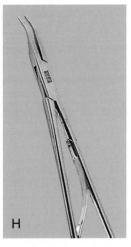

H

I

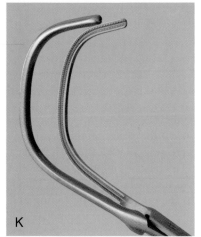

K

L

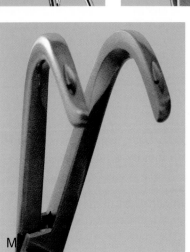

M

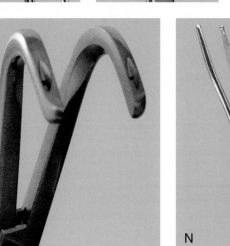

N

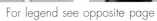

For legend see opposite page

Figure 33-6, cont'd *E,* *Top, left to right,* 1 tubing clamp; 1 Parsonnet epicardial (self-retaining spring) retractor, sharp, 3 × 3 prongs; 1 safety pin with rings. *Bottom, left to right,* 1 Snowden-Pencer scissors, straight; 1 Yasargil scissors, bayonet handle, 125-degree angle; 1 You-Potts scissors, fine, thin 10-mm blades, 45-degree angle; 2 Snowden-Pencer dressing forceps, 8 inch; 3 Garrett dilators: 2 mm, 1 mm, and 1.5 mm; 2 metal coronary suction tubes with tips. *F, Left to right,* 1 Ankeney sternal retractor; 1 Himmelstein sternal retractor. *G, Top,* 1, hemoclip cartridge base. *Bottom, left to right,* 5 Weck EZ Load hemoclip appliers: 2 medium, 7.75 inch; 2 small, 7.75 inch; 1 large, 10.75 inch and tip. *H,* Close-up of Weck hemoclip applier. *I,* Semb ligature-carrying forceps, 9 inch; *J, Left to right,* 1 Semb ligature-carrying forceps, 9 inch; 1 Lambert-Kay aorta clamp; 1 Fogarty clamp-applying forceps, angled; 1 bulldog clamp applier. *K,* Lambert-Kay aorta clamp. *L,* Fogarty clamp-applying forceps, angled. *M,* Semb ligature-carrying forceps, close-up of tip. *N,* Bulldog clamp applier. *(From Tighe SM: Instrumentation for the operating room, ed 6, St Louis, 2003, Mosby.)*

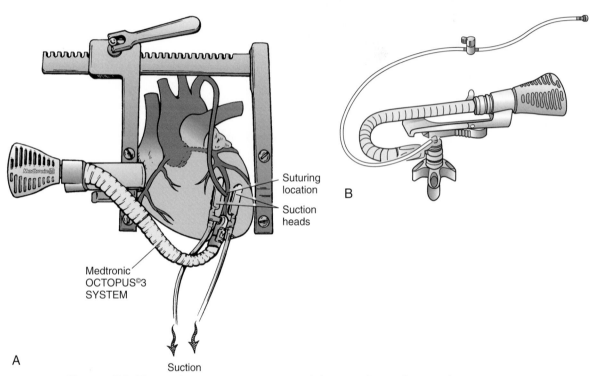

Figure 33-7 **A,** The Octopus 3 coronary stabilizer attaches to the sternal retractor proximally and immobilizes the coronary artery. The device uses suction pads to minimize tissue motion at the anastomosis site. **B,** The Starfish left ventricular suction device holds the left ventricle apex and allows it to be retracted for access to lateral and posterior coronary arteries. *(From Seifert PC: Cardiac surgery: perioperative patient care, St Louis, 2002, Mosby.)*

Disposable, adhesive defibrillator patches may be used during repeat sternotomy or minimally invasive procedures.

Fibrillator

The temporary pacing wires attached to the alligator cables (used for temporary pacing) may also be used with a fibrillator to create fine fibrillation of the heart. The wires are connected to the fibrillator power source, and the heart is fibrillated (causing it to quiver) during repair of a leaking anastomosis. After the air is removed or the repair is completed, the heart is defibrillated.

Cardiopulmonary Bypass

The heart-lung machine takes the place of the heart and lungs by pumping and perfusing blood, which has been shunted outside the body. The heart-lung pump collects the blood, removes excess carbon dioxide, oxygenates the blood, and returns it to the body (Figure 33-11). The tubing and oxygenator for the heart-lung machine are assembled and primed by a perfusionist (pump technician). Sterile cannulas, which **shunt** the blood away from the heart, are delivered to the scrub, who prepares them for surgical insertion into the heart.

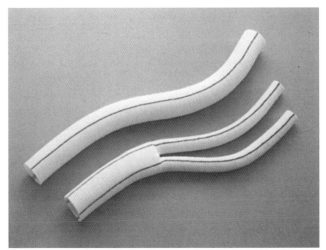

Figure 33-8 Straight and bifurcated arterial tube grafts. *(From Rothrock JC: Alexander's care of the patient in surgery, ed 12, St Louis, 2003, Mosby.)*

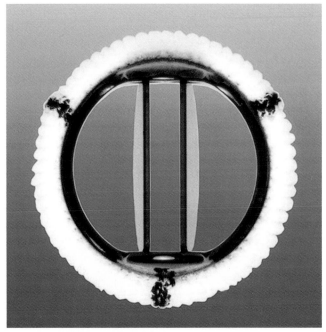

Figure 33-9 St. Jude Medical bileaflet valve prosthesis. *(From Rothrock JC: Alexander's care of the patient in surgery, ed 12, St Louis, 2003, Mosby.)*

The surgical technologist should be familiar with the basic function and operation of the pump. This includes the size of the pump lines and how they connect to the patient. The scrub should also know which lines infuse blood and which remove blood, as well as the types of cannulas and catheters.

- *Venous cannula:* Straight ended and has multiple holes in the distal tip. This type of cannula is used to shunt blood from the heart. A two-stage venous cannula also has openings in the midportion of the catheter.
- *Aortic cannula:* May have a straight or an angled tip to direct the blood toward the descending thoracic aorta. This cannula carries oxygenated (arterial) blood.
- *Femoral arterial cannula:* Also carries oxygenated (arterial) blood, is tapered to match the size of the artery, and has a beveled end to allow easier insertion.
- *Coronary antegrade perfusion cannula:* Has a cuff near its tip to prevent the cannula from being inserted too far into the coronary arteries. It is used to infuse cardioplegic solution directly into the heart; a retrograde cannula is placed in the great cardiac vein.
- *Left ventricular sump (vent) catheter:* Drains air and blood within the heart and prevents the accumulation of blood, which can cause distention of the ventricle and injure the heart muscle.
- *Right superior pulmonary vent catheter:* Also used to decompress the left ventricle and remove intracardiac air.

DRUGS

Heparin

Heparin sodium is an anticoagulant that prevents the conversion of fibrinogen to fibrin, an essential part of the body's clotting mechanism. The drug does not dissolve blood clots, but only prevents them from forming. It is administered through a large vein or the right atrium before cannulation for cardiopulmonary bypass or before a blood vessel is occluded. It prevents clot formation in the bypass circuit while the patient is on the heart-lung machine. The drug dosage is calculated according to body weight. Heparin also is distributed to the surgical technologist for local use on the field.

Protamine Sulfate

Protamine sulfate is administered to reverse the anticoagulant effects of heparin. Intravenous protamine is administered after bypass has been completed and the cannulas have been removed. Some patients have a reaction to protamine, and the surgeon may elect to allow heparin reversal to proceed without it.

Lidocaine

Lidocaine (Xylocaine) 1% is commonly used in the treatment of ventricular **arrhythmia**. This drug controls particular rhythmic patterns, including premature ventricular contractions and ventricular **tachycardia**. These arrhythmias can develop into ventricular fibrillation in which the heart stops beating and instead quivers without coordination, effectively stopping circulation.

Epinephrine

Epinephrine has many actions, including cardiac stimulation. Under normal circumstances, it cannot start a heart that has stopped beating, but it can stimulate the adrenergic receptors in the heart.

Cardioplegic Solution

Cardioplegia is the intentional interruption of the heart's pumping action. A cardioplegic solution may contain a

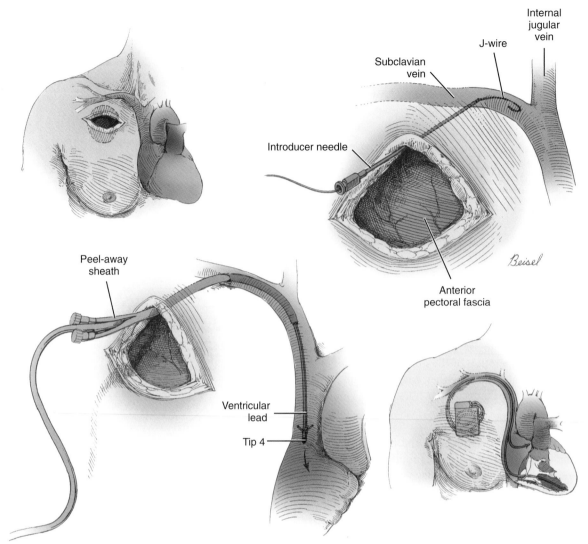

Figure 33-10 Insertion of a pacemaker. **A,** A transverse incision is made for the skin pocket. **B,** Needle insertion into the subclavian vein is performed to introduce the J-tip guide wire. **C,** The pacing electrode is introduced and advanced into the right ventricle. **D,** Completion of the pacemaker procedure, with the pulse generator placed in the pocket. (Modified from Waldhausen JA, Pierce WS, Campbell DB: Surgery of the chest, ed 6, St Louis, 1996, Mosby.)

mixture of potassium chloride, lidocaine, dextrose, insulin, albumin, tromethamine, and Plasmanate. The exact type and amount of the drugs in the solution vary. The solution may be cooled or warmed for administration.

A cardioplegic solution is administered by two methods. In antegrade cardioplegic infusion (after the aortic **cross-clamp** has been applied), a needle is placed in the aorta (proximal to the aortic clamp) where it exits the left ventricle (the aortic "root"). The cardioplegic solution is infused into the aorta. It then flows into the right and left coronary openings and into the coronary circulation. In retrograde cardioplegic infusion, a catheter is placed in the coronary sinus of the right atrium and into the great cardiac vein. The cardioplegic solution is then infused into the coronary venous system.

SURGICAL PROCEDURES

MEDIAN STERNOTOMY

Surgical Goal

A median sternotomy is a midline incision used for surgical procedures of the heart and great vessels in the thoracic cavity.

Technique

Thoracotomy

1. The surgeon makes a midline thoracic incision.
2. The xyphoid is divided.
3. The sternum is divided.

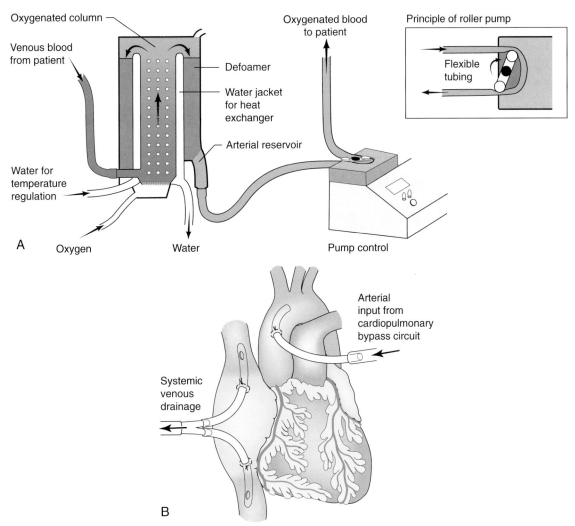

Figure 33-11 **A,** Schematic of cardiac bypass (heart-lung machine). **B,** Cannulation of the heart. *(From Garden O, Bradbury A, Forsythe J, Parks R: Principles and practice of surgery, ed 5, Edinburgh, 2007, Elsevier/Churchill Livingstone.)*

Discussion

The patient is placed in the supine position, prepped, and draped for a midline thoracic incision. The surgeon makes a midline incision from the sternal notch to 2 to 3 inches (5 to 7.5 cm) below the xyphoid. The subcutaneous tissue and linea alba (the fascial layer distal to the xyphoid) is divided with the knife or electrosurgical unit (ESU). The surgeon digitally separates the underlying tissue from the sternal notch and xyphoid. The xyphoid then is divided on the midline with heavy curved scissors. A sternal saw is placed in the center of the xyphoid or sternal notch, and the bone is divided.

The assistant elevates the raw edges of the sternum with handheld retractors (e.g., Army-Navy retractors) while the surgeon coagulates bleeders with the ESU. A small amount of bone wax may be applied to the bone edges.

Before placing a self-retaining retractor, the surgeon protects the edges of the incision with towels or moist laparotomy sponges. The retractor then is opened slowly. This exposes the pericardium, which is incised with the ESU or scissors.

The surgeon elevates the pericardium with vascular forceps or a clamp to prevent injury to the heart. The pericardium is

incised to expose the heart and ascending aorta. Lateral incisions are made as needed.

If the procedure requires bypass, traction sutures may be placed through the edges of the pericardium and sewn to the periosteum. An umbilical tape or vessel loop is used to encircle and retract the aorta. The heart and aorta are then cannulated for cardiopulmonary bypass. If an **off-pump procedure** is to be performed (i.e., cardiopulmonary bypass is not needed), cannulation is not required. However, the scrub should be prepared to institute bypass if the patient's condition deteriorates. A median sternotomy is illustrated in Figure 33-12.

Technique
Closing
1. Wires are placed through the sternum.
2. The sternal edges are approximated.
3. The fascia and periosteum are approximated.
4. The subcutaneous tissue and skin are closed.

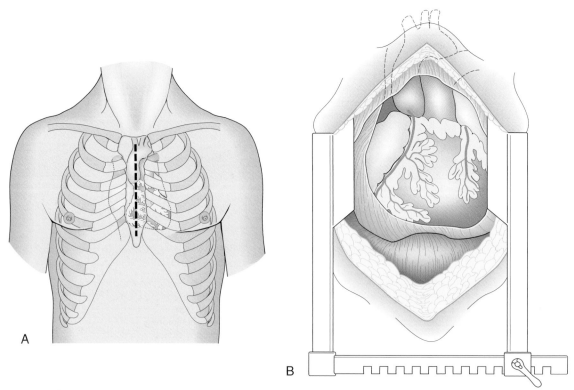

Figure 33-12 Median sternotomy. **A,** Incision. **B,** Right atrium and ascending aorta exposed with the retractor in place. *(From Garden O, Bradbury A, Forsythe J, Parks R: Principles and practice of surgery, ed 5, Edinburgh, 2007, Elsevier/Churchill Livingstone.)*

Discussion

After the surgical procedure, drainage catheters are inserted to remove blood, fluid, and air from the pericardium and the pleural spaces (if they have been entered). Temporary pacing wires are placed on the epicardial surface of the heart. The surgeon places six to eight #5 wire sutures through each sternal edge. When passing stainless steel sutures, the scrub holds the free ends of the wire to control the ends and protect them from contamination. The surgeon tightens the wires and twists each one to bring the sternal edges together. The surgeon uses a wire twister to make a final twist, burying the ends in the periosteum.

When Wolvek sternal-approximation fixation instruments are used, the ends of the wires are threaded through small metal plates. The surgeon then tightens the ends and locks the wire into position by crimping the plate. The excess wire is cut with wire cutters, and sharp tips are buried in the periosteum with the wire twister. Other approximation systems also are available.

The surgeon approximates the fascia and periosteum with interrupted sutures, such as size 0 polyester sutures.

CARDIOPULMONARY BYPASS

Cardiopulmonary bypass diverts blood away from the heart and lungs so that surgery can be performed. An increasing number of cardiac procedures are performed without the use of cardiopulmonary bypass. However many types of surgery,

such as valve replacement and aneurysm repair, do require bypass.

The pump tubing is connected to cannulas that are inserted into the venae cavae and ascending aorta through a median sternotomy incision. The femoral artery and femoral vein occasionally are used when the great vessels are not accessible because of disease. Before cannulation, the anesthesia care provider administers heparin.

Cardiopulmonary bypass may be total or partial. The surgeon performs total bypass by tightening umbilical tapes around the venae cavae and cannulas. This forces all blood returning to the right side of the heart into the cannula and pump. It also prevents air from entering the venous line and obstructing the flow of blood to the pump when the right side of the heart is open. Total bypass also is used for procedures such as mitral valve replacement, repair of septal defects, and resection of a left ventricular aneurysm. In partial bypass, blood can escape around the cannula and enter the heart. Partial bypass often is used during aortic valve replacement. It also is used to support a patient in emergencies such as cardiac arrest or a ruptured aneurysm. Figure 33-13 illustrates caval-aortic bypass.

In both types of bypass, blood returns to the pump through the cannula by gravity drainage and is pumped back into the circulation by a roller head (or a centrifugal pump) on the bypass machine. When the right side of the heart is open and the patient is on bypass, the risk exists that air will enter the venous line. This can cause an

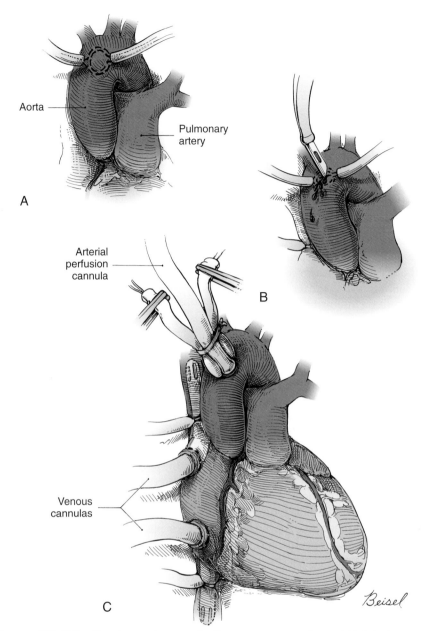

Aorta

Pulmonary artery

A

B

Arterial perfusion cannula

Venous cannulas

C

Beisel

Figure 33-13 Caval-aortic bypass. **A,** The insertion site is located high in the ascending aorta. **B,** A purse-string suture is placed around the adventitia, and a stab wound is made for insertion of the aortic cannula. **C,** The purse-string sutures are tightened to secure the aortic cannula with rubber keepers, which are held to the cannula with a heavy ligature. Venous cannulae are inserted through purse-string sutures into the upper and lower portions of the right atrium. (*Modified from Waldhausen JA, Pierce WS, Campbell DB: Surgery of the chest, ed 6, St Louis, 1996, Mosby.*)

"air lock" (a large amount of air in the venous line), which may obstruct the flow of blood to the pump. The vacuum created by the pump draws the air away from the heart and into the pump.

The surgical technologist must always watch for the presence of air in the heart or pump lines and alert the surgeon immediately if air is noticed. Air must be removed immediately to prevent an air embolus.

The technologist should have a needle and syringe readily available for evacuating air. A 10-cc syringe with a 19-gauge needle can be used for both adult and pediatric patients.

Cannulation Techniques in Cardiopulmonary Bypass

Aorta

A purse-string suture is placed on the anterior portion of the ascending aorta, and the ends are pulled through a Rumel tourniquet. A stab incision is made into the aorta, and the incision is dilated with an aortic dilator or clamp. The surgeon controls bleeding by holding one finger over the hole as the cannula is inserted. The assistant controls the top end of the cannula, which is occluded by a tube-occluding clamp. The surgeon positions the cannula, and the assistant tightens the suture to form a tourniquet. The tourniquet then is tied to the cannula with heavy silk suture. The surgeon clamps and unclamps the cannula to allow it to fill with blood and to remove the air. The cannula then is connected to the arterial perfusion line from the pump.

Superior and Inferior Venae Cavae

If two cannulas are to be inserted, the surgeon uses vascular forceps to grasp the right atrial appendage (a small muscular pouch attached to the atrium) and places a curved partial occlusion vascular clamp (Beck or Glover clamp) across it. A purse-string suture of 2-0 polyester or polypropylene is placed through the occluded portion of the appendage. The assistant snares the ends of the suture through a piece of tubing and tags them with a hemostat.

The surgeon excises the tip of the atrial appendage with scissors and applies clamps or forceps to the two edges of the atrial wall. The assistant controls the vascular clamp and retracts the atrial wall as the surgeon inserts the cannula. The technologist should control the end of the cannula during this procedure. The assistant removes the vascular clamp and controls the suture to prevent bleeding from the atrium.

The surgeon introduces the cannula into the superior vena cava. The assistant forms a tourniquet around the suture as previously described. The surgeon ties the cannula and tourniquet together with a heavy silk tie and then allows blood to fill the cannula by gravity or by lung inflation. The assistant places a tube-occluding clamp across the cannula. Care must be taken not to clamp the wire-reinforced portion of the cannula.

The inferior vena cava is cannulated through a similar technique. The major difference is that the cannula is inserted through the atrial wall instead of through the appendage. A knife blade and scissors may be used to open the atrium. The cannulas are connected to the venous return line from the pump.

Two-Stage Cannulation

Two-stage cannulation is similar to bicaval cannulation except that only one cannula is used. The cannula has holes both in the distal end (which is inserted into the inferior vena cava to drain the lower body) and in the midportion of the cannula (which lies in the atrium to drain blood from the superior vena cava).

Femoral Artery and Vein

Cannulation of the femoral artery and vein is performed when partial bypass is needed to support the patient's circulation in an emergency or during surgical resection of the descending thoracic aorta and ascending aorta. The femoral artery also is cannulated whenever the ascending aorta cannot be cannulated and in some minimally invasive cardiac procedures.

After heparin has been given, the surgeon makes an incision in the groin over the femoral vessels with the knife. The subcutaneous tissue and fascial layers are divided with scissors. A self-retaining retractor is placed in the incision. The surgeon then isolates the common femoral artery with Metzenbaum scissors. The vessel is encircled with umbilical tape and secured in the jaw of a right-angle clamp. The assistant places a tube tourniquet over the ends of the tapes. The femoral vein is isolated using the same technique.

The surgeon occludes the femoral artery with small angled vascular clamps (e.g., a Glover or Cooley clamp). An arteriotomy is performed in the occluded segment with a #11 knife, and the incision is extended with Potts scissors. The opening may be dilated with a clamp. The surgeon inserts the cannula as the assistant removes the superior vascular clamp. The assistant tightens the umbilical tape to hold the cannula in place. The surgeon ties a heavy silk suture around the cannula and the tape and releases the tube-occluding clamp to allow blood to fill the cannula and evacuate air. The cannula then is connected to the arterial perfusion line.

In patients with pulmonary emboli, partial cardiopulmonary bypass using the femoral vein and the femoral artery can be used. Left heart bypass may be used to perfuse the lower body when the descending aorta is cross-clamped.

SUMP CATHETERIZATION

Surgical Goal

A sump catheter is inserted into the left ventricle soon after cardiopulmonary bypass has been established to suction blood and air and maintain cardiac decompression. By venting air, a sump catheter reduces the risk of air embolism in the systemic circulation.

Insertion of the Catheter: Left Ventricle

As soon as bypass is initiated, the surgeon elevates the **apex** of the left ventricle with a laparotomy sponge. A purse-string suture is placed in the apex and snared through a tube tourniquet. The technologist connects the sump catheter to the pump line.

The surgeon makes a stab incision in the apex with a #11 knife blade and dilates the opening with a Schnidt clamp or similar clamp. The catheter is inserted and secured with the tourniquet. The surgeon ties the catheter and tourniquet together with heavy silk suture and lowers the apex into normal position.

Insertion of the Sump Catheter: Right Superior Pulmonary Vein

A right superior pulmonary vein catheter is used more often than a left ventricular apical catheter, which can damage the ventricular muscle.

The assistant retracts the right atrium to expose the right superior pulmonary vein as the surgeon places a purse-string suture. A tourniquet is placed over the suture ends. The surgeon makes a stab incision in the vein with a #11 knife blade, dilates the incision with a clamp, and inserts the catheter into the vein. The catheter is manipulated into the left atrium, across the mitral valve, and into the left ventricle. The tourniquet is then snugged down, and a tube-occluding clamp is put in place across the catheter. The surgeon ties the catheter to the tourniquet with heavy silk suture and connects it to the pump suction line.

INFUSION OF A CARDIOPLEGIC SOLUTION

Surgical Goal

A cardioplegic solution is used to stop the heart; this reduces the energy required by the cardiac muscle by eliminating the energy requirements of contraction. The process of infusing a cardioplegic solution into the coronary arteries protects the cardiac muscle from damage while the aorta is occluded and the blood supply is interrupted. The solution may be infused directly into the coronary artery or transatrially into the coronary sinus. A cardioplegic solution can be infused indirectly into the aortic root just above the aortic valve.

Technique

Direct Coronary Artery Infusion (Antegrade)

1. The ascending aorta is occluded and opened below the clamp.
2. The openings of the coronary arteries are identified and cannulated.
3. Solution is infused, and the cannulas are removed immediately after each infusion.
4. The aorta is closed when the surgery has been completed.

Direct coronary artery infusion and the transatrial retrograde method (discussed later) are the methods most commonly used. The surgeon places a polypropylene purse-string suture in the aorta below the site of the cross-clamp. The ascending aorta is then occluded, and an indwelling catheter (e.g., a 14-gauge Angiocath) is inserted into the aorta below the clamp. The assistant connects the tubing from the cardioplegic solution to the catheter. A Y-connector can be inserted into the cardioplegic tubing, and a suction line can be inserted to vent air from the aorta. Each line from the Y (cardioplegic solution and vent) can be occluded. When cardioplegic solution is being infused, the suction line is occluded; when the suction line is opened, the cardioplegic solution line is occluded.

The surgeon occludes the ascending aorta and opens it below the clamp. The coronary openings are located, and the correct cannulas are determined. The technologist connects the cannulas to the tubing. The surgeon then gently inserts the cannulas into the opening of the coronary arteries and holds them in position until the pump perfusionist or anesthesia care provider completes the infusion. Solution is infused until the heart stops beating (Figure 33-14). The technologist should keep the cannulas and tubing secure in a towel until they are needed for subsequent infusions. The surgeon closes the aorta at the completion of surgery.

Technique

Indirect Coronary Artery Infusion (Antegrade)

1. The ascending aorta is occluded.
2. An indwelling catheter is inserted into the aortic root above the valve.
3. The catheter is connected to the tubing and filled with cardioplegic solution.
4. The solution is infused.

5. The indwelling catheter is removed immediately before the aorta is unclamped.
6. The defect made by the catheter is repaired with suture.

Cardioplegic solution is infused as often as necessary during the procedure. The surgeon withdraws the indwelling catheter and removes the clamp from the aorta. Air in the aorta is suctioned through the vent line. After removal of the catheter, the surgeon closes the defect with 5-0 polypropylene suture.

Transatrial Cardioplegia via the Coronary Sinus (Retrograde)

Technique

1. A small purse-string suture is placed in the atrial wall, and an incision is made in the center.
2. A retrograde cardioplegia catheter is passed through the atrial stab wound, inserted into the opening of the coronary sinus, and positioned in the coronary vein.
3. The proximal end of the catheter is connected to a line leading to the source of the cardioplegic solution.
4. The cardioplegic solution is infused to stop the heart.
5. When cardioplegia is no longer needed, the catheter is removed and the purse-string is tied to close the wound.
6. Cardioplegic solution often is infused by the retrograde route (into the coronary venous system) rather than by the arterial antegrade route. The cardioplegic solution flows from the coronary veins through the capillaries and into the coronary arteries, stopping the heart.
7. After placing a 5-0 polypropylene purse-string suture in the atrial wall, the surgeon incises the atrium with a #11 or #15 blade. The retrograde cardioplegia catheter is inserted into the atrium and guided to the entrance of the coronary sinus. Palpating the outer atrial wall, the surgeon positions the catheter in the sinus opening and advances it into the vein. The catheter is attached to tubing connected to the source of the cardioplegic solution in the bypass circuit.
8. When cardioplegia is no longer needed, the catheter is removed and the atrial incision is closed.

Decannulation

Technique

Decannulation of the Ventricle, Venae Cavae, and Aorta

1. A tube-occluding clamp is placed across the catheter or cannula.
2. Suture ties are removed from the catheter.
3. The catheter is withdrawn, and the suture is tied.

Discussion

The left ventricular catheter usually is removed from the ventricle before bypass is discontinued. The catheter is occluded with a tube-occluding clamp, and the silk suture and tourniquet are removed. The catheter is withdrawn, and the suture is tied securely to occlude the cannulation site. Additional sutures (often on pledgets) may be used for hemostasis. Decannulation of the venae cavae and aorta uses the same technique after bypass has been discontinued.

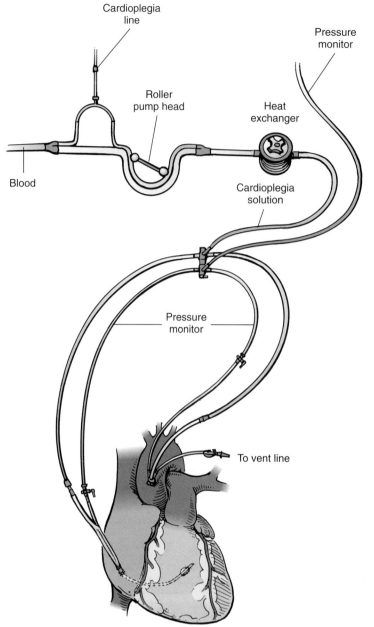

Figure 33-14 Infusion of a cardioplegic solution. *(Modified from Waldhausen JA, Pierce WS, Campbell DB: Surgery of the chest, ed 6, St Louis, 1996, Mosby.)*

Technique

Decannulation of the Femoral Artery and Vein
1. The cannula is occluded.
2. The umbilical tape is released.
3. The cannula is withdrawn, and the femoral vein is occluded with a vascular clamp.
4. The venotomy is closed, and all clamps and tapes are removed.
5. The artery is decannulated using the same technique.

At the conclusion of bypass, the surgeon occludes the femoral vein cannula. The assistant releases the cannula from the drapes and other attachments on the field. The surgeon then withdraws the cannula and occludes the vein with a vascular clamp. The venotomy is closed with a continuous suture of 5-0 or 6-0 polypropylene. All clamps are removed, and the artery is decannulated with the same technique.

Postoperative Considerations

Bleeding or hemorrhage can occur if cannulation sites have not been closed securely, if heparin has not been adequately reversed with protamine, if dissection of the cannulated blood vessel occurs, or if surrounding tissue has been damaged. Atelectasis may persist because of lung deflation during bypass. Temporary cognitive, sensory, and perceptual changes may occur as a result of the effects of extracorporeal circulation.

CORONARY ARTERY BYPASS GRAFTING

Surgical Goal

Coronary artery bypass (CAB) of a narrow segment of one or more coronary arteries is performed to improve circulation to the heart. An autograft (tissue from the patient's own body) usually is used as the bypass graft. The procedure is commonly known by its acronym, CABG, for coronary artery bypass grafting.

Pathology

The inner and outer walls of the heart may be affected by coronary artery disease (CAD). CAD is caused by the buildup of cholesterol deposits in the arterial lining, a condition called atherosclerosis. This can affect any artery. A closely related disease is arteriosclerosis, which is loss of elasticity in and hardening of the arteries. Arteriosclerosis often is the result of diet and other environmental causes. When the flow of coronary blood is reduced, the myocardial cells are deprived of oxygen and other nutrients. This in turn can produce a weakening of the heart muscle or a myocardial **infarction**, resulting in tissue death.

Technique

1. A median sternotomy incision is made.
2. A segment of the saphenous vein is removed. The internal mammary artery (IMA) is dissected from its retrosternal bed.
3. The heart is cannulated for cardiopulmonary bypass unless an off-pump procedure is planned.
4. The aorta is occluded, and cardioplegic solution is administered into the aortic root.
5. The coronary artery is incised, and the vein, IMA, or other graft conduit is anastomosed to the coronary arteriotomy.
6. The aorta is unclamped.
7. Venous and other free grafts are anastomosed to the ascending aorta. These may be anastomosed while the cross-clamp is applied.
8. Cardiopulmonary bypass is discontinued, and decannulation is performed.
9. Pacing wires and chest tubes are inserted, and the wound is closed.

Discussion

The surgeon performs a median sternotomy and cannulates for cardiopulmonary bypass. However, an increasing number of coronary bypass procedures are performed without the use of cardiopulmonary bypass. In patients with very complex, multivessel disease, bypass often is required. The assistant removes the greater saphenous vein from the leg, or the left or right radial artery may be harvested for use as a free graft. (This procedure is described and illustrated in Chapter 31.) Video-assisted endoscopic vein harvesting may be performed.

Preparation of the Internal Mammary Artery

The internal mammary artery (IMA) is dissected free from the retrosternal bed (Figure 33-15). The sternal edge may be elevated with a self-retaining retractor attached to the side from which the IMA is dissected. The left IMA commonly is used, although the right IMA also may be used.

After cardiopulmonary bypass has been instituted (if used), the surgeon identifies the segment of coronary artery to which the bypass graft will be anastomosed. Excess epicardial fat is removed from the arteriotomy site with a #64 Beaver blade or a #15 blade. The surgeon then occludes the ascending aorta and inserts the indwelling catheter for infusion of the cardioplegic solution and venting of air.

Next, the coronary artery is opened with a #11 knife blade (or Beaver blade), and the incision is extended with Diethrich or fine Potts coronary scissors. A Garrett dilator may be inserted into the lumen of the artery to assess its size. The technologist places the vein in a small basin with heparinized blood solution to keep the graft moist. The surgeon bevels the free end of the vein with Potts scissors. The vein then is sutured to the coronary artery with continuous or interrupted sutures (e.g., 6-0 or 7-0 polypropylene). When the anastomosis is complete, the assistant inflates the vein with a physiological solution to test for leaks and to determine the diameter and length of the graft when it is filled.

The surgeon performs all other anastomoses using the same technique. Size 8-0 polypropylene may be used for the anastomosis (Figure 33-16). The aorta then is unclamped, and the indwelling catheter is removed. A portion of the aorta is occluded with a vascular clamp (e.g., Lambert-Kay clamp). A #11 knife blade and aortic punch are used to create a hole in the occluded portion.

The surgeon inflates the vein to make sure it is not twisted and does not have any leaks and to determine the length needed to reach the aorta. The vein is then cut to the appropriate length, and the end is beveled with Potts scissors. The anastomosis is performed between the vein and the hole in the aorta. The surgeon completes each anastomosis and removes the clamp from the aorta. When the procedures are performed off-pump, a small horseshoe retractor is positioned over the coronary arteriotomy to minimize cardiac movement during the distal anastomosis. The proximal aortic anastomosis is performed with partial occlusion of the aorta. In some patients, both distal and proximal anastomoses are created with the aorta cross-clamped.

Air is evacuated from the vein grafts with a 25- or 27-gauge needle. The surgeon inspects each anastomosis for leaks, and any found are repaired before bypass is discontinued. The cannulas are removed, and a pacemaker electrode may be sutured to the heart. Metal rings or radiopaque material may be placed around each vein graft on the aorta. These mark the veins in the event cardiac catheterization is performed in the postoperative period. The completed anastomosis is shown in Figure 33-17.

Off-Pump Coronary Artery Bypass

Off-pump coronary artery bypass (OPCAB) is performed through a median sternotomy. The Octopus retractor and left ventricular suction apparatus are commonly used to expose the coronary arteries.

A special rib retractor with endoscope is used to harvest the left IMA. The rib retractor is exchanged for another small

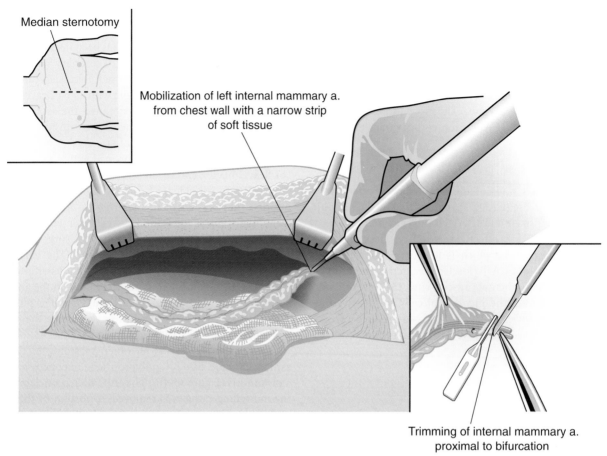

Median sternotomy

Mobilization of left internal mammary a.
from chest wall with a narrow strip
of soft tissue

Trimming of internal mammary a.
proximal to bifurcation

Figure 33-15 Harvesting of the internal mammary artery for coronary artery bypass. *(From Jones RH: Coronary artery bypass grafts. In Sabiston DC Jr, editor: Atlas of cardiothoracic surgery, Philadelphia, 1995, WB Saunders.)*

thoracotomy retractor positioned to expose the anastomosis site. A stabilizing device is used to minimize cardiac movement during suturing. The anastomosis is performed in the traditional manner.

Postoperative Considerations

Complications include hemorrhage, atrial and/or ventricular arrhythmias, stroke, infection, **ischemia**, and death. Arterial grafts may spasm, producing changes in the electrocardiogram that can signal ischemia. A sufficiently normal blood pressure should be maintained for arterial grafts to function properly. CABG grafts may clot, causing a myocardial infarction.

TRANSMYOCARDIAL REVASCULARIZATION

Surgical Goal

In transmyocardial revascularization (TMR) a series of small-bore, transmural channels are created with the carbon dioxide or holmium–yttrium-aluminum-garnet (holmium:YAG) laser to perfuse the myocardium. The goal is to increase blood flow to the heart in patients in whom bypass surgery or medical management is not feasible. TMR may be used in conjunction with standard CAB.

Technique

1. In patients not undergoing coronary artery bypass (CAB), a minithoracotomy is made on the side of the affected coronary artery.
2. The pericardium is opened to expose the heart.
3. The sterile laser probe is used to create channels into the heart muscle.
4. A chest tube may be inserted.
5. The incision is closed.

Discussion

If TMR is performed in conjunction with CAB, only laser-specific instruments and supplies should be used. If TMR is to be performed through a thoracotomy, chest instruments in addition to the laser supplies and equipment are used. External defibrillator patches are applied to all

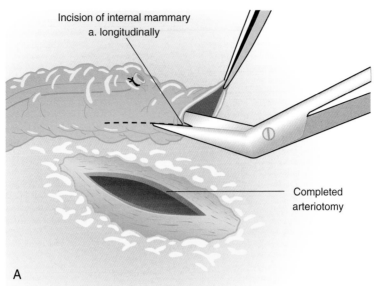

Incision of internal mammary
a. longitudinally

Completed
arteriotomy

A

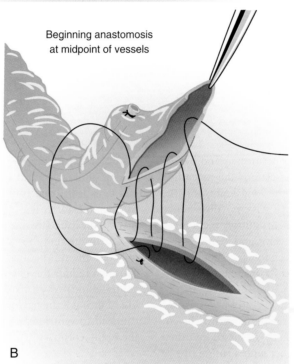

Beginning anastomosis
at midpoint of vessels

B

Figure 33-16 Coronary artery bypass. **A,** Potts scissors are used to open the vein graft. **B,** Anastomosis of the vein graft. *(From Townsend CM: Sabiston textbook of surgery, ed 17, Philadelphia, 2001, WB Saunders.)*

patients; pediatric internal defibrillator paddles may also be requested.

The surgeon uses a sterile laser probe to make the myocardial channels from the epicardium to the endocardium. Both the scrub and the circulating personnel keep track of the number of channels formed.

RESECTION OF A LEFT VENTRICULAR ANEURYSM

Surgical Goal

Resection of a left ventricular aneurysm reduces the risk of rupture and embolism.

Pathology

An aneurysm of the left ventricle most often is caused by a reduced blood supply from an infarcted coronary artery.

Technique

1. A median sternotomy is performed.
2. Cannulation and total cardiopulmonary bypass are initiated.
3. A left ventriculotomy is performed, and the aneurysm is resected.
4. The ventricle is closed.
5. The cannulas are removed.
6. Pacer electrodes are sutured to the heart, chest tubes are inserted, and the wound is closed.

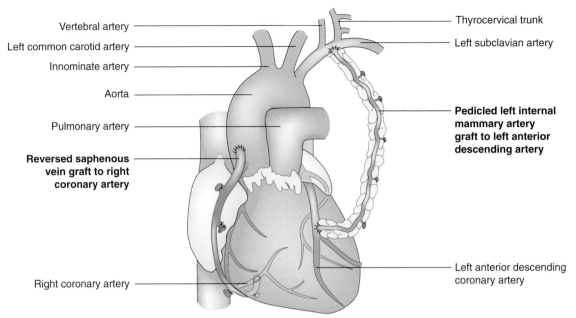

Vertebral artery
Left common carotid artery
Innominate artery
Aorta
Pulmonary artery
Reversed saphenous vein graft to right coronary artery
Right coronary artery

Thyrocervical trunk
Left subclavian artery
Pedicled left internal mammary artery graft to left anterior descending artery
Left anterior descending coronary artery

Figure 33-17 Completed coronary bypass with venous and left internal mammary artery grafts in place. *(From Garden O, Bradbury A, Forsythe J, Parks R: Principles and practice of surgery, ed 5, Edinburgh, 2007, Elsevier/Churchill Livingstone.)*

Discussion

After a median sternotomy has been performed and bypass has been initiated, the surgeon cross-clamps the ascending aorta. The ventricle is incised with the long knife, and the incision is extended with curved Mayo scissors. Allis clamps may be applied to the edges of the aneurysm for traction.

The surgeon assesses the mitral valve and removes any clots with forceps or suction. The technologist should keep the instruments clean to prevent clots from entering the bloodstream.

The aneurysm tissue is excised with curved Mayo scissors, and a Dacron patch is inserted to repair the ventricle. An alternate technique is to resect the aneurysm tissue and then bring the edges of the ventricle together with a suture of size 0 polypropylene or polyester. Strips of Teflon felt or pledgets are incorporated with the suture. A second or third row of sutures is placed through the ventricular edges for a more secure closure. The surgeon decompresses the ventricle using the sump catheter from the heart-lung machine. The catheter is removed before the final suture is placed. The apex of the ventricle may be aspirated with a 19-gauge needle. The wound then is prepared for closure as previously described, and the incision is closed. Resection of a left ventricular aneurysm is illustrated in Figure 33-18.

AORTIC VALVE REPLACEMENT

Surgical Goal

The aortic valve maintains one-way blood flow from the left ventricle to the aorta. Aortic valve replacement involves the replacement of a diseased valve.

Pathology

Common causes of valve insufficiency are endocarditis, congenital anomalies, and calcification. A leaking valve allows blood to leak back into the left ventricle instead of going through the aorta. The left ventricle eventually fails as a result increased cardiac work.

Calcification of the valves also can occur. The valve leaflets may become stiff because of calcification or other thickening. This can reduce the opening of the valve to a small slit. The ventricle must work harder to pump a sufficient amount of blood through the narrowed orifice of the stenotic valve. This can lead to ventricular failure and insufficient blood flow to the brain, coronary arteries, and other organs.

Technique

1. A median sternotomy and cardiopulmonary bypass usually are performed with a two-stage venous cannulation.
2. The ascending aorta is occluded, and cardioplegic solution is infused through the aortic root or through the coronary sinus and into the coronary circulation.
3. A transverse incision is made in the anterior aortic wall.
4. A prosthetic valve is selected and sutured in place.
5. The aortotomy is closed, and the aorta is unclamped.
6. Cardiopulmonary bypass is discontinued, and the cannulas are removed.
7. Pacing wires and chest tubes are inserted, and the wound is closed.

Discussion

The surgeon performs a median sternotomy and cannulates for cardiopulmonary bypass. A retrograde cardioplegic catheter is inserted into the coronary sinus. The ascending aorta

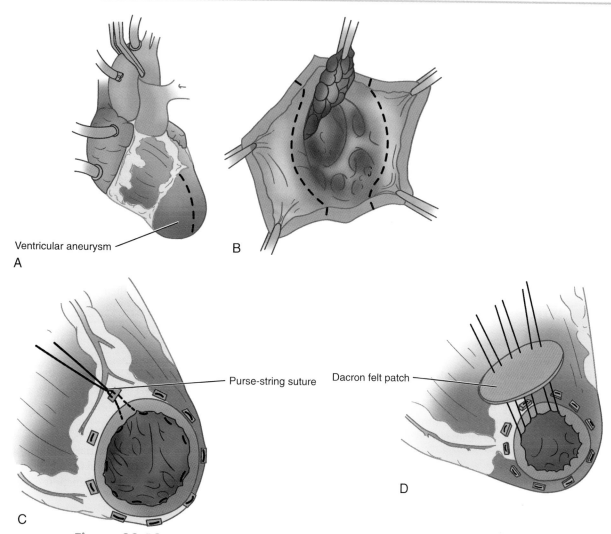

Ventricular aneurysm

A

B

Purse-string suture

C

Dacron felt patch

D

Figure 33-18 Repair of a ventricular aneurysm. **A,** Left ventricular apical aneurysm. **B,** The aneurysm is opened, and clots are removed. **C.** A purse-string suture is used. **D,** A Dacron patch is sutured to the edge of the defect. *(Modified from Waldhausen JA, Pierce WS, Campbell DB: Surgery of the chest, ed 6, St Louis, 1996, Mosby.)*

is occluded, and the cardioplegic solution is infused. The route through which the cardioplegic solution is delivered depends on the valve pathology. If aortic **stenosis** is present, the cardioplegic solution initially is infused through the aortic root. After the aorta is opened, subsequent cardioplegic infusions are given through the retrograde catheter. If aortic insufficiency is present, cardioplegic solution infused into the aortic root preferentially flows into the left ventricle. Fluid in the ventricular chamber distends and damages the ventricular wall. In these situations, retrograde cardioplegic solution is infused. Direct coronary perfusion rarely is required.

The surgeon opens the aorta with a transverse incision or, occasionally, a vertical incision. The valve cusps are incised with forceps and scissors or a long knife. If the valve leaflets are extensively calcified, the surgeon may debride the calcium with rongeurs. The technologist should keep the instruments clean with a damp sponge to prevent calcium particles and other materials from dropping back into the wound, where they might cause an embolus.

The annulus is measured with obturators. Different types of valve prostheses have their own unique sizing obturators. The scrub obtains the correct size of prosthesis from the circulating nurse. The surgeon places interrupted sutures through the annulus of the prosthetic sewing ring. Some surgeons prefer to use a continuous suture of 2-0 or 3-0 polypropylene. Interrupted sutures in the aortic valve may be inserted in three series, corresponding to the three cusps of the valve. The distal suture ends are tagged with mosquito clamps or placed in a suture holder. When biological valves are used, they must be rinsed to remove the glutaraldehyde storage solution; the valve must be kept moist with saline before it is implanted. If the leaflets become dry, the prosthesis can be damaged.

The surgeon seats the valve in position and ties all sutures. The aortotomy is closed with two 2-0 or 3-0 polypropylene sutures. One suture begins on the left side, and the other suture begins on the right side. The sutures are tied in the middle portion of the aortotomy. Before tying the sutures, the surgeon allows air to escape from the suture line. The sutures are then tied securely. The surgeon may oversew the initial closure to enhance hemostasis. The aortic clamp is removed, and the aortic vent line is turned on to aspirate air. The surgeon also may elevate the left ventricular apex and insert a 19-gauge needle into the chamber to allow air to escape.

Bypass is discontinued, and the cannulas are removed. Temporary pacemaker electrodes may be sutured to the heart. Chest tubes are inserted, and the wound is closed in layers.

Postoperative Considerations

Complications include hemorrhage, atrial and/or ventricular arrhythmias, stroke, infection, ischemia, and death. Additional complications include valve failure or malfunction. Aortic valve replacement is illustrated in Figure 33-19.

MITRAL VALVE REPAIR AND REPLACEMENT

Surgical Goal

In mitral valve repair and replacement, a diseased mitral valve is replaced to open a constricted valve (stenosis) or to prevent blood from regurgitating into the left atrium. The valve is repaired with an annuloplasty (or other reparative techniques). If the valve is severely damaged, it is replaced.

Pathology

The mitral valve is situated between the left atrium and left ventricle. Over time, a stenotic valve causes the left atrium to become dilated and can lead to arrhythmias, such as atrial fibrillation. Mitral valve disease may be caused by rheumatic heart disease, dilation of the annulus, ischemic heart disease, trauma, or changes in the tissue that produces regurgitation

Technique

1. A midline sternotomy is performed.
2. Cannulation of the superior and inferior venae cavae is performed for total cardiopulmonary bypass.
3. The ascending aorta is occluded, and cardioplegic solution is infused through the aortic root and into the coronary arteries.
4. A left atriotomy is performed, and the mitral valve is excised.
5. A prosthetic valve is sutured in place.
6. The atriotomy is closed, and the aorta is unclamped.
7. Cardiopulmonary bypass is discontinued, and the cannulas are removed.
8. Chest tubes and pacing wires are inserted, and the wound is closed.

Discussion

Mitral Valve Replacement

A median sternotomy is performed, and both venae cavae are cannulated for total cardiopulmonary bypass. The ascending aorta is occluded, and a cardioplegic solution is infused through the aortic root and into the coronary arteries.

The surgeon opens the left atrium with the long knife, extends the incision with scissors, and inserts an atrial retractor, which the assistant uses to expose the valve. The surgeon grasps the valve with a valve hook or long Allis clamp and excises the cusps with valve scissors or the knife. The chordae tendineae and papillary muscles of the anterior leaflet are cut; the posterior leaflet chordae often are left intact.

The annulus then is measured so that the technologist can obtain the correct size of prosthetic valve from the circulator. The surgeon places the sutures through the annulus and the prosthetic sewing ring using the same technique as described for aortic valve replacement. The valve is seated in position, and the sutures are tied.

The atriotomy is closed with continuous 3-0 polypropylene suture. Before tying the sutures, the surgeon temporarily releases the vena cava tourniquets and allows the heart to fill with blood. The blood is allowed to spill out of the heart to remove air bubbles. The surgeon then ties the sutures securely. The aortic clamp is removed, and the aorta is aspirated with a vent catheter to ensure that no air remains in the heart.

Cardiopulmonary bypass is discontinued, and the cannulas are removed. A temporary pacemaker electrode may be sutured to the heart. Chest tubes are inserted, and the wound is closed. Mitral valve replacement is illustrated in Figure 33-20.

Postoperative Considerations

Complications include hemorrhage, atrial and/or ventricular arrhythmias, stroke, infection, ischemia, and death. Additional complications are failure or malfunction of the prosthetic valve.

Mitral Commissurotomy

Occasionally a mitral commissurotomy (opening of the commissures that bring the cusps of the valve together) is performed rather than valve replacement. This technique can be used to relieve stenosis when the valve leaflets are sufficiently flexible to allow it. The procedure is performed during bypass. The surgeon incises the commissures with a knife or breaks them apart with a mitral valve dilator (e.g., Gerbode or Tubbs dilator) to separate the cusps. The atrium then is closed as described for mitral valve replacement.

Mitral Ring Annuloplasty

A dilated mitral valve annulus can be repaired by placement of an annuloplasty ring in the annulus to allow the valve leaflets to come together more efficiently. Sutures are placed in the annulus and the annuloplasty ring and are tied. This procedure reduces the annular orifice, allowing the valve leaflets to close properly.

Related Procedure

Tricuspid Valve Replacement or Repair

In replacement procedures, the tricuspid valve is excised and replaced with a prosthetic valve through a right atriotomy. Total cardiopulmonary bypass is required. Tricuspid ring annuloplasty (similar to mitral valve annuloplasty) often is preferred over replacement.

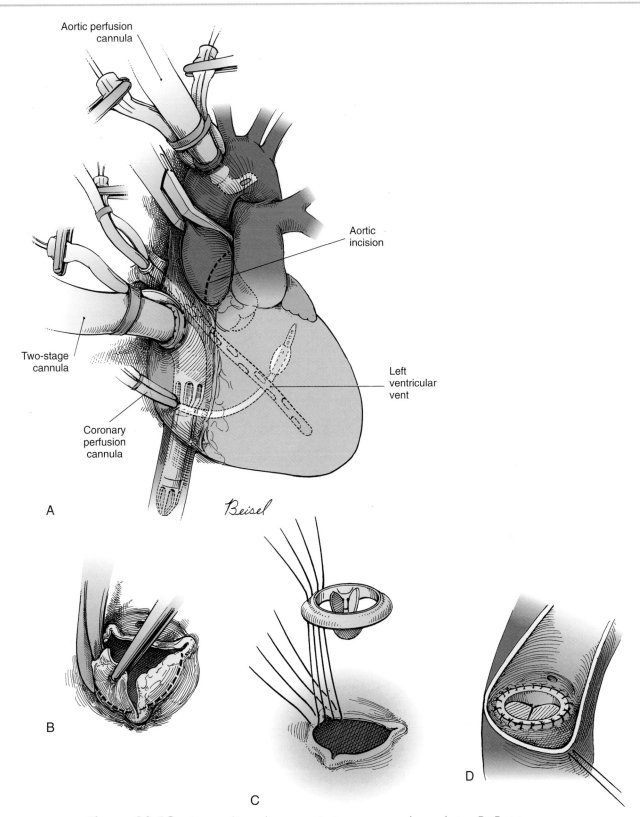

Aortic perfusion cannula

Aortic incision

Two-stage cannula

Left ventricular vent

Coronary perfusion cannula

Beisel

A

B

C

D

Figure 33-19 Aortic valve replacement. **A,** Incision site and cannulation. **B,** Excision of the valve. **C,** Valve replacement and placement of sutures. **D,** Completed suture line. *(Modified from Waldhausen JA, Pierce WS, Campbell DB: Surgery of the chest, ed 6, St Louis, 1996, Mosby.)*

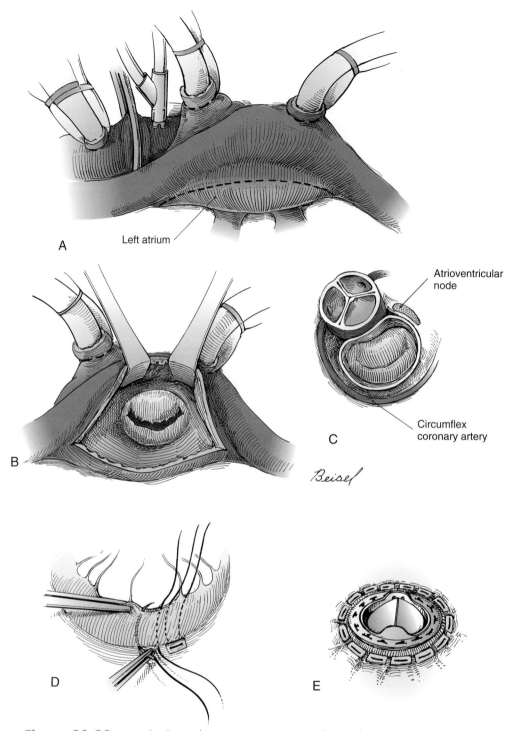

Figure 33-20   Mitral valve replacement. **A,** Incision and cannulation sites. **B,** Exposure of the valve. **C,** Anatomical relationship between the mitral and aortic valves. **D,** Pledgets are placed with double-arm sutures. **E,** Completed valve replacement. *(Modified from Waldhausen JA, Pierce WS, Campbell DB: Surgery of the chest, ed 6, St Louis, 1996, Mosby.)*

RESECTION OF AN ANEURYSM OF THE ASCENDING AORTA

Surgical Goal

An aneurysm or dissection of the ascending aorta can rupture or prevent the aortic valve leaflets from closing properly. The goal of resection of an aneurysm of the ascending aorta is to repair the aneurysm and restore function to the valve.

Pathology

An aortic aneurysm is a potentially life-threatening condition in which the walls of the aorta (or any other vessel or heart chamber) balloons out because of cardiovascular disease (Figure 33-21). Aneurysms can be classified as saccular or fusiform. A **saccular aneurysm** is a ballooning out of a localized area in the artery. A **fusiform aneurysm** involves the

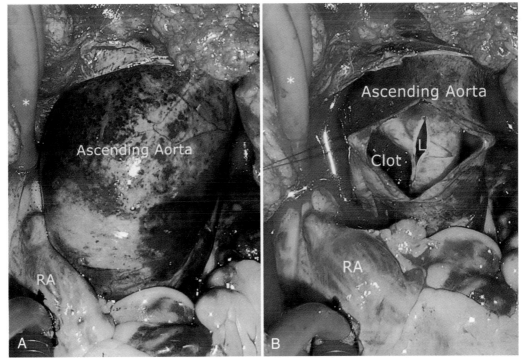

Figure 33-21 Ascending aortic aneurysm. **A,** Acute aortic dissection. **B,** The aorta has been opened, showing the true lumen. *(From Townsend CM: Sabiston textbook of surgery, ed 17, Philadelphia, 2001, WB Saunders.)*

entire circumference of the artery. Arteriosclerosis and atherosclerosis both contribute to these conditions. As the disease progress, the walls of the aorta become increasingly stiff and blocked by fatty deposits. The walls of the segment *distal to* the blockage (in the direction of blood flow) become weak and distended. Finally, the ballooning vessel begins to delaminate (the intimal layer separates), and blood is forced between the layers, resulting in rupture. This delamination is called *dissection,* and the aneurysm then is referred to as a *dissecting aneurysm.* The condition requires immediate surgery to prevent rupture.

Technique

1. A median sternotomy is performed.
2. The femoral artery is isolated and cannulated.
3. The venae cavae are cannulated.
4. Total cardiopulmonary bypass is initiated, and a vent catheter of the right superior pulmonary vein is inserted.
5. The aorta is occluded distal to the aneurysm or dissection, and the aortic wall is opened.
6. Retrograde cardioplegic solution is infused (the coronary arteries rarely are directly perfused).
7. A prosthetic graft is anastomosed to the proximal and distal aorta, and the aorta is unclamped.
8. Cardiopulmonary bypass is discontinued, and the cannulas are removed.
9. Chest tubes are inserted, and the wound is closed.

Discussion

A median sternotomy may be performed, after the femoral artery and vein have been isolated for cannulation, if the risk exists that the aorta may rupture when the chest is opened.

After cannulation has been completed and the right superior pulmonary vein sump catheter has been inserted, the surgeon occludes the aorta distal to the aneurysm. The aneurysm is opened with scissors, and all clots and debris are removed. If the aorta is dissected, the location of the aortic tear is identified.

Retrograde cardioplegic solution is administered through the coronary sinus. The surgeon examines the aortic valve to determine the extent of injury and to replace it if necessary. The technologist should have valve instruments available on the setup tray to prevent delay. Valve suture should be ready for immediate opening if needed.

The surgeon obtains the appropriate-size graft from the technologist and performs the distal anastomosis with a continuous suture of 3-0 polypropylene. When the anastomosis is complete, the surgeon occludes the graft with a vascular clamp and temporarily releases the aortic clamp to test the suture line. Additional sutures are placed as needed. Teflon felt pledgets are used to reinforce the suture line.

The surgeon cuts the graft to an appropriate length and performs the proximal anastomosis. Before tying the suture, the surgeon temporarily releases the aortic clamp to fill the graft and flush out air and clots. The right superior pulmonary vein sump catheter is the removed. After cardiopulmonary bypass has been discontinued, the cannulas are removed. The surgeon may cover the graft with aneurysm tissue. The assistant closes the groin incision while the surgeon inserts chest tubes and closes the sternotomy.

The surgeon occasionally must replace both the aorta and the aortic valve. Special composite graft-valve prostheses are available for these procedures. If the coronary opening is

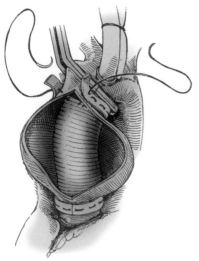

Figure 33-22   Resection and repair of an ascending aortic aneurysm. *(From Rothrock J: Alexander's care of the patient in surgery, ed 17, Philadelphia, 2007, Mosby.)*

obscured by the composite graft, the surgeon must reimplant the coronary opening or create bypass grafts that attach proximally to the aortic graft. Coronary bypass instruments should be available.

Postoperative Considerations

Complications include hemorrhage, stroke, infection, and death. Graft anastomoses may require repair if persistent bleeding arises. Neurological deficit or paralysis may be a complication of surgery on the descending thoracic aorta. Figure 33-22 illustrates the resection of an ascending aortic aneurysm.

RESECTION OF AN ANEURYSM OF THE AORTIC ARCH

Surgical Goal

An aneurysm or dissection of the aortic arch can impair blood flow to the brain and the upper body because of the frequent involvement of the aortic branches (i.e., the brachiocephalic artery, the left carotid artery, and the left subclavian artery). The goal of resection of an aortic arch aneurysm is to repair the aneurysm and restore adequate blood flow to the aorta and its branches.

Pathology

Refer to the Pathology section in the previous procedure.

Discussion

An aneurysm that extends or is limited to the aortic arch may require resection and anastomosis of both the aorta and its branching arch vessels using a graft. The femoral vein and artery are cannulated as for aneurysms of the ascending aorta. In some cases, the branch vessels cannot be clamped because of their location or because of their involvement in the aneurysm. In these cases, the surgeon may elect to turn off the

pump for the period required to anastomose the arch vessels. Once the anastomoses are complete, the pump is started again and the remainder of the procedure is performed under bypass. Figure 33-23 illustrates the repair of an aortic arch aneurysm.

RESECTION OF AN ANEURYSM OF THE DESCENDING THORACIC AORTA

Surgical Goal

The goal of surgical repair of an aneurysm of the descending thoracic aorta is to prevent rupture and life-threatening hemorrhage.

Pathology

Refer to *Resection of an Aneurysm of the Ascending Aorta* above.

Technique

1. A thoracotomy is performed.
2. The mediastinal pleura is incised.
3. The aneurysm or dissection is mobilized from the surrounding tissue.
4. Vascular occluding clamps are applied to the aorta, and the aneurysm or dissection is resected.
5. The intercostal arteries are ligated.
6. A prosthetic graft is implanted.
7. The occluding clamps are removed from the aorta.
8. The graft may be enclosed by the remaining vascular wall.
9. The mediastinal pleura is closed.
10. Chest tubes are inserted, and the wound is closed.

Discussion

The patient is placed in the lateral position, prepped, and draped for a thoracotomy. A thoracotomy incision is performed as described previously. After the chest has been opened and the retractors placed, the surgeon retracts the edges of the pleura with 2-0 silk sutures.

The surgeon begins to free the aneurysm from the surrounding tissue. Femoral vein–femoral artery cardiopulmonary bypass may be used to perfuse the kidneys and the rest of the lower body. If bypass is not used, speed is essential at this time because there is no flow to the lower body. The technologist must be alert and avoid unnecessary movements and loss of time while handling instruments.

The surgeon occludes the aorta proximal and distal to the aneurysm. The knife is then used to make a longitudinal incision into the aneurysm, and the incision is extended with scissors. The outer layer of the aneurysm is preserved and retracted with 2-0 or 3-0 silk sutures. These flaps are used later in the procedure to cover the grafts and prevent them from adhering to the lung.

The surgeon removes all debris and blood clots inside the aneurysm using suction and tissue forceps. The technologist should have a small basin to receive loose debris and blood clots and a moist sponge to wipe debris from the surgeon's instruments. The surgeon ligates the intercostal vessels along the posterior wall of the aneurysm with polyester sutures.

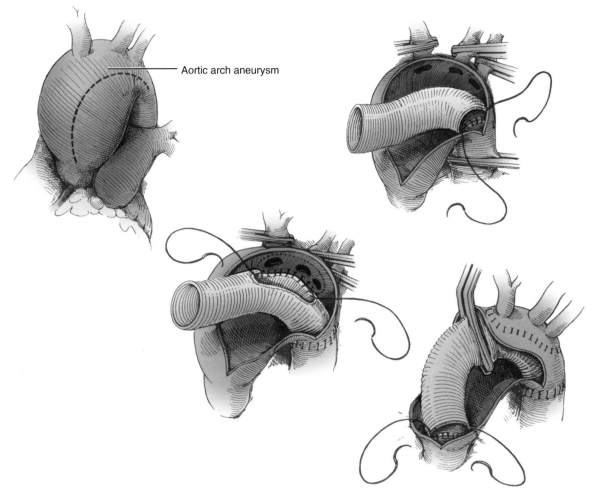

Figure 33-23 Repair of an aortic arch aneurysm. **A,** Incision. **B,** Distal anastomosis. **C,** Anastomosis of the graft below the arch vessels. **D,** Proximal anastomosis. *(Modified from Waldhausen JA, Pierce WS, Campbell DB: Surgery of the chest, ed 6, St Louis, 1996, Mosby.)*

Identifying the origin of these vessels may be difficult. To aid identification, the surgeon may irrigate the area with warm saline solution and look for bleeding points, indicating an open vessel. When hemostasis is secured, the graft is anastomosed to the aorta.

The surgeon transects the aorta immediately above and below the aneurysm and removes the middle segment. A graft then is implanted to replace the diseased segment.

Anastomosing the Graft

The surgeon performs the proximal anastomosis with a continuous suture of 3-0 or 4-0 polypropylene or polyester. A straight vascular clamp may be placed across the graft while the surgeon releases the proximal aortic clamp briefly to check for leaks. The surgeon reapplies the aortic clamp, removes the graft clamp, and places any additional sutures needed to control leakage. Teflon pledgets may be used to bolster the sutures.

After completing the proximal anastomosis, the surgeon trims the graft to the appropriate length and performs the distal anastomosis. Before the suture is tied, the graft is flushed to clear it of clots and debris. The suture is then tied, and all clamps are removed, restoring blood flow to the lower body.

If cardiopulmonary bypass has been used, it is discontinued at this stage, and the cannulas are removed. To complete the procedure, the surgeon covers the graft with remaining aneurysm tissue (if it has not been excised) using absorbable continuous or interrupted 2-0 or 3-0 suture. The mediastinal pleura is closed, chest tubes are inserted, and the wound is closed in layers.

ENDOVASCULAR REPAIR OF A THORACIC ANEURYSM

Endovascular repair of a descending thoracic aneurysm is now frequently used for the treatment of descending thoracic aortic aneurysm (DTAA). Devices currently used are the TAG Device (L. Gore and Associates, Flagstaff, Ariz). Others are under investigation at this time. A discussion on endovascular repair of abdominal aneurysm (EVAR) is found in Chapter 32 and clarifies the principles of endovascular repair.

Discussion

Endovascular repair of descending aortic aneurysms are performed on patients with fusiform type aneurysms, which are at least double the normal size of the aorta. Computed tomography angiography is used to measure and evaluate the extent of disease to determine whether the patient is suitable for endovascular repair.

The surgical approach may be through an incision into the femoral artery or percutaneous insertion (without incision) may be possible. Like endovascular repair of abdominal aneurysm, a wire stent graft is deployed through the femoral artery and positioned at the level of the aneurysm. This is done under fluoroscopy and intraoperative angiography using the opposite groin for entry of angiocatheters.

For femoral surgery, a needle is inserted into the femoral artery and a guide wire is threaded into the thoracic portion of the aorta. The needle is removed. , Because the guide wires may be over 6 feet long, the surgical technologist should take precautions to avoid contaminating the wire by anchoring the distal end of the wire with sterile towels or another weighted sterile object.

Dilators of increasing size are inserted over the guide wire; each dilator is inserted and removed in succession and replaced with a larger guide wire in order to enlarge the femoral artery.

An angiographic catheter is inserted into the patient's opposite femoral artery in order to visualize the inside of the aorta, to perform intraoperative angiograms, and to guide and verify the placement of the deployed stent. The surgeon uses fluoroscopy to identify the location of the arch vessels and to identify normal proximal and distal aortic tissue into which the endovascular stent graft will be secured. Intravascular ultrasound may be used to measure internal diameters and to note anatomic angles that can affect placement of the device(s). More than one device may be deployed when there is an extensive aneurismal lesion.

When the target area is reached, the device is positioned and opened in the aorta. The surgeon confirms the proper placement of the endostent(s) and the absence of endoleaks. If hemostasis is not achieved, the surgeon may reposition the graft or replace the existing graft with another stent. If there is acute hemorrhage that cannot be repaired endoscopically, the technologist should be prepared for open surgery to complete the repair.

Recovery is considerably shorter after endovascular repair than after thoracotomy. Possible complications include bleeding and migration of the device, requiring adjustment and/or insertion of another device.

INSERTION OF AN ARTIFICIAL CARDIAC PACEMAKER

Surgical Goal

An artificial pacemaker is implanted in the body to correct cardiac arrhythmia caused by a disease of the conduction system. A pulse generator provides electrical impulses through the device's cardiac leads, which are implanted in conductive tissue of the heart.

Pathology

Cardiac arrhythmia is an abnormal pattern of conductivity in the heart. Healthy individuals may have an arrhythmia.

However, when the heart's conduction mechanism is affected by disease, certain arrhythmias can be life-threatening. Arrhythmias are named by type and origin (e.g., atrial flutter). Some common arrhythmias are:

- *Ventricular tachycardia*: A heart rate over 120 beats per minute.
- *Atrial flutter*: A heart rate of 240 to 450 beats per minute.
- *Ventricular fibrillation*: Chaotic, disorganized stimulation of one or both ventricles that does not pump the blood.
- *Atrial fibrillation*: Chaotic, disorganized stimulation of one or both atria that prevents atrial contraction (which normally to fill the ventricle with blood).
- *Bradycardia*: A heart rate below 40 to 60 beats per minute.

Conduction disease can arise from ischemic heart disease, which can be caused by atherosclerosis, infection, or congenital defects.

Temporary Pacemaker

Technique

1. An electrode is sutured to the right atrium and/or the right ventricle or can be inserted transvenously.
2. The free end of the electrode is brought through the skin and secured with a suture.
3. The electrode is connected to an alligator cable attached to a temporary external pacemaker generator.

Discussion

A pacemaker may be implanted in the cardiac catheterization suite or in the perioperative period. Postsurgically, a pacemaker can be implanted via the transvenous route (a temporary pacer is used until it is replaced by a permanent pacing system).

A pacemaker may be implanted temporarily, such as during cardiac procedures, or the implantation may be permanent. Three approaches are used for permanent implantation: the transvenous, epicardial, and subxyphoid approaches. The transvenous and subxyphoid procedures, which do not require a thoracotomy, are commonly performed with the patient under local anesthesia with monitored anesthesia care. When the transvenous approach is used, the electrodes are placed with the aid of fluoroscopy.

A right or left subclavian venotomy is performed, and the electrode is advanced into the right atrium, through the tricuspid valve, and into the right ventricle, where it is placed in the right ventricular apex. The pulse generator then is placed within the superficial tissues of the chest wall. An atrial electrode also may be placed in the atrial appendage for dual-chamber (atrial and ventricular) pacing.

Implantation of both permanent and temporary pacemakers through a thoracotomy is less common than placement through the transvenous approach (the procedures are discussed in the next section).

Temporary pacemaker leads are implanted before cardiopulmonary bypass is discontinued, because the field is more accessible with the lungs deflated (as occurs on bypass).

Another reason the leads are implanted before bypass is discontinued is that if touching the heart during lead attachment causes an arrhythmia, perfusion to the body is not compromised. The surgeon sutures the metal wire electrode to the heart with 5-0 silk. Only the tip of the electrode is exposed wire; the remaining section is insulated.

The technologist prepares the electrode on a needle holder before or after bypass is discontinued. The assistant cuts the needle off the electrode after the surgeon places it through the myocardium. The surgeon then secures the electrode with 5-0 silk sutures. The surgeon brings the opposite end of the electrode through the skin and secures it with 2-0 silk sutures. The electrode is connected to an alligator cable and pacemaker generator. The anesthesia care provider then can pace the heart as necessary. Insertion of a transvenous pacemaker is shown in Figure 33-10.

Epicardial Pacemaker

Although permanent epicardial pacemakers are inserted less frequently than transvenous pacers, the intravenous route is not feasible in some cases, such as with stenosis of the subclavian vein. A sternotomy for cardiac surgery is not necessarily an indication for epicardial lead attachment, because leads may be inserted transvenously after sternotomy when temporary pacing is sufficient to maintain an acceptable heart rate.

The techniques for implanting the permanent pacemaker through a thoracotomy or short transverse incision are similar. Using the skin knife, the surgeon makes a short transverse incision below the xyphoid and across the diaphragm. The subcutaneous, fascial, and muscle layers are divided with the scalpel or ESU. A self-retaining retractor (e.g., a small Finochietto or a large Weitlaner retractor) is placed in the wound.

The surgeon exposes the right ventricle by opening the pericardium with the knife or dissecting scissors. Size 2-0 silk sutures are placed on the edges of the pericardium so that the assistant can put traction on the tissue. The surgeon then places several sutures of 4-0 silk or polyester through the ventricle and into the electrode's Silastic casing. The coiled metal tip of the electrode is placed in the myocardium, and the sutures are tied. Additional sutures may be needed to secure the electrode. The coiled (pigtail) lead usually is inserted into the ventricle; the harpoonlike lead generally is attached to the atrium.

To test the electrode, the surgeon connects it to an alligator cable attached to the temporary external pacemaker generator. The circulator or anesthesia care provider activates the battery. If the electrode functions normally, it is connected to the permanent battery. The surgeon makes a pocket for the battery beneath the fascia of the chest or, less often, the abdomen. The battery is inserted into the pocket, which is closed with interrupted size 0 or 2-0 nonabsorbable sutures. Size 0 or 2-0 absorbable sutures are used to approximate the subcutaneous tissue, and the skin is closed with the surgeon's suture of choice.

REPLACEMENT OF A PACEMAKER BATTERY

Surgical Goal

A malfunctioning pacemaker generator is replaced to produce continuous pacing.

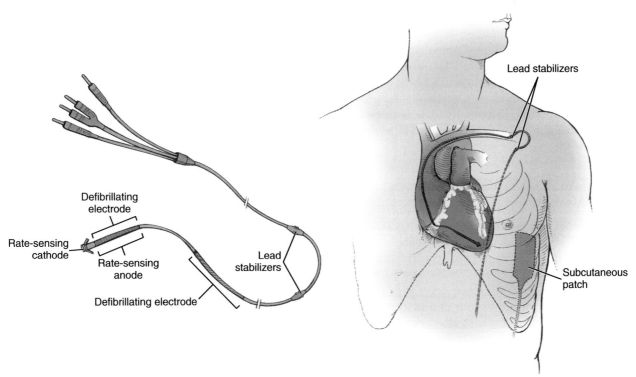

Figure 33-24   Internal cardioverter defibrillator (ICD). *(From Rothrock J: Alexander's care of the patient in surgery, ed 17, Philadelphia, 2007, Mosby.)*

Pathology

Pacemaker batteries have a limited lifespan and must be replaced periodically. A warning system, built into the battery, and routine patient assessment is normally sufficient to provide a wide measure of safety to prevent complete and sudden battery failure. Besides normal wear due to age, a battery may become damaged by trauma (such as a direct blow to the patient and battery), or a fault in the circuitry.

Technique

1. Skin and subcutaneous tissue over the generator are incised.
2. The tissue layers are divided to expose the generator and electrode or electrodes.
3. The generator is removed from the tissue pocket.
4. The electrode is connected to an alligator cable and tested.
5. The electrode is inserted into the new generator.
6. The new generator is inserted into the tissue pocket, and the wound is closed.

Discussion

The surgeon incises the skin over the generator. The underlying tissue layers are divided with sharp dissection to expose the electrodes and generator. The generator is removed from the tissue pocket, and the electrodes are disconnected. The surgeon immediately connects the electrodes to the alligator cable of an external pacer generator so that the heart can be paced continually during the exchange of generators. The electrodes are then connected to the new generator. The surgeon places the new generator in the tissue pocket. Interrupted sutures of 3-0 absorbable suture are used to approximate the tissues over the generator. The skin is then closed with interrupted 4-0 sutures.

Postoperative Considerations

Complications include malfunction or failure of the device. Frequent shocking by an implanted defibrillator can wear out the battery; patients are monitored for excessive "shocks." Injury to blood vessels used for insertion of the device (e.g., the subclavian vein) is possible, as is infection of the generator pocket. Patients are observed for injury to the heart by assessing electrocardiogram and blood pressure and other hemodynamic parameters.

IMPLANTABLE CARDIOVERTER DEFIBRILLATOR

The implantable cardioverter defibrillator (ICD) (Figure 33-24) is an electronic cardiac defibrillating and monitoring device used in patients susceptible to ventricular fibrillation or ventricular tachycardia. Most ICDs also have pacing functions to treat bradycardia, which may occur after an episode of defibrillation. The device consists of a generator, sensing electrodes, and defibrillation/pacing electrodes. Newer, transvenous ICD catheters have largely replaced the older models that used epicardial patch electrodes applied during open procedures.

The ICD may be implanted through a thoracotomy, subxyphoid, or median sternotomy incision, although most are inserted transvenously. The sensing leads are commonly placed in the right ventricle through a transvenous approach. The ventricular defibrillation leads are inserted into the heart transvenously, and the generator is placed in the superficial tissue of the chest or abdominal wall. A subcutaneous thoracic patch occasionally is used to optimize defibrillation.

SURGERY FOR ATRIAL FIBRILLATION (CARDIAC ABLATION)

Surgical Goal

Cardiac ablation is the selective destruction of diseased conductive tissue to correct atrial fibrillation (AF). Other conduction disorders include Wolff-Parkinson-White syndrome, which is characterized by multiple atrioventricular conduction pathways. By creating small areas of scar tissue in the cardiac muscle, electrical impulses are forced to follow an alternative conduction path or "maze." Ablation is commonly performed through a cardiac catheter, which delivers radiofrequency (RF) energy or cryoenergy. The procedure also may be performed through an open sternotomy.

Pathology

Atrial fibrillation is an abnormal heart rhythm. It may cause only minor discomfort, or it may result in the pooling of blood in the atria. This can lead to insufficient cardiac output and thrombus (clotting), which in turn can lead to cerebrovascular accident or pulmonary embolism.

Discussion

Interventional Cardiac Ablation

Depending on the anticipated origin of the problem, the electrophysiologist inserts a catheter percutaneously into the femoral vein or artery and threads the catheter retrograde to the right or left atrium and ventricle. The electrophysiologist tests various areas of the heart in an attempt to reproduce the dysrhythmia and then ablates the area of the heart where the rhythm disturbance originates. Postoperative considerations are similar to those for atrial fibrillation surgery.

Sternotomy Approach

Technique

1. The surgeon performs a midline sternotomy. Cannulation of the superior and inferior venae cavae is performed for total cardiopulmonary bypass.
2. The ascending aorta is occluded, and cardioplegic solution is infused through the aortic root and into the coronary arteries.
3. A right atriotomy is performed, and the right atrial targets are ablated.
4. A left atriotomy is performed, and the left atrial targets are ablated.
5. The atriotomies are closed, and the aorta is unclamped.
6. Cardiopulmonary bypass is discontinued, and the cannulas are removed.
7. Chest tubes and pacing wires are inserted, and the wound is closed.

Postoperative Considerations

Postoperatively, patients are monitored for heart rhythm problems. In patients treated for AF, it may take up to 3 months for the heart to resume beating in the normal manner. Additional postoperative considerations include monitoring for bleeding, infection, and other potential complications related to heart surgery.

PERICARDIAL WINDOW

Surgical Goal

Accumulated blood or fluid in the pericardium can compress the heart and impede filling of the ventricles. This reduces the amount of blood ejected into the systemic circulation. Removal of the fluid, through the creation of a pericardial window, improves cardiac function.

Pathology

Pericardial effusion is caused by inflammation related to an infectious disease or a tumor. It may also be a result of a fluid shift related to homeostasis. Occasionally, a postoperative chest tube may become obstructed with clotted blood, causing drainage fluid to back up into the pericardium.

Discussion

The patient is placed in the supine position with a small roll under the left chest, and the chest is prepped and draped. External defibrillator patches should be applied in case fibrillation occurs. A small incision is made in the fourth or fifth intercostal space, and a retractor is inserted. The pericardium is exposed, and a small portion (a "window") of the pericardial tissue is excised to allow fluid to leave the pericardium. The surgeon inserts a suction catheter and removes the excess fluid. One or more chest tubes are inserted, and the incision is closed.

PERICARDIECTOMY

Surgical Goal

Chronic inflammation of the pericardium can produce a fibrotic (and often calcified) coating over the heart that constricts the ventricles. Removal of the adherent scar tissue improves cardiac function.

Pathology

Constrictive pericarditis may develop because of viral infection, tuberculosis, or chronic pericarditis. The heart becomes encased within an adherent layer of scar tissue.

Technique

1. A median or bilateral transverse sternotomy is performed.
2. Fibrous tissue is removed over the left ventricle between the parietal pericardium and the epicardium (visceral pericardium).
3. Both ventricles, atria, and venae cavae are decorticated.
4. Hemostasis is maintained.
5. Chest drainage tubes are inserted.
6. The sternum is approximated with wire.
7. The incision is closed.

Discussion

The patient is placed in the supine position, and the anterior chest is prepped and draped. External defibrillator pads should be applied in case of ventricular fibrillation resulting from manipulation of the heart during dissection. A median sternotomy is performed with a sternal saw. Dissection of the dense adhesions can cause increased bleeding; suture ligatures of 4-0 or 5-0 polypropylene or silk, on pledgets if desired, may be used. Cardiopulmonary bypass often is available on a standby basis.

Basic sternotomy instruments are used in addition to lung retractors. An ultrasound debridement system occasionally is used for very dense calcification. Portions of adherent scar may be left in place if the risk of injury to underlying structures is great. Common examples are areas of the right and left coronary artery. Bilateral dissection is performed to the phrenic nerves (which are identified and preserved).

HEART FAILURE

Surgical techniques to support a failing heart are available for temporary, long-term, or permanent support. When mechanical devices cannot reverse the decline of heart function, cardiac transplantation may be required.

INSERTION AND REMOVAL OF AN INTRAAORTIC BALLOON CATHETER

Surgical Goal

An intraaortic balloon catheter reduces the workload of the heart after myocardial infarction or in patients who cannot be taken off bypass. The intraaortic balloon catheter is inserted into the descending thoracic aorta in a retrograde direction via the femoral artery. The distal tip of the catheter is positioned just below the left subclavian artery. The balloon increases the supply of oxygen to the heart by increasing coronary blood flow during diastole and improves distal perfusion of the body's organs. When the ventricle contracts, the balloon deflates, creating a vacuum that lowers the pressure in the aorta. When the ventricle relaxes, the balloon inflates, increasing the volume of blood into the coronary arteries and distal organs (Figure 33-25). This produces additional blood flow to the brain, kidneys, and other organs. The size of the balloon is determined by the size of the femoral artery.

Pathology

Myocardial infarction, described above in *Coronary Artery Bypass Grafting,* is caused by obstruction of the coronary artery and results in death of cardiac tissue. An intra-aortic balloon catheter reduces the workload of a damaged heart following myocardial infarction. This also reduces the oxygen requirements of heart tissue and compensates for the loss of coronary artery function.

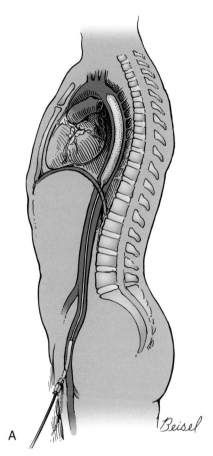

A

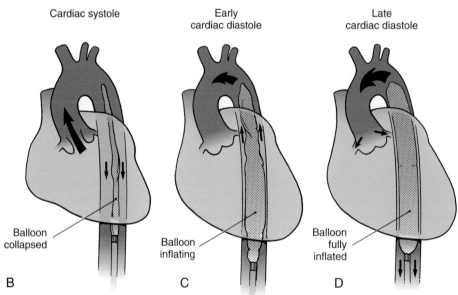

Cardiac systole | Early cardiac diastole | Late cardiac diastole

Balloon collapsed

B

Balloon inflating

C

Balloon fully inflated

D

Figure 33-25   Phases of balloon pumping. **A,** Placement of the balloon in the descending aorta. **B,** Deflation of the balloon. **C,** Early inflation of the balloon. **D,** Inflated balloon. *(Modified from Waldhausen JA, Pierce WS, Campbell DB: Surgery of the chest, ed 6, St Louis, 1996, Mosby.)*

Technique

Insertion

1. The femoral artery is exposed and isolated through a groin incision.
2. A heavy silk suture is tied around the proximal end of the balloon catheter to mark the level of insertion.
3. The femoral artery and branches are occluded, and the artery is incised.
4. The catheter is inserted into the femoral artery and advanced into the descending thoracic aorta up almost to the left subclavian artery.

Removal

1. The groin is reopened, and the femoral artery is isolated.
2. The balloon catheter is withdrawn, and the artery is occluded.
3. The femoral artery is unclamped, and the wound is closed.

Discussion

Insertion

The patient is placed in the supine position, prepped, and draped for a bilateral femoral incision. This is a precaution in case the first attempt to insert the balloon percutaneously is not successful because of aortoiliac stenosis. The procedure is performed with the patient under local anesthesia or during cardiac surgery if the heart requires support.

The groin is incised, and the incision is carried to the femoral artery and branches with sharp and blunt dissection. A small self-retaining retractor is placed in the wound. The common femoral artery and branches are mobilized with dissecting scissors, and umbilical tapes or vessel loops are placed around the vessels for traction. Bolsters may be inserted over the loops and the ends tagged.

The surgeon measures the catheter against the distance between the patient's subclavian artery and the femoral artery and then marks this level by tying a suture around the proximal end of the catheter. The catheter is deflated with a syringe before insertion.

The femoral arteries are occluded with vascular clamps (e.g., Glover or DeBakey peripheral vascular clamps), or the umbilical tapes are used as tourniquets. The surgeon makes an incision in the common femoral artery with a #11 blade. Potts scissors are used to extend the incision as needed.

The scrub moistens the balloon with saline solution. The proximal clamp is removed from the artery, and the surgeon inserts the catheter into the arteriotomy. The catheter is advanced to the level of the suture mark. The assistant controls bleeding while holding tension on the umbilical tape.

The pump technician evacuates the atmospheric air from the catheter with a 50-cc syringe, and the pump is activated. The surgeon secures the catheter to the patient's leg with 2-0 silk suture. The wound may be irrigated with antibiotic solution.

The wound is closed in layers with absorbable and nonabsorbable sutures. A pressure dressing is applied to prevent the formation of a hematoma.

Removal

The previous wound is reopened, and the femoral artery is isolated. The balloon is deflated, and the catheter is slowly withdrawn. The femoral artery is occluded, and the incision is over-sewn with continuous 5-0 polypropylene suture. Two sutures may be used. One suture is started at one side of the incision, and the other suture is started on the opposite side; the two sutures are tied in the center of the femoral artery incision.

VENTRICULAR ASSIST DEVICE

Surgical Goal

A ventricular assist device (VAD) is used to wean patients from the cardiopulmonary bypass when other means are ineffective. Patients awaiting heart transplantation also may be candidates for a VAD, which may consist of a polyurethane blood sac, flexible diaphragm, and pump assembly. The VAD maintains perfusion through cannulas placed in the chambers of the heart and the great vessels according to the patient's need. Power is provided by pneumatic, electrical, or battery-powered pumps.

VADs may be use as a bridge to transplantation (supporting the heart until an organ donor becomes available). Some newer left ventricular devices can be used as end-destination therapy (the device remains permanently implanted).

Pathology

Patients may not regain sufficient cardiac capacity to sustain full circulatory perfusion in spite of cardiac surgery with cardiopulmonary bypass. Blood must be pumped throughout the circulatory system in order to sustain life. The ventricular assist device is used when the heart is unable to fully perform this function.

Discussion

In left ventricular assistance, blood is directed from the left ventricle through the inflow cannula into the assist device and returned to the ascending aorta through the outflow cannula (Figure 33-26). Inflow and outflow are distinguished by the direction of the blood flow relative to the VAD pump. Some VAD pumps can be implanted in the chest cavity. Drivelines from the pump exit through incisions in the chest.

In right ventricular assistance, blood is directed from the right atrium into the pump and into the pulmonary artery. The outflow cannula is sutured to the pulmonary artery. In biventricular assistance, left ventricular and right ventricular devices support the two ventricles simultaneously.

An extracorporeal VAD is used for temporary short-term assistance. The pump is connected to inflow and outflow cannulas, which are passed into the thoracic cavity through the chest wall. The pump itself is secured to the outer chest wall and covered with an occlusive dressing. An implantable VAD, which is used for long-term support, uses a pump that is surgically implanted in the chest or abdomen. If a battery pack is used, it is external and its cannulas are passed through the abdomen. VADs may be used as a bridge to transplantation, as an investigational tool, or as end-stage therapy.

Postoperative Considerations

Complications include malfunction of the device, infection, and stroke. Additional complications include hemorrhage and death. Graft anastomoses within the device may require repair if persistent bleeding develops.

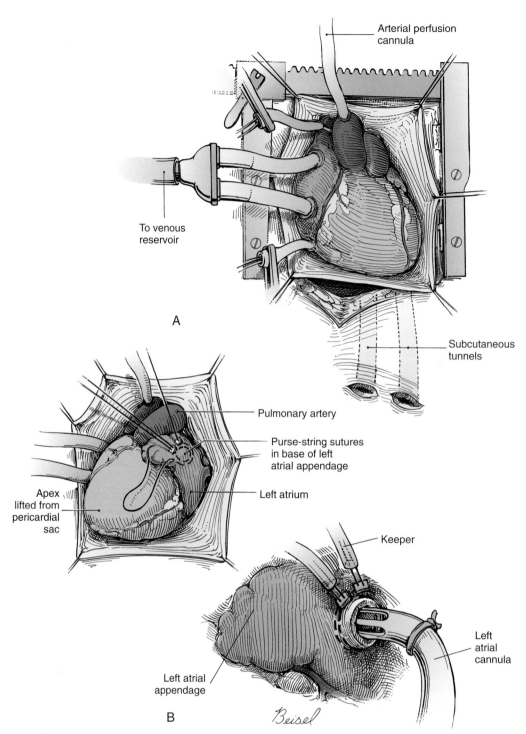

Arterial perfusion
cannula

To venous
reservoir

Subcutaneous
tunnels

A

Pulmonary artery

Purse-string sutures
in base of left
atrial appendage

Left atrium

Apex
lifted from
pericardial
sac

Keeper

Left
atrial
cannula

Left atrial
appendage

Beisel

B

Figure 33-26 Left ventricular assistance. **A,** Tunnels are developed from the pericardial
space to the skin in preparation for placement of the arterial and atrial cannulas. **B,** Two
purse-string sutures are placed at the neck of the left atrial appendage, the atrium is incised,
and the atrial cannula is inserted.

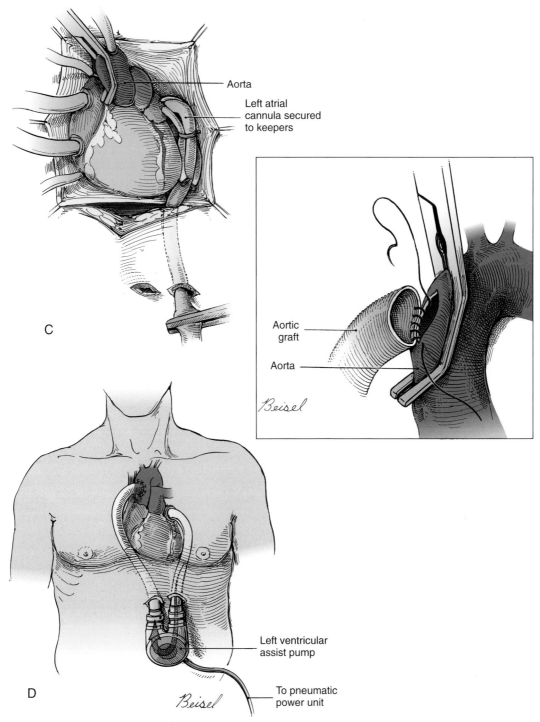

Aorta

Left atrial
cannula secured
to keepers

C

Aortic
graft

Aorta

Beisel

Left ventricular
assist pump

To pneumatic
power unit

D   *Beisel*

Figure 33-26, cont'd **C,** The Dacron graft portion of the composite arterial cannula is anastomosed to the side of the ascending aorta. The cannula is clamped and passed through the medial subcostal tunnel. **D,** Attachment of the pump. *(Modified from Waldhausen JA, Pierce WS, Campbell DB: Surgery of the chest, ed 6, St Louis, 1996, Mosby.)*

HEART TRANSPLANTATION

Surgical Goal

The goal of heart transplantation is to replace a diseased heart with a healthy donor heart.

Pathology

Heart transplant may be performed in suitable patients with end-stage cardiac disease. Patients suitable for heart transplant include those with:

- Coronary artery disease
- Congenital heart disease
- Valve disease
- Coronary artery disease
- Rejection of previously transplanted heart

Heart Procurement

Technique

1. The donor is prepped from chin to knees.
2. A median sternotomy is performed.
3. A sternal retractor is inserted.
4. The pericardium is divided.
5. Umbilical tapes are placed around the aorta and the superior and inferior venae cavae.
6. Heparin is given.
7. The aorta, the superior and inferior venae cavae, and the main pulmonary artery are dissected.
8. The superior vena cava is ligated with heavy silk ties.
9. Cardioplegic solution is infused through the proximal aorta into the heart via the coronary arteries.
10. The venae cavae and the aorta are divided; the heart is lifted to expose the pulmonary veins. The veins are divided.
11. The pulmonary artery is divided just distal to the bifurcation.
12. The heart is removed and placed in a sterile bag containing cold preservative solution.

The native (recipient) heart is not removed until the donor procurement team has confirmed that the donor heart is acceptable. Tissue-matching protocols are scrupulously followed to prevent donor-recipient mismatch.

Native Heart Excision

Technique

1. The patient is placed in the supine position and prepped from chin to knees.
2. A median sternotomy incision is made to expose the heart and great vessels.
3. Heparin is given.
4. Bicaval cannulation for cardiopulmonary bypass is performed.
5. Caval tapes are placed around each vena cava.
6. The patient is cooled, the aorta is cross-clamped, and the caval tapes are tightened around the venae cavae.
7. The pulmonary trunk and aorta are divided.
8. The atria are incised to leave intact the posterior portions of the right and left atrial walls and the interatrial septum.
9. The recipient's native heart is excised.

Two types of cardiac transplantation can be performed: orthotopic transplantation is performed more often and is the replacement of one heart with another (Figure 33-27); heterotopic ("piggy back") transplantation is the insertion of a second (donor) heart into the recipient patient's right pleural cavity. The donor heart works in tandem with the recipient's native heart. This procedure occasionally is performed when a significant size mismatch exists between a small donor and a large recipient. Combined heart-lung procedures also may be performed.

As with other transplantation procedures, it is important to minimize any delay in removing the donor heart and transporting it to the recipient.

Donor Heart Implantation

Technique

1. The donor heart is removed from the transport container and placed in a basin on the back table.
2. The surgeon inspects the heart and trims the atrial walls and great vessels in preparation for the anastomoses.
3. The donor heart is placed in the pericardial cavity and aligned with the remnant interatrial septum and the right and left atrial wall remnants of the recipient's heart.
4. The donor left atrial wall is anastomosed with a running 3-0 polypropylene suture (suture size and type may vary according to the surgeon's preference).
5. The right atrial wall is anastomosed with a running 3-0 polypropylene suture, followed by pulmonary artery anastomosis with a 4-0 polypropylene suture.
6. The aorta is anastomosed with a 3-0 running polypropylene suture.
7. Air is removed from the heart.
8. Chest drainage tubes and epicardial pacing wires are inserted.
9. The chest incision is closed.

A modification of the orthotopic implantation technique has been developed that reduces some of the cardiac rhythm problems that can occur after transplantation. End-to-end anastomoses between the superior vena cava and the inferior vena cava are performed rather than the traditional atrial-to-atrial anastomoses. A cuff of the recipient left atrium is sewn to the donor left atrium; pulmonary artery and aorta anastomoses are performed in the usual manner. A pulmonary pressure monitoring line may be inserted before the patient leaves the operating room.

Postoperative Considerations

Complications of heart transplantation include rejection and infection. Transplant anastomoses may require repair if persistent bleeding develops. Rhythm changes may occur if retained conduction tissue from both the native and donor hearts is present.

Myocardial biopsies are required after surgery to detect possible rejection. Postoperatively, the transplant patient is placed on lifelong therapy with immunosuppressive medications to prevent rejection of the donor heart. Endomyocardial biopsies are taken regularly to monitor for rejection. Patients who have undergone cardiac surgery are commonly

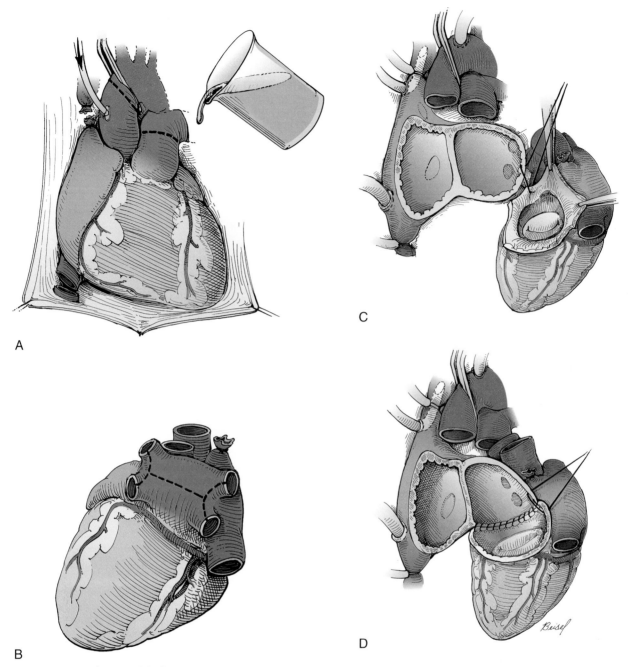

Figure 33-27 Orthotopic heart transplantation. **A,** Incision lines in the donor heart. **B,** Posterior portion of the heart incision lines connecting the pulmonary veins. **C** and **D,** Left atrial anastomosis.

Continued

transported to a cardiovascular intensive care unit (CVICU) for intensive monitoring of blood pressure, heart rate, cardiac rhythm, chest tube drainage, and temperature.

Chest tube management is especially important to remove fluid from the pericardium; fluid buildup can compress the heart, causing tamponade. If the pleural cavities have been entered, chest tubes recreate a negative pressure environment in the pleural cavity or cavities so that lung expansion (and gas exchange) can occur.

The endotracheal tube may be removed within a few hours after arrival in the CVICU, or it may remain in place until the patient is able to breathe independently. The patient's neurological, renal, pulmonary, and pain status are also closely observed and treated as necessary. Complications can include hemorrhage, prolonged ventilation, renal failure, infection, cardiac arrest, stroke, and death. Patients often are discharged from the hospital within 5 to 7 days unless complications develop.

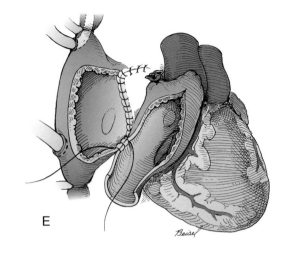

E

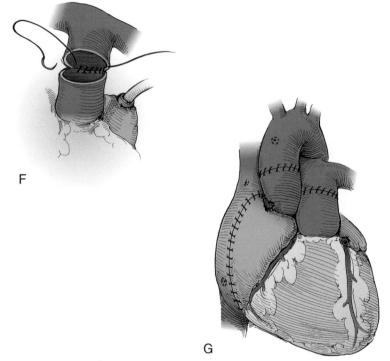

F

G

Figure 33-27, cont'd   E, Right atrial anastomosis. **F,** Pulmonary artery anastomosis. **G,** Completed transplantation. *(Modified from Waldhausen JA, Pierce WS, Campbell DB: Surgery of the chest, ed 6, St Louis, 1996, Mosby.)*

CHAPTER SUMMARY

- Cardiac surgery includes procedures of the heart and associated great vessels performed to treat acquired or congenital disease.
- The heart is a muscular organ that consists of four hollow spaces, or chambers. The two upper chambers are the right atrium and the left atrium; the two lower chambers are the right ventricle and the left ventricle.
- The walls of the heart have three layers: the outer epicardium, the middle myocardium, and the inner endocardium.

- The heart's own blood supply is delivered by the coronary artery circulation
- The valves of the heart maintain unidirectional blood flow. The atria are separated from the ventricles by the atrioventricular valves. The tricuspid valve lies on the right side, and the bicuspid (mitral) valve lies on the left side.
- The large vessels of the heart also have valves. The semilunar valves connect the ventricles to the large vessels. The pulmonary valve connects the right ventricle with the pulmonary artery. The left

aortic valve connects the left ventricle to the aorta.

- The cardiac cycle is the pumping action of the heart from one beat to the next. The cycle occurs in two phases, systole and diastole.
- During systole, the ventricles contract; during diastole, they relax and fill with blood.
- The electrical conduction system contains a network of specialized cells, which generate electrical activity along conduction pathways.
- In coronary artery disease, scarring of the arterial wall, calcification, thrombosis, and uptake of cholesterol results in decreased blood flow to the heart muscle. This can cause myocardial infarction, angina, conduction defects, and death.
- Blockage in one or more coronary arteries can produce myocardial infarction. This is vascular blockage to an area of the heart, resulting in tissue death and cessation of effective heart contraction.
- Fibrillation is ineffective quivering of the heart muscle rather than coordinated muscular action that results in effective pumping.
- In cardiac catheterization, the heart chambers and great vessels are cannulated by percutaneous insertion of a catheter. Specific tests are then performed from within the cardiac system.
- Cardiac procedures are commonly performed through a median sternotomy or lateral incision.
- A number of implants are used in cardiac surgery, including valves, vessel grafts, and repair patches for the heart and vessels.
- A pacemaker is a device that produces electrical impulses that stimulate the heart muscle. This process is called *pacing the heart*.
- The heart-lung machine takes the place of the heart and lungs by pumping and perfusing blood, which has been shunted outside the body. The heart-lung pump collects the blood, removes excess carbon dioxide, oxygenates it, and returns it to the body.
- Median sternotomy is a midline incision used for surgical procedures of the heart and great vessels in the thoracic cavity.
- Cardioplegic solution is used to stop the heart; this reduces the energy required by the cardiac muscle by eliminating the energy requirements of contraction during surgery.
- During coronary artery bypass, an autograft artery commonly is used to bypass a diseased coronary artery to increase blood flow to the heart muscle.
- In transmyocardial revascularization, a series of small-bore transmural channels are created with the carbon dioxide or holmium:YAG laser to perfuse the myocardium.
- The aortic valve maintains one-way blood flow from the left ventricle to the aorta. A diseased valve may be replaced to restore blood flow. Common causes of valve insufficiency are endocarditis, congenital anomalies, and calcification.
- An aneurysm is a potentially life-threatening condition in which the walls of a vessel or heart chamber weaken because of cardiovascular disease, leading to thinning and ballooning. This can lead to separation of the vessel or chamber walls or complete rupture.
- A saccular aneurysm is a ballooning out of a localized area in the artery. A fusiform aneurysm involves the entire circumference of the artery.
- A ballooning vessel begins to delaminate (the intimal layer separates), and blood is forced between the layers, resulting in rupture. Delamination is also called *dissection*, and the aneurysm then is referred to as a *dissecting aneurysm*.
- An implantable cardioverter-defibrillator is an electronic cardiac defibrillating and monitoring device used in patients susceptible to ventricular fibrillation or ventricular tachycardia. Most ICDs also have pacing functions to treat bradycardia, which may occur after an episode of defibrillation.
- Cardiac ablation is the selective destruction of diseased conductive tissue to correct atrial fibrillation and other conduction disorders.
- Constrictive pericarditis may develop because of viral infection, tuberculosis, or chronic pericarditis. The heart becomes encased within an adherent layer of scar tissue. Pericardiectomy is performed to relieve the stricture.
- An intraaortic balloon catheter reduces the workload of the heart after myocardial infarction or in patients who cannot be taken off bypass.
- Removal of the native heart and replacement with a donor heart is indicated for patients with end-stage cardiac disease.
- The ductus arteriosus is a normal anatomical opening in the fetal heart. During fetal development, blood is pumped from the right ventricle into the systemic circulation by way of the ductus, which connects the pulmonary artery and descending thoracic aorta. At birth, the lungs expand and the ductus closes spontaneously within a short time. A patent ductus is one that does not close spontaneously.
- Coarctation of the thoracic aorta is a congenital stenosis that usually occurs near the junction of the fetal ductus arteriosus and the aorta. Severe narrowing obstructs the normal flow of blood through the thoracic aorta and to the lower body.
- An atrial septal defect is a congenital anomaly in which a hole in the interatrial septum allows blood from the left atrium to flow to the right atrium. The goal of surgery is to close the defect and reduce excessive blood flow to the pulmonary system.
- A ventricular septal defect causes increased pulmonary pressure by allowing blood from the left ventricle to flow into the right ventricle and to the lungs, leading to

congestive heart failure. The septal defect is repaired to restore normal cardiac circulation.

- Tetralogy of Fallot is a combination of congenital defects that includes pulmonary stenosis, ventricular septal defect, right ventricular hypertrophy, and dextroposition (displacement) of the aorta. Surgical repair is performed to correct cyanosis and restore normal blood flow.

REVIEW QUESTIONS

1. What is the cause of endocarditis?
2. Define tetralogy of Fallot.
3. What is the difference between atherosclerosis and arteriosclerosis?
4. What is a cardioplegic solution?
5. What is the primary significance of coronary artery disease?
6. Define a dissecting aneurysm.
7. Define commissurotomy.
8. What are the effects of ischemic heart disease on the heart's ability to conduct electrical impulses?
9. What is the purpose of atrial ablation?

BIBLIOGRAPHY

Carabello BA: Aortic stenosis: two steps forward, one step back, *Circulation* 115:2799, 2007.

Cohn LH, editor: *Cardiac surgery in the adult*, New York, 2008, McGraw-Hill.

Conrad MF, Cambria RP: Contemporary management of descending thoracic and thoracoabdominal aortic aneurysms: endovascular versus open, *Circulation* 117:841, 852, 2008.

Crum BGL: Thoracic surgery. In Rothrock JC, editor: *Alexander's care of the patient in surgery*, ed 13, St Louis, 2007, Elsevier/Mosby.

Damiano RJ: Robotics in cardiac surgery: the emperor's new clothes, *Journal of Thoracic and Cardiovascular Surgery* 134:559, 2007.

Denholm B: Clinical issues: implant documentation, *AORN Journal* 87:433, 2008.

Fedak PWM, McCarthy PM, Bonow RO: Evolving concepts and technologies in mitral valve repair (review), *Circulation* 117:963, 2008.

Fuster V, editor: *The heart*, ed 12, New York, 2007, McGraw-Hill.

Goksel OS, Tireli E, Kalko Y et al: Mid-term outcome with surgery for type B aortic dissections: a single center experience, *Journal of Cardiac Surgery* 23:27, 2008.

Grube E, Schuler G, Buellesfeld L et al: Percutaneous aortic valve replacement for severe aortic stenosis in high-risk patients using the second- and current third-generation self-expanding CoreValve prosthesis: device success and 30-day clinical outcomes, *Journal of the American College of Cardiology* 50:69, 2007.

Haywood PAR, Buxton BF: Contemporary graft patency: 5-year observational data from a randomized trial of conduits, *Annals of Thoracic Surgery* 84:795, 2007.

Jeong SM, Hahn KD, Jeong YB et al: Warming of intravenous fluids prevents hypothermia during off-pump coronary artery bypass graft surgery, *Journal of Cardiothoracic and Vascular Anesthesia* 22:67, 2008.

Kouchoukos NT, Blackstone EH, Doty DB et al: *Kirklin/Barratt-Boyes cardiac surgery*, ed 3, vol 1 and 2, Philadelphia, 2003, Churchill Livingstone.

Levy MN, Pappano A: *Cardiovascular physiology*, ed 9, St Louis, 2007, Mosby.

Nagelhout JJ, Zaglaniczny KL: *Nurse anesthesia*, ed 3, St Louis, 2005, Elsevier/Saunders.

Oakley RE, Kleine P, Bach DS: Choice of prosthetic heart valve in today's practice, *Circulation* 117:253, 2008.

Pagana KD, Pagana TJ: *Mosby's diagnostic and laboratory test reference*, ed 7, St Louis, 2005, Elsevier/Mosby.

Paul S, Vollano L: Care of patients with acute heart failure. In Moser DK, Riegel B, editors: *Cardiac nursing: a companion to Braunwald's heart disease*, St Louis, 2008, Elsevier/Saunders.

Pelter MM: Electrocardiography: normal electrocardiogram. In Moser DK, Riegel B, editors: *Cardiac nursing: a companion to Braunwald's heart disease*, St Louis, 2008, Elsevier/Saunders.

Rubertone JA: Anatomy of the cardiovascular system. In Moser DK, Riegel B, editors: *Cardiac nursing: a companion to Braunwald's heart disease*, St Louis, 2008, Elsevier/Saunders.

Seeley RR, Stephens TD, Tate P: *Anatomy and physiology*, ed 8, Boston, 2008, McGraw-Hill.

Seifert PC: Cardiac surgery. In Rothrock JC, editor, *Alexander's care of the patient in surgery*, ed 13, St Louis, 2007, Elsevier/Mosby.

Seifert PC, Collins J, Ad N: Surgery for atrial fibrillation, *AORN Journal* 86:23, 2008.

Stewart S: Epidemiology of coronary artery disease. In Moser DK, Riegel B, editors: *Cardiac nursing: a companion to Braunwald's heart disease*, St Louis, 2008, Elsevier/Saunders.

Thompson J, Bertling G: *Endovascular leaks: perioperative nursing implications, AORN Journal* 89: 839, 2009.

Trupp RJ, Bubien RS: Care of patients with implanted cardiac rhythm management devices. In Moser DK, Riegel B, editors: *Cardiac nursing: a companion to Braunwald's heart disease*, St Louis, 2008, Elsevier/Saunders.

Wagner GS: *Marriott's practical electrocardiography*, ed 11, Philadelphia, 2008, Lippincott Williams & Wilkins.

Pediatric Surgery

CHAPTER OUTLINE

LEARNING OBJECTIVES

After studying this chapter the reader will be able to:

- Discuss terms associated with congenital birth anomalies
- Describe the basic physiological and anatomical differences between children and adults
- Discuss important aspects of pediatric anesthesia
- Identify the developmental stages of pediatric groups
- Apply developmental features to the care of the pediatric patient

- Discuss the special equipment and supplies used in pediatric surgery
- Explain the strategies and role of the surgical technologist in pediatric patient safety
- Identify common pediatric procedures by specialty and organ system

TERMINOLOGY

Acquired abnormality: A physiological or anatomical defect that develops in fetal life as a result of environmental factors, such as exposure to infection or certain drugs or poor nutrition.

Atresia: The absence or closure of an orifice or tubular structure.

Bolus: A compact substance (e.g., undigested food, fecal material) which occurs normally in the digestive tract.

Child life specialist: A trained professional who specializes in the psychosocial care of and communication with pediatric patients and their families.

Choanal: A term that describes the communicating passageways between the nasal fossae and the pharynx.

Coarctation: Narrowing of the passageway of a blood vessel, such as coarctation of the aorta, a congenital condition.

Congenital: A condition or an anomaly that develops during fetal life.

Ductus arteriosus: A normal fetal structure that allows blood to bypass circulation to the lungs. If this structure remains open after birth, it is called a *patent ductus arteriosus.*

Embryonic life: The first 8 weeks of gestational development.

Exstrophy: The eversion, or turning out, of an organ.

Fetus: Gestational life after 8 weeks.

Gastroschisis: A herniation of abdominal contents through the abdominal wall that is present at birth.

Genetic abnormality: A birth anomaly that is inherited.

Homeostasis: The balance of physiological processes that maintain life.

Intussusception: The telescoping of one portion of the intestine into another.

Isolette: An infant-size "bed" and transport unit that is environmentally controlled and equipped with monitoring devices.

Magical thinking: A psychological process in which a person attributes intention and will to inanimate objects. Magical thinking may also include a patient who believes that an event will happen because he or she wills it or wishes it. This is a normal developmental stage of toddlers.

Mutagenic substance: A chemical or other agent which causes permanent change in the cell's genetic material.

Nephroblastoma: Wilms' tumor.

Neural tube defect: A congenital abnormality resulting from failure of the neural tube to close in embryonic development.

Omphalocele: A protrusion of abdominal contents through an opening at the navel, especially when it occurs as a congenital defect.

Prewarming: A procedure in which the patient is warmed before surgery, which is done as a separate process in perioperative care.

Pyloric stenosis: A narrowing of the part of the stomach (pylorus) that leads to the small intestine.

Teratogen: A chemical or agent that can injure the fetus or cause birth defects.

Thyroglossal duct: A transitory endodermal tube in the embryo that carries thyroid-forming tissue at its caudal end. The duct normally disappears after the thyroid has moved to its ultimate location in the neck. The point of origin of the thyroglossal duct is regularly marked on the base of the adult tongue by the foramen cecum.

INTRODUCTION

Pediatric surgery is a multidisciplinary field that encompasses many surgical specialties. Most procedures can be classified in one of three groups:

- Surgery for treatment of **congenital** anomalies
- Procedures for treatment of disease
- Trauma surgery

Innovative techniques in fetal surgery are also being developed and refined as a separate specialty of pediatric medicine.

Pediatrics includes the care of the child from neonate to late adolescence. Because many surgical procedures are an integral part of the child's growth and development, the patient often is followed into adulthood.

Pediatric surgery includes a variety of pathologies, which are not restricted to one body system. However many pediatric surgeons specialize in a particular system or area of medicine, such as pediatric cardiac, maxillofacial, or trauma surgery.

An important dynamic of pediatric surgery is the family's experience in the perioperative process. The family and patient cannot be separated in this specialty, and they require equal consideration in communication and psychosocial care.

The purpose of this chapter is to provide an overview of the physiological and psychological needs of the pediatric patient and to present *common* procedures. Procedures that are performed in both adult and pediatric patients are presented in that specialty chapter (e.g., hernia surgery is presented in Chapter 23 because it is performed on adults and children while omphalocele, which also an abdominal wall defect, is presented in this chapter). The procedures included in this chapter are performed most often in pediatric patients only.

The reader should refer to specialty chapters to review the *Surgical Anatomy* associated with each procedure presented in this chapter. Important physiological and psychosocial considerations are provided to highlight special needs of pediatric patients in the perioperative environment.

PHYSIOLOGICAL AND ANATOMICAL CONSIDERATIONS

The body's mechanisms for maintaining **homeostasis** (physiological balance) in a pediatric patient are different from those in an adult in many ways. Some of these differences create increased risks for the pediatric surgical patient.

THERMOREGULATION

All patients are at risk of hypothermia during surgery. However, pediatric patients, especially infants and neonates, are particularly vulnerable to hypothermia and hyperthermia. Important facts to remember are:

1. Physiological mechanisms that normally regulate temperature in an adult are absent or undeveloped in the infant. Infants and children tend to lose more heat than they generate.
2. Infants' relatively large skin surface area and low body weight can contribute to rapid lowering of the core temperature.
3. Children and infants have extensive peripheral circulation, which contributes to relatively rapid cooling.
4. Infants lack adequate insulation (fatty tissue) to maintain the core temperature in a cold environment.
5. Infants and children shown a wide range in temperature variation compared to adults.

Hypothermia

Environmental factors are an important cause of hypothermia in pediatric patients:

- Loss of body heat can occur through conduction when the patient's skin comes in contact with cold surfaces (e.g., a cold operating table or transport crib).
- Heat loss by radiation occurs as the patient's own body heat is given up to cold air in the operating room. Heat loss by radiation is intensified when body tissues are exposed during open procedures.
- Prep solutions contribute to hypothermia in two ways. Water absorbs heat from the body much more rapidly

than air. Consequently, cool prep solutions lower the body temperature by both conduction and evaporation.

- Wet linens, drapes, and bedclothes are a source of body cooling during the perioperative period.
- Anesthetics have a profound hypothermic effect in children. This is an added burden to the physiological stress of poor thermoregulation.

Hypothermia can result in a chain of physiological events that place the pediatric patient at risk for cardiac problems, apnea, and hypoglycemia. Pediatric patients, especially infants, have little metabolic tolerance for cold. They have little reserve fat, and blood vessels are close to the skin, causing rapid heat loss. Approximately 60% to 75% of body heat is lost through radiation of body heat to the air. As the core temperature begins to drop, metabolism slows (approximately 50% at 82.4° F [28° C]). Heart rate and stroke volume decrease, and systemic blood pressure falls. A drop in circulating blood and respiratory rate causes a decrease of up to 6% in normal oxygen intake. In the pediatric patient, this can be a critical level.

Shivering, a compensatory reaction to cold normally occurs with hypothermia in adults. However, infants lack this mechanism. When an infant is cold, brown fat, found only in babies, is metabolized, using up oxygen and glucose. The result is hypoxemia and hypoglycemia. Electrolyte balance is disturbed, leading to loss of intravascular fluids into the skin. The effects of these physiological events can be rapid and severe. Cardiac arrhythmias leading to arrest may occur.

Hyperthermia

Environmental hyperthermia is less of a risk to pediatric surgical patients. However, elevated core temperatures can occur with misuse of warming devices. Warm light from the operating microscope may generate enough heat to raise an infant's core temperature, especially when the light is directed into a body cavity. Hyperthermia also can be induced in the perioperative period by too much covering. Waterproof drapes trap heat and may contribute to hyperthermia.

Physiological hyperthermia, such as malignant hyperthermia (MH), is a greater risk in pediatric patients than in adults. (Chapter 12 presents a complete discussion of malignant hyperthermia, its causes, and the emergency response.)

PERIOPERATIVE INTERVENTIONS TO MAINTAIN NORMOTHERMIA

Steps to maintain the pediatric patient's temperature are implemented throughout the perioperative period. If the patient becomes chilled, it may be difficult to re-establish warmth, which must be done by active warming methods.

Transport and Prewarming

Interventions to maintain the patient's temperature begin during transport to the surgical department. Infants and children may become chilled during transport therefore personnel must make sure that adequate blankets are available before transport. Neonates may arrive in a heated **Isolette** (an infant-size transport unit that is environmentally controlled and equipped with monitoring devices). Infants and neonates should wear a head covering at all times. On arrival in the operating room, the patient is taken to a preheated holding area. A period of **prewarming** may be done in the holding area of the operating room. The patient is covered with a warm air blanket composed of connecting air tubes or placed on a warm air mattress for prewarming.

Intraoperative Warming

During surgery, a number of methods are used to maintain the core temperature (see Chapter 12).

- The operating room is prewarmed before the patient arrives. The anesthesia care provider and surgeon agree on the correct temperature for preparation of the patient.
- A warm air blanket may remain in use during the procedure. Upper and lower body mattresses are available for this purpose.
- A water-filled blanket may be used underneath the patient during surgery. Warm or cool water can be used to treat hyperthermia or to prevent hypothermia. Water blankets are programmable to maintain a constant temperature and have alarms in case flow is occluded.
- Heating lamps or overhead heating panels are used during the preoperative prep or anytime supplemental warming is needed. These are commonly used in neonatal and infant care in the surgical environment. Portable overhead lamps must be adjusted to prevent patient burns. A safe distance based on light aperture and intensity is established by the manufacturer. These parameters must be followed precisely, and the patient must be continuously monitored to prevent injury. Dehydration is a risk when overhead heating lamps are used.
- A solution warmer is used during surgical procedures to maintain the correct temperature of irrigation solutions. Intravenous solutions are also prewarmed before administration.
- Surgical sponges are moistened with warm saline before use.

Monitoring

Pediatric biophysical monitoring uses many of the same techniques as in adult care. Esophageal and rectal probes assess the precise core body temperature. For short procedures, external measuring devices (axillary probes) are used.

FLUID BALANCE

Fluid balance (maintaining the correct amount and types of fluids in body spaces) is an important goal in the care of pediatric patients. Infants and children can become rapidly dehydrated, requiring intravenous (IV) replacement. Before surgery begins, an IV line is inserted to maintain access to the circulatory system. Renal output is measured carefully and if needed, tests can be done for specific electrolyte balance at any time. The body to surface area ratio in young children and infants contributes to an increased risk of acid-base imbalance in the blood. Arterial blood gas determinations (ABGs; see chapters 12 and 20) can rapidly detect acid-base imbalance. Certain surgical procedures, such as those of the gastrointestinal system, increase the risk of dehydration and electrolyte shifts. The anesthesia care provider maintains constant monitoring to ensure that electrolyte imbalance is quickly brought under control.

Hemostasis is a critical element in pediatric surgery. Infants and children have little blood reserve and cannot tolerate persistent bleeding. All members of the surgical team are jointly responsible for monitoring blood loss as efficiently and accurately as possible. The scrubbed technologist must report the cumulative amount of irrigation fluid used during surgery so that this can be subtracted from the amount of fluid in each suction canister. Used sponges are maintained carefully, according to facility protocol, and weighed to determine blood loss.

The surgical technologist should have appropriate clamps, suture, and hemostatic materials and agents available according to the requirements of the procedure. The importance of the scrub's role during critical moments of hemorrhage cannot be overstated. The technologist should plan for such emergencies before surgery and mentally rehearse the steps needed to act quickly and correctly. Consulting with the surgeon on specific instruments and supplies *before surgery* reinforces learning.

RESPIRATORY SYSTEM AND AIRWAY

An important anatomical difference between the adult and pediatric respiratory systems is the structure airway. Failure to manage a pediatric patient's airway is among the leading causes of death in medical and traumatic emergency. The following are some of the important features of the pediatric airway:

- The tongue is large in proportion to the oral cavity.
- Infants less than 8 weeks of age are obligate nose breathers; this means that obstruction of the nasal passages may cause severe respiratory compromise.
- In infants and children, the trachea is much shorter and smaller than in adults.
- The airway is more delicate and less rigid than in an adult.
- The thoracic wall is weak and unstable in children. The costal and suprasternal muscles are prominent with airway obstruction or lung disease (e.g., pneumonia).
- Lung residual capacity is much lower in children than in adults. This contributes to much more rapid hypoxia if the airway is lost.

PATHOLOGY

During early **embryonic life,** organ systems develop from one of three cellular layers: the endoderm, the ectoderm, or the mesoderm (Figure 34-1). Each layer gives rise to a specific set of organs through a complex process. Figure 34-2 illustrates weekly developmental events as the embryo devel-

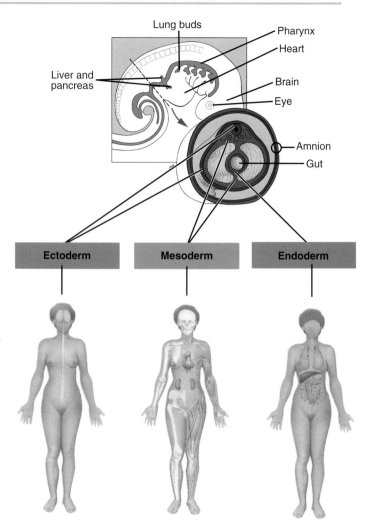

Figure 34-1 Embryonic membranes. In early embryonic life, three germ layers begin to develop into specific organ systems. *(Thibodeau G, Patton K:* Anatomy and physiology, *ed 6, Philadelphia, Mosby, 2007.)*

ops into a **fetus** in the first 3 months. Disturbances during the critical stages of germ cell differentiation and organ development can result in errors or defects in a structure or organ system.

Much of pediatric surgery is performed to correct structural defects that develop during fetal life; these are called *congenital or genetic abnormalities.* The cause of the abnormality may be **genetic** (inherited) or **acquired.** An *acquired* defect is the result of one or more *environmental agents* or conditions to which the fetus is exposed. The most vulnerable period in fetal life is the first 60 days. This is a period of rapid cellular and tissue differentiation.

An environmental agent (a chemical or drug) that injures the embryo or fetus is called a **teratogen.** Examples of teratogens are environmental mercury and alcohol. Certain drugs are also known to cause severe developmental defects. These include some recreational and prescription drugs.

Mutagenic substances cause gene mutation, a chemical change in the genetic structure. Mutation can cause retardation, skeletal deformity, or microcephaly (severely diminished

TIMETABLE OF HUMAN PRENATAL DEVELOPMENT
1 TO 6 WEEKS

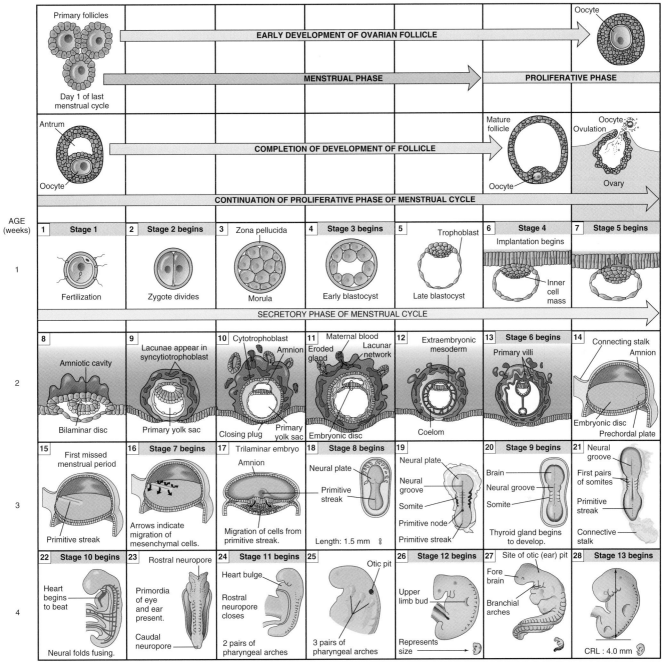

Figure 34-2 Embryonic development in the first trimester of life. Disturbances during the critical stages of germ cell differentiation and organ development can result in errors or defects in a structure or organ system. (*Thibodeau G, Patton K: Anatomy and physiology, ed 6, Philadelphia, Mosby, 2007.*)

Continued

brain development). Gamma radiation (x-rays) is both mutagenic and teratogenic.

The maternal diet is an important source of congenital birth defects. For example, lack of folic acid in the mother's diet causes specific spinal cord (neural tube) defects, such as spina bifida and anencephaly (absence of a cranial vault). A low-protein diet results in poor fetal development.

Certain *infectious agents* are also known be teratogenic. The following infectious microorganisms cause significant congenital abnormalities (listed in parenthesis):

- *Toxoplasma gondii* (cerebral calcifications, microcephaly, heart defects)
- Rubella virus—the causative agent of measles (cataract, glaucoma, deafness, heart defects, retinal defects)
- Cytomegalovirus (hydrocephalus, deafness)
- Herpes virus (microcephaly, microphthalmia, retinal defect)
- Varicella-zoster virus—the causative agent of chickenpox (muscle atrophy, mental retardation)

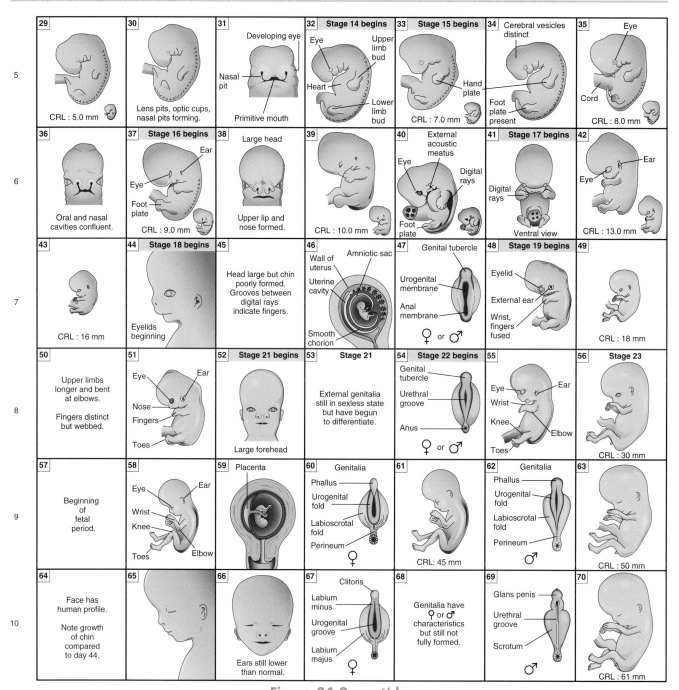

Figure 34-2, cont'd.

- *Treponema pallidum*—the causative agent of syphilis (hydrocephalus, deafness, bone defects)

Table 34-1 presents important congenital and inherited abnormalities.

Note: Congenital defects of the skull and facial bones are presented in Chapters 28 and 35.

ANESTHESIA

Many procedures that otherwise could be carried out using regional anesthesia or monitored sedation are performed in the pediatric patient using general anesthesia. This is partly because general anesthesia allows the anesthesia care provider to secure the airway and maintain full respiratory control during the procedure. General anesthesia is also necessary because children are unable to cooperate during regional anesthesia.

The differences between adult and pediatric anesthesia are related to mainly physiological and anatomical variations between the two populations. (A complete discussion of anesthesia is presented in Chapter 12.) Important considerations in learning about pediatric anesthesia are:

1. Anesthesia (and surgery) involves the entire family, not just the patient.
2. Children are much more sensitive to small variations in drug doses than are adults.

Table 34-1

Congenital and Genetic Abnormalities

Condition	Description	Considerations
Ancephaly	Congenital anomaly in which large parts of the brain fail to development. Occurs in 3 out of 10,000 births.	Neonates with this lethal neural tube defect do not survive.
Atrial septal defect	Congenital cardiac defect in which a hole in the interatrial septum allows blood from the left atrium to flow into the right atrium.	Surgical repair is necessary to close the defect. See *Closure of an Atrial Septal Defect.*
Branchial cleft cysts and clefts	These are embryonic reminents or slits in the neck region which persist as cysts or fistulas after birth. They may not be diagnosed unless they interfere with structural function or become infected.	Surgical removal may be necessary.
Chest wall deformities	Two common chest wall deformities are *pectus excavatum* (PE) and *pectus carinatum* (PC). In PE the sternum is concave and may impinge on thoracic structures. In PC the sternum protrudes.	Surgical reconstruction is performed for cosmetic purposes or to relieve pressure on thoracic structures. See *Repair of Pectus Excavatum.*
Choanal atresia	Choanal atresia is a congenital anomaly characterized by a stricture or blockage of the passage between the nasal sinus and the pharyngonasal airways. Bilateral choanal atresia (both sides of the nasal passage are blocked) is a neonatal emergency; immediate treatment is required to maintain oxygen perfusion in the newborn.	Surgical repair is performed at birth in emergency cases. Endoscopic surgery and splinting of airways may be performed in non-emergency cases.
Cleft lip or palate	Partial or complete division of the lip or palate prevents the infant from suckling effectively. The defect occurs in about 1 in 700 live births.	Surgical reconstruction is performed in stages beginning at about 12 weeks of age. See *Repair of a Cleft Lip* and *Repair of a Cleft Palate*
Coarctation of the aorta	Congenital narrowing of the thoracic aorta which restricts blood flow to the lower body.	Surgical treatment is necessary to restore circulation. See *Correction of Coractation of the Aorta*
Esophageal atresia	Complete or partial absence of the esophagus. The defect is associated with tracheoesophageal fistula (see below).	Surgical reconstruction of the esophagus is necessary for nutritional intake. See *Correction of Esophageal Atresian and Tracheoesophogeal Fistula.*
Gastroschisis	An abominal wall defect in which the viscera form outside the body. In this defect there is no sac surrounding the viscera. The cause is unknown.	Immediate surgical repair is required to preserve the viscera. See *Abdominal Wall Defects.*
Hirschsprung disease (megacolon)	Congenital absence of ganglion cells, which control the relaxation and contraction that occur in peristalsis of the bowel. This causes chronic bowel obstruction.	Surgery is performed to remove the disease bowel. See *Resection and Pull-Through for Hirschsprung Disease.*
Infantile hypertrophic pyloric stenosis (IHPS)	Also called *pyloric stenosis;* a congenital anomaly in which the longitudinal and circular muscles of the gastric pylorus are thickened. This results in obstruction at the pylorus.	Surgical treatment is performed to release the thickened bands of muscle and release the stricture. See *Pyloromyotomy.*
Omphalocele	A type of abdominal wall deformity in which the viscera develop outside the body, contained within a peritoneal sac.	Surgery is performed as soon as possible after birth to conserve the tissues involved. See *Repair of an Omphalocele.*
Patent ductus arteriosus	The ductus arteriosus is a fetal heart structure that shunts blood from the right ventrical into the systemic circulation. The ductus normally closes shortly after birth. A persistent or patent ductus arteriosus may result in heart failure	Surgical repair is necessary to close a patient ductus arteriosus. See *Closure of a Patent Ductus Arteriosus.*
Pulmonary valve stenosis	Congenital cardiac defect in which the pulmonary valve leaflets are fused, restricting circulation of blood from the right ventricle to the lungs.	Surgical repair is necessary to restore circulation. See *Correction of Pulmonary Valve Stenosis.*
Spina bifida	A congenital anomaly which includes several types neural tube defects including incomplete closure of the bony spinal column around the spinal cord. The deformity often causes lower extremity paralysis and loss of bladder and bowel function. Spina bifida is associated with folic acid deficiency during pregnancy.	Surgical repair to close the superficial tissue layers is possible. However, nerve damage is not reversible. See *Repair of Myelomeningocele.*

Continued

Table 34-1

Congenital and Genetic Abnormalities—cont'd

Condition	Description	Considerations
Syndactyly	Webbing of the fingers or toes as a result of incomplete separation of the digits in embryonic life.	See *Correction of Syndactyly*
Tetralogy of Fallot	A combination of congenital defects. The anomalies include pulmonary stenosis, ventricular septal defect, right ventricular hypertrophy, and transposition of the aorta.	Treatment is surgical repair of the defects. See *Repair of Tetralogy of Fallot.*
Tracheoesophageal fistula	A fistula connecting the esophagus with the trachea. The defect results in aspiration of liquid and food particles into the trachea.	The defect is surgically closed to prevent aspiration. See *Correction of Esophageal Atresia and Tracheoesophageal Fistula.*
Ventricular septal defect	Congenital cardiac defect in which blood from the left ventricle flows into the right ventricle and lungs, leading to congestive heart failure.	Surgical repair is necessary to close the defect. See *Closure of a Ventricular Septal Defect.*
Wilms' tumor (nephroblastoma)	The most common primary renal malignancy of children. The tumor can become very large and spread from the abdomen to the lungs.	Surgical en bloc resection is performed when possible. The kidney, ureter, and adrenal gland are removed. More extensive dissection and resection may be required.

3. IV fluids are commonly administered with micro drip tubing and a burette chamber. This provides accurate measurement of fluids.

4. Pediatric patients often are induced and maintained with inhalation anesthesia by mask or by laryngeal or endotracheal tube. Inhalation anesthetics are taken up quickly by the brain, allowing rapid induction.

5. IV access is usually obtained after induction to avoid patient struggling and anxiety.

6. Oral intake is restricted preoperatively in pediatric patients to reduce the risk of aspiration and during anesthesia. As a general rule, clear liquids are withheld for 2 hours before surgery and breast milk for 4 hours. Solid food is withheld for 6 hours before surgery.[1]

7. Children are unable to cooperate fully during procedures that could otherwise be performed under regional anesthesia and therefore require a general anesthetic more often.

PREPARATION FOR ANESTHESIA

Pediatric patients are assessed and prepared for anesthesia using methods similar to those for adults. However, the psychological preparation must take into consideration the child's more extreme fears, especially the trauma of separation. Whenever possible, the family is prepared for the experience of anesthesia at least 4 days before surgery. Age-appropriate preparation may include familiarizing the child with anesthesia devices, surgical attire, and other objects that can cause anxiety. (Chapter 12 presents a complete discussion of the preoperative assessment of a patient.) A brief review of preoperative preparation as it applies to pediatric patients is presented here:

1. A preoperative history is taken, including current health status, chronic and acute conditions, history of past diseases, and previous surgery.

2. The patient's current medications, anesthesia history, and allergies are recorded.

3. A review of systems is performed (i.e., routine physical assessment of each system).

4. The results of routine laboratory tests are reviewed.

5. Additional tests are requested as needed.

6. The preoperative medication and induction method are discussed with the family.

7. Special considerations for children are taken into account (e.g., loose or missing teeth, cardiac defects, croup, history of apnea, recent respiratory infection).

PREOPERATIVE MEDICATION AND INDUCTION

Pediatric patients may be given an anxiolytic (anxiety reducing) medication before surgery. However, this practice varies from institution to institution and among anesthesia care providers. Preoperative sedation may delay recovery from anesthesia, and the method of administration (injection or a bitter-tasting oral medication) may increase anxiety in the child. Other drawbacks include an increased risk of falls and adverse physiological events, such as respiratory depression. If preoperative medication is required, a number of drugs are available (Table 34-2).

Induction

Allowing one or both parents to be present during induction now is an accepted practice in many health care facilities. This has proved to reduce the need for preoperative medication in

Table 34-2

Common Preoperative Medications Used in Pediatric Surgery

Agent/Drug	Route	Comments
H₂ blocker (ranitidine, famotidine)	Oral, intravenous (IV)	• Prevents gastrin-stimulated acid secretion
Ketamine	Intramuscular (IM) injection Oral	• Produces anesthesia within 3 minutes • May be combined with midazolam for mask induction
Lidocaine 2.5% and prilocaine 2.5% (EMLA cream)	Topical	• Applied to the skin before insertion of an IV cannula to reduce the pain of insertion
Methohexital (Brevital)	Rectal	• Produces sleep within about 10 minutes
Metoclopramide (Reglan)	Oral or IV	• Antiemetic
Midazolam (Versed)	Oral Intranasal Sublingual Rectal	• May be administered by the parent • Produces peak effect in 30 minutes • May prolong anesthesia recovery • Causes antegrade amnesia after 10 minutes
Oral transoral fentanyl citrate	Oral transmucosal	• May be used in lollipop form for pain relief in short procedures

many pediatric patients. Parents who are not fearful themselves may stay with the patient from the time of arrival in the surgical department through the entire induction process. Patients older than 4 years are the best candidates for parental presence during induction. Infants and young children may be induced in the parent's or nurse's arms. The method of induction depends on the following conditions:

- The child's age
- Whether there is IV access
- The presence of a parent
- The preference and skill of the anesthesia care provider
- The American Society of Anesthesiologists' (ASA) case classification (see Chapter 12)

Anesthesia may be induced by a combination of methods or by a single method:

- Mask inhalation
- Intramuscular injection
- Rectal administration
- Oral administration
- IV administration

If the child already has an IV line, intravenous induction with thiopental or Propofol (Diprivan) is often administered for rapid, safe induction. Inhalation induction is easily performed with a cooperative child. The child can be asked to try on a mask and is praised for compliance. Even if the child refuses the mask, it can be held below the face. As soon as the child becomes sleepy, the mask can be fitted over the face. A child who arrives asleep may be administered an anesthetic through this "blow by" method and quickly induced during sleep.

Anesthesia Maintenance

After induction or just before, the precordial stethoscope, pulse oximeter, and cardiac electrodes are placed. IV access is secured when the child is unconscious. Inhalation anesthesia is maintained through an endotracheal tube. Continuous inhalation anesthesia by mask can be used for short proce-

dures (lasting less than 1 hour). Intraoperative monitoring is carried out as in adults and includes a minimum of electrocardiography, pulse oximetry, respiratory function, and blood pressure.

Emergence and Recovery

When anesthetic agents are withdrawn or reversed the patient experiences increased physiological stress from pain and other strong stimuli. The child's response during emergence from anesthesia depends on whether opioids, sedatives, or benzodiazepines were given. These can prolong emergence but also contribute to a smoother recovery. Patients who have had a routine surgical procedure without complications may remain in the operating room until the airway reflexes are intact and the endotracheal tube is removed. If the patient is to be transported to the intensive care unit (ICU), the endotracheal tube may be left in place and the patient maintained on ventilation. After the patient is admitted to the postanesthesia care unit (PACU), parents usually are permitted to remain with the child for comfort and reassurance.

The most common postanesthesia complications in pediatric patients are postoperative nausea and vomiting (PONV), which occur in 40% to 50% of children. Other, less common events include respiratory depression and delirium during emergence. (Chapter 12 presents a complete discussion of postanesthesia complications.)

PSYCHOSOCIAL CARE OF THE PEDIATRIC PATIENT

Psychosocial care of the pediatric patient is a process that involves the child, parents or guardians, and perioperative staff. The goal of psychosocial care is to help patients and families develop strategies that can help them cope with the perioperative experience. The child's developmental stage, emotional state, and social support system are considered in planning for a safe, smooth surgical outcome. Planning for surgery usually includes a preoperative visit or counseling session involving the patient, family, and child life specialist. The **child life specialist,** who is trained in providing age-appropriate counseling to children about to undergo surgery, can explain the perioperative procedures. This helps reduce anxiety and allows both the patient and family to ask questions before surgery. One of the most important goals of preoperative planning is to provide patient and family education. Allowing the child to ask questions in an informal setting demystifies the fearful aspects of surgery and engenders trust.

Pediatric patients tend to react to their environment in predictable ways according to their developmental age. This may or may not match the child's actual numerical age (Box 34-1), but it provides a basis on which to communicate with and help orient the child to his or her surroundings in surgery.

It is important for all staff members to understand the basic developmental stages *and their significance in the perioperative setting.* The greatest fears of young children undergoing surgery are:

1. Fear of the unknown
2. Fear of separation from the primary caregivers

Children appreciate supportive, positive statements about their perioperative experience. Trust in caregivers begins with honest but careful descriptions of what will happen to them. Certain words and phrases are avoided (Box 34-2) so that the patient does not develop a sense of fear or dread.

DEVELOPMENTAL STAGES OF THE CHILD

Childhood development traditionally is divided into age categories in which children display distinct social and cognitive characteristics (Erikson's stages of psychosocial development).

Box 34-1

Pediatric Age Groups

Neonate	Birth to 1 month
Infant	1 month to 1 year
Toddler	1 to 3 years
Preschooler	3 to 6 years
School age	6 to 10 years
Adolescent	11 to 18 years

Box 34-2

Terms to Avoid (and Substitutes) in Caring for Pediatric Patients

Avoid	**Substitute**
Bad, no good	Good, good job!
Gas	Breeze, air
Stick, poke	Pinch
Strap in	Put on the safety belt
Stink	Smells funny
Feels strange	Feels funny
Cold water	Feels cool
Put to sleep	Nap

Infants (Birth to 18 Months)

Between birth and 18 months of age, children begin to develop trust in others. They require tactile comfort and are unable to tolerate sudden environmental changes. Loud noises may cause anxiety and fear. Between 7 months and 1 year, the child begins to fear separation from the parent or caregiver and usually has a strong mistrust of strangers. Transitional objects, such as a soft toy or blanket, are very comforting at this stage of development, and some facilities allow these to be brought into the surgical environment (they are labeled and returned to the parent or guardian for safekeeping). Parents may be allowed into the operating room during induction and may be present in the PACU, depending on the facility's policy.

Toddlers and Preschoolers (3 to 6 Years)

Toddlers and preschoolers understand their environment in very literal terms and believe that they are personally responsible for events. A 3- or 4-year old may believe that surgery is a form of punishment or that the illness is the result of something the child did. Children in this age group have a strong fear of the unknown and show **magical thinking,** in which ordinary or inanimate objects have intentions (harmful or benevolent). When communicating with the toddler or preschooler, health care professionals should give simple explanations and should avoid words that imply harm or injury. Children in this age group usually respond well to distraction as a means of soothing and calming.

Early and Middle School Age (6 to 12 Years)

Children in the middle school years use concrete reasoning (immediate experience) rather than complex abstract thinking; they are curious about objects and events in their environment. Children in this group fear harm and pain but are able to comprehend simple explanations of cause and effect. Patients in this age group and can be comforted by knowing what to expect. All children have a need for privacy; however, children in this age group may have a heightened sense of invasion when exposed.

Adolescence (12 to 18 Years)

Patients between 12 and 18 years are able to project the significance of current events into the future. They understand the consequences of their illness but often focus on the social rather than the physical aspects. Among their greatest concerns are separation from their peers (including rejection by peers), and loss of mobility. A change in body image caused by a perceived disfigurement can be very disturbing. Disruption of their normal routines, especially those that contribute to socialization are also upsetting. Fear of exposure and loss of privacy are extremely important in this age group, especially in middle adolescence.

Adolescents often reject or are mistrustful of care by strangers and need to demonstrate personal independence. This aspect of development increases their stoicism, and they may refuse to take pain medication or to report pain, even when it is severe. Patients in this age group often find it difficult to admit fear, but they usually are grateful for straightforward, "no nonsense" explanations of what is happening in their environment and why.

SAFETY OF THE PEDIATRIC PATIENT

Pediatric specialization involves the same domains of safety required in surgery of the adult. The surgical technologist maintains a safe environment in collaboration with other members of the perioperative team. Pediatric patients *are particularly vulnerable* to risks related to their age, size, and stage of development. The student should review environmental risks that apply to all patients, which are covered in previous chapters. Specific risks and concerns are described in Table 34-3.

SAFE HANDLING OF DRUGS

Because of their small size and undeveloped organ systems, pediatric patients are at high risk of adverse events from overdosing. The surgical technologist participates in the medication process while in the scrubbed role. Pediatric medications are prescribed according to the child's weight in kilograms, and the correct dose must be verified by the surgeon, circulating registered nurse, and technologist. Cumulative amounts of drugs, such as local anesthetic, vasoconstriction agents, given throughout the procedure must be recorded and tracked

in real time to prevent an overdose. All safety precautions discussed in Chapter 13 apply to the pediatric patient, with special emphasis on the potential risks of errors made in measuring, dispensing, and documentation.

TRANSPORTATION OF THE PEDIATRIC PATIENT

Neonates and infants usually are transported to the operating room in a heated Isolette. Occasionally, a neonate may be carried to the operating room by a parent. Young children may walk to the surgical department (for outpatient cases) and are placed on a stretcher in the holding area for transportation to the operating suite. Transporting an inpatient toddler can present challenges because of this age group's innate curiosity and agility. The hospital crib is equipped with side and bottom pads, and a flexible top may be used over the crib. During transport, a child may attempt to climb over the crib or stretcher rails. Also, it is critical to ensure that the child does not extend a limb through the rails.

POSITIONING THE PATIENT

The principles of safe patient positioning apply to pediatric patients as well as adults. (A complete discussion of appropriate techniques is presented in Chapter 10.) Although the

Table 34-3

Risks in the Perioperative Care of Pediatric Patients

Domain of Care	Specific Risk	Precautions/Prevention	Rationale
Electrosurgery	Burns	• Use pediatric-size patient return electrode (PRE) according to the manufacturer's specifications. • Never cut a PRE.	A PRE must be the correct size to properly disperse electricity flowing from the active electrode through the patient's body
Patient transport	Falls	• Never turn your attention away from the patient during transport. • Do not abandon the patient *for any reason.* • Make sure that crib rails are secure.	Children (especially toddlers) are curious and extremely active. A child can quickly climb over the top of a crib or over stretcher rails.
Skin prep	Chemical burn Hypothermia	• Prep solutions may be diluted to prevent skin burns. • Follow the surgeon's orders for solution strength. • Use warmed solutions to prevent loss of body heat.	Infants and toddlers have very delicate skin. About 60% to 75% of body heat is lost through radiation. Additional cooling by evaporation can rapidly cause hypothermia.
Positioning	Skeletal injury	• Follow all the usual precautions for positioning the patient. • Pay careful attention to moving the patient's body within the normal range of motion. • Provide ample padding over skin, nerves, and blood vessels.	Children's joints are very flexible but fragile. Limbs and joints may be overstretched, causing injury because of the patient's small stature and apparent flexibility.
Surgical technique	Injury to body tissue	• Do not put any pressure on the patient's body (e.g., from heavy instruments, tension from power cords, or leaning over the patient during surgery).	Bruising and other injury can result from weight or pressure, not directly observed because drapes hide the patient's body. Pressure on the thorax may result in respiratory compromise.

principles are the same for adults and children, it is important to use appropriate-size padding to fit the pediatric patient. Gel and foam pads are appropriate for infants and children, whose delicate skin must be protected from shearing pressure injury at all times. When creating a surgical position, the surgical technologist must keep in mind that a child's joints are extremely flexible. Care must be taken to move the patient's body within the normal range of motion and to consider anatomical restrictions related to injury or congenital defect. Adhesive tape should not be used when positioning children, because it can cause severe skin injury. Instead, soft Velcro straps designed for use with foam pads and supports should be used.

ELECTROSURGERY

All types of electrosurgical units (ESUs) are used in pediatric procedures, including monopolar and bipolar (high frequency or radiofrequency) units. The safety principles for adult electrosurgery are the same for pediatric patients. The primary differences are the size of the active electrodes and the patient return electrodes (PREs). Active electrodes are selected according to the tissue and location in the body. Special pediatric-size PREs are used on children according to the child's weight. The parameters for size are established by the manufacturer of the electrode and must be followed. A PRE must *never* be cut or trimmed, because this can result in patient injury. (Chapter 19 presents a complete discussion of electrosurgery hazards for adults and pediatric patients.)

INSTRUMENTS

Pediatric instrument sets are assembled for a specialty such as cardiac, genitourinary, or gastrointestinal surgery. The instruments themselves may be smaller in all dimensions, or only the tips (working ends) may be smaller. For example, adult microsurgical instruments and those used in eye surgery often are used in pediatric plastic and genitourinary procedures. Fine scissors, needle holders, forceps, and calipers are found across these specialties. Pediatric instruments used in general surgery include a greater number of mosquito forceps (to replace Kelly and Crile clamps), and short Babcock and Allis clamps. Smaller retractors (e.g., narrow Deaver, small Richardson, and "baby Balfour" retractors) are suited to children older than toddlers. Smaller self-retraining retractors are useful in pediatric general surgery, such as the small Weitlaner and various small spring retractors from thyroid and vascular surgery.

Minimally invasive techniques use very small trocars and endoscopes, which are designed in proportion to an infant or a child's body size. The instruments themselves are shorter and have finer tips than the adult-size versions.

SPONGES

Sponges used in open pediatric procedures usually (but not always) are smaller than those used in adult procedures. Radiopaque 4 × 4 sponges and 4 × 18 lap sponges are commonly used in pediatric procedures. Dissecting sponges must be mounted on a clamp, as in adult surgery; however, smaller

shorter clamps are used. For example, short ring forceps (sponge clamps) are used for 4 × 4 sponges. Mayo clamps, rather than long Péan clamps, are used for sponge dissectors. The guidelines and protocols for using only radiopaque sponges in the body cavity apply in pediatric surgery, just as in adult surgery.

SUTURES

Pediatric sutures naturally are smaller to meet the needs of more delicate tissues. In general, suture materials more often are absorbable than synthetic, except in cardiac, orthopedic, and reconstructive surgery. Nylon, Prolene, and other monofilament sutures are commonly used for skin and other connective tissues, because they are the least reactive and rarely tear when pulled through tissue. The size of sutures depends on the patient's age and the tissue involved. Skin most often is closed with subcuticular sutures and colloidal skin adhesive.

SURGICAL PROCEDURES

REPAIR OF A CLEFT LIP

Surgical Goal
Repair of a cleft lip involves the closure of a cleft defect in the lip.

Pathology
The *philtrum* (the groove that extends from the upper lip to the nose) is formed during embryonic development by the joining of the median nasal processes. The lateral portions of the upper lip are formed by the maxillary processes. These formations occur during the first 8 weeks of development. Interruption of normal development and closure of these structures may result in a cleft lip. The cleft may be complete or incomplete and unilateral or bilateral. Bilateral cleft lip often is associated with clefts of the soft palate. An infant with a cleft lip is referred to a surgeon immediately after birth. The cleft is repaired in stages, and the initial repair is performed at 10 to 12 weeks of age (Figure 34-3).

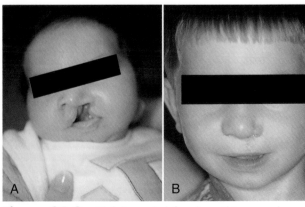

Figure 34-3   Cleft lip and cleft palate. This anomaly occurs in the first 8 weeks of embryonic life as a result of incomplete closure of the maxilla. *Left,* Three-month-old patient. *Right,* Patient at 5 years. *(From Townsend CM, Beauchamp DR, Evers MB, Mattox KL: Sabiston textbook of surgery, ed 18, Philadelphia, 2007, WB Saunders.)*

Technique

1. The incision and anatomical landmarks are marked.
2. Incisions are made along the marked incision lines.
3. Dissection is performed.
4. The defect is closed.
5. Splints or dressings are applied.

Discussion

Pediatric plastic instruments are used to repair facial abnormalities. The patient is placed in the supine position with the head on a doughnut headrest and the arms at the sides. Before the prep, the surgeon draws the anatomical landmarks and the planned incisions on the skin with a skin scribe. If local anesthetic is to be used, it is injected at this time. The patient is prepped with Betadine solution and then draped for a head and neck procedure.

The incision is made with a #11 blade along the vermilion border toward the cleft-side midline. Double- or single-prong skin hooks are used for retraction, and the mucosa is separated off the orbicularis oris muscle with a #11 knife or tenotomy scissors. The surgeon then detaches the medial lip from the maxilla by incising the cleft at the top of the labial sulcus. This releases the medial lip.

A Z-plasty incision is made through the skin, muscle, and mucosa with a #11 or #15 blade. Hemostasis is maintained with the ESU. The procedure is repeated on the lateral portion of the cleft. When the dissection has been completed and the Z-plasty flaps have been created, the wound is ready to be closed. The mucosa is closed with interrupted absorbable sutures. The muscle then is closed with subcuticular absorbable sutures through the tips of the Z-plasty flaps. The vermilion border is closed with a subcuticular suture. The skin then is closed with absorbable suture (Figure 34-4).

REPAIR OF A CLEFT PALATE

Surgical Goal

Repair of a cleft palate involves closure of the palate to restore normal function.

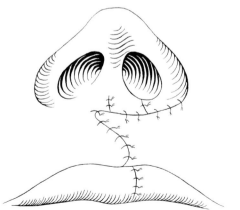

Figure 34-4 Repair of cleft lip. Rotation-advancement technique. (From Cummings C, Flint P, Haughey B, Robbins K, Thomas J, et al: Otolaryngology: head and neck surgery, ed 4, Philadelphia, 2005, Mosby.)

Pathology

In the development of the midface, the palate arises from the joining of the medial nasal prominences on each side of the oral cavity to the maxillary prominence. Failure of these structures to meet results in a cleft palate. The degree of clefting can be complete or incomplete, depending on the level of fusion that occurred during embryonic development. Although cleft palate sometimes is seen in conjunction with cleft lip, they are separate malformations and are rarely related to one another. Infants with this condition are referred to a surgeon shortly after birth. However, the defects usually are not repaired until the infant is 11 to 12 months old to avoid interference with facial growth.

Before surgical repair of the palate, the infant may require myringotomy with tube placement, because cleft palate often is associated with chronic ear infection and partial deafness. The infant also may be fitted with a palatal prosthesis to allow for easier feeding until the time of repair.

Technique

1. The incision is injected with a local anesthetic.
2. Incisions are made in the palate and the muscle.
3. The flaps are prepared.
4. The palatal incisions are closed.
5. The flaps are closed.
6. Dressings are applied.

Discussion

The patient is placed in the supine position with the head on a doughnut headrest and with a shoulder roll to hyperextend the head. The surgeon may insert the cleft palate mouth gag, or Dingman mouth gag, before the prep. The palate is injected with a local anesthetic with epinephrine. This injection is given before the prep so that the hemostatic effects of the epinephrine have time to begin working before the initial incision. The patient then is prepped with Betadine scrub and paint. If the mouth gag is already in place, it also must be prepped.

The surgeon first suspends the mouth gag from the Mayo stand. Once the gag is attached, the scrub must avoid jarring the Mayo stand because this can severely injure the patient.

The surgeon makes the initial incisions along the borders of the mucosa with a #15 blade. The incisions are extended through the oral mucosa, muscle, and nasal mucosa with a cleft palate blade (#6910 Beaver blade). After making the incisions, the surgeon elevates the nasal mucosa off the underlying muscle with the cleft palate blade and a Freer or Cottle elevator. This step is performed on both sides of the cleft. Figure 34-5 shows a rotation flap approach.

Next, the surgeon separates the oral mucosa from the overlying muscle. This step is performed in the same fashion as in the nasal mucosa. This creates three layers for closure.

After the mucosa has been elevated to the most lateral edges, the incisions are closed. The nasal mucosa is closed first with 4-0 absorbable suture on a 6-inch (15 cm) Crile-Wood needle holder and DeBakey forceps. The muscle is

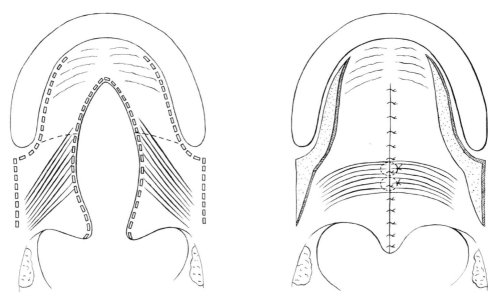

Figure 34-5 Repair of cleft palate using rotation closure. Dotted lines show lines of incision. *(From Cummings C, Flint P, Haughey B, Robbins K, Thomas J, et al: Otolaryngology: head and neck surgery, ed 4, Philadelphia, 2005, Mosby.)*

closed with 4-0 absorbable suture. The oral mucosa is closed with 4-0 or 5-0 absorbable suture. After closing the palate, the surgeon examines the wound and releases any areas under tension. The wound then is irrigated, and the mouth gag is removed.

Postoperative Considerations

Infants can begin to take liquids by sippy cup shortly after surgery. Any feeding method that involves sucking (bottles, straws, cups with valves) is not used because this can disrupt the repair. Some surgeons require their postoperative patients to wear arm restraints for several weeks. This prevents the infant from putting anything in the mouth, which might disturb the repair.

OTOPLASTY

Surgical Goal

Otoplasty is performed to reconstruct the external ear after a traumatic injury or to correct protruding ears.

Pathology

Otoplasty can be performed in children or adults. In children, it usually is performed to reattach the ear closer to the head. This condition usually is the result of the absence or small size of the antihelical fold in the external ear (Figure 34-6). The repairs usually are performed before the patient starts school. The external ear may also be reconstructed after traumatic injury caused by fire, animal bites, or other accidents. Loss of the external ear or protruding ears can cause great anxiety and stress in children and can affect their social development and body image. A procedure for protruding ears is presented here; reconstruction of the ear is discussed later in the chapter.

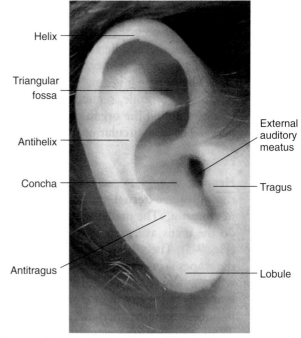

Figure 34-6 External ear. *(Thibodeau G, Patton K: Anatomy and physiology, ed 6, Philadelphia, Mosby, 2007.)*

Technique

1. The antihelical fold is marked.
2. The posterior ear is injected with epinephrine, and an ellipse of skin is excised.
3. Cartilage near the antihelical fold is incised, and the anterior surface is scored.
4. Suture is placed in the cartilage.
5. The skin is closed.
6. Dressings are applied.

Discussion

The patient is placed in the supine position with the affected ear up and the unaffected ear heavily padded to cushion pressure. The arms are tucked at the sides to give the surgeon full access to the head. The patient is prepped, and a body and head drape is applied. If both ears are affected, a Mayfield headrest, which allows access to both ears, may be useful for positioning the head.

The antihelical fold is marked by the placement of 22-gauge needles that have been dipped in methylene blue. The surgeon performs this step by folding the external ear against the head and then inserting and withdrawing the needles from anterior to posterior. This procedure produces marks through all layers of the tissue. The scrub should have calipers available for this part of the procedure. The surgeon then injects the posterior ear with epinephrine, with or without a local anesthetic, and excises an ellipse of skin with a #15 blade and Adson toothed forceps or Brown-Adson forceps. Double-prong skin hooks are used to retract the skin flaps, and the underlying tissue is elevated with a Freer elevator.

The cartilage can be scored with a #15 blade, making it more pliable, and then sutured in the postauricular area close to the head. An alternative technique is to excise the cartilage to create an antihelical fold, or it can be thinned with a power shaver to allow it to be molded. A 4-0 nonabsorbable suture (e.g., Mersilene, clear nylon, or polydioxanone surgical [PDS] suture) may be used to hold the cartilage in place.

The skin incision is closed with 3-0 absorbable suture. A bulky mastoid dressing consisting of Telfa, Kerlix fluffs, and Kerlix rolls is applied to the ear. This gives the newly formed ear adequate support and protection.

RECONSTRUCTION OF THE EAR

Surgical Goal

Congenital anomalies, which often accompany defects of the outer ear structure, require extensive surgical repair. In this procedure, only the cosmetic defect is addressed.

Pathology

Microtia is a congenital defect in which all or part of the external ear is missing. The deformity also affects the inner ear, resulting in deafness. Reconstructive surgery is performed in childhood before the patient reaches school age. Microtia may be present at birth or can be caused by accidents such as fire, dog bite, or other trauma.

Discussion

Reconstruction of the ear is performed in multiple stages with several operations. The technique varies, depending on the type and severity of the defect. A common method of reconstruction is to raise the skin where the ear normally would lie and insert a graft taken from the patient's costal cartilage. The tragus then is elevated in stages, and the folds and ear lobe are created using grafts and skin flap techniques.

When an autograft is to be used, the patient is placed in the supine position. The surgeon creates a template (pattern) for the graft by placing a sheet of transparent material over the unaffected ear and tracing its outline on the material. The template then is placed over the affected ear, and the ear remnants are traced on the template.

The surgeon makes an incision over the seventh, eighth, or ninth intercostal space. The template is placed over the costal cartilage, and the tissue is excised, following the outline of the template. The incision is closed in layers in routine fashion.

The graft is shaped to form the basis of the pinna and helix. This is done with a power drill and small bur attachments. The surgeon may choose to work at the back table or at a separate draped table. The technologist should make sure that carving instruments, burrs, and elevators are neatly assembled for the surgeon's use. Clear nylon or fine stainless steel sutures are used to assemble the graft components. After the graft has been prepared, it is preserved in a safe location on the back table.

To prepare the implant site for the graft, the surgeon outlines the postauricular area where the graft will be inserted. The skin is incised, and small bleeders are controlled with a needle-tip ESU. The skin is undermined, and the graft is inserted into the skin pocket. The surgeon pulls the skin over the graft and sutures it in place. The lobe is transferred from the existing ear remnant. This completes the first stage of the reconstruction.

When the first stage has healed, subsequent operations are done to raise the frame of the ear and to construct the folds and recesses of the outer ear. These steps are performed by incising flaps of adjacent skin and rotating them into position. Fine sutures of nylon, Prolene, or other synthetic material are used to suture the flaps in place. Bulky dressings are used after ear repair to protect the reconstructed tissues from injury during healing. Figures 34-7 and 34-8 illustrate the techniques involved in ear reconstruction.

CORRECTION OF ESOPHAGEAL ATRESIA AND TRACHEOESOPHAGEAL FISTULA

Surgical Goal

The goal of surgical repair of esophageal atresia (EA) is to restore continuity of the esophagus. In repair of a tracheoesophageal fistula (TEF), an abnormal opening between the trachea and the esophagus is closed to prevent the flow of food and saliva from the esophagus to the lungs.

Pathology

Esophageal **atresia** (the absence or closure of a normal anatomical orifice) is a nongenetic defect in which the esophagus is interrupted. The upper or proximal portion terminates in a blind pouch that does not communicate with the distal esophagus. Numerous variations of the anomaly can be seen, including, often, a tracheoesophageal fistula (Figure 34-9). A TEF is a direct passageway or duct between either esophageal section (distal or proximal) and the trachea.

Esophageal atresia prevents the normal passage of food and saliva to the stomach. A TEF between the proximal esophageal

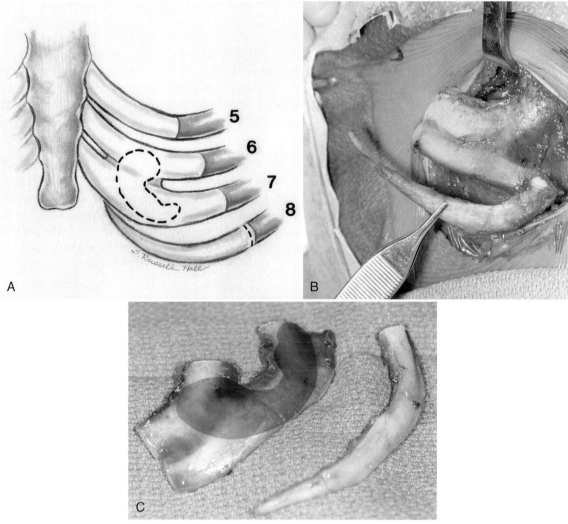

Figure 34-7   Reconstruction of the ear for microtia. **A,** A template is placed over the costal cartilage, and an autograft is removed from the tissue. **B,** and **C,** Two separate graft components are required, for the pinna and the helix. *(From Cummings C, Flint P, Haughey B, Robbins K, Thomas J, et al: Otolaryngology: head and neck surgery, ed 4, Philadelphia, 2005, Mosby.)*

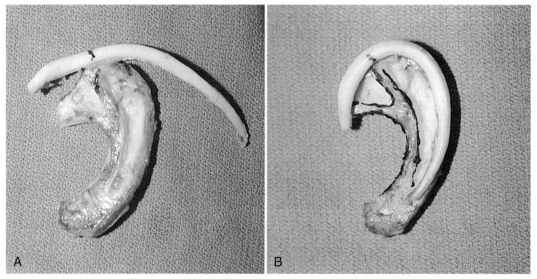

Figure 34-8   Construction of the implant taken from the costal cartilage. **A,** The framework is shaped with cutting burrs and carving instruments. **B,** The components are assembled using clear nylon or fine stainless steel sutures. *(From Cummings C, Flint P, Haughey B, Robbins K, Thomas J, et al: Otolaryngology: head and neck surgery, ed 4, Philadelphia, 2005, Mosby.)*

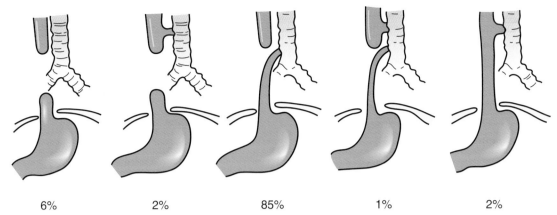

6%   2%   85%   1%   2%

Figure 34-9 Variations of esophageal atresia and tracheoesophageal fistula with the percent incidence of each type of defect. *(From Townsend CM, Beauchamp DR, Evers MB, Mattox KL: Sabiston textbook of surgery, ed 18, Philadelphia, 2007, WB Saunders.)*

segment and the trachea causes aspiration of saliva and milk into the trachea and lungs; a TEF in the distal esophageal segment causes gastric secretions to flow into the lungs. EA may exist as a single anomaly or, more commonly, with TEF.

EA/TEF is associated with a number of other birth defects, some of which are lethal. These include:

- Imperforate anus
- Ventricular and atrial septal defect
- Tetralogy of Fallot
- Limb deformities
- Neural tube defect

In addition to these and other anomalies, the fetus with EA/TEF is prevented from swallowing amniotic fluid, a source of nutrition in fetal life. This results in low neonatal birth weight and size.

Surgical options for the correction of EA/TEF depend on the type and severity of the defect. Staged or delayed repair may be necessary if other life-threatening conditions (e.g., cardiac defects) take precedence or to allow normal growth and elongation of the esophagus. A colon graft may be used to elongate the esophagus, although primary closure is preferred when possible. Primary repair (anastomosis of the two esophageal segments) is performed when the two segments can be brought together and the infant's general physiological condition is good. An isolated TEF without EA can be repaired through a cervical approach. Primary closure of EA is described here.

Technique

1. A right posterolateral thoracotomy is performed.
2. The TEF is identified and retracted.
3. The TEF is divided and closed.
4. The proximal and distal esophageal pouches are mobilized.
5. The esophageal ends are excised and trimmed.
6. An end-to-end or end-to-side anastomosis is performed.
7. A chest tube may be placed.
8. The wound is closed.

Discussion

The technologist should have pediatric general surgical and thoracic instruments available. Silastic vessel loops and sponge dissectors should also be available. A pediatric Finochietto retractor is commonly used for retraction. The infant is placed in thoracotomy position with the head of the operating table slightly elevated. The prep extends from the neck to the iliac crest and includes the anterior and posterior chest.

The knife is used to make a transverse, posterolateral thoracotomy incision, and the ESU is used to extend it into the latissimus muscles. Rake retractors can be used to retract the skin and subcutaneous layers while the muscle and fascia are divided. The scapula is retracted, and the chest cavity is entered by incising the intercostal muscles. The ESU is used to divide the muscles. This exposes the pleura, which is dissected from the chest wall with small sponge dissectors. A Finochietto retractor is placed in the wound, and pleural dissection continues to expose the azygos vein. This is clamped, ligated with 4-0 silk suture, and divided.

The esophageal defect is assessed. The anesthesia care provider advances the preplaced Replogle tube (nasogastric decompression tube). This demonstrates the blind proximal esophageal pouch. The TEF is located and encircled with a Silastic vessel loop. The fistula then is excised with fine dissecting scissors. The tracheal opening is closed with interrupted sutures of 4-0 or 5-0 absorbable synthetic suture. The surgeon tests the closure with warm saline irrigation solution. Bleeders are controlled with the ESU.

The proximal and distal esophageal segments are grasped with Babcock clamps, and the anastomosis site is examined. The surgeon excises the proximal pouch with fine dissecting scissors and smooth forceps. The distal portion, which is larger, is also excised to fit the proximal segment. An end-to-end anastomosis may be planned, or the proximal segment may be implanted in a circular incision made in the distal portion of the esophagus. The Replogle tube is advanced across the anastomosis site, and traction sutures are placed through the esophageal segments. Absorbable 5-0 or 6-0 synthetic suture is used to create a single-layer anastomosis. Surgical alternatives include a double-layer closure and variations in the anastomosis to prevent tension on the esophagus. The Replogle tube may be left in place or withdrawn.

The wound is irrigated with warm saline, and bleeders are controlled with the ESU. A small chest tube maybe placed in the extrapleural space. The wound then is closed in layers with absorbable synthetic sutures.

Postoperative Considerations

Care of the infant immediately after surgery focuses mainly on the airway. Pharyngeal secretions are suctioned frequently for the first few days until the infant is able to swallow. The chest tubes are securely maintained, and the incision sites are monitored for leakage or blockage. Oral feeding begins 2 to 6 days after surgery, after contrast studies have shown that the anastomosis is secure. Complications include infection, recurrent TEF, and leakage of the anastomosis.

PYLOROMYOTOMY

Surgical Goal

Pyloromyotomy is surgery to correct infantile hypertrophic pyloric stenosis (IHPS), or simply **pyloric stenosis,** a thickening of the pylorus that results in stricture at the gastric outlet. The goal of surgery is to release the pyloric muscle fibers by incising them. This relaxes the gastric opening and allows food to pass normally out of the stomach into the intestine.

Pathology

Pyloric stenosis is a congenital anomaly involving the longitudinal and circular muscle fibers of the gastric outlet. The pylorus (or gastric outlet) of the stomach is enlarged and edematous, causing food to be regurgitated almost immediately after intake. This leads to dehydration and failure to thrive. The condition is about four times more common in male children. In the Ramstedt procedure, the muscle of the hypertrophic pylorus is split, and the mucosa is left intact.

Technique

1. A right upper (subcostal) transverse incision is made.
2. The greater curvature of the stomach (near the pylorus) is grasped with a noncrushing clamp and brought out through the incision.
3. The anterior pylorus is incised.
4. A blunt instrument is used to split the muscle fibers.
5. The wound is closed.
6. The skin is closed with subcuticular suture.

Discussion

Ramstedt pyloromyotomy is commonly performed to treat pyloric stenosis. Either an open or a minimally invasive technique may be used. The open procedure is described here.

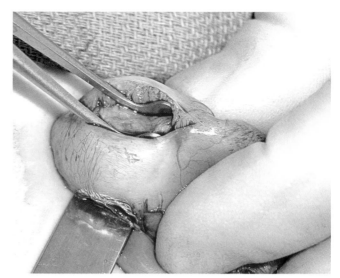

Figure 34-10 Pyloromyotomy. The pylorus is delivered from the wound, and a short incision is made through the muscle layers. Here a pyloric spreader is used to release the muscle tissue. *(From Townsend CM, Beauchamp DR, Evers MB, Mattox KL: Sabiston textbook of surgery, ed 18, Philadelphia, 2007, WB Saunders.)*

The infant is placed in the supine position. The chest and abdomen are prepped with an iodophor-povidone solution and draped for a laparotomy.

A 1- to 1.2-inch (2.5 to 3 cm) transverse incision is made in the right upper quadrant over the right rectus muscle. The fascial layers are divided transversely, but the rectus muscle is either retracted laterally or split in the middle. The edge of the liver is retracted superiorly, exposing the greater curvature of the stomach (near the pylorus), which is grasped with a noncrushing clamp and brought out through the incision. A damp gauze sponge is used to grasp the stomach, and with traction inferiorly and laterally, the pylorus is delivered from the incision. The ESU or knife is used to incise the serosa on the anterior wall of the pylorus to the level of the submucosa. A curved hemostat or pyloric spreader may be used to open out the muscle fibers and enlarge the pylorus (Figure 34-10). The pylorus is returned to the abdomen, and the abdominal incision is closed with 3-0 and 4-0 absorbable sutures. A flat dressing is placed over the wound.

RESECTION AND PULL-THROUGH FOR HIRSCHSPRUNG DISEASE

Surgical Goal

The goal of pull-through surgery for Hirschsprung disease (megacolon) is resection and reconstruction of the distal colon to restore functional peristalsis and prevent bowel obstruction.

Pathology

The normal intestine provides absorption, motility, secretion, and blood flow through a set of complex nerve plexuses that are nearly independent of the central nervous system. Reflexes for stool motility are located in the distal rectum. A **bolus** in this region causes the bowel to contract above the bolus and relax below it, moving stool through the sphincter. Hirschsprung disease is characterized by a congenital absence of ganglion cells, which control the relaxation and contraction that occur in peristalsis. The affected tissue begins at the anus and may extend proximally, causing functional obstruction in both the aganglionic and normal portions of the bowel. Severe distention, or megacolon, occurs in the bowel and abdomen.

Diagnosis of Hirschsprung disease is confirmed by rectal biopsy. The problem should be recognized soon after birth in neonates who have not passed meconium within the first 24 to 48 hours. Delayed diagnosis may result in necrotizing enterocolitis, which often is fatal if not treated promptly.

A colostomy may be performed soon after birth and intestinal correction delayed, or a single-stage procedure (without colostomy) may be performed in the first 48 hours of life. Many variations are possible for the procedure, which involves resection of the diseased bowel and endorectal pull-through of the distal colon and anastomosis to the rectal musculature. This technique is similar to reconstruction after abdomino-perineal resection (see Chapter 23).

Technique

1. A left paramedian incision is made, and if a colostomy is present, it is excised.
2. The sigmoid colon is mobilized, and the superior hemorrhoidal vessels are divided.
3. Frozen section specimens may be taken to determine the presence of ganglia.
4. The pelvis is entered, the lateral rectal ligaments are divided, and the rectum is further mobilized
5. A long clamp (e.g., Babcock or ring forceps) is inserted transanally, and a segment of the dissected colon is grasped.
6. Using counterpressure from the pelvis, the colon is everted and "pulled through" the anus.
7. The layers of the everted bowel are circumferentially incised, and absorbable suture is used to anchor the rim of the retained portion of the colon to the rectum.
8. The diseased portion of bowel is divided, and the anastomosis is performed with absorbable synthetic suture.
9. At the completion of this portion of the procedure, gowns, gloves, and setup are changed in preparation for the abdominal portion of the procedure.
10. The proximal edge of the muscular cuff is approximated to the seromuscular layer of the colon, completing the abdominal anastomosis.
11. The abdomen is irrigated and closed.

BOWEL RECONSTRUCTION FOR IMPERFORATE ANUS

Surgical Goal

Repair of an imperforate anus provides continuity of the lower intestinal tract to the outside of the body.

Pathology

An imperforate anus is a congenital malformation of the anorectal system in which the rectum and anus do not communicate with the outside of the body. This is one of many types of anorectal malformations that can occur during embryonic development. An imperforate anus may occur alone or in association with other anomalies of the genitourinary system. The defect may present in a variety of forms and is graded as high or low, depending on the severity and the location of rectal tissue in the distal gut. In the low form, which is the easier type to repair, the rectum has descended through the sphincter system. In more complex presentations, the rectum does not descend through the sphincter mechanism, and the malformation can include rectovaginal and rectourethral fistulas. A colostomy is performed on the neonate for diversion of feces until surgical repair is complete and the rectum and anus are functional.

Technique

The techniques used to repair these anomalies depend on the type and severity of the defect. A low defect can be corrected with a pull-through procedure similar to that described previously. Combined laparoscopic-perineal surgery now is performed in many pediatric surgery centers. The technique described here is for a simple pull-through procedure.

1. The anus is located through a fistulous tract or by imaging studies.
2. The fistula is incised circumferentially.
3. The rectum is pulled through the anal structure and sutured to the skin.

Discussion

A Foley catheter is inserted during or before the skin prep. The prone position is used for a posterior approach. The hips are elevated on a soft pad. A change in position may be necessary during the procedure. A pediatric gastrointestinal set is required. A fine nerve stimulator is used throughout dissection to locate the anal structures.

A low imperforate anus is located through a fistulous tract that develops during embryonic life between the rectum and the anal structure. This fistula may or may not penetrate the perineal skin. If it is not visible, it can be approached through a combined transverse and midline perineal incisions. The nerve stimulator is used to identify the exact location of the anus on the midline and to preserve the nerves necessary for continence. The tract is mobilized proximally with dissecting scissors and fine-tooth forceps. This dissection frees the rectum. Silk traction sutures may be placed through the edge of the distal fistula to aid mobilization of the tissue.

The mobilized rectum is grasped with Babcock forceps and delivered at the true rectum through a midline perineal incision. The edges of the rectum are carefully trimmed with fine dissecting scissors. The edges then are sutured to the skin at the site of the true anus. Multiple interrupted 4-0 or 5-0 synthetic absorbable sutures are used to create the anus.

REDUCTION OF AN INTUSSUSCEPTION

Surgical Goal

Intussusception, or the telescoping of one portion of the intestine into another, can be reduced with hydrostatic pressure (usually a barium enema) or by manual manipulation through a laparotomy incision. Nonoperative reduction is successful in about 50% of cases when performed within 24 to 48 hours.

Pathology

Intussusception is the most common cause of intestinal obstruction in children 3 months to 6 years of age and therefore among the most common surgical emergencies in this age group. A gangrenous bowel may rupture, leading to peritonitis.

Technique

1. A transverse or low right paramedian incision is made, and the peritoneum is entered.
2. The entire bowel is carefully inspected to determine whether the bowel wall at the intussusception is viable.
3. Manual manipulation is attempted to reduce the intussusception.
4. The bowel may require fixation after reduction to prevent recurrence.
5. Alternatively, if the viability of the bowel is in question, a resection with possible colostomy is performed.
6. The abdomen is closed.

Discussion

In this procedure a routine laparotomy is performed as described in Chapter 23, using pediatric instruments. The surgeon locates the area of intussusception and reduces the obstruction by manually easing the bowel tissue into normal position. In cases when manual reduction is not possible, or if the bowel has perforated, a resection and end-to-end anastomosis is performed as described in Chapter 23. The wound is closed in routine manner.

REDUCTION OF A VOLVULUS

Surgical Goal

Reduction of a volvulus is performed to relieve intestinal obstruction by untwisting (counterclockwise detorsion) of the affected bowel. Depending on the viability of the affected bowel, a resection with anastomosis, ileostomy, or colostomy may be required.

Pathology

Volvulus is rotation of the intestine around itself or the attached mesentery. This can lead to strangulation of the blood vessels, ischemia in the bowel, and eventual gangrene of the affected portion. Volvulus is a rare condition; it affects children most often but can occur at any age. The developmental anomaly that causes volvulus is called *malrotation*. The central part of the intestine normally rotates into its final posi-

tion in about week 10 of pregnancy. Occasionally this part of the intestine does not rotate fully, leaving the bowel predisposed to later twisting. Volvulus requires emergency surgery to prevent bowel perforation and peritonitis.

Technique

1. The patient is placed in the supine position, and the abdomen is prepped and draped.
2. A supraumbilical right transverse incision is made, extending from the midline laterally.
3. The bowel is thoroughly assessed.
4. The volvulus is reduced, and any restrictive tissue bands are divided.
5. A resection and anastomosis, colostomy, or ileostomy may be performed.
6. The wound is closed.

Discussion

A routine laparotomy is performed as described in Chapter 23 and the volvulus is manually "untwisted." A bowel resection may be required if necrosis or perforation has occurred (refer to Chapter 23).

REPAIR OF AN OMPHALOCELE

Surgical Goal

An **omphalocele** is a congenital anomaly in which the abdominal viscera develop outside the body, contained within a peritoneal sac. The goal of surgery is to replace the contents of the abdomen in phases until the abdominal wall can be closed.

Pathology

An omphalocele is covered by a clear sac or membrane composed of peritoneum and amnion (Figure 34-11, *A*). The size of the omphalocele can range from very small, containing only a small portion of the intestine, to extremely large (*giant omphalocele*), including the intestine and other abdominal viscera such as the liver and spleen (Figure 34-12). The anomaly is associated with genetic defects, including trisomies 13, 18, and 21 in 30% of cases. Cardiac, musculoskeletal, and genitourinary defects are also associated with omphalocele.

Discussion

Surgical options for repair of an omphalocele depend on the size of the defect. Small defects (less than 0.8 inch [2 cm]) can be reduced in one step. In such cases, a primary abdominal closure is performed soon after birth.

Larger defects require multiple-stage procedures in which portions of the viscera are replaced in the abdominal cavity over a period of days or weeks. To prevent hypothermia, infection, and dehydration, a Silastic, Dacron-reinforced silo is sutured to the abdominal wall. The silo is reduced gradually, over a period of days, while the infant is in intensive care. When the omphalocele has been sufficiently reduced, the infant is taken to the operating room for complete closure of

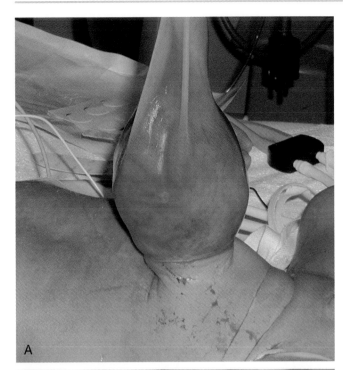

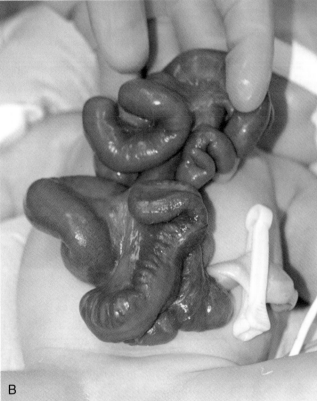

Figure 34-11 Defects of the abdominal wall.
A, *Omphalocele:* The infant is born with the abdominal viscera outside the body; the organs are encased in a membrane.
B, *Gastroschisis:* The abdominal viscera are not covered by a membrane. *(From Townsend CM, Beauchamp DR, Evers MB, Mattox KL: Sabiston textbook of surgery, ed 18, Philadelphia, 2007, WB Saunders.)*

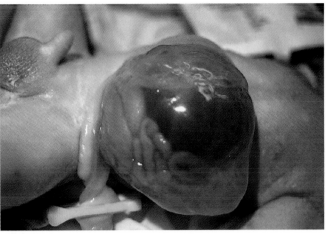

Figure 34-12 Giant omphalocele, with organs clearly visible. *(From Clark DA, Thompson JE, Barnemeyer BM: Atlas of neonatology, ed 7, Philadelphia, 2000, WB Saunders.)*

the abdominal wall. If the contents cannot be reduced completely, skin closure alone is performed. This results in a large abdominal wall hernia, which may be repaired later in childhood.

In some cases, the skin cannot be closed over the defect. In these patients, the abdominal contents are covered with a scarification agent, such as silver sulfadiazine. Granulation tissue leading to epithelialization (growth of skin tissue) occurs over a period of months, and repair is delayed for 1 to 2 years.

Shortly after birth, the omphalocele is protected with moist sponges, and the infant prepared for surgery. General anesthesia is induced, and the abdomen, umbilical cord, and sac are prepped and draped. A Foley catheter is inserted. A small defect is closed with 3-0 nonabsorbable suture.

Phased reduction of the omphalocele takes placed in the neonatal ICU. Final closure is performed as for a laparotomy.

Gastroschisis

Gastroschisis is similar to an omphalocele defined above, except no peritoneal sac or membrane covers the abdominal viscera (Figure 34-11, *B*). Unlike with an omphalocele, associated anomalies are rare. Intestinal atresia (narrowing of the lumen) may be present. The exposed bowel often is thickened and edematous and may be abnormally short. This may be related to exposure to amniotic fluid or during fetal life. The cause of gastroschisis is not known.

Surgical treatment for gastroschisis is similar to that for an omphalocele, involving the use of a Silastic silo and phased reduction. However, repair is more urgent because of the absence of a protective peritoneum.

Postoperative Considerations

The primary risks of an omphalocele and gastroschisis are infection and bowel necrosis. A silo is closed as soon as possible after birth to prevent infection. Fluid loss from the exposed bowel can be significant; therefore the tissue is kept covered and moist during staged closure. Increased intraabdominal pressure, which occurs after repair, may result in difficult ventilation and decreased urinary output. Adequate pain relief is provided by continuous infusion of morphine.

REPAIR OF BLADDER EXSTROPHY/ EPISPADIAS

Surgical Goal

The surgical goal of reconstruction is to restore the normal functions of the lower urinary tract.

Pathology

Bladder **exstrophy**/epispadias is a complex set of congenital anomalies involving the lower genitourinary tract and skeletal system. The anomalies arise from the same developmental defect, which occurs in the first trimester of fetal life. The anomalies associated with the defect are:

- Bladder exstrophy (the anterior bladder wall is exposed on the outside of the body through an abdominal wall defect)
- Epispadias (the urethra is fully exposed or terminates on the dorsum of the penis)
- Shortening of the penis, which also demonstrates chordee (bands of tissue that cause an upward curvature)
- Opening out of the glans and absence of the dorsal foreskin
- Anterior displacement of the vagina and anus
- Exposure of the bladder neck
- Possible presence of an omphalocele
- Divergence of the rectus muscles and widening of the pubic symphysis

Discussion

Reconstruction usually is performed in three stages, although this varies with the individual patient and with the surgical strategy chosen by the surgeon:

- First stage: Closure of the bladder and abdomen (24 to 48 hours of life)
- Second stage: Repair of epispadias (2 to 3 years old)
- Third stage: Achieving urinary continence (4 to 5 years old)

Repair of an exstrophic bladder in the male is described here.

Technique

1. The patient is placed in the supine position. A wide area is prepped, including the entire body anteriorly and posteriorly below the level of the nipple so that turning is possible, and the area is draped.
2. Traction sutures of 5-0 Prolene are placed in the glans penis, and ureteral catheters are secured in each ureteral orifice.
3. The surgeon incises and completely dissects around the periphery of the bladder and urethral plate.

4. The incision is extended distally to the area where the ejaculatory ducts join the urethra, on both sides.
5. The umbilical cord is excised, and an umbilicoplasty is performed during or after the initial procedure.
6. A paraexstrophy flap may be created if any question exists about the urethral length.
7. The bladder is completely mobilized, with preservation of its blood supply.
8. Inversion of the bladder plate and approximation of the corpora are the first stage of epispadias repair.
9. The corpora are approximated carefully in the midline to promote penile elongation.
10. The surgeon approximates the skin at the urethral plate inferiorly
11. The urethral plate is made tubular, and ureteral catheters are placed bilaterally and brought out on each side of the bladder.
12. After two-layer closure of the bladder and urethral plate, the bladder is reduced into the pelvis and fixed with suture.
13. Sutures are placed to approximate the pubic halves. The drainage tubes are brought out superiorly, and the fascia, subcutaneous tissue, and skin are approximated.

Figure 34-13 illustrate bladder exstrophy and epispadias and procedures for their repair.

ORCHIOPEXY FOR AN UNDESCENDED TESTICLE

Surgical Goal

The goal of surgery for congenital undescended testicle is to restore the testicle to its normal position in the scrotum. The procedure sometimes is called an *orchiopexy*; however, this term actually refers only to the surgical attachment of the testicle to the scrotal wall. Orchiopexy is performed for a variety of conditions, including surgical attachment for the prevention and treatment of testicular torsion.

Pathology

During normal fetal life, the testicles are retained within the abdomen. Just before birth, the testicles should descend into the scrotum. Occasionally one or both testicles fail to descend into the scrotum. This can result in sterility because of the testicles' exposure to the increased temperature in the abdominal cavity.

Technique

1. The surgeon enters and explores the inguinal region.
2. The testicle is identified.
3. The spermatic cord is mobilized.
4. The testicle is mobilized by sharp and blunt dissection.
5. A tunnel is made through the inguinal canal into the scrotum.
6. The testicle is brought through the tunnel and secured with sutures.
7. The inguinal layers are closed.

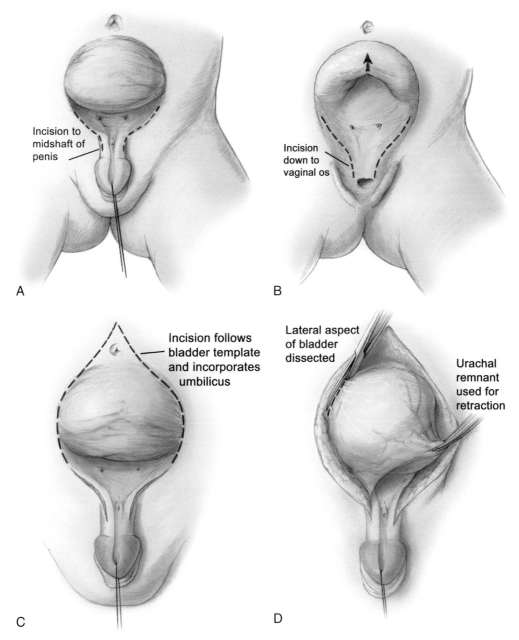

Figure 34-13   Surgical reconstruction for bladder exstrophy and epispadias. **A,** The bladder plate is dissected from the abdominal wall. **B,** Incision in the female. **C** and **D,** Continuation of the incision.

Continued

Discussion

The patient is placed in the supine position, prepped, and draped with the inguinal, groin, and scrotal areas on the affected side exposed. The surgeon makes an incision over the external ring as for a hernia repair. The incision is carried into the deep inguinal tissues with sharp dissection.

Small bleeders are coagulated with the ESU or clamped with mosquito hemostats and ligated with fine absorbable sutures. The spermatic cord is identified and dissected with blunt and sharp dissection. The cord is dissected high in the internal ring to create sufficient slack to bring the testicle into the scrotum; the processus vaginalis is ligated.

The surgeon uses a finger or a blunt clamp (e.g., Mayo or sponge forceps) to create a tunnel for the testicle. The clamp is advanced through the external oblique fascia, and the tissue is manually separated, forming a pocket in the scrotum.

The testicle is brought through the tunnel, and the scrotum is incised to expose the scrotal septum. Several 3-0 or 4-0 absorbable sutures are placed through the septum and testicle, securing the testicle in place (Figure 34-14).

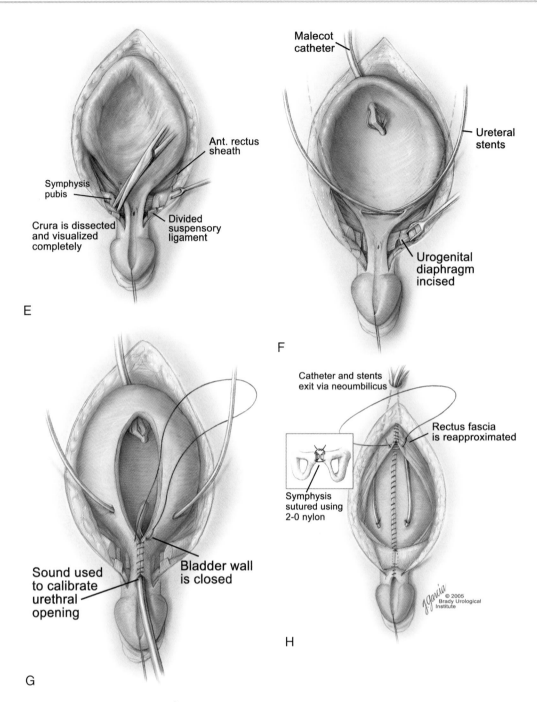

Figure 34-13, cont'd **E,** Dissection of muscles from the symphysis pubis. **F,** Stents are placed in the bladder. **G,** A sound is placed in the urethra and closure begins. **H,** The symphysis, bladder, and rectus fascia are closed. *(From Wein AJ, editor:* Campbell-Walsh urology, *Philadelphia, 2007, WB Saunders.)*

CLOSURE OF A PATENT DUCTUS ARTERIOSUS

Surgical Goal

Surgical closure of a patent **ductus arteriosus** (PDA) is performed to prevent arterial blood from recirculating through the pulmonary circulation. The ductus may be approached by an open incision or by the endoscopic route.

Pathology

The ductus arteriosus is a normal anatomical opening in the fetal heart. During fetal development, blood is pumped from the right ventricle into the systemic circulation by way of the ductus, which connects the pulmonary artery and descending thoracic aorta (Figure 34-15, *A*). At birth, the lungs expand and the ductus closes spontaneously within a short time (Figure 34-15, *B*). If the ductus fails to close, arterial blood returns to the lungs, putting an added burden on the lungs

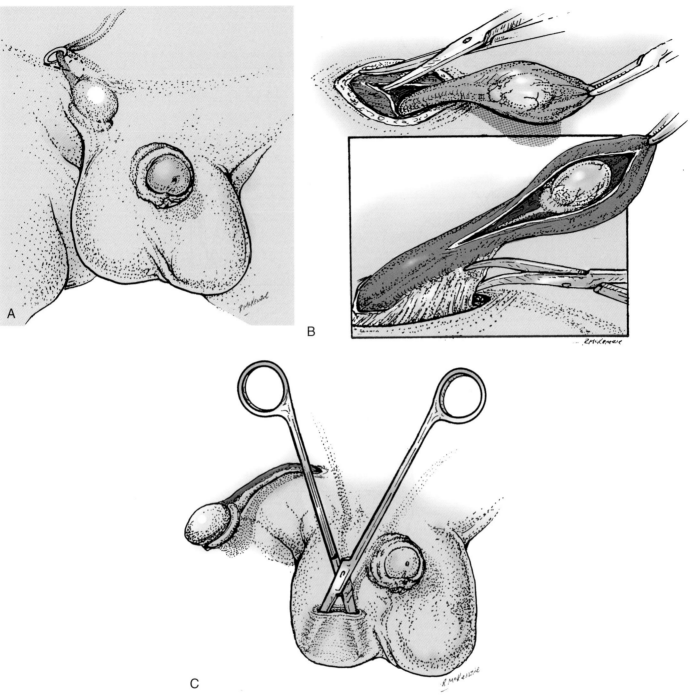

Figure 34-14 Orchiopexy for an undescended testicle. **A,** The testicle is approached through a transverse inguinal incision. **B,** The external ring is opened, and the cremaster fibers are mobilized from the cord. **C,** Formation of the pouch.

Continued

and heart. The heart becomes enlarged and may fail. The ductus is closed surgically to correct this defect, usually during infancy.

Technique

1. A left thoracotomy is performed.
2. The mediastinal pleura is incised.
3. The ductus is isolated.
4. The ductus is closed.
5. A chest tube is inserted, and the chest is closed.

Discussion

Surgical repair of a PDA may be performed by minimally invasive surgery. An open procedure is described here.

The patient is placed in the supine position, prepped, and draped for a thoracotomy. A thoracotomy is performed as previously described. To begin the repair, the surgeon places a traction suture through the edges of the pleura (usually with 3-0 silk suture). The ends are tagged with a hemostat. The assistant retracts the pleura with the suture. The surgeon then carefully dissects the aorta and pulmonary

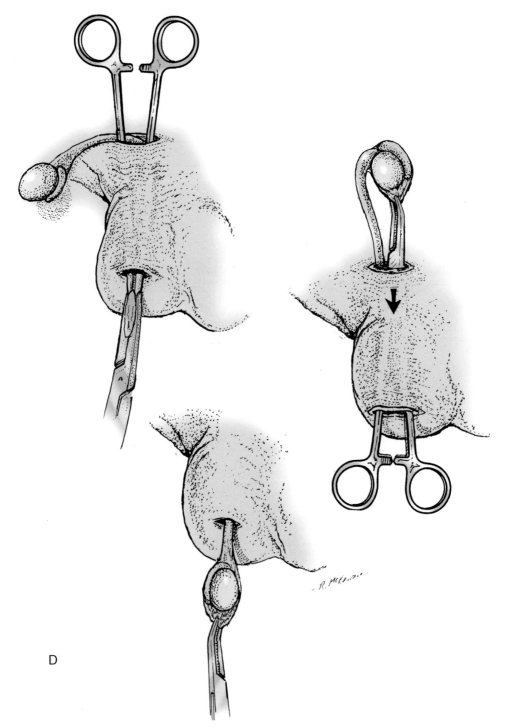

D

Figure 34-14, cont'd   D, The testicle is brought through the tunnel. *(From Wein AJ, editor:* Campbell-Walsh urology, *Philadelphia, 2007, WB Saunders.)*

artery with fine dissecting scissors to expose the ductus (Figure 34-16, *A*). A heavy silk suture may be passed around the ductus.

The surgeon continues the dissection until the ductus is fully isolated. Straight or angled vascular clamps are placed across the ductus, one close to the aorta and the other close to the pulmonary artery (Figure 34-16, *B*). In a newborn or a small infant, the surgeon may simply tie the ductus with

size 0 silk, because the ductus is small and may not allow placement of the vascular clamps. Vascular clips also may be used.

In other situations, the surgeon may divide and oversew the cut edges. The surgeon cuts halfway through the ductus with Potts scissors or a knife. A 5-0 or 6-0 polypropylene suture is used to begin the closure of the ductus on the aortic side. The surgeon continues to incise the ductus and contin-

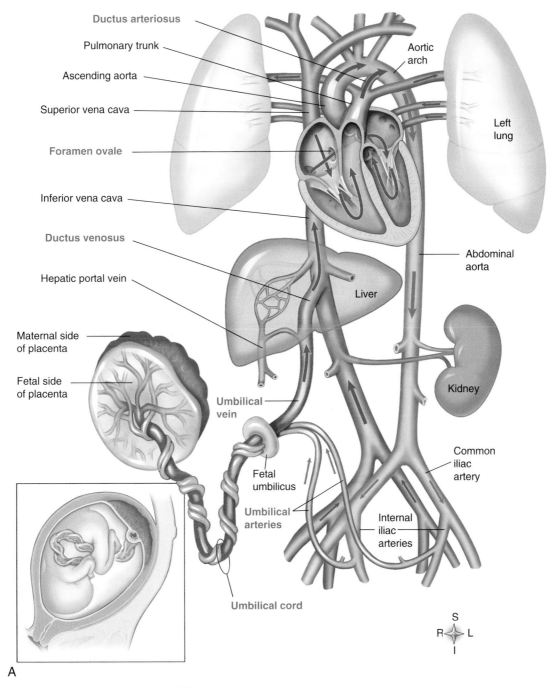

Ductus arteriosus

Pulmonary trunk

Ascending aorta

Superior vena cava

Foramen ovale

Inferior vena cava

Ductus venosus

Hepatic portal vein

Maternal side
of placenta

Fetal side
of placenta

Aortic
arch

Left
lung

Abdominal
aorta

Liver

Kidney

Umbilical
vein

Fetal
umbilicus

Umbilical
arteries

Common
iliac
artery

Internal
iliac
arteries

Umbilical cord

S
R ✦ L
I

A

Figure 34-15 **A,** Fetal circulation.

Continued

ues the suture to close the defect on the aortic side. The vascular clamp then is slowly released. Additional sutures are placed if needed. The end of the ductus closest to the pulmonary artery is sutured in the same manner. A topical hemostatic agent can be used to control bleeding at the anastomosis.

The mediastinal pleura is closed with a continuous suture of 3-0 or 4-0 silk or chromic gut. An appropriate-size chest tube is inserted, and the wound is closed in layers (Figure 34-16, *C*).

CORRECTION OF A COARCTATION OF THE THORACIC AORTA

Surgical Goal

Correction of a coarctation of the thoracic aorta is performed to restore blood flow to the lower body and reduce cardiac workload.

Pathology

Coarctation of the thoracic aorta is a congenital stenosis that usually occurs near the junction of the fetal ductus

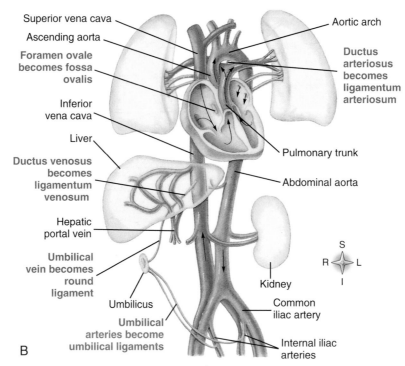

Superior vena cava
Ascending aorta
Foramen ovale becomes fossa ovalis
Inferior vena cava
Liver
Ductus venosus becomes ligamentum venosum
Hepatic portal vein
Umbilical vein becomes round ligament
Umbilicus
Umbilical arteries become umbilical ligaments

Aortic arch
Ductus arteriosus becomes ligamentum arteriosum
Pulmonary trunk
Abdominal aorta
Kidney
Common iliac artery
Internal iliac arteries

B

Figure 34-15, cont'd   B, Changes in fetal circulation at birth. (Thibodeau G, Patton K: *Anatomy and physiology, ed 6, Philadelphia, Mosby, 2007.*)

arteriosus and the aorta. Severe narrowing obstructs the normal flow of blood through the thoracic aorta and to the lower body. The heart becomes enlarged as a result of the increased work required to pump blood through a stricture. The lower body may be underdeveloped as a result of the defect.

Technique

1. A thoracotomy is performed.
2. The mediastinal pleura is incised.
3. The ligamentum arteriosum is ligated and divided.
4. The aorta is occluded proximal and distal to the coarctation.
5. The aorta is transected and anastomosed, or a prosthetic graft is inserted.
6. The aorta is unclamped.
7. The wound is closed.

Discussion

The patient commonly is placed in the lateral position, prepped, and draped for a thoracotomy. The thoracic cavity is entered through a posterolateral thoracotomy. A moist laparotomy sponge is placed over the lung, which is retracted by the assistant. The surgeon incises the mediastinal pleura and places 3-0 or 4-0 silk traction sutures in the edges. This exposes the aorta. Moist umbilical tape is placed around the aorta for mobilization and retraction.

The intercostal arteries are mobilized. Fine dissecting scissors are used to dissect the aorta in the area of the coarctation.

The surgeon ligates and divides the ductus (a ductus that has closed naturally is called the *ligamentum arteriosum*) to free the aorta and prevent bleeding from the ductus or ligamentum if it is still patent. Additional sutures of 4-0 silk are placed in the ductus if needed.

The surgeon occludes the aorta proximal and distal to the coarctation with straight or angled vascular clamps. The arteries that supply the coarctated segment also are ligated, and bulldog clamps may be placed on other vessels that lie between the coarctated segment and the cross-clamps of the aorta. The aorta then is transected, and the stricture is removed.

The two ends of the aorta are anastomosed with 5-0 or 6-0 continuous suture. Interrupted sutures often are used in pediatric patients to allow growth. (In adults, 3-0 or 4-0 polypropylene suture is used.) If the two limbs of the aorta cannot be brought together easily (often the case in adults), a synthetic tube graft may be inserted, or a proximal portion of the left subclavian artery may be used to form a patch. In this technique, a part of the artery wall is swung around and anastomosed to the resected coarctation. The distal artery then is ligated.

All clamps are removed from the aorta and intercostal arteries. Blood flow to the lower body is restored. The surgeon inspects all suture lines for hemostasis, and additional sutures are placed as needed. A topical hemostatic agent may be applied to control bleeding.

The mediastinal pleura is closed with 3-0 or 4-0 suture. A chest tube is inserted, and the wound is closed in layers. Figure 34-17 illustrates the repair of a coarctation of the thoracic aorta.

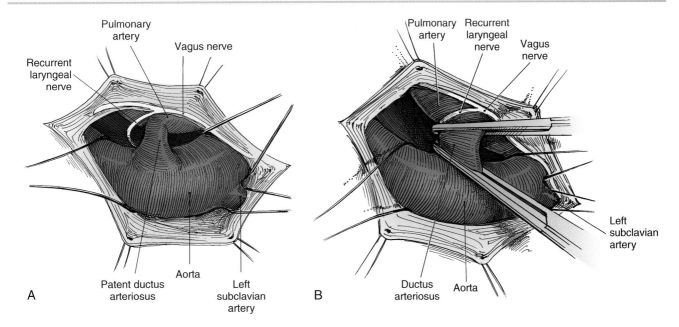

A — Recurrent laryngeal nerve, Pulmonary artery, Vagus nerve, Patent ductus arteriosus, Aorta, Left subclavian artery

B — Pulmonary artery, Recurrent laryngeal nerve, Vagus nerve, Ductus arteriosus, Aorta, Left subclavian artery

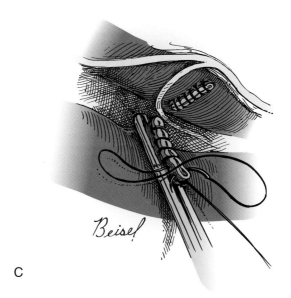

C

Beisel

Figure 34-16 Surgery for patent ductus arteriosus. **A,** Exposure of the patent ductus. **B,** Vascular clamps are placed across the ductus. **C,** Continuous suture closure. *(Modified from Waldhausen JA, Pierce WS, Campbell DB: Surgery of the chest, ed 6, St Louis, 1996, Mosby.)*

CORRECTION OF PULMONARY VALVE STENOSIS

Surgical Goal

Valvulotomy is performed to release fused valve leaflets and restore circulation from the right ventricle to the lungs. Most cases are treated by balloon catheterization.

Pathology

Pulmonary valve stenosis usually is a congenital anomaly in which the pulmonary valve is narrowed. Severe stenosis may require emergency treatment.

Technique

1. Cardiopulmonary bypass is initiated through a median sternotomy.
2. The venae cavae are encircled with umbilical tapes.
3. The pulmonary artery is opened, and the fused leaflets are separated.
4. The pulmonary artery is closed.
5. Cardiopulmonary bypass is discontinued, and the wound is prepared for closure.
6. The wound is closed.

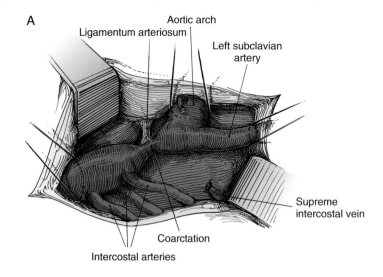

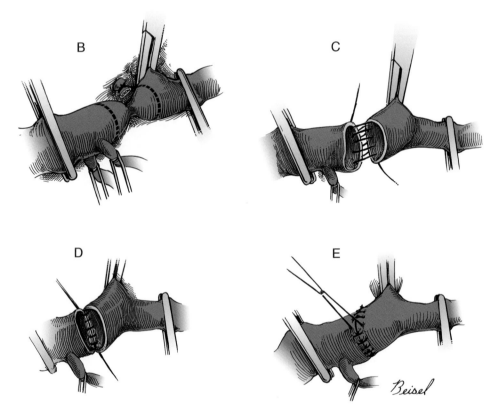

Figure 34-17 **A,** Coarctation of the aorta. **B,** Arterial clamps are applied above and below the constriction, and the vessel is resected. **C** and **D,** Continuous absorbable suture is used in closure. **E,** Closure of the anterior wall is completed with interrupted or continuous sutures. *(Modified from Waldhausen JA, Pierce WS, Campbell DB: Surgery of the chest, ed 6, St Louis, 1996, Mosby.)*

Discussion

The surgeon enters the chest through a median sternotomy. The pericardial sac is incised with scissors, and the incision is extended downward to the diaphragm and upward to the innominate vein. Cannulas of the correct size are obtained, and bypass is initiated.

An umbilical tape is placed on the aorta, and a purse-string suture of 4-0 polypropylene or polyester is placed. The assistant brings the ends of the suture through a bolster (a short vinyl or Silastic tube that holds the suture ends together) and holds the suture with a hemostat. Heparin is administered to the patient. Bicaval venous cannulation and aortic cannula-

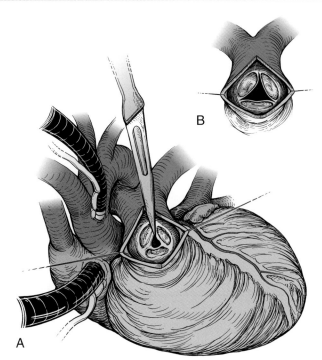

Figure 34-18 Pulmonary valvulotomy. **A,** The fused valve is incised. **B,** Completed valvulotomy. *(Modified from Mavroudis C, Backer DL: Pediatric cardiac surgery, ed 3, St Louis, 2003, Mosby.)*

tion are performed as described previously. Cardiopulmonary bypass is started.

To begin the repair, the surgeon isolates the vena cava with umbilical tape, and a tourniquet is placed as previously described. The pulmonary artery above the valve is opened with scissors. The aorta may be occluded temporarily to create a drier field. The fused leaflets are separated with a knife, Metzenbaum scissors, or Potts scissors (Figure 34-18). The surgeon closes the pulmonary artery with 5-0 continuous suture. If the pulmonary artery is stenotic, a patch graft may be inserted to enlarge the artery.

CLOSURE OF AN ATRIAL SEPTAL DEFECT

Surgical Goal
An atrial septal defect is a congenital anomaly in which a hole in the interatrial septum allows blood from the left atrium to flow into the right atrium. The goal of surgery is to close the defect and reduce excessive blood flow to the pulmonary system.

Pathology
Blood normally flows from the left atrium into the left ventricle before entering the systemic circulation. An atrial septal defect causes the blood to shunt from the left atrium to the right atrium. This creates increased pressure on the right ventricle and lungs, causing the heart to enlarge and eventually fail. An atrial septal defect usually is closed during childhood. However, some patients reach adulthood before developing symptoms that require surgical repair.

Technique
1. Cardiopulmonary bypass is initiated through a median sternotomy.
2. The aorta is occluded.
3. A right atriotomy is performed, the defect is closed, and the atriotomy is closed.
4. Cardiopulmonary bypass is discontinued, and the wound is prepared for closure.
5. The wound is closed.

Discussion
The patient is prepped and draped for a median sternotomy. The sternotomy is performed, and bypass is initiated. The surgeon may fibrillate the heart and occlude the aorta before performing a right atriotomy. A Richardson (pediatric) retractor is placed in the wound, and the surgeon examines the defect. Additional supplies may be needed, depending on this assessment.

The surgeon may repair the defect with a primary closure or by inserting a patch or pericardial graft. Large defects require a patch graft, which is cut to size and sutured in place with polypropylene or nylon sutures. Air is removed from the left side of the heart before the final sutures are placed and tied. Bypass is discontinued, and the wound is prepared for closure. The incision is closed in layers. Figure 34-19 illustrates the procedure for closure of an atrial septal defect.

CLOSURE OF A VENTRICULAR SEPTAL DEFECT

Surgical Goal
A ventricular septal defect is incomplete closure of the septum between the right and left ventricle which normally occurs during fetal life. This causes increased pulmonary pressure by allowing blood from the left ventricle to flow into the right ventricle and to the lungs, leading to congestive heart failure after birth. The septal defect is repaired to restore normal cardiac circulation.

Pathology
A ventricular septal defect is a hole in the intraventricular septum. It can occur in a variety of locations. Increased pressure in the left ventricle causes blood to flow through the defect into the area of lower pressure, the right ventricle.

Technique
1. Cardiopulmonary bypass is initiated through a median sternotomy.
2. The aorta is occluded, and a cardioplegic solution is infused into the coronary arteries.
3. A ventriculotomy is performed, and the defect is closed.
4. The aorta is unclamped, and the ventricle is closed.
5. Bypass is discontinued, and the cannulas are removed.
6. A temporary pacemaker electrode is sutured to the heart.
7. Chest tubes are inserted, and the wound is closed.

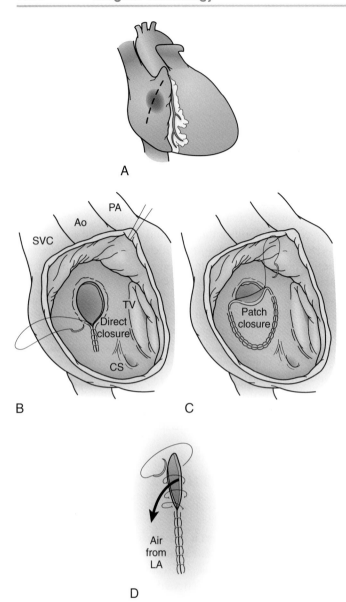

Figure 34-19 Repair of an atrial septal defect. **A,** The atrium is incised. **B,** Direct closure of the defect. *AO,* Aorta; *CS,* coronary sinus; *PA,* pulmonary artery; *SVC,* superior vena cava; *TV,* tricuspid valve. **C,** Patch closure. **D,** Air is removed from the left atrium. *(From Nichols DG, Ungerleider RM, Spevak PJ et al, editors: Critical heart disease in infants and children, Philadelphia, 2006, Mosby.)*

Discussion

The surgeon performs a median sternotomy and cannulates for total cardiopulmonary bypass as described in Chapter 33. The surgeon occludes the aorta with a pediatric vascular clamp and infuses a retrograde cardioplegic solution through the coronary sinus. A right ventriculotomy is performed with the knife or Mayo scissors. The surgeon may place sutures through the edges of the ventricle for traction.

The defect is assessed, and a patch graft is sutured into place. Teflon pledgets may be used to reinforce the suture line. Air is removed from the left ventricle before final closure.

After removing the aortic clamp, the surgeon closes the ventricle with continuous suture. Bypass is discontinued, and the cannulas are removed. A temporary pacemaker lead may be sutured to the right ventricle and right atrium. Chest tubes are inserted, and the wound is closed.

TOTAL CORRECTION OF TETRALOGY OF FALLOT

Surgical Goal

Tetralogy of Fallot is a combination of congenital defects that includes pulmonary stenosis, ventricular septal defect, right ventricular hypertrophy, and dextroposition (displacement) of the aorta. Surgical repair is performed to correct cyanosis and restore normal blood flow.

Pathology

Tetralogy of Fallot causes reduced pulmonary blood flow and right to left shunting (from the right ventricle to the left ventricle) of blood. This shunting mixes deoxygenated blood with oxygenated blood, and the mixture is pumped into the systemic circulation. The right ventricle becomes hypertrophied (enlarged) because of the work needed to pump the blood through the obstructed pulmonary system. The patient is cyanotic, and increased oxygen demand results in reduced pulmonary blood flow. If delayed repair is necessary, a systemic-pulmonary shunt may be performed to increase blood flow to the lungs. This shunt improves oxygenation and allows the baby to develop to a stage at which total correction is possible.

Technique

1. A median sternotomy is performed, and bypass is initiated.
2. Cardioplegia is performed.
3. A right ventriculotomy is performed, the infundibular muscle is resected, and a pulmonary valvulotomy is performed.
4. The ventricular septal defect is closed, and the right ventricle is closed with a patch.
5. Bypass is discontinued.
6. A temporary pacemaker lead is inserted.
7. Chest tubes are inserted, and the wound is closed.

Discussion

The incision used for this procedure depends on whether a palliative shunt previously was performed. Total correction in the absence of a previous shunt is performed through a median sternotomy. After the chest has been opened, bypass is initiated. Cardioplegia then is performed as described previously.

The surgeon performs the right ventriculotomy with a knife and curved Mayo scissors. Retractors are inserted, and a portion of the infundibular muscle is excised. The technologist should wipe all instruments clean after use to prevent emboli from forming.

A pulmonary valvulotomy then is performed, and the ventricular septal defect is closed as previously described. After air is evacuated from the left ventricle, the clamp is removed from the aorta.

The surgeon closes the ventricle with a continuous suture of 4-0 polypropylene. A patch of woven Dacron or Teflon is used to enlarge the right ventricular outflow tract (the area beneath the pulmonary valve). The pulmonary artery also may be enlarged with a patch, using a smaller size suture.

The pulmonary artery pressure and right ventricular pressure are measured to determine whether the surgery was successful. If the results indicate that additional surgery is required, additional surgical supplies are needed.

If the surgery is successful, bypass is discontinued and the wound is prepared for closure as described previously. Chest tubes are inserted, and the wound is closed. Complete repair of teratology of Fallot is illustrated in Figure 34-20.

REPAIR OF PECTUS EXCAVATUM

Surgical Goal

Pectus excavatum, or funnel chest, is a nongenetic defect of the chest wall marked by overgrowth of the costal cartilages, a sunken appearance in the anterior chest, and a restricted sternum. The goal of surgery is to reconstruct the chest wall to restore normal inspiratory function and improve body image.

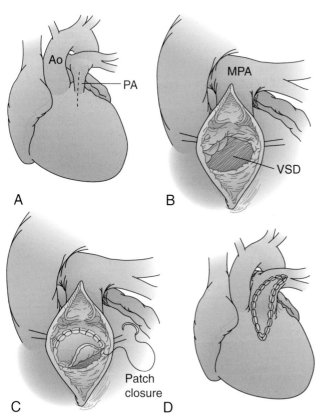

Figure 34-20 Repair of tetralogy of Fallot. **A,** Enlargement of the right ventricle; main pulmonary artery (MPA) connection. *Ao,* Aorta. **B,** Resection of muscle from the ventricular septal defect (VSD). **C,** Closure of the VSD. **D,** Patch graft. *(From Townsend CM, Beauchamp DR, Evers MB, Mattox KL: Sabiston textbook of surgery, ed 18, Philadelphia, 2007, WB Saunders.)*

Pathology

Pectus excavatum does not have a genetic component, but it may be associated with Marfan syndrome. Children born with the acquired defect may have mild to moderate paradoxical movement of the sternum with inhalation. Children have a typical slouching appearance, and older children may experience shortness of breath. Surgery is performed in adolescence or preadolescence.

In the Nuss procedure, a metal bar is placed under the sternum to lift the chest wall. The bar is left in place for 2 years or longer until growth is complete. The bar then is removed, a procedure for which local anesthesia is used.

Technique

1. The defect is measured, and the skin is marked for insertion of the pectus bar.
2. The pectus bar is prepared using a plate bender.
3. Two 0.8-inch (2 cm) incisions are made in the midaxillary line following the skin marks.
4. Under thoracoscopic visualization, a curved introducer is inserted through one of the incisions and a tunnel is made.
5. The bar is inserted in inverted position and advanced to the opposite incision.
6. When the bar is in place, it is inverted to evert the sternum, creating a convex chest wall.
7. The bar may be stabilized with #3 steel wire and stabilizers.
8. The ends of the bar are buried in the subcutaneous tissue.
9. The wound is checked for bleeding and to ensure that the bar is stabilized.
10. The wounds are closed with synthetic absorbable sutures and flat dressings or Steri-Strips.

Postoperative Considerations

As the child emerges from anesthesia, the PACU team ensures that the patient remains in the supine position to prevent the bar from being dislodged. Patients are kept in the hospital for at least 3 to 4 days for pain control and to ensure that the bar is stable. Epidural catheterization for continuous pain control is used in selected patients. Limited activity may be resumed 6 weeks after surgery.

NEURAL TUBE DEFECTS

The neural tube is an embryonic structure that gives rise to the central nervous system (i.e., the spinal cord and the brain). During embryonic development, a variety of environmental conditions can cause defects in the neural tube. Normally, the embryonic spinal cord develops from a flat area, which then rolls into a tubal structure at about 28 days after conception. A **neural tube defect** occurs when the tube fails to close completely. The most common defects are spina bifida, anencephaly, and encephalocele. These are called *open defects* because the neural tissue is exposed at birth and leakage of cerebrospinal fluid (CSF) occurs.

- *Spina bifida* is an anomaly that includes several types of defects. The most common is a myelomeningocele. A myelomeningocele is an exposed portion of the spinal cord and nerves that is contained within a membranous sac, which may rupture at birth. Hydrocephalus, paralysis, bowel and bladder incontinence, and severe mental retardation are associated with a myelomeningocele. The defect can be closed, but nerve damage is permanent.

- *Anencephaly* is the absence of a cranial vault. The defect is incompatible with life and the neonate dies soon after birth. The defect can be diagnosed during routine prenatal ultrasound.
- *Encephalocele* is an anomaly in which meninges, CSF, and sometimes brain tissue are contained within a herniated sac. The incidence is 1 to 4 in 10,000 births, with a 50% survival rate.

Repair of a myelomeningocele is described here.

REPAIR OF A MYELOMENINGOCELE

Surgical Goal

The surgical goal of repair of a myelomeningocele is to close a dural and cutaneous defect and preserve neural function. Immediate surgical repair is essential if the defect is leaking CSF; otherwise, the procedure is performed within 48 hours of birth to prevent infection.

Pathology

Spina bifida is a birth defect associated with incomplete closure of a section of the vertebral column. Spina bifida may occur at any point in the vertebral column but is most common in the lumbar and sacral spine. The defect may be small (spina bifida occulta) and not cause any neurological deficit for the infant, or it may cause herniation of the meninges and leakage of CSF (meningocele). The most significant form of spina bifida causes the spinal cord, meninges, and nerve roots to herniate through the skin (Figure 34-21). The structures generally are contained within a cyst or saclike enclosure. The neural tissue in the myelomeningocele is abnormal, and even with repair, the patient still has some degree of neurological deficit, such as paralysis or loss of sensation below the level of the defect. A myelomeningocele often is accompanied by birth defects such as heart and urinary system problems, which may complicate the infant's care.

Hydrocephalus (excessive accumulation of cerebrospinal fluid within the ventricles of the brain) is discussed in Chapter 35. It often is associated with a myelomeningocele. If the hydrocephalus is significant, the surgeon may elect to place a ventricular shunt at the time of myelomeningocele repair. If the hydrocephalus is less of a concern, the surgeon may postpone the shunt placement to allow the infant to recover from the primary surgery.

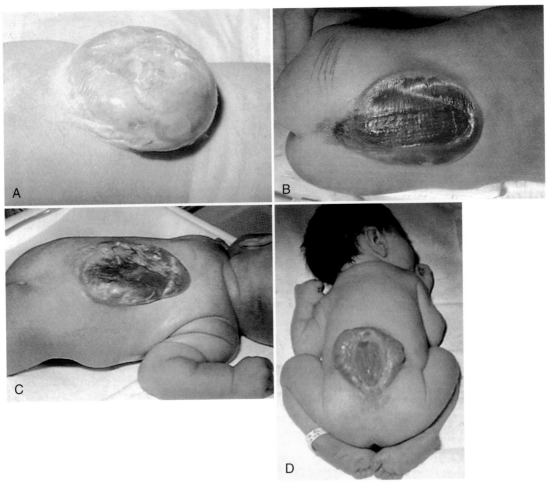

Figure 34-21 Myelomeningocele. **A,** A lesion covered by membrane. **B,** A flat lesion. **C,** A thoracolumbar lesion. **D,** Exposed spinal cord. *(From Rothrock J: Alexander's care of the patient in surgery, ed 17, Philadelphia, 2007, Mosby.)*

Technique

1. The infant is positioned prone on small chest and hip rolls.
2. Fluid is aspirated from the sac and submitted for culture.
3. An incision is made around the circumference of the defect.
4. The tissue around the defect is explored and dissected free.
5. The dura is separated from the fascia and closed.
6. The fascia is separated from the muscle and closed.
7. The muscle and skin are closed.

Discussion

Infants with a myelomeningocele often undergo many surgical procedures to address the primary defect and associated birth defects. Consequently, latex sensitization often develops in these patients. Many institutions that routinely treat infants with a myelomeningocele use a latex-free protocol to minimize exposure and reduce sensitization. The surgical technologist should be familiar with the facility's policies and procedures for latex allergy to ensure that a safe environment is maintained for the patient.

Infants with a myelomeningocele are more vulnerable to hypothermia because of the exposure of their skin and neural structures to the ambient room temperature. The technician must ensure that the solutions used during the procedure are warm. Because of the delicate nature of this procedure and the patient's size, small, fine instruments are used.

The patient is placed in the prone position using small chest and hip rolls. If the neural sac is intact, the surgeon decompresses it with a 20-gauge needle attached to a syringe. The fluid is sent for culture and analysis.

The surgeon begins the procedure by making a circumferential incision around the defect with a #15 blade on a #3 knife handle. The technician should be prepared with bipolar ESU and 4 × 4 sponges to assist the surgeon with hemostasis. The incision is carried through the subcutaneous tissue until the fascia or dura is visualized.

The surgeon uses Metzenbaum scissors to remove the tissue over the exposed spinal cord and dissects along the side of the cord to reach the dura. The technician should be prepared with the bipolar ESU and moistened cottonoids, as necessary, for hemostasis during the dissection. Metzenbaum scissors are used to separate the dura from the fascia, and the dura is closed over the spinal cord with 4-0 braided nylon or silk suture.

The fascia is dissected from the muscle layer with Metzenbaum scissors and a #11 blade as necessary. The fascial layer is closed over the dura with nonabsorbable suture. The wound is irrigated with warm saline. The muscle layer is closed with absorbable synthetic sutures. If the defect is small, the surgeon may be able to reapproximate the skin edges easily; larger defects may require Z-plasty or flap closure with interrupted sutures of synthetic nonabsorbable material.

CORRECTION OF SYNDACTYLY

Surgical Goal

Surgery is performed to separate the fingers, which are joined at birth.

Pathology

During weeks 6 and 8 of gestation, the paddle-shaped hands and feet normally differentiate into separate fingers and toes. Syndactyly results when this separation fails to occur. It is the most common malformation of the limbs and is associated with at least 28 other specific syndromes, occurring in 1 per 2,000 births. The cause is unknown. The condition is classified as incomplete or complete, depending on whether the fingers are joined from the base (web) to the tip. In complex syndactyly, bone and soft tissue are shared by two fingers, whereas in simple syndactyly, only superficial tissues and skin are involved. Surgery is performed before school age. Simple syndactyly is shown in Figure 34-22.

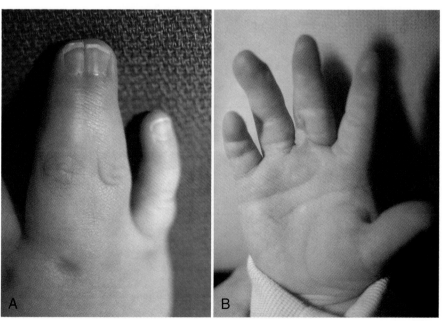

Figure 34-22 Syndactyly before and after surgical correction. (From Canale S, Beaty J: Campbell's operative orthopaedics, ed 11, Philadelphia, 2008, WB Saunders.)

Technique

1. The skin incisions are marked.
2. A graft site is prepared, and an inguinal graft is removed.
3. Skin flaps are raised.
4. The web space is reconstructed using primary Z-closure on one side.
5. A skin graft is sutured in place.
6. Dressings are applied.

Discussion

The patient is placed in the supine position with the operative arm on a hand board. General anesthesia is induced. A tourniquet is applied, and the arm is prepped from the elbow to the hand. If a skin graft is required, the groin is prepped and draped separately.

To begin the procedure, the surgeon plans the incisions and draws them on the hand. If a graft is to be taken, this is done first. A small amount of skin is removed from the groin crease using the free-hand method and scalpel. The skin is handed to the surgical technologist to be kept moist until needed. The site is covered with a towel to protect it from contamination.

The skin incisions are made with a #15 knife and plastic surgery forceps. A Z-shaped or modified Z-incision is used. The tourniquet is released momentarily, and bleeders are controlled with a needle point bipolar ESU. The tourniquet can then be reinflated. The triangular flaps are closed on one finger with anchor sutures of 5-0 nylon and interrupted sutures to complete the repair.

The graft is positioned over the denuded area of the other finger and trimmed as needed. Tenotomy scissors or iris scissors may be used for this. The graft is sutured in placed with 4-0 or 5-0 interrupted nylon or absorbable synthetic sutures.

A Xeroform dressing can be placed over the graft site, and a stent dressing can be used to maintain close contact between the graft and finger. (Stent dressings are described in detail in Chapter 17.) The opposite finger is dressed with Xeroform and gauze. Webril is applied around each site while the fingers are widely separated. Many surgeons apply a hard cast to maintain the repair during healing. A simple syndactyly repair is shown in Figure 34-23.

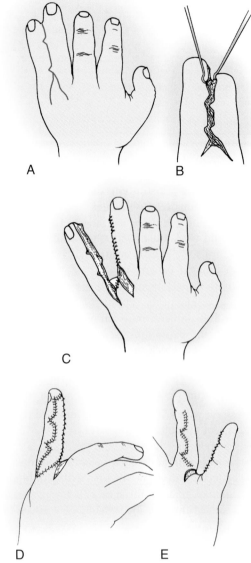

Figure 34-23   Syndactyly repair. **A** and **B,** Skin incisions. **C,** Reconstruction of the ring finger. **D** and **E,** Closure of the little finger and web space graft. *(From Canale S, Beaty J: Campbell's operative orthopaedics, ed 11, Philadelphia, 2008, WB Saunders.)*

CHAPTER SUMMARY

- Much of pediatric surgery is performed to correct physical defects that develop during fetal life. These are called *congenital abnormalities.*
- Abnormalities may be genetic (inherited) or acquired through environmental exposure during fetal life.
- An environmental agent (chemical or drug) that injures the embryo or fetus is called a *teratogen.*
- Mutagenic substances cause gene mutation, a chemical change in the genetic structure.
- The maternal diet is an important cause of congenital birth defects.

- Certain infectious agents are also known be teratogenic.
- Pediatric patients, especially infants and neonates, are particularly vulnerable to hypothermia and hyperthermia.
- Physiological mechanisms that normally regulate temperature in an adult are absent or undeveloped in the infant. Infants and children tend to lose more heat than they generate.
- A relatively large skin surface area and low body weight can contribute to rapid lowering of an infant's core temperature.

- Children and infants have extensive peripheral circulation, which contributes to relatively rapid cooling.
- Loss of body heat occurs through radiation, conduction, and evaporation. Anesthetics also lower the core temperature.
- Shivering is a compensatory reaction to cold that normally occurs during hypothermia in adults; infants lack this mechanism.
- Environmental hyperthermia is less of a risk to pediatric surgical patients. However, an elevated core temperature can occur with misuse of warming devices.
- Steps to maintain the pediatric patient's temperature are implemented throughout the perioperative period. If the patient becomes chilled, it may be difficult to re-establish warmth, which must be done with active warming methods.
- Warm air blankets, water-filled mattresses, and overhead heat lamps are used to maintain a safe core temperature in the pediatric patient.
- Fluid balance (maintaining the correct amount and types of fluids in body spaces) is an important goal in the care of pediatric patients.
- Hemostasis is a critical element in pediatric surgery. Infants and children have little blood reserve and cannot tolerate persistent bleeding. All members of the surgical team are jointly responsible for monitoring blood loss as efficiently and accurately as possible.
- The importance of the scrub's role during critical moments of hemorrhage cannot be overstated. The technologist should plan for such emergencies before surgery and mentally rehearse the steps needed to act quickly and correctly.
- An important anatomical difference between the adult and the pediatric respiratory system is the airway. Failure to manage the pediatric patient's airway is among the leading causes of death in medical and traumatic emergency.
- Pediatric patients are assessed and prepared for anesthesia using similar methods as for adults. However, the psychological preparation must take into consideration the child's more extreme fears, especially the trauma of separation.
- Age-appropriate preparation may include familiarizing the child with anesthesia devices, surgical attire, and other objects that can cause anxiety.
- Pediatric patients may be given an anxiolytic (anxiety reducing) medication before surgery. However, this practice varies from institution to institution and among anesthesia care providers.
- The presence of the parent or parents during induction is now an accepted practice in many health care facilities. This has been shown to reduce the need for preoperative medication in many pediatric patients.
- Psychosocial care of the pediatric patient is a process involving the child, parents or guardians, and perioperative staff. The goal of psychosocial care is to help patients and families develop strategies that help them cope with the perioperative experience.
- Pediatric patients tend to react to their environment in predictable ways according to their developmental age.
- The greatest fears of young children undergoing surgery are fear of the unknown and fear of separation from family or caregivers.
- Childhood development traditionally is separated into age categories in which children display distinct social and cognitive characteristics (Erikson's stages of psychosocial development).
- Pediatric specialization involves the same domains of safety required in surgery of the adult. The surgical technologist maintains a safe environment in collaboration with the perioperative registered nurse in specific areas.
- Because of their small size and immature organ systems, pediatric patients are at high risk of adverse effects from overdosing. The surgical technologist participates in the medication process while in the scrubbed role.
- Pediatric patients *are particularly vulnerable* to risks related to their age, size, and stage of development.
- Neonates and babies usually are transported to the operating room in a heated Isolette (infant-size transport unit), which is environmentally controlled and equipped with monitoring devices.
- Toddlers may walk to the surgical department (for outpatient cases) and are placed on a stretcher in the holding area, or they may be transported in a crib.
- The safety principles that apply to adult electrosurgery are the same for pediatric patients. The primary differences are the size of the active and patient return electrodes.
- Although the principles for positioning are the same for adults and children, it is important to use appropriate-size padding to fit the pediatric patient. Gel and foam pads are appropriate for infants and children, whose delicate skin must be protected from shearing pressure injury at all times.
- Cleft lip and cleft palate occur within the first 8 weeks of embryonic development when the philtrum and palate fail to close normally.
- Although cleft palate sometimes is seen in conjunction with cleft lip, they are separate malformations and are rarely related to one another.
- The term *branchial* refers to "gills" and is derived from the science of embryology. When these clefts and pouches (gills) fail to develop, they may persist as cysts or fistulas and are diagnosed sometime in childhood, usually during infancy.
- A thyroglossal duct cyst or fistula is the result of incomplete closure of the thyroglossal duct, which forms during development of the thyroid gland during embryonic life.

- Choanal atresia is a congenital anomaly of the anterior skull base characterized by a stricture or blockage of the passage between the nasal sinuses and the pharyngeal nasal airways.
- A graft taken from the intercostal cartilage is used to create or reconstruct the external ear.
- In pyloromyotomy, the pyloric outlet muscles are divided and released to allow normal passage of food into the intestine.
- Esophageal atresia is the absence of or a gap in the esophagus. The goal of surgery is to join the two sections and provide continuity of the structure.
- Tracheoesophageal fistula often is associated with EA. This is a defect in which a fistula or tract develops between the esophagus and trachea, causing saliva, stomach contents, and food to enter the trachea and lungs of the neonate.
- Omphalocele is a congenital anomaly in which the abdominal viscera develop outside the body, contained within a peritoneal sac. Gastroschisis is similar to omphalocele except there is no peritoneal covering over the abdominal viscera.
- Hirschsprung disease is congenital absence of ganglionic cells in the colon. This results in the bowel's failure to function in peristalsis. Severe obstruction and distention occur in the colon and abdomen.
- The pull-through procedure for Hirschsprung disease involves removal of the diseased portion of the bowel and anastomosis to the rectal muscles.
- Intussusception is an emergency in which the bowel telescopes into itself, causing obstruction and ischemia.
- Volvulus is rotation of the bowel around the mesenteric attachment, or twisting on itself. An emergency medical response is required to prevent gangrene and peritonitis.

- Bladder exstrophy is part of a complex congenital defect in which the bladder develops outside the body in open configuration. The defect also involves other structures of the genitourinary tract, skeletal system, and other systems.
- Orchiopexy is surgical correction for an undescended testicle.
- Patent ductus arteriosus occurs when the duct fails to close normally after birth, causing arterial blood to continue its fetal path back to the lungs.
- Coarctation of the aorta is a congenital narrowing that obstructs the normal flow of blood through the thoracic aorta to the lower body.
- An atrial septal defect is a congenital anomaly in which a hole in the interatrial septum allows blood from the left atrium to flow to the right atrium.
- A ventricular septal defect causes increased pulmonary pressure by allowing blood from the left ventricle to flow into the right ventricle and to the lungs, leading to congestive heart failure. The septal defect is repaired to restore normal cardiac circulation.
- Tetralogy of Fallot is a combination of congenital defects that includes pulmonary stenosis, ventricular septal defect, right ventricular hypertrophy, and dextroposition (displacement) of the aorta.
- Pectus excavatum is a defect of the chest wall marked by overgrowth of the costal cartilages and a sunken appearance in the sternum. The defect may be repaired using the Nuss minimally invasive surgical technique.
- Spina bifida is a birth defect associated with incomplete closure of a section of the vertebral column. The most significant form of spina bifida causes the spinal cord, meninges, and nerve roots to herniate through the skin; this is referred to as a *myelomeningocele*.

REVIEW QUESTIONS

1. What are the disadvantages of administering a preoperative anxiolytic to a pediatric patient?
2. List at least five reasons infants are at risk for hypothermia.
3. Explain magical thinking and how this affects a toddler's view of the perioperative environment.
4. Explain the difference between an omphalocele and gastroschisis.
5. List at least six reasons pediatric patients should not be considered "small adults." Give examples from your knowledge of pediatric physiology.
6. What are the specific risks associated with transporting a pediatric patient?
7. What are the responsibilities of the scrubbed surgical technologist in maintaining fluid balance in the pediatric patient? Hint: Include blood loss, irrigation, tissue dehydration, and other factors.
8. What are the risks to tissue which is left exposed to the environment in conditions such as omphalocele and spina bifida?
9. Why might the presence of a parent upset a child during induction?
10. Explain the anatomical aspects of tetralogy of Fallot.

REFERENCE

1. American Society of Anesthesiologists: Practice guidelines for preoperative fasting and the use of pharmacologic agents to reduce the risk of pulmonary aspiration: application to healthy patients undergoing elective procedures—a report by the American Society of Anesthesiologists Task Force on Preoperative Fasting, *Anesthesiology* 90:3, 1999.

BIBLIOGRAPHY

Association of periOperative Registered Nurses (AORN): Pediatric medication safety, *AORN Journal* 83:1, 2006.

Busen N: Perioperative preparation of the adolescent surgical patient, *AORN Journal* 73:2, 2001.

Cartwright CC, Jimenez DF, Barone CM et al: Endoscopic strip craniectomy: a minimally invasive treatment for early correction of craniosynostosis, *Journal of Neuroscience Nursing* 35:3, 2003.

Dreger V, Tremback T: Management of preoperative anxiety in children, *AORN Journal* 84:5, 2006.

Golden L, Pagala M, Sukhavasi S, Nagpal D, Ahmad A et al: Giving toys to children reduces their anxiety about receiving premedication for surgery, *Anesthesia and Analgesia* 102:1070, 2006.

Hommertzheim R, Steinke E: Malignant hyperthermia: the perioperative nurse's role, *AORN Journal* 83:1, 2006.

Ingoe R, Lange P: The Ladd's procedure for correction of intestinal malrotation with volvulus in children, *AORN Journal* 85:2, 2007.

Phippen ML, Papanier Wells M: *Patient care during operative and invasive procedures,* Philadelphia, 2000, WB Saunders.

Swoveland B, Medvick C, Thompson G: The Nuss procedure for pectus excavatum correction, *AORN Journal* 74:6, 2001.

Touloukian RJ, Smith EI: Disorders of rotation and fixation. In: *Pediatric surgery,* ed 5, vol 2, St Louis, 1998, Mosby.

Viitanen H, Paivi A, Viitanen M, Tarkkila P: Premedication with midazolam delays recovery after ambulatory sevoflurane anesthesia in children, *Anesthesia and Analgesia* 90:498, 2000.

Neurosurgery

CHAPTER OULINE

LEARNING OBJECTIVES

After studying this chapter the reader will be able to:

- Identify important anatomical and physiological features of the central and peripheral nervous systems
- Identify the equipment and supplies used during neurosurgery
- Discuss the surgical techniques used during a craniotomy
- Identify the basic surgical techniques used during spinal surgery
- Discuss the safety precautions taken when prepping a patient for neurosurgery

- List the instrument sets used for cranial surgery, spinal surgery, and peripheral nerve surgery
- Discuss the positioning, skin prep, and draping used in different types of neurosurgery
- Identify important neurological diseases, especially those correctable by surgery
- Discuss the surgical goals of common neurosurgical procedures

TERMINOLOGY

Acoustic neuroma: A benign tumor of the eighth cranial nerve; more accurately referred to as a *schwannoma,* because it is composed of Schwann cells, which produce myelin.

Adenoma: A benign tumor consisting of glandular tissue.

Aneurysm: Dilation or ballooning of an artery wall as a result of injury, disease, or a congenital condition.

Arteriovenous: Relating to both arteries and veins.

Arteriovenous malformation (AVM): A collection of blood vessels with abnormal communication between the arteries and veins. It may be the result of injury, infection, or a congenital condition.

Astrocytes: Cells that support the nerve cells (neurons) of the brain and spinal cord by providing nutrients and insulation.

Bone flap: A section of bone removed from the skull during craniotomy procedures.

Central nervous system (CNS): The part of the nervous system comprising the brain and spinal cord.

Embolization: A technique used to occlude a blood vessel. A variety of materials, including platinum coils and microscopic plastic particles, are injected into the vessel under fluoroscopic control to stop active bleeding or prevent bleeding.

Intracranial pressure (ICP): The pressure within the skull exerted by the brain tissue, blood, and cerebrospinal fluid.

Stereotactic: A computerized method of locating a point in space or in tissue, using coordinates in three-dimensions. During stereotactic surgery, the precise location of a tumor or other tissue can be identified from outside the body. The tissue can then be targeted for destruction. The term originates from the Greek words *stereo*, meaning three dimensional, and *tactos*, meaning touched.

INTRODUCTION

Neurosurgery is a specialized field of medicine that focuses on the surgical treatment of diseases and functional disorders of the brain, spine, and peripheral nerves. The surgical technologist assisting in neurosurgery should have a solid foundation in the anatomy and pathology of the nervous system. Access to the brain and spinal anatomy often requires penetration or removal of bony tissue. Therefore many procedures require both soft tissue and orthopedic instruments.

SURGICAL ANATOMY

The nervous system is a communication center for the body. It receives, processes, and interprets information from the environment. It then coordinates appropriate sensory and motor responses. The nervous system is divided structurally into two parts: the **central nervous system (CNS)**, which includes the brain and spinal cord, and the peripheral nervous system (PNS), which includes the cranial and spinal nerves and their branches.

CELLS OF THE NERVOUS SYSTEM

Neurons

The neuron is the primary cell type of the nervous system located throughout the body. It transmits information to other neurons, muscle, and glandular tissue. The neuron has three main parts: the body (or soma), the axon, and the dendrites (Figure 35-1).

- The *soma* acts as the sending and receiving area for nerve impulses and is the energy center for the cell.
- The *axon* carries nerve impulses away from the cell.
- The *dendrites* carry nerve impulses toward the cell.

Neuroglia and Schwann Cells

Neuroglia and Schwann cells provide support to the neurons. Brain and spinal cord tissue is composed primarily of neuroglia. **Astrocytes**, the most common type of neuroglia, fill the spaces between the neurons. Oligodendrocytes form myelin, the fatty sheath that provides insulation for the dendrites. Microglia are specialized immune cells that remove cellular debris. Ependymal cells line the brain ventricles and are involved in the production of cerebrospinal fluid (CSF). Schwann cells are found in the peripheral nervous system. Their main functions are the production of myelin and the removal of cellular debris.

CENTRAL NERVOUS SYSTEM

Skull (Cranium)

The skull covers and protects the brain. It is composed of bony plates that are connected by a thin membrane called a *suture*. The major bones of the skull (Figure 35-2) are as follows:

- One *frontal bone*, which provides structure for the forehead and orbits.
- Two parietal bones on either side of the skull, which provide structure for the sides and roof of the cranium.
- Two temporal bones on either side of the skull, which contribute to the structure for the sides of the cranium.
- One occipital bone, which provides structure to the back of the skull and a portion of the floor of the cranium.

The skull is covered by the multilayered scalp, which is composed of skin and highly vascular subcutaneous tissue. The *pericranium* is the periosteal layer of the skull bones. The pericranium is covered by muscle and the galea, a tough, fibrous tissue sheet. The skin of the scalp is very thick and highly vascular and contains numerous hair follicles.

Meninges

Directly beneath the skull lie the three protective coverings of the brain, the meninges. The outermost layer, the dura mater, is composed of very dense, fibrous tissue. The middle layer is the arachnoid mater. The arachnoid mater is a very delicate, serous membrane that has the appearance of a spider web. Beneath the arachnoid mater is the subarachnoid space, which is filled with CSF. The pia mater is the layer closest to the brain. This is a vascular membrane that contains portions of areolar connective tissue. This membrane dips down into the various crevices and convolutions of the brain. The layers of the scalp, superficial brain, and associated structures are illustrated in Figure 35-3.

BRAIN

The brain itself is divided into three main sections: the cerebrum, cerebellum, and brainstem. Each of these sections is further subdivided (Figure 35-4).

Cerebrum

The cerebrum, or forebrain, controls all motor activity and sensory impulses. It is divided into halves, the right and left cerebral hemispheres. Each hemisphere is subdivided into four lobes:

- The *frontal lobe* is responsible for thought and behavior.

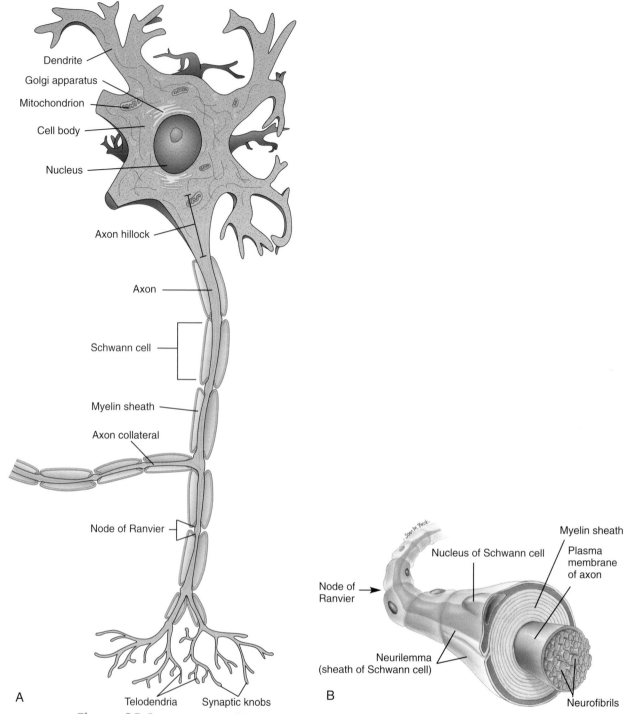

Figure 35-1 **A,** Structure of the neuron. Note the three main sections: the cell body, dendrites, and axon. **B,** Structure of the axon. The myelinated sheath of some neurons affects the speed of nerve transmission. *(A from Thibodeau G, Patton K:* Anatomy and physiology, *ed 6, St. Louis, Mosby, 2007; B courtesy Brenda Russell, PhD, University of Illinois at Chicago.)*

- The *temporal lobe* controls memory, the senses, language, and emotions.
- The *parietal lobe* primarily controls language.
- The *occipital lobe* controls vision.

The cerebrum is the largest part of the brain, accounting for almost 88% of the total weight of the organ. The surface of the cerebrum is convoluted, having small bulges that occur throughout. These bulges are called *gyri* (sing., gyrus). Between the bulges are shallow indentations, called *sulci* (sing., sulcus). Larger, deeper furrows in this area are known as *fissures.*

The outer tissue layer of the cerebrum is known as the *cerebral cortex.* This layer is composed of gray matter and is divided into lobes, which are named for the bones that overlie them. The gray matter is composed of nerve cells and blood

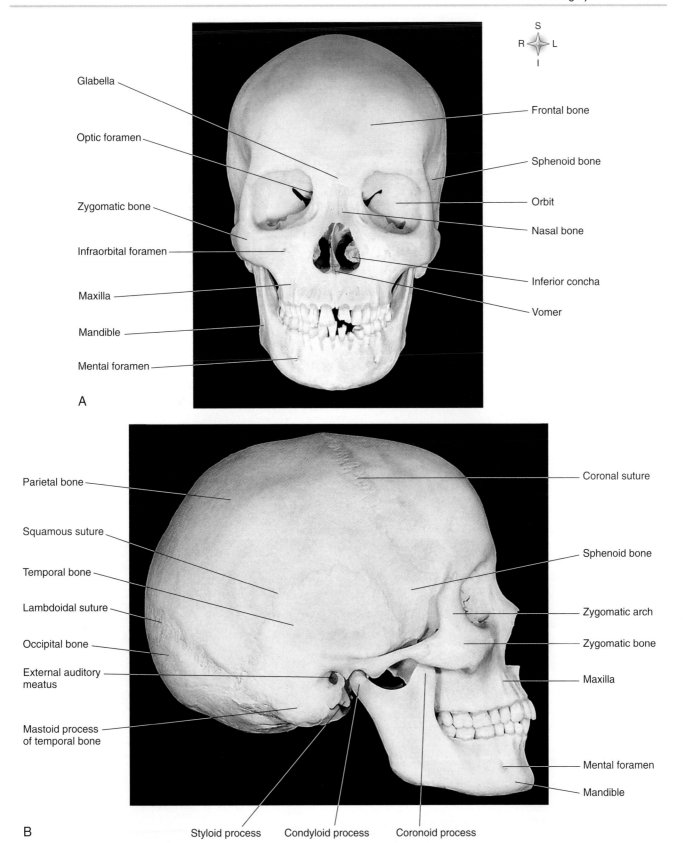

Figure 35-2 Bones of the cranium. **A,** Front view. **B,** Side view. *(From Vidic B, Suarez FR: Photographic atlas of the human body, St Louis, 1984, Mosby.)*

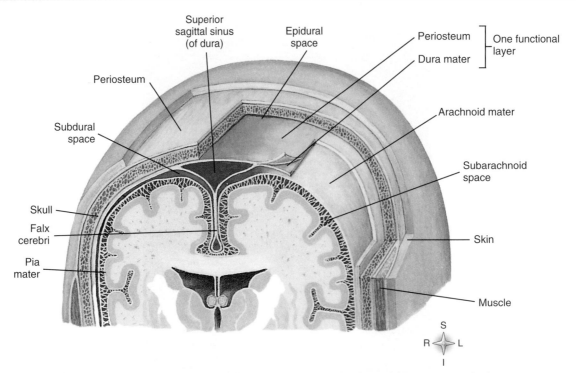

Figure 35-3 Surgical layers of the scalp, galea, meninges, and brain. *(From Abrahams P, Hutchings RT, Marks SC: McKinn's color atlas of human anatomy, ed 4, St Louis, 1999, Mosby.)*

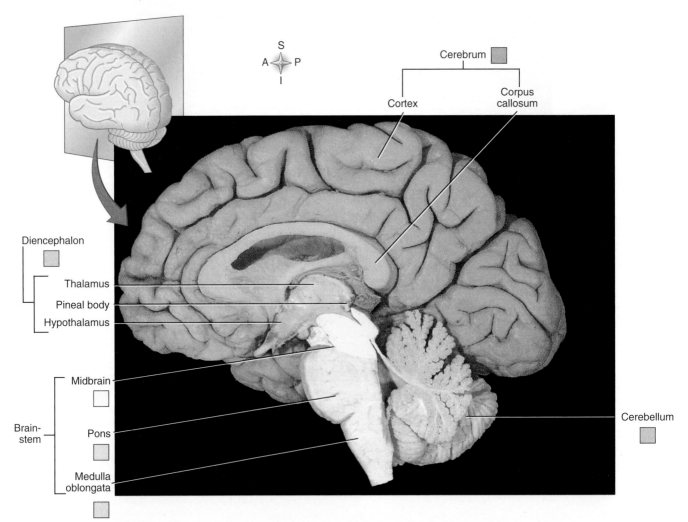

Figure 35-4 Divisions of the brain. *(From Vidic B, Suarez FR: Photographic atlas of the human body, St Louis, 1984, Mosby.)*

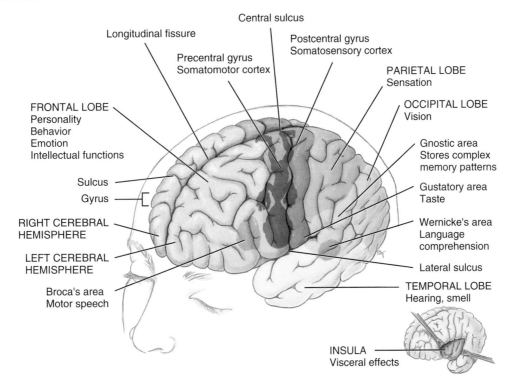

Figure 35-5 Lobes of the cerebrum. *(From Applegate E: The anatomy and physiology learning system, ed 2, St Louis, 2000, WB Saunders.)*

vessels. The lobes and functional areas of the cerebrum are illustrated in Figure 35-5.

Cerebellum

The cerebellum, or hindbrain, lies under the posterior cerebrum and is the second largest area of the brain (Figure 35-6). Like the cerebrum, it is covered by a cortex composed of gray matter and is divided into lobes by fissures. The cerebellar lobes are the anterior, posterior, and flocculonodular lobes. The anterior and posterior lobes help control coordination and movement. The flocculonodular lobe helps control equilibrium. Coordination between the cerebrum and cerebellum is necessary for the "planning" and execution of movement. The sensory information provided by the cerebrum guides the coordinated movement of muscles and balance.

Brainstem

The brainstem is composed of three sections: the medulla oblongata, midbrain, and pons (Figure 35-7). The medulla oblongata is a continuous connection between the spinal cord and the pons. It is made up primarily of gray matter and closely resembles the spinal cord in internal structure except that it is much thicker. Lines of white matter are interspersed within the gray matter, and all impulses into and out of the spinal cord are located here. The medulla is responsible for vital functions such as control of the circulatory system, respiration, and heart rate.

The midbrain is situated between the forebrain and the hindbrain. The major structures of the midbrain are the thalamus, hypothalamus, posterior pituitary gland, and pineal gland. On the ventral side of the midbrain are two masses of

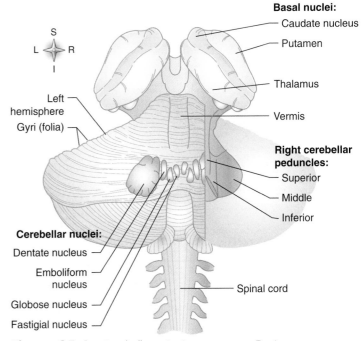

Figure 35-6 Cerebellum. **A,** Posterior view. **B,** Anterior view. *(From Abrahams P, Hutchings RT, Marks SC: McKinn's color atlas of human anatomy, ed 4, St Louis, 1999, Mosby.)*

white matter called the *cerebral peduncles.* White matter contains millions of myelinated nerve fibers that carry impulses between the neurons. On the dorsal side are four rounded tissue masses called the *corpora quadrigemina.* This section is responsible for relaying auditory and visual impulses.

The pons lies between the midbrain and the medulla, in front of the cerebellum. It consists mainly of white matter and serves as a relay between the medulla and the cerebral peduncles. The fifth, sixth, seventh, and eighth cranial nerves originate in this portion of the hindbrain.

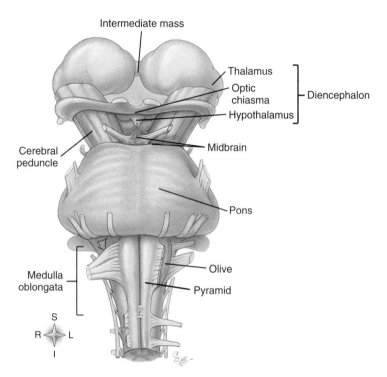

Figure 35-7 Brainstem and diencephalon. *(From Thibodeau G, Patton K: Anatomy and physiology, ed 6, St Louis, 2007, Mosby.)*

VENTRICULAR SYSTEM

The ventricles are four cavities that are found between the various sections within the brain. They are filled with CSF, which bathes and nourishes the brain. Two lateral ventricles occupy the two halves of the cerebrum. These are connected by the interventricular foramen, which leads to the third ventricle. This ventricle opens into a narrow path, called the *cerebral aqueduct,* which leads directly into the fourth ventricle, lying near the base of the brain. The CSF leaves the fourth ventricle through three openings and then circulates around the brainstem and cord. The ventricles are illustrated in Figure 35-8.

BLOOD SUPPLY TO THE BRAIN

The brain requires 20% more oxygen than the other organs in the body to function adequately. It receives arterial blood from two systems, the internal carotid arteries and the vertebral arteries. These systems communicate through a structure called the *circle of Willis,* which is located at the base of the brain (Figure 35-9). The circle of Willis gives rise to the other arteries that supply blood to the cerebral hemispheres and ensures continuity of the blood supply to the brain if any of the arteries are compromised. Blood is carried away from the brain by the cerebral veins that drain into the dural sinuses and internal jugular veins.

VERTEBRAL COLUMN

The vertebral column provides structure and protects the spinal cord. The vertebral column is composed of 24 bones, or vertebrae in addition to the sacrum and coccyx, which are separate in childhood but become fused in adulthood. (Figure 35-10):

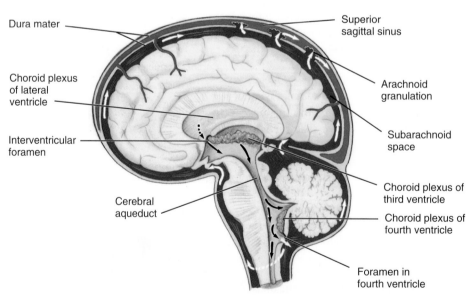

Figure 35-8 Ventricles of the brain. *(From Applegate E: The anatomy and physiology learning system, ed 2, St Louis, 2000, WB Saunders.)*

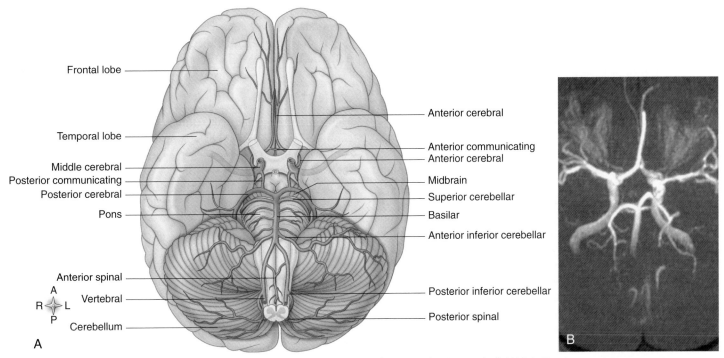

Frontal lobe

Temporal lobe

Middle cerebral
Posterior communicating
Posterior cerebral
Pons

Anterior spinal
Vertebral
Cerebellum

A
R — L
P

Anterior cerebral

Anterior communicating
Anterior cerebral

Midbrain
Superior cerebellar
Basilar
Anterior inferior cerebellar

Posterior inferior cerebellar

Posterior spinal

A

B

Figure 35-9   Arteries of the brain. *(From Drake R, Vogl AW, Mitchell AWM: Gray's anatomy for students, Edinburgh, 2005, Elsevier; and Abrahams P, Hutchings RT, Marks SC: McKinn's color atlas of human anatomy, ed 5, St Louis, 2003, Mosby.)*

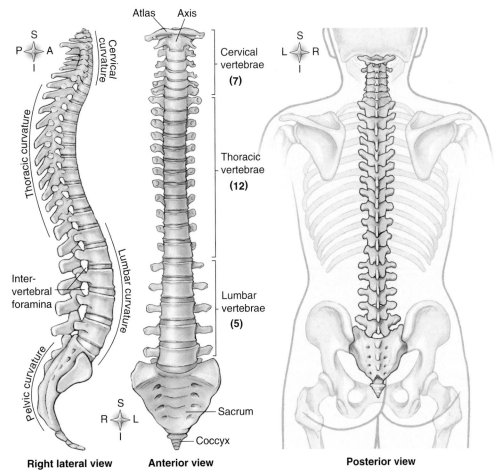

Atlas   Axis

S
P — A
I

Cervical curvature

Thoracic curvature

Inter-vertebral foramina

Lumbar curvature

Pelvic curvature

S
R — L
I

Cervical vertebrae
(7)

Thoracic vertebrae
(12)

Lumbar vertebrae
(5)

Sacrum

Coccyx

S
L — R
I

Right lateral view   **Anterior view**   **Posterior view**

Figure 35-10   Spinal column. *(From Thibodeau G, Patton K: Anatomy and physiology, ed 6, St Louis, Mosby, 2007 and Standring S: Gray's anatomy: 38e, Edinburgh, Churchill Livingstone, 2004.)*

- 7 cervical vertebrae
- 12 thoracic vertebrae
- 5 lumbar vertebrae
- 5 sacral vertebrae (fused as one)
- 1 coccygeal vertebra, which also is a fused structure containing 1 to 3 separate vertebrae

The vertebrae are referred to by a numerical designation preceded by the first letter of the region where they are located (e.g., the first cervical vertebra is C-1; the first thoracic vertebra is T-1).

The atlas, or first cervical vertebra (C-1), supports the skull and is fused with the second vertebra, the axis (C-2), to provide rotational movement of the neck. The remaining vertebrae are similar in structure and appearance. Each vertebra has a body with a circular opening through which the spinal cord passes. Two pedicles extend backward from the body and form the transverse processes. The transverse processes project laterally and support the articulating surfaces, known as the *facets.* Each vertebra has openings (intervertebral foramina) for the passage of spinal nerves. Muscles and ligaments hold the vertebral column together.

The vertebrae are separated by cartilaginous cushions called *intervertebral discs.* The tough outer layer of the disc is the annulus fibrosis, and the jellylike center layer is the nucleus pulposus (Figure 35-11).

SPINAL CORD

The spinal cord is located within the vertebral canal and is continuous with the medulla oblongata of the hindbrain. The cord originates at the foramen magnum, a large opening at the base of the skull, and terminates in the cauda equina at the first and second lumbar vertebrae. The spinal cord has 31 segments—8 cervical, 12 thoracic, 5 lumbar, 5 sacral, and 1 coccygeal.

Structurally, the spinal cord is somewhat flat on the dorsoventral side. It has an outer layer of white matter and an inner body of gray matter. A cross section of the cord reveals that the gray matter forms a rough H shape. The two dorsal portions of the H are called the *dorsal horns,* and the two ventral portions are called the *ventral horns.* The cross portion of the H is called the *gray commissure,* and this portion encom-

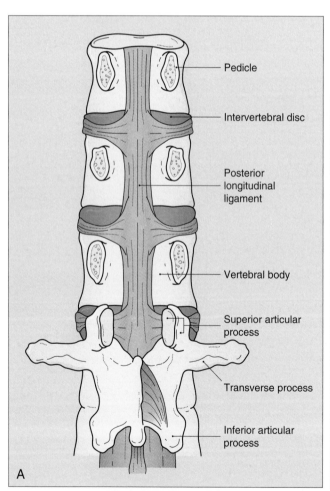

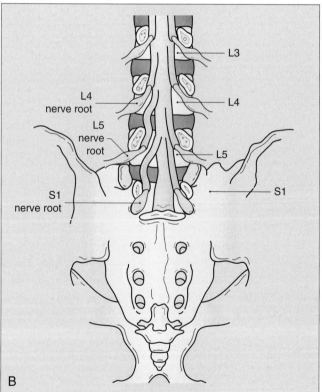

Figure 35-11   A, Posterior view of the lumbar spine, showing the intervertebral discs and bony processes. Note that the upper processes have been cut away to show the deeper structures. **B,** Lumbar spine, illustrating the nerve roots. *(From Rengachary S, Ellenbogen R: Principles of neurosurgery, ed 2, St Louis, 2005, Mosby.)*

Table 35-1

Common Conditions of the Neurological System—cont'd

TRAUMATIC CRANIAL CONDITIONS

Condition	Description	Considerations
Closed head injury	Any injury to the brain that leaves the skull intact. The brain may be injured directly by a direct blow, resulting in bleeding, concussion (i.e., transient loss of brain function), or contusion (i.e., bruising), or it may be damaged indirectly by lack of oxygen, swelling, or interruption of blood flow. A direct blow results in damage to the underlying tissue. A blow to a moving head results in a *countercoup injury*. In this type of injury, the damage occurs to the side opposite the impact and is caused by the brain moving in the skull in response to the force of the injury.	Surgical treatment may be indicated to manage any fractures or bleeding. (See *Burr Holes.*)

CONGENITAL SPINAL DISEASE

Condition	Description	Considerations
Spina bifida	Incomplete closure of the spine. *Spina bifida occulta* is the mildest form of the defect and often does not cause any disability or change in functional status; the defect is confined to the bone of the vertebra and does not extend externally. *Spina bifida cystica (myelomeningocele)* is characterized by protrusion of the spinal cord and meninges through the vertebral column and the skin. This defect is associated with varying degrees of disability. *Meningocele* is the least common form of spina bifida. In this form, the meninges protrude through the skin, but the spinal cord and nerves are not involved.	Surgical intervention is aimed at preserving nerve function while closing the defect in patients with myelomeningocele or meningocele. Surgery generally is performed in the first 24 to 48 hours of life to reduce the risk of a central nervous system (CNS) infection. Hydrocephalus is a frequent complication of spina bifida. (Spina bifida is discussed in Chapter 34 and see also *Ventriculoperitoneal/Ventricular Shunt)* in this chapter.
Sacrococcygeal teratoma	The most common sacral tumor in newborns. The tumor sac is visible in the sacral area and may contain skin, teeth, hair, and tissue from the gastrointestinal tract.	Surgical correction is necessary and in some cases may be performed in utero.
Scoliosis	Abnormal curvature of the spine, resulting in an **S**- or a **C**-shaped curve in the vertebral column. The typical age of onset is 10 to 15 years old. The disease tends to be more severe in females.	Some cases may respond to bracing. Surgery is required for more severe cases to prevent complications. (See Correction of Scoliosis.)

FUNCTIONAL SPINAL CONDITIONS

Condition	Description	Considerations
Degenerative spine conditions	A variety of degenerative conditions may adversely affect the vertebral column. Any of these can cause pressure on the spinal cord, pain, and disabling symptoms. *Osteoarthritis* occurs from wear and tear on the spine and is characterized by the loss of cartilage and bony changes in the joints. *Spondylolisthesis* is the slippage of one vertebra over the top of another. *Spondylosis* causes narrowing of the spinal canal through overgrowth of bone. In *spinal stenosis,* the joint spaces in the spine and foramina are severely narrowed, causing compression injury to the spinal cord and nerve roots.	Surgery may be indicated to relieve pressure on the spinal cord and adjacent structures. (See Lumbar Laminectomy and Discectomy; Lumbar Fusion; and Anterior Cervical Discectomy and Fusion.)
Intervertebral disc disease	Problems with the intervertebral discs are a common neurological condition. The terms *herniated disc* and *ruptured disc* often are used interchangeably and refer to the extension of the nucleus pulposus beyond its capsule to the margin of the annulus. Mechanical forces (e.g., twisting, trauma, excess weight) often are responsible for changes in the discs.	Treatment may include conservative measures or surgery. (See Lumbar Laminectomy and Discectomy; Microdiscectomy; and Anterior Cervical Discectomy and Fusion.)

Continued

<u>Table 35-1</u>

Common Conditions of the Neurological System—cont'd

FUNCTIONAL SPINAL CONDITIONS

Condition	Description	Considerations
Pain disorders	Chronic pain may be the result of metastatic lesions, intervertebral disc disorders, postlaminectomy syndrome (e.g., failed back syndrome), or peripheral nerve disorders.	A multidisciplinary approach is used for patients with pain disorders. Treatment involves medication, behavioral therapy and, in some cases, surgery to disrupt nerve pathways or implant medication pumps or pain stimulators. (See Cordotomy; Rhizotomy; and Dorsal Column Stimulator.)

NEOPLASTIC SPINAL CONDITIONS

Condition	Description	Considerations
Spinal cord tumors	Spinal cord tumors are most commonly the result of metastasis from cancer elsewhere in the body, but they may be benign (e.g., meningiomas, schwannomas, lipomas). Symptoms vary according to the location and size of the tumor. Tumors are classified as *extradural* (i.e., outside the dura mater) or *intradural* (i.e., inside the dura mater)	See Spinal Tumors.

INFECTIOUS SPINAL CONDITIONS

Condition	Description	Considerations
Epidural abscess	A collection of pus between the dura mater and spinal cord. The lumbar spine is affected more often than the cervical or thoracic spine. An abscess threatens the spinal cord by compression and vascular compromise.	Emergency decompression of the spinal cord and drainage of the abscess is indicated. (See Lumbar Laminectomy and Discectomy.)

SPINAL TRAUMA

Condition	Description	Considerations
Vertebral fractures	Vertebral fractures may be the result of trauma, degenerative diseases (e.g., osteoporosis, osteoarthritis [via compression]), metastatic disease, or certain infections.	Minor fractures that do not cause instability of the vertebral column are managed with rest, physical therapy, bracing, and pain medication. Fractures that cause instability may be managed surgically. The goals of surgery are to decompress the spinal cord canal and stabilize the vertebral column. Cervical spine fractures may require halo bracing in conjunction with surgery. (See Lumbar Laminectomy and Discectomy; Lumbar Fusion; Posterior Cervical Laminectomy; and Application of a Halo Brace.)
Cord injury	The spinal cord is very vulnerable to injury. Trauma (with or without a fracture) is a frequent cause of spinal cord injury, but other conditions (e.g., tumors, degenerative diseases, vascular ischemia) may also injure the cord. A cord injury is referred to as *complete* when no level of functioning exists below the site of injury. A person with an *incomplete* injury retains some degree of functioning below the site of injury. Cord injuries at the C-1 or C-2 level can result in loss of the ability to breathe. Lower injuries in the cervical level may result in loss of function in the upper extremities or trunk, as well as in the lower extremities (e.g., quadriplegia). Injuries to the thoracic area and below may result in some degree of paraplegia.	Steroid medications are given before surgery to reduce inflammation. Stabilization of the vertebral column at the level of injury often is necessary to prevent further damage. Cervical spine injuries may require halo bracing in conjunction with surgery. (See Lumbar Laminectomy and Discectomy; Lumbar Fusion; Posterior Cervical Laminectomy; and Application of a Halo Brace.)

Table 35-2

Cranial Nerve Evaluation

Cranial Nerve	Method of Testing
I (Olfactory)	Patient is asked to identify a smell.
II (Optic)	Patient is asked to describe an object. Neurosurgeon evaluates visual field by asking when the patient first sees an object (e.g., the surgeon's finger) moving into the line of vision.
III (Oculomotor)	Surgeon examines the patient's pupils for size, shape, equality, and reaction to light.
IV (Trochlear)	Tested in conjunction with CN III.
V (Trigeminal)	Patient is asked to identify sensations of hot and cold, pinpricks. Also asked to clench teeth and move jaw from side to side.
VI (Abducens)	Surgeon has patient follow an object visually from side to side and up and down.
VII (Facial)	Patient is asked to close eyes, smile, and frown.
VIII (Vestibulocochlear)	Patient's response to verbal questions indicates that the nerve is grossly intact. Surgeon may also use a tuning fork to check bone and air conduction.
IX (Glossopharyngeal)	Surgeon tests the patient's gag reflex with a tongue blade and asks the patient to swallow.
X (Vagus)	Tested in conjunction with CN IX.
XI (Spinal accessory)	Patient is asked to rotate the head and shrug the shoulders against resistance.
XII (Hypoglossal)	Patient is asked to stick out the tongue.

Digital Subtraction Angiography

Digital subtraction angiography (DSA) is an imaging technique used with standard angiography to selectively isolate vascular structures. Images are obtained before and after injection of the contrast medium. The precontrast image is "subtracted" from the data, revealing the vascular structure only. This technology is used less routinely since the advent of three-dimensional CT angiography.

Three-Dimensional CT Angiography

In three-dimensional CT angiography, a contrast medium is used to provide images of the intracranial vasculature, which later are reconstructed in a three-dimensional view by the CT program software. This technology is less invasive than DSA.

Myelography

Although myelography largely has been replaced by MRI, some surgeons use x-rays to visualize the spinal cord. For these imaging studies, a contrast medium is injected into the subarachnoid space of the cervical or lumbar spine. Plain x-rays are then taken to record the images produced by the contrast medium.

Discography

Discography is an imaging technique used to evaluate pathology of an intervertebral disc (e.g., herniation). In this procedure, a small amount of contrast dye is injected directly into the disc, and the patient's response is monitored in terms of the intensity and location of the pain resulting from the injection. Fluoroscopy is used for real-time assessment of the disc during the test. A CT scan may be performed afterward for a more detailed anatomical view of the disc.

Ultrasound

Ultrasound technology often is used before neurosurgery to assess the blood flow in the cerebral blood vessels. It is used intraoperatively for real-time imaging of cysts, tumors, and other structures in the brain or spinal cord.

Electroencephalogram

An electroencephalogram (EEG) measures the electrical activity of the brain. It typically is obtained to evaluate seizure disorders, head injuries, dementia, and metabolic conditions affecting the brain. In the perioperative setting, it can be used during a procedure to monitor the depth of anesthesia or to monitor brain activity in procedures that require occlusion of the carotid artery.

Electromyography

Electromyography (EMG) measures the conduction rate of motor nerves. During this test, needle electrodes are placed in the muscle, and a low-voltage current is delivered. The period between stimulus and muscle contraction is measured. This test often is used to evaluate loss of nerve conduction caused by a herniated disc, spondylosis, or other types of impingement disorders.

Somatosensory Evoked Potentials

The somatosensory evoked potentials (SSEP) test measures sensory impulses from the body to the brain. This test may be performed preoperatively to assess nerve damage, or it may be performed intraoperatively to monitor changes in the nerves in spinal, carotid artery, or cerebral aneurysm surgery. Electrodes or fine needles are used to stimulate selected nerves, and function is determined by the elapsed time between stimulus and response.

PERIOPERATIVE CONSIDERATIONS

PSYCHOLOGICAL CONSIDERATIONS

All patients undergoing surgery arrive in the OR with concerns about their safety and the surgical outcome. Because of the delicate nature of neurosurgery and the risk of impaired function after the surgery, neurosurgical patients often are very fearful or anxious. Patients facing cranial surgery may fear they will not awaken after the surgery or that they will lose their sight, hearing, or mobility. The fear of losing cognitive ability is very strong in many patients.

Patients who appear to be unaware or even unconscious often are highly aware of their surroundings. Although voluntary movement may be impaired, their sensory perception may be fully intact. The perioperative team can provide important emotional and psychological support to the patient.

ROOM SETUP AND EQUIPMENT

Because of the highly technical nature of neurosurgery procedures, a great deal of specialized equipment and accessories may be required. The surgical technologist shares responsibility for ensuring that all needed equipment and supplies are available and ready to be used.

Standard Equipment

Standard furniture and equipment for the neurosurgery OR include the following:

- OR bed with specialized headrests
- Monopolar electrosurgical unit (ESU), bipolar ESU, or combined unit
- Nitrogen (inline or tank)
- Two suction units
- Surgeons' sitting stools
- Imaging equipment
- Operating microscope

A special overhead table (Mayfield table) often is used in place of the Mayo stand during neurosurgical procedures (Figure 35-13). The Mayfield table can be positioned over the patient during cranial surgery so that instruments and equipment can be passed to the surgeons, who stand at the patient's head. During spinal surgery, the table can be placed over the patient's lower body. The table is large enough to accommodate the many supplies and solutions needed during a neurosurgical procedure. In many cases, the Mayfield table is draped

continuously with the patient to produce one large sterile field. The technologist usually stands on a lift (platform) to reach both the table and the surgical site.

INSTRUMENTS

Hand Instruments

General surgery instruments are used for soft tissue access to neurological structures. Once exposure is accomplished, specialty instruments are used to provide retraction and exposure, remove bone, extract disc fragments, and manipulate the delicate tissue of the brain and spinal cord.

Basic neurosurgical instruments are listed in Box 35-1. Instrumentation specific to the neurosurgical procedure is discussed in the surgical techniques section. Commonly used instruments are illustrated in Figures 35-14 through 35-17.

Microsurgical instruments are used in both cranial and spinal surgery. These instruments are very delicate and must be handled with care. When the surgeon is using an instrument under the microscope, the surgical technologist must be very mindful of the procedure and the fact that the surgeon is working within a very limited visual field. The scrub must anticipate which instrument will be needed next and pass it correctly so that the surgeon does not have to look away from the field to receive it. (Chapter 16 contains illustrations demonstrating this technique.)

Decontamination and sterilization processing for neurosurgical instruments generally is identical to processing for other hand instruments. However, special processing is indicated for instruments used in known or suspected cases of Creutzfeldt-Jakob disease (CJD). CJD is a fatal disease of the nervous system that is caused by a prion, which cannot be destroyed by normal disinfection and sterilization methods. Although guidelines for decontamination vary by institution,

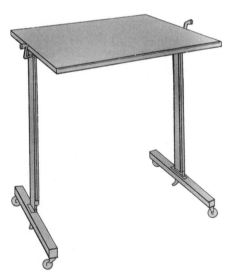

Figure 35-13 *Mayfield instrument table. (From Rothrock J: Alexander's care of the patient in surgery, ed 12, St Louis, 2003, Mosby.)*

<u>Box 35-1</u>

Neurosurgical Instruments

- Assorted bone rongeurs
- Assorted pituitary rongeurs
- Penfield dissectors
- Self-retaining retractors (e.g., Weitlaner, Adson-Beckman, Gelpi)
- Cranial self-retaining retractor systems (e.g., Greenburg, Budde, Leyla-Yasargil)
- Handheld retractors (e.g., Army-Navy, Richardson, Meyerding, Cushing, malleable, Senn retractors; skin hooks)
- Toothed and untoothed forceps (e.g., bayonet, Cushing, Adson, Gerald)
- Periosteal elevators
- Osteotomes and gouges
- Dural hooks, nerve hooks
- Scalp clip appliers or clip applier gun
- Bone curettes
- Bipolar forceps
- Frazier suction tips (assorted sizes)
- Microsurgical instruments as requested

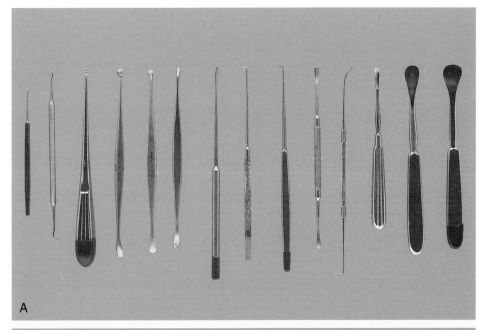

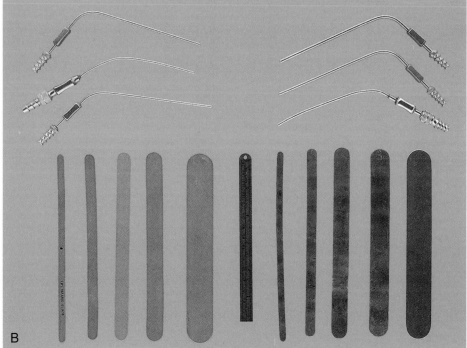

Figure 35-14 Neurosurgical instruments. **A,** *Left to right,* 1 dura hook; 1 Woodson dura separator; 1 Brun curette; 4 Penfield dissectors; 1 Adson dura hook, 1 nerve hook; 1 Freer elevator; 1 Kistner probe; 1 Joker elevator; 2 Hoen periosteal elevators. **B,** *Top,* Frazer suction tips. *Bottom,* Silicone retractors, metal spatulas.

recommendations include the use of disposable instruments, which are isolated and incinerated upon disposal. (A discussion of prion disease can be found in Chapter 7.) Further information on isolation and sterilization measures is available on the Web sites for the Centers for Disease Control and Prevention (CDC, at http://www.cdc.gov) and the Association of periOperative Registered Nurses (AORN, at http://www.aorn.org).

Power Instruments

Power instruments are used to remove and shape bone. Power drills and saws are used for cutting and remolding bone. Neurosurgical power equipment can be pneumatic (air powered) or battery or electrically powered. The surgical technologist is responsible for the safe handling of power instruments on the surgical field. Switches must always be in the safety position, except during use, to prevent injury

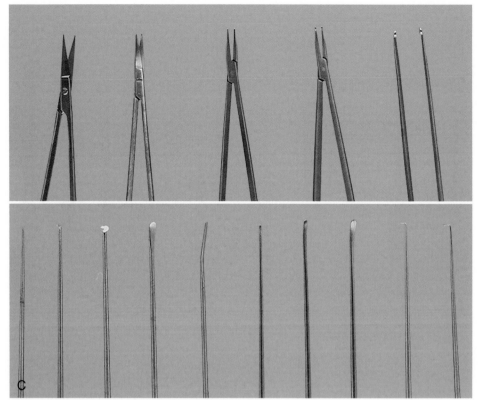

Figure 35-14, cont'd   C, Microsurgical instruments. *(From Tighe SM: Instrumentation for the operating room, ed 6, St Louis, 2003, Mosby.)*

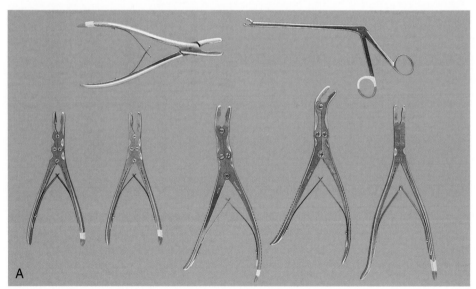

Figure 35-15 Bone and laminectomy instruments. **A,** *Top left,* Adson rongeur; cup forceps. *Left to right,* 2 Ruskin; 2 Leksell; 1 Smith-Peterson cup forceps.

in the event of inadvertent activation. The surgical technologist also is responsible for irrigating the tip of the drill when it is in use to prevent overheating of tissue. Commonly used power systems are the Midas Rex system, the Hall perforator, and the Codman craniotome (a craniotomy saw) (Figure 35-18). A complete discussion on the care and use of power drills, including craniotomies, is covered in Chapter 30.

During a craniotomy, a perforator bit is used to drill holes in the cranial bones. The perforator is used with a power drill, called a craniotome, which is equipped with a safety clutch that stops the drill bit before it touches the dura.

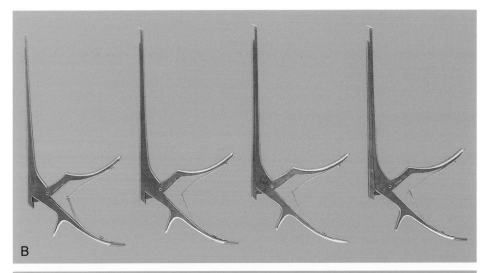

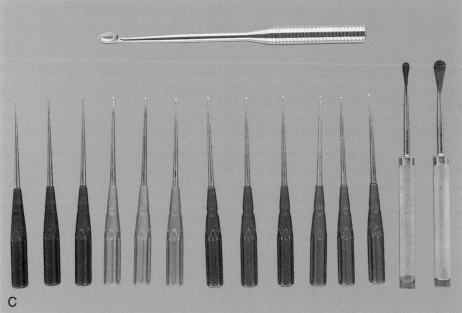

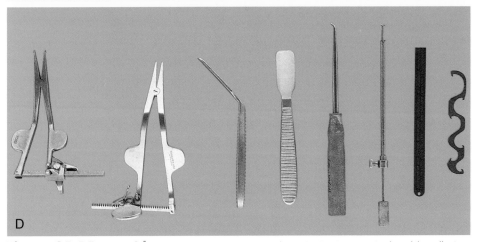

Figure 35-15, cont'd   B, Kerrison rongeurs (upbiting). **C,** Curettes (colored handles) and Cobb elevators. **D,** *Left to right,* 2 Cloward vertebra spreaders; 2 Cloward blade retractors; 1 osteophyte elevator; 1 depth gauge; 1 ruler; 1 spanner wrench. *(From Tighe SM:* Instrumentation for the operating room, *ed 6, St Louis, 2003, Mosby.)*

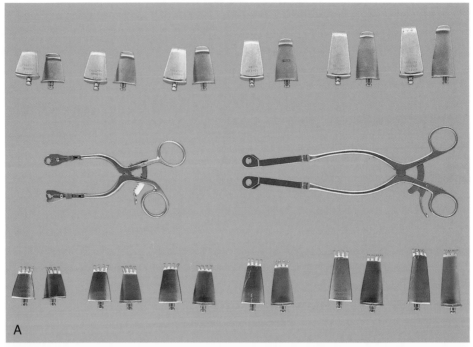

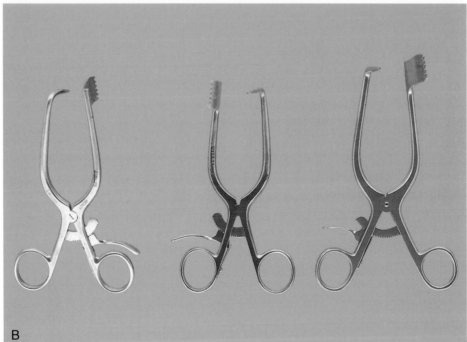

Figure 35-16 Laminectomy retractors. **A,** Cloward retractor with blunt and sharp blades. **B,** Williams retractors.

IMPLANTS

A variety of materials are implanted in the course of many neurosurgical procedures. Implants include tissue, bone, plates, screws, rods, clips, shunts, coils, chemotherapeutic wafers, and generators. Specific devices are discussed as applicable in the Surgical Procedures section. In general, surgical technologists must take care in handling any implantable device to ensure its sterility and integrity. The scrub must also be mindful about reporting regulations for implantable

devices and retain any serial numbers, labels, or other information contained in the sterile packaging for the circulating nurse to process and record. When multiple devices are implanted, the scrub must ensure their correct locations are noted by the circulating nurse.

The U.S. Food and Drug Administration (FDA) regulates the tracking of certain implantable devices and requires that manufacturers have processes in place to locate devices in the event of a recall. The FDA regulations govern devices for which failure would result in serious, adverse health conse-

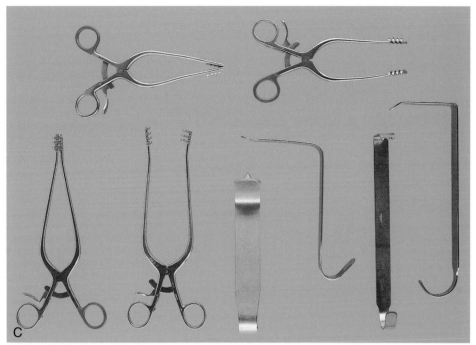

Figure 35-16, cont'd C, *Top,* Adson retractors. *Bottom, left to right,* 2 Weitlaner retractors; 2 Taylor retractors; 2 Hibbs retractors. *(From Tighe SM: Instrumentation for the operating room, ed 6, St Louis, 2003, Mosby.)*

quences; those that are intended to be left in the human body for at least 1 year; and any implantable device that is life sustaining or life supporting and is used outside of a health care facility. Facilities may develop policies and procedures for tracking any implantable device, but at minimum they must track the devices identified by the FDA. Typical information used in tracking includes the following:

- Device identification (e.g., lot number, serial number, model or batch number)
- Date of manufacture and shipping
- Name, address, telephone number, and social security number of the patient in whom the device was implanted
- Location where the device was implanted
- Name, address, and telephone number of the physician who implanted the device

On occasion, a previously implanted device is removed during a procedure. This process is known as *explantation.* Surgical technologists should be familiar with their facility's policies regarding explanted devices; most explanted devices are sent for pathological examination before their final disposition.

WOUND MANAGEMENT

Sponges

Radiopaque 4 × 4 sponges are used in neurosurgical procedures to absorb blood and fluid and control bleeding. In addition to these, the neurosurgeon uses small, square, felted sponges made of cotton or rayon to control bleeding on neural and vascular tissue. These are commonly referred to as

"patties" or "cottonoids" (see Chapter 17). Radiopaque threads are sewn into the body of each sponge, which also has a strong string, colored green, for visibility in the wound. Patties are supplied in a variety of sizes. The felted consistency allows the surgeon to use the sponge as a filter when suction is applied to the neural tissue. The suction tip is kept in contact with the patty so that the tissue underneath is not damaged.

Small cotton balls with radiopaque markers and strings also are used in neurosurgery. Cottonoids and cotton balls are always offered moist. The surgeon may place a cottonoid or cotton ball on top of the tissue and suction through it to avoid damaging the tissue. All sponges are counted on all neurosurgical procedures.

Drugs and Irrigation

Drugs used intraoperatively during neurosurgery include:

- Hemostatic agents
- Irrigation fluid
- Antibiotics in solution with injectable saline

The temperature of the irrigation solution is very important. To prevent tissue damage, the temperature should be below 120° F (48.9°C). Fluid that is too cold may contribute to hypothermia. A piston syringe is used to irrigate the tissue. A catheter or needle-tip irrigator similar to that used in eye surgery may also be used during microsurgery or nerve repair.

Among the more important drugs administered during cranial procedures is the osmotic diuretic, which removes fluid from tissue and prevents swelling as a result of surgical trauma. Drugs commonly used in neurosurgery are listed in Table 35-3.

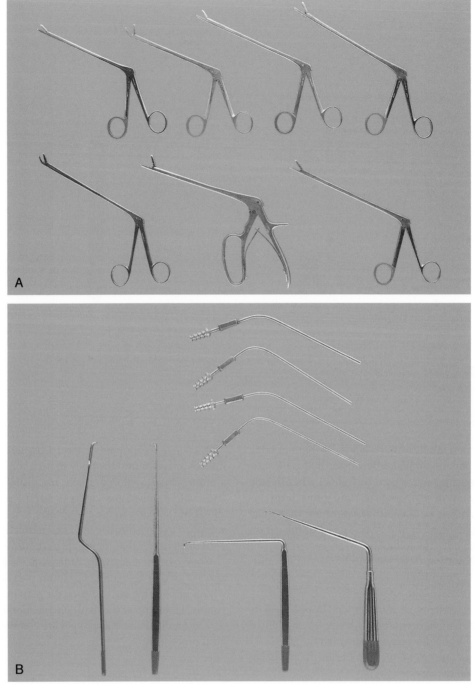

Figure 35-17 Discectomy instruments. **A,** Cushing pituitary rongeurs, straight and angled. **B,** Frazier suction tips *(top)* and nerve root retractors. *(From Tighe SM: Instrumentation for the operating room, ed 6, St Louis, 2003, Mosby.)*

Drains

A variety of drains are used in neurosurgery to evacuate blood, serum, and fluid and to eliminate dead space in the surgical wound. A lumbar drain may be placed in the subarachnoid space before a surgical procedure to remove CSF from the spinal canal or brain; this decompresses the tissue. A lumbar drain also can be used to monitor **intracranial pressure (ICP).** As an alternative, a ventricular drain may be placed for the same purpose. The surgical technologist must make sure

strict sterility is maintained during the placement of this type of drain, because the drain acts as a direct conduit to the CNS, providing a portal of entry for infection. A separate surgical field should be set up for placement of the lumbar or ventricular drain.

Suture

Silk and nylon sutures are commonly used on neural tissue for dural retraction, closure, and repair. Peripheral nerve

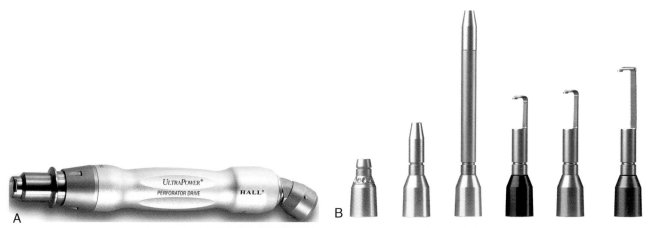

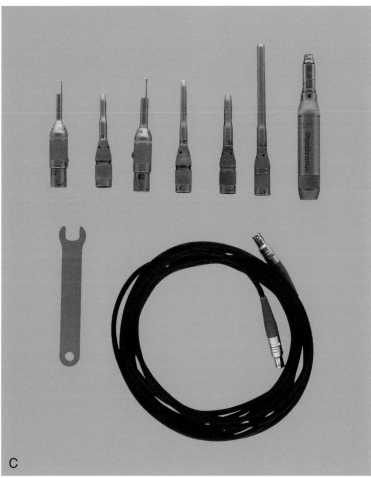

Figure 35-18 Neurosurgical power instruments. **A,** Hall perforator drill. **B,** Burr guards. L-shaped guards prevent the drill tip from penetrating the cranial meninges. **C,** Midas Rex drill and guards (Medtronic, Minneapolis, MN). *(From Tighe SM: Instrumentation for the operating room, ed 6, St Louis, 2003, Mosby.)*

anastomosis usually is performed with fine nylon or Prolene suture. Wire is used to suture the cranial bones in place following craniotomy. Staples generally are used for skin closure in the scalp and back.

Cements and Adhesives

Bone cements and adhesives are used in neurosurgical procedures. Methylmethacrylate (see Chapter 30) is used in cranioplasty procedures and to construct antibiotic beads, which are used in cases of vertebral column infection. (The Cranioplasty section, later in the chapter, presents more information on techniques used to prepare methylmethacrylate in cranial surgery.) Octylcyanoacrylate, an adhesive, may be used to close the skin edges of incisions that are not under pressure.

Dressings

Wound dressings are applied at the end of a neurosurgical procedure to protect the incision and provide an environment

Table 35-3

Medications Used in Neurosurgery

Agent	Form	Mechanism of Action	Special Considerations
Lidocaine with epinephrine	Injectable	Inhibits the conduction of nerve impulses and constricts blood vessels.	Must be clearly labeled when used on the sterile field to avoid confusion with other medications. Surgical technician must track the amount administered by the surgeon.
Mannitol	Injectable	Acts on the kidneys to move fluid from the tissues.	Given by the anesthesia care provider to prevent increased intracranial pressure and reduce cerebral or spinal cord edema.
Papaverine	Injectable/Topical	Relaxes the blood vessel wall.	May be applied topically to the vessels feeding a cerebral aneurysm to prevent spasm.
Topical thrombin	Powder for reconstitution; packaged with diluent and spray pump, or diluent and spray tip syringe with diluent only	Catalyzes the conversion of fibrinogen to fibrin.	For external use only; must be refrigerated.
Gelatin matrix (FloSeal)	Gelatin matrix granules and topical thrombin packaged as a kit with syringes and mixing bowl	Matrix particles form a composite clot that seals the bleeding site; thrombin component converts the fibrinogen in the patient's blood to fibrin.	Product reaches maximum expansion at approximately 10 minutes. Excess product should be removed with gentle irrigation.
Absorbable gelatin sponge (Gelfoam)	Film, powder, and topical forms	Absorbs and holds blood and fluid within its interstices; exerts physical hemostatic effect.	Should not be used in the closure of skin incisions, because it may interfere with healing of skin edges. Often moistened with saline or topical thrombin before use.
Collagen hemostat (Avitene, Helistat, Instat)	Pads, powder, sheets, sponges	When in contact with a bleeding surface, attracts platelets, which aggregate into thrombi, initiating the formation of a physiological platelet plug.	Applied dry; excess material should be removed from the wound before closure.
Oxidized regenerated cellulose (Surgicel)	Fibrous, knitted, or sheer weave fabric	Allows platelets and aggregates of thrombin and particulate blood elements to cling and form a coagulum that can act as a patch.	Store at room temperature.

Modified from Ferrera D: Neurosurgery. In Rothrock JC, editor: *Alexander's care of the patient in surgery*, ed 14, St Louis, 2007, Mosby.

for wound healing. Radiopaque sponges should never be used as dressing materials. Spinal incisions are dressed with non-adherent Telfa and absorbent gauze pads secured with tape. Cranial dressings tend to be more complex and more difficult to secure. A single, nonadherent strip (Telfa or mesh) is placed over the incision. Square gauze and bulky fluff gauze are added, followed by soft, rolled gauze, which is wrapped around the head to secure the dressings. If an external brace is required, it is applied over the dressing.

ANESTHESIA

Neurosurgery of the cranium and back usually is performed using general (inhalation) anesthesia. Selected procedures, such as the placement of brain electrodes, can be performed with the patient awake or under light sedation. Depending on the patient's condition, an "awake" intubation may be required for safety in some procedures of the cervical spine.

Regional anesthesia can be used in peripheral nerve repair. The Bier block (see Chapter 12) is commonly used for nerve repair or transposition in the arm. The scalp incision site routinely is injected with a vasoconstrictive drug in a local anesthetic carrier (lidocaine) to maintain local vasoconstriction and a dryer surgical field.

Extensive physiological monitoring is carried out during cranial procedures.

Thermoregulation is an important consideration for neurosurgical patients undergoing general anesthesia because most procedures are lengthy. Hypothermia can interfere with clotting, alter the metabolism of drugs, and impair wound healing. The anesthesia care provider implements a variety of measures to minimize the patient's risk of developing intraoperative hyperthermia, such as warming the anesthetic gases and fluids and using warm blankets and forced air warming blankets. Infants undergoing neurosurgical procedures are very vulnerable to the effects of hypothermia. An infrared light system often is used to keep the infant warm and reduce the risk of hypothermia.

In addition to standard anesthetic goals, specific areas of monitoring and care are required during neurosurgery. The patient's blood pressure is maintained within a normal or below normal range to prevent bleeding and increases in ICP. Smooth emergence from anesthesia is extremely important to minimize the risk of laryngospasm and struggling. Often the surgical dressing is applied before the reversal agents are given to avoid overstimulating the patient, which might increase the blood pressure.

PATIENT POSITIONING

The long duration of neurosurgical procedures increases the risk of injury related to positioning. The surgeons and anesthesia care provider check any possible pressure points and make sure the areas are adequately padded. Because cranial procedures often use the prone position, respiratory clearance for expansion of the thorax is very important. (These points and others are covered in Chapter 10.)

Specialized Positioning Aids
Headrests

During cranial surgery, a variety of specialized positioning devices are used, including headrests and fixation devices that attach to the operating bed. Many different types of headrests are available, some designed with disposable or reusable detachable pins that are inserted into the patient's skull. The patient first is positioned with the headrest in place, and the pins then are reattached to the headrest to immobilize the head completely.

Two types of headrests commonly used are the Mayfield headrest, and the three-pin fixation headrest (Figure 35-19). Skull tongs (e.g., Gardner-Wells tongs) may also be used to secure the patient's head in a particular position and as a means for attaching traction devices. The surgical technologist establishes a small sterile field on a prep table for the neurosurgeon to use when inserting the fixation pins or tongs (Figure 35-20). The scrub may also assist the surgeon with insertion or removal of the device.

❖ *When assisting the surgeon during patient positioning, the surgical technologist must take care to prevent injury to the spine, shoulders, and head. Make sure the head is cradled securely and in anatomical position at all times to prevent hyperextension of the neck or sudden movement.*

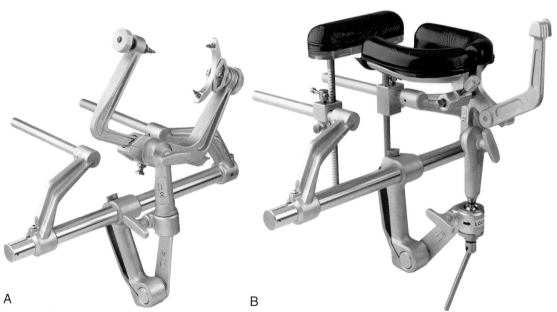

A   B

Figure 35-19 Cranial headrests. **A,** Three-pin suspension skull clamps. **B,** Mayfield headrest. *(From Rothrock J: Alexander's care of the patient in surgery, ed 12, St Louis, 2003, Mosby.)*

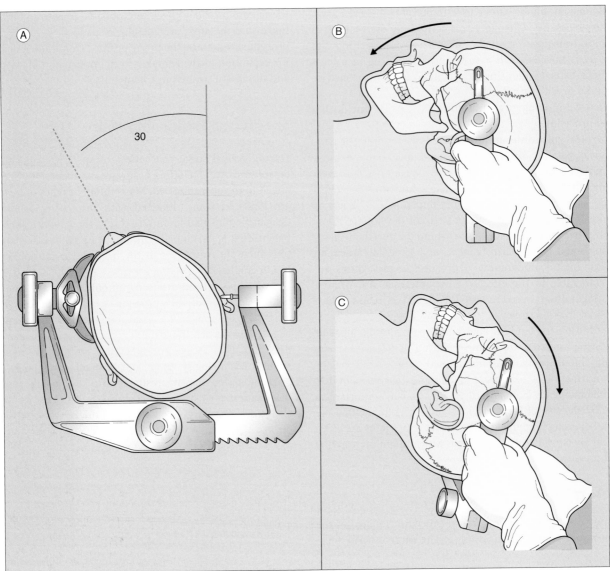

Figure 35-20   Three-pin suspension clamps allow rotation and flexion for secure positioning. *(From Rengachary S, Ellenbogen R: Principles of neurosurgery, ed 2, St Louis, 2005, Mosby.)*

Operating Table

A specialty operating table is used in neurosurgery, especially for spinal and cranial procedures. These beds come with many accessories to optimize safe positioning. The Andrews bed and the Jackson spinal table are two examples of specialized OR beds. These specialized tables allow a wide variety of customized positions with clearance for C-arm fluoroscopy. An alternate to a dedicated spinal table is a laminectomy frame (e.g., the Wilson frame), which is positioned on the operating table and adjusted to elevate the thorax. (Chapter 10 presents a complete discussion of positioning.)

Cranial Surgery

Accurate positioning of the patient's head is crucial in cranial surgery. The location of the lesion determines the exact position and whether fixation is needed. Venous drainage and maintaining a low ICP are other important considerations when positioning patients for cranial procedures.

Risks Associated with Fowler Position

A significant risk of air embolisms is associated with sitting positions (e.g., Fowler or beach chair position). Air embolism can occur when air enters the vascular system through an open blood vessel, the exposed occipital muscles, or the sinuses of the brain. Air embolism is a surgical emergency for which all team members must be prepared. If an embolism occurs through the wound, the surgeon needs copious irrigation and sponges to cover the open vessels. This prevents any more air from entering the wound while attempts are made to locate the source of air entry. Another action the surgeon may take is to reposition the patient in a left lateral decubitus position. This prevents air that might have entered the heart from forming an air lock. The scrubbed surgical technologist should protect the sterile field and quickly move sterile equipment out of the way so that the patient can be positioned. When the patient is secured, the equipment is again moved into place.

Spinal Surgery

Procedures of the anterior cervical spine are performed with the patient in the supine position, often with the individual's head in a three-pin skull fixation device to maintain stability. Traction also may be used, with a chin harness attached to a weight to open the spaces between the cervical vertebrae. Procedures of the posterior cervical spine are performed with the patient in either the prone or sitting position.

Procedures of the thoracic spine may use the supine, lateral, or prone position or even a combination of positions, which may require an intraoperative position change. The prone or knee-chest position is used for surgery on the lumbar spine. The knee-chest position spreads the lamina, decompresses the epidural veins, minimizes wound depth, and allows the great vessels of the abdomen to drop away from the spine

PREPPING AND DRAPING

Once the patient has been positioned, the skin prep is performed: If the body hair substantially interferes with the incision site, the hair is removed before the skin prep. When necessary, hair removal should be done as close to the time of surgery as possible. A small table should be set up for hair removal with an electrical or battery-powered clippers, razor, prep sponges, and solutions. If the patient is to be prepped for a craniotomy procedure, the hair is first shaved with electrical clippers (this should be done outside the OR suite) and then with a razor. Generally, hair removal is limited to the amount necessary to facilitate the incision and ensure a clean surgical field; rarely is the entire head shaved. The patient's hair must be saved and returned to the patient as personal property. In preparation for procedures of the cervical spine, the surgeon may order the patient's nape to be shaved to the level of the ears. If the patient's hair is long, it should be secured to the top of the head with an elastic band.

Certain neurosurgical procedures, such as those involving harvesting of a bone or fat graft, may require a second surgical prep. A separate prep setup is used for the second prep site. (See Chapter 11 for a complete discussion of the skin prep.)

Because most surgeries involving the brain require complex draping routines, the surgeons may direct and complete the draping themselves. Drapes may be sewn directly to the scalp with silk sutures, adhesive drapes may be used, or surgical skin staples may be used. In any case involving the head, it is wise to have extra drapes available to secure a large sterile field. A specialized craniotomy drape with an attached fluid collection system often is used for cranial surgery.

Draping for spinal procedures is fairly straightforward and uses towels and a fenestrated drape.

TEAM POSITIONING

For cranial procedures, the surgeon and assistant stand at the patient's head and the scrub stands to the surgeon's right or at the overhead table. During spinal procedures, a right-handed surgeon usually stands at the patient's left side and the assistant stands on the patient's right side. The scrub should stand to the patient's left unless otherwise directed. Peripheral nerve procedures on a patient's upper extremities may be performed with the surgical team seated around a hand table. Team positioning during procedures with the patient in the high Fowler position may need to be altered to accommodate standing platforms for scrubbed personnel to ensure safe access to the surgical field. Other considerations for team positioning include the presence of equipment such as the C-arm, surgical microscopes, Cavitron Ultrasonic Surgical Aspirator (CUSA) console, and other items.

CRANIAL PROCEDURES

BURR HOLES

Surgical Goal

In cranial surgery, holes are drilled in the cranium with a neurosurgical drill (craniotome). The procedure is performed most often to relieve pressure on the brain caused by the accumulation of fluid beneath the dura mater. Burr holes are also used when the skull is opened for a craniotomy.

Pathology

Traumatic head injury often causes blood to accumulate under the dura. The resulting hematoma causes pressure on the brain tissue, causing injury and alterations in consciousness or motor function. A skull fracture may or may not have occurred during the injury. Trauma usually is the result of a motor vehicle accident, sports injury, or intentional violence. Suspicion of a hematoma is treated as an emergency. CT scans are obtained quickly, and a craniotomy often is performed as an emergency procedure to evacuate accumulated blood or infectious exudate from a brain abscess.

Technique

1. The patient is placed in the supine position, and the head is stabilized.
2. The incision line is marked and injected with lidocaine with epinephrine. 3. The scalp is incised and the pericranium elevated.
4. A craniotome with a perforating bit is used to drill a hole through the skull.
5. The dura is incised.
6. The clot, tissue debris, and fluid are evacuated.
7. Drains may be placed.
8. The wound is closed in layers.

Discussion

Before the procedure begins, the CT scans showing the location of the hematoma should be placed on the view boxes.

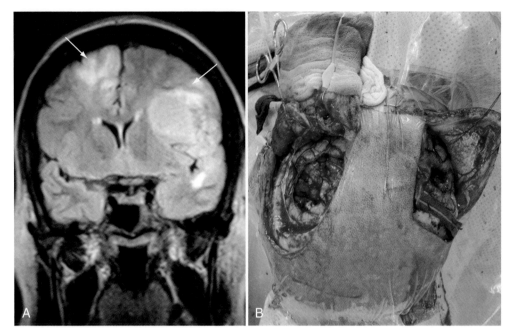

Figure 35-21   A, MRI showing a metastatic brain tumor. **B,** Simultaneous craniotomies for resection of tumors. *(From Townsend CM: Sabiston textbook of surgery, ed 17, Philadelphia, 2001, WB Saunders.)*

The patient is prepped and draped for a routine craniotomy. A surgical marker is used to mark the position of each burr hole. Some surgeons infiltrate the scalp with lidocaine with epinephrine to control bleeding, which usually is brisk. However, if the procedure is an emergency, this step may be omitted.

To begin the procedure, the surgeon makes a linear incision over the site of the purposed burr hole. The scrub should have the ESU and numerous 4 × 4 sponges available.

After the scalp is incised, a periosteal elevator is used to separate the pericranium from the skull.

A craniotome with a perforator bit is used to create the burr holes. The scrub must irrigate the perforator bit during drilling to prevent friction and thermal injury to the underlying tissue. Suction is applied adjacent to the irrigation stream to remove any bone particles from the field. The surgical technologist should have bone wax prepared in case of bleeding from the bone edges. Two or more burr holes may be drilled to evacuate the hematoma or fluid collection. The number of holes placed and their location depend on the size of the hematoma and its orientation. Typically, the first burr hole is placed in the temporal region immediately above the zygomatic arch, and subsequent holes are placed in the parietal or frontal regions.

The surgeon uses a dura hook to elevate the dura and then incises it with a knife with a #15 blade. Metzenbaum scissors are used to create a larger opening.

Irrigation fluid is used to evacuate the clot. The scrub provides copious amounts of warm irrigation fluid. Several bulb syringes can be used simultaneously. Irrigation continues until the clot is evacuated and the irrigation return is clear.

Hemostasis is maintained with the ESU. In some cases, a drain may be inserted into the subdural or epidural space to promote complete evacuation of the hematoma. The dura is closed with braided nylon or silk. The galea is closed with absorbable suture, and the skin is closed with staples or nylon suture.

CRANIOTOMY: TUMOR REMOVAL

Surgical Goal

A craniotomy is an incision into the cranium to permit access to the brain and intracranial structures. Intracranial access is achieved by creating a **bone flap** (a removable section of the cranium). Tumor removal is an indication for a craniotomy.

Pathology

A craniotomy may be required to provide access for treatment of a variety of intracranial conditions, such as a neoplasm, cerebral aneurysm, arteriovenous malformation, or hemorrhage. Implantation of electrodes and stimulators also is performed through a craniotomy.

The presence of any type of tumor presents a risk, because the skull is a fixed space, and any tumor can impinge on surrounding tissue (Figure 35-21). Tumors that require resection are listed in Table 35-4.

Technique

1. The patient is positioned using the horseshoe headrest or pin fixation.
2. The incision line is marked and injected with lidocaine with epinephrine to promote vasoconstriction of the wound edges.
3. The incision is carried through the galea.
4. Scalp clips are applied to the scalp edges with a clip applier or clip gun to provide hemostasis.

Table 35-4

Common Brain Tumors Resected During a Craniotomy

Tumor Type	Special Considerations
Ependymoma: A cancerous tumor composed of the ependymal cells that line the brain ventricles and spinal cord.	Commonly located in the fourth ventricle of the brain. Often slower growing than other brain tumors. More common in children.
Astrocytoma: A cancerous tumor composed of astrocytes, the most prominent glial cell.	A four-tiered grading system, established by the World Health Organization (WHO), is used to rank the severity of the tumor and prognosis. Grade I tumors have a more favorable outcome than grade IV tumors. Glioblastoma multiforme (GBM), a type of grade IV tumor, is extremely aggressive that commonly occurs in the sixth and seventh decades of life.
Oligodendroglioma: A cancerous tumor composed of oligodendrocytes (cells that produce myelin).	Occurs primarily in adults and usually is located in the cerebral hemispheres.
Meningioma: A benign tumor composed of cells from the arachnoid.	More common in females than in males.

5. The scalp flap is retracted, and the pericranium is stripped off the skull with periosteal elevators.
6. Burr holes are placed and widened with rongeurs and curettes.
7. A Penfield or Woodson dissector is used to release the dura from the bone.
8. The burr holes are connected; a craniotome with a dura guard and cutting blade is used to produce the bone flap.
9. The bone flap is elevated from the dura and removed or retracted.
10. Retraction sutures are placed in the dura, which is opened.
11. The resection site is irrigated, and hemostasis is achieved.
12. The dura is closed to form a watertight seal.
13. The bone flap is replaced and secured with wire or mini-plates and miniscrews.
14. The muscle is approximated, and the galea is closed.
15. The skin is closed with staples or suture.

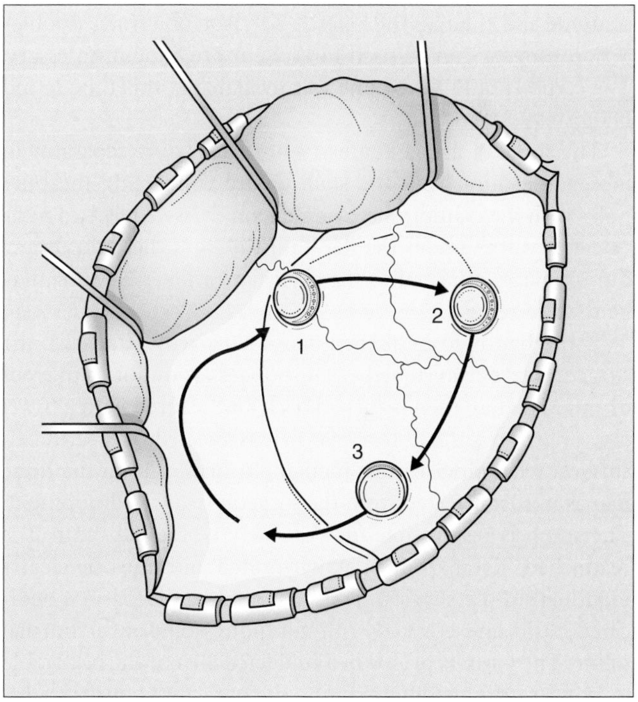

Figure 35-22 Craniotomy. An incision is made to the cranial bone, and scalp clips are applied. Two burr holes are drilled, and the bone is cut between the holes. *(From Rengachary S, Ellenbogen R: Principles of neurosurgery, ed 2, St Louis, 2005, Mosby.)*

Discussion

The craniotomy approach depends on the location of the pathology; it may be made through the anterior, middle, or posterior fossa. In addition, a craniotomy may be classified as frontal, parietal, temporal, or occipital, depending on the planned location of the incision. The patient is placed in the supine, prone, or sitting position. During a craniotomy, a section of the cranium (i.e., a bone flap) is removed. The size of the flap is determined by the size and location of the tumor. A superficial tumor is easier to access and requires a smaller flap than a deep, large tumor. The bone flap is created by drilling multiple burr holes in the skull and then "connecting" them with a protected saw blade (Figure 35-22). This provides a safe method of making an incision into the cranium. The bone flap can be folded back and secured during the procedure or removed completely (a free flap). In either case, the bone is reattached at the close of the procedure.

After infiltrating the incision site with local anesthetic for hemostasis, the surgeon makes a curved incision in the scalp. The surgical assistant applies digital pressure to the wound edges, therefore the scrub should make sure that numerous folded 4 × 4 sponges are available. The monopolar ESU is used for hemostasis.

The surgeon uses scalp clips to secure the edges of the scalp and provide continuous hemostasis during the procedure. Scalp clips are supplied in a disposable, preloaded applier, or the scrub may be required to load them onto a manual applier. If manual loading is performed, two appliers should be used for rapid delivery. One is used while the other is loaded.

Blunt and sharp dissection are used to free the galea from the skull. The scalp flap, with the scalp clips in place, is secured to the drapes with silk suture, towel clips, hemostats, or scalp hooks attached to rubber bands tethered by a hemostat. A self-retaining retractor (e.g., a Weitlaner retractor) may also be used to hold the scalp back. A moistened 4 × 4 sponge may be placed over the flap to prevent the tissue from drying.

A periosteal elevator is used to remove the periosteum from the bone and prepare it for drilling of the burr holes. To create a bone flap, the surgeon "connects" the burr holes by dividing the bone between each hole with a saw. This frees the cranial segment, which is removed to provide access to the brain tissue below. The flap is turned back or removed.

During the procedure to create a bone flap, the scrub should provide a continuous stream of irrigation fluid over the drill tip or saw during drilling. This prevents the bone tissue from heating as a result of friction. After each burr hole is made, the surgeon removes the bone debris and dust with a curette and enlarges the holes. A Kerrison or a small, double-action rongeur can be used to excise more bone if necessary. The scrub should have bone wax available at this time to aid hemostasis.

The surgeon uses a Penfield #3 or Sachs dura separator to loosen the dura from the skull before connecting the burr holes with the craniotome. The surgeon then wedges two periosteal elevators under the flap to lift it from the dura. If any dura remains attached to the skull flap, a joker elevator may be used to release it.

If the flap is to be turned back (left partly attached), the surgeon places moistened 4 × 4 sponges around it to prevent drying. The flap then is turned back and secured with a towel clip or nylon suture. If a free flap is created, the scrubbed surgical technologist must maintain a firm grip on the bone flap as it is transferred from the surgeon to avoid dropping it. The scrub is responsible for the safety of the flap until it is reattached. The flap must stay hydrated and must be clearly identified in the surgical field. It should be placed in a dedicated basin and covered with antibiotic solution or normal saline. The basin is placed in a protected area of the back table to protect it from contamination or contact with instruments and supplies. The flap must be clearly identified to anyone scrubbing in during the case.

After the flap is created, Gelfoam and cottonoid sponges are placed at the periphery of the open dura. A self-retaining retractor system may be placed at this time. In preparation for entry into the brain tissue, the scrub should have a bipolar ESU and a #5 or #6 Frazier suction tip available. The surgeon uses a dura hook to lift the dura away from the brain and incises it with a #15 knife blade mounted on a #7 handle. The incision is extended with Frazier dura scissors or Lahey-Metzenbaum scissors and toothed Adson or Cushing tissue forceps. The technologist should prepare traction sutures of 4-0 silk on a fine controlled-release needle. These are used to secure the dura away from the wound. The brain then is exposed.

A surgical microscope may be used to magnify the tumor bed. The surgeon uses brain spoons, curettes, and delicate rongeurs to remove the tumor. The CUSA also can be used to fragment and debulk neurological tumors.

The scrub should have irrigation fluid available at all times during the procedure. A 30- or 50-mL syringe or bulb syringe is used. A variety of cottonoid sponges and topical hemostatic material also should be available throughout the dissection of the brain tissue. A tissue specimen may be submitted for frozen section during the procedure. All specimens are identified as soon as they are received and passed off the sterile field.

Whenever possible, the entire tumor is removed. If the size or location of the tumor prevents complete removal (e.g., if the tumor is too close to a vital speech or vision center), the surgeon debulks it. In debulking, the surgeon removes as much of the tumor as possible while preserving function in the adjacent areas. Debulking relieves pressure on remaining brain tissue and may make any postoperative radiation or chemotherapy more effective.

After removing the tumor, the surgeon irrigates the wound with antibiotic solution. The dura then may be closed with fine silk sutures or left unsutured.

If the tumor is identified as a high-grade astrocytoma (e.g., glioblastoma multiforme), the surgeon may implant Gliadel wafers in the tumor bed before closing the dura. The Gliadel wafer is impregnated with an antineoplastic agent that delivers chemotherapy directly to the tumor site. The surgical technologist and surgeons must double glove when handling the wafers for protection from the chemicals. The surgeon places up to eight wafers in the tumor bed and secures them in place with ½-inch (1.25 cm) strips of Surgicel before closing the dura. The scrub should ensure that any instruments used in placing the wafers are passed off the sterile field so that they do not come in contact with healthy cranial tissue. Any opened but unused wafers should be disposed of according to the facility's policy and procedure for disposal of chemotherapeutic agents. The team regloves before proceeding with cranial closure.

The surgeon then prepares the bone flap for reattachment to the cranium. When transferring the free flap back to the surgeon at the end of the procedure, the scrub should verify that the surgeon has a firm grip on the flap before releasing it. The surgeon reattaches the flap with wire sutures. A craniotome drill is used to place small holes in the bone flap and the edges of the skull. Short lengths of #28 steel wire are passed through the holes to attach the flap. A wire twister is used to secure the suture ends to the bone.

Alternately, the surgeon may attach the bone flap with cranial plates and screws. The loose pericranium and galea are attached over the burr holes and bone flap with absorbable synthetic or silk sutures. The scalp clips then are removed, and the muscle and subcutaneous layers are approximated with 3-0 absorbable or silk sutures. The skin is closed with 4-0 nylon suture or staples.

Postoperative Considerations

Any surgical manipulation of the brain raises the possibility of postoperative seizures, swelling, and increased ICP. Intraoperative swelling may necessitate leaving the bone flap off and loosely closing only the skin to give the brain space to expand. Should this occur, the bone flap may be packaged sterilely according to the facility's policy and procedure and frozen for later reimplantation (see the Cranioplasty section). Because of the risk of increased ICP and seizure activity, patients undergoing a craniotomy are monitored in the intensive care unit (ICU) postoperatively. Increased ICP usually is manifested by changes in the patient's neurological status, such as a decreased level of consciousness, changes in pupil size and reaction, and changes in the ability to move the extremities on command. The surgeon assesses the patient's pupil size and neurological status after transfer from the operating bed to the transport device. Any change from the patient's baseline may necessitate immediate removal of the bone flap or re-exploration of the wound, therefore the scrub must maintain the integrity of the sterile field and instrumentation until the patient is transferred from the operating suite.

Longer term complications from a craniotomy include infection of the bone flap or brain tissue, persistent seizure activity (e.g., epilepsy), and unresolved neurological deficits.

CRANIECTOMY

Surgical Goal

A craniectomy is the removal of cranial bone to access the structure below it. This procedure differs from a craniotomy, because the bone that is removed is not replaced.

Pathology

A craniectomy may be done to remove bone from any region of the skull for decompression of the brain or evacuation of epidural or subdural hematomas. More commonly, a craniectomy is performed to remove tumors in the posterior fossa. Tumors in this region may occur in the cerebellum, fourth ventricle, or brainstem. A posterior fossa craniectomy is described in this section.

Technique

1. The patient is placed in the sitting position.
2. An occipital burr hole is made for placement of a ventricular catheter.
3. The incision line is marked and injected with lidocaine with epinephrine to promote vasoconstriction of the wound edges.
4. The incision is made.
5. Hemostasis is maintained.
6. A skin flap is created and retracted.
7. One or more burr holes are placed.
8. A Penfield or Woodson dissector is used to release the dura from the bone.
9. Rongeurs are used to enlarge the burr holes and remove an adequate amount of bone for exposure.
10. The dura is opened.
11. The brain is explored for tumor or other pathology and resected if necessary.
12. The dura is closed.
13. The muscle is reapproximated, and the skin is closed.
14. The patient is placed in the supine position. The skull fixation is removed before the individual emerges from anesthesia.

Discussion

The patient is prepped and placed in a sitting or beach chair position with the head stabilized at the forehead with pin fixation or tongs. A tall Mayfield table is used, and standing platforms are required so that the surgical technologist is accessible to the surgeons without compromise to the sterile field. The procedure may also be performed with the patient prone.

To lower the ICP and provide an additional means of decompression, the surgeon may place a ventricular drain through a burr hole before beginning the craniectomy. If this is done before the main procedure, the technologist prepares a separate surgical field and assists as necessary. The burr hole is made as previously described. The burr hole may also be made concurrently with the procedure.

After infiltrating the incision site with a local anesthetic for hemostasis, the surgeon makes a midline or upwardly curved incision between the mastoid tips. The surgical assistant applies digital pressure to the wound edges, therefore folded 4 × 4 sponges should be available. The monopolar and bipolar ESUs are used for hemostasis.

The skin flap is retracted with Weitlaner retractors. A Key periosteal elevator is used to free the muscles, which are then divided with the monopolar ESU.

One or more holes are drilled into the occipital bone, and the holes are widened with a large rongeur or a craniotome burr. The dura mater is stripped from the underside of the bone, and a double-action rongeur (e.g., Kerrison or Leksell rongeur) is used to enlarge the craniectomy to the desired size and to smooth the bone edges. The scrub should anticipate that bone bleeding may occur and be prepared to supply the surgeon with bone wax to help control the bleeding. Moistened cottonoid strips and Gelfoam are also placed to prevent air embolism.

The surgeon tents the dura with a dura hook and opens it with a #15 blade in a #7 knife handle. A cottonoid strip may be placed on the brain tissue to protect the brain as the dural incision is widened with a pair of Metzenbaum scissors.

The extent to which the posterior fossa is explored depends on the nature of the disease. The exploration may include opening of the cisterna magna, draining of the spinal fluid, and inspection of the cerebellar hemispheres.

When the brain has been exposed, brain retractors are placed over cottonoid strips to increase exposure. The surgical technologist must keep the handles of the handheld retractors dry to prevent them from slipping in the surgeon's hand; however, the inserted edge should be kept wet to prevent damage to the brain. During the procedure, cranial nerves may be identified with a nerve stimulator.

After removal of the lesion, the surgeon must check for adequate hemostasis because of the increased venous pressure in the patient's head. The dura mater may be partly or fully closed, and the muscle, fascia, and skin are closed as for a craniotomy. The patient must remain anesthetized until returned to a supine position and the pin fixation or tongs are removed.

Postoperative Considerations

The formation of an intracerebral hematoma is a risk after craniectomy. A hematoma can contribute to increased ICP and damage the cerebral tissue. Longer term complications that may occur include those previously discussed in the craniotomy section and CSF leakage.

CEREBRAL ANEURYSM SURGERY

Surgical Goal
Aneurysm surgery is performed to isolate a cerebral aneurysm from the normal circulation while preserving flow to the nearby vessels.

Pathology
An intracranial aneurysm is the bulging of an artery within the cerebral circulation. Aneurysms can take many forms and shapes. They are caused by a weakening of the arterial wall, which occurs as a congenital defect or as a result of trauma or infection. As blood flows through the vessel, the weakened aneurysm wall becomes thin (Figure 35-23). This creates a high risk of sudden rupture and hemorrhage, which can be quickly fatal. Types of cerebral aneurysms are listed in Table 35-5.

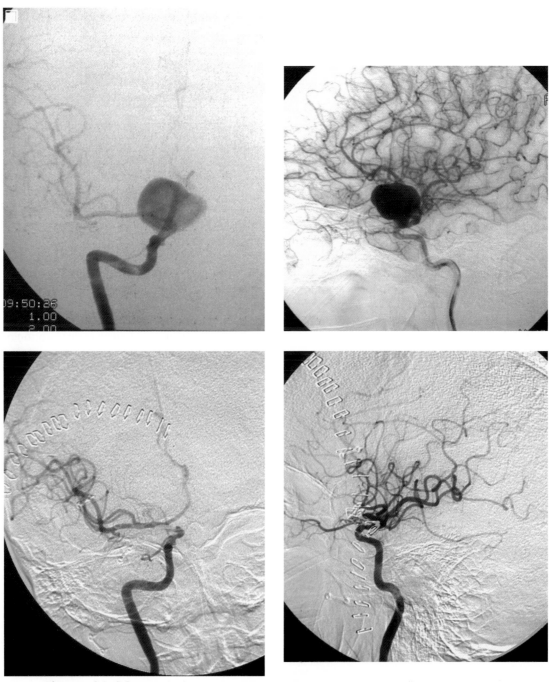

Figure 35-23 Cerebral aneurysm. *(From Le Roux P, Winn H, Newell D: Management of cerebral aneurysms, Philadelphia, 2004, WB Saunders.)*

Table 35-5

Types of Cerebral Aneurysms

Type	Description	Special Considerations
Saccular	Any aneurysm with a saclike outpouching that comes off a stem or neck. Many saccular aneurysms are referred to as *berry aneurysms* because they resemble a berry.	This is the most common type of aneurysm. It appears at a branch in the arterial system, usually in the circle of Willis or the middle cerebral artery. Multiple aneurysms may be present.
Fusiform	An aneurysm that does not have a stem or neck; also known as an *atherosclerotic aneurysm.*	Typically occurs in older patients. Most commonly located in the vertebrobasilar system.
Giant	Any saccular or fusiform aneurysm larger than 25 mm.	Commonly located on the internal carotid artery.

Technique

1. A lumbar drain may be placed before the patient is positioned.
2. The patient's head is placed in a three-point pin fixation device, and the patient is positioned according to the anatomical location of the aneurysm.
3. The incision line is marked and injected with lidocaine with epinephrine to promote vasoconstriction of the wound edges.
4. A craniotomy is performed to expose the dura.
5. The operating microscope is brought to the field and adjusted.
6. The arachnoid webs and other tissue are dissected away as necessary to allow visualization of key intracranial structures.
7. The arteries supplying the aneurysm are identified.
8. One or more clips are applied to the base of the aneurysm.
9. A needle is used to aspirate the aneurysm sac after the clip is placed.
10. Hemostasis is achieved
11. The dura is closed.
12. The muscle is reapproximated, and the skin is closed.

Discussion

Aneurysms vary in size, shape, and location, and the surgical treatment is adjusted to each individual case. The goal is to prevent rupture. This may require application of a surgical clip (small clamp), wrapping, or a combination of techniques. In selected cases, an endovascular coil can be placed inside the vessel under fluoroscopic guidance. This procedure can be performed as an interventional radiology procedure using a minimally invasive approach. The coil occludes the vessel and may be inserted before open surgery to prevent rupture until surgery can be safely performed.

A lumbar drain, connected to a drainage bag with a stopcock, may be placed by the neurosurgeon before the patient is prepped or positioned. The drain is used to control the volume of CSF in the ventricles, if needed, during the procedure. The anesthesia care provider opens the stopcock and releases CSF into the drainage bag to promote brain relaxation and reduce the ICP. The surgical technologist should ensure that the lumbar drain is prepared and isolated in separate sterile field. Drains are supplied in a prepackaged kit with all the necessary components for insertion. The scrub may be responsible for assisting the surgeon in the insertion of the drain.

The patient is always placed in a three-point pin cranial fixation system to ensure absolute head stability and immobility. After the pins are placed and attached to the fixation device, the patient is positioned. The approach for most cerebral aneurysms is a frontal, bifrontal, or frontotemporal (i.e., pterional) craniotomy. The craniotomy is performed as previously described.

A self-retaining brain retractor system is placed after the dura is opened and tacked back from the surgical field. Moistened cottonoids or Gelfoam strips are placed beneath the retractor blades for cushioning and hydration. The retractors are essential for gentle, consistent retraction of the cerebral tissue. The system allows for placement of retractors in almost any direction. Each system is configured differently, but all are designed to be secured to the patient's head, to the skull pin fixation device, or to a post and coupling attached to the operating bed. The surgeon may periodically adjust the retractor blades to ensure that the tissue beneath remains perfused and the brain is not bruised.

The draped operating microscope is brought to the field and positioned. At this point, the surgeon may request a draped sitting stool with an arm rest. The arachnoid is opened with microscissors, hooks, dissectors, and a microbipolar ESU. As the arachnoid is opened, CSF is released, which further relaxes the brain.

Dissection continues until the surgeon visualizes the aneurysm. Dissection is meticulous to avoid undue manipulation of the aneurysm. The surgeon needs an adequate supply of moistened cottonoids and working suction during this phase of the procedure. The microscopic suction tips can easily become occluded with blood and debris. The scrub should have several suction tips available on the field so that the tips can be changed out quickly with minimal interruption to the flow of the procedure.

The aneurysm is occluded at its base with one or more aneurysm clips. Aneurysm clips are available from a variety of manufacturers but share common characteristics (Figure 35-24). The clip is composed of a body, a pivot point, and two blades. The blades of the clip come in different lengths and are configured in a variety of ways, including straight, curved, and angled up, down, or sideways, to allow for anatomical variation.

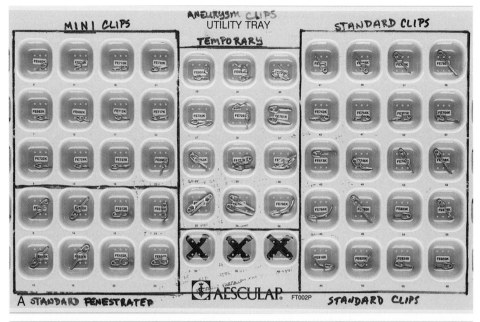

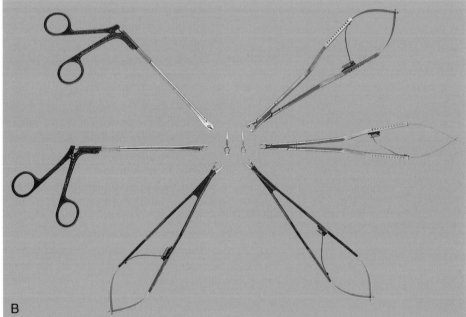

Figure 35-24   Yasargil aneurysm clips with assorted appliers. *(From Tighe SM: Instrumentation for the operating room, ed 6, St Louis, 2003, Mosby.)*

The scrub must be familiar with the basic aneurysm clips and clip appliers available for use. Clips are supplied as permanent or temporary devices. Temporary clips have blades that open wider than permanent clips, and they also have less closing force. They are used to occlude the arterial source to the aneurysm temporarily or to test-occlude the base of the aneurysm before the permanent clip is applied. Temporary clips generally are gold colored, for easy identification, and should be discarded after use.

Permanent clips have a greater closing force and are designed to remain in place as a permanent implant. Fenestrated clips have an open blade. These clips may be used for indirect access to the aneurysm. A Sundt-type clip has a Teflon-lined lumen and is used to encircle the vessel completely when bleeding is encountered. Clip appliers may have a spring-loaded configuration or a pistol grip. They may have a hinged shaft to improve visualization. The scrub must make sure that at least two clip appliers are available for each type of clip used.

When handling aneurysm clips, the scrub must not compress the clips or manipulate them in any way while loading them in the applier. The clip should be compressed only by the surgeon immediately before placement, because opening and closing the clip alters its closing force, and the clip may not seat securely.

The surgeon prepares the aneurysm for occlusion by continuing to isolate and identify the proximal and distal vasculature. This phase of the surgery requires careful handling of

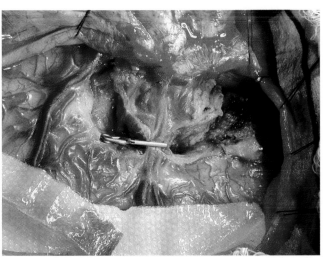

Figure 35-25 Aneurysm clip applied over a defect. *(From Rengachary S, Ellenbogen R: Principles of neurosurgery, ed 2, St Louis, 2005, Mosby.)*

Pathology

An arteriovenous malformation is an abnormal communication or fistula between the arteries and veins. AVMs are commonly diagnosed in adults between 20 and 40 years of age. As the connection becomes larger under pressure, blood is diverted from surrounding brain tissue. When this occurs, multiple hemorrhages from the dilated blood vessels can cause seizures and subarachnoid hemorrhage.

Technique

1. The patient's head is placed in a three-point pin fixation device, and the patient is positioned according to the anatomical location of the arteriovenous malformation (AVM).
2. The incision line is marked and injected with lidocaine with epinephrine to promote vasoconstriction of the wound edges.
3. A craniotomy is performed.
4. Using techniques discussed in the section on aneurysm surgery, the surgeon isolates the AVM and applies aneurysm clips to the feeder vessels.
5. The AVM is dissected further and resected.
6. Closure is as described for a craniotomy.

Discussion

Some AVMs may be very complex and involve many vessels, making surgical resection risky. A multidisciplinary approach often is used in treating these patients. An interventional radiologist may be involved in the patient's care before surgery to embolize the AVM and reduce its size. During **embolization**, platinum coils, glue, or microscopic plastic particles are placed in the vessels feeding the AVM. The materials close off the feeder vessels, reducing the vascularity of the AVM to reduce the chance of rupture. Embolization may also be used after craniotomy for AVM resection, if required, to secure additional vessels not accessible during open surgery. Radiosurgery with the gamma knife is another option that may be used as an adjunct to surgery.

The procedure to resect an AVM is similar to the procedure for clipping a cerebral aneurysm. A craniotomy approach is used, and the AVM is exposed using the same techniques described in the previous section. Because of the complexity of the vascular structure of most AVMs, microscopic dissection to identify the feeder vessels can be prolonged. A microtipped bipolar ESU is used extensively during this dissection. The scrub must have several microbipolar forceps available to allow for rapid exchange when the tips become coated with eschar. The scrub should observe the dissection on the video monitor to anticipate when the bipolar instrument will need to be exchanged and to make sure that the flow of instruments, sponges, and other materials is seamless and that the surgeon does not have to look away from the microscope.

Once the AVM is exposed, the surgeon uses the bipolar ESU to occlude smaller vessels. Multiple aneurysm clips are placed on the larger feeder vessels. The AVM then is resected with the bipolar ESU. The scrub should be prepared with strips of Surgicel and Gelfoam to line the AVM cavity. The wound is closed as described for cerebral aneurysm clipping.

tissues, because handling of the aneurysm, especially the dome, could cause it to rupture. Rupture can occur at any time during the procedure but is more likely to happen during dissection. The scrub should always be prepared for the possibility of rupture by having a temporary clip loaded on a clip applier. If rupture occurs, suction and moistened cottonoids are needed immediately.

The surgeon places the clip across the neck of the aneurysm (Figure 35-25). Additional clips are used as necessary to ensure that the aneurysm and its feeder vessels are occluded. Once the aneurysm is occluded, the surgeon requires a 30-gauge needle attached to the syringe to aspirate the aneurysm sac. This maneuver removes any blood in the aneurysm and allows the surgeon to establish that there is no filling of the aneurysm and the clip is secure. In cases of giant aneurysms, the surgeon may open the dome of the aneurysm (aneurysmectomy) after the clips are placed to evacuate blood, clots, or tissue debris. If a clip cannot be applied to occlude the aneurysm, the surgeon may attempt to occlude it by wrapping or coating the vessel with a piece of the galea, methylmethacrylate, or cyanoacrylate.

After clip placement, the surgeon may request a cottonoid moistened with papaverine to apply to the vessels surrounding the aneurysm. Papaverine is used to prevent vessel spasm. Wound closure follows as outlined for a craniotomy. The pin fixation device is removed before the patient emerges from anesthesia.

ARTERIOVENOUS MALFORMATION RESECTION

Surgical Goal

Arteriovenous malformation (AVM) resection is performed to correct the fistula that occurs when an abnormal communication exists between the cerebral arteries and veins.

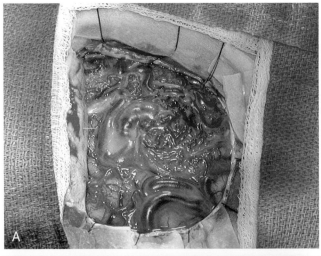

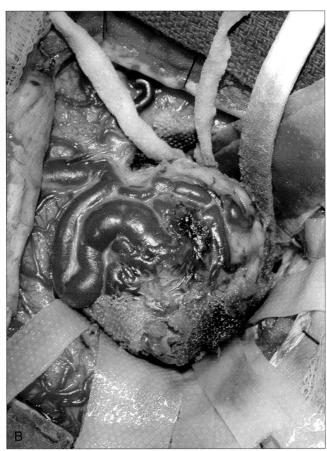

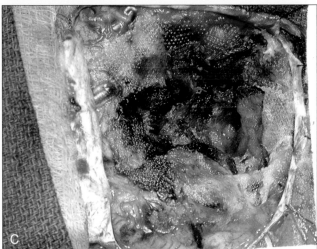

Figure 35-26 Arteriovenous malformation (AVM). **A,** The surface of the AVM before resection. **B,** The AVM has been separated from the surrounding area of the brain. **C,** Appearance of the resection cavity after resection. *(From Rengachary S, Ellenbogen R: Principles of neurosurgery, ed 2, St Louis, 2005, Mosby.)*

Figure 35-26 illustrates the techniques used in the treatment of an AVM.

CORRECTION OF CRANIOSYNOSTOSIS

Surgical Goal
A linear strip craniectomy is performed to correct the premature closure of an infant's cranial suture lines by separating the involved bones and treating the bones to prevent resealing until the brain has completed most of its growth.

Pathology
Craniosynostosis is a congenital deformity of the skull that results from premature closure of one or more of the cranial sutures of the skull. Fusion of each of the major cranial vault sutures can have different types of effects on the skull, generally causing growth restriction perpendicular to the suture (Figure 35-27). Fusion of multiple sutures can lead to increased ICP as the brain grows. Surgery usually is performed when the infant is 6 weeks to 6 months of age,

because the skull bones are more malleable and a better cosmetic result can be achieved. The following procedure is used to treat sagittal hypostasis, the most common form of craniosynostosis.

Technique
1. The patient is positioned supine with the head in a headrest.
2. The incision line is marked and injected with lidocaine with epinephrine to promote vasoconstriction of the wound edges.
3. An incision is made at the midpoint between the anterior and posterior fontanelles and is extended from ear to ear.
4. The scalp is separated from the skull with blunt dissection, leaving the pericranium intact. Scalp clips are applied to the wound edges.
5. Burr holes are made in the cranium.
6. The burr holes are connected to form strips of bone.
7. The dura is dissected from the bone strips.
8. Hemostasis is maintained.

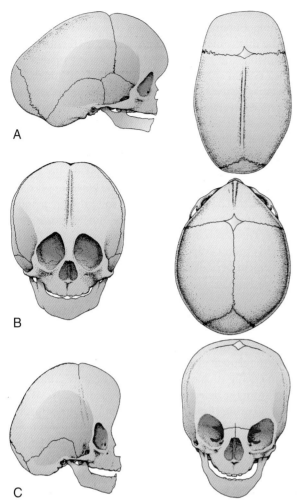

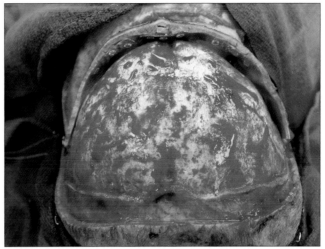

Figure 35-28 Craniosynostosis. Absorbable plates are applied to cranial strips after repair. *(From Rengachary S, Ellenbogen R: Principles of neurosurgery, ed 2, St Louis, 2005, Mosby.)*

Figure 35-27 Craniosynostosis. Effects on the skull resulting from fusion of major vault sutures. **A,** Sagittal sutures. **B,** Metopic suture. **C,** Coronal suture. *(From Choux M, DiRocco C, Hockley A et al: Pediatric neurosurgery, London, 1999, Churchill Livingstone.)*

9. The bone strips are reshaped and replaced to correct the defect.
10. Absorbable plates and screws are placed to anchor the strips in their new configuration.
11. Closure proceeds as described for a craniotomy.

Discussion

Preoperative preparation of a pediatric patient includes protection against hypothermia. The operating room temperature is increased, and extra draping layers may be used. The scrub must ensure that irrigation solutions are warm to prevent the loss of heat through exposed tissues.

The scalp is incised over the area where the premature closure of the suture line has caused the deformity. The surgical assistant applies digital pressure to the wound edges, therefore the scrub should ensure that an ample supply of folded 4 × 4 sponges is available. A zigzag incision may be made to provide a more cosmetic result.

Scalp clips are applied (see the craniotomy procedure for special considerations when using scalp clips), and the scalp is secured away from the field with a towel clip, suture, or hooks attached to rubber bands. The scrub should have moistened 4 × 4 sponges available to place over the scalp surface to prevent it from drying during the procedure.

The periosteum is lifted from the bone with a small Key elevator. A small, round burr on a drill is used to place a series of burr holes, which are connected with a bone saw to form bone strips. The number of strips cut depends on how extensive the correction needs to be. The calvarial bone is soft and cuts easily but is still vulnerable to heat damage from the burrs and cutting blades; the scrub therefore must be ready to provide gentle irrigation during cutting to prevent heat buildup.

The dura mater is stripped from the underside of the skull using blunt dissection with a nerve hook. The bone strips are then removed with a heavy scissors, a craniotome, or a small Kerrison rongeur. Bone wax should be available for hemostasis of the bone edges.

The surgeon reshapes the bone strips by bending them or shaving them with a fine burr. After the pieces have been reshaped, the surgeon places them back on the head, usually in an altered configuration, and secures them in place with absorbable suture, plates, and screws (Figure 35-28). Hemostasis is achieved using the bipolar and monopolar ESUs, Gelfoam strips, and Surgicel as needed. The scalp clips are removed, and closure proceeds as described for a craniotomy.

CRANIOPLASTY

Surgical Goal

In this procedure, an area of bone in the skull is replaced with a bone graft or prosthetic material to restore the continuity of the skull, protect the brain, and improve the patient's cosmetic appearance.

Pathology

Deformities of the skull resulting from trauma or disease may leave a portion of the brain and dura mater exposed. More commonly, cranial defects may occur as a result of an infection of the bone flap after elective craniotomy.

If the cranial defect is clean (e.g., in closed trauma), the repair may be performed immediately. If the wound is contaminated (e.g., bone flap infection, open trauma), repair is delayed. The bone flap created by craniotomy may have been removed and stored under sterile conditions to allow the brain to expand and to reduce the ICP. In other circumstances, calvarial bone strips are used to cover the exposed area, protect it from injury, and improve the patient's appearance. Methylmethacrylate most often is used for prosthetic replacement. However, some surgeons use an acrylic prosthesis that is customized for the patient with three-dimensional imaging and computer-aided design (CAD). The following description is for the process of methylmethacrylate cranioplasty.

Technique

1. The patient is positioned according to the location of the defect.
2. The incision line is marked and injected with lidocaine with epinephrine to promote vasoconstriction at the wound edges.
3. An incision is made through the existing scar.
4. Scalp clips are applied.
5. Blunt dissection is used to separate the scalp from the skull.
6. The bone edges are trimmed, and a bony ledge is created.
7. The methylmethacrylate is prepared, allowed to cure to the desired consistency, and placed in the bag provided by the manufacturer.
8. The bag containing the methylmethacrylate is molded to the defect.
9. The bag is removed from the wound and allowed to cool.
10. The cooled prosthesis is placed back in the wound and trimmed and smoothed as necessary to fit.
11. The prosthesis is secured in place with wire.
12. Closure proceeds as previously described for a craniotomy.

Discussion

The patient is positioned, prepped, and draped for access to a particular area of the skull. The scalp is incised over the defect as for a craniotomy. The surgeon may excise the scar overlying the defect.

Depending on the nature of the previous injury or disease, remnants of bone may be present in the affected area. If bone fragments are present, the surgeon may use a rongeur to trim them away. If the affected area is completely devoid of bone, the surgeon trims the periphery of the area with rongeurs to form a saucerlike ledge. This prevents the prosthesis from slipping below the level of the skull and helps seat it in place. The scrub should retain all the bits of trimmed bone as specimens.

When the surgeon has completed this procedure, the wound is irrigated with warm saline solution. An antibiotic irrigant also may be used at this time.

The scrub uses a commercially prepared cranioplasty kit containing a premeasured amount of powder and solvent to form the methylmethacrylate prosthesis. Methylmethacrylate is flammable and must be mixed in a well-ventilated area. A vacuum system specifically designed for methylmethacrylate mixing may be used to minimize the fumes released as part of the chemical reaction. A single dose is supplied in each cranioplasty kit. If additional material is needed, it should be mixed separately. Double-gloving is recommended for mixing and handling the cement.

The entire package of powder is emptied into a stainless steel mixing bowl or a disposable sterile bowl supplied by the manufacturer. The entire volume of solvent is then added. A spatula is used to mix the substances for approximately 30 seconds. The scrub should cover the bowl after the initial mixing to prevent evaporation and should test the consistency of the cement periodically. The cement becomes doughy and pulls away from the walls of the mixing bowl within 5 minutes.

While the cement is still doughy, the scrub places it in the plastic bag provided in the kit and passes it to the surgeon. The surgeon then flattens and molds the bag over the cranial defect until it fits. This step must be performed quickly, because the cement gives off heat as it hardens and can damage the underlying tissue. The surgeon removes the molded cement from the defect to allow the cement to cure. While the cement is curing (usually 15 to 20 minutes), the surgeon may assess the wound for any small bleeders. During this time, the scrub should prepare a dental drill or similar drill and a fine drill point.

When the cement plate has hardened, the surgeon drills several holes in its edge. Similar holes are drilled at the periphery of the skull defect. Any rough spots in the cement plate are smoothed with a large burr attached to a power drill or craniotome. The surgeon then fits the cement plate into the defect and secures it by passing fine stainless steel wires through the holes. The wound is irrigated and closed in routine fashion.

Postoperative Considerations

Because cranioplasty does not involve the manipulation of brain tissue, neurological complications are rare. Infection involving the scalp or replanted bone may occur, and resorption of the bone may occur if calvarial bone strips are used.

VENTRICULOPERITONEAL/ VENTRICULAR SHUNT

Surgical Goal

Ventricular shunting is used to divert the cerebrospinal fluid away from the ventricles of the brain to another location in the body, such as the peritoneal cavity, pleural space, or atrium of the heart, where the CSF can be absorbed. This reduces intracranial pressure.

Pathology

Hydrocephalus is a condition involving an inappropriate amount of CSF in the intracranial space at an inappropriate pressure. CSF is produced by the epidermal cells in the lateral

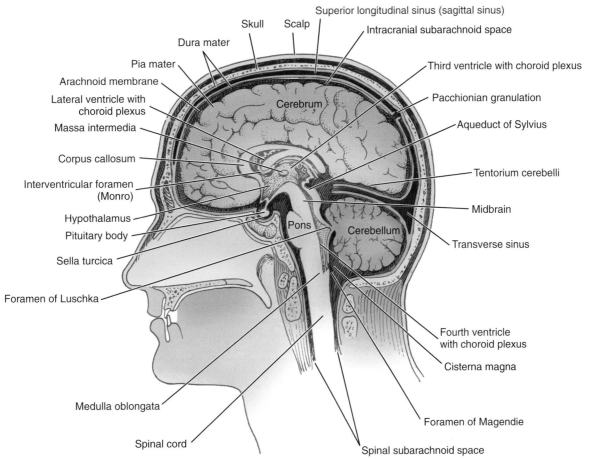

Figure 35-29 Normal flow of cerebrospinal fluid in the brain. *(From Applegate E: The anatomy and physiology learning system, ed 2, St Louis, 2000, WB Saunders.)*

third and fourth ventricles. CSF circulates through the foramen of Monro into the third ventricle, through the cerebral aqueduct (aqueduct of Sylvius), into the fourth ventricle. From the fourth ventricle, it flows through the cerebromedullary cistern down the spinal cord and over the cerebral hemispheres (Figure 35-29). Hydrocephalus can occur as a result of an overproduction of CSF, or it may be the result of a condition that interferes with the normal absorption of fluid. Hydrocephalus can develop in children and adults. Persistent hydrocephalus can interfere with cerebral blood flow and cause enlargement of the skull in infants. In selected cases, surgical intervention is aimed at removing the excess fluid to relieve pressure on the brain. A ventriculoperitoneal shunt most often is used to divert CSF.

Technique

1. The patient is positioned supine with the head slightly rotated opposite the side of the shunt and the neck extended in a straight line to the abdomen.
2. A scalp incision is made, and hemostasis is achieved.
3. A small scalp flap is created and retracted.
4. A burr hole is made.
5. The ventricular catheter is placed through the burr hole into the lateral ventricle.

6. The reservoir and valve are connected to the ventricular catheter.
7. A subcutaneous tunnel is created from the burr hole to the neck. The end of the tunnel is marked, and the neck incision is made at that site.
8. The peritoneal catheter is connected to the reservoir and valve.
9. An abdominal incision is made.
10. A second subcutaneous tunnel is created from the neck incision to the abdomen.
11. The peritoneal catheter is threaded through the abdominal incision.
12. Flow of cerebrospinal fluid through the end of the peritoneal catheter is verified.
13. The peritoneal catheter is placed in the peritoneal cavity and secured with a purse-string suture.
14. The incisions are closed.

Discussion

Shunt systems vary by manufacturer, but common components include a ventricular catheter, a CSF reservoir, a valve, and a peritoneal catheter (Figure 35-30). Valves are designed for one-way flow and are supplied with a variety of pressure

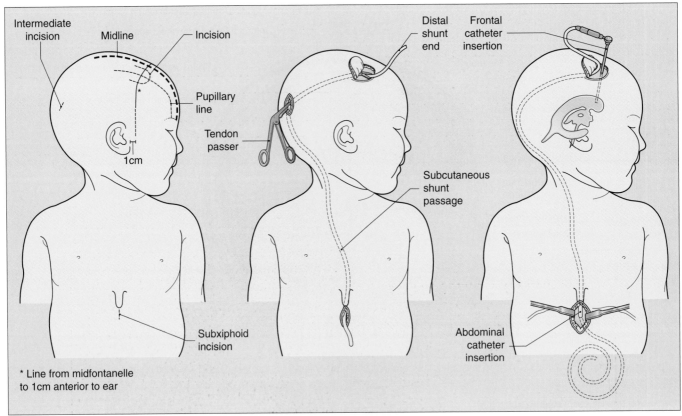

Figure 35-30　Ventriculoperitoneal shunt. The patient is positioned, and exact positions are marked. A subcutaneous tunnel is created for the shunt, and the catheter is inserted. *(From Rengachary S, Ellenbogen R: Principles of neurosurgery, ed 2, St Louis, 2005, Mosby.)*

and flow settings. The scrub should read the manufacturer's specifications and instructions before the procedure is performed. As with all Silastic or other implant materials, the shunt should be handled carefully and protected from contamination by lint, dust, or glove powder. The shunt components should be soaked in antibiotic solution before they are implanted. The scrub is responsible for priming the assembly with saline and ensuring that no air is present in the system. Because ventricular shunting may be performed on adults or children, the scrub should ensure that the instruments and sutures selected are appropriate for the age and size of the patient.

The surgeon may choose a frontal, parietal, or occipital approach to place the ventricular catheter. The patient is positioned in a flat plane, according to the approach chosen, to facilitate insertion of the tunneling device from the neck to the abdomen.

After the patient is prepped and draped, the surgeon makes a curved incision in the scalp over the area where the burr hole will be drilled. The burr hole is placed as previously described, and the dura is incised.

A bipolar ESU is used to open the pia. Intraoperative ultrasound may be used to confirm the location of the ventricle before catheter insertion is attempted. The scrub loads the ventricular catheter on an introducer, and the surgeon inserts it through the burr hole into the lateral ventricle. The introducer is removed, and CSF flow through the catheter is con-

firmed. If no CSF flow is present, the catheter is removed, the introducer is replaced, and the procedure is attempted again. When CSF flow is confirmed, the reservoir and valve are attached to the ventricular catheter and secured with 2-0 silk sutures.

A tendon passer is used to create a subcutaneous tunnel from the burr hole to the neck. The surgeon makes a small neck incision and completes any dissection using the Metzenbaum scissors. The catheter is brought through the tunnel, and the surgeon confirms that CSF is still flowing through the valve before connecting the peritoneal catheter.

The surgeon makes a small abdominal incision and dissects through the subcutaneous tissue and fascia to reach the peritoneum. The scrub should be prepared for this step with Senn retractors, monopolar ESU, and Metzenbaum scissors. A tunneling device is used to create space in the soft tissues from the abdominal incision to the neck incision.

The peritoneal catheter is brought through the tunnel, and CSF flow is confirmed. The catheter may be flushed with normal saline to ensure that it has not become occluded with blood or debris. The upper valve can also be pumped to confirm that the shunt is working. After confirming patency, the surgeon uses 3-0 absorbable synthetic sutures to secure the catheter to the peritoneum.

The incisions are closed with absorbable synthetic suture. The scalp and abdominal skin incisions are closed with staples or with interrupted 4-0 nylon suture. The neck incision can be closed with a running subcuticular stitch or interrupted sutures.

Postoperative Considerations

The most common complication after ventricular shunt placement is shunt malfunction as a result of blockage of the valve or catheter. This complication can occur shortly after placement or at any time after the shunt is in place. Overdrainage or underdrainage also can occur and can cause patients to exhibit a variety of symptoms ranging from headache to neurological deficits. Shunts placed in infants and children need to be replaced periodically to accommodate their growth.

TRANSSPHENOIDAL HYPOPHYSECTOMY

Surgical Goal

The goal of hypophysectomy is to remove all or a part of the pituitary gland. This procedure may be performed to slow the growth and spread of endocrine-dependent malignant tumors or to excise a pituitary tumor. The surgical approach is through the sphenoid.

Pathology

The pituitary gland is responsible for the storage, release, and secretion of a variety of hormones. The gland is attached by a stalk to the hypothalamus and rests in the sella turcica. It is adjacent to critical structures such as the optic chiasma and cavernous sinuses. The cavernous sinuses contain several cranial nerves and the internal carotid arteries. Because the gland is uniquely located, symptoms from a tumor often are noticed as visual field anomalies or may be related to pressure on cranial nerves III through VI. Tumors may damage the adjacent brain tissue through mass effect by displacing structures, blocking CSF flow, or creating pressure.

Technique

1. The patient is positioned in a semisitting position with the head secured with three-point pin fixation.
2. Preoperative fluoroscopy is used to confirm the correct position.
3. Topical and infiltration anesthetic is applied to the nasal mucosa.
4. The patient's face, mouth, nasal cavity, and a small abdominal area are prepped and draped.
5. The gingiva and nasal mucosa are incised and lifted from the septum.
6. Bone and nasal cartilage is resected and preserved.
7. The sphenoid sinus is examined.
8. The sinus is opened, and the floor of the sella turcica is identified.
9. The sella turcica is opened with a pneumatic drill.
10. The microscope is used to visualize the pituitary tumor.
11. The tumor and gland are resected.
12. The sella turcica is packed with fatty tissue, and the floor is reconstructed with cartilage from the nasal septum.
13. The nasal mucosa is sutured, and the gingival incision is closed.
14. Nasal packing and splints are inserted.

Discussion

Transsphenoidal hypophysectomy requires an interdisciplinary approach. An otorhinolaryngologist participates in the surgery during access to the sella turcica. An open or endoscopic approach may be used (see Chapter 27 for a discussion of endoscopic sinus techniques). The scrub should have combined sinus instrumentation available. Specialized pituitary instrumentation, which includes self-retaining specula, long pituitary spoons and scoops, rongeurs, and curettes, should also be available. The operating microscope may be prepared and draped before the start of surgery.

Before the start of surgery, the scrub should prepare a side table that includes supplies needed for injection and application of a local anesthetic. Supplies include nasal specula, cottonoids, syringes, and several 25-gauge needles. The circulating nurse dispenses topical cocaine and lidocaine with epinephrine to this nonsterile field. Before beginning the procedure, the surgeon injects the nasal and gingival mucosa to provide hemostasis.

The scrub also is responsible for preparing a separate sterile field with a few basic instruments for obtaining a fat graft from the abdomen. The fat graft is harvested before the transsphenoidal procedure begins to maintain the flow from a clean to a contaminated area.

The patient is placed in the three-point pin fixation device and positioned in a semisitting position with the neck flexed toward the left and the head rotated to the right. The surgical approach is from the patient's right side. After the patient has been positioned, the C-arm is used to confirm that the positioning is accurate for access to the sella. Often the floor is marked with a piece of tape where the C-arm's wheels are placed so that it can be repositioned in the same location during the procedure. Because the patient is in a semisitting position, the risk of air embolism exists. Refer to the posterior fossa craniectomy procedure for information about intraoperative air embolism.

To secure hemostasis before the incision, the otorhinolaryngologist injects the nasal submucosa and gingival mucosa with lidocaine with epinephrine. Cottonoids saturated with cocaine solution are used to pack the nose. The anesthesia care provider may insert a throat pack so that any blood or fluid from the procedure does not enter the patient's stomach.

❖ *The scrub should note the number of cottonoids placed in the nose for reconciliation during the sponge count. Although a counted sponge is not typically used for the throat pack, the scrub should note its presence and remind the anesthesia care provider to remove it at the end of the procedure.*

The procedure begins with the harvesting of the fat graft from the abdomen. The surgeon makes a small incision below the belt line. A small amount of subcutaneous fat is removed with the monopolar ESU and Metzenbaum scissors. The fat may be harvested from any location in the abdomen, but the site usually is chosen for a cosmetic result. Alternately, muscle may be removed from the patient's thigh for use as packing material. The surgical technologist should keep the tissue graft in a basin filled with saline or wrapped in a moistened 4 × 4 on the back table until it is needed. The surgeon uses 2-0 polyglactin suture to close the subcutaneous tissue. The skin can be closed with staples or a running subcuticular stitch of 3-0 or 4-0 nylon or polypropylene suture. The scrub should protect the incision with a sterile towel for the remainder of the procedure.

Next, the otolaryngologist exposes the sella. This may be done endoscopically (see Chapter 27 for details) or by incising the septal cartilage with a #15 blade and elevating the mucous membrane with a septal elevator. The otorhinolaryngologist removes nasal bone and cartilage until the sella is exposed. If necessary, the otorhinolaryngologist may open a window in the patient's gingiva to gain exposure. The scrub should retain any pieces of bone and cartilage in an irrigation basin on the surgical field for reimplantation at the end of the procedure.

The surgical technologist drapes the C-arm with a sterile drape, and the radiology technician moved it into place, aligning it with the tape placed on the floor earlier. Fluoroscopy is used at this stage to confirm exposure of the sphenoid sinus and the floor of the sella.

Once exposure is confirmed, a drill or rongeur is used to enter the sphenoid sinus. The surgeon removes the mucosa covering the sphenoid with a pituitary rongeur. The surgical microscope is positioned. With the microscope in place, the surgeon opens the roof of the sphenoid with a narrow osteotome. Small pieces of bone are removed with a rongeur to expose the dura. The surgeon uses a #11 blade with a bayonet knife handle to open the dura and then dissects the dura off the pituitary gland with a dura hook. Angled microscissors are used to further open the dura and separate it from the gland. The microbipolar ESU is used to control any bleeding.

Before tumor resection begins, the tumor mass is biopsied and sent for frozen section identification to confirm the presence of pituitary tissue. After positive identification, the surgeon uses microblunt ring curettes, enucleators, suction, and microdissectors to remove the tumor mass. Bleeding is controlled with the ESU, cottonoids, and Gelfoam packing.

Using the fat graft or muscle tissue obtained at the start of the procedure, the surgeon packs the floor of the sella and reinforces the graft with pieces of nasal cartilage and bone to prevent a CSF leak. The otorhinolaryngologist closes the gingival incision (if used) with polyglactin suture, reapproximates the nasal mucosa, and places flexible polyethylene splints in the patient's nose to maintain septal alignment. The splints are secured anteriorly with nylon or polypropylene suture. Gauze, Telfa strips, or nasal tampons coated with antibiotic ointment may be packed into the nasal cavity after the splints are placed. The patient is returned to a supine position and the pin fixation device is removed before the patient emerges from anesthesia.

Postoperative Considerations

Patients who have undergone transsphenoidal hypophysectomy are monitored in the ICU postoperatively for changes in neurological status and CSF leakage. Leakage of CSF indicates that the sella is not sealed and the patient is at risk for infection. Because the pituitary gland has been manipulated or partly resected, patients may experience symptoms related to underproduction or overproduction of the various hormones controlled by the gland. These symptoms may be present immediately postoperatively or may manifest in the weeks or months after the procedure. Some patients require lifelong hormonal replacement after hypophysectomy.

RESECTION OF A VESTIBULAR SCHWANNOMA (ACOUSTIC NEUROMA)

Surgical Goal

Resection of a vestibular schwannoma is performed to remove tumors from the vestibular branch of cranial nerve VIII while preserving the function of the nerve. A suboccipital, translabyrinth, or middle fossa approach can be used. Vestibular schwannomas may also be treated with radiosurgery. Each approach is associated with particular advantages and disadvantages. The choice of one approach over another is based on the surgeon's preference and the size and location of the tumor. The translabyrinth approach is discussed here.

Pathology

A schwannoma, also called an *acoustic neuroma,* is a benign, slow-growing tumor composed of Schwann cells. As the tumor grows, it impinges on cranial nerve VIII, causing one-sided hearing loss, ringing in the ears, dizziness, and problems with balance. The tumor also can cause pressure on the nearby seventh cranial nerve, causing facial numbness and pain. If the tumor is left untreated and continues to grow, it eventually may cause deafness.

Technique

1. The patient is positioned supine with the head turned.
2. The postauricular incision line is marked and injected with lidocaine with epinephrine.
3. A tissue graft is obtained.
4. The incision is made, and hemostasis is achieved.
5. The periosteum is stripped from the mastoid bone.
6. A cutting burr is used to open the mastoid.
7. The operating microscope is used to visualize the inner ear.
8. Select structures of the inner ear are removed.
9. Bone is removed from the structures around the inner ear.
10. The dura is opened.
11. The tumor is removed.
12. The mastoid cavity is packed.
13. The wound is closed.

Discussion

Resection of a vestibular schwannoma involves a multidisciplinary team approach. The neurosurgeon partners with an otologic surgeon to ensure that the patient receives optimum care.

The patient is positioned supine with the head at the foot of the table so that the surgeon can be seated for the procedure. A facial nerve monitor may be used to assess the functioning of the facial nerve during the procedure. The surgeon injects the postauricular incision line and continues the injection into the internal auditory canal.

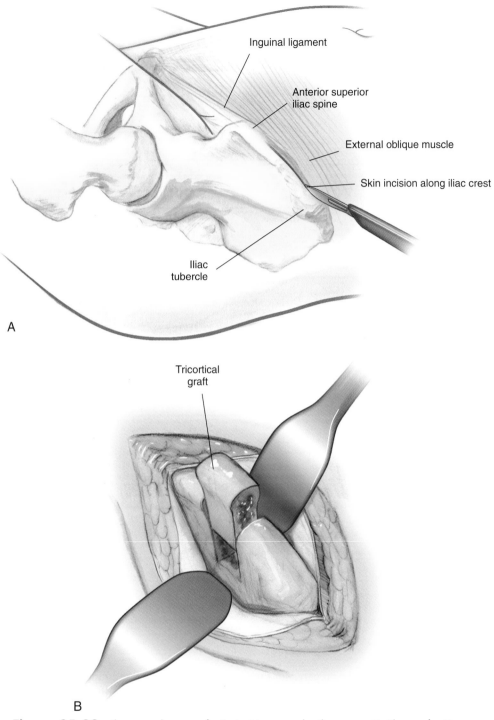

Figure 35-32 Iliac crest bone graft. **A,** Incision over the iliac crest. **B,** Plug graft. *(From Miller MD, Chhabra AB, Hurwitz SR, Mihalko WM: Orthopaedic surgical approaches, Philadelphia, 2008, WB Saunders.)*

edge of the sternocleidomastoid muscle. This plane of dissection is carried laterally between the carotid artery and medially between the esophagus and trachea. A small self-retaining retractor is placed in the wound. Hemostasis is maintained with the monopolar and bipolar ESUs and cottonoid sponges.

The surgeon incises the muscle fibers to expose the vertebrae (Figure 35-33). A layer of fascia overlying the vertebra is incised with a #15 knife blade mounted on a #7 handle. A small handheld retractor may be needed by the assistant to help retract the muscle to expose the vertebra. Next, the surgeon incises and removes the anterior longitudinal ligament. With the disc then clearly visible, radiographs are taken to verify the diseased the disc. The surgeon may insert a hypodermic needle into the disc body for identification during the

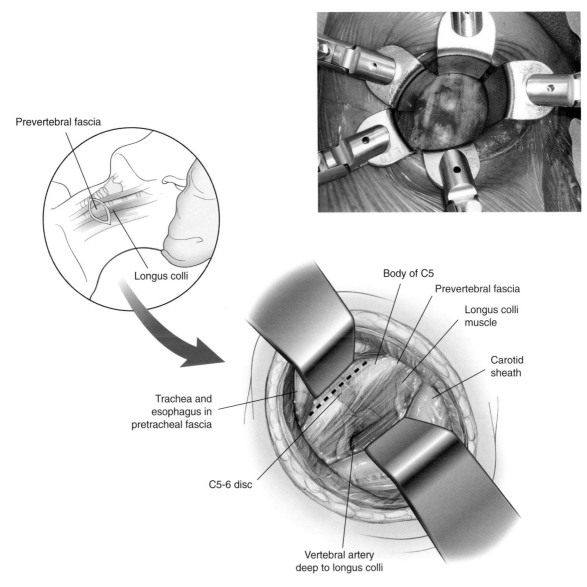

Figure 35-33 Anterior cervical fusion and discectomy. *(From Miller MD, Chhabra AB, Hurwitz SR, Mihalko WM: Orthopaedic surgical approaches, Philadelphia, 2008, WB Saunders.)*

radiographic procedure. The scrub should be prepared for this and provide a sterile radiographic cassette cover if needed. In some cases, the C-arm may be used for real-time confirmation by fluoroscopy.

Once the anatomy has been confirmed, the surgeon places a self-retaining retractor (e.g., a Cloward or Caspar retractor) in the wound. Care is taken in placing these retractors to avoid damaging the carotid artery and esophagus. Usually a combination of sharp and dull blades is used. The retractor systems allow for customization with a variety of blade curvatures, lengths, and retraction surfaces.

With the retractors in place, the surgeon incises the disc with a #15 knife blade. Pituitary rongeurs and fine curettes are used to remove the disc. The disc is removed piece by piece, and the surgical technologist must retrieve the bits of disc from the rongeur or curette with a moistened 4 × 4 sponge.

The surgeon may use an intervertebral spreader to expose the disc. A small drill bit or burr may be used to expose the dura within the interspace. The dura then is elevated with a sharp nerve hook or dura hook and incised with a #15 knife blade. When the interspace has been adequately enlarged and all traces of disc have been removed, the surgeon uses a depth gauge and calipers to measure the defect. These measurements are used to size the bone graft.

While the bone graft is being prepared, the neck wound should be covered with a saline-soaked 4 × 4 sponge to prevent tissue drying and with a sterile towel to protect it from contamination. The surgeon examines the graft and cuts it to the appropriate size to fit into the intervertebral space. Any extra bits of bone from the graft must be saved, because they may be used later to fill the interspace. The surgeon places the graft in the interspace and taps it with a mallet so that it fits snugly between the vertebrae. If the Cloward dowel cutter has been used, the Cloward impactor is used to place the graft. Cervical plates and screws may be used to secure the bone graft in place. In this instance, the surgeon drills pilot holes in the vertebrae on either side of the graft. The scrub must be prepared with irrigation to cool the drill bit while the holes are drilled. The surgeon places the plate in position and secures it with screws. An intraoperative radiograph may be taken to confirm the position of the bone graft, plate, and screws.

The wound then is irrigated with normal saline or antibiotic solution. Bleeding vessels are controlled with the monopolar and bipolar ESUs or a topical hemostatic agent. If it was not closed at the start of the procedure, the hip wound is closed at this time. The surgeon closes the cervical incision in layers with 3-0 polyglactin and staples. Both wounds are dressed in routine fashion, and a rigid cervical collar is placed to help support the neck and maintain cervical alignment.

When the patient is moved from the operating table to the stretcher, particular care is taken to keep the head in alignment with the body to prevent dislodgement of the graft.

Postoperative Considerations

Postoperative hemorrhage, edema, and CSF leakage are possible after any surgery on the spine. Hemorrhage or edema can damage the spinal cord and cause the patient to exhibit neurological changes such as inability to move the extremities or numbness or weakness. The surgeon assesses the patient's neurological status immediately after transfer from the operating bed to the transfer device by testing the patient's ability to follow commands and move the extremities. The surgical technologist should maintain the integrity of the sterile field until the patient has been transferred from the operating room in case re-exploration of the surgical site is necessary.

Longer term complications after spinal surgery include wound infection or meningitis, hardware failure (if used), and nonunion of the bone graft (if used).

POSTERIOR CERVICAL LAMINECTOMY

Surgical Goal

Posterior cervical laminectomy is performed to access the cervical spinal cord and to remove a portion of the cervical lamina.

Pathology

Posterior cervical laminectomy may be required to access neurological tumors. Tumors may occur in the cervical spinal cord or form in the vertebral elements of the cervical spine. Metastatic tumors are common in the bone. Patients with cervical spinal cord tumors typically experience neck pain and numbness and weakness in the upper extremities.

Cervical stenosis is a common condition in older adults that may affect the spinal cord. Cervical stenosis occurs when the discs degenerate and bone spurs form on or between the vertebral surfaces, or the ligaments in the spine buckle, causing pressure on the spinal cord. Symptoms vary, depending on the amount of compression and the location of the stenosis. Most often, symptoms include pain and numbness that radiate down the patient's arm. Cervical stenosis left untreated can seriously damage the spinal cord.

Traumatic injury may result in fracture of the cervical spine and damage to the spinal cord, resulting in a variety of neurological deficits, depending on the level of injury. Decompression laminectomy may be necessary to remove bone fragments and fuse or fixate the spine to prevent ongoing damage to the cord.

Technique

1. The patient is positioned prone on a laminectomy frame with the head in pin fixation, or in the sitting position with the head in pin fixation.
2. The incision is marked and infiltrated with lidocaine and epinephrine. If a bone graft is required, an additional site is marked and infiltrated. (The section on the procedure for anterior cervical discectomy provides details on obtaining the bone graft.)
3. A midline incision is made, and the soft tissue and muscle are retracted.
4. Intraoperative radiographs are taken to confirm the correct vertebral level.
5. Bone is removed from the lamina to reduce pressure.
6. Disc is removed as necessary.
7. If indicated, a fusion or fixation is performed to stabilize the neck.
8. The wound is closed in layers.
9. Bupivacaine may be injected into the soft tissue and musculature to reduce postoperative pain.
10. A rigid cervical collar or external cervical brace system (e.g., halo brace) is placed before the patient emerges from anesthesia.

Discussion

The patient may be positioned in the sitting position or prone on chest rolls or a laminectomy frame for this procedure (Figure 35-34). The position used depends on the surgeon's preference and the pathological condition. The sitting position may provide better exposure for the higher vertebrae. A three-point pin fixation clamp is used in both positions to ensure that the patient's head and cervical spine remain as immobile as possible during the procedure. Immobilization is especially critical in traumatic injuries to the spine.

The surgeon marks the incision site and infiltrates it with lidocaine with epinephrine. If a fusion is planned, an additional site on the patient's hip is marked and infiltrated. Both sites are prepped and draped in routine fashion.

If necessary, a bone graft is harvested from the patient's hip. Alternatively, cadaver bone may be used. The surgeon's preference and the patient's condition determine which method is used. Harvesting of the bone graft may be done at the start of the procedure or after the laminectomy is performed. The scrub should always be prepared for the possibility that a bone graft may be needed and ensure that the proper draping material and instrumentation is available.

After palpating the cervical spinous processes to determine the location of the incision, the surgeon makes a midline incision and begins to expose the musculature of the neck. A monopolar ESU is used for hemostasis, along with 4 × 4s. The

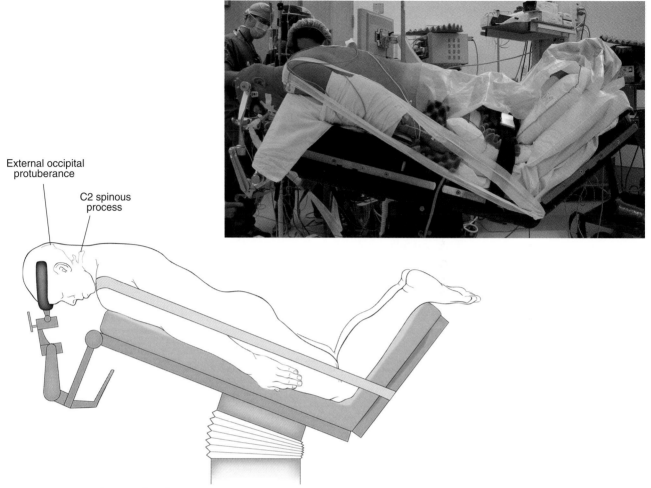

External occipital
protuberance

C2 spinous
process

Figure 35-34 Posterior cervical laminectomy. The patient is placed in the prone position. *(From Miller MD, Chhabra AB, Hurwitz SR, Mihalko WM: Orthopaedic surgical approaches, Philadelphia, 2008, WB Saunders.)*

surgeon uses sharp dissection with Metzenbaum scissors and blunt finger dissection to separate the muscle layers. A self-retaining retractor (e.g., Weitlaner or Adson Beckman retractor) is placed to help maintain exposure. Dissection continues until the spinous processes are visualized. The surgeon uses a variety of periosteal elevators (e.g., Cobb or Key elevator) to clean the periosteum off the bone and gain exposure. Moistened cottonoids and Gelfoam may be used to aid hemostasis.

An intraoperative radiograph is obtained after exposure is completed. The surgeon places a towel clip on the vertebral process or inserts a spinal needle into the disc space to provide a marker, and the radiograph is taken. The scrub should provide a sterile cassette cover or sterile draping over the radiograph cassette holder. Depending on the patient's position, C-arm fluoroscopy may be used for real-time imaging.

The term *laminectomy* refers to the removal of the bony roof of the spinal canal. In a laminectomy, additional bone may also be removed from one or both sides of the vertebra to open up the spinal canal as needed. The surgeon begins the laminectomy with a Leksell rongeur to remove the spinous process and then uses Kerrison rongeurs in a variety of sizes

to remove smaller pieces of bone (Figure 35-35). The scrub should be prepared to assist in removing the pieces of bone from the instrument with a moistened 4 × 4 sponge. Any bone fragments retrieved should be placed in a small bowl filled with saline. The surgeon may also use a high-speed drill (e.g., the Midas Rex) to perform the laminectomy. A variety of cutting and shaping burrs are available. If necessary, the disc is removed with pituitary rongeurs and curettes, as described for an anterior discectomy.

In cases of cervical fracture, the surgeon may fuse the vertebra with a bone graft or with a variety of internal fixation methods, including plates, screws, and cables. The method of fixation varies, depending on the level of fracture and the severity of injury. (Chapter 30 presents a discussion of techniques of internal fixation.)

When the laminectomy and discectomy are completed, the surgeon irrigates the wound with antibiotic solution and secures hemostasis with the ESU. The wound is closed in layers with size 0 or 1-0 polyglactin suture on a cutting needle. The skin usually is closed with staples.

The wound is dressed with a simple gauze dressing. A rigid cervical collar is applied before the patient emerges from anes-

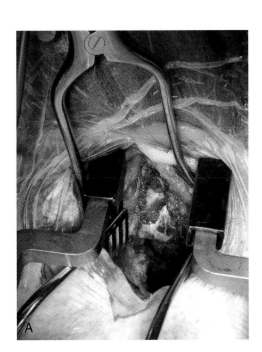

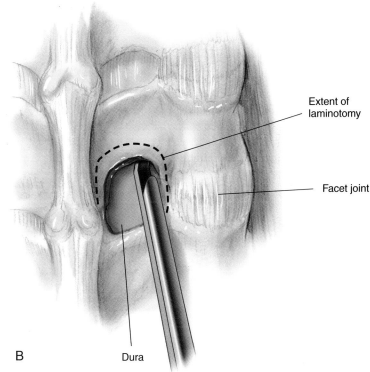

Extent of
laminotomy

Facet joint

Dura

Figure 35-35 Posterior cervical laminectomy. **A,** With self-retaining retractors in place, the lamina is exposed. **B,** A Kerrison upbiting rongeur is used to remove bone. *(From Miller MD, Chhabra AB, Hurwitz SR, Mihalko WM: Orthopaedic surgical approaches, Philadelphia, 2008, WB Saunders.)*

thesia. The collar provides stabilization while the laminectomy heals. Patients who have undergone fusion and instrumentation may require additional stabilization with a halo brace.

APPLICATION OF A HALO BRACE

Surgical Goal

A halo brace is used to provide traction and restore spinal alignment to the cervical spine. It may also be used to provide initial decompression of the spinal cord after injury.

Pathology

Fracture of the cervical spine requires immobilization to prevent displacement of the bone and impingement on the spinal cord. A halo traction brace is applied to maintain alignment during healing after traumatic injury and selected cervical spine procedures.

Technique

1. The patient is placed in the supine position.
2. A local anesthetic is injected into the pin sites.
3. Four to six people log-roll the patient, and the back panel of the vest is placed.
4. The posterior bars are attached to the back panel of the vest.
5. The halo pins are placed and tightened.
6. The halo ring is attached to the posterior bars.
7. The front panel of the vest is placed, and the anterior bars are secured to the vest.
8. The halo ring is attached to the anterior bars.
9. The pins are adjusted as needed for optimum immobilization.

Discussion

Cervical halo systems may vary by manufacturer but commonly consist of a halo ring that surrounds the head and is held in place by pins, a frame made of four upright bars and connectors to attach the bars to the halo, and a vest, which is a plastic structure that covers the chest and acts as a foundation for the brace.

The patient is positioned supine with the head extending over the edge of the bed and manually stabilized by the surgical assistant. The surgeon injects the pin sites with local anesthetic for hemostasis. Most systems use a four-pin configuration. The surgeon injects two sites on either side of the patient's eyes over the orbital ridge and two sites just behind the ears.

The patient is log-rolled onto the side, and the surgeon slides the back panel of the halo vest into place. The posterior bars are secured to the back panel of the vest by sliding them through the connectors and tightening the connectors with an Allen wrench.

An appropriate-size ring is selected, and the pins are placed through the pin sockets in the ring. The surgeon positions the ring over the patient's head until the tips of the pins just touch the skin. Each pin is tightened by hand, starting with a front pin, then the diagonally opposite back pin, until all the pins pierce the skin and are secure in the outer layer of the skull bone. The front panel of the vest is placed over the chest, and the anterior bars are placed through the connectors and tightened. The halo ring is attached to the bars with connectors in the front and back. A torque wrench is used to tighten the pins to 6 to 8 pounds (2.7 to 3.6 kg) of tightness. Once the ring and bars are secured, the straps on the side of the vest are buckled. The scrub must ensure that the wrenches that come with the vest are sent with the patient after the procedure, in case the halo device must be removed in an emergency. Often the wrenches are taped to the front of the vest for easy access.

LUMBAR LAMINECTOMY AND DISCECTOMY

Surgical Goal

Lumbar laminectomy is performed to access the lumbar spinal cord and remove a portion of the lumbar lamina. Discectomy is performed to excise and remove a portion of the intervertebral disc.

Pathology

Lumbar laminectomy as a stand-alone procedure most often is performed to decompress the spinal column in cases of spinal stenosis; to gain access to a spinal cord tumor; or as a step in a more extensive surgery to correct a spinal deformity.

Discectomy is used to treat a herniation of the intervertebral disc. Disc herniation refers to a tear in the outer ring (annulus fibrosis) that allows the softer middle portion of the disc (nucleus pulposus) to bulge out (Figure 35-36). Disc herniation occurs most frequently between the fourth and fifth lumbar vertebrae or between the fifth lumbar vertebra and the sacrum. Disc herniation may be the result of general wear and tear or of a traumatic event, such as lifting while bent at the waist.

Technique

1. The patient is positioned prone on a laminectomy frame or in the knee-chest position on a spinal table.
2. The incision is marked and infiltrated with lidocaine and epinephrine.
3. A midline incision is made, and hemostasis is maintained as the tissue is dissected to the level of the fascia.
4. The fascia is incised, and the spinous processes are exposed.
5. Intraoperative radiographs are taken to confirm the correct vertebral level.
6. Bone is removed from the lamina.
7. Disc is removed as necessary.
8. The wound is closed in layers.
9. Bupivacaine may be injected into the soft tissue and musculature to reduce postoperative pain.

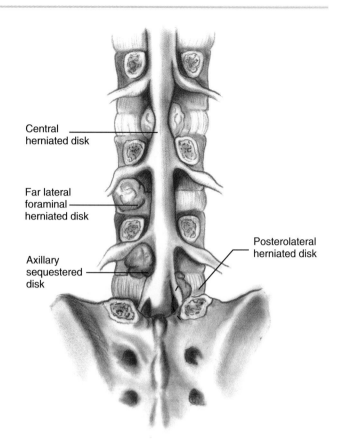

Figure 35-36 Lumbar laminectomy. Locations of possible disc hernias. *(From Vaccaro AR, Betz RR, Zeidman SM: Principles and practice of spine surgery, St Louis, 2003, Mosby.)*

Central herniated disk

Far lateral foraminal herniated disk

Axillary sequestered disk

Posterolateral herniated disk

Discussion

After induction and placement of an endotracheal tube, the patient is placed in the prone position on a laminectomy frame (e.g., Wilson or Jackson frame) or a specialized spinal operating bed.

To begin the procedure, the surgeon may inject the incisional site with a small amount of local anesthetic with epinephrine to aid hemostasis. A midline vertical incision is made over the spine with a #20 knife blade. The surgeon deepens the wound with the knife or monopolar ESU to the level of the fascia and incises the fascia with toothed forceps and the monopolar ESU. Two angled Weitlaner retractors are inserted into the wound for better exposure.

The scrub should have a large number of unfolded 4 × 4 sponges available at this time. The surgeon packs the sponges along the vertebra with periosteal elevators. This is done both to aid hemostasis and to expose the vertebrae by retracting the larger back muscles. Because the wound is now deep, the surgeon may replace the Weitlaner retractors with Beckman-Adson, Meyerding, or Taylor retractors (Figure 35-37). If Taylor retractors are used, the surgical technologist should have roller gauze available. The surgeon wraps the gauze around the tail of the retractor and drops the opposite end to the circulating nurse, who secures it to the table frame or a sandbag to keep the retractor in place.

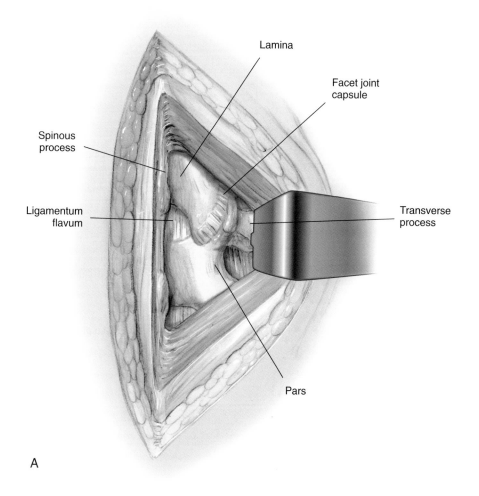

Spinous process

Ligamentum flavum

Lamina

Facet joint capsule

Transverse process

Pars

A

Figure 35-37 **A,** Lumbar laminectomy. Exposure of the vertebrae with a Hibbs retractor in place.

Continued

Intraoperative radiographs are obtained to confirm the correct vertebral level. The surgeon may request a spinal needle to mark the level or may clamp a towel clip through the spinous process. Generally, the radiographic cassette is loaded into a portable radiograph stand draped by the scrub. C-arm fluoroscopy may also be used.

The surgeon uses a large rongeur to remove small pieces of the spinous process and expose the lamina. Up-biting and down-biting Kerrison rongeurs then are used to excise the lamina and create access to the disc. The surgeon may also use a high-speed drill with a cutting burr to remove the bone. Any bone chips removed must be retained as specimens. After the lamina has been removed, cottonoid sponges are used instead of 4 × 4 sponges. To prevent the dura from tearing, the surgeon uses a dental probe or Freer-type elevator to loosen any dura attached to the lamina. The surgical technologist should be prepared with a small piece of bone wax on the end of a Penfield elevator or on the edge of a small medicine glass to aid hemostasis.

The surgeon identifies the yellowish ligamentum flavum (the ligament that connects each vertebra to the next) and

incises it with a #15 knife blade mounted on a #7 handle. Down-biting Kerrison rongeurs are used to remove any ligament that obstructs the surgeon's view of the disc. The disc is now approachable.

The assistant retracts the vertebral nerve with a Love retractor or similar nerve root retractor as the surgeon snips off pieces of the bulging disc with a Takahashi or pituitary rongeur. As the disc is removed, the surgeon may use a curette for further evacuation. The scrub must clean the tips of the instrument with each bite and keep the fragments as specimens. These specimens should be kept separate from the bone fragments previously retrieved. The scrub must remain alert during this maneuver, because the surgeon cannot turn away from the wound (because the risk of spinal cord damage is great).

After the herniated disc has been removed, the surgeon closes the wound. The fascial layer usually is closed with size 0 absorbable synthetic sutures and a large cutting needle. Before closing the muscle layer, the surgeon may inject a local anesthetic to control postoperative pain. The muscle and subcutaneous layers are closed with 2-0 sutures. The skin is

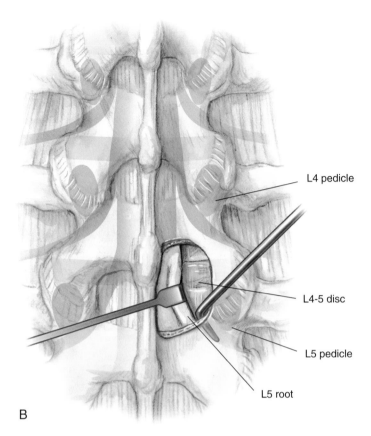

L4 pedicle

L4-5 disc

L5 pedicle

L5 root

B

Figure 35-37, cont'd   B, A Kerrison rongeur is used to decompress the lamina. *(From Miller MD, Chhabra AB, Hurwitz SR, Mihalko WM: Orthopaedic surgical approaches, Philadelphia, 2008, WB Saunders.)*

closed according to the surgeon's preference (a variety of materials may be used), and the wound is dressed in routine fashion.

FORAMINOTOMY

Foraminotomy is performed to relieve pressure on the spinal nerves. The spinal nerves pass through the intervertebral foramina as they branch off the spinal cord. When the nerves are compressed by bone, herniated disc, scarring, or ligament hypertrophy, the patient may experience symptoms of pain, numbness, or weakness in the area served by that particular nerve.

Foraminotomy often is an adjunct procedure to laminectomy, but it may also be performed as a minimally invasive, stand-alone procedure through a small incision. The surgeon widens the foramen with a high-speed drill or fine-tip rongeurs.

MICRODISCECTOMY

Surgical Goal

During microdiscectomy, a small window is made in the lamina for access to an intervertebral disc. This is a minimally invasive approach to lumbar laminectomy and discectomy.

Pathology

See Lumbar Laminectomy and Discectomy.

Technique

1. The patient is positioned prone on a laminectomy frame or in the knee-chest position on a spinal operating bed.
2. The incision is marked and infiltrated with lidocaine and epinephrine.
3. A guide needle is inserted through the skin under fluoroscopic visualization.
4. A guide wire is placed through the needle to confirm the correct vertebral level fluoroscopically.
5. Dilators in progressively larger sizes are placed over the guide wire to separate the muscles and expose the intralaminar space.
6. A tubular retractor is placed, and the dilating tubes are removed.
7. The operating microscope (or an endoscopic telescope) is used to visualize the spinal anatomy.
8. Bone is removed, and the nerve root is retracted.
9. The disc is removed.
10. The incision is closed if necessary.
11. A small dressing is applied.

Discussion

Microdiscectomy may be performed using general anesthesia, local anesthesia, or local anesthesia with sedation. The patient may be positioned in the lateral decubitus position, the prone position on a laminectomy frame, or in the knee-chest position on an Andrews table. If general anesthesia is used, induction and intubation take place before positioning. Some surgeons prefer using local anesthesia, because they feel they can better monitor the patient's responses to pain.

The surgeon injects the incision line with lidocaine with epinephrine to promote hemostasis. The C-arm is used to confirm placement of a guide needle through the skin to the level of the affected lamina. The surgeon passes a guide wire through the needle and removes the needle, leaving the guide wire in place. The scrubbed scrub should be prepared with a Crile clamp to secure the guide wire while the needle is removed.

A dilating tube is placed over the guide wire to separate the soft tissue and muscle. The surgeon removes the guide wire and leaves the dilating tube in place. A sequence of progressively larger tubes is placed over the existing tube to further dilate the space.

A tubular retractor is placed over the dilating tubes and docked on the lamina. The retractor is secured to a post that clamps onto the operating bed for stability. The dilating tubes are removed, leaving the retractor in place. The operating microscope is positioned and adjusted. Alternately, an endoscope attached to a camera and monitoring system may be used.

The scrub places a long electrode on the monopolar ESU, and the surgeon uses it through the tubular retractor to remove any remaining muscle or soft tissue overlying the lamina. A small window of bone is removed through the retractor with a Kerrison or Leksell rongeur. Some surgeons prefer to use a high-speed powered drill with a long cutting burr for removing the bone. The surgeon removes a window of bone, preserving the ligamentum flavum underneath to protect the dura.

A nerve root retractor is passed through the tubular retractor, and the nerve root is gently retracted. The epidural veins are coagulated with the bipolar ESU and dissected off the disc space. A special endoscopic knife is used to incise the disc surface. The surgeon uses standard disc rongeurs to remove any extruded portions of the disc. The nerve root retractor is removed, and the area is inspected visually. The surgeon irrigates the wound with normal saline to ensure that all debris is cleared and to visualize any bleeding areas. Any necessary hemostasis is accomplished with the bipolar ESU and Gelfoam pledgets soaked in topical thrombin.

The tubular retractor is removed. Because the wound is very small, minimal closure is necessary. The surgeon may use size 0 and 3-0 polyglactin for a layered closure and then 4-0 polyglactin for subcuticular closure. The wound edges are approximated with Steri-Strips or Dermabond glue.

LUMBAR FUSION

Surgical Goal

Lumbar fusion is performed to stabilize the spine using a bone graft or metal implant. The graft stimulates the growth of new bone between the vertebral elements, causing the area to fuse.

If necessary, metal implants are used to further stabilize the spine and offer greater support.

Pathology

A fusion may be required after laminectomy or as a means to stabilize traumatic or pathological fractures. Fusion may also be indicated after removal of a tumor or as a corrective procedure for spinal deformities. The technique described here details the procedure for a posterior lumbar interbody fusion with pedicle screws and rods.

Technique

1. A lumbar laminectomy is performed, and a bone graft is obtained.
2. The area where the screws will be placed is identified.
3. A high-speed drill with a cutting burr is used to remove the cortical surface of the bone.
4. The screw entrance hole is identified.
5. The screw hole is tapped and widened.
6. The pedicle screws are placed on either side of the vertebra, and guide pins are attached to the screw heads.
7. The bone graft is placed between the vertebrae.
8. An appropriate-size rod is selected, and connectors are placed over the rod.
9. The rod-connector assembly is threaded over the guide pins and secured.
10. Hemostasis is maintained, and a drain is placed.
11. The wound is closed in layers.
12. An external brace may be placed before the patient emerges from anesthesia.

Discussion

Two types of fusion are commonly used in the lumbar spine, posterolateral fusion and interbody fusion. Both types may be used independently or in conjunction with one another. In posterolateral fusion, the bone graft is placed between the transverse processes and fixed in place with screws (or wire) placed through the vertebral pedicles and attached to metal rods. In interbody fusion, the surgeon places the bone graft between the vertebrae in the area normally occupied by the intervertebral disc. The graft may or may not be secured with instrumentation.

The surgeon performs a laminectomy to prepare the area for fusion (refer to the discussion of lumbar laminectomy for the procedural steps). Using external landmarks and radiographic confirmation, the surgeon identifies the pedicle canal entry site and removes the cortical layer over the bone with a high-speed cutting burr. The scrub should be prepared with irrigation and suction while the surgeon is using the drill. Next, the surgeon places a bone probe through the entry site to determine its depth.

Pedicle markers are placed in the canal, and the proposed screw path is confirmed with real-time fluoroscopy with the C-arm or a lateral radiograph. After confirming the path, the surgeon taps the hole and widens it as appropriate for the screw configuration. The screw is placed in the pedicle until the base of the screw head makes contact with the bone. The process is repeated until the desired number of pedicle screws has been placed on either side of the spine.

A guide pin guide is positioned over the screw head, and a guide pin is threaded through it. The guide pin is tightened onto the screw, and the guide pin guide is removed. The process is repeated for each screw. When the screws are in place, the surgeon places the bone graft between the vertebrae.

The surgeon selects the rod to be used. Rods are available in a variety of diameters and lengths and can be customized for the patient with a rod bender and rod cutter. The surgeon places lateral connectors on to the rods and tightens the connector screws to secure the connectors to the rods. The connector-rod assembly is slid over the guide pins down to the pedicle screws. A lock nut is placed over the guide pin and secured over the connector. The guide pin is removed, and the process is repeated until all the connectors are secured to the pedicle screws. A screwdriver is used to tighten the lock nuts into place.

Hemostasis is maintained with the ESU, and the wound is irrigated with antibiotic solution. Gelfoam strips and Surgicel may also be used to aid hemostasis. The surgeon closes the wound in layers with size 0 or 1-0 absorbable synthetic suture and skin staples. To further immobilize the spine and promote patient comfort, the surgeon may place an external lumbar brace or jacket on the patient before the individual emerges from anesthesia.

CORRECTION OF SCOLIOSIS

Surgical Goal
Surgical correction of scoliosis is performed to restore anatomical alignment to the spine, prevent further curvature, and provide stability.

Pathology
Scoliosis is a three-dimensional spinal deformity. Typically, the spine is curved from side to side in an S or C concave-convex configuration. It also may have a degree of rotation. Scoliosis may occur in patients with muscular dystrophy or cerebral palsy, but in most cases the cause is unknown. The condition is familial and occurs more frequently in females than in males. Scoliosis usually is diagnosed during childhood or adolescence. Patients with scoliosis can have varying degrees of cosmetic deformity and may experience back pain and difficulty breathing as a result of rib cage compression. Many surgical procedures are available to provide correction and stabilization. Surgery involves the implantation of metal rods or other implants through an anterior or posterior approach and fusion with bone grafting. The hardware is designed to distract the spine and realign it to a more normal curvature, and fusion is used to maintain the new alignment. A basic posterior segmental rodding technique with hooks is described here.

Technique

1. The patient is positioned prone on a spinal operating bed. A bone graft will be obtained, therefore the position may be altered to provide access to the iliac crest.

2. The incisions are marked and infiltrated with lidocaine and epinephrine.
3. The bone graft is obtained.
4. A midline lumbar incision is made, and hemostasis is maintained.
5. The spinous processes are exposed, and the anatomical level is confirmed by radiographs.
6. Curettes and elevators are used to clear the soft tissue and ligament attachments over the vertebrae.
7. A facetectomy is performed, and a bone graft is placed.
8. The hook sites are prepared, and the hooks are placed.
9. The rods are prepared and attached to the hooks with connectors.
10. Distraction of the curves is achieved by bending the rods and securing them in the new position with the connectors and cross-links.
11. The bone graft is placed.
12. The wound is closed in layers; staples are used for skin closure.

Discussion
The patient is positioned prone on a spinal operating bed, and the surgeon marks the incision lines for a midline lumbar incision and an iliac crest bone graft. A bone graft is obtained and prepared as described in the procedure for an anterior cervical discectomy.

The surgeon performs a midline lumbar incision and maintains hemostasis with the monopolar ESU and digital pressure with 4×4 sponges. The incision is extended into deep tissue, and Weitlaner retractors are placed for exposure. A Cobb elevator is used to strip the periosteum off the spinous processes. The scrub should be prepared to provide a spinal needle or towel clamp to the surgeon for radiographic localization of the anatomical levels after the spinous processes have been prepared.

Once the anatomical levels have been confirmed, the surgeon uses curettes and pituitary rongeurs to clean the surface of the vertebrae. Larger self-retaining retractors are placed as needed to maintain exposure and aid visualization. The surgeon may use a high-speed drill with a cutting burr to decorticate the bone further in preparation for the fusion and instrumentation.

A thoracic facetectomy is performed by placing a cut through the facet at the base of the lamina and carrying it along the transverse processes, leaving the fragment hinged. An additional cut is made in the upper articular facet with a Cobb gouge to produce another hinged fragment. The surgeon places cancellous bone chips in the defects.

Next, the surgeon prepares the hook sites. Two types of hooks are used, *pedicle* and *laminar*. Pedicle hooks are used in the thoracic spine, and laminar hooks are used in other areas of the spine. The surgeon introduces a pedicle finder into the facet joint and enlarges the space as necessary with a drill. The pedicle hook is inserted and secured. The laminar hooks are temporarily placed on either the superior or inferior edge of the lamina, depending on the direction of distraction needed for correction of the curvature. The surgeon removes the laminar hooks and performs a lumbar facetectomy as previously described. The laminar hooks are replaced, and the surgeon prepares the rods.

The rods are available in a variety of lengths and curvatures. The surgeon can also customize the curvature using rod benders if necessary. After choosing and modifying the rods, if necessary, the surgeon places the rods into the hooks. The hooks are top loading. The surgeon places a set screw into the first hook where the rod is securely seated. If necessary, a rod cam or ratcheted rod reducer is used to manipulate the rods into place over the hooks. Once the rods are in place, the surgeon uses set screws to secure them to the hooks. At this point, the surgeon evaluates the distraction and compression by attaching cross-links to the rods and tightening the connectors.

A high-speed drill or Cobb elevator is used to decorticate the vertebral surfaces to prepare them for the bone graft. The bone graft is placed, and the wound is closed in layers as previously described for other spinal procedures. An external brace may be placed before the patient emerges from anesthesia to help maintain alignment and provide comfort.

SPINAL TUMORS

Surgical Goal

A spinal tumor is removed surgically to restore circulation of spinal fluid and increase patient mobility and also for pain management.

Pathology

Tumors of the spinal cord may be primary (the tumor is composed of cells derived from the nervous system) or secondary (arising from a distant or metastatic location). Primary tumors may be malignant or benign. Secondary tumors are always malignant.

Spinal tumors are differentiated according to their location; they are either extradural (outside the dura mater) or intradural (inside the dura mater). Intradural tumors can be further identified by their proximity to the spinal cord. Intramedullary tumors are found within the spinal cord, and extramedullary tumors are found inside the dura mater but outside the spinal cord.

Extradural tumors include sarcomas, carcinomas from a metastasis, lipomas, neurofibromas, chondromas, angiomas, granulomas, and abscesses. Intradural extramedullary tumors usually are benign tumors that originate either from the dura mater or from the arachnoid space around the spinal cord. Gliomas are the most common intramedullary tumors; they have a very poor prognosis because of their ability to infiltrate the cord, making them difficult to remove.

Technique

1. A laminectomy is performed, and the dura is exposed (see the lumbar laminectomy procedure for details).
2. The dura is incised and retracted with sutures.
3. The tumor is excised.
4. The dura is closed.
5. Wound closure proceeds as described for a laminectomy.

Discussion

During spinal surgery for tumor removal, a variety of materials or a dural graft may be needed to restore continuity of the dura. This is necessary for large, invasive tumors. Graft materials include a portion of the patient's pericranium, bovine pericardium, or biosynthetic dura substitutes. Handling techniques for the dural replacement materials vary, depending on the material and amount used. The scrub should anticipate the possibility of dural replacement in this procedure and ensure that the surgeon's preferred material is available, along with any items needed to prepare it.

The surgeon performs a laminectomy and then removes the ligamentum flavum with scissors, a scalpel, or Kerrison or Cloward rongeur. The epidural fat is removed, and the dura mater is exposed. The dura mater is elevated with a nerve hook, and the surgeon uses a #15 blade to nick it. Using a groove director, the surgeon extends the dural incision. The dural edges are retracted with 4-0 silk and dural needles. The cord then is exposed.

The tumor is identified, gently dissected free, and removed. Dissection can be performed with suction, bipolar ESU forceps, pituitary scoops, curettes, rongeurs, or the CUSA. Hemostasis is maintained with the bipolar ESU, cottonoids, hemostatic clips, Gelfoam, and topical hemostatic agents. The wound is irrigated, and the dura is tightly closed or a duraplasty is performed to ensure a watertight seal. Once the dura has been closed, wound closure progresses as described for a laminectomy.

NEUROSURGICAL PAIN MANAGEMENT

CORDOTOMY

Surgical Goal

The goal of cordotomy (or chordotomy) is to disable pain-conducting tracts in the spinal cord.

Pathology

A variety of conditions may cause severe or intractable pain. In these conditions, the nerve fibers may be damaged or injured, resulting in incorrect neural transmission and pain. Cordotomy is performed primarily on patients with somatic or visceral pain related to cancer. Somatic pain arises from pressure on ligaments, tendons, fascia, muscles, bone, and blood vessels. Patients with tumors in the legs, hips, chest, or abdominal space may report somatic pain. Visceral pain in cancer patients is characterized by cramping and aching and generally is related to extensive involvement of the pancreas, colon, or reproductive organs. Somatic cancer pain may be treated with an anterolateral cordotomy, whereas visceral pain requires a bilateral cordotomy.

Other conditions less commonly treated with a cordotomy include phantom limb pain (pain perceived to be located in an amputated limb), severe spinal cord injury, and pain associated with peripheral nerve injury.

A percutaneous cordotomy may be performed as a minimally invasive technique using stereotactic guidance to locate the tracts associated with enervated tissue and destruction of the nerve bundle with a thermoregulated cordotomy electrode. Open cordotomy is used if percutaneous cordotomy is not feasible or was previously unsuccessful. Regardless of the method used, cordotomy may require repeat surgery, because the effect of surgery diminishes over the first 6 months after the procedure.

Technique

1. A laminectomy is performed, and the dura is exposed.
2. The dura is incised and retracted with sutures.
3. The operating microscope is used to locate the nerve tract.
4. A specialized ball electrode is placed against the nerve tract, and radiofrequency current is applied.
5. The dura is closed.
6. The wound is closed.

Discussion

Electrophysiological nerve monitoring may be used in the procedure to monitor the spinal nerve responses to manipulation. The surgical technologist should be aware of the location of any electrodes placed in the patient before surgery to avoid dislodging them during the draping procedure. The operating microscope should be draped before the start of surgery.

The surgeon performs a laminectomy and opens the dura as previously described. The operating microscope is used to visualize the nerve tract and determine the depth for the electrode placement. Using careful blunt dissection with microsurgical instruments, the surgeon frees the dorsal root branches from the cord. The spinal cord must be slightly rotated to provide safe access to the nerve tracts. The surgeon places a silk suture through a clip and attaches the clip to the dentate ligament of the cord. The suture is used to gently put traction on the cord and rotate it approximately 45 degrees. A dental mirror is used to visualize the anterior spinal artery and other vascular structures. Blunt dissection continues until the correct spinal tract is identified.

A specialized ball electrode is inserted at the cordotomy site, and a grounding needle electrode is placed in the nearby paraspinal muscle. A radiofrequency signal is generated, causing a lesion in the area in direct contact with the ball electrode. The lesion prevents the transmission of pain signals to the area beyond it. If bilateral cordotomies are required, the procedure is repeated on the opposite side. When the procedure has been completed, the surgeon the wound is closed as described in the procedure for a spinal cord tumor.

RHIZOTOMY

Surgical Goal

Rhizotomy is performed to selectively sever nerve roots in the spinal cord to relieve severe pain or symptoms related to neuromuscular conditions, such as multiple sclerosis, or spasticity arising from cerebral palsy or spinal cord injury.

Pathology

(Refer to the Pathology section in the cordotomy procedure for a discussion of pain syndromes that may be amenable to rhizotomy.) Spasticity refers to a form of increased tone or tension in the muscles that occurs as a result of damage to the motor pathways from the CNS. Spasticity may occur in patients with cerebral palsy, multiple sclerosis, spinal cord injuries, and other disorders.

Technique

1. A laminectomy is performed, and the dura is exposed.
2. Ultrasound is used to locate the tip of the spinal cord where the separation of sensory and motor nerves occurs.
3. The dura is incised and retracted with sutures.
4. The operating microscope is used to expose and isolate the sensory nerves.
5. The nerves are tested with EMG for the degree of spasticity.
6. Selective nerves are severed.
7. The dura is closed
8. The wound is closed.

Discussion

The patient is positioned for a lumbar laminectomy. Electromyographic (EMG) electrodes are placed and tested before the skin prep is performed. The surgeon performs a multilevel lumbar laminectomy, as described in previous sections of the text, and exposes the spinal cord and spinal nerves.

Intraoperative ultrasound is used to identify the area where the sensory and motor nerves arise from the spinal cord. Only the sensory nerves are severed in a rhizotomy. The operating microscope is brought to the field, and the surgeon carefully identifies and isolates the sensory nerves using blunt dissection with microsurgical probes. The surgeon uses a Silastic pad to separate the sensory nerves from the motor nerves. It is important that the spinal cord and nerve roots stay moist. The scrub should be prepared with moistened cottonoids and periodic irrigation.

After the sensory nerves have exposed, the surgeon divides the nerve root into three to five rootlets and tests each one with the EMG. The EMG helps the surgeon identify which rootlets are responsible for the pain or spasticity response, because these rootlets show increased activity on the EMG recording. The surgeon uses microscissors to sever the nerve roots that show abnormal activity. The dura is closed, and the wound is irrigated with saline. Wound closure proceeds as described for lumbar laminectomy.

DORSAL COLUMN STIMULATOR

Surgical Goal

Implanted dorsal column stimulators are used to manage chronic pain. The device generates an electrical impulse that causes a tingling sensation, which alters the perception of pain by the patient.

Pathology

Dorsal column stimulators may be used to treat a variety of chronic pain conditions, such as intractable back pain, complex regional pain syndrome, phantom limb pain, and postherpetic neuralgia (severe localized pain that occurs after an attack of shingles).

Technique

1. A needle is placed into the epidural space, and the electrode is threaded through the needle and connected to a stimulator.
2. The patient is awakened, and the trial stimulator is activated.
3. The electrode is repositioned as necessary, and the stimulator is adjusted according to the patient's responses.
4. The stimulator is disconnected, and additional local anesthetic is infiltrated into the surrounding area.
5. The electrode is anchored and tunneled through the skin.
6. Any incisions are closed, and the electrode is reconnected to the trial stimulator.
7. The patient is discharged to home for 4 to 7 days to use the stimulator and determine whether the treatment will be effective.
8. The patient returns for phase 2 and is positioned and sedated as previously described.
9. The stimulator site is infiltrated with lidocaine and epinephrine.
10. A subcutaneous pocket is created, and the stimulator is placed in the pocket.
11. A tunneling tool is used to create a pathway from the stimulator to the previously implanted electrode.
12. The electrode is connected to the stimulator, and the incision is closed in layers.

Discussion

The dorsal column stimulator procedure is performed in two phases to allow for a trial period in which to determine whether the device will be effective at relieving the patient's pain. The procedure frequently is performed with the patient sedated, because the surgeon must be able to awaken the patient and ask questions during placement of the electrode.

During both phases, the patient is positioned prone on a fluoroscopic table and sedated. The procedure can be lengthy, therefore the patient is made as comfortable as possible and sedated. The surgeon infiltrates the patient's back with lidocaine with epinephrine. A 3-mL syringe filled with saline is attached to a 15-gauge Tuohy needle, and the needle is inserted through the skin and ligaments and maneuvered into the epidural space. During the placement, the surgeon gently presses the plunger of the syringe and notes the resistance of the saline solution to the pressure. Loss of resistance is considered an indication of entry into the epidural space.

The surgeon threads the electrode through the needle under fluoroscopic guidance. A stylet is included in the electrode to assist the surgeon in placement. Once the electrode is placed at the anatomical target, it is anchored and attached to a temporary cable, which is passed off the sterile field and attached to a trial stimulator. The patient is awakened, and the stimulator is activated. The patient is questioned about the presence or absence of sensations and their locations as the stimulator settings are adjusted.

After confirming the functioning of the device, the surgeon disconnects the electrode from the cable and makes a small vertical incision over the site of the Tuohy needle. The monopolar ESU is used for hemostasis, and Metzenbaum scissors are used to undermine the subcutaneous tissue. The surgeon

removes the Tuohy needle and electrode stylet, leaving the electrode in place. Next, the electrode is anchored with an anchoring device supplied by the manufacturer to prevent it from migrating.

The surgeon attaches the electrode to a percutaneous extension lead and tunnels it under the skin. The electrode remains under the skin, and a portion of the extension lead is brought out through the skin. The subcutaneous layers and skin are closed with polyglactin and staples. The externalized lead is attached to a temporary stimulator for a trial period of 4 to 7 days.

At the end of the trial period, the patient is questioned about the success of pain reduction. A 50% reduction of pain is considered an indicator of success and qualifies the patient to move to phase 2. If the trial was not successful, the electrode and extension lead are removed.

For the phase 2 procedure, the patient is positioned prone and sedated. The surgeon opens the previous midline incision and disconnects the extension lead from the electrode. Next, the site for stimulator placement is chosen. A variety of anatomical locations are suitable for the implantation, including the buttocks, abdomen, lateral chest, or subaxillary space.

The surgeon makes a horizontal incision over the proposed stimulator site and, using blunt and sharp dissection, creates a pocket large enough to house the stimulator. The monopolar ESU and 4 × 4 sponges are used for hemostasis. The pocket is purposely made shallow so that the stimulator can be easily programmed through a device held over the skin.

A small tunneler is used to connect the midline incision to the pocket. A new extension lead is attached to the electrode and passed through the tunneler to the pocket. The stimulator is placed in the pocket and connected to the extension lead. The surgeon closes the wound in layers with 3-0 polyglactin and staples. The device is activated after the procedure has been completed and the wound dressing applied.

PERIPHERAL NERVE PROCEDURES

CARPAL TUNNEL RELEASE

Surgical Goal
The goal of surgical carpal tunnel release is to free an entrapped median volar nerve and restore mobility of the wrist.

Pathology
Carpal tunnel syndrome occurs when the median nerve in the carpal tunnel of the wrist is compressed. A variety of factors may contribute to nerve compression, including an anatomical decrease in the size of the carpal tunnel, wrist fracture, posttraumatic arthritis, and inflammatory diseases such as rheumatoid arthritis. External conditions such as vibration, prolonged direct pressure, and repetitive movement may contribute to or trigger the condition.

Carpal tunnel syndrome most often occurs in adults 30 to 60 years of age and is more common in women than in men. Patients experience numbness and tingling in the fingers and pain in the hand that often radiates up the forearm.

Technique

1. A curvilinear or longitudinal incision is made in the palm and extended to the wrist.
2. The carpal ligament is retracted and divided.
4. Hemostasis is maintained.
5. The wound is closed.
6. A compression bandage and splint are applied.

Discussion

The patient is positioned supine on the operating room bed with the affected arm resting on a hand table. The procedure is performed using local infiltration, a regional nerve block (Bier block), or general anesthesia. A pneumatic tourniquet is used to create a bloodless field. (The procedure for application and use of a pneumatic tourniquet is discussed fully in Chapter 17.)

The surgeon uses a #15 blade to create a longitudinal or curvilinear incision in the skin. Blunt dissection with small Metzenbaum scissors is used to expose the fascia. The fascia is retracted with small Weitlaner retractors, skin hooks, or sharp Senn retractors. The flexor tendon is exposed and retracted. The surgeon identifies both the flexor tendon and the neurovascular bundle that lies close to the tendon. The carpal ligament then is well visualized, and the midsection is cut with either scissors or a knife blade to release the carpal ligament. The incision is irrigated with sterile saline.

Tourniquet pressure is released, and the wound is checked for bleeders, which are controlled with the bipolar ESU. The surgeon may inject the incision with bupivacaine to control postoperative pain. The skin is closed with an absorbable subcuticular suture. A bulky compression dressing using gauze fluffs and a splint is applied.

Carpal tunnel release may also be performed as minimally invasive surgery using Endo wrist instruments. The anesthesia considerations, prepping, draping, and tourniquet use are as described for the open carpal tunnel release. An advantage to the endoscopic approach is that it uses one or two small incisions over the palm of the hand instead of the extensive incision described for the open approach. The carpal ligament is directly below the incisions, in the distal area of the palm just below the wrist. The carpal ligament is cut longitudinally. This releases the pressure on the nerve as it passes through the ligament. The wound closure and dressing application are as described previously.

Postoperative Considerations

Carpal tunnel release most often is performed in the outpatient setting, and the patient is discharged within hours of the procedure. Immediate and long-term postoperative complications are rare, and the surgery generally has a high success rate.

ULNAR NERVE TRANSPOSITION

Surgical Goal

The surgical goal of an ulnar nerve transposition is to free the ulnar nerve from a groove on the medial epicondyle, thereby restoring function and eliminating desensitization of the affected arm.

Pathology

The ulnar nerve is a peripheral nerve that travels through the groove of the medial epicondyle from the upper to the lower arm. The ulnar nerve can be injured by trauma, elbow fractures and dislocations, and repeated bending of the elbow as part of occupational or recreational activities. Symptoms generally include reduced sensation in the affected arm, hand atrophy or, in severe cases, a claw hand deformity.

Technique

1. A long incision is made over the lateral elbow.
2. The muscles are divided.
3. The ulnar nerve is freed from the surrounding soft tissues.
4. The nerve is repositioned.
5. Hemostasis is maintained.
6. The wound is closed.

Discussion

The patient is placed in the supine position with the operative arm on an arm table, suspended over the patient, or laid across the patient's body, depending on the surgeon's preference. A pneumatic tourniquet is applied to the upper arm, and the procedure for exsanguination performed.

The surgeon makes the skin incision over the median epicondyle. Using blunt and sharp dissection with Metzenbaum scissors, the surgeon mobilizes the ulnar nerve. Delicate scissors are used to free a section of the nerve, and moist umbilical tapes, vessel loops, or a Penrose drain is looped around the nerve to aid manipulation.

The surgeon continues the dissection around the nerve to free a portion extending from above the elbow to below the elbow. A flap of fascia over the medial epicondyle is created with scissors. The nerve then is transposed (moved) from the groove at the back of the medial epicondyle of the humerus to the front of the epicondyle and positioned under the fascial flap. The fascial flap is loosely reapproximated with 2-0 Dexon suture to protect the nerve. The tourniquet pressure is released, and the wound is checked for bleeders. The bipolar ESU is used for hemostasis as needed. The wound is irrigated with sterile saline or an antibiotic solution and closed in layers with Dexon suture and dressed with gauze. A splint or cast is applied to the arm.

PERIPHERAL NERVE RESECTION AND REPAIR

Surgical Goal

In peripheral nerve repair, a severed nerve, usually in the hand or forearm, is anastomosed to restore function.

Pathology

Peripheral nerve injuries are commonly caused by industrial or home accidents involving tools or machinery. Successful repair depends on the patient's age, the extent of injury to adjacent tissue, and the type of injury to the nerve. An injury may be a clean-cut type (e.g., caused by a sharp object such as a knife or glass shard) or an injury that causes the nerve to shatter. If the nerve is severely damaged, it may be replaced with a nerve graft taken from another location in the body. The procedure described here is an upper extremity nerve repair.

Technique

1. The patient is prepared for routine hand or forearm surgery.
2. The wound is debrided if necessary.
3. The nerve is anastomosed.
4. The wound is closed and dressed with supportive material.

Discussion

The procedure to repair a severed peripheral nerve usually is performed as an emergency. If nerve repair is delayed, the risk of a poor outcome increases. Two common methods of peripheral nerve repair are the funicular suture technique and the epineural suture technique. In the funicular technique, the funiculi (the fibers that make up the nerve) are joined individually. In the epineural technique, the epineurium (the component of connective tissue that surrounds the nerve) is anastomosed, and the individual funiculi are not sutured together.

In preparation for peripheral nerve repair, the scrub should have microinstruments or eye instruments available, as well as an operating microscope or surgical loupes, bipolar ESU, nerve stimulator, and a physiological saline solution, such as that used in eye surgery. Fine 6-0, 7-0, and 10-0 sutures swaged to small cutting needles also are needed. The choice of suture material and size depends on the surgeon's preference, but monofilament nylon usually is used.

The patient is positioned supine with the affected arm or hand resting on a hand table. A pneumatic tourniquet is used as previously described. The procedure may be performed using general or regional anesthesia.

If the limb has been extensively damaged, the surgeon may want to debride (excise any devitalized or ragged tissue) before beginning the nerve repair. Debridement usually takes place in conjunction with the skin prep or immediately after it. If the surgeon wants to perform the skin prep and debridement, the scrub or circulator should supply the surgeon with copious amounts of sterile saline solution, sponges, antiseptic soap, a fine scalpel, tissue forceps, and dissecting scissors.

When debridement has been completed, the limb is draped in routine fashion and the tourniquet is inflated. Some surgeons drape the limb first and then perform the debridement. The first step of the actual procedure is the mobilization of the injured nerve. The surgeon uses fine dissecting scissors and thumb forceps to gently free the severed nerve from its surrounding tissue.

Before the anastomosis is started, the jagged ends of the nerve must be severed. Two fine traction sutures are placed through each end of the nerve and are used to bring the nerve ends into approximation. The surgeon incises the ends of the nerve with a #15 blade to ensure that the damaged fibers are removed and clean edges are available for the anastomosis. A moistened wooden tongue blade may be used as a firm surface on which to place the nerve. The nerve ends are cut serially in 1-mm slices under the operating microscope until the ends appear satisfactory for anastomosis (Figure 35-38).

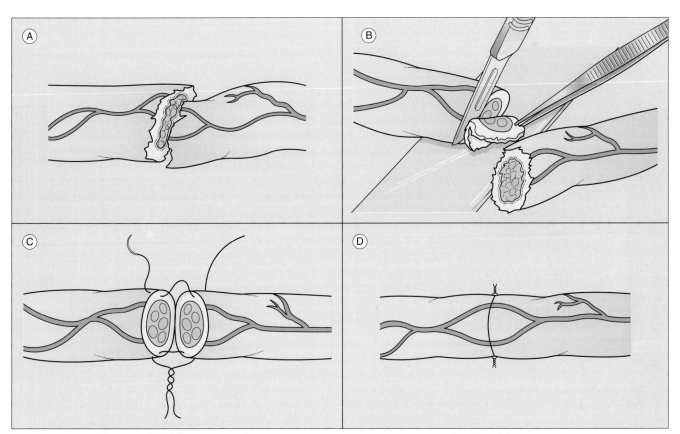

Figure 35-38 End-to-end nerve anastomosis. **A,** Tear injury. **B,** Debriding of the nerve. **C,** Placement of sutures through the epineurium. **D,** Completed repair. *(From Rengachary S, Ellenbogen R: Principles of neurosurgery, ed 2, St Louis, 2005, Mosby.)*

In the epineural technique, the surgeon places several 6-0 or 7-0 nylon sutures, one through each quadrant of the nerve. For funicular repair, each individual funiculus is joined with interrupted sutures of 10-0 nylon. During the anastomosis, the scrub should irrigate the nerve frequently with balanced saline solution, such as that used in eye surgery, to prevent the nerve from drying out.

After the repair, the tourniquet is released and the wound bed is inspected for bleeders. Hemostasis is maintained with the bipolar ESU, Gelfoam strips, and topical thrombin as necessary. The tissue layers are approximated with 3-0 and 4-0 polyglactin interrupted sutures. A dressing of cotton gauze and plaster splints or other casting material is used to immobilize the limb until healing is complete.

CHAPTER SUMMARY

- The nervous system is a communication center for the body; it receives, processes, and interprets information from the environment.
- The neuron is the main cell type in the nervous system.
- The skull covers the brain and protects it. It is composed of bony plates connected by a membrane called a *suture*.
- Directly beneath the skull lie the three protective coverings of the brain, the meninges. The outermost layer, the dura mater, is composed of very dense, fibrous tissue. The middle layer is the arachnoid mater.
- The brain is divided into three main sections: the forebrain, midbrain, and hindbrain.
- The ventricles are cavities within the brain. These four cavities lie between the various sections of the brain and are filled with cerebrospinal fluid, which bathes and nourishes the brain.
- The vertebral column provides structure and protects the spinal cord. There are 24 vertebra: 7 cervical, 12 thoracic, and 5 lumbar vertebrae. There are also 5 sacral and several coccygeal vertebrae, which are articulated in childhood but become fused in adulthood. The spinal cord is located within the vertebral canal and is continuous with the medulla oblongata of the hindbrain.
- The peripheral nervous system is composed of structures outside the CNS, such as the cranial and spinal nerves. It is further subdivided into the autonomic nervous system and the somatic nervous system.
- There are 35 pairs of spinal nerves that originate from the cord and are attached at various points along the length of the entire cord.
- The autonomic nervous system is an involuntary system that transmits signals for vital functions such as the heart rate, respiration, and digestion. It connects the CNS to the visceral organs via the cranial and spinal nerves.
- The somatic nervous system connects the CNS to the skin and skeletal muscles via the cranial and spinal nerves.
- Instruments used in neurosurgery include general surgery instruments, microinstruments, and neurovascular instruments.
- Powered instruments, such as the pneumatic drill and craniotomy, are used in neurosurgery because the brain and spinal cord are protected by bone.

- Specialty sponges used in neurosurgery are accounted for, as in all surgical procedures in which the risk exists that an item can be lost in the wound.
- Patient positioning for cranial and back procedures requires specialty equipment to stabilize the operative site and provide clear visualization of the wound.
- The Andrews table is often used in back surgery. The patient is placed in the prone kneeling position.
- Cranial surgery may require removal of the some of the patient's hair. The head is not fully shaved except in rare circumstances.
- Burr holes are drilled into the cranium to release intracranial pressure and to create a bone flap for access to the brain. An incision into the cranium for any reason is called a craniotomy. Craniotomy often is performed as an emergency procedure after head trauma.
- A bone flap is created in the cranium by drilling burr holes and making cuts in the bone between the holes. The flap may be left in placed by a hinge of tissue or completely removed during surgery.
- Cerebral aneurysms are surgically removed when they cannot be managed by interventional radiological means.
- Surgical procedures involving the vascular system of the brain require advanced surgical technological skills. Neurovascular procedures are extremely delicate and carry a high risk of an intraoperative emergency.
- Brain tissue does not have sensory nerves, therefore procedures can be performed under local anesthesia with monitored sedation.
- The scalp bleeds profusely when incised. It therefore is injected with a vasoconstrictor (e.g., epinephrine) in a local anesthetic before a craniotomy. Scalp clips are placed on the edges of the wound to prevent bleeding during surgery.
- Methylmethacrylate cement commonly is used to form a replacement implant for cranial bone. The fumes given off during mixing are highly toxic, therefore a closed system device is required for mixing.
- Hemostasis is meticulously maintained during a craniotomy. The cranium is a closed cavity, and any pressure from excess fluid, such as blood, can impinge on brain tissue, causing injury and permanent damage.

- Surgical procedures of the pituitary gland are approached from the sphenoid bone intranasally. The surgical team therefore includes an otorhinolaryngologist to assist.
- Procedures of the pituitary require techniques and instruments across two specialties, neurosurgery and nasal surgery.
- Surgery of the spinal column commonly is performed to release pressure on the spinal cord and nerves that exit the cord within the bony lamina.
- Techniques used in back surgery require orthopedic and neurosurgical skills. Microinstruments are used during most procedures.
- Positioning of the patient for back surgery may be done after induction of anesthesia and intubation. Maneuvering of an unconscious patient requires adequate, trained staff to prevent serious injury.

- Stabilization of the spinal column may be achieved with bone grafts, plates, or rods.
- A diseased intervertebral disc is removed (discectomy) if the disc impinges on nerves, causing pain and dysfunction. Surgery is performed only when conservative measures have failed.
- External stabilization of the cervical spine is required after trauma to the spine or in surgical procedures. The most common type is the halo brace.
- Peripheral nerve repair is performed to restore function and relieve chronic pain. Surgery of the hand and forearm can be vital for returning the patient to normal activities and livelihood.
- Industrial and home injuries to large peripheral nerves often require emergency surgery to prevent permanent loss of nerve function.

REVIEW QUESTIONS

1. Why is hemostasis particularly important during cranial surgery?
2. How is excess cerebrospinal fluid surgically shunted out of the brain?
3. What precautions should be taken to prevent loss or damage of the bone flap during craniotomy?
4. Why are burr holes required to remove a bone flap?
5. Name several specialty instrument sets that might be needed during neurosurgery (e.g., orthopedic set).
6. Neurosurgical procedures can be quite lengthy. What safety and environmental precautions are particularly important to protect the patient from injury during a long procedure?
7. Fowler position carries a high risk of embolism. Explain why.
8. Why is a subdural hematoma an emergency condition?
9. What methods of hemostasis are used during cranial surgery?
10. During laminectomy, small bits of bone are removed from the lamina in rapid succession. What is the role of the scrub during this part of the procedure?
11. In what cranial procedures might a fat graft be needed?
12. Describe the supplies that might be needed for debridement of a hand after an industrial accident.

BIBLIOGRAPHY

Asthagiri A, Pouratian N, Sherman J, Ahmed G, Shaffrey M: Advances in brain tumor surgery, *Neurologic Clinics* 25:975, 2007.

Baron EM: Cervical spondylosis: diagnosis and management. Accessed July 13, 2008, at http://www.emedicine.com/neuro/topic564.htm.

Brackmann DE, Green JD: Translabyrinth approach for acoustic tumor removal, *Neurosurgery Clinics of North America* 19:251, 2008.

Brown JA: Principles of pain management. In Rengachary SS, Ellenbogen RG, editors: *Principles of neurosurgery*, ed 2, St Louis, 2005, Mosby.

Drake JM, Iantosca MR: Cerebrospinal fluid shunting and management of pediatric hydrocephalus. In Schmidek HH, Roberts DW, editors: *Operative neurosurgical techniques: indications, methods and results*, ed 5, Philadelphia, 2006, WB Saunders.

Drummond JC, Patel PM: Neurosurgical anesthesia. In Miller RD: *Miller's anesthesia*, ed 6, Philadelphia, 2005, Churchill Livingstone.

Fanciullo GJ, Ball PA: Spinal cord stimulation and intraspinal infusions for pain. In Schmidek HH, Roberts DW, editors: *Operative neurosurgical techniques: indications, methods and results*, ed 5, Philadelphia, 2006, WB Saunders.

Freeman BL: Scoliosis and kyphosis. In Canale ST, Beaty JH, editors: *Campbell's operative orthopaedics*, ed 11, Philadelphia, 2008, Mosby.

Harrop JH: Spinal cord tumors: management of intradural intramedullary neoplasms. Accessed July 18, 2008, at http://www.emedicine.com/Med/topic2905.htm.

Jobe MT, Martinez SF: Peripheral nerve injuries. In Canale ST, Beaty JH, editors: *Campbell's operative orthopaedics*, ed 11, Philadelphia, 2008, Mosby.

Kolaski K: Myelomeningocele. Accessed June 28, 2008, at http://www.emedicine.com/pmr/TOPIC83.HTM.

Lonser RR, Apfelbaum RI: Neurovascular decompression in surgical disorders of cranial nerves V, VII, IX, and X. In Schmidek HH, Roberts DW, editors: *Operative neurosurgical techniques: indications, methods and results*, ed 5, Philadelphia, 2006, WB Saunders.

MGI Pharma: How to use Gliadel wafers. Accessed July 4, 2008, at http://www.gliadel.com/hcp/about/how.aspx.

Polletti CE: Open cordotomy and medullary tractotomy. In Schmidek HH, Roberts DW, editors: *Operative neurosurgical techniques: indications, methods and results*, ed 5, Philadelphia, 2006, WB Saunders.

Qureshi NH, Harsh G: Skull fracture. Accessed June 28, 2008, at http://www.emedicine.com/med/TOPIC2894.HTM.

Roberts GA, Dacey RG: General techniques of aneurysm surgery. In LeRoux PD, Winn HR, Newell DW, editors: *Management of cerebral aneurysms*, Philadelphia, 2004, WB Saunders.

Schmidek HH, Roberts DW: Schmidek and Sweet's *Operative neurosurgical techniques: indications, methods and results*, ed 5, Philadelphia, 2006, WB Saunders.

Seidel HM, Ball JW, Dains JE, Benedict GW, editors: *Mosby's guide to physical examination*, ed 6, St Louis, 2007, Mosby.

Shen FH, Samartzis D, Khanna AJ, Anderson DG: Minimally invasive techniques for lumbar interbody fusions, *Orthopedic Clinics of North America* 38:373, 2007.

St-Arnaud D, Paquin M: Safe positioning for neurosurgical patients, *AORN Journal* 87:1156, 2008.

Sugarman RA: Structure and function of the neurologic system. In McCance KL, Huether SE, editors: *Pathophysiology: the biologic basis for disease in adults and children,* ed 5, St Louis, 2006, Mosby.

Sutton LN: Spinal dysraphism. In Rengachary SS, Ellenbogen RG, editors: *Principles of neurosurgery,* ed 2, St Louis, 2005, Mosby.

Tarlov EC, Magge SN: Microsurgery of ruptured lumbar intervertebral disc. In Schmidek HH, Roberts DW, editors: *Operative neurosurgical techniques: indications, methods and results,* ed 5, Philadelphia, 2006, WB Saunders.

US Food and Drug Administration, Medical Device Reporting (website). Accessed June 29, 2008, at http://www.fda.gov/cdrh/devadvice/.

Wang PP, Avellino AA: Hydrocephalus in children. In Rengachary SS, Ellenbogen RG, editors: *Principles of neurosurgery,* ed 2, St Louis, 2005, Mosby.

Wright PE: Carpal tunnel, ulnar tunnel, and stenosing tenosynovitis. In Canale ST, Beaty JH, editors: *Campbell's operative orthopaedics,* ed 11, Philadelphia, 2008, Mosby.

Yaremchuk MJ: Surgical repair of major defects of the scalp and skull. In Schmidek HH, Roberts DW, editors: *Operative neurosurgical techniques: indications, methods and results,* ed 5, Philadelphia, 2006, WB Saunders.

Yeung AT, Yeung CA: Minimally invasive techniques for the management of lumbar disc herniation, *Orthopedic Clinics of North America* 38:363, 2007.

Glossary

AAMI: Association for the Advancement of Medical Instrumentation. The AAMI is an authoritative source of standards for sterilization and disinfection.

Abandonment: A health professional's failure to provide care to a patient, especially when there is an implied contract to do so. Examples include leaving the operating room during a surgical case without transferring care to another person, and leaving a patient on a stretcher alone in the hallway.

Abdominal adhesions: Bands of scar tissue on the outer membranes of the abdomen and the abdominal wall.

Abdominal peritoneum: The serous membrane lining the walls of the abdominal cavity. The *retroperitoneum* is the posterior aspect. In surgical discussions, *abdominal* usually refers to the anterior aspect.

Abduction: Movement of a joint or body part away from the body.

Ablate: To remove or destroy tissue.

Ablation: The complete destruction of tissue.

ABO blood groups: Inherited antigens found on the surface of an individual's red blood cells. These antigens identify the blood group (i.e., type A blood has type A antigens). Also known as blood types.

Absorbable suture: Suture material that is broken down and digested by the cell's lysosomal enzymes. It is then absorbed by the body.

Accommodation: A process in which the lens continually changes shape to maintain the focus of an image on the retina.

Accreditation: The process by which a hospital is evaluated by an independent organization, which examines the hospital's practices, records, procedures, and outcomes.

Accupuncture: An alternative health therapy in which fine needles are inserted into energy "meridians" of the body for the treatment of disease.

Acoustic neuroma: A benign tumor of the eighth cranial nerve; more accurately referred to as a *schwannoma,* because it is composed of Schwann cells, which produce myelin.

Acquired abnormality: A physiological or anatomical defect that develops in fetal life as a result of environmental factors, such as exposure to infection or certain drugs or poor nutrition.

Acquired immunity: Disease immunity established through cellular memory following exposure to the disease antigen.

ACS: American College of Surgeons. A professional organization that establishes educational standards for surgeons and surgical residency programs.

Active electrode: In electrosurgery, the point of the electrosurgical instrument that delivers current to tissue.

Active electrode monitoring (AEM): A method of reducing the risk of patient burns during monopolar electrosurgery. AEM systems monitor the impedance of the instruments and stop the flow of electricity when it reaches a critical level.

Active immunity: Production of antibodies that combat a specific disease. Acquired by contracting the disease or by vaccination.

Activities of daily living (ADLs): Basic activities and tasks necessary for day-to-day care, such as dressing, bathing, toileting, and meal preparation.

Acute illness: Sudden onset of disease or trauma or disease of short duration, usually 3 weeks or less.

Adduction: Movement of a body part toward the midline.

Adenoma: A benign tumor consisting of glandular tissue.

Adhesion: Scar formation, particularly of the abdominal viscera.

Administrative law: A law created by an agency or a department of the government.

Adnexa: A collective term for the ovaries, fallopian tubes, and their connective and vascular attachments.

Advance directive: A document in which a person gives instructions about his or her medical care in the event that the individual cannot speak for himself or herself. Examples are a living will and a medical power of attorney.

Adverse reaction: An unexpected reaction to a drug that is not related to dose.

Aerobes: Organisms that favor an environment with oxygen. Strict aerobes cannot live without oxygen.

Aerosol droplet: A droplet of moisture small enough to remain suspended in the air; it can carry microorganisms within it.

Aesthetic surgery: Surgery that is performed to improve appearance but not function; also called *cosmetic surgery.*

Aggression: The exertion of power over others through intimidation, loudness, sarcasm, or bullying.

Agonist: A drug that potentiates the release or uptake (or both) of a particular neurotransmitter.

Air exchange: The exchange of fresh air for air that has been recirculated in a closed area.

Airborne contamination: An incident of contamination in which microorganisms carried in the air by moisture droplets or dust particles make contact with a sterile surface.

Airborne transmission precautions: Precautions that prevent airborne transferral of disease organisms in the environment.

Airway: The anatomical passageway or artificial tube through which the patient breathes.

Aldrete scale: A numerical scale used to measure physiological and neurological criteria for discharge to the hospital unit (ward).

Allergy: Hypersensitivity to a substance, a response produced by the immune system.

Allied health profession: A profession that follows the principles of medicine and nursing but that focuses on an expertise set apart from those practices.

Allograft: A tissue graft in which the donor and recipient are of the same species.

Alloys: Substances that are mixtures of pure metals.

Alternating current (AC): A type of electrical current in which electricity changes direction to complete its circuit.

Amnesia: The loss of recall of events or sensations.

Amniotic fluid: Water around the fetus in the uterus.

Amniotic membranes: Two membranes that encase the fetus, amniotic fluid, and placenta during pregnancy.

Amplification: In wave science, the phenomenon of increasing wave height by lining up the peaks and troughs of individual waves.

Amplitude: In electromagnetic wave energy, the height of a wave.

Anaerobes: Organisms that prefer an oxygen-poor environment. Strict anaerobes cannot survive in the presence of oxygen.

Analgesia: The absence of pain, produced by specific drugs.

Anaphylactic shock: A type I hypersensitive immune reaction that occurs in response to previous sensitization to a substance, usually a protein. Anaphylactic shock can be quickly fatal.

Anaphylaxis: A life-threatening allergic reaction to a drug or substance.

Anastomosis: The surgical creation of an opening between two blood vessels, hollow organs, or ducts.

Anesthesia: The absence of sensory awareness or medically induced unconsciousness.

Anesthesia care provider (ACP): A professional who is licensed to administer anesthetic agents and manage the patient throughout the period of anesthesia.

Anesthesia machine: A biotechnical device used to deliver anesthetic gases or volatile liquids and provide physiological monitoring.

Anesthesia technician: An allied health professional trained to assist the anesthesia care provider.

Anesthesiologist: A physician specialist in the administration of anesthetics and pain management.

Anesthetic: A drug that reduces or blocks sensation or induces unconsciousness.

Aneurysm: Dilation or ballooning of an artery wall as a result of injury, disease, or a congenital condition. It may be caused by atherosclerosis, infection, or a hereditary defect in the vascular system.

Angioplasty: Dilation of an artery using endovascular techniques (i.e., an arterial catheter); may include insertion of a supportive stent inside the artery to maintain blood flow.

Antagonist: A drug that counteracts the effects of another agent or physiological process.

Antegrade amnesia: In anesthesia, the patient's inability to recall events that occur after the administration of specific drugs. After the drug is metabolized and cleared from the body, normal recall returns.

Antibiotic: A chemical agent used specifically for the treatment of bacterial infection.

Antibiotic resistant: A microorganism that is able to resist destruction by antimicrobial therapy.

Antibodies: Complex glycoproteins produced by the immune system that are formed in response to antigens. An antibody makes contact with an antigen to destroy or control it.

Anticoagulant: A drug that prolongs blood clotting time.

Antigens: Macromolecules (e.g., proteins, glycoproteins, lipoproteins, and polysaccharides) on the surface of cells that identify them as part of the organism ("self") or foreign ("nonself"). Antigens can trigger a response by the immune system, which seeks out and destroys the marked cell.

Antisepsis: A process that greatly reduces the number of microorganisms on skin or other tissue.

Antiseptics: Chemical agents approved for use on the skin that inhibit the growth and reproduction of microorganisms. Antiseptics are used to cleanse and paint the surgical site to reduce the number of microorganisms to an absolute minimum.

Anxiolytic: A drug that reduces anxiety.

AORN: Association of periOperative Registered Nurses. The professional organization for surgical nurses; originally known as the Association of Operating Room Nurses.

Apex: The lower left tip of the left ventricle of the heart; also, the rounded upper portion of each lung.

APGAR score: Method of assessing neonate according to respiratory rate, color, reflex response, heart rate, and body tone.

Apnea: A period of cessation of breathing.

Aponeurosis: A tendinous sheet that separates muscles or attaches a muscle to bone.

Approximate: To bring tissue together by sutures or other means.

ARC/STSA: Accreditation Review Council on Education in Surgical Technology and Surgical Assisting. The ARC/STSA establishes, maintains, and promotes quality standards for education programs in surgical technology and surgical first assisting.

Argon: An inert gas used in electrosurgery to direct and shroud the electrical current.

Arrhythmia: An abnormal heartbeat (also called *dysrhythmia*).

Arterial blood gases (ABGs): A blood test that measures the level of oxygen and carbon dioxide and the pH of the blood.

Arteriosclerosis: A disease characterized by thickening, hardening, and loss of elasticity of the arterial wall.

Arteriotomy: An incision made in an artery, usually to perform an anastomosis with a graft or another artery or to remove plaque or a thrombus.

Arteriovenous: Relating to both arteries and veins.

Arteriovenous fistula (or shunt [AV shunt]): Surgical creation of vascular access for patients undergoing hemodialysis.

Arteriovenous malformation (AVM): A collection of blood vessels with abnormal communication between the arteries and veins. It may be the result of injury, infection, or a congenital condition.

Arthrodesis: Surgical fusion of a joint.

Arthroscopy: Endoscopic assessment and surgery of a joint.

Articulated: A jointed structure. In mechanics, an articulated arm is one with joints to allow movement of the structure.

Asepsis: The absence of pathogenic microorganisms on an animate surface or on body tissue. Literally, *asepsis* means "without infection." In surgery, asepsis is a state of minimal or zero pathogens. Asepsis is the goal of many surgical practices.

Aseptic technique: Methods or practices in health care that reduce infection.

Aspiration: Inhalation of fluid or solid matter.

Assertiveness: A quality in people with self-esteem; assertive behavior seeks to protect one's own rights while respecting those of others.

Assignment board: A large, erasable board that lists scheduled surgical cases and assigned personnel. The board is kept in a central location in the restricted area of the surgical department.

Assisted suicide: Intentional harm to a person, at their request, in order to cause death.

AST: Association of Surgical Technologists. The professional association for surgical technologists (Web site: http://www.ast.org).

Astrocytes: Cells that support the nerve cells (neurons) of the brain and spinal cord by providing nutrients and insulation.

Asystole: The absence of a heartbeat; cardiac standstill.

Atherosclerosis: The most common form of arteriosclerosis, which causes plaque to form on the inner surface of an artery.

Atom: A discrete unit made of matter consisting of charged particles.

Atomic number: The number of protons in an atom of a specific element.

Atomic weight: The combined weight of an atom's protons and neutrons.

Atresia: The absence or closure of an orifice or tubular structure.

Augment: To enlarge a structure.

Auscultation: Listening to the lungs, heart, or abdomen through the stethoscope.

Autoclave: A small steam sterilizer used in low volume clinical settings.

Autograft: A tissue graft taken from the patient. Autograft sites are usually prepped at the same time as the primary operative site.

Autoinfection: The spread of infection from one part of the body to another part.

Auxiliary water channel: A channel in the flexible endoscope used to deliver irrigation fluid at the tip.

Bacilli: Rod-shaped bacteria that occur in pairs, chains, or filaments.

Bactericidal: Able to kill bacteria.

Bacteriology: The study of bacteria.

Bacteriophage: A virus that invades bacterial cells and can replicate from within the cell.

Bacteriostatic: Chemical agent capable of inhibiting the growth of bacteria.

Bacterium (sing); bacteria (pl): A unicellular microorganism with a rigid cell wall.

Balanced anesthesia: A somewhat outdated term used to describe the use of multiple drugs to produce sedation, analgesia, amnesia, and muscle relaxation during general anesthesia.

Balloon dissector: A balloon device used to separate tissue planes during minimally invasive surgery.

Barium sulfate: An opaque contrast medium used in imaging studies of the gastrointestinal tract.

Barrier drape: A drape intended to separate a contaminated area from the incision site. For example, a barrier drape is placed across the perineum between the vagina and anus during gynecological procedures.

Basic metabolic panel: Blood test commonly performed to measure metabolic markers such as electrolytes and other essential elements.

Benign: A term used to characterize a tumor that does not have the capability to spread to other parts of the body and usually is composed of tissue similar to its tissue of origin.

Benign prostatic hypertrophy (BPH): Nonmalignant enlargement of the prostate gland, which occurs mainly in men over age 40.

Bicoronal incision: An incision made between the frontal and the parietal bones bilaterally.

Bicortical screws: Screws that penetrate both cortical layers and the intervening spongy layer of the bone.

Bier block: Regional anesthesia in which the anesthetic agent is injected into a vein.

Bifurcation: A tube, duct, or other hollow structure that forms a Y split.

Bile: A digestive substance produced by the liver. Its main function is to emulsify fats (i.e., break them into small particles) so that the body can digest them.

Biliary system: The organ system that includes the gallbladder, hepatic ducts, common bile duct, and cystic duct.

Billroth I procedure: A gastroduodenostomy, or surgical anastomosis, of the stomach and the duodenum.

Billroth II procedure: A gastroduodenostomy, or surgical anastomosis, of the stomach and the jejunum.

Bilobate: Having two lobes.

Bioactive implant: An orthopedic implant which releases calcium to enhance healing.

Bioavailability: The extent and rate at which a drug or its metabolites (products of breakdown) enter the systemic circulation and reach the site of action.

Biocompatibility: A term that describes a material that is compatible with tissue (i.e., causes no toxic or inflammatory effect).

Biofilm: A matrix of extracellular polymers produced by microorganisms. These substances bind the microorganisms tightly to a living or nonliving surface, making them highly resistant to antimicrobial action. Biotin increases the risk of disease transmission on internal medicine devices such as catheters and endoscopic instruments.

Biological graft: A graft derived from live tissue, whether human or animal.

Biological indicator: A quality control mechanism used in the process of sterilization. It consists of a closed system containing harmless, spore-forming bacteria that can be rapidly cultured after the sterilization process.

Biomechanics: The relationship between movement and biological or anatomical structures.

Biomedical technologists: Professionals who specialize in the maintenance, repair, and safe operation of devices used in medicine, including surgical equipment.

Biopsy: Removal of a sample of tissue for pathological analysis.

Biopsy channel: A channel that extends the full length of a flexible endoscope and is used to retrieve biopsy tissue.

Bipolar circuit: An electrosurgical circuit in which current travels from the source of electricity through an instrument containing two opposite poles in contact with the tissue and then returns directly to the energy source.

Birth canal: The maternal pelvis and soft structures through which the baby passes during birth.

Bispectral index system (BIS): A monitoring method used to determine the patient's level of consciousness and prevent intraoperative awareness.

Bladder flap: A peritoneal fold between the bladder and the uterus.

Blebs: Areas of overdistention in the lung tissue.

Bleeder: A bleeding vessel.

Blended mode: The electrosurgical waveform in which current is intermittently pulsed on and off and combined with intermediate high-frequency energy.

Blood-borne pathogens: Harmful microorganisms that may be present in and transmitted through human blood and body fluids (e.g., the hepatitis B virus [HBV] and the human immunodeficiency virus [HIV]).

Blunt dissection: The technique of separating tissue layers by teasing them apart with a rough sponge dissector.

Blunt needle: A curved, tapered needle with a blunt point that is used for highly vascular organs, such as the liver.

Body image: The way individuals perceive themselves physically in the eyes of others.

Boggy: Soft, doughy; a characteristic of diseased tissue.

Boiling point: The temperature of a substance when its state changes from a liquid to a gas.

Bolsters: Tubing through which retention sutures are threaded to prevent them from cutting into the patient's skin.

Bolus: A compact substance (e.g. undigested food, fecal material) which occurs normally in the digestive tract.

Bolus injection: A single dose of medication administered all at one time.

Bolus: A compact substance (e.g. undigested food, fecal material) which occurs normally in the digestive tract.

Bone flap: A section of bone removed from the skull during craniotomy procedures.

Bone wax: A pliable, waxy dough made from synthetic material used to control capillary bleeding on the surface of bone.

Bowel technique: A method of preventing cross-contamination between the bowel contents and the abdominal cavity.

Box lock: The hinge point of many surgical instruments.

Brachytherapy: The implantation of small pellets of radioactive material to destroy tumors.

Bradycardia: A slow heart rate (usually a heart rate under 60 beats per minute).

Breathing bag: The reservoir breathing apparatus of the anesthesia machine. Gases are titrated and shunted into the breathing bag, which is connected to the patient's airway.

Breech presentation: Presentation of the baby in which the buttocks or feet deliver first.

Bridle suture: In ophthalmic surgery, a temporary traction suture placed through the sclera and used to pull the globe laterally for exposure of the posterolateral surface. It is called a *bridle suture* because of its resemblance to the reins of a horse's bridle.

Broach: A fin-shaped rasp used to enlarge the medullary canal for insertion of an implant. The broach is the same shape as the implant.

Bronchospasm: An involuntary smooth muscle spasm of the bronchi. Also, the partial or complete closure of the bronchial tubes.

Brown and Sharp (B & S) sizing system: A sizing standard used to measure the diameter of wire or stainless steel.

Burn intensive care unit (ICU): A critical care unit for severely burned patients.

CAAHEP: Commission on Accreditation of Allied Health Education Programs. The CAAHEP is an organization that accredits health science programs, including those for surgical technology.

Calculi: Stones caused by the precipitation of minerals, such as calcium, and other substances from the urine or kidney filtrate.

Camera control unit (CCU): The main control source for the video camera. The unit captures video signals from the camera head and processes them for display on the monitor.

Canalplasty: A procedure in which the external auditory canal is reconstructed.

Cannula: In minimally invasive surgery, a cannula is a slender tube inserted through the body wall and used to receive and stabilize telescopic instruments.

Cannulated: A device having a hollow core; for example, an instrument with a central channel that can be fitted over a guide wire or pin.

Capacitive-coupled return electrode: A design of patient return electrode in which the patient is in contact with the capacitive-coupled system.

Capacitive coupling: In minimally invasive surgery, the unintended transmission of electrical current to pass randomly through a nonconductive medium and across a conductive material, sometimes resulting in a patient burn.

Capacitor: A point in an electrical circuit where energy (usually heat or light) builds up or is stored between insulators.

Capillary action: The ability of suture material to absorb fluid.

Capsule: With regard to cells, a surface layer on some cells that resists chemicals and the invasion of viruses; also called a slime layer.

Carbon dioxide: An inert gas used as a lasing medium during laser surgery.

Cardioplegia: Intentional stopping of the heart during cardiac surgery. This is achieved with a cardioplegic solution, which often contains a mixture of potassium chloride, lidocaine, dextrose, insulin, albumin, tromethamine, and Plasmanate.

Carrier: An individual who harbors disease microbes and is capable of transmitting the disease to others but may not show signs of the infection.

Case cart system: Organizational method of preparing equipment and instruments for a specific surgery. Equipment is prepared by the central services or supply department and sent to the operating room.

Case planning: The process of organizing the tasks and equipment required for a surgical procedure. Case planning requires the ability to prioritize, organizational skills, and a knowledge of the procedure.

Case setup: A time-related set of procedures in which sterile supplies are distributed and arranged on the sterile table.

Casting: A method of immobilizing a limb by the application of rigid or semi-rigid material along the length of the limb. A cast can be fully or partially circumferential.

Cataract: Clouding of the eye, caused by a disease in which the crystalline lens of the eye, its capsule, or both become opaque. This prevents light from focusing on the retina, resulting in visual distortion. Cataracts may develop as a result of disease or injury.

Cauterization: The use of a hot object to burn tissue to achieve coagulation.

Cavitation: A process in which air bubbles are imploded (burst inward), releasing particles of soil or tissue debris.

Cell theory: An early hypothesis in biology that stated that cells are the basic unit of all living things, cells are derived from other cells, and all living things are composed of cells.

Cell wall: A rigid structure surrounding certain types of cells.

Centers for Disease Control and Prevention (CDC): The U.S. government agency that researches public health issues and educates the lay public and professionals about disease transmission, origin, and prevention.

Central core: The restricted area of the operating room, where sterile supplies and flash sterilizers are located.

Central nervous system (CNS): The part of the nervous system comprising the brain and spinal cord.

Central Service department: The area of the hospital where medical devices and equipment are processed; also called *Central Surgical Supply,* the *Surgical Processing department,* and the *Central Processing department.*

Cerclage: A procedure in which a suture ligature is placed around the cervix to prevent spontaneous abortion.

Certification: Acknowledgment by a private agency that a person has achieved a minimum level of knowledge and skill. Certification usually is established by graduation from an accredited institution and passing a written examination. Certification does not confer legal status.

Certified Registered Nurse Anesthetist (CRNA): A registered nurse trained and qualified to administer anesthesia.

Cerumen: A substance produced by the cerumen glands of the ear (i.e., ear wax).

Chain of command: A hierarchy of personnel positions that establishes both vertical and horizontal relationships between positions.

Chemical barrier: The barrier formed by the action of an antiseptic; it not only reduces the number of microorganisms on a surface, but also prevents recolonization (regrowth) for a limited period.

Chemical energy: The energy contained in the bonds of atomic particles and between molecules. When these bonds are broken, energy is released.

Chemical indicator: A method of testing a sterilization parameter. Chemicals sensitive to physical conditions, such as temperature, are placed with the item being sterilized and change color when the parameter is reached.

Chemical name: The name of a drug that reflects its molecular structure.

Chemical sterilization: A process that uses chemical agents to achieve sterilization.

Chemistry study: Usually a blood or urine analysis that provides information on the metabolism and function of the body.

Child life specialist: A trained professional who specializes in the psychosocial care of and communication with pediatric patients and their families.

Chisel: An orthopedic instrument used to slice bone; one side is straight and the other is beveled.

Choanal: A term that describes the communicating passageways between the nasal fossae and the pharynx.

Cholesteatoma: A benign tumor of the middle ear caused by shedding of keratin in chronic otitis media.

Chromatin: A protein substance containing the genetic code of the cell.

Chromic salt: A chemical used to treat surgical gut to make it resistant to absorption by tissue.

Chromosomes: Double strands of specifically paired proteins that contain the genetic code of a cell.

Chronic illness: An illness that has continued for months, weeks, or years.

Chronic infection: An infection that is unusually prolonged, usually months beyond the normal healing period.

–cidal: A suffix indicating death. For example, bactericidal means "able to kill bacteria."

Circuit: The path of free electrons as they move through conductive material. In a *closed circuit,* the electrons proceed unhindered and electrical energy is maintained; in an *open circuit,* the path of the electrons is interrupted, which stops the flow of current.

Circulator: The nonsterile team member who assists in gathering additional supplies and equipment needed during the surgical procedure and advocates for the patient.

Circumcision: Removal of all or part of the prepuce (foreskin) of the penis.

Circumference: The circular path of an object.

Cirrhosis: A disease of the liver in which the tissue hardens and the venous drainage becomes blocked. It usually is caused by chronic alcoholism but may result from other disease conditions.

Clamp: An instrument designed to occlude or to hold tissue, objects, or fabric between its jaws.

Cleaning: A process that removes organic or inorganic soil or debris using detergent and mechanical or hand washing.

Closed chest drainage: A system of removing air from the thoracic cavity and restoring negative pressure so that the lungs can expand properly after thoracic surgery or trauma to the chest wall.

Closed gloving: A technique of gloving in which the bare hand does not come in contact with the outside of the glove. The sterile glove is protected from the nonsterile hand by the cuff of a surgical gown.

Closed reduction: Alignment of bone fragments into anatomical position by manipulation or traction.

Coagulum: A sticky, semiliquid substance that forms when tissue is altered by electrical or ultrasonic energy.

Coarctation: Narrowing of the passageway of a blood vessel, such as coarctation of the aorta, a congenital condition.

Cobalt-60 radiation: A method of sterilizing prepackaged equipment using ionizing radiation.

Cocci: Round or spherical bacteria that occur in chains, pairs, or clusters.

Cognitive impairment: A physiological condition in which a person is unable to carry out normal cognitive tasks, such as rational decision making.

Coherency: A quality of laser light in which all light waves are lined up with troughs and peaks matching.

Coitus: Sexual intercourse.

Collagen: The protein matrix of connective tissue.

Colonization: The process of a group of bacteria living together.

Colposcopy: Microscopic examination of the cervix.

Commensalism: The relationship between two organisms in which one uses the other for physiological needs but causes it no harm.

Comminuted: A fracture in which there are multiple bone fragments.

Condyle: The rounded end of a long bone. A condyle plate is a contoured implant which fits over the condyle and also extends along the shaft of the bone, used to repair a fracture of the condyle.

Common bile duct exploration (CBDE): A procedure to detect stones or strictures in the common bile duct. It usually is performed endoscopically before surgery.

Common law: Binding decisions made by a court judge and based on the precedent of a similar case.

Compartment syndrome: Severe swelling and tissue injury caused by constriction of the blood and lymph. Compartment syndrome can progress to tissue necrosis.

Complete blood count (CBC): A blood test that measures specific components of the blood, including the hemoglobin, hematocrit, red blood cells, and white blood cells.

Compression: Mechanical force in which a structure is compacted or pressed together. Compression is used to repair tissue. A compression injury (e.g., compression fracture) results when bone or other tissue is compacted.

Compression injury: Tissue injury caused by continuous pressure over an area.

Computed tomography (CT): An imaging technique that allows physicians to obtain cross-sectional radiographic views of the patient. The result is a CT scan or computed axial tomography (CAT) scan.

Concave lens: A type of lens that is thinner at the middle than at the edges. A concave lens bends light rays away from the center.

Concentration: A measure of the quantity of a substance by volume or weight.

Conduction: The transfer of heat from one substance to another by the natural movement of molecules, which sets other molecules in motion.

Conductive: The quality of a material to give up electrons easily and thus transmit electrical current.

Conductivity: The relative ability of a substance to transmit free electrons or electricity.

Conformer: A device placed in the socket after enucleation or evisceration to fill the orbital space.

Congenital: A condition or an anomaly present at birth.

Consensus: Agreement among members of a group.

Constitutional law: The supreme law of the nation in the United States.

Contaminate: To render nonsterile and unacceptable for use in critical areas of the body.

Contaminated: The condition of instruments, supplies, or items that have been exposed to a nonsterile item, particle, or surface through physical or airborne contact.

Contamination: The consequence of physical contact between a sterile surface and a nonsterile surface in surgery. Contamination also can result from airborne dust, moisture droplets, or fluids that act as a vehicle for transporting contaminants from a nonsterile surface to a sterile one.

Content: The substance or actual information contained in a message.

Continuing education: More formally called professional development. It demonstrates an ongoing learning process in an individual's profession. Continuing education credits are provided by a professional organization. Credits are earned by attending lectures and in-service presentations or by study and examination. Usually only peer-reviewed professional literature qualifies for CE credits.

Continuous wave lasers: Lasers that emit the laser light continuously rather than in pulses.

Contracture: Tissue that heals without scar formation, causing limited mobility.

Contraindication: A protocol, drug, or procedure that is medically inadvisable because it increases the risk of injury or harm.

Contrast medium: A radiopaque solution (i.e., not penetrated by x-rays) that is introduced into body cavities to outline their inside surfaces.

Control head: The proximal section of a flexible endoscope where the controls are located.

Controlled hypothermia: Deliberate lowering of the patient's core body temperature during general anesthesia.

Controlled substances: Drugs that have the potential for abuse. Controlled substances are rated according to their risk potential; these ratings are called *schedules.*

Control-release: A suture-needle combination designed to release the suture easily.

Convalescence: The stage of disease in which damaged cells are repaired and the patient recovers from the effects of the illness or operation.

Convection: The displacement of cool air by warm air. Convection usually creates currents as the warm air rises and the cool air falls.

Convex lens: A ground segment of glass, plastic, or sapphire that is thicker at the middle than at the edges. A convex lens is used to focus light rays on a small area.

Coroner's case: A patient death that requires investigation by the coroner, as well as an autopsy on the deceased.

Count: A systematic method of accounting for all sponges, needles, instruments, and other items that can be retained in the patient. Counts are performed in all cases in which a possibility of leaving an item in the surgical wound exists.

Court trial: A trial in which a judge determines the factual evidence and makes the final judgment.

CPU: Central processing unit; the component of a computer that contains the circuitry, memory, and power controls.

Crest: The greatest point of disturbance in a medium such as water or air.

Cricoid pressure: Direct manual pressure on the cricoid cartilage to prevent aspiration and facilitate intubation.

Critical items: In medicine, items that must be sterilized for use on patients. A critical item is any device that enters body tissue, including the vascular system.

Critical thinking: The process of analyzing information about the patient, comparing it with similar previous experience, and responding to the unique needs of that patient.

Cross-clamp: To place a clamp across a structure (usually a blood vessel) to occlude it.

Cross-contamination: The spread of infection from one person to another or from an object to a person.

Cruciate: Cross shaped.

Cryosurgery: The use of extremely low temperature to destroy diseased tissue.

Cryotherapy: A technique in which a cold probe is used to freeze tissue, such as the sclera, ciliary body (for glaucoma), or retinal layers, after detachment.

CST: Certified surgical technologist. A surgical technologist who has successfully passed the National Board of Surgical Technology and Surgical Assisting certification examination.

CST-CFA: Certified surgical technologist–certified first assistant. A surgical technologist with advanced training who has successfully passed the certification examination for surgical first assistants and is credentialed by the National Board of Surgical Technology and Surgical Assisting.

Cultural competence: The ability to provide support and care to individuals of cultures and belief systems different from one's own.

Culture: A process in which a sample of exudate, pus, or fluid is grown in culture media and analyzed for the presence of infectious microorganisms. If microorganisms colonize the sample, they are examined for type and sensitivity to specific antibiotics. This procedure is called a *culture and sensitivity* (C & S).

Culture and sensitivity (C & S): A microbiological study in which cells or fluid are allowed to incubate and then are tested for infectivity and sensitivity to an antibacterial agent.

Curettage: The removal of tissue by scraping with a surgical curette.

Current: The rate of electrical flow through a conductive material.

Current density: The concentration of current at any given point in the electrical circuit.

Cursor: The visual marker, in the form of an arrow or some other symbol that indicates an entry point on the computer screen.

CUSA: Cavitron Ultrasonic Surgical Aspirator; this instrument destroys tumors through the use of high-frequency sound waves (ultrasound).

Cutting instruments: Instruments with a sharp edge that is used to cut and dissect tissue. This group includes scissors, scalpels, osteotomes, curettes, chisels, biopsy punches, saws, drills, and needles.

Cutting mode: In electrosurgery, the use of high voltage and relatively low frequency to cut through tissue.

Cyanosis: A blue or dusky hue of the skin that results from inadequate perfusion of tissue.

Cycle: In alternating current, electrons change direction in the path of the circuit. The cycle is one complete change.

Cystocele: A herniation of the bladder into the vaginal wall.

Cystoscope: A fiberoptic instrument used to assess the lower genitourinary tract and in transurethral surgery. Also called a *cystourethroscope.*

Cystoscopy assistant: A trained surgical technologist or nurse whose primary specialty is transurethral surgery. The cystoscopy assistant functions in circulating and scrub roles.

Damages: Money awarded in a civil lawsuit to compensate the injured party.

Database: In computer technology, a compilation of information, usually lists or numerical information, that can be manipulated or calculated.

Debridement: The removal of devitalized tissue, debris, and foreign objects from a wound. Debridement is performed on trauma injuries, burns, and infected wounds either before surgery or as part of the surgical procedure.

Decompression: A technique or process in which the stomach contents are continually drained into a collection device. Decompression is required after gastric surgery or disease. Can also be the removal of air or fluid from an organ.

Decontamination: A process in which recently used and soiled medical devices, including instruments, are rendered safe for personnel to handle.

Decontamination area: A room or small department in which soiled instruments and equipment are cleaned of gross matter and decontaminated to remove microorganisms.

Defamation: A derogatory statement concerning another person's skill, character, or reputation.

Dehiscence: Separation of the layers of a surgical wound; it may be partial or involve the full thickness of the wound.

Delayed drug sensitivity: Allergic reaction to a drug occurring up to 12 hours after exposure. This type of reaction is mediated by T lymphocytes.

Delegation: The transfer of responsibility for an activity from one person to another.

Delirium: A state of confusion and disorientation.

Delivery: The way in which a message is conveyed.

Dentition: The number, type, and pattern of the teeth.

Dependent areas of the body: Areas of the body subject to pressure from gravity and weight. For example, the sacrum is a dependent area when a person is in the supine position.

Dependent tasks: In medicine, nursing, and allied health, those tasks that are performed with the collaborative oversight of another professional. For example, the surgeon provides oversight to the surgical assistant during surgery.

Deposition: The testimony of a witness given under oath and transcribed by a court reporter during the pretrial phase of a civil lawsuit.

Dermoid cyst: A mass arising from the germ layers of the embryo that contains tissue remnants, including hair and teeth.

Desiccation: The removal of water from tissue, causing it to die. Alcohol is a desiccating skin prep solution. It destroys tissue protein and therefore is never used around the eyes or on mucous membranes.

Detergent: A chemical that breaks down organic debris by emulsification (separation into small particles) to aid in cleaning.

Determination of death: A formal medical process to determine brain death.

Diagnostic endoscopy: A diagnostic procedure in which a long, flexible, fiberoptic tube is inserted into a body cavity for viewing and diagnosis.

Diastolic pressure: The lowest pressure exerted on the arterial wall during the resting phase of the cardiac cycle (**diastole**).

Diathermy: Low-power cautery used to mark the sclera over an area of retinal detachment.

Differential count: A test that determines the number of each type of white blood cell in a specimen of blood.

Diffusion: The molecular passage of oxygen across the alveoli and into the bloodstream.

Digital output recorder: During video-assisted surgery, digital signals are captured from the video camera and transmitted to a monitor. The digital output recorder processes these signals.

Dilation: Opening of the cervix during labor (measured in centimeters).

Dilators: Graduated, smooth instruments that are used to increase the diameter of an anatomical opening in tissue.

Direct coupling: The transfer of electrical current from an active electrode to another conductive instrument by accident or as part of the electrosurgical process.

Direct current (DC): A type of low voltage electrical current in which electrons flow in one direction to complete a circuit. Battery power uses direct current.

Direct inguinal hernia: A hernia that results from an acquired weakness in the inguinal floor.

Direct transmission: The transfer of microbes from their source to a new host by direct physical contact with the microbes; for example, a water droplet containing respiratory virus is exhaled by one person and inhaled by another.

Discharge against medical advice (AMA): Self-discharge by a patient who has not necessarily met discharge criteria.

Discharge criteria: Objective criteria used to determine whether a patient is safe for discharge from the health care facility.

Disinfection: Destruction of microorganisms by heat or chemical means. Spores usually are not destroyed by disinfection.

Dislocation: Displacement of a joint from its normal position.

Dispersive electrode: The part of the electrosurgical system that delivers current and heat directly to the tissue.

Distraction (distractor): A mechanical process in which a structure is elongated. Distraction can be used to suspend a limb (and thereby stretch the soft tissue) and bones during surgery. A distraction injury is caused by the pulling apart or stretching of tissue (the opposite of a compression injury).

Diuresis: Increased formation of urine by the kidneys.

DNAR: "Do not attempt resuscitation." Emphasizes the patient's desire to refuse intervention to resuscitate.

DNR: "Do not resuscitate." An official request to refrain from certain types of resuscitation, usually cardiopulmonary resuscitation.

Docking: In robotic surgery, the process of positioning the robotic instruments in the exact location over the patient so that instruments can be safely attached from their ports in the body cavity.

Doppler duplex ultrasonography: A type of ultrasonography that amplifies sounds that pass through tissue and produces a visual image of blood flow.

Doppler effect: The effect perceived when the origin or receiver of sound waves moves. The perception is an increase in the frequency of the waves and corresponding pitch.

Doppler studies: A technique that uses ultrasonic waves to measure blood flow in a vessel.

Doppler ultrasound: A medical device that uses the Doppler effect and ultrasonic waves to measure and record tissue density and shape.

Dosage: The regulated administration of prescribed amounts of a drug. Dosage is expressed as a quantity of drug per unit of time.

Dose: The quantity of a drug to be taken at one time or the stated amount of drug per unit of distribution (e.g., 0.5 mg per milliliter of solution).

Double-action rongeur: A cutting instrument with two hinges in the middle. This provides greater leverage and cutting strength than a single-action instrument. Usually used to describe an orthopedic rongeur.

Double-armed suture: Suture-needle combination that contains a needle at each end of the suture; it is used to join circular or tubular structures.

Drapes: Sterile materials, including towels and sheets that are placed around the prepared incision site to create a sterile field.

Droplet nuclei: Dried remnants of previously moist secretions containing microorganisms. Droplet nuclei are an important source of disease transmission.

Drug: A chemical substance that, when taken into the body, changes one or more of the body's functions.

Drug administration: The giving of a drug to a person by any route.

Ductus arteriosus: A normal fetal structure that allows blood to bypass circulation to the lungs. If this structure remains open after birth, it is called a *patent ductus arteriosus*.

Duty cycle: In electrosurgery, the duration of current flow sometimes is referred to as the duty cycle. The duty cycle can intermittently be applied to produce the desired effect on tissue.

Dye: Colored substance used to stain tissue or verify the patency of a hollow or tubular structure (e.g., fallopian tube, ureter) under direct visualization.

Dyspnea: Difficulty breathing.

Eclampsia: A seizure during pregnancy, usually as a result of pregnancy-induced hypertension.

Ectopic pregnancy: Implantation of the fertilized ovum outside the uterus.

Efficiency: The economic use of time and energy to prevent unnecessary expenditure of work, materials, and time.

Effusion: Fluid in the middle ear.

Electric generator: A device used to convert mechanical power into electricity. A generator consists of a rotating shaft covered with a coil of conductive material. This shaft is passed through a set of magnets, creating an electrical current.

Electrocardiogram (ECG): A noninvasive assessment of the heart's electrical activity. In the United States, electrocardiogram is abbreviated correctly as ECG. EKG is the European abbreviation.

Electrocardiograph machine: A medical device that receives signals from the heart's electrical activity through conductive pads and displays the activity on a graph in real time.

Electroencephalogram (EEG): A diagnostic tool that measures the electrical activity of the brain. During vascular surgery, an EEG may be used to determine the patient's neurophysiological response.

Electrolytic media: Fluids that contain electrolytes and therefore can transmit an electrical current.

Electromagnetic field: A three-dimensional pattern of force created by the attraction and repelling of charged particles around a magnet.

Electromagnetic waves: The natural phenomenon of wave energy, such as electricity, light, and radio broadcasts. The type of energy is determined by the frequency of the waves.

Electron: A negatively charged particle that orbits the nucleus of an atom.

Electronic probe thermometer: A digital thermometer commonly used in the clinical setting.

Electrostatic discharge: The sudden release of electrical energy from surfaces where charged particles have accumulated because of friction.

Electrosurgical unit (ESU): Medical device commonly used in surgery to coagulate blood vessels and cut tissue.

Electrosurgical vessel sealing: A type of bipolar electrosurgery in which tissue is welded together using low voltage, low temperature, and a high-frequency current.

Electrosurgical waveforms: The transduced or actual waves generated when frequency, voltage, and power are delivered in different combinations during electrosurgery.

Element: A pure substance composed of atoms, each with the same number of protons (e.g., iron, copper, and uranium).

Elevator: A nonhinged, sharp, or dull-tipped instrument. An elevator is used to separate tissues or to bluntly remodel tissue.

Elevator channel: A channel that extends the full length of a flexible endoscope and receives biopsy forceps or other instruments.

Elimination: The physiological process of removing cellular and chemical waste products from the body.

Embolism: A clot of blood, air, organic material, or a foreign body that moves freely in the vascular system. An embolus travels from larger to smaller vessels until it cannot pass through a vessel. At that level, it interrupts the flow of blood and may result in severe disease or death.

Embolization: A technique used to occlude a blood vessel. A variety of materials, including platinum coils and microscopic plastic particles, are injected into the vessel under fluoroscopic control to stop active bleeding or prevent bleeding.

Embolus: A moving substance in the vascular system. An embolus may consist of air, a blood clot, atherosclerotic plaque, or fat.

Embryonic life: The first 8 weeks of gestational development.

Emergence: The stage in general anesthesia in which the anesthetic agent is withdrawn and the patient regains consciousness.

Empyema: A pus-filled area of the lung.

En bloc: A term meaning "in one piece." In surgery, it describes the technique of removing tissue.

Endarterectomy: The surgical removal of plaque from inside an artery.

Endocoupler: A device that connects the endoscope to the camera.

Endocytosis: A process by which the cell engulfs large particles in the environment.

End of life: A period within which death is expected, usually days to months.

Endometriosis: The growth of endometrial tissue outside the uterine cavity.

Endoplasmic reticulum: An extension of the nuclear membrane in the cell that facilitates the movement of protein out of the nucleus.

Endoscope: A telescopic instrument with serial lenses that is used to view anatomical structures inside the body.

Endoscopic procedures: Medical assessment of body cavities using a fiberoptic lensed instrument (endoscope).

Endospore (spore): The dormant stage of some bacteria that allows them to survive without reproducing in extreme environmental conditions, including heat, cold, and exposure to many disinfectants. When conditions are favorable for reproduction, the spore again becomes active and produces bacterial colonies.

Endotoxins: Bacterial toxins that are associated with the outer membrane of certain gram-negative bacteria. Endotoxins are not secreted but are released when the cells are disrupted or broken down.

Endotracheal tube: An artificial airway (tube) that is inserted into the patient's trachea to maintain patency.

Endovascular repair: Endoscopic surgery of the vascular system.

Energy: Power or force generated by various types of natural occurrences.

Entry site: In microbial transmission, the sites where microorganisms enter the body.

Enucleation: The removal of tissue or an organ without previous fragmentation or dissection. In ophthalmic surgery, the surgical removal of the globe and accessory attachments.

Enzymatic cleaner: A specific chemical used in detergents and cleaners to penetrate and break down biological debris, such as blood and tissue.

Epidural: A type of anesthesia in which the anesthetic is delivered through a small tube in the patient's back to relieve pain in labor. The patient usually is in bed and catheterized during labor in which this form of anesthesia is used.

Epigastric: A term referring to the region of the abdomen above the umbilicus.

Episiotomy: A perineal incision made during the second stage of labor to prevent the tearing of tissue.

Epispadias: A rare congenital abnormality in which the opening of the urethra is on the dorsum of the penis. This anomaly does not usually occur in isolation but is part of a more complex set of defects of the urogenital system.

Epistaxis: Bleeding arising from the nasal cavity.

Eschar: Burned tissue fragments that can accumulate on the electrosurgical tip during surgery; eschar can cause sparking and become a source of ignition.

Esmarch bandage: A rolled bandage made of rubber or latex that is used to exsanguinate blood from a limb.

Esophageal varices: Distended veins of the esophagus, caused by advanced liver disease. The condition occurs as a result of portal vein obstruction arising from fibrosis of the liver. Esophageal varices may bleed profusely.

Ethical dilemmas: Situations in which ethical choices involve conflicting values.

Ethics: Standards of behavior that are accepted within groups.

Ethylene oxide: A highly flammable, toxic gas that is capable of sterilizing an object.

Eukaryote: The basic type of cell; it is surrounded by a membrane and contains complex organs for metabolism and reproduction.

Event-related sterility: A wrapped sterile item may become decontaminated by environmental conditions or events, such as a puncture in the wrapper. Event-related sterility refers to sterility based on the absence of such events. The shelf life of a sterilized pack is event related, not time related.

Evert: To turn outward or inside out.

Evisceration: The protrusion of an internal organ through a wound or surgical incision.

Examination under anesthesia (EUA): Fracture and dislocation may be fully assessed when general anesthesia is used.

Excimer: A type of lasing energy that is created when electrons are removed from the lasing medium.

Excisional biopsy: The removal of a tissue mass for pathological examination.

Excitation source: In laser technology, the energy that causes the atoms of a lasing medium (gas or solid) to vibrate.

Exenteration: Removal of the entire contents of the orbit.

Exotoxins: Toxic substances produced by microorganisms and excreted outside the bacterial cell. Exotoxins differ in the particular tissues of the host that they may affect.

Expiration: The act of breathing out (exhalation).

Exploratory laparotomy: A laparotomy performed to examine the abdominal cavity when less invasive measures fail to confirm a diagnosis.

Exstrophy: The eversion, or turning out, of an organ.

External fixation: A method of stabilizing bone fragments in anatomical position from outside the body. A cast is an example of an external fixation device.

Extracorporeal: A term meaning "outside the body." In minimally invasive surgery, it refers to a technique for placing sutures in which the knots are formed outside the body and then tightened after they have been introduced into the surgical wound. In extracorporeal hemodialysis, the blood is shunted outside the body for filtering and cleansing.

Extracorporeal shockwave lithotripsy (ESWL): A procedure in which ultrasonic sound waves are used to pulverize kidney or gallbladder stones.

Extravasation: The absorption of the fluid into the vascular system, leading to increased blood pressure and possible death related to fluid overload. This occurs during surgery when distension fluid used during endoscopic procedures is absorbed through large blood vessels in the bladder or uterus.

Extubation: Withdrawal of an artificial airway.

Eyepiece: The proximal portion of the endoscopic lens.

Facultative: The ability of some organisms to live with or without oxygen.

Fascia: In the abdomen, a tough, fibrous tissue layer between the parietal peritoneum and muscle layers.

Fasciotomy: A surgical treatment for compartment syndrome in which the fascia is incised to release severe tissue swelling.

Feedback: The physical response to a message; a component of effective communication.

Fenestrated drape: A sterile body sheet with a hole or "window" (fenestration) that exposes the incision site. The fenestrated drape is positioned after other drapes and towels have been placed in keeping with the procedure. Fenestrated drapes are differentiated by type (e.g., laparotomy, thyroid, kidney, eye, ear, and extremity drapes).

Fetal demise: Death of the fetus.

Fetus: Gestational life after 8 weeks.

Fibrillation: Uncoordinated muscular activity in the heart muscle, which results in "quivering" rather than pumping action. This results in pooling of blood.

Fibrin: A component of whole blood that promotes clotting.

Fibroid: See Leiomyoma.

Fistula: A complication of wound infection in which one or more hollow, skin-lined tracts form at the wound site and continue to drain pus and fluid. This prevents the wound from healing.

Five rights of medication: Requirements for safe administration of drugs: right drug, right dose right route, right patient, right time.

Flaming: Sending an inflammatory message or statement by e-mail. Flaming is a violation of e-mail etiquette and is an inappropriate use of the technology.

Floor grade instruments: Surgical instruments manufactured from inferior metal that can bend and break easily. Fittings and joints are poorly constructed and fittings are poor quality.

Fluoroscopy: A radiological technique that provides real-time images of an anatomical region.

Focal point: The exact location where light rays converge after passing through a convex lens.

Focused assessment: An assessment of the patient that focuses on specific organ systems or regions of the body.

Focus ring: A device fitted on the endoscopic camera to focus the image seen through the lens system.

Foley catheter: A retention catheter with an expandable balloon at the distal end.

Fomite: An intermediate, inanimate source in the process of disease transmission. Any object, such as a contaminated surgical instrument or medical device, can become a fomite in disease transmission.

Force: In physics, the pushing or pulling of objects (e.g., gravity and magnetism).

Fowler position: The sitting position, which is used for cranial, facial, and some reconstructive breast procedures.

Frequency: In physics, the number of waves that pass a point in one second. The unit of measurement for frequency is the hertz (Hz).

Friable: Tearing or fragmenting easily when handled (tissue characteristic).

Frozen section: A microscopic slice of frozen anatomical tissue that is evaluated for the presence of abnormal cells. Frozen section analysis is performed during surgery to diagnose malignancy.

Fulcrum: The area on an instrument where the lever moves.

Fulguration: A process of tissue surface destruction used in electrosurgery.

Full-thickness skin graft (FTSG): A skin graft composed of the epidermis and dermis.

Fungicidal: Able to kill fungi.

Fusiform aneurysm: A type of aneurysm that involves the entire circumference of a blood vessel.

Gain: In electronics, the intensity of the signal.

Gas scavenging: The capture and safe removal of extraneous anesthetic gases from the anesthesia machine.

Gastroesophageal reflux disease (GERD): A condition in which the gastroesophageal sphincter allows gastric contents to backflow (reflux) into the esophagus, causing irritation and mucosal burning and possibly leading to cancer of the esophagus.

Gastroschisis: A herniation of abdominal contents through the abdominal wall that is present at birth.

Gastrostomy: A surgical opening through the stomach wall connecting to the outside of the body or another hollow anatomical structure.

General anesthesia: Anesthesia associated with a state of unconsciousness. General anesthesia is not a fixed state of unconsciousness, but rather ranges along a continuum from semiresponsiveness to profound unresponsiveness.

Generation: In pharmacology, refers to a drug group that was developed from a previous prototype (e.g., first generation cephalosporin).

Generic name: The formulary name of a drug that is assigned by the U.S. Adapted Names Council.

Genetic abnormality: A birth anomaly that is inherited.

Genetic mutation: A permanent change in the DNA makeup of a gene.

Germicidal: Able to kill germs.

Gestational age: The age of the baby as measured in the number of weeks from conception.

Glasgow Coma Scale (GCS): A standardized method of measuring a patient's response to external stimuli.

Glaucoma: A group of diseases characterized by elevation of the intraocular pressure. Sustained pressure on the optic nerve and other structures may result in ischemia and blindness.

Glomerular filtration rate (GFR): An indication of kidney function in which serum creatinum (normally filtered by the kidney) is measured.

Goiter: Benign enlargement of the thyroid gland.

Golgi apparatus: An extension of the endomembrane of the cell that stores, modifies, and transports large molecules.

Gossip: The telling and retelling of events of another's personal life, professional life, or physical condition.

Gouge: A V-shaped bone chisel.

Gram staining: A method of differential staining of bacteria that separates them into one of two groups, gram positive (accepts the stain) or gram negative (is not stained). Each group has common characteristics that identify its members and aid in diagnosis and treatment.

Gravitational energy: The natural attractive force of masses in the universe.

Gravity displacement sterilizer: A type of sterilizer that removes air by gravity.

Gross contamination: Contamination of a large area of tissue by a highly infective source.

Ground wire: In electrical circuits, the ground wire in a plug or receptacle captures current that has escaped from its intended pathway and discharges it into the ground.

Grounding pad: An alternate name for the patient return electrode.

Groupthink: In sociology and group behavior theory, the conformity of a group to one way of thinking and behaving. Groupthink creates two factions, those who agree (in-group) and those who disagree (out-group). This generates resentment and conflict in the workplace.

Half-life: The time required for one half of a drug to be cleared from the body.

Hand antisepsis: A technique for removing transient flora from the hands using alcohol-based hand rub or surgical hand scrub.

Hand washing: A specific technique used to remove debris and dead cells from the hands. Hand washing with an antiseptic also reduces the number of microorganisms on the skin.

Handover (hand-off): A verbal and written report from one nurse to another to provide updated patient information.

Haptic feedback: Tactile feedback, conveyed from tissue to the hand when a hand instrument is used. Robotic instruments do not provide any tactile feedback.

Hard copy: In computer technology, the paper form of data, records, or reports.

Hard drive: The component of a computer's CPU where most of the data are stored, including information the computer uses to operate.

Head drape: A turban-style drape created with two surgical towels that covers the patient's head and eyes. The ability to prepare and place this drape is a valuable draping skill.

Head to toe assessment: A complete assessment of the patient, one that includes all systems.

Heartbeating cadaver: A cadaver maintained on cardiopulmonary support to provide tissue perfusion. This is done to maintain viability in organs for donation.

Hematocrit (Hct): The ratio of red blood cells to plasma.

Hematuria: Blood in the urine.

Hemodialysis: A process in which blood is shunted out of the body and passed through a complex set of filters for the treatment of end-stage renal disease (and in some cases, poisoning); also called *renal replacement therapy* (RRT).

Hemodynamic: A term referring to the pressure, flow, and resistance in the cardiovascular system.

Hemoglobin (Hgb): The oxygen-carrying molecule found in red blood cells.

Hemoptysis: Bloody sputum or bleeding arising from the respiratory tract.

Hemorrhage: Continuous bleeding from a pathological cause.

Hemostat: A surgical clamp most often used to occlude a blood vessel.

Hemothorax: The presence of blood in the thoracic cavity or between the pleural sac and lungs, usually caused by trauma.

Herbal therapy: The use of medicinal herbs for the treatment of disease.

Hernia: A protrusion of tissue under the skin through a weakened area of the body wall.

Hesselbach triangle: The area bounded by the rectus abdominis muscle, the inguinal ligament, and the inferior epigastric vessels. This region is most commonly associated with inguinal hernias.

Hiatus: An opening in the diaphragm where the esophagus passes from the abdominal cavity.

High definition (HD): In video technology, the clarity of an image based on the number of signals (pixels) emitted by the camera. A high-definition format displays 1280×721 pixels in a rectangular image.

High-efficiency particulate air (HEPA) filters: Filters installed in the operating room ventilation system that remove 99.97% of particles equal to or larger than 0.3 micrometers (μm).

High level disinfection (HLD): A process that reduces the bioburden to an absolute minimum.

High vacuum sterilizer: A type of steam sterilizer that removes air in the chamber by vacuum and refills the chapter with pressurized steam. Also known as a prevacuum sterilizer.

Histology: The study of the structure of tissue.

Holmium:YAG: A solid crystal lasing medium that penetrates a wide variety of substances, including renal and biliary stones and soft tissue.

Homeostasis: A state of balance in physiological functions.

Honed: Sharpened.

Hook wire: A device used to pinpoint the exact location of a non-palpable mass detected during a mammogram. A fine needle is inserted into the mass during the examination, and the tissue around the needle is removed for pathological examination and definitive diagnosis.

Horizontal abuse: Verbal abuse or sabotage among people of equal job or professional ranking.

Hospital policy: A set of rules or regulations that hospital employees are required to follow. They are created to protect patients and employees from harm and to ensure smooth operation of the hospital.

Host: The organism that harbors or nourishes another organism (parasite).

Hot wire: In electrical circuits, the hot wire is the one that carries the electrical current.

Hydrodressing: A dressing impregnated with a water-based gel. This type of dressing prevents the wound from drying and encourages healing.

Hydronephrosis: Distension of the renal pelvis and proximal ureter caused by an obstruction in the ureter and reflux of kidney filtrate.

Hyperextension: Extension of a joint beyond its normal anatomical range.

Hyperflexion: Flexion of a joint beyond its normal anatomical range.

Hyperlinks: In computer technology, electronic links between files and the electronic addresses for data associated with those links. Hyperlinks allow data to be obtained electronically and quickly from another computer through a computer network.

Hyperplasia: An excessive proliferation of tissue.

Hypersensitivity: Allergic immune to a substance causing a range of symptoms from mild inflammation to anaphylactic shock and death.

Hypertension: An abnormal increase in blood pressure.

Hypertrophy (Hypertrophic): Enlargement of an organ or tissue.

Hypocalcemia: An abnormally low serum calcium.

Hypogastric: A term referring to the region of the abdomen below the stomach.

Hypokalemia: An abnormally low serum potassium.

Hyponatremia: An abnormally low serum sodium.

Hyponaturemia: Low serum sodium. Severe hyponaturemia and death can result from the use of hypotonic distension fluids used during hysteroscopy.

Hypospadias: A congenital abnormality in which the urethra opens inferior to its normal location. It is normally seen in males, when the urethra opens on the undersurface of the penis.

Hypotension: Decreased blood pressure.

Hypothermia: A subnormal body temperature.

Hypoventilation: Inadequate respirations.

Hypoxia: Lack of oxygen in the tissue.

Hysteroscopy: The use of a special endoscope for diagnostic procedures and interventional surgery of the uterus.

Icon: A visual cue on the computer screen. The icon is a small picture or graphic that is linked or connected electronically to data in the computer.

Imaging studies: Diagnostic tests that produce a picture or image.

Imaging system: The combined components of the endoscopic system, which create the image captured in the focal view of the endoscope.

Immediate drug sensitivity: An allergic reaction mediated by antibodies that are released as shortly after the drug enters the circulation.

Immunity: The body's ability to defend itself from "nonself" substances.

Impedance: In direct current, impedance is the opposition or interruption of current.

Impervious: Waterproof.

Implant: A synthetic or metal replacement for an anatomical structure, such as a joint or cranial bone.

Implanted electronic device (IED): An electronic device that monitors and corrects physiological conditions. Electrosurgery may interfere with the function of such devices, which include pacemakers, internal defibrillators, deep brain stimulators, ventricular assist devices, and others.

Inactive electrode: An alternate term for the patient return electrode.

Inanimate: Nonliving.

Incarcerated hernia: Herniated tissue that is trapped in an abdominal wall defect. Incarcerated tissue requires emergency surgery to prevent ischemia and tissue necrosis.

Incise drape: A plastic, self-adhesive drape that is positioned over the incision site after the surgical skin prep. The incise drape creates a sterile surface over the skin. The incision is made directly through the incise drape and skin.

Incisional hernia: The postoperative herniation of tissue into the tissue layers around an abdominal incision. This may occur in the immediate postoperative period or later, after the incision has healed.

Incompetent cervix: A condition in which previous cervical injury results in repeated spontaneous abortions.

Incomplete abortion: The demise of the embryo or fetus and expulsion of the tissue.

Independent tasks: In medicine, nursing, and allied health, tasks for which a professional has full responsibility and accountability without the oversight of another professional.

Indicator: A device used in the sterilization process to verify that a parameter of the process (e.g., temperature) has been achieved. Indicators are not used to verify that an item is sterile, only that a parameter has been achieved.

Indirect inguinal hernia: A hernia that protrudes into the membranous sac of the spermatic cord. This condition usually is due to a congenital defect in the abdominal wall.

Induced hypotension: The deliberate lowering of blood pressure during surgery to control hemorrhage, producing a more bloodless operative field, or control intracranial pressure.

Induction: Initiation of general anesthesia with a drug that causes unconsciousness.

Indwelling catheter: A urethral or ureteral catheter that is left in place.

Inert: Causing little or no reaction in tissue or with other materials.

Infarction: A blockage in an artery that leads to ischemia and tissue death.

Infection: The state or condition in which the body or body tissues are invaded by pathogenic microorganisms that multiply and produce injurious effects.

Inflammation: The body's nonspecific reaction to injury or infection that causes redness, heat, swelling, and pain.

Informed consent: A process and a legal document that states the patient's surgical procedure and the risks, consequences, and benefits of that procedure. It must be signed by the patient or the patient's representative before surgery can proceed. Also known as a patient operative consent form.

Infusion: Gradual administration of a drug over a specified period.

Innervation: The supplying of a body part or organ with nerves or nervous stimuli.

Insertion tube: The long, narrow portion of the flexible endoscope that is inserted into the body.

In situ: A term meaning "in the natural position or normal place, without disturbing or invading surrounding tissues."

Inspiration: The act of taking a breath (inhalation).

Instrument channel: A channel that extends the full length of a flexible endoscope and receives instruments during flexible endoscopy.

Insufflation: In minimally invasive surgery, inflation of the abdominal or thoracic cavity with carbon dioxide gas.

Insufflation unit: A device that regulates the flow and amount of carbon dioxide gas during insufflation.

Insulate: To cover or surround a conductive substance with nonconductive material.

Insulator: A substance that does not conduct electrical current and is used to prevent electricity from seeking an alternate path.

Insurance: A contract in which the insurance company agrees to defend the policy holder if that individual is sued for acts covered by the policy and to pay any damages up to the policy limit.

Internal fixation: A method of surgically repairing a fracture by inserting an implant a device that holds the bone fragments in place. Metal plates, rods, pins, and screws are examples of internal fixation devices.

Internet: A network of computers that are connected by wires, fiber-optic cables, or satellite signals. Computers connected to this system can receive and transmit data to other computers in the system.

Interrupted sutures: A technique of bringing tissue together by placing individual sutures close together.

Interstitial needle: A fine needle used to instill a radioactive isotope into a tumor.

Interventional radiology: Medical assessment procedures in which irradiation is used; usually requires invasive procedures combined with radiographic technology.

Intracorporeal: A term meaning "inside the body." In minimally invasive surgery, it refers to a suture technique in which sutures are knotted and secured inside the patient.

Intracranial pressure (ICP): The pressure within the skull exerted by the brain tissue, blood, and cerebrospinal fluid.

Intranet: A computer network within a facility or an organization that can be accessed only by those employed or affiliated with the organization.

Intraoperative awareness (IOA): A rare condition in which a patient undergoing general anesthesia is able to feel pain and other noxious stimuli but unable to respond.

Intraosseous: Refers to administration of a drug directly into the bone marrow.

Intrathecal: Refers to administration of a drug into the spinal canal.

Intravasation: The unintended absorption of irrigation fluids into the body.

Intravascular ultrasound: A diagnostic tool in which a transducer is introduced into an artery and ultrasound is used to translate the physical characteristics of the lumen into a visible image.

Intubation: The process of inserting an invasive artificial airway.

Intussusception: The telescoping of one portion of the intestine into another.

Iodinated contrast medium (ICM): A radiopaque liquid injected or infused into a hollow structure to allow radiographic study of the structure.

Ion: A charge particle created when an atom loses or gains an electron.

Ischemia: Loss of blood supply to a body part either by compression or as a result of a blockage in the blood vessels. Prolonged ischemia causes tissue death from lack of oxygen to the tissue.

Isolated circuit: An electrical circuit that has no ground reference or method of conducting current into the ground at the site of use. Current is directed from the energy source, through the patient, and back to the source.

Isolette: An infant-size "bed" and transport unit that is environmentally controlled and equipped with monitoring devices.

Isotope: An atom of a specific element with the correct number of electrons and protons but a different number of neutrons.

Jackknife (Kraske) position: A type of prone position in which the patient lies on the abdomen with the hips flexed into an inverted V.

Joint Commission: The accrediting organization for hospitals and other health care facilities in the United States.

Jury trial: A trial in which a case is presented to a selected jury, and the facts and final judgment are determined by the jury.

Keith needle: A straight cutting needle used on superficial tissue.

Keloid: Excessive scar formation, which can result in a cosmetic or functional defect.

Keratin: A substance created by the squamous epithelium.

Keratoplasty: Surgery of the cornea. The term *penetrating keratoplasty* refers to corneal transplantation.

Kinetic energy: Energy derived from electromagnetic waves (e.g., electricity and light).

Knee-chest position: A familiar term that describes the patient position used for administration of spinal anesthetics and for access to the rectum in patient (nursing) care. The patient lies in the lateral position with the knees drawn toward the abdomen and the spine flexed outward.

Knot pusher: A device used to secure suture knots during minimally invasive surgery.

Kübler-Ross, Elisabeth: A Swiss psychiatrist who proposed a theory of developmental or psychological stages of the dying experience.

Labor: The process of regular contraction of the uterine muscle that results in birth.

Laminar airflow (LAF) system: A ventilation system that moves a contained volume of air in layers at a continuous velocity, with 800 to 900 air exchanges per hour.

Laparoscopy: Minimally invasive surgery of the abdomen.

Laparotomy: A procedure in which the abdominal cavity is surgically opened. The techniques used for laparotomy are used for all open surgical procedures of the abdomen.

Laryngeal mask airway (LMA): An airway consisting of a tube and small mask that is fitted internally over the patient's larynx.

Laryngoscope: A lighted instrument used to assist endotracheal intubation.

Laryngospasm: Muscular spasm of the larynx, resulting in obstruction.

Laser: Acronym for light amplification by stimulated emission of radiation.

Laser classification: Industry and international standards for grading laser energy according to its ability to cause injury.

Laser head: The component of the laser system that holds the lasing medium.

Laser medium: A solid or gas that is sensitive to atomic excitation by an energy source, which creates intense laser light and energy.

Lateral heat: The unintentional heating of tissue outside the direct area of electrosurgical application. Also called *thermal spread.*

Lateral (Sims) position: The position in which the patient lies on his or her side on the operating table or bed.

Latex: A naturally occurring sap obtained from rubber trees that is used in the manufacture of medical devices and other commercial goods.

Latex allergy: Sensitivity to latex, which can cause itching, rhinitis, conjunctivitis, and anaphylactic shock leading to death. Personnel and patients with latex allergy must not come in contact with any articles that contain latex.

Law of inertia: Newton's first law of motion.

Laws: Standards that apply to all people in a given society.

LCD: Liquid crystal display; a type of computer monitor that is thin and flat.

LEEP: Loop electrode excision procedure. In this technique, an electrosurgical loop is used to remove a core of tissue from the cervical canal.

Leiomyoma: A fibrous, benign tumor of the uterus that usually arises from the myometrium.

Liable: Legally responsible and accountable.

Libel: Defamation in writing.

Licensed personnel: Health care workers who have been given the right to practice by a government agency.

Licensure: Professional status, granted by state government that defines the limits (scope) of practice and regulates those who hold a license. Licensure is provided to protect the public and to ensure a legal minimum standard of professional and ethical conduct.

Ligate: A loop or tie placed around a blood vessel or duct.

Ligation loop: A commercially prepared suture loop used to secure structures during minimally invasive surgery.

Light cable: The fiberoptic light cable that transmits light from the source to the endoscopic instrument. Sometimes called a *light guide.*

Light source: A device that controls and emits light for endoscopic procedures.

Linea alba: A strip of avascular tissue that follows the midline and extends from the pubis to the xyphoid process.

Liquid: One of the three states or properties of a substance; a liquid results when the temperature of the substance reaches the melting point.

Lithotomy position: The position used for vaginal, perineal, and rectal surgery. The patient's legs are positioned on stirrups.

Lithotripsy: A procedure in which stones are crushed within a body cavity, such as the bladder.

Living will: A legal document signed by the patient stating the conditions and limitations of medical assistance in the event of near death or a prognosis of death.

Livor mortis: A red and purple discoloration of the face that appears soon after death.

Lobectomy: Surgical removal of one or more anatomical sections of the liver.

Log roll: A technique for moving the patient in which a bed sheet or draw sheet is used to roll the patient onto his or her side.

Lumen: The inside of a hollow structure, such as a blood vessel.

Lysogenesis: The process whereby viruses replicate their genetic material and then cause the host cell to rupture, releasing the genetic material and forming new virions.

Lysosome: An organelle capable of releasing enzymes to kill the cell.

Magical thinking: A psychological process in which a person attributes intention and will to inanimate objects. Magical thinking may also include a patient who believes that an event will happen because he or she wills it or wishes it. This is a normal developmental stage of toddlers.

Magnetic resonance imaging (MRI): A diagnostic technique that uses radiofrequency signals and magnetic energy to produce images.

Magnetism: The natural attraction of unlike charges.

Malignant: A term used to characterize tissue that shows disorganized, uncontrolled growth (cancer). Malignant tissue has the potential to spread locally or to distant areas of the body. It is then termed metastatic.

Malignant hyperthermia (MH): A potentially fatal syndrome of hypermetabolism that results in an extremely high body temperature, cardiac dysrhythmia, and respiratory distress.

Malpractice: Negligence committed by a professional. Malpractice also may be committed if a person deliberately acts outside of his or her scope of practice or while impaired.

Maslow's hierarchy of human needs: A model of human achievement and self-actualization developed by psychologist Abraham Maslow.

Mastectomy: A procedure in which breast tissue, including the skin, areola, and nipple, is removed, but the lymph nodes are not removed. Also called a *simple mastectomy.*

Master controllers: In robotic surgery, the nonsterile hand controls that manipulate surgical instruments.

Mastication: Chewing.

Maxillomandibular fixation (MMF): Also called application of arch bars, a procedure in which the maxilla and mandible are placed in their normally closed position (jaw closed) and fixed with wires.

Mayo stand: A stainless tray mounted on a floor stand, which is draped and placed within the immediate sterile field during surgery. Instruments and lightweight equipment are placed on the Mayo stand for immediate use. These are exchanged for others on the back table as required during the surgery.

McBurney incision: An incision in which the oblique right muscle is manually split to allow removal of the appendix.

Mean arterial pressure (MAP): The average amount of pressure exerted throughout the cardiac cycle.

Meatotomy: A procedure in which a small incision is made in the urethral meatus to relieve a stricture. A topical anesthetic is used.

Mechanics: In physics, the study of objects and motion; that is, how they behave and the natural laws that govern their behavior.

Meconium: A nearly sterile fecal waste that accumulates while the fetus is in the uterus. It is passed within the first few days after birth.

Mediastinum: An enclosed cavity in the chest that contains the heart, large vessels, trachea, esophagus, and lymph nodes.

Medical devices: Any equipment, instrument, implant, material, or apparatus used for the diagnosis, treatment, or monitoring of patients.

Medical ethics: A branch of ethics concerned with the practice of medicine.

Medical power of attorney: A legal document signed by a person who is giving another individual the power to make health care decisions for the first person if he or she becomes incompetent, unconscious, or unable to make decisions for himself or herself.

Medical practice acts: State laws that define the practice of medicine.

Memory: In suture material, the tendency of suture to recoil to its original shape during packaging.

Menarche: Menstruation, menses.

Menorrhagia: Excessive bleeding during menses.

Menu: In computer technology, a list of tasks displayed on the monitor. Tasks are selected and executed from the menu.

Mesh: A pliable synthetic or biosynthetic material used to bridge the tissue edges of the abdominal wall. It is used during hernia repair.

Metastasis: The spread of malignant or cancerous cells to a local or distant area of the body.

Microbiology: The study of microbes, or organisms that require a microscope for observation.

Micturition: Urination.

Minimally invasive surgery (MIS): Surgery performed through small incisions using telescopic instruments.

Missed abortion: An abortion in which the products of conception are no longer viable but are retained in the uterus.

Mission statement: A written declaration that defines the central goal of the health care institution and reflects the organization's ethical and moral beliefs in broad terms.

Mitochondrion (sing); mitochondria (pl): An organelle that synthesizes adenosine triphosphate (ATP) to provide cellular energy.

Mixter clamp: A type of hemostat with a straight shank and a right-angle tip.

Mobility: The ability of an organism to move. As a protective mechanism, mobility allows an organism to move away from harmful stimuli.

Mobilize: To surgically free up an organ or other structure by dissecting its attachments to other tissue. Most tissues of the body are attached by serous membranes or connective tissue. Whenever tissue is removed or remodeled, these attachments must be freed up. This often includes dividing and ligating attached blood vessels. This is called *tissue mobilization.*

Modified radical mastectomy: A procedure in which the entire breast, nipple, and areolar region are removed. The lymph nodes also are usually removed.

Sentinel lymph node biopsy (SLNB): A procedure in which one or more lymph nodes are removed to determine whether a tumor has metastasized. Other lymph nodes may be removed periodically to determine whether metastasis has occurred.

Molecule: A specific substance made up of elements that are bonded together.

Momentum: The mathematical relationship between the weight and velocity of a mass.

Monitor: The computer screen.

Monitored anesthesia care (MAC): Monitoring of vital functions during regional anesthesia to ensure the patient's safety and comfort.

Monochromatic: A characteristic of laser light in which the frequency of each wave is the same.

Monofilament suture: Extruded suture of a single fiber.

Monopolar circuit: In electrosurgery, a continuous path of electricity that flows from the electrosurgical unit to the active electrode, through the patient and the return electrode, back to the electrosurgical unit.

Morbid obesity: A condition in which the patient's body mass index (BMI) is 40 or higher, and the individual is at least 100 pounds (45 kg) over the ideal weight despite aggressive attempts to lose weight.

Morcellization: A surgical technique in which tissue is fragmented to permit removal through an endoscopic cannula.

Multifilament suture: Braided or twisted suture.

Muscle recession: Surgery in which the eye muscle is moved back to release the globe.

Mutagenic substance: A chemical or other agent which causes permanent change in the cell's genetic material.

Mycotic: Referring to fungi.

Nasogastric (NG) tube: A flexible tube inserted through the nose and advanced into the stomach. The NG tube is used to decompress the stomach or to provide a means of feeding the patient liquid nutrients and medication.

Nasolaryngoscope: A flexible endoscope that is passed through the nose to visualize the larynx.

National Certifying Examination for Surgical Technologists: A comprehensive written examination required for official certification by the Association of Surgical Technologists.

NBSTSA: National Board of Surgical Technology and Surgical Assisting. The NBSTSA (formerly the Liaison Council on Certification for the Surgical Technologist) is responsible for all decisions related to certification such as eligibility, renewal, and revocation.

NCCT: National Center for Competency Testing. A nonprofit organization that provides a certification examination for military and other trained surgical technologists whose programs are not recognized by the Association of Surgical Technologists.

Necrosis: Tissue death.

Needleless system: A system of parenteral access that does not use needles for the collection or withdrawal of body fluids through venous puncture.

Negligence: Negligence can occur in two ways: it can be a failure to do something that a reasonable person, guided by the ordinary considerations that regulate human affairs, would do; or, it can be the act of doing something that a reasonable and prudent person would not do.

Neodymium:YAG: A solid lasing medium known for its attraction to protein and deep penetration into tissue.

Neoplasm: A tumor, which may be benign or malignant.

Nephroblastoma: Wilms tumor.

Nephroscopy: Endoscopic surgery of the kidney.

Neural tube defect: A congenital abnormality resulting from failure of the neural tube to close in embryonic development.

Neuromuscular blocking agent: A drug that blocks nerve conduction in striated muscle tissue.

Neuropathy: Permanent or temporary nerve injury that results in numbness or loss of function of a part of the body.

Neurotransmitters: Chemicals that bind to target cells to produce a specific neurological effect.

Neutral electrode: An alternate term for the patient return electrode.

Neutral zone (no-hands) technique: A method of transferring sharp instruments on the surgical field without hand-to-hand contact. A neutral zone is identified, and sharps are exchanged in this zone.

Neutron: A subatomic particle located in the nucleus of the atom. It has no electrical charge.

Newton's laws of motion: A set of hypotheses concerning the behavior of objects in motion, proposed by Sir Isaac Newton in the 1600s. Some of these laws are used in modern physics.

Nonabsorbable sutures: Suture materials that resist breakdown in the body.

Nonconductive: The quality of a substance that resists the transfer of electrons and therefore electrical current.

Noncritical items: Items that are not required to be sterile because they do not penetrate intact tissues. Patient care items such as a blood pressure cuff and a stethoscope are noncritical.

Nonelectrolytic: Nonconductive; nonelectrolytic solutions must be used for bladder distension or continuous irrigation whenever the electrosurgical unit (ESU) is used.

Nonheartbeating cadaver: A cadaver in which perfusion at and after death was not possible. Only certain tissues may be procured for donation.

Nonpathogenic: Refers to an organism that does not cause disease in a healthy individual. About 95% to 97% of all bacteria are nonpathogenic.

Nonsterile team members: Surgical team members who handle only nonsterile equipment, supplies, and instruments.

Nonwoven: A fabric or material that is bonded together as opposed to a process of interweaving individual threads.

Normal spontaneous vaginal delivery (NSVD): A normal delivery of the fetus, without the need for medical intervention. The normal birth process.

Norms: Behaviors that are accepted as part of the environment and culture of a group. Norms usually are established by custom and popular acceptance rather than by law, although the two may not be mutually exclusive.

Nosocomial infection: Another term for hospital-acquired infection (HAI) or health care-acquired infection; an infection acquired as a result of being in a health care facility.

Nuchal cord: A complication of pregnancy in which the umbilical cord is wrapped around the fetus' neck. This may lead to obstructed blood flow to the fetus.

Nuclear energy: The energy derived when subatomic particles are separated from the atom.

Nuclear medicine: Medical procedures that use radioactive particles to track target tissue in the body.

Nucleolus: An organelle inside the nucleus that contains proteins necessary for cell reproduction.

Nucleus: The organ structure in the cell that contains the genetic material for replication and reproduction of the cell. The center of an atom.

Nurse practice acts: State laws that define the practice of nursing.

Nutrition: Usually refers to the intake of food. On a cellular and tissue level, it may include the availability of nutrients, fluid, and electrolytes.

Nystagmus: Rapid oscillation of the eye, a symptom of certain nervous system diseases.

Obligate aerobe: A microorganism that requires oxygen to live and grow.

Obligate anaerobe: An organism that must live in the absence of oxygen to survive.

Obturator: A blunt-nosed instrument that is inserted through the sheath of a rigid endoscope or hysteroscope to protect the tissue as the instrument is advanced.

Occupational exposure: Exposure to hazards in the workplace; for example, exposure to hazardous chemicals or contact with potentially infected blood and body fluids.

Odontectomy: Tooth extraction.

Off-pump procedure: A procedure performed without a cardiopulmonary bypass (i.e., "the pump").

Omphalocele: A protrusion of abdominal contents through an opening at the navel, especially when it occurs as a congenital defect.

Oophorectomy: Removal of the ovary.

Open gloving: A gloving technique in which the bare skin does not touch any part of the outside of the glove. Open gloving generally is used when a health care worker does not wear a sterile gown.

Open reduction: Surgical access (through an incision) to bring bone fragments into anatomical alignment.

Open surgery: Standard surgery in which an incision is made and standard instruments are used.

Operative report: A patient record of the surgery, which is maintained and submitted by the attending circulating nurse.

Optical angle: The angle at which light is transmitted at the distal end of a fiberoptic or video endoscope.

Optical resonant cavity: The component of a laser system in which the lasing medium is contained and light is transformed.

Organizational chart (organigram): A graphic depiction of an organization's chain of command that shows the lines of vertical (higher and lower) and horizontal (equal) administrative authority.

Oromaxillofacial surgery: Surgery involving the bones of the face, primarily for repair of fractures and reconstruction for congenital anomalies.

Orthopedic system: A specific (usually patented) set of instruments and implants used for an orthopedic technique. For example, arthroplasty implants are marketed as systems that include the joint components and instruments that are designed for use with that implant.

Orthostatic (postural) blood pressure: A technique used to check the patient's blood pressure in the upright or recumbent position.

ORTs: Operating room technicians. Former title of the surgical technologist (the title was changed in the early 1970s).

OSHA: Occupational Safety and Health Administration. The agency of the U.S. Department of Labor that establishes rules and standards to protect the safety of employees in the workplace.

Ossicles: The bones of the middle ear that conduct sound (i.e., the malleus, incus, and stapes).

Osteophytes: Bony outgrowths found in an arthritic joint.

Osteotomy: A surgical cut into bone tissue.

-Ostomy: A suffix that refers to an opening between two hollow organs; for example, *gastroduodenostomy,* a surgical procedure that joins the stomach and duodenum.

Ostomy: A technique in which a new opening is made between a tubular structure such as the intestine or ureter and the outside of the body or another hollow structure or organ.

Otitis media: Middle ear infection.

Ototoxic: A substance that can injure the ear.

Outcome-oriented care: Care based on the predicted result of particular tasks and duties.

Oxygen-enriched atmosphere (OEA): An environment that contains a high percentage of oxygen and presents a high risk for fire.

Pacemaker: A device that stimulates the heart muscle to contract.

Packing: A method of applying a dressing to a body cavity. In nasal procedures, 1/4- or 1/2-inch (0.63 or 1.25 cm) gauze strips are inserted into the nasal cavity to absorb drainage, control bleeding, or expose the mucosa to topical medication. "Packing" a wound may refer to any dressing that is introduced into an anatomical space or cavity.

Palpating: Assessing a part of the body by feeling the outline, density, movement, or other attributes.

Papanicolaou (PAP) test: A diagnostic test in which epithelial cells are taken from the endocervical canal and examined for abnormalities that can lead to cervical cancer.

Papilloma: A benign epithelial tumor characterized by a branching or lobular tumor. Also called a *papillary tumor*.

Paramedian incision: An abdominal incision lying parallel to the midline.

Paranasal sinuses: Air cells surrounding or on the periphery of the nasal cavities. These are the maxillary, ethmoid, sphenoid, and frontal sinuses.

Parasite: An organism that lives on or within another organism and gains an advantage at the expense of that organism.

Parasympathetic nervous system: Part of the autonomic nervous system that is responsible for energy conservation and rest, including relaxation of muscle groups, dilation of blood vessels, and decreased blood pressure.

Parenteral: Refers to administration of a drug by injection.

Paresis: Paralysis of a structure (e.g., vocal cord paresis).

Partial thromboplastin time (PTT): A test of blood coagulation used in patients receiving heparin to determine the correct level of anticoagulation.

Parturition: Birth.

Patency: The condition of being open; an unobstructed passageway (e.g., a patent fallopian tube).

Pathogen: A disease-causing (pathogenic) microorganism.

Pathogenic: Having the potential to cause disease.

Pathogenicity: An organism's biological and chemical mechanisms that cause disease.

Pathology: The study of disease.

Patient-centered care: Therapeutic care, communication, and intervention provided according to the unique needs of the patient.

Patient return electrode (PRE): A critical component of the monopolar electrosurgical circuit. The PRE is a conductive pad that captures electricity and shunts it safely out of the body and back to the electrosurgical unit.

Peak effect: The period of maximum effect of a drug.

Pelvic cavity: The lower abdominal cavity, which contains the bladder, uterus, and adnexa.

Peracetic acid: A chemical used in the sterilization of critical items.

Percutaneous: A term that literally means "through the skin." In a percutaneous approach in surgery, an incision is not made; rather, a catheter or other device is introduced through a puncture site.

Percutaneous endoscopic gastrostomy (PEG): The insertion of a tube into the stomach for enteral feedings or gastric decompression.

Perforation: A defect in the tympanic membrane caused by trauma or infection.

Perfusion (oxygen): The distribution of oxygen to tissues.

Perichondrium: Tissue overlying the cartilage that provides its vascular and nervous supply.

Perineum: The anatomical area between the posterior vestibule and the anus.

Periosteum: Tissue overlying the bone that provides its vascular and nervous supply.

Perjury: The crime of intentionally lying or falsifying information during court testimony after a person has sworn to tell the truth.

Personal protective equipment (PPE): Approved attire worn during the reprocessing of medical devices and the cleaning of patient areas. PPE protects the wearer from contamination by microorganisms.

Personnel policy: A policy that sets forth the health care facility's job descriptions, role delineations, requirements for employment, and rules of conduct for personnel.

Pfannenstiel incision: A transverse incision below the umbilicus and just above the pubis; it generally is used for pelvic surgery.

Phacoemulsification: A process whereby high-frequency sound waves are used to emulsify tissue, such as a cataract.

Phagocyte: Any cell capable of ingesting particulate matter and microorganisms.

Phagocytosis: A defensive mechanism in which a cell engulfs a substance or another cell.

Pharmacodynamics: The biochemical and physiological effects of drugs and their mechanisms of action in the body.

Pharmacokinetics: The movement of a drug through the tissues and cells of the body, including the processes of absorption, distribution, and localization in tissues, biotransformation, and excretion by mechanical and chemical means.

Pharmacology: The study of drugs and their action in the body.

Phase change thermometer: A disposable adhesive strip impregnated with temperature-sensitive dots that indicate the surface temperature of skin.

Philtrum: The vertical groove in the center of the upper lip.

Phonation: Vibration of the vocal cords during speaking or vocalization.

Photodamage: Damage to the skin caused by ultraviolet light.

Photon: In physics, the name given to a light particle. The particle theory is disputed by many scientists, who believe that light is wave energy.

Physical barrier: In surgery, a barrier that separates a sterile surface from a nonsterile surface. Examples are sterile surgical gloves, gowns, and drapes. A physical barrier, such as a clean surgical cap, also can prevent a bacteria-laden surface, such as the hair, from shedding microorganisms.

Physiological: A term that refers to the biochemical, mechanical, and physical processes of life.

PID: Pelvic inflammatory disease; PID is caused by a sexually transmitted disease or some other source of infection. It causes scarring of the fallopian tubes and adhesions in the abdominal and pelvic cavity.

Pili: A rodlike attachment extending from the cell membrane that is capable of attaching to another cell to transfer genetic material.

Pixel: An element within each silicone chip contained within a device which produces electronic images such as those seen on a surgical monitor used in minimally invasive surgery. One pixel is represented as a signal. As the number of signals (pixels) increases, the quality of the image is enhanced.

Placenta: The organ that transfers selected nutrients to the baby during pregnancy.

Placenta abruption: Premature separation of the placenta from the uterine wall after 20 weeks' gestation and before the fetus is delivered.

Placenta previa: A complication of pregnancy in which the placenta implants completely or partly over the cervical os. In this position, the placenta begins to bleed as it separates from the cervix during labor.

Plasma sterilization: A process that uses the form of matter known as plasma (e.g., hydrogen peroxide plasma) to sterilize an item.

Plastic and reconstructive surgery: Surgery performed to restore form and function that have been lost because of trauma, radical surgery, or congenital anomaly.

Pleur-Evac: The prototype of single-use, closed chest drainage systems, introduced in 1967.

Pleuritis: Inflammation of the pleural membrane, usually caused by an infection or a tumor.

Pliability: The flexibility of a suture material.

Plicate: To fold tissue and secure it in place surgically.

Pneumatic tourniquet: An air-filled tourniquet used to prevent blood flow to an extremity during surgery.

Pneumoperitoneum: An abdomen insufflated or distended with carbon dioxide gas during laparoscopy.

Pneumothorax: Air in the chest cavity, which prevents the lungs from expanding and may displace the mediastinal structures.

Points: The tips of a surgical instrument.

Policy manual: Operational guidelines, procedures, and protocols contained in written or electronic documents. Employees are required to follow the policies of the department in which they are employed and to be familiar with procedures for emergency and general safety.

Polyp: Excessive proliferation of the mucosal epithelium.

Positron emission tomography (PET): A type of medical imaging that measures a specific type of metabolic activity in the target tissue.

Postanesthesia care unit (PACU): The critical care area where patients are taken after surgery for monitoring, evaluation, and response to emergencies.

Postexposure prophylaxis (PEP): Recommended procedures to help prevent the development of blood-borne diseases after an exposure incident such as a needle stick injury.

Postmortem care: Physical care of the body to prepare it for viewing by the family and for mortuary procedures.

Potassium-titanyl-phosphate (KTP): A low-power lasing medium that produces a very small diameter beam well-suited to microsurgery.

Potential energy: Energy stored in the form of gravity, chemical bonds, nuclear particles, and mechanical springs.

Preclotting: The process of soaking a graft or patch of synthetic graft material in the patient's blood or plasma before insertion. Most grafts no longer need preclotting.

Prenatal: The period of pregnancy before birth.

Preoperative medication: One or more drugs administered before surgery to prevent complications related to the surgical procedure or anesthesia.

Prep: The use of antiseptic solutions to clean the skin, reduce the microbial count, and prevent unnecessary contamination of an area for a sterile invasive procedure (e.g., skin incision) or a sterile noninvasive procedure (e.g., urinary catheterization).

Prescription: An order for a drug written by a qualified medical staff member.

Presentation: A term that refers to the part of the baby that comes down the birth canal first.

Press-fit: To impact or press a joint implant into position. Press-fitted implants do not require bone cement.

Prewarming: A procedure in which the patient is warmed before surgery, which is done as a separate process in perioperative care.

Primary intention (wound healing): The healing process after a clean surgical repair.

Prion: An infectious protein substance that is resistant to common sterilization methods.

Professional ethics: Ethical behavior established by authoritative peers of a particular profession, such as medicine or law.

Professional license: Governmental permission to perform specified actions.

Prognosis: A prediction of the patient's medical outcome (e.g., poor prognosis, good prognosis).

Projectile motion: The path of an object in motion in which gravity acts to pull the object downward.

Prokaryotes: Cellular organisms that lack a true nucleus or nuclear membrane. Prokaryotes include only bacteria and the Archaea, a smaller primitive group of single-cell organisms.

Prolapsed cord: Complication of pregnancy in which the umbilical cord emerges from the uterus during labor and may be compressed against the material pelvis or the vagina. This can cause obstructed blood supply to the fetus.

Prone position: The position in which the front of the body is in contact with the operating table.

Proprietary name: The patented name given to a drug by its manufacturer.

Proprietary school: Private, for-profit school.

Protective mechanisms: Nervous system responses to harmful environmental stimuli, such as pain, obstruction of the airway, and extreme temperature. Coughing, blinking, shivering, and withdrawal (from pain) are protective mechanisms.

Prothrombin time (PT): A measurement of the time required for blood to clot.

Proton: A subatomic particle that is part of the nucleus of an atom. It has a positive charge.

Pterygium: A triangular membrane that arises from the medial canthus; the tissue may extend over the cornea, causing blindness.

Ptosis: Drooping or sagging of any anatomical structure.

Pulmonary function tests (PFTs): Tests performed to measure the function and strength of the pulmonary system.

Pulse oximeter: A monitoring device that measures the patient's hemoglobin oxygen saturation by means of spectrometry.

Pulsed wave lasers: Lasers that apply the laser light intermittently to the target tissue.

Punitive: Actions intended to punish a person who has violated the law.

Purse-string: A suturing technique in which a continuous strand is passed in and out of the circumference of a lumen and then is pulled tight, like a drawstring.

Pyeloplasty: Reconstruction of the ureter in the renal pelvis. This procedure usually is performed to repair a distended ureter caused by a ureteral obstruction and backward flow of urine.

Pyloric stenosis: A narrowing of the part of the stomach (pylorus) that leads to the small intestine.

Pyrexia: Fever.

Q-switched lasers: An alternate name for pulsed wave lasers.

Quadrants: Four designated regions of the abdomen.

Radiant exposure: In laser technology, the combination of the concentration of laser energy and the length of time tissue is exposed to it.

Radiation: The transfer of heat by electromagnetic waves.

Radioactive seeds: Small "seeds" of radioactive material that are implanted for cancer treatment.

Radiofrequency: Electromagnetic energy in which the frequency is in the area of radio transmission. In electrosurgery, radiofrequency electromagnetic waves are used to produce the desired surgical effect.

Radiofrequency ablation (RFA): The use of radiofrequency waves to destroy a tissue mass or surface.

Radionuclides or isotopes: In nuclear medicine, radioactive particles are directed at the nucleus of a selected element to create energy. These special elements are referred to as *radionuclides or isotopes*.

Radiopaque: Any object that is not penetrable by x-rays (gamma radiation).

RAM: Random access memory; the memory capacity of a computer.

Range of motion: The normal anatomical movement of an extremity.

Ream: To enlarge a pre-existing hole, depression, or channel, such as the medullary canal.

Receiver: The person to whom a message is communicated by a sender.

Receptacle: An outlet in an electrical circuit that receives a plug containing live current, completing the circuit.

Rectocele: A bulging of intestinal tissue into a weakened posterior vaginal wall.

Reduce: To replace or push herniated tissue back into its normal anatomical position.

Reduction: The process of manipulating a bone t structure to restore anatomical position.

Reflection: The behavior of a wave when it reaches a nonabsorbent material. The wave reverses and is directed back toward the source. Also, communication with the patient that helps the individual connect current emotions with events in the environment.

Reflux: Backward (opposite of its normal direction) flow of a body fluid. Urinary reflux is backward flow of urine into the ureter or kidney.

Refraction: A phenomenon of physics in which light rays are bent as they pass through a transparent medium that is denser than air. In the eye, refraction occurs as light enters the front of the eye and passes through the cornea, lens, aqueous humor, and vitreous.

Refractive index: A measurement of a substance's ability to absorb light waves. The refractive index is higher in substances that light can pass through easily (e.g., glass, plastics).

Regional block: Anesthesia in a specific area of the body, achieved by injection of an anesthetic around a major nerve or group of nerves.

Regression: An abnormal return to a former or earlier state, particularly infantile patterns of thought or behavior. In patients, this can result from feelings of helplessness and dependency.

Relational: A term that refers to a person's interactions with other individuals.

Replantation (reimplantation): Surgical attachment of the hand, thumb, or fingers after traumatic amputation.

Reprocessing: Activities or tasks that prepare used medical devices for use on another patient; these activities include cleaning, disinfection, and sterilization.

Required request law: A law requiring medical personnel to request organ procurement from a deceased's family.

Resection: A surgical technique in which a portion of tissue or an organ is removed and rejoined in another configuration.

Resectoscope: A cutting instrument used to remove and coagulate tissue piece by piece. It is used in conjunction with endoscopic procedures to remove tumors or other tissue, such as the prostate or endometrium.

Resident flora: Microorganisms that are normally present in specific tissues. Resident flora are necessary to the regular function of these tissues or structures. Also called *normal flora*.

Resident microorganisms: The microorganisms that normally live in certain tissues of the body; also called normal flora.

Residual activity: The "–cidal" activity of an antiseptic or a disinfectant that continues after the solution has dried.

Resistance: In electricity, the measurement of a substance's ability to conduct electricity. Also, the restriction of electron flow in a direct current circuit.

Respiration: Oxygen exchange at the cellular and molecular levels and the process of ventilation.

Restricted area: The area of the operating room where only personnel wearing surgical attire, including masks, shoe coverings, and head coverings, are allowed. Doors are kept closed, and the air pressure is greater than that in areas outside the restricted area.

Retained object: An item that is inadvertently left inside the patient during surgery.

Retention catheter: A urinary catheter with an inflatable balloon that is used to drain the bladder continuously during surgery. It is inserted before the surgical skin prep. Also called an *indwelling* or a *Foley catheter*.

Retention sutures: Heavy, nonabsorbable sutures that are placed behind the skin sutures and through all tissue layers to give added strength to the closure. Also called a *secondary suture line*.

Retrograde pyelography: Imaging studies of the renal pelvis in which a contrast medium is instilled through a transurethral catheter. *Retrograde* refers to flow, which is opposite (or backwards from) the normal direction.

Return electrode monitoring (REM): A safety system used in electrosurgery in which the PRE transmits continuous feedback on the quality of impedance in the electrode and stops the current when it becomes dangerously high.

Reusable: A designation used by manufacturers to indicate that a medical device can be reprocessed for use on more than one patient.

Reverse cutting needle: A curved surgical needle with three honed edges, one on the outside curve of the needle.

Reverse Trendelenburg position: The position in which a prone or supine patient is tilted with the feet down.

Revision arthroplasty: A repeat arthroplasty in which previously implanted joint components are replaced.

Rigor mortis: The natural stiffening of the body that starts approximately 15 minutes after death and lasts about 24 hours.

Risk: The statistical probability of a given event based on the number of such events that have already occurred in a certain population.

Risk management: The process of tracking, evaluating, and studying accidents and incidents to protect patients and employees. Risk management produces change in policy or enforcement of policy if the risk reaches an unacceptable level.

Robot: A mechanical device that can be programmed to perform tasks.

Role confusion: Lack of clarity about one's job duties and requirements.

Rongeur: A hinged instrument with sharp, cup-shaped tips that is used to extract pieces of bone or other connective tissue.

Running suture: A method of suturing that uses one continuous suture strand for tissue approximation.

Saccular aneurysm: A type of aneurysm in which a saclike formation with a narrow neck projects from the side of the artery.

Safe Medical Device Act: A federal regulation that requires the reporting of any incident causing death or injury that is suspected to be the result of a medical device.

Sanitation: A method that reduces the number of bacteria in the environment to a safe level.

Satellite facilities: Community health care offices that are administered by a single institution but are located in communities in surrounding urban or rural areas. These facilities offer primary and preventive health care services in general medicine and other specialties.

Save (data): Data are stored on the computer after they are created and before the computer is turned off; this is called *saving data.*

Scar: The formation of permanent connective tissue at the site of tissue trauma.

Scrub: Role and name commonly applied to the surgical technologist or perioperative nurse who is part of the sterile team. The scrub participates in surgery and handles only sterile supplies, instruments, and equipment.

Scrubbed personnel: In surgery, members of the surgical team who work within the sterile field. Also called *sterile personnel.*

Secondary intention (wound healing): Natural healing of a wound without sutures or other means of approximating tissue.

Sedative: A drug that induces a range of unconscious states. The effects are dose dependent. At low doses, sedatives cause some drowsiness. Increasing the dose causes central nervous system depression, ending in loss of consciousness.

Segmental resection: An anatomical resection of the liver in which segments divided by specific blood vessels and biliary ducts are removed.

Selective absorption: The absorption of a lasing medium by the distinct color and density of a substance.

Self-actualization: An individual's ability to express and achieve personal goals.

Self-determination: The right of an individual to determine the direction and path of his or her life.

Semicritical items: Items that are required to be free of most pathogenic organisms, including *Mycobacterium tuberculosis*, because these items come in contact with mucous membranes (e.g., respiratory equipment, endoscopes).

Semi-Fowler position: A semisitting position, which is used for surgery on the neck and thyroid.

Semirestricted area: A designated area in which only personnel wearing scrub suits and hair caps that enclose all facial hair are allowed.

Sender: The person who communicates a message to another.

Sensation: The ability to feel stimuli in the environment (e.g., pain, heat, touch, visual stimuli, and sound).

Sensorineural hearing loss: Hearing impairment arising from the cochlea, auditory nerve, or central nervous system.

Sentinel event: An unexpected incident resulting in serious physical injury, psychological harm, or death. The risk of injury or harm is also considered a sentinel event.

Sentinel lymph node biopsy (SLNB): A procedure in which one or more lymph nodes are removed to determine whether a tumor has metastasized. Other lymph nodes may be removed periodically to determine whether metastasis has occurred.

Serial lenses: An optical system in which several lenses are lined up to produce a clear, well-defined image. Surgical endoscopes use serial lenses.

Serosa: The delicate outer layer of tissue of most organs.

Sexual harassment: Sexual coercion; sexual innuendoes; or unwanted sexual comments, gestures, or touch.

Shank: The area of a surgical instrument between the box lock and the finger ring.

Sharps: Any objects used in health care that are capable of penetrating the skin, causing injury.

Shear injury: Tissue injury or necrosis that results when two tissue planes are forcefully pulled in opposite directions. Shearing usually occurs when the body is pulled or slides by gravity across a high-friction surface, such as a bed sheet. Shearing can lead to a decubitus ulcer.

Shelf life: The length of time a wrapped item remains sterile after it has been subjected to a sterilization process.

Shunt: To bypass a structure or carry fluid from one anatomical location to another.

Side effects: Anticipated effects of a drug other than those intended. Side effects may be uncomfortable for the patient or may have a positive outcome.

Single action rongeur: A cutting instrument that has one hinge.

Single-use items: Instruments and devices intended for use on one patient only; sometimes called disposable items.

Skeletal traction: Traction device in which is connected by pins or rods which are surgically inserted into the bone.

Skeletonization: Surgical dissection to separate vessels or other small structures from the surrounding connective tissue attachments.

Skin flap: A flap that is created by incising the skin and cutting it away from the underlying tissue to which it is attached. The flap can be increased in size or "raised" as it is enlarged by dissection.

Skin traction: Taping a traction system to the skin, used as a temporary measure only (e.g., Buck traction). Skin traction is seldom used in adults in modern medicine.

Slander: Spoken defamation.

Slap hammer: A type of impactor used primarily in arthroplasty to seat a joint component into the bone.

Smoke plume: Smoke created during the use of an electrosurgical unit (ESU) or laser. This smoke contains toxic chemicals, vapors, blood fragments, and viruses.

Software: Computer programs or applications that allow the user to perform different kinds of function and tasks, such as data or word processing.

Solid: A state of matter in which the molecules are bonded very tightly. Characteristics of solids are hardness and the ability to break apart into other solid pieces.

Spatula needle: A side cutting with flat top and bottom, used in ophthalmic surgery.

Spaulding system: A system used to determine the level of microbial destruction on medical devices and supplies based on the risk of infection associated with the area of the body where the device is used. Categories include critical, semi-critical, and non-critical.

Specific gravity: The ratio of the density of a fluid compared to water. The specific gravity of urine is an important diagnostic tool.

Speed (wave): In wave energy, the number of waves that pass a point in 1 second.

Sphygmomanometer: An instrument used to measure blood pressure.

Spirochetes: Curved or spiral-shaped bacteria.

Split-thickness (or partial-thickness) skin graft (PTSG): A skin graft that consists of the epidermis and a portion of the papillary dermis.

Spore: The highly resistant dormant stage of some bacteria. Spores can live in extreme environmental conditions, sometimes indefinitely; also called an endospore.

Sporicidal: Able to kill spores.

Spray coagulation: An alternate term for fulguration.

Staghorn stone: A large, jagged kidney stone that forms in the renal pelvis.

Staging: A complex method of determining the severity of a malignant tumor. Lymph node involvement and the tumor's size, location, and type are considered.

Stain: A substance applied directly to anatomical surfaces to differentiate normal cells from abnormal ones.

Staining: The process of coloring microbial specimens so that they can be seen with the optical microscope.

Standard definition (SD): A type of video format. The clarity of an image is based on the number of signals (pixels) emitted by the camera. A standard definition format displays 640×480 pixels in a rectangular image.

Standard Precautions: Guidelines recommended by the Centers for Disease Control and Prevention (CDC) to reduce the risk of transmission of blood-borne and other pathogens.

Stasis (venous): Pooling of blood in the veins caused by inactivity or disease. Stasis can cause distension of the veins.

States of matter: The physical forms of matter. The four states of matter are gas, liquid, solid, and plasma.

Statutes: Laws passed by legislative bodies.

Stenosis: The narrowing of a hollow structure such as a blood vessel or duct.

Stent: A surgical method of providing support to an anatomical structure; the term may also refer to the support device itself. In plastic surgery, a stent dressing is used to maintain contact between a skin graft and the graft site.

Stereoscopic viewer: In robotic surgery, the binocular lens system of the surgeon console.

Stereotactic: A computerized method of locating a point in space or in tissue, using coordinates in three-dimensions. During stereotactic surgery, the precise location of a tumor or other tissue can be identified from outside the body. The tissue can then be targeted for destruction. The term originates from the Greek words *stereo*, meaning three dimensional, and *tactos*, meaning touched.

Sterile: Completely free of all microorganisms.

Sterile field: An area that includes the draped patient, all sterile tables, and sterile equipment in the immediate area of the patient. The patient is considered the center of the sterile field.

Sterile item: Any item that has been subjected to a process that renders it free of all microbial life, including spores.

Sterility: A state in which an inanimate or animate substance harbors absolutely no viable microorganisms.

Sterilization: A process by which all microorganisms, including spores, are destroyed.

Sternotomy: An incision made into the sternum.

Stoma: An opening created in a hollow organ and sutured to the skin to drain the organ's contents (e.g., an intestinal or ureteral stoma). A stoma may be a temporary or permanent method of bypass.

Stoma appliance: A two- or three-piece medical device used to collect drainage from a stoma. The appliance is attached to the patient's skin and completely covers the stoma. This allows free drainage into a collection device or bag.

Strabismus: Inability to coordinate the extraocular muscles, which prevents binocular vision.

Straight catheter: A urinary nonretaining catheter used for one-time drainage of the bladder. It may be called a "red Robinson" or simply a "Robinson" catheter.

Strangulated hernia: A hernia in which abdominal tissue has become trapped between the layers of an abdominal wall defect. The strangulated tissue usually becomes swollen as a result of venous congestion. Lack of blood supply can lead to tissue necrosis.

Strike-through contamination: An event in which fluid from a nonsterile surface or air penetrates the protective wrapper of a sterile item, potentially contaminating the item.

Subatomic particles: The physical components of an atom. The most common are the neutron, proton, and electron.

Subcostal: A term referring to the area of the abdomen that follows the slope of the tenth costal cartilage. A subcostal incision is made in this area.

Subcutaneous mastectomy: A procedure in which the breast is removed, but the skin, nipple, and areola are left intact. Also called a **lumpectomy**.

Subcutaneous tissue: The fatty (adipose) tissue layer lying directly under the skin of the abdominal wall and other areas of the body.

Sublingual: A term for the region under the tongue, which is highly vascular. Specific medications may be administered sublingually, because they are rapidly absorbed through the mucous membrane.

Subphrenic area: The area under or below the liver.

Subpoena: A court order requiring its recipient to appear and testify at a trial or deposition. Medical records also can be the subject of subpoenas.

Summons: A court-issued document that is received by a person being sued, notifying the person that he or she is a defendant in the lawsuit.

Supine position: The position in which the patient lies on the back, facing upward.

Suppurative: Having developed pus and fluid.

Suprapubic catheter: A bladder catheter inserted through the skin in the suprapubic area of the abdomen.

Suprapubic pressure: Pressure that is applied downward on the patient's abdomen just above the pubic bone.

Surfactant: A surface agent such as soap that lowers surface tension, allowing greater permeability.

Surgeon console: In robotic surgery, the nonsterile control unit used by the surgeon to manipulate instruments.

Surgical conscience: In surgery, the ethical motivation to practice excellent aseptic technique to protect the patient from infection. Surgical conscience implies that the professional practices excellent technique regardless of whether others are observing.

Surgical hand rub: The systematic application of antiseptic foam or cream on the hands before gowning and gloving for a sterile procedure. The surgical hand rub may be used as an alternative to the surgical hand scrub under certain conditions.

Surgical hand scrub: A specific technique for washing the hands before donning a surgical gown and gloves before surgery. The scrub is performed with timed or counted strokes using detergent-based antiseptic. The surgical hand scrub is designed to remove dirt, oils, and transient microorganisms and reduce the number of resident microorganisms.

Surgical site infection (SSI): Postoperative infection of the surgical wound, most commonly caused by the normal bacteria found on the patient's skin or shed from the skin or hair from members of the surgical team.

Swage: The area of an atraumatic suture where the suture strand is fused to the needle. Also called an atraumatic suture.

Symbiosis: The environmental relationship between two or more organisms in which each benefits from the other.

Sympathetic nervous system: Part of the autonomic nervous system responsible for "fight or flight" response to danger and stress. Physiologic reactions include diversion of blood to essential organs, increased heart rate, and blood pressure.

Synapse: The synapse is the small space in which the neurotransmitter passes from one nerve cell to another.

Syncope: A temporary loss of consciousness caused by an interruption of or a decrease in the flow of blood to the brain.

Synergistic: The interaction of agents or conditions such that the total effect is greater than the sum of the individual effects.

Synthetic graft: A graft derived from synthetic material compatible with body tissue. Synthetic grafts may be soft, semisolid, or liquid.

Systolic pressure: The highest pressure exerted on the inside arterial wall during contraction of the heart (**systole**).

Table break: The hinged joint between sections of the operating table that can be flexed in any direction.

Tachycardia: A fast heart rate (usually over 120 beats per minute).

Tamper-evident seal: A latching mechanism or lock that secures a container and is designed so that it cannot be resealed after opening.

Tamponade: An instrument or other device that puts pressure on tissue, usually to stop bleeding.

Task bar: In graphics-based computer platforms, a horizontal or vertical block that contains small pictures or menus that activate tasks.

Technetium-99: A radioactive substance used to identify sentinel lymph nodes.

Telescopic instruments: Long, narrow instruments used during endoscopic surgery.

Telesurgery: A type of robotic surgery in which surgery is performed from a nearby location through computer-mediated instruments. In telesurgery, no direct physical contact with the instruments occurs.

Tenaculum: A grasping instrument with sharp pointed tips, generally used to manipulate or grasp tissue such as the thyroid or cervix.

Tensile strength: The amount of force or stress a suture can withstand without breaking.

Teratogen: A chemical or agent that can injure the fetus or cause birth defects.

Therapeutic communication: A purposeful method of communication in which the caregiver responds to explicit or implicit needs of the patient.

Therapeutic touch: The purposeful touching of another person to convey empathy, care, and tenderness.

Therapeutic window: The difference in drug dose between the therapeutic level and toxic level.

Thermal conductivity: The ability of a substance to conduct heat. Different substances have different abilities to conduct or transmit heat.

Thermoregulation: A complex physiological process in which the body maintains a temperature that is optimal for survival.

Third intention (wound healing): Delayed primary wound closure. Routine wound closure after a period of healing.

Thoracic outlet syndrome: A group of disorders attributed to compression of the subclavian vessels and nerves. Such compression can cause permanent injury to the arm and shoulder.

Thoracoscopy: Minimally invasive surgery of the thoracic cavity; also referred to as video assisted thoracoscopic surgery or VATS.

Thoracotomy: Open chest surgery in which the thoracic cavity is entered; literally, an incision into the chest wall.

Thromboembolus: A blood clot that breaks loose and enters the systemic circulation, causing obstruction or occlusion of a blood vessel. Also referred to as a *thrombus*.

Thrombus: Any organic or nonorganic material blocking an artery; generally refers to a blood clot or atherosclerotic plaque but also includes fat or air.

Thyroglossal duct: A transitory endodermal tube in the embryo that carries thyroid-forming tissue at its caudal end. The duct normally disappears after the thyroid has moved to its ultimate location in the neck. The point of origin of the thyroglossal duct is regularly marked on the base of the adult tongue by the foramen cecum.

Tie on a passer: A strand of suture material attached to the tip of an instrument.

Timeout: A procedure for verifying the patient's identity, correct surgical procedure, site, and side. Timeout takes place after the patient has been positioned, prepped, draped, but before the first incision.

Tissue drag: A characteristic of some suture material that results in friction between the suture and the tissue.

TM: The tympanic membrane.

TNM classification system: An international system for determining the extent of cancer spread and the level of cell differentiation, two attributes that determine treatment and prognosis.

Tone: The expression of emotion or opinion contained in the delivery of a message. It is not explicit but is implied by intonation, emphasis on certain words, or measured delivery of words. Tone also is established by nonverbal communication.

Toolbar: Similar to a taskbar, a block or bar containing icons that represent packets of data.

Topical: Refers to application of a drug to the skin or mucous membranes.

Topical anesthesia: Anesthesia of superficial nerves of the skin or mucous membranes.

Topical antiseptics: Agents applied to skin or mucous membranes that temporarily reduce or prevent the growth of microorganisms.

Torsion: Twisting of an organ or a structure on itself. Torsion may cause local ischemia and necrosis.

Tort: A wrong, independent of contract law violations, perpetrated by one person against another person or another person's property. Any act of negligence or fraud compensable by money damages. Torts may be intentional or negligent in nature.

Touch screen: A computer screen on which tasks or commands are executed by touching an image on the screen. Touch screens are commonly used in computer-assisted and robotic surgery.

Trabeculectomy: Surgical removal of a portion of the trabecula to improve the outflow of aqueous humor for the treatment of glaucoma.

Traction: A mechanical method of applying pulling force to fractured bone.

Traction injury: A nerve injury caused by stretching or compression of the nerve.

Trade name: The name given to a drug by the company that produces and sells it.

Traffic patterns: The movement of people and equipment into, out of, and within the operating room.

Transcervical: Literally, "through the cervix." In surgery, a transcervical approach means that surgery is performed by passing instruments through the cervix.

Transcutaneous: Literally "through the skin"; it refers to a procedure in which a needle or other medical device is inserted from the outside of the body to the inside.

Transdermal: Refers to administration of a drug through a skin patch impregnated with the drug.

Transect: To surgically divide or cut into sections of tissue or an organ by sharp dissection.

Transfer board: A thin Plexiglas, fiberglass, or roller board that is placed under the patient to move the person from the operating table to the stretcher or bed.

Transformer: A device that steps up or steps down the voltage in an electrical circuit.

Transient flora: Microorganisms that do not normally reside in the tissue of an individual. Transient microorganisms are acquired through skin contact with an animate or inanimate source colonized by microbes. Transient flora may be removed by routine methods of skin cleaning (see Hand washing and Surgical hand scrub).

Transitional area: An area in which surgical personnel or visitors prepare to enter the semirestricted and restricted areas. Transitional areas include the locker rooms and changing rooms.

Transmission-based precautions: Standards and precautions to prevent the spread of infectious disease by patients known to be infected.

Transsphenoidal: Literally, "across or through the sphenoid bone." Surgery of the pituitary gland may be performed by approaching it through the sphenoid bone.

Transurethral: Surgical access through the urethral orifice. The term also may describe an instrument that enters the bladder through the urethral meatus.

Transverse incision: An incision that is perpendicular to the midline of the body.

Trendelenburg position: The position in which a prone or supine patient is tilted with the head down.

Trisegmentectomy: In hepatic surgery, the removal of the right lobe of the liver and a portion of the left. In practice, this is a multiple segmental resection.

Trocar: A sharp, rod-shaped instrument used to puncture the body wall.

Trough: The negative or lowest point on a wave.

TS-C (NCCT): Tech in surgery–certified. A qualification awarded by the National Center for Competency Testing that is achieved by examination and specific entry requirements.

Tumor margins: The edges of a tumor between the tumor mass and healthy tissue. When the surgical goal is to completely remove a tumor, the margins must be clear of any cancer cells in order to prevent recurrence of the tumor.

Tumor marker: An antigen present on the tumor cell, or a substance (protein, hormone, or other chemical) released by the cancer cells into the blood.

Tunable dye laser: A type of laser formed by the combination of argon gas and specific dyes that alter tissue absorption of the lasing beam.

Tympanic membrane thermometer: A type of thermometer that measures the patient's core temperature by scanning the tympanic membrane.

Tympanostomy tube: A tube that is placed in a myringotomy to produce aeration of the middle ear.

Ultrasound: A technology that uses high-frequency wave energy to identify anatomical structures and anomalies. In ultrasound imaging, sound waves are transformed into visual images on a screen.

Ultrasonic cleaner: Equipment that cleans instruments using ultrasonic waves.

Ultrasonic energy: High-frequency energy created by vibration or excitation of molecules. This type of energy destroys tissue by breaking molecular bonds.

Umbilical tape: A length of mesh tape used to loop around a blood vessel for retraction. See *vessel loop*.

Unconsciousness: A neurological state in which the person is unable to respond to external stimuli. Unconsciousness can be induced with drugs or may be caused by trauma or disease.

Undermine: A surgical technique in which a plane of tissue is created or an existing tissue plane is lifted, such as skin from the fascia.

Underwriters Laboratories: A nonprofit agency that tests and certifies electrical equipment in the United States.

Unrestricted area: An area that people dressed in street clothes may enter.

Urethrotomy: A small incision made in the urethra to reduce scarring or relieve a stricture.

U.S. Pharmacopeia (USP): An organization that establishes standards for drugs approved by the U.S. Food and Drug Administration (FDA) for their labeled use. All approved drugs have been tested for consumer safety, and written information is available about their pharmacological action, use, risks, and dosage.

Uterus: The muscular organ that holds the baby and the placenta during pregnancy.

Uvulopalatopharyngoplasty (UPP): A procedure in which the tonsils, uvula, and a portion of the soft palate are removed to reduce and stiffen excess oropharyngeal and oral cavity tissue in patients with obstructive sleep apnea.

Vacuoles: Cellular compartments formed by the "pinching off" of the endomembrane.

Valsalva maneuver: Voluntary closure of the epiglottis and contraction of the intraabdominal muscles, which results in increased thoracic pressure. Action used during "breath holding" and "bearing down."

Values: Beliefs, customs, behaviors, and norms that a person defends and upholds.

Varicosity: Thinning and enlargement of veins as a result of stasis (pooling of blood in the vessel).

Vasoconstriction: Narrowing of blood vessels, which can be caused by hormones, drugs, or some other factor.

Vector: A living intermediate carrier of microorganisms from one host to another. An example is the transmission of the bubonic plague. The vector is a flea, and the bacterium is transmitted to the human through a bite from an infected flea.

Ventilation: The physical act of taking air into the lungs by inflation and releasing carbon dioxide from the lungs by deflation.

Ventral hernia: A weakness in the abdominal wall, usually resulting in protrusion of abdominal viscera against the peritoneum and abdominal fascia.

Veress needle: A spring-loaded needle used to deliver carbon dioxide gas during insufflation.

Vertigo: A symptom rather than a disease, *vertigo* is a general term referring to sensory disturbances in which the patient is unable to maintain balance or has the perception of spinning, falling, or the environment turning.

Vessel loop: A device used to retract a vessel during surgery. A length of thin Silastic tubing or cotton tape (umbilical tape) is passed around the vessel. The ends can be threaded through a bolster (a 1/8- to 1/4-inch [0.3 to 0.6 cm] length of rubber or Silastic tubing) to secure the loop against the blood vessel.

Video cable: In video-assisted endoscopy, the cable that transmits digital data from the camera head to the camera control unit and from the monitor to the output recorder.

Video printer: A device that stores and prints output data viewed through the video endoscope.

Viricidal: Able to kill viruses.

Virion: A complete virus particle.

Virology: The study of viruses.

Virulence: The degree to which a microorganism is capable of causing disease.

Virus: A genetic element containing either deoxyribonucleic acid (DNA) or ribonucleic acid (RNA) that replicates in cells but is characterized by an extracellular state. It is parasitic in that it is entirely dependent on nutrients inside cells for its metabolic and reproductive needs. Viruses are different from other microbes in that they cannot reproduce their genetic material but must produce within a living host.

Viscera: The organs or tissue of the abdominal cavity.

Vital signs: Cardinal signs of well being: temperature, pulse, respiration, and blood pressure. These are measured to assess a patient's status.

Volt: The unit of measurement of electrical force.

Voltage: The electrical force in a circuit, measured as the amount of force that passes a given point over a stated period. Voltage is measured in amperes (A).

Washer-sterilizer/disinfector: Equipment that washes and decontaminates instruments after an operative procedure.

Wave: In physics, a naturally occurring phenomenon in which energy is transmitted in the form of peaks (high points) and troughs (low points).

Wavelength: The distance between peaks in a complete wave cycle.

White balance: A procedure for adjusting the light color of the video camera to other components of the system.

Window: In graphics-based computer platforms, the basic visual image within which tasks are performed.

Win-lose solution: In conflict resolution, a solution that leaves one party satisfied but the other party dissatisfied.

Win-win solution: In conflict resolution, a solution that allows both parties in a conflict to gain.

Wire localization biopsy: A procedure in which a hooked wire is inserted under fluoroscopy into tissue suspected of being cancerous. The tissue surrounding a hook wire is removed.

Word processing: A type of computer software in which documents can be created.

World Wide Web: In computer technology, a network of links to data via an Internet system. The Web uses a special computer language protocol and is only one of many types of systems for transmitting data through a computer network.

Index